DIAGNOSTIC AND STATISTICAL MANUAL OF MENTAL DISORDERS

FIFTH EDITION

DSM-5®

DIAGNOSTIC AND STATISTICAL MANUAL OF MENTAL DISORDERS

FIFTH EDITION

DSM-5®

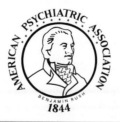

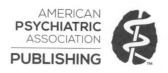

AMERICAN
PSYCHIATRIC
ASSOCIATION
PUBLISHING

Correspondence regarding copyright permissions should be directed to DSM Permissions, American Psychiatric Publishing, 1000 Wilson Boulevard, Suite 1825, Arlington, VA 22209-3901.

Manufactured in the United States of America on acid-free paper.

ISBN 978-0-89042-554-1 (Hardcover) 2nd printing June 2013

ISBN 978-0-89042-555-8 (Paperback) 4th printing July 2017

American Psychiatric Association
1000 Wilson Boulevard
Arlington, VA 22209-3901
www.psych.org

The correct citation for this book is American Psychiatric Association: Diagnostic and Statistical Manual of Mental Disorders, Fifth Edition. Arlington, VA, American Psychiatric Association, 2013.

Library of Congress Cataloging-in-Publication Data
Diagnostic and statistical manual of mental disorders : DSM-5. — 5th ed.
    p. ; cm.
DSM-5
DSM-V
Includes index.
ISBN 978-0-89042-554-1 (hardcover : alk. paper) — ISBN 978-0-89042-555-8 (pbk. : alk. paper)
I. American Psychiatric Association. II. American Psychiatric Association. DSM-5 Task Force.
III. Title: DSM-5. IV. Title: DSM-V.
[DNLM: 1. Diagnostic and statistical manual of mental disorders. 5th ed. 2. Mental Disorders—classification. 3. Mental Disorders—diagnosis. WM 15]
RC455.2.C4
616.89'075—dc23

                                                                    2013011061

British Library Cataloguing in Publication Data
A CIP record is available from the British Library.

Text Design—Tammy J. Cordova

Manufacturing—LSC Communications

Contents

Section I
DSM-5 Basics

Section II
Diagnostic Criteria and Codes

Section III
Emerging Measures and Models

Appendix

DSM-5 Task Force

DAVID J. KUPFER, M.D.
Task Force Chair

DARREL A. REGIER, M.D., M.P.H.
Task Force Vice-Chair

William E. Narrow, M.D., M.P.H.,
Research Director

Dan G. Blazer, M.D., Ph.D., M.P.H.
Jack D. Burke Jr., M.D., M.P.H.
William T. Carpenter Jr., M.D.
F. Xavier Castellanos, M.D.
Wilson M. Compton, M.D., M.P.E.
Joel E. Dimsdale, M.D.
Javier I. Escobar, M.D., M.Sc.
Jan A. Fawcett, M.D.
Bridget F. Grant, Ph.D., Ph.D. *(2009–)*
Steven E. Hyman, M.D. *(2007–2012)*
Dilip V. Jeste, M.D. *(2007–2011)*
Helena C. Kraemer, Ph.D.
Daniel T. Mamah, M.D., M.P.E.
James P. McNulty, A.B., Sc.B.
Howard B. Moss, M.D. *(2007–2009)*

Susan K. Schultz, M.D., *Text Editor*
Emily A. Kuhl, Ph.D., *APA Text Editor*

Charles P. O'Brien, M.D., Ph.D.
Roger Peele, M.D.
Katharine A. Phillips, M.D.
Daniel S. Pine, M.D.
Charles F. Reynolds III, M.D.
Maritza Rubio-Stipec, Sc.D.
David Shaffer, M.D.
Andrew E. Skodol II, M.D.
Susan E. Swedo, M.D.
B. Timothy Walsh, M.D.
Philip Wang, M.D., Dr.P.H. *(2007–2012)*
William M. Womack, M.D.
Kimberly A. Yonkers, M.D.
Kenneth J. Zucker, Ph.D.
Norman Sartorius, M.D., Ph.D., *Consultant*

APA Division of Research Staff on DSM-5

Darrel A. Regier, M.D., M.P.H.,
Director, Division of Research
William E. Narrow, M.D., M.P.H.,
Associate Director
Emily A. Kuhl, Ph.D., *Senior Science
Writer; Staff Text Editor*
Diana E. Clarke, Ph.D., M.Sc., *Research
Statistician*

Lisa H. Greiner, M.S.S.A., *DSM-5 Field
Trials Project Manager*
Eve K. Moscicki, Sc.D., M.P.H.,
Director, Practice Research Network
S. Janet Kuramoto, Ph.D. M.H.S.,
*Senior Scientific Research Associate,
Practice Research Network*

Amy Porfiri, M.B.A.
Director of Finance and Administration

Jennifer J. Shupinka, *Assistant Director,
DSM Operations*
Seung-Hee Hong, *DSM Senior Research
Associate*
Anne R. Hiller, *DSM Research Associate*
Alison S. Beale, *DSM Research Associate*
Spencer R. Case, *DSM Research Associate*

Joyce C. West, Ph.D., M.P.P.,
*Health Policy Research Director, Practice
Research Network*
Farifteh F. Duffy, Ph.D.,
*Quality Care Research Director, Practice
Research Network*
Lisa M. Countis, *Field Operations
Manager, Practice Research Network*

Christopher M. Reynolds,
Executive Assistant

APA Office of the Medical Director

JAMES H. SCULLY JR., M.D.
Medical Director and CEO

Editorial and Coding Consultants

DSM-5 Work Groups

ADHD and Disruptive Behavior Disorders

Anxiety, Obsessive-Compulsive Spectrum, Posttraumatic, and Dissociative Disorders

Childhood and Adolescent Disorders

Eating Disorders

DSM-5 Study Groups

Diagnostic Spectra and DSM/ICD Harmonization

STEVEN E. HYMAN, M.D.
Chair (2007–2012)

William T. Carpenter Jr., M.D.
Wilson M. Compton, M.D., M.P.E.
Jan A. Fawcett, M.D.
Helena C. Kraemer, Ph.D.
David J. Kupfer, M.D.

William E. Narrow, M.D., M.P.H.
Charles P. O'Brien, M.D., Ph.D.
John M. Oldham, M.D.
Katharine A. Phillips, M.D.
Darrel A. Regier, M.D., M.P.H.

Lifespan Developmental Approaches

ERIC J. LENZE, M.D.
Chair

SUSAN K. SCHULTZ, M.D.
Chair Emeritus

DANIEL S. PINE, M.D.
Chair Emeritus

Dan G. Blazer, M.D., Ph.D., M.P.H.
F. Xavier Castellanos, M.D.
Wilson M. Compton, M.D., M.P.E.

Daniel T. Mamah, M.D., M.P.E.
Andrew E. Skodol II, M.D.
Susan E. Swedo, M.D.

Gender and Cross-Cultural Issues

KIMBERLY A. YONKERS, M.D.
Chair

ROBERTO LEWIS-FERNÁNDEZ, M.D., M.T.S.
Co-Chair, Cross-Cultural Issues

Renato D. Alarcon, M.D., M.P.H.
Diana E. Clarke, Ph.D., M.Sc.
Javier I. Escobar, M.D., M.Sc.
Ellen Frank, Ph.D.
James S. Jackson, Ph.D.
Spiro M. Manson, Ph.D. *(2007–2008)*
James P. McNulty, A.B., Sc.B.

Leslie C. Morey, Ph.D.
William E. Narrow, M.D., M.P.H.
Roger Peele, M.D.
Philip Wang, M.D., Dr.P.H. *(2007–2012)*
William M. Womack, M.D.
Kenneth J. Zucker, Ph.D.

Psychiatric/General Medical Interface

LAWSON R. WULSIN, M.D.
Chair

Ronald E. Dahl, M.D.
Joel E. Dimsdale, M.D.
Javier I. Escobar, M.D., M.Sc.
Dilip V. Jeste, M.D. *(2007–2011)*
Walter E. Kaufmann, M.D.

Richard E. Kreipe, M.D.
Ronald C. Petersen, Ph.D., M.D.
Charles F. Reynolds III, M.D.
Robert Taylor Segraves, M.D., Ph.D.
B. Timothy Walsh, M.D.

Impairment and Disability
JANE S. PAULSEN, PH.D.
Chair

J. Gavin Andrews, M.D.
Glorisa Canino, Ph.D.
Lee Anna Clark, Ph.D.
Diana E. Clarke, Ph.D., M.Sc.
Michelle G. Craske, Ph.D.

Hans W. Hoek, M.D., Ph.D.
Helena C. Kraemer, Ph.D.
William E. Narrow, M.D., M.P.H.
David Shaffer, M.D.

Diagnostic Assessment Instruments
JACK D. BURKE JR., M.D., M.P.H.
Chair

Lee Anna Clark, Ph.D.
Diana E. Clarke, Ph.D., M.Sc.
Bridget F. Grant, Ph.D., Ph.D.

Helena C. Kraemer, Ph.D.
William E. Narrow, M.D., M.P.H.
David Shaffer, M.D.

DSM-5 Research Group
WILLIAM E. NARROW, M.D., M.P.H.
Chair

Jack D. Burke Jr., M.D., M.P.H.
Diana E. Clarke, Ph.D., M.Sc.
Helena C. Kraemer, Ph.D.

David J. Kupfer, M.D.
Darrel A. Regier, M.D., M.P.H.
David Shaffer, M.D.

Course Specifiers and Glossary
WOLFGANG GAEBEL, M.D.
Chair

Ellen Frank, Ph.D.
Charles P. O'Brien, M.D., Ph.D.
Norman Sartorius, M.D., Ph.D.,
  Consultant
Susan K. Schultz, M.D.

Dan J. Stein, M.D., Ph.D.
Eric A. Taylor, M.B.
David J. Kupfer, M.D.
Darrel A. Regier, M.D., M.P.H.

DSM-5 Classification

Before each disorder name, ICD-9-CM codes are provided, followed by ICD-10-CM codes in parentheses. Blank lines indicate that either the ICD-9-CM or the ICD-10-CM code is not applicable. For some disorders, the code can be indicated only according to the subtype or specifier.

ICD-9-CM codes are to be used for coding purposes in the United States through September 30, 2015. ICD-10-CM codes are to be used starting October 1, 2015. For DSM-5 coding and other updates, see the DSM-5® Update on www.PsychiatryOnline.org.

Following chapter titles and disorder names, page numbers for the corresponding text or criteria are included in parentheses.

Note for all mental disorders due to another medical condition: Indicate the name of the other medical condition in the name of the mental disorder due to [the medical condition]. The code and name for the other medical condition should be listed first immediately before the mental disorder due to the medical condition.

Neurodevelopmental Disorders (31)

Intellectual Disabilities (33)

___.__ (___.__)   Intellectual Disability (Intellectual Developmental Disorder) (33)
Specify current severity:

317	**(F70)**	Mild
318.0	**(F71)**	Moderate
318.1	**(F72)**	Severe
318.2	**(F73)**	Profound
315.8	**(F88)**	Global Developmental Delay (41)
319	**(F79)**	Unspecified Intellectual Disability (Intellectual Developmental Disorder) (41)

Communication Disorders (41)

315.32	**(F80.2)**	Language Disorder (42)
315.39	**(F80.0)**	Speech Sound Disorder (44)
315.35	**(F80.81)**	Childhood-Onset Fluency Disorder (Stuttering) (45)

Note: Later-onset cases are diagnosed as 307.0 (F98.5) adult-onset fluency disorder.

315.39	**(F80.82)**	Social (Pragmatic) Communication Disorder (47)
307.9	**(F80.9)**	Unspecified Communication Disorder (49)

Autism Spectrum Disorder (50)

Attention-Deficit/Hyperactivity Disorder (59)

Specific Learning Disorder (66)

Motor Disorders (74)

Tic Disorders

Schizophrenia Spectrum and Other Psychotic Disorders (87)

The following specifiers apply to Schizophrenia Spectrum and Other Psychotic Disorders where indicated:

[a]*Specify* if: The following course specifiers are only to be used after a 1-year duration of the disorder: First episode, currently in acute episode; First episode, currently in partial remission; First episode, currently in full remission; Multiple episodes, currently in acute episode; Multiple episodes, currently in partial remission; Multiple episodes, currently in full remission; Continuous; Unspecified

[b]*Specify* if: With catatonia (use additional code 293.89 [F06.1])

[c]*Specify* current severity of delusions, hallucinations, disorganized speech, abnormal psychomotor behavior, negative symptoms, impaired cognition, depression, and mania symptoms

Bipolar and Related Disorders (123)

The following specifiers apply to Bipolar and Related Disorders where indicated:
[a]*Specify:* With anxious distress (*specify* current severity: mild, moderate, moderate-severe, severe); With mixed features; With rapid cycling; With melancholic features; With atypical features; With mood-congruent psychotic features; With mood-incongruent psychotic features; With catatonia (use additional code 293.89 [F06.1]); With peripartum onset; With seasonal pattern

301.13 (F34.0)   Cyclothymic Disorder (139)
   Specify if: With anxious distress

___.__ (___.__)   Substance/Medication-Induced Bipolar and Related Disorder (142)
   Note: See the criteria set and corresponding recording procedures for
      substance-specific codes and ICD-9-CM and ICD-10-CM coding.
   Specify if: With onset during intoxication, With onset during withdrawal

293.83 (___.__)   Bipolar and Related Disorder Due to Another Medical Condition
            (145)
   Specify if:
   (F06.33)   With manic features
   (F06.33)   With manic- or hypomanic-like episode
   (F06.34)   With mixed features

296.89 (F31.89)   Other Specified Bipolar and Related Disorder (148)

296.80 (F31.9)   Unspecified Bipolar and Related Disorder (149)

Depressive Disorders (155)

The following specifiers apply to Depressive Disorders where indicated:
[a]*Specify:* With anxious distress (*specify* current severity: mild, moderate, moderate-severe,
   severe); With mixed features; With melancholic features; With atypical features; With mood-
   congruent psychotic features; With mood-incongruent psychotic features; With catatonia
   (use additional code 293.89 [F06.1]); With peripartum onset; With seasonal pattern

296.99 (F34.81)   Disruptive Mood Dysregulation Disorder (156)

___.__ (___.__)   Major Depressive Disorder[a] (160)
___.__ (___.__)   Single episode
296.21 (F32.0)   Mild
296.22 (F32.1)   Moderate
296.23 (F32.2)   Severe
296.24 (F32.3)   With psychotic features
296.25 (F32.4)   In partial remission
296.26 (F32.5)   In full remission
296.20 (F32.9)   Unspecified
___.__ (___.__)   Recurrent episode
296.31 (F33.0)   Mild
296.32 (F33.1)   Moderate
296.33 (F33.2)   Severe
296.34 (F33.3)   With psychotic features
296.35 (F33.41)   In partial remission
296.36 (F33.42)   In full remission
296.30 (F33.9)   Unspecified

300.4 (F34.1)   Persistent Depressive Disorder (Dysthymia)[a] (168)
   Specify if: In partial remission, In full remission
   Specify if: Early onset, Late onset
   Specify if: With pure dysthymic syndrome; With persistent major depres-
      sive episode; With intermittent major depressive episodes, with current

Anxiety Disorders (189)

Dissociative Disorders (291)

Somatic Symptom and Related Disorders (309)

Feeding and Eating Disorders (329)

Elimination Disorders (355)

Sleep-Wake Disorders (361)

The following specifiers apply to Sleep-Wake Disorders where indicated:
[a]*Specify* if: Episodic, Persistent, Recurrent
[b]*Specify* if: Acute, Subacute, Persistent
[c]*Specify* current severity: Mild, Moderate, Severe

307.42 (F51.01)   Insomnia Disorder[a] (362)
        Specify if: With non–sleep disorder mental comorbidity, With other
            medical comorbidity, With other sleep disorder

307.44 (F51.11)   Hypersomnolence Disorder[b, c] (368)
        Specify if: With mental disorder, With medical condition, With another
            sleep disorder

___.__ (___.__)   Narcolepsy[c] (372)
        Specify whether:
347.00 (G47.419)   Narcolepsy without cataplexy but with hypocretin deficiency
347.01 (G47.411)   Narcolepsy with cataplexy but without hypocretin deficiency
347.00 (G47.419)   Autosomal dominant cerebellar ataxia, deafness, and
            narcolepsy
347.00 (G47.419)   Autosomal dominant narcolepsy, obesity, and type 2 diabetes
347.10 (G47.429)   Narcolepsy secondary to another medical condition

Breathing-Related Sleep Disorders (378)

327.23 (G47.33)   Obstructive Sleep Apnea Hypopnea[c] (378)

___.__ (___.__)   Central Sleep Apnea (383)
        Specify whether:
327.21 (G47.31)   Idiopathic central sleep apnea
786.04 (R06.3)   Cheyne-Stokes breathing
780.57 (G47.37)   Central sleep apnea comorbid with opioid use
        Note: First code opioid use disorder, if present.
        Specify current severity

___.__ (___.__)   Sleep-Related Hypoventilation (387)
        Specify whether:
327.24 (G47.34)   Idiopathic hypoventilation
327.25 (G47.35)   Congenital central alveolar hypoventilation
327.26 (G47.36)   Comorbid sleep-related hypoventilation
        Specify current severity

___.__ (___.__)   Circadian Rhythm Sleep-Wake Disorders[a] (390)
        Specify whether:
307.45 (G47.21)   Delayed sleep phase type (391)
        Specify if: Familial, Overlapping with non-24-hour sleep-wake type
307.45 (G47.22)   Advanced sleep phase type (393)
        Specify if: Familial
307.45 (G47.23)   Irregular sleep-wake type (394)
307.45 (G47.24)   Non-24-hour sleep-wake type (396)

Sexual Dysfunctions (423)

Gender Dysphoria (451)

Disruptive, Impulse-Control, and Conduct Disorders (461)

Substance-Related and Addictive Disorders (481)

The following specifiers and note apply to Substance-Related and Addictive Disorders where indicated:

[a]*Specify* if: In early remission, In sustained remission

[b]*Specify* if: In a controlled environment

[c]*Specify* if: With perceptual disturbances

[d]The ICD-10-CM code indicates the comorbid presence of a moderate or severe substance use disorder, which must be present in order to apply the code for substance withdrawal.

Substance-Related Disorders (483)

Alcohol-Related Disorders (490)

___.__	(___.__)	Alcohol Use Disorder[a, b] (490)
		Specify current severity:
305.00	(F10.10)	Mild
303.90	(F10.20)	Moderate
303.90	(F10.20)	Severe
303.00	(___.__)	Alcohol Intoxication (497)
	(F10.129)	With use disorder, mild
	(F10.229)	With use disorder, moderate or severe
	(F10.929)	Without use disorder
291.81	(___.__)	Alcohol Withdrawal[c, d] (499)
	(F10.239)	Without perceptual disturbances
	(F10.232)	With perceptual disturbances
___.__	(___.__)	Other Alcohol-Induced Disorders (502)
291.9	(F10.99)	Unspecified Alcohol-Related Disorder (503)

Caffeine-Related Disorders (503)

305.90	(F15.929)	Caffeine Intoxication (503)
292.0	(F15.93)	Caffeine Withdrawal (506)
___.__	(___.__)	Other Caffeine-Induced Disorders (508)
292.9	(F15.99)	Unspecified Caffeine-Related Disorder (509)

Cannabis-Related Disorders (509)

___.__	(___.__)	Cannabis Use Disorder[a, b] (509)
		Specify current severity:
305.20	(F12.10)	Mild
304.30	(F12.20)	Moderate
304.30	(F12.20)	Severe

304.60 (F18.20) Moderate
304.60 (F18.20) Severe

292.89 (___.__) Inhalant Intoxication (538)
(F18.129) With use disorder, mild
(F18.229) With use disorder, moderate or severe
(F18.929) Without use disorder
___.__ (___.__) Other Inhalant-Induced Disorders (540)
292.9 (F18.99) Unspecified Inhalant-Related Disorder (540)

Opioid-Related Disorders (540)

___.__ (___.__) Opioid Use Disorder[a] (541)
Specify if: On maintenance therapy, In a controlled environment
Specify current severity:
305.50 (F11.10) Mild
304.00 (F11.20) Moderate
304.00 (F11.20) Severe

292.89 (___.__) Opioid Intoxication[c] (546)
Without perceptual disturbances
(F11.129) With use disorder, mild
(F11.229) With use disorder, moderate or severe
(F11.929) Without use disorder
With perceptual disturbances
(F11.122) With use disorder, mild
(F11.222) With use disorder, moderate or severe
(F11.922) Without use disorder
292.0 (F11.23) Opioid Withdrawal[d] (547)
___.__ (___.__) Other Opioid-Induced Disorders (549)
292.9 (F11.99) Unspecified Opioid-Related Disorder (550)

Sedative-, Hypnotic-, or Anxiolytic-Related Disorders (550)

___.__ (___.__) Sedative, Hypnotic, or Anxiolytic Use Disorder[a, b] (550)
Specify current severity:
305.40 (F13.10) Mild
304.10 (F13.20) Moderate
304.10 (F13.20) Severe

292.89 (___.__) Sedative, Hypnotic, or Anxiolytic Intoxication (556)
(F13.129) With use disorder, mild
(F13.229) With use disorder, moderate or severe
(F13.929) Without use disorder

292.0 (___.__) Sedative, Hypnotic, or Anxiolytic Withdrawal[c, d] (557)
(F13.239) Without perceptual disturbances
(F13.232) With perceptual disturbances

292.9 (___.__)   Unspecified Stimulant-Related Disorder (570)
 (F15.99)   Amphetamine or other stimulant
 (F14.99)   Cocaine

Tobacco-Related Disorders (571)

___.__ (___.__)   Tobacco Use Disorder[a] (571)
               Specify if: On maintenance therapy, In a controlled environment
               Specify current severity:
305.1 (Z72.0)   Mild
305.1 (F17.200)   Moderate
305.1 (F17.200)   Severe
292.0 (F17.203)   Tobacco Withdrawal[d] (575)
___.__ (___.__)   Other Tobacco-Induced Disorders (576)
292.9 (F17.209)   Unspecified Tobacco-Related Disorder (577)

Other (or Unknown) Substance–Related Disorders (577)

___.__ (___.__)   Other (or Unknown) Substance Use Disorder[a, b] (577)
               Specify current severity:
305.90 (F19.10)   Mild
304.90 (F19.20)   Moderate
304.90 (F19.20)   Severe

292.89 (___.__)   Other (or Unknown) Substance Intoxication (581)
 (F19.129)   With use disorder, mild
 (F19.229)   With use disorder, moderate or severe
 (F19.929)   Without use disorder
292.0 (F19.239)   Other (or Unknown) Substance Withdrawal[d] (583)
___.__ (___.__)   Other (or Unknown) Substance–Induced Disorders (584)
292.9 (F19.99)   Unspecified Other (or Unknown) Substance–Related Disorder (585)

Non-Substance-Related Disorders (585)

312.31 (F63.0)   Gambling Disorder[a] (585)
               Specify if: Episodic, Persistent
               Specify current severity: Mild, Moderate, Severe

---

Neurocognitive Disorders (591)

___.__ (___.__)   Delirium (596)
               [a]**Note:** See the criteria set and corresponding recording procedures for
                 substance-specific codes and ICD-9-CM and ICD-10-CM coding.
               Specify whether:
___.__ (___.__)   Substance intoxication delirium[a]
___.__ (___.__)   Substance withdrawal delirium[a]
292.81 (___.__)   Medication-induced delirium[a]
293.0 (F05)   Delirium due to another medical condition

293.0 (F05)   Delirium due to multiple etiologies
                             Specify if: Acute, Persistent
                             Specify if: Hyperactive, Hypoactive, Mixed level of activity

780.09 (R41.0)   Other Specified Delirium (602)

780.09 (R41.0)   Unspecified Delirium (602)

Major and Mild Neurocognitive Disorders (602)

Specify whether due to: Alzheimer's disease, Frontotemporal lobar degeneration, Lewy body
   disease, Vascular disease, Traumatic brain injury, Substance/medication use, HIV infection,
   Prion disease, Parkinson's disease, Huntington's disease, Another medical condition, Multiple etiologies, Unspecified

[a]*Specify:* Without behavioral disturbance, With behavioral disturbance. *For possible major neurocognitive disorder and for mild neurocognitive disorder, behavioral disturbance cannot be coded but
   should still be indicated in writing.*

[b]*Specify* current severity: Mild, Moderate, Severe. *This specifier applies only to major neurocognitive disorders (including probable and possible).*

Note: As indicated for each subtype, an additional medical code is needed for probable major
neurocognitive disorder or major neurocognitive disorder. An additional medical code should
not be used for possible major neurocognitive disorder or mild neurocognitive disorder.

Major or Mild Neurocognitive Disorder Due to Alzheimer's Disease (611)

___.__ (__.__)   Probable Major Neurocognitive Disorder Due to Alzheimer's
                             Disease[b]
                             Note: Code first **331.0 (G30.9)** Alzheimer's disease.

294.11 (F02.81)   With behavioral disturbance

294.10 (F02.80)   Without behavioral disturbance

331.9 (G31.9)   Possible Major Neurocognitive Disorder Due to Alzheimer's
                             Disease[a, b]

331.83 (G31.84)   Mild Neurocognitive Disorder Due to Alzheimer's Disease[a]

Major or Mild Frontotemporal Neurocognitive Disorder (614)

___.__ (__.__)   Probable Major Neurocognitive Disorder Due to Frontotemporal
                             Lobar Degeneration[b]
                             Note: Code first **331.19 (G31.09)** frontotemporal disease.

294.11 (F02.81)   With behavioral disturbance

294.10 (F02.80)   Without behavioral disturbance

331.9 (G31.9)   Possible Major Neurocognitive Disorder Due to Frontotemporal
                             Lobar Degeneration[a, b]

331.83 (G31.84)   Mild Neurocognitive Disorder Due to Frontotemporal Lobar
                             Degeneration[a]

Major or Mild Neurocognitive Disorder With Lewy Bodies (618)

___.__ (__.__)   Probable Major Neurocognitive Disorder With Lewy Bodies[b]
                             Note: Code first **331.82 (G31.83)** Lewy body disease.

294.11 (F02.81)   With behavioral disturbance

294.10 (F02.80)   Without behavioral disturbance

331.9 (G31.9) Possible Major Neurocognitive Disorder With Lewy Bodies[a, b]

331.83 (G31.84) Mild Neurocognitive Disorder With Lewy Bodies[a]

Major or Mild Vascular Neurocognitive Disorder (621)

___.__ (___.__) Probable Major Vascular Neurocognitive Disorder[b]
Note: No additional medical code for vascular disease.

290.40 (F01.51) With behavioral disturbance

290.40 (F01.50) Without behavioral disturbance

331.9 (G31.9) Possible Major Vascular Neurocognitive Disorder[a, b]

331.83 (G31.84) Mild Vascular Neurocognitive Disorder[a]

Major or Mild Neurocognitive Disorder Due to Traumatic Brain Injury (624)

___.__ (___.__) Major Neurocognitive Disorder Due to Traumatic Brain Injury[b]
Note: For ICD-9-CM, code first **907.0** late effect of intracranial injury without skull fracture. For ICD-10-CM, code first **S06.2X9S** diffuse traumatic brain injury with loss of consciousness of unspecified duration, sequela.

294.11 (F02.81) With behavioral disturbance

294.10 (F02.80) Without behavioral disturbance

331.83 (G31.84) Mild Neurocognitive Disorder Due to Traumatic Brain Injury[a]

Substance/Medication-Induced Major or Mild Neurocognitive Disorder[a] (627)
Note: No additional medical code. See the criteria set and corresponding recording procedures for substance-specific codes and ICD-9-CM and ICD-10-CM coding.
Specify if: Persistent

Major or Mild Neurocognitive Disorder Due to HIV Infection (632)

___.__ (___.__) Major Neurocognitive Disorder Due to HIV Infection[b]
Note: Code first **042 (B20)** HIV infection.

294.11 (F02.81) With behavioral disturbance

294.10 (F02.80) Without behavioral disturbance

331.83 (G31.84) Mild Neurocognitive Disorder Due to HIV Infection[a]

Major or Mild Neurocognitive Disorder Due to Prion Disease (634)

___.__ (___.__) Major Neurocognitive Disorder Due to Prion Disease[b]
Note: Code first **046.79 (A81.9)** prion disease.

294.11 (F02.81) With behavioral disturbance

294.10 (F02.80) Without behavioral disturbance

331.83 (G31.84) Mild Neurocognitive Disorder Due to Prion Disease[a]

Major or Mild Neurocognitive Disorder Due to Parkinson's Disease (636)

___.__ (___.__) Major Neurocognitive Disorder Probably Due to Parkinson's Disease[b]
Note: Code first **332.0 (G20)** Parkinson's disease.

294.11 (F02.81) With behavioral disturbance

294.10 (F02.80) Without behavioral disturbance

331.9 (G31.9)   Major Neurocognitive Disorder Possibly Due to Parkinson's
                      Disease[a, b]

331.83 (G31.84)   Mild Neurocognitive Disorder Due to Parkinson's Disease[a]

Major or Mild Neurocognitive Disorder Due to Huntington's Disease (638)

___.__ (___.__)   Major Neurocognitive Disorder Due to Huntington's Disease[b]
                   Note: Code first **333.4 (G10)** Huntington's disease.
294.11 (F02.81)   With behavioral disturbance
294.10 (F02.80)   Without behavioral disturbance

331.83 (G31.84)   Mild Neurocognitive Disorder Due to Huntington's Disease[a]

Major or Mild Neurocognitive Disorder Due to Another Medical Condition (641)

___.__ (___.__)   Major Neurocognitive Disorder Due to Another Medical
                   Condition[b]
                   Note: Code first the other medical condition.
294.11 (F02.81)   With behavioral disturbance
294.10 (F02.80)   Without behavioral disturbance

331.83 (G31.84)   Mild Neurocognitive Disorder Due to Another Medical
                      Condition[a]

Major or Mild Neurocognitive Disorder Due to Multiple Etiologies (642)

___.__ (___.__)   Major Neurocognitive Disorder Due to Multiple Etiologies[b]
                   Note: Code first all the etiological medical conditions (with the exception
                   of vascular disease).
294.11 (F02.81)   With behavioral disturbance
294.10 (F02.80)   Without behavioral disturbance

331.83 (G31.84)   Mild Neurocognitive Disorder Due to Multiple Etiologies[a]

Unspecified Neurocognitive Disorder (643)

799.59 (R41.9)   Unspecified Neurocognitive Disorder[a]

Personality Disorders (645)

Cluster A Personality Disorders

301.0 (F60.0)   Paranoid Personality Disorder (649)

301.20 (F60.1)   Schizoid Personality Disorder (652)

301.22 (F21)   Schizotypal Personality Disorder (655)

Cluster B Personality Disorders

301.7 (F60.2)   Antisocial Personality Disorder (659)

301.83 (F60.3)   Borderline Personality Disorder (663)

301.50 (F60.4)   Histrionic Personality Disorder (667)

301.81 (F60.81)   Narcissistic Personality Disorder (669)

Cluster C Personality Disorders

301.82 (F60.6)   Avoidant Personality Disorder (672)

301.6   (F60.7)   Dependent Personality Disorder (675)

301.4   (F60.5)   Obsessive-Compulsive Personality Disorder (678)

Other Personality Disorders

310.1   (F07.0)   Personality Change Due to Another Medical Condition (682)
            Specify whether: Labile type, Disinhibited type, Aggressive type, Apathetic
                type, Paranoid type, Other type, Combined type, Unspecified type

301.89 (F60.89)   Other Specified Personality Disorder (684)

301.9   (F60.9)   Unspecified Personality Disorder (684)

Paraphilic Disorders (685)

The following specifier applies to Paraphilic Disorders where indicated:
[a]*Specify* if: In a controlled environment, In full remission

302.82 (F65.3)   Voyeuristic Disorder[a] (686)

302.4   (F65.2)   Exhibitionistic Disorder[a] (689)
            Specify whether: Sexually aroused by exposing genitals to prepubertal
                children, Sexually aroused by exposing genitals to physically mature
                individuals, Sexually aroused by exposing genitals to prepubertal chil-
                dren and to physically mature individuals

302.89 (F65.81)   Frotteuristic Disorder[a] (691)

302.83 (F65.51)   Sexual Masochism Disorder[a] (694)
            Specify if: With asphyxiophilia

302.84 (F65.52)   Sexual Sadism Disorder[a] (695)

302.2   (F65.4)   Pedophilic Disorder (697)
            Specify whether: Exclusive type, Nonexclusive type
            Specify if: Sexually attracted to males, Sexually attracted to females, Sexu-
                ally attracted to both
            Specify if: Limited to incest

302.81 (F65.0)   Fetishistic Disorder[a] (700)
            Specify: Body part(s), Nonliving object(s), Other

302.3   (F65.1)   Transvestic Disorder[a] (702)
            Specify if: With fetishism, With autogynephilia

302.89 (F65.89)   Other Specified Paraphilic Disorder (705)

302.9   (F65.9)   Unspecified Paraphilic Disorder (705)

Other Mental Disorders (707)

294.8   (F06.8)   Other Specified Mental Disorder Due to Another Medical
                Condition (707)

294.9   (F09)   Unspecified Mental Disorder Due to Another Medical Condition
                (708)

300.9   (F99)   Other Specified Mental Disorder (708)

300.9   (F99)   Unspecified Mental Disorder (708)

Medication-Induced Movement Disorders and Other Adverse Effects of Medication (709)

Other Conditions That May Be a Focus of Clinical Attention (715)

Relational Problems (715)

Abuse and Neglect (717)

Child Maltreatment and Neglect Problems (717)

Child Physical Abuse (717)

Child Physical Abuse, Confirmed (717)

995.54 (T74.12XA)   Initial encounter

995.54 (T74.12XD)   Subsequent encounter

Child Physical Abuse, Suspected (717)

995.54 (T76.12XA)   Initial encounter

995.54 (T76.12XD)   Subsequent encounter

Other Circumstances Related to Child Physical Abuse (718)

V61.21 (Z69.010)   Encounter for mental health services for victim of child abuse by parent

V61.21 (Z69.020)   Encounter for mental health services for victim of nonparental child abuse

V15.41 (Z62.810)   Personal history (past history) of physical abuse in childhood

V61.22 (Z69.011)   Encounter for mental health services for perpetrator of parental child abuse

V62.83 (Z69.021)   Encounter for mental health services for perpetrator of nonparental child abuse

Child Sexual Abuse (718)

Child Sexual Abuse, Confirmed (718)

995.53 (T74.22XA)   Initial encounter

995.53 (T74.22XD)   Subsequent encounter

Child Sexual Abuse, Suspected (718)

995.53 (T76.22XA)   Initial encounter

995.53 (T76.22XD)   Subsequent encounter

Other Circumstances Related to Child Sexual Abuse (718)

V61.21 (Z69.010)   Encounter for mental health services for victim of child sexual abuse by parent

V61.21 (Z69.020)   Encounter for mental health services for victim of nonparental child sexual abuse

V15.41 (Z62.810)   Personal history (past history) of sexual abuse in childhood

V61.22 (Z69.011)   Encounter for mental health services for perpetrator of parental child sexual abuse

V62.83 (Z69.021)   Encounter for mental health services for perpetrator of nonparental child sexual abuse

Child Neglect (718)

Child Neglect, Confirmed (718)

995.52 (T74.02XA)   Initial encounter

995.52 (T74.02XD)   Subsequent encounter

Child Neglect, Suspected (719)

995.52 (T76.02XA)   Initial encounter
995.52 (T76.02XD)   Subsequent encounter

Other Circumstances Related to Child Neglect (719)

V61.21 (Z69.010)   Encounter for mental health services for victim of child neglect by parent
V61.21 (Z69.020)   Encounter for mental health services for victim of nonparental child neglect
V15.42 (Z62.812)   Personal history (past history) of neglect in childhood
V61.22 (Z69.011)   Encounter for mental health services for perpetrator of parental child neglect
V62.83 (Z69.021)   Encounter for mental health services for perpetrator of nonparental child neglect

Child Psychological Abuse (719)

Child Psychological Abuse, Confirmed (719)

995.51 (T74.32XA)   Initial encounter
995.51 (T74.32XD)   Subsequent encounter

Child Psychological Abuse, Suspected (719)

995.51 (T76.32XA)   Initial encounter
995.51 (T76.32XD)   Subsequent encounter

Other Circumstances Related to Child Psychological Abuse (719)

V61.21 (Z69.010)   Encounter for mental health services for victim of child psychological abuse by parent
V61.21 (Z69.020)   Encounter for mental health services for victim of nonparental child psychological abuse
V15.42 (Z62.811)   Personal history (past history) of psychological abuse in childhood
V61.22 (Z69.011)   Encounter for mental health services for perpetrator of parental child psychological abuse
V62.83 (Z69.021)   Encounter for mental health services for perpetrator of nonparental child psychological abuse

Adult Maltreatment and Neglect Problems (720)

Spouse or Partner Violence, Physical (720)

Spouse or Partner Violence, Physical, Confirmed (720)

995.81 (T74.11XA)   Initial encounter
995.81 (T74.11XD)   Subsequent encounter

Spouse or Partner Violence, Physical, Suspected (720)

995.81 (T76.11XA)   Initial encounter
995.81 (T76.11XD)   Subsequent encounter

Other Circumstances Related to Spouse or Partner Violence, Physical (720)

V61.11 (Z69.11)   Encounter for mental health services for victim of spouse or partner violence, physical

V15.41 (Z91.410) Personal history (past history) of spouse or partner violence, physical

V61.12 (Z69.12) Encounter for mental health services for perpetrator of spouse or partner violence, physical

Spouse or Partner Violence, Sexual (720)

Spouse or Partner Violence, Sexual, Confirmed (720)

995.83 (T74.21XA) Initial encounter

995.83 (T74.21XD) Subsequent encounter

Spouse or Partner Violence, Sexual, Suspected (720)

995.83 (T76.21XA) Initial encounter

995.83 (T76.21XD) Subsequent encounter

Other Circumstances Related to Spouse or Partner Violence, Sexual (720)

V61.11 (Z69.81) Encounter for mental health services for victim of spouse or partner violence, sexual

V15.41 (Z91.410) Personal history (past history) of spouse or partner violence, sexual

V61.12 (Z69.12) Encounter for mental health services for perpetrator of spouse or partner violence, sexual

Spouse or Partner, Neglect (721)

Spouse or Partner Neglect, Confirmed (721)

995.85 (T74.01XA) Initial encounter

995.85 (T74.01XD) Subsequent encounter

Spouse or Partner Neglect, Suspected (721)

995.85 (T76.01XA) Initial encounter

995.85 (T76.01XD) Subsequent encounter

Other Circumstances Related to Spouse or Partner Neglect (721)

V61.11 (Z69.11) Encounter for mental health services for victim of spouse or partner neglect

V15.42 (Z91.412) Personal history (past history) of spouse or partner neglect

V61.12 (Z69.12) Encounter for mental health services for perpetrator of spouse or partner neglect

Spouse or Partner Abuse, Psychological (721)

Spouse or Partner Abuse, Psychological, Confirmed (721)

995.82 (T74.31XA) Initial encounter

995.82 (T74.31XD) Subsequent encounter

Spouse or Partner Abuse, Psychological, Suspected (721)

995.82 (T76.31XA) Initial encounter

995.82 (T76.31XD) Subsequent encounter

Other Circumstances Related to Spouse or Partner Abuse, Psychological (721)

V61.11 (Z69.11) Encounter for mental health services for victim of spouse or partner psychological abuse

V15.42 (Z91.411)   Personal history (past history) of spouse or partner
                         psychological abuse
V61.12 (Z69.12)   Encounter for mental health services for perpetrator of spouse
                         or partner psychological abuse

Adult Abuse by Nonspouse or Nonpartner (722)

Adult Physical Abuse by Nonspouse or Nonpartner, Confirmed (722)
995.81 (T74.11XA)   Initial encounter
995.81 (T74.11XD)   Subsequent encounter

Adult Physical Abuse by Nonspouse or Nonpartner, Suspected (722)
995.81 (T76.11XA)   Initial encounter
995.81 (T76.11XD)   Subsequent encounter

Adult Sexual Abuse by Nonspouse or Nonpartner, Confirmed (722)
995.83 (T74.21XA)   Initial encounter
995.83 (T74.21XD)   Subsequent encounter

Adult Sexual Abuse by Nonspouse or Nonpartner, Suspected (722)
995.83 (T76.21XA)   Initial encounter
995.83 (T76.21XD)   Subsequent encounter

Adult Psychological Abuse by Nonspouse or Nonpartner, Confirmed (722)
995.82 (T74.31XA)   Initial encounter
995.82 (T74.31XD)   Subsequent encounter

Adult Psychological Abuse by Nonspouse or Nonpartner, Suspected (722)
995.82 (T76.31XA)   Initial encounter
995.82 (T76.31XD)   Subsequent encounter

Other Circumstances Related to Adult Abuse by Nonspouse or Nonpartner (722)
V65.49 (Z69.81)   Encounter for mental health services for victim of nonspousal
                         adult abuse
V62.83 (Z69.82)   Encounter for mental health services for perpetrator of
                         nonspousal adult abuse

Educational and Occupational Problems (723)

Educational Problems (723)
V62.3 (Z55.9)   Academic or Educational Problem (723)

Occupational Problems (723)
V62.21 (Z56.82)   Problem Related to Current Military Deployment Status (723)
V62.29 (Z56.9)   Other Problem Related to Employment (723)

Housing and Economic Problems (723)

Housing Problems (723)
V60.0 (Z59.0)   Homelessness (723)
V60.1 (Z59.1)   Inadequate Housing (723)

Other Circumstances of Personal History (726)

Problems Related to Access to Medical and Other Health Care (726)

Nonadherence to Medical Treatment (726)

Preface

The American Psychiatric Association's *Diagnostic and Statistical Manual of Mental Disorders* (DSM) is a classification of mental disorders with associated criteria designed to facilitate more reliable diagnoses of these disorders. With successive editions over the past 60 years, it has become a standard reference for clinical practice in the mental health field. Since a complete description of the underlying pathological processes is not possible for most mental disorders, it is important to emphasize that the current diagnostic criteria are the best available description of how mental disorders are expressed and can be recognized by trained clinicians. DSM is intended to serve as a practical, functional, and flexible guide for organizing information that can aid in the accurate diagnosis and treatment of mental disorders. It is a tool for clinicians, an essential educational resource for students and practitioners, and a reference for researchers in the field.

Although this edition of DSM was designed first and foremost to be a useful guide to clinical practice, as an official nomenclature it must be applicable in a wide diversity of contexts. DSM has been used by clinicians and researchers from different orientations (biological, psychodynamic, cognitive, behavioral, interpersonal, family/systems), all of whom strive for a common language to communicate the essential characteristics of mental disorders presented by their patients. The information is of value to all professionals associated with various aspects of mental health care, including psychiatrists, other physicians, psychologists, social workers, nurses, counselors, forensic and legal specialists, occupational and rehabilitation therapists, and other health professionals. The criteria are concise and explicit and intended to facilitate an objective assessment of symptom presentations in a variety of clinical settings—inpatient, outpatient, partial hospital, consultation-liaison, clinical, private practice, and primary care—as well in general community epidemiological studies of mental disorders. DSM-5 is also a tool for collecting and communicating accurate public health statistics on mental disorder morbidity and mortality rates. Finally, the criteria and corresponding text serve as a textbook for students early in their profession who need a structured way to understand and diagnose mental disorders as well as for seasoned professionals encountering rare disorders for the first time. Fortunately, all of these uses are mutually compatible.

These diverse needs and interests were taken into consideration in planning DSM-5. The classification of disorders is harmonized with the World Health Organization's *International Classification of Diseases* (ICD), the official coding system used in the United States, so that the DSM criteria define disorders identified by ICD diagnostic names and code numbers. In DSM-5, both ICD-9-CM and ICD-10-CM codes (the latter scheduled for adoption in October 2015) are attached to the relevant disorders in the classification.

Although DSM-5 remains a categorical classification of separate disorders, we recognize that mental disorders do not always fit completely within the boundaries of a single disorder. Some symptom domains, such as depression and anxiety, involve multiple diagnostic categories and may reflect common underlying vulnerabilities for a larger group of disorders. In recognition of this reality, the disorders included in DSM-5 were reordered into a revised organizational structure meant to stimulate new clinical perspectives. This new structure corresponds with the organizational arrangement of disorders planned for ICD-11 scheduled for release in 2015. Other enhancements have been introduced to promote ease of use across all settings:

- **Representation of developmental issues related to diagnosis.** The change in chapter organization better reflects a lifespan approach, with disorders more frequently diagnosed in childhood (e.g., neurodevelopmental disorders) at the beginning of the manual and disorders more applicable to older adulthood (e.g., neurocognitive disorders) at the end of the manual. Also, within the text, subheadings on development and course provide descriptions of how disorder presentations may change across the lifespan. Age-related factors specific to diagnosis (e.g., symptom presentation and prevalence differences in certain age groups) are also included in the text. For added emphasis, these age-related factors have been added to the criteria themselves where applicable (e.g., in the criteria sets for insomnia disorder and posttraumatic stress disorder, specific criteria describe how symptoms might be expressed in children). Likewise, gender and cultural issues have been integrated into the disorders where applicable.
- **Integration of scientific findings from the latest research in genetics and neuroimaging.** The revised chapter structure was informed by recent research in neuroscience and by emerging genetic linkages between diagnostic groups. Genetic and physiological risk factors, prognostic indicators, and some putative diagnostic markers are highlighted in the text. This new structure should improve clinicians' ability to identify diagnoses in a disorder spectrum based on common neurocircuitry, genetic vulnerability, and environmental exposures.
- **Consolidation of autistic disorder, Asperger's disorder, and pervasive developmental disorder into autism spectrum disorder.** Symptoms of these disorders represent a single continuum of mild to severe impairments in the two domains of social communication and restrictive repetitive behaviors/interests rather than being distinct disorders. This change is designed to improve the sensitivity and specificity of the criteria for the diagnosis of autism spectrum disorder and to identify more focused treatment targets for the specific impairments identified.
- **Streamlined classification of bipolar and depressive disorders.** Bipolar and depressive disorders are the most commonly diagnosed conditions in psychiatry. It was therefore important to streamline the presentation of these disorders to enhance both clinical and educational use. Rather than separating the definition of manic, hypomanic, and major depressive episodes from the definition of bipolar I disorder, bipolar II disorder, and major depressive disorder as in the previous edition, we included all of the component criteria within the respective criteria for each disorder. This approach will facilitate bedside diagnosis and treatment of these important disorders. Likewise, the explanatory notes for differentiating bereavement and major depressive disorders will provide far greater clinical guidance than was previously provided in the simple bereavement exclusion criterion. The new specifiers of anxious distress and mixed features are now fully described in the narrative on specifier variations that accompanies the criteria for these disorders.
- **Restructuring of substance use disorders for consistency and clarity.** The categories of substance abuse and substance dependence have been eliminated and replaced with an overarching new category of substance use disorders—with the specific substance used defining the specific disorders. "Dependence" has been easily confused with the term "addiction" when, in fact, the tolerance and withdrawal that previously defined dependence are actually very normal responses to prescribed medications that affect the central nervous system and do not necessarily indicate the presence of an addiction. By revising and clarifying these criteria in DSM-5, we hope to alleviate some of the widespread misunderstanding about these issues.
- **Enhanced specificity for major and mild neurocognitive disorders.** Given the explosion in neuroscience, neuropsychology, and brain imaging over the past 20 years, it was critical to convey the current state-of-the-art in the diagnosis of specific types of disorders that were previously referred to as the "dementias" or organic brain diseases. Biological markers identified by imaging for vascular and traumatic brain disorders and

specific molecular genetic findings for rare variants of Alzheimer's disease and Huntington's disease have greatly advanced clinical diagnoses, and these disorders and others have now been separated into specific subtypes.

- **Transition in conceptualizing personality disorders.** Although the benefits of a more dimensional approach to personality disorders have been identified in previous editions, the transition from a categorical diagnostic system of individual disorders to one based on the relative distribution of personality traits has not been widely accepted. In DSM-5, the categorical personality disorders are virtually unchanged from the previous edition. However, an alternative "hybrid" model has been proposed in Section III to guide future research that separates interpersonal functioning assessments and the expression of pathological personality traits for six specific disorders. A more dimensional profile of personality trait expression is also proposed for a trait-specified approach.

- **Section III: new disorders and features.** A new section (Section III) has been added to highlight disorders that require further study but are not sufficiently well established to be a part of the official classification of mental disorders for routine clinical use. Dimensional measures of symptom severity in 13 symptom domains have also been incorporated to allow for the measurement of symptom levels of varying severity across all diagnostic groups. Likewise, the WHO Disability Assessment Schedule (WHODAS), a standard method for assessing global disability levels for mental disorders that is based on the International Classification of Functioning, Disability and Health (ICF) and is applicable in all of medicine, has been provided to replace the more limited Global Assessment of Functioning scale. It is our hope that as these measures are implemented over time, they will provide greater accuracy and flexibility in the clinical description of individual symptomatic presentations and associated disability during diagnostic assessments.

- **Online enhancements.** DSM-5 features online supplemental information. Additional cross-cutting and diagnostic severity measures are available online (www.psychiatry.org/dsm5), linked to the relevant disorders. In addition, the Cultural Formulation Interview, Cultural Formulation Interview—Informant Version, and supplementary modules to the core Cultural Formulation Interview are also included online at www.psychiatry.org/dsm5.

These innovations were designed by the leading authorities on mental disorders in the world and were implemented on the basis of their expert review, public commentary, and independent peer review. The 13 work groups, under the direction of the DSM-5 Task Force, in conjunction with other review bodies and, eventually, the APA Board of Trustees, collectively represent the global expertise of the specialty. This effort was supported by an extensive base of advisors and by the professional staff of the APA Division of Research; the names of everyone involved are too numerous to mention here but are listed in the Appendix. We owe tremendous thanks to those who devoted countless hours and invaluable expertise to this effort to improve the diagnosis of mental disorders.

We would especially like to acknowledge the chairs, text coordinators, and members of the 13 work groups, listed in the front of the manual, who spent many hours in this volunteer effort to improve the scientific basis of clinical practice over a sustained 6-year period. Susan K. Schultz, M.D., who served as text editor, worked tirelessly with Emily A. Kuhl, Ph.D., senior science writer and DSM-5 staff text editor, to coordinate the efforts of the work groups into a cohesive whole. William E. Narrow, M.D., M.P.H., led the research group that developed the overall research strategy for DSM-5, including the field trials, that greatly enhanced the evidence base for this revision. In addition, we are grateful to those who contributed so much time to the independent review of the revision proposals, including Kenneth S. Kendler, M.D., and Robert Freedman, M.D., co-chairs of the Scientific Review Committee; John S. McIntyre, M.D., and Joel Yager, M.D., co-chairs of the Clinical and Public Health Committee; and Glenn Martin, M.D., chair of the APA Assembly review process. Special thanks go to Helena C. Kraemer, Ph.D., for her expert statistical consultation; Michael B. First, M.D., for his valuable input on the coding and review of criteria; and Paul S. Appelbaum, M.D., for feedback on forensic issues. Maria N. Ward, M.Ed., RHIT, CCS-P, also helped in verifying all ICD coding. The Summit Group, which included these consultants, the chairs of all review groups, the task force chairs, and the APA executive officers, chaired by Dilip V. Jeste, M.D., provided leadership and vision in helping to achieve compromise and consensus. This level of commitment has contributed to the balance and objectivity that we feel are hallmarks of DSM-5.

We especially wish to recognize the outstanding APA Division of Research staff— identified in the Task Force and Work Group listing at the front of this manual—who worked tirelessly to interact with the task force, work groups, advisors, and reviewers to resolve issues, serve as liaisons between the groups, direct and manage the academic and routine clinical practice field trials, and record decisions in this important process. In particular, we appreciate the support and guidance provided by James H. Scully Jr., M.D., Medical Director and CEO of the APA, through the years and travails of the development process. Finally, we thank the editorial and production staff of American Psychiatric Publishing—specifically, Rebecca Rinehart, Publisher; John McDuffie, Editorial Director; Ann Eng, Senior Editor; Greg Kuny, Managing Editor; and Tammy Cordova, Graphics Design Manager—for their guidance in bringing this all together and creating the final product. It is the culmination of efforts of many talented individuals who dedicated their time, expertise, and passion that made DSM-5 possible.

David J. Kupfer, M.D.
DSM-5 Task Force Chair

Darrel A. Regier, M.D., M.P.H.
DSM-5 Task Force Vice-Chair
December 19, 2012

SECTION I
DSM-5 Basics

This section is a basic orientation to the purpose, structure, content, and use of DSM-5. It is not intended to provide an exhaustive account of the evolution of DSM-5, but rather to give readers a succinct overview of its key elements. The introductory section describes the public, professional, and expert review process that was used to extensively evaluate the diagnostic criteria presented in Section II. A summary of the DSM-5 structure, harmonization with ICD-11, and the transition to a non-axial system with a new approach to assessing disability is also presented. "Use of the Manual" includes "Definition of a Mental Disorder," forensic considerations, and a brief overview of the diagnostic process and use of coding and recording procedures.

Introduction

The creation of the fifth edition of *Diagnostic and Statistical Manual of Mental Disorders* (DSM-5) was a massive undertaking that involved hundreds of people working toward a common goal over a 12-year process. Much thought and deliberation were involved in evaluating the diagnostic criteria, considering the organization of every aspect of the manual, and creating new features believed to be most useful to clinicians. All of these efforts were directed toward the goal of enhancing the clinical usefulness of DSM-5 as a guide in the diagnosis of mental disorders.

Reliable diagnoses are essential for guiding treatment recommendations, identifying prevalence rates for mental health service planning, identifying patient groups for clinical and basic research, and documenting important public health information such as morbidity and mortality rates. As the understanding of mental disorders and their treatments has evolved, medical, scientific, and clinical professionals have focused on the characteristics of specific disorders and their implications for treatment and research.

While DSM has been the cornerstone of substantial progress in reliability, it has been well recognized by both the American Psychiatric Association (APA) and the broad scientific community working on mental disorders that past science was not mature enough to yield fully validated diagnoses—that is, to provide consistent, strong, and objective scientific validators of individual DSM disorders. The science of mental disorders continues to evolve. However, the last two decades since DSM-IV was released have seen real and durable progress in such areas as cognitive neuroscience, brain imaging, epidemiology, and genetics. The DSM-5 Task Force overseeing the new edition recognized that research advances will require careful, iterative changes if DSM is to maintain its place as the touchstone classification of mental disorders. Finding the right balance is critical. Speculative results do not belong in an official nosology, but at the same time, DSM must evolve in the context of other clinical research initiatives in the field. One important aspect of this transition derives from the broad recognition that a too-rigid categorical system does not capture clinical experience or important scientific observations. The results of numerous studies of comorbidity and disease transmission in families, including twin studies and molecular genetic studies, make strong arguments for what many astute clinicians have long observed: the boundaries between many disorder "categories" are more fluid over the life course than DSM-IV recognized, and many symptoms assigned to a single disorder may occur, at varying levels of severity, in many other disorders. These findings mean that DSM, like other medical disease classifications, should accommodate ways to introduce dimensional approaches to mental disorders, including dimensions that cut across current categories. Such an approach should permit a more accurate description of patient presentations and increase the validity of a diagnosis (i.e., the degree to which diagnostic criteria reflect the comprehensive manifestation of an underlying psychopathological disorder). DSM-5 is designed to better fill the need of clinicians, patients, families, and researchers for a clear and concise description of each mental disorder organized by explicit diagnostic criteria, supplemented, when appropriate, by dimensional measures that cross diagnostic boundaries, and a brief digest of information about the diagnosis, risk factors, associated features, research advances, and various expressions of the disorder.

Clinical training and experience are needed to use DSM for determining a diagnosis. The diagnostic criteria identify symptoms, behaviors, cognitive functions, personality traits, physical signs, syndrome combinations, and durations that require clinical expertise to differentiate from normal life variation and transient responses to stress. To facilitate a thorough examination of the range of symptoms present, DSM can serve clinicians as a guide to identify the most prominent symptoms that should be assessed when diagnosing a disorder. Although some mental disorders may have well-defined boundaries around symptom clusters, scientific evidence now places many, if not most, disorders on a spectrum with closely related disorders that have shared symptoms, shared genetic and environmental risk factors, and possibly shared neural substrates (perhaps most strongly established for a subset of anxiety disorders by neuroimaging and animal models). In short, we have come to recognize that the boundaries between disorders are more porous than originally perceived.

Many health profession and educational groups have been involved in the development and testing of DSM-5, including physicians, psychologists, social workers, nurses, counselors, epidemiologists, statisticians, neuroscientists, and neuropsychologists. Finally, patients, families, lawyers, consumer organizations, and advocacy groups have all participated in revising DSM-5 by providing feedback on the mental disorders described in this volume. Their monitoring of the descriptions and explanatory text is essential to improve understanding, reduce stigma, and advance the treatment and eventual cures for these conditions.

A Brief History

The APA first published a predecessor of DSM in 1844, as a statistical classification of institutionalized mental patients. It was designed to improve communication about the types of patients cared for in these hospitals. This forerunner to DSM also was used as a component of the full U.S. census. After World War II, DSM evolved through four major editions into a diagnostic classification system for psychiatrists, other physicians, and other mental health professionals that described the essential features of the full range of mental disorders. The current edition, DSM-5, builds on the goal of its predecessors (most recently, DSM-IV-TR, or Text Revision, published in 2000) of providing guidelines for diagnoses that can inform treatment and management decisions.

DSM-5 Revision Process

In 1999, the APA launched an evaluation of the strengths and weaknesses of DSM based on emerging research that did not support the boundaries established for some mental disorders. This effort was coordinated with the World Health Organization (WHO) Division of Mental Health, the World Psychiatric Association, and the National Institute of Mental Health (NIMH) in the form of several conferences, the proceedings of which were published in 2002 in a monograph entitled *A Research Agenda for DSM-V*. Thereafter, from 2003 to 2008, a cooperative agreement with the APA and the WHO was supported by the NIMH, the National Institute on Drug Abuse (NIDA), and the National Institute on Alcoholism and Alcohol Abuse (NIAAA) to convene 13 international DSM-5 research planning conferences, involving 400 participants from 39 countries, to review the world literature in specific diagnostic areas to prepare for revisions in developing both DSM-5 and the *International Classification of Diseases*, 11th Revision (ICD-11). Reports from these conferences formed the basis for future DSM-5 Task Force reviews and set the stage for the new edition of DSM.

In 2006, the APA named David J. Kupfer, M.D., as Chair and Darrel A. Regier, M.D., M.P.H., as Vice-Chair of the DSM-5 Task Force. They were charged with recommending chairs for the 13 diagnostic work groups and additional task force members with a multidisciplinary range of expertise who would oversee the development of DSM-5. An additional vetting process was initiated by the APA Board of Trustees to disclose sources of income and thus avoid conflicts of interest by task force and work group members. The full disclosure of all income and research grants from commercial sources, including the pharmaceutical industry, in the previous 3 years, the imposition of an income cap from all commercial sources, and the publication of disclosures on a Web site set a new standard for the field. Thereafter, the task force of 28 members was approved in 2007, and appointments of more than 130 work group members were approved in 2008. More than 400 additional work group advisors with no voting authority were also approved to participate in the process. A clear concept of the next evolutionary stage for the classification of mental disorders was central to the efforts of the task force and the work groups. This vision emerged as the task force and work groups recounted the history of DSM-IV's classification, its current strengths and limitations, and strategic directions for its revision. An intensive 6-year process involved conducting literature reviews and secondary analyses, publishing research reports in scientific journals, developing draft diagnostic criteria, posting preliminary drafts on the DSM-5 Web site for public comment, presenting preliminary findings at professional meetings, performing field trials, and revising criteria and text.

Proposals for Revisions

Proposals for the revision of DSM-5 diagnostic criteria were developed by members of the work groups on the basis of rationale, scope of change, expected impact on clinical management and public health, strength of the supporting research evidence, overall clarity, and clinical utility. Proposals encompassed changes to diagnostic criteria; the addition of new disorders, subtypes, and specifiers; and the deletion of existing disorders.

In the proposals for revisions, strengths and weaknesses in the current criteria and nosology were first identified. Novel scientific findings over the previous two decades were considered, leading to the creation of a research plan to assess potential changes through literature reviews and secondary data analyses. Four principles guided the draft revisions: 1) DSM-5 is primarily intended to be a manual to be used by clinicians, and revisions must be feasible for routine clinical practice; 2) recommendations for revisions should be guided by research evidence; 3) where possible, continuity should be maintained with previous editions of DSM; and 4) no a priori constraints should be placed on the degree of change between DSM-IV and DSM-5.

Building on the initial literature reviews, work groups identified key issues within their diagnostic areas. Work groups also examined broader methodological concerns, such as the presence of contradictory findings within the literature; development of a refined definition of mental disorder; cross-cutting issues relevant to all disorders; and the revision of disorders categorized in DSM-IV as "not otherwise specified." Inclusion of a proposal for revision in Section II was informed by consideration of its advantages and disadvantages for public health and clinical utility, the strength of the evidence, and the magnitude of the change. New diagnoses and disorder subtypes and specifiers were subject to additional stipulations, such as demonstration of reliability (i.e., the degree to which two clinicians could independently arrive at the same diagnosis for a given patient). Disorders with low clinical utility and weak validity were considered for deletion. Placement of conditions in "Conditions for Further Study" in Section III was contingent on the amount of empirical evidence generated on the diagnosis, diagnostic reliability or validity, presence of clear clinical need, and potential benefit in advancing research.

DSM-5 Field Trials

The use of field trials to empirically demonstrate reliability was a noteworthy improvement introduced in DSM-III. The design and implementation strategy of the DSM-5 Field Trials represent several changes over approaches used for DSM-III and DSM-IV, particularly in obtaining data on the precision of kappa reliability estimates (a statistical measure that assesses level of agreement between raters that corrects for chance agreement due to prevalence rates) in the context of clinical settings with high levels of diagnostic comorbidity. For DSM-5, field trials were extended by using two distinctive designs: one in large, diverse medical-academic settings, and the other in routine clinical practices. The former capitalized on the need for large sample sizes to test hypotheses on reliability and clinical utility of a range of diagnoses in a variety of patient populations; the latter supplied valuable information about how proposed revisions performed in everyday clinical settings among a diverse sample of DSM users. It is anticipated that future clinical and basic research studies will focus on the validity of the revised categorical diagnostic criteria and the underlying dimensional features of these disorders (including those now being explored by the NIMH Research Domain Criteria initiative).

The medical-academic field trials were conducted at 11 North American medical-academic sites and assessed the reliability, feasibility, and clinical utility of select revisions, with priority given to those that represented the greatest degree of change from DSM-IV or those potentially having the greatest public health impact. The full clinical patient populations coming to each site were screened for DSM-IV diagnoses or qualifying symptoms likely to predict several specific DSM-5 disorders of interest. Stratified samples of four to seven specific disorders, plus a stratum containing a representative sample of all other diagnoses, were identified for each site. Patients consented to the study and were randomly assigned for a clinical interview by a clinician blind to the diagnosis, followed by a second interview with a clinician blind to previous diagnoses. Patients first filled out a computer-assisted inventory of cross-cutting symptoms in more than a dozen psychological domains. These inventories were scored by a central server, and results were provided to clinicians before they conducted a typical clinical interview (with no structured protocol). Clinicians were required to score the presence of qualifying criteria on a computer-assisted DSM-5 diagnostic checklist, determine diagnoses, score the severity of the diagnosis, and submit all data to the central Web-based server. This study design allowed the calculation of the degree to which two independent clinicians could agree on a diagnosis (using the intraclass kappa statistic) and the agreement of a single patient or two different clinicians on two separate ratings of cross-cutting symptoms, personality traits, disability, and diagnostic severity measures (using intraclass correlation coefficients) along with information on the precision of these estimates of reliability. It was also possible to assess the prevalence rates of both DSM-IV and DSM-5 conditions in the respective clinical populations.

The routine clinical practice field trials involved recruitment of individual psychiatrists and other mental health clinicians. A volunteer sample was recruited that included generalist and specialty psychiatrists, psychologists, licensed clinical social workers, counselors, marriage and family therapists, and advanced practice psychiatric mental health nurses. The field trials provided exposure of the proposed DSM-5 diagnoses and dimensional measures to a wide range of clinicians to assess their feasibility and clinical utility.

Public and Professional Review

In 2010, the APA launched a unique Web site to facilitate public and professional input into DSM-5. All draft diagnostic criteria and proposed changes in organization were posted on www.dsm5.org for a 2-month comment period. Feedback totaled more than 8,000 submissions, which were systematically reviewed by each of the 13 work groups, whose members, where appropriate, integrated questions and comments into discussions of draft revisions and plans for field trial testing. After revisions to the initial draft criteria and proposed chapter organization, a second posting occurred in 2011. Work groups considered feedback from both Web postings and the results of the DSM-5 Field Trials when drafting proposed final criteria, which were posted on the Web site for a third and final time in 2012. These three iterations of external review produced more than 13,000 individually signed comments on the Web site that were received and reviewed by the work groups, plus thousands of organized petition signers for and against some proposed revisions, all of which allowed the task force to actively address concerns of DSM users, as well as patients and advocacy groups, and ensure that clinical utility remained a high priority.

Expert Review

The members of the 13 work groups, representing expertise in their respective areas, collaborated with advisors and reviewers under the overall direction of the DSM-5 Task

Force to draft the diagnostic criteria and accompanying text. This effort was supported by a team of APA Division of Research staff and developed through a network of text coordinators from each work group. The preparation of the text was coordinated by the text editor, working in close collaboration with the work groups and under the direction of the task force chairs. The Scientific Review Committee (SRC) was established to provide a scientific peer review process that was external to that of the work groups. The SRC chair, vice-chair, and six committee members were charged with reviewing the degree to which the proposed changes from DSM-IV could be supported with scientific evidence. Each proposal for diagnostic revision required a memorandum of evidence for change prepared by the work group and accompanied by a summary of supportive data organized around validators for the proposed diagnostic criteria (i.e., antecedent validators such as familial aggregation, concurrent validators such as biological markers, and prospective validators such as response to treatment or course of illness). The submissions were reviewed by the SRC and scored according to the strength of the supportive scientific data. Other justifications for change, such as those arising from clinical experience or need or from a conceptual reframing of diagnostic categories, were generally seen as outside the purview of the SRC. The reviewers' scores, which varied substantially across the different proposals, and an accompanying brief commentary were then returned to the APA Board of Trustees and the work groups for consideration and response.

The Clinical and Public Health Committee (CPHC), composed of a chair, vice-chair, and six members, was appointed to consider additional clinical utility, public health, and logical clarification issues for criteria that had not yet accumulated the type or level of evidence deemed sufficient for change by the SRC. This review process was particularly important for DSM-IV disorders with known deficiencies for which proposed remedies had neither been previously considered in the DSM revision process nor been subjected to replicated research studies. These selected disorders were evaluated by four to five external reviewers, and the blinded results were reviewed by CPHC members, who in turn made recommendations to the APA Board of Trustees and the work groups.

Forensic reviews by the members of the APA Council on Psychiatry and Law were conducted for disorders frequently appearing in forensic environments and ones with high potential for influencing civil and criminal judgments in courtroom settings. Work groups also added forensic experts as advisors in pertinent areas to complement expertise provided by the Council on Psychiatry and Law.

The work groups themselves were charged with the responsibility to review the entire research literature surrounding a diagnostic area, including old, revised, and new diagnostic criteria, in an intensive 6-year review process to assess the pros and cons of making either small iterative changes or major conceptual changes to address the inevitable reification that occurs with diagnostic conceptual approaches that persist over several decades. Such changes included the merger of previously separate diagnostic areas into more dimensional spectra, such as that which occurred with autism spectrum disorder, substance use disorders, sexual dysfunctions, and somatic symptom and related disorders. Other changes included correcting flaws that had become apparent over time in the choice of operational criteria for some disorders. These types of changes posed particular challenges to the SRC and CPHC review processes, which were not constructed to evaluate the validity of DSM-IV diagnostic criteria. However, the DSM-5 Task Force, which had reviewed proposed changes and had responsibility for reviewing the text describing each disorder contemporaneously with the work groups during this period, was in a unique position to render an informed judgment on the scientific merits of such revisions. Furthermore, many of these major changes were subject to field trial testing, although comprehensive testing of all proposed changes could not be accommodated by such testing because of time limitations and availability of resources.

A final recommendation from the task force was then provided to the APA Board of Trustees and the APA Assembly's Committee on DSM-5 to consider some of the clinical utility and feasibility features of the proposed revisions. The assembly is a deliberative body of the APA representing the district branches and wider membership that is composed of psychiatrists from throughout the United States who provide geographic, practice size, and interest-based diversity. The Committee on DSM-5 is a committee made up of a diverse group of assembly leaders.

Following all of the preceding review steps, an executive "summit committee" session was held to consolidate input from review and assembly committee chairs, task force chairs, a forensic advisor, and a statistical advisor, for a preliminary review of each disorder by the assembly and APA Board of Trustees executive committees. This preceded a preliminary review by the full APA Board of Trustees. The assembly voted, in November 2012, to recommend that the board approve the publication of DSM-5, and the APA Board of Trustees approved its publication in December 2012. The many experts, reviewers, and advisors who contributed to this process are listed in the Appendix.

Organizational Structure

The individual disorder definitions that constitute the operationalized sets of diagnostic criteria provide the core of DSM-5 for clinical and research purposes. These criteria have been subjected to scientific review, albeit to varying degrees, and many disorders have undergone field testing for interrater reliability. In contrast, the classification of disorders (the way in which disorders are grouped, which provides a high-level organization for the manual) has not generally been thought of as scientifically significant, despite the fact that judgments had to be made when disorders were initially divided into chapters for DSM-III.

DSM is a medical classification of disorders and as such serves as a historically determined cognitive schema imposed on clinical and scientific information to increase its comprehensibility and utility. Not surprisingly, as the foundational science that ultimately led to DSM-III has approached a half-century in age, challenges have begun to emerge for clinicians and scientists alike that are inherent in the DSM structure rather than in the description of any single disorder. These challenges include high rates of comorbidity within and across DSM chapters, an excessive use of and need to rely on "not otherwise specified" (NOS) criteria, and a growing inability to integrate DSM disorders with the results of genetic studies and other scientific findings.

As the APA and the WHO began to plan their respective revisions of the DSM and the *International Classification of Disorders* (ICD), both considered the possibility of improving clinical utility (e.g., by helping to explain apparent comorbidity) and facilitating scientific investigation by rethinking the organizational structures of both publications in a linear system designated by alphanumeric codes that sequence chapters according to some rational and relational structure. It was critical to both the DSM-5 Task Force and the WHO International Advisory Group on the revision of the ICD-10 Section on Mental and Behavioral Disorders that the revisions to the organization enhance clinical utility and remain within the bounds of well-replicated scientific information. Although the need for reform seemed apparent, it was important to respect the state of the science as well as the challenge that overly rapid change would pose for the clinical and research communities. In that spirit, revision of the organization was approached as a conservative, evolutionary diagnostic reform that would be guided by emerging scientific evidence on the relationships between disorder groups. By reordering and regrouping the existing disorders, the revised structure is meant to stimulate new clinical perspectives and to encourage researchers to identify the psychological and physiological cross-cutting factors that are not bound by strict categorical designations.

The use of DSM criteria has the clear virtue of creating a common language for communication between clinicians about the diagnosis of disorders. The official criteria and disorders that were determined to have accepted clinical applicability are located in Section II of the manual. However, it should be noted that these diagnostic criteria and their relationships within the classification are based on current research and may need to be modified as new evidence is gathered by future research both within and across the domains of proposed disorders. "Conditions for Further Study," described in Section III, are those for which we determined that the scientific evidence is not yet available to support widespread clinical use. These diagnostic criteria are included to highlight the evolution and direction of scientific advances in these areas to stimulate further research.

With any ongoing review process, especially one of this complexity, different viewpoints emerge, and an effort was made to consider various viewpoints and, when warranted, accommodate them. For example, personality disorders are included in both Sections II and III. Section II represents an update of the text associated with the same criteria found in DSM-IV-TR, whereas Section III includes the proposed research model for personality disorder diagnosis and conceptualization developed by the DSM-5 Personality and Personality Disorders Work Group. As this field evolves, it is hoped that both versions will serve clinical practice and research initiatives.

Harmonization With ICD-11

The groups tasked with revising the DSM and ICD systems shared the overarching goal of harmonizing the two classifications as much as possible, for the following reasons:

- The existence of two major classifications of mental disorders hinders the collection and use of national health statistics, the design of clinical trials aimed at developing new treatments, and the consideration of global applicability of the results by international regulatory agencies.
- More broadly, the existence of two classifications complicates attempts to replicate scientific results across national boundaries.
- Even when the intention was to identify identical patient populations, DSM-IV and ICD-10 diagnoses did not always agree.

Early in the course of the revisions, it became apparent that a shared organizational structure would help harmonize the classifications. In fact, the use of a shared framework helped to integrate the work of DSM and ICD work groups and to focus on scientific issues. The DSM-5 organization and the proposed linear structure of the ICD-11 have been endorsed by the leadership of the NIMH Research Domain Criteria (RDoC) project as consistent with the initial overall structure of that project.

Of course, principled disagreements on the classification of psychopathology and on specific criteria for certain disorders were expected given the current state of scientific knowledge. However, most of the salient differences between the DSM and the ICD classifications do not reflect real scientific differences, but rather represent historical by-products of independent committee processes.

To the surprise of participants in both revision processes, large sections of the content fell relatively easily into place, reflecting real strengths in some areas of the scientific literature, such as epidemiology, analyses of comorbidity, twin studies, and certain other genetically informed designs. When disparities emerged, they almost always reflected the need to make a judgment about where to place a disorder in the face of incomplete—or, more often, conflicting—data. Thus, for example, on the basis of patterns of symptoms, comorbidity, and shared risk factors, attention-deficit/hyperactivity disorder (ADHD) was placed with neurodevelopmental disorders, but the same data also supported strong arguments to place ADHD within disruptive, impulse-control, and conduct disorders. These issues were settled with the preponderance of evidence (most notably validators approved by the DSM-5 Task Force). The work groups recognize, however, that future discoveries might change the placement as well as the contours of individual disorders and, furthermore, that the simple and linear organization that best supports clinical practice may not fully capture the complexity and heterogeneity of mental disorders. The revised organization is coordinated with the mental and behavioral disorders chapter (Chapter V) of ICD-11, which will utilize an expanded numeric–alphanumeric coding system. However, the official coding system in use in the United States at the time of publication of this manual is that of the *International Classification of Diseases, Ninth Revision, Clinical Modification* (ICD-9-CM)—the U.S. adaptation of ICD-9. *International Classification of Diseases, Tenth Revision, Clinical Modification* (ICD-10-CM), adapted from ICD-10, is scheduled for implementation in the United States in October 2015. Given the impending release of ICD-11, it was decided that this iteration, and not ICD-10, would be the most relevant on which to focus harmonization. However, given that adoption of the ICD-9-CM coding system will remain at the time of the DSM-5 release, it will be necessary to use the ICD-9-CM codes. Furthermore, given that DSM-5's organizational structure reflects the anticipated structure of ICD-11, the eventual ICD-11 codes will follow the sequential order of diagnoses in the DSM-5 chapter structure more closely. At present, both the ICD-9-CM and the ICD-10-CM codes have been indicated for each disorder. These codes will not be in sequential order throughout the manual because they were assigned to complement earlier organizational structures.

Dimensional Approach to Diagnosis

Structural problems rooted in the basic design of the previous DSM classification, constructed of a large number of narrow diagnostic categories, have emerged in both clinical practice and research. Relevant evidence comes from diverse sources, including studies of comorbidity and the substantial need for not otherwise specified diagnoses, which represent the majority of diagnoses in areas such as eating disorders, personality disorders, and autism spectrum disorder. Studies of both genetic and environmental risk factors, whether based on twin designs, familial transmission, or molecular analyses, also raise concerns about the categorical structure of the DSM system. Because the previous DSM approach considered each diagnosis as categorically separate from health and from other diagnoses, it did not capture the widespread sharing of symptoms and risk factors across many disorders that is apparent in studies of comorbidity. Earlier editions of DSM focused on excluding false-positive results from diagnoses; thus, its categories were overly narrow, as is apparent from the widespread need to use NOS diagnoses. Indeed, the once plausible goal of identifying homogeneous populations for treatment and research resulted in narrow diagnostic categories that did not capture clinical reality, symptom heterogeneity within disorders, and significant sharing of symptoms across multiple disorders. The historical aspiration of achieving diagnostic homogeneity by progressive subtyping within disorder categories no longer is sensible; like most common human ills, mental disorders are heterogeneous at many levels, ranging from genetic risk factors to symptoms.

Related to recommendations about alterations in the chapter structure of DSM-5, members of the diagnostic spectra study group examined whether scientific validators could inform possible new groupings of related disorders within the existing categorical framework. Eleven such indicators were recommended for this purpose: shared neural substrates, family traits, genetic risk factors, specific environmental risk factors, biomarkers, temperamental antecedents, abnormalities of emotional or cognitive processing, symptom similarity, course of illness, high comorbidity, and shared treatment response. These indicators served as empirical guidelines to inform decision making by the work groups and the task force about how to cluster disorders to maximize their validity and clinical utility.

A series of papers was developed and published in a prominent international journal (*Psychological Medicine,* Vol. 39, 2009) as part of both the DSM-5 and the ICD-11 developmental processes to document that such validators were most useful for suggesting large groupings of disorders rather than for "validating" individual disorder diagnostic criteria. The regrouping of mental disorders in DSM-5 is intended to enable future research to enhance understanding of disease origins and pathophysiological commonalities between disorders and provide a base for future replication wherein data can be reanalyzed over time to continually assess validity. Ongoing revisions of DSM-5 will make it a "living document," adaptable to future discoveries in neurobiology, genetics, and epidemiology.

On the basis of the published findings of this common DSM-5 and ICD-11 analysis, it was demonstrated that clustering of disorders according to what has been termed *internalizing* and *externalizing* factors represents an empirically supported framework. Within both the internalizing group (representing disorders with prominent anxiety, depressive, and somatic symptoms) and the externalizing group (representing disorders with prominent impulsive, disruptive conduct, and substance use symptoms), the sharing of genetic and environmental risk factors, as shown by twin studies, likely explains much of the systematic comorbidities seen in both clinical and community samples. The adjacent placement of "internalizing disorders," characterized by depressed mood, anxiety, and related physiological and cognitive symptoms, should aid in developing new diagnostic approaches, including dimensional approaches, while facilitating the identification of biological markers. Similarly, adjacencies of the "externalizing group," including disorders exhibiting antisocial behaviors, conduct disturbances, addictions, and impulse-control disorders, should encourage advances in identifying diagnoses, markers, and underlying mechanisms.

Despite the problem posed by categorical diagnoses, the DSM-5 Task Force recognized that it is premature scientifically to propose alternative definitions for most disorders. The organizational structure is meant to serve as a bridge to new diagnostic approaches without disrupting current clinical practice or research. With support from DSM-associated training materials, the National Institutes of Health other funding agencies, and scientific publications, the more dimensional DSM-5 approach and organizational structure can facilitate research across current diagnostic categories by encouraging broad investigations within the proposed chapters and across adjacent chapters. Such a reformulation of research goals should also keep DSM-5 central to the development of dimensional approaches to diagnosis that will likely supplement or supersede current categorical approaches in coming years.

Developmental and Lifespan Considerations

To improve clinical utility, DSM-5 is organized on developmental and lifespan considerations. It begins with diagnoses thought to reflect developmental processes that manifest early in life (e.g., neurodevelopmental and schizophrenia spectrum and other psychotic disorders), followed by diagnoses that more commonly manifest in adolescence and young adulthood (e.g., bipolar, depressive, and anxiety disorders), and ends with diagnoses relevant to adulthood and later life (e.g., neurocognitive disorders). A similar approach has been taken, where possible, within each chapter. This organizational structure facilitates the comprehensive use of lifespan information as a way to assist in diagnostic decision making.

The proposed organization of chapters of DSM-5, after the neurodevelopmental disorders, is based on groups of internalizing (emotional and somatic) disorders, externalizing disorders, neurocognitive disorders, and other disorders. It is hoped that this organization will encourage further study of underlying pathophysiological processes that give rise to diagnostic comorbidity and symptom heterogeneity. Furthermore, by arranging disorder clusters to mirror clinical reality, DSM-5 should facilitate identification of potential diagnoses by non–mental health specialists, such as primary care physicians.

The organizational structure of DSM-5, along with ICD harmonization, is designed to provide better and more flexible diagnostic concepts for the next epoch of research and to serve as a useful guide to clinicians in explaining to patients why they might have received multiple diagnoses or why they might have received additional or altered diagnoses over their lifespan.

Cultural Issues

Mental disorders are defined in relation to cultural, social, and familial norms and values. Culture provides interpretive frameworks that shape the experience and expression of the symptoms, signs, and behaviors that are criteria for diagnosis. Culture is transmitted, revised, and recreated within the family and other social systems and institutions. Diagnostic assessment must therefore consider whether an individual's experiences, symptoms, and behaviors differ from sociocultural norms and lead to difficulties in adaptation in the cultures of origin and in specific social or familial contexts. Key aspects of culture relevant to diagnostic classification and assessment have been considered in the development of DSM-5.

In Section III, the "Cultural Formulation" contains a detailed discussion of culture and diagnosis in DSM-5, including tools for in-depth cultural assessment. In the Appendix, the "Glossary of Cultural Concepts of Distress" provides a description of some common cultural syndromes, idioms of distress, and causal explanations relevant to clinical practice.

The boundaries between normality and pathology vary across cultures for specific types of behaviors. Thresholds of tolerance for specific symptoms or behaviors differ across cultures, social settings, and families. Hence, the level at which an experience becomes problematic or pathological will differ. The judgment that a given behavior is abnormal and requires clinical attention depends on cultural norms that are internalized by the individual and applied by others around them, including family members and clinicians. Awareness of the significance of culture may correct mistaken interpretations of psychopathology, but culture may also contribute to vulnerability and suffering (e.g., by amplifying fears that maintain panic disorder or health anxiety). Cultural meanings, habits, and traditions can also contribute to either stigma or support in the social and familial response to mental illness. Culture may provide coping strategies that enhance resilience in response to illness, or suggest help seeking and options for accessing health care of various types, including alternative and complementary health systems. Culture may influence acceptance or rejection of a diagnosis and adherence to treatments, affecting the course of illness and recovery. Culture also affects the conduct of the clinical encounter; as a result, cultural differences between the clinician and the patient have implications for the accuracy and acceptance of diagnosis as well as for treatment decisions, prognostic considerations, and clinical outcomes.

Historically, the construct of the culture-bound syndrome has been a key interest of cultural psychiatry. In DSM-5, this construct has been replaced by three concepts that offer greater clinical utility:

1. *Cultural syndrome* is a cluster or group of co-occurring, relatively invariant symptoms found in a specific cultural group, community, or context (e.g., *ataque de nervios*). The syndrome may or may not be recognized as an illness within the culture (e.g., it might be labeled in various ways), but such cultural patterns of distress and features of illness may nevertheless be recognizable by an outside observer.
2. *Cultural idiom of distress* is a linguistic term, phrase, or way of talking about suffering among individuals of a cultural group (e.g., similar ethnicity and religion) referring to shared concepts of pathology and ways of expressing, communicating, or naming essential features of distress (e.g., *kufungisisa*). An idiom of distress need not be associated with specific symptoms, syndromes, or perceived causes. It may be used to convey a wide range of discomfort, including everyday experiences, subclinical conditions, or suffering due to social circumstances rather than mental disorders. For example, most cultures have common bodily idioms of distress used to express a wide range of suffering and concerns.
3. *Cultural explanation or perceived cause* is a label, attribution, or feature of an explanatory model that provides a culturally conceived etiology or cause for symptoms, illness, or distress (e.g., *maladi moun*). Causal explanations may be salient features of folk classifications of disease used by laypersons or healers.

These three concepts (for which discussion and examples are provided in Section III and the Appendix) suggest cultural ways of understanding and describing illness experiences that can be elicited in the clinical encounter. They influence symptomatology, help seeking, clinical presentations, expectations of treatment, illness adaptation, and treatment response. The same cultural term often serves more than one of these functions.

Gender Differences

Sex and gender differences as they relate to the causes and expression of medical conditions are established for a number of diseases, including selected mental disorders. Revisions to DSM-5 included review of potential differences between men and women in the expression of mental illness. In terms of nomenclature, *sex differences* are variations attributable to an individual's reproductive organs and XX or XY chromosomal complement. *Gender differences* are variations that result from biological sex as well as an individual's self-representation that includes the psychological, behavioral, and social consequences of one's perceived gender. The term *gender differences* is used in DSM-5 because, more commonly, the differences between men and women are a result of both biological sex and individual self-representation. However, some of the differences are based on only biological sex.

Gender can influence illness in a variety of ways. First, it may exclusively determine whether an individual is at risk for a disorder (e.g., as in premenstrual dysphoric disorder). Second, gender may moderate the overall risk for development of a disorder as shown by marked gender differences in the prevalence and incidence rates for selected mental disorders. Third, gender may influence the likelihood that particular symptoms of a disorder are experienced by an individual. Attention-deficit/hyperactivity disorder is an example of a disorder with differences in presentation that are most commonly experienced by boys or girls. Gender likely has other effects on the experience of a disorder that are indirectly relevant to psychiatric diagnosis. It may be that certain symptoms are more readily endorsed by men or women, and that this contributes to differences in service provision (e.g., women may be more likely to recognize a depressive, bipolar, or anxiety disorder and endorse a more comprehensive list of symptoms than men).

Reproductive life cycle events, including estrogen variations, also contribute to gender differences in risk and expression of illness. Thus, a specifier for postpartum onset of mania or major depressive episode denotes a time frame wherein women may be at increased risk for the onset of an illness episode. In the case of sleep and energy, alterations are often normative postpartum and thus may have lower diagnostic reliability in postpartum women.

The manual is configured to include information on gender at multiple levels. If there are gender-specific symptoms, they have been added to the diagnostic criteria. A gender-related specifier, such as perinatal onset of a mood episode, provides additional information on gender and diagnosis. Finally, other issues that are pertinent to diagnosis and gender considerations can be found in the section "Gender-Related Diagnostic Issues."

Use of Other Specified and Unspecified Disorders

To enhance diagnostic specificity, DSM-5 replaces the previous NOS designation with two options for clinical use: *other specified disorder* and *unspecified disorder*. The other specified disorder category is provided to allow the clinician to communicate the specific reason that the presentation does not meet the criteria for any specific category within a diagnostic class. This is done by recording the name of the category, followed by the specific reason. For example, for an individual with clinically significant depressive symptoms lasting 4 weeks but whose symptomatology falls short of the diagnostic threshold for a major depressive episode, the clinician would record "other specified depressive disorder, depressive episode with insufficient symptoms." If the clinician chooses not to specify the reason that the criteria are not met for a specific disorder, then "unspecified depressive disorder" would be diagnosed. Note that the differentiation between other specified and unspecified disorders is based on the clinician's decision, providing maximum flexibility for diagnosis. Clinicians do not have to differentiate between other specified and unspecified disorders based on some feature of the presentation itself. When the clinician determines that there is evidence to specify the nature of the clinical presentation, the other specified diagnosis can be given. When the clinician is not able to further specify and describe the clinical presentation, the unspecified diagnosis can be given. This is left entirely up to clinical judgment.

For a more detailed discussion of how to use other specified and unspecified designations, see "Use of the Manual" in Section I.

The Multiaxial System

Despite widespread use and its adoption by certain insurance and governmental agencies, the multiaxial system in DSM-IV was not required to make a mental disorder diagnosis. A nonaxial assessment system was also included that simply listed the appropriate Axis I, II, and III disorders and conditions without axial designations. DSM-5 has moved to a nonaxial documentation of diagnosis (formerly Axes I, II, and III), with separate notations for important psychosocial and contextual factors (formerly Axis IV) and disability (formerly Axis V). This revision is consistent with the DSM-IV text that states, "The multiaxial distinction among Axis I, Axis II, and Axis III disorders does not imply that there are fundamental differences in their conceptualization, that mental disorders are unrelated to physical or biological factors or processes, or that general medical conditions are unrelated to behavioral or psychosocial factors or processes." The approach of separately noting diagnosis from psychosocial and contextual factors is also consistent with established WHO and ICD guidance to consider the individual's functional status separately from his or her diagnoses or symptom status. In DSM-5, Axis III has been combined with Axes I and II. Clinicians should continue to list medical conditions that are important to the understanding or management of an individual's mental disorder(s).

DSM-IV Axis IV covered psychosocial and environmental problems that may affect the diagnosis, treatment, and prognosis of mental disorders. Although this axis provided helpful information, even if it was not used as frequently as intended, the DSM-5 Task Force recommended that DSM-5 should not develop its own classification of psychosocial and environmental problems, but rather use a selected set of the ICD-9-CM V codes and the new Z codes contained in ICD-10-CM. The ICD-10 Z codes were examined to determine which are most relevant to mental disorders and also to identify gaps.

DSM-IV Axis V consisted of the Global Assessment of Functioning (GAF) scale, representing the clinician's judgment of the individual's overall level of "functioning on a hypothetical continuum of mental health–illness." It was recommended that the GAF be dropped from DSM-5 for several reasons, including its conceptual lack of clarity (i.e., including symptoms, suicide risk, and disabilities in its descriptors) and questionable psychometrics in routine practice. In order to provide a global measure of disability, the WHO Disability Assessment Schedule (WHODAS) is included, for further study, in Section III of DSM-5 (see the chapter "Assessment Measures"). The WHODAS is based on the International Classification of Functioning, Disability and Health (ICF) for use across all of medicine and health care. The WHODAS (version 2.0), and a modification developed for children/adolescents and their parents by the Impairment and Disability Study Group were included in the DSM-5 field trial.

Online Enhancements

It was challenging to determine what to include in the print version of DSM-5 to be most clinically relevant and useful and at the same time maintain a manageable size. For this reason, the inclusion of clinical rating scales and measures in the print edition is limited to those considered most relevant. Additional assessment measures used in the field trials are available online (www.psychiatry.org/dsm5), linked to the relevant disorders. The Cultural Formulation Interview, Cultural Formulation Interview—Informant Version, and supplementary modules to the core Cultural Formulation Interview are also available online at www.psychiatry.org/dsm5.

DSM-5 is available as an online subscription at PsychiatryOnline.org as well as an e-book. The online component contains modules and assessment tools to enhance the diagnostic criteria and text. Also available online is a complete set of supportive references as well as additional helpful information. The organizational structure of DSM-5, its use of dimensional measures, and compatibility with ICD codes will allow it to be readily adaptable to future scientific discoveries and refinements in its clinical utility. DSM-5 will be analyzed over time to continually assess its validity and enhance its value to clinicians.

Use of the Manual

The introduction contains much of the history and developmental process of the DSM-5 revision. This section is designed to provide a practical guide to using DSM-5, particularly in clinical practice. The primary purpose of DSM-5 is to assist trained clinicians in the diagnosis of their patients' mental disorders as part of a case formulation assessment that leads to a fully informed treatment plan for each individual. The symptoms contained in the respective diagnostic criteria sets do not constitute comprehensive definitions of underlying disorders, which encompass cognitive, emotional, behavioral, and physiological processes that are far more complex than can be described in these brief summaries. Rather, they are intended to summarize characteristic syndromes of signs and symptoms that point to an underlying disorder with a characteristic developmental history, biological and environmental risk factors, neuropsychological and physiological correlates, and typical clinical course.

Approach to Clinical Case Formulation

The case formulation for any given patient must involve a careful clinical history and concise summary of the social, psychological, and biological factors that may have contributed to developing a given mental disorder. Hence, it is not sufficient to simply check off the symptoms in the diagnostic criteria to make a mental disorder diagnosis. Although a systematic check for the presence of these criteria as they apply to each patient will assure a more reliable assessment, the relative severity and valence of individual criteria and their contribution to a diagnosis require clinical judgment. The symptoms in our diagnostic criteria are part of the relatively limited repertoire of human emotional responses to internal and external stresses that are generally maintained in a homeostatic balance without a disruption in normal functioning. It requires clinical training to recognize when the combination of predisposing, precipitating, perpetuating, and protective factors has resulted in a psychopathological condition in which physical signs and symptoms exceed normal ranges. The ultimate goal of a clinical case formulation is to use the available contextual and diagnostic information in developing a comprehensive treatment plan that is informed by the individual's cultural and social context. However, recommendations for the selection and use of the most appropriate evidence-based treatment options for each disorder are beyond the scope of this manual.

Although decades of scientific effort have gone into developing the diagnostic criteria sets for the disorders included in Section II, it is well recognized that this set of categorical diagnoses does not fully describe the full range of mental disorders that individuals experience and present to clinicians on a daily basis throughout the world. As noted previously in the introduction, the range of genetic/environmental interactions over the course of human development affecting cognitive, emotional and behavioral function is virtually limitless. As a result, it is impossible to capture the full range of psychopathology in the categorical diagnostic categories that we are now using. Hence, it is also necessary to include "other specified/unspecified" disorder options for presentations that do not fit exactly into the diagnostic boundaries of disorders in each chapter. In an emergency department setting, it may be possible to identify only the most prominent symptom expressions associated with a particular chapter—for example, delusions, hallucinations, mania, depression, anxiety, substance intoxication, or neurocognitive symptoms—so that an "unspecified" disorder in that category is identified until a fuller differential diagnosis is possible.

Definition of a Mental Disorder

Each disorder identified in Section II of the manual (excluding those in the chapters entitled "Medication-Induced Movement Disorders and Other Adverse Effects of Medication" and "Other Conditions That May Be a Focus of Clinical Attention") must meet the definition of a mental disorder. Although no definition can capture all aspects of all disorders in the range contained in DSM-5, the following elements are required:

> A mental disorder is a syndrome characterized by clinically significant disturbance in an individual's cognition, emotion regulation, or behavior that reflects a dysfunction in the psychological, biological, or developmental processes underlying mental functioning. Mental disorders are usually associated with significant distress or disability in social, occupational, or other important activities. An expectable or culturally approved response to a common stressor or loss, such as the death of a loved one, is not a mental disorder. Socially deviant behavior (e.g., political, religious, or sexual) and conflicts that are primarily between the individual and society are not mental disorders unless the deviance or conflict results from a dysfunction in the individual, as described above.

The diagnosis of a mental disorder should have clinical utility: it should help clinicians to determine prognosis, treatment plans, and potential treatment outcomes for their patients. However, the diagnosis of a mental disorder is not equivalent to a need for treatment. Need for treatment is a complex clinical decision that takes into consideration symptom severity, symptom salience (e.g., the presence of suicidal ideation), the patient's distress (mental pain) associated with the symptom(s), disability related to the patient's symptoms, risks and benefits of available treatments, and other factors (e.g., psychiatric symptoms complicating other illness). Clinicians may thus encounter individuals whose symptoms do not meet full criteria for a mental disorder but who demonstrate a clear need for treatment or care. The fact that some individuals do not show all symptoms indicative of a diagnosis should not be used to justify limiting their access to appropriate care.

Approaches to validating diagnostic criteria for discrete categorical mental disorders have included the following types of evidence: antecedent validators (similar genetic markers, family traits, temperament, and environmental exposure), concurrent validators (similar neural substrates, biomarkers, emotional and cognitive processing, and symptom similarity), and predictive validators (similar clinical course and treatment response). In DSM-5, we recognize that the current diagnostic criteria for any single disorder will not necessarily identify a homogeneous group of patients who can be characterized reliably with all of these validators. Available evidence shows that these validators cross existing diagnostic boundaries but tend to congregate more frequently within and across adjacent DSM-5 chapter groups. Until incontrovertible etiological or pathophysiological mechanisms are identified to fully validate specific disorders or disorder spectra, the most important standard for the DSM-5 disorder criteria will be their clinical utility for the assessment of clinical course and treatment response of individuals grouped by a given set of diagnostic criteria.

This definition of mental disorder was developed for clinical, public health, and research purposes. Additional information is usually required beyond that contained in the DSM-5 diagnostic criteria in order to make legal judgments on such issues as criminal responsibility, eligibility for disability compensation, and competency (see "Cautionary Statement for Forensic Use of DSM-5" elsewhere in this manual).

Criterion for Clinical Significance

There have been substantial efforts by the DSM-5 Task Force and the World Health Organization (WHO) to separate the concepts of mental disorder and disability (impairment in social, occupational, or other important areas of functioning). In the WHO system, the International Classification of Diseases (ICD) covers all diseases and disorders, while the International Classification of Functioning, Disability and Health (ICF) provides a separate classification of global disability. The WHO Disability Assessment Schedule (WHODAS) is based on the ICF and has proven useful as a standardized measure of disability for mental disorders. However, in the absence of clear biological markers or clinically useful measurements of severity for many mental disorders, it has not been possible to completely separate normal and pathological symptom expressions contained in diagnostic criteria. This gap in information is particularly problematic in clinical situations in which the patient's symptom presentation by itself (particularly in mild forms) is not inherently pathological and may be encountered in individuals for whom a diagnosis of "mental disorder" would be inappropriate. Therefore, a generic diagnostic criterion requiring distress or disability has been used to establish disorder thresholds, usually worded "the disturbance causes clinically significant distress or impairment in social, occupational, or other important areas of functioning." The text following the revised definition of a mental disorder acknowledges that this criterion may be especially helpful in determining a patient's need for treatment. Use of information from family members and other third parties (in addition to the individual) regarding the individual's performance is recommended when necessary.

Elements of a Diagnosis

Diagnostic Criteria and Descriptors

Diagnostic criteria are offered as guidelines for making diagnoses, and their use should be informed by clinical judgment. Text descriptions, including introductory sections of each diagnostic chapter, can help support diagnosis (e.g., providing differential diagnoses; describing the criteria more fully under "Diagnostic Features").

Following the assessment of diagnostic criteria, clinicians should consider the application of disorder subtypes and/or specifiers as appropriate. Severity and course specifiers should be applied to denote the individual's current presentation, but only when the full criteria are met. When full criteria are not met, clinicians should consider whether the symptom presentation meets criteria for an "other specified" or "unspecified" designation. Where applicable, specific criteria for defining disorder severity (e.g., mild, moderate, severe, extreme), descriptive features (e.g., with good to fair insight; in a controlled environment), and course (e.g., in partial remission, in full remission, recurrent) are provided with each diagnosis. On the basis of the clinical interview, text descriptions, criteria, and clinician judgment, a final diagnosis is made.

The general convention in DSM-5 is to allow multiple diagnoses to be assigned for those presentations that meet criteria for more than one DSM-5 disorder.

Subtypes and Specifiers

Subtypes and specifiers (some of which are coded in the fourth, fifth, or sixth digit) are provided for increased specificity. *Subtypes* define mutually exclusive and jointly exhaustive phenomenological subgroupings within a diagnosis and are indicated by the instruction "*Specify* whether" in the criteria set. In contrast, *specifiers* are not intended to be mutually exclusive or jointly exhaustive, and as a consequence, more than one specifier may be given. Specifiers are indicated by the instruction "*Specify*" or "*Specify* if" in the criteria set. Specifiers provide an opportunity to define a more homogeneous subgrouping of individuals with the disorder who share certain features (e.g., major depressive disorder, with mixed features) and to convey information that is relevant to the management of the individual's disorder, such as the "with other medical comorbidity" specifier in sleep-wake disorders. Although a fifth digit is sometimes assigned to code a subtype or specifier (e.g., 294.11 [F02.81] major neurocognitive disorder due to Alzheimer's disease, with behavioral disturbance) or severity (296.21 [F32.0] major depressive disorder, single episode, mild), the majority of subtypes and specifiers included in DSM-5 cannot be coded within the ICD-9-CM and ICD-10-CM systems and are indicated only by including the subtype or specifier after the name of the disorder (e.g., social anxiety disorder [social phobia], performance type). Note that in some cases, a specifier or subtype is codable in ICD-10-CM but not in ICD-9-CM. Accordingly, in some cases the 4th or 5th character codes for the subtypes or specifiers are provided only for the ICD-10-CM coding designations.

A DSM-5 diagnosis is usually applied to the individual's current presentation; previous diagnoses from which the individual has recovered should be clearly noted as such. Specifiers indicating *course* (e.g., in partial remission, in full remission) may be listed after the diagnosis and are indicated in a number of criteria sets. Where available, *severity specifiers* are provided to guide clinicians in rating the intensity, frequency, duration, symptom count, or other severity indicator of a disorder. Severity specifiers are indicated by the instruction "*Specify* current severity" in the criteria set and include disorder-specific definitions. *Descriptive features specifiers* have also been provided in the criteria set and convey additional information that can inform treatment planning (e.g., obsessive-compulsive disorder, with poor insight). Not all disorders include course, severity, and/or descriptive features specifiers.

Medication-Induced Movement Disorders and Other Conditions That May Be a Focus of Clinical Attention

In addition to important psychosocial and environmental factors (see "The Multiaxial System" in the "Introduction" elsewhere in this manual), these chapters in Section II also contain other conditions that are not mental disorders but may be encountered by mental health clinicians. These conditions may be listed as a reason for clinical visit in addition to, or in place of, the mental disorders listed in Section II. A separate chapter is devoted to medication-induced disorders and other adverse effects of medication that may be assessed and treated by clinicians in mental health practice such as akathisia, tardive dyskinesia, and dystonia. The description of neuroleptic malignant syndrome is expanded from that provided in DSM-IV-TR to highlight the emergent and potentially life-threatening nature of this condition, and a new entry on antidepressant discontinuation syndrome is provided. An additional chapter discusses other conditions that may be a focus of clinical attention. These include relational problems, problems related to abuse and neglect, problems with adherence to treatment regimens, obesity, antisocial behavior, and malingering.

Principal Diagnosis

When more than one diagnosis for an individual is given in an inpatient setting, the principal diagnosis is the condition established after study to be chiefly responsible for occasioning the admission of the individual. When more than one diagnosis is given for an individual in an outpatient setting, the reason for visit is the condition that is chiefly responsible for the ambulatory care medical services received during the visit. In most cases, the principal diagnosis or the reason for visit is also the main focus of attention or treatment. It is often difficult (and somewhat arbitrary) to determine which diagnosis is the principal diagnosis or the reason for visit, especially when, for example, a substance-related diagnosis such as alcohol use disorder is accompanied by a non-substance-related diagnosis such as schizophrenia. For example, it may be unclear which diagnosis should be considered "principal" for an individual hospitalized with both schizophrenia and alcohol use disorder, because each condition may have contributed equally to the need for admission and treatment. The principal diagnosis is indicated by listing it first, and the remaining disorders are listed in order of focus of attention and treatment. When the principal diagnosis or reason for visit is a mental disorder due to another medical condition (e.g., major neurocognitive disorder due to Alzheimer's disease, psychotic disorder due to malignant lung neoplasm), ICD coding rules require that the etiological medical condition be listed first. In that case, the principal diagnosis or reason for visit would be the mental disorder due to the medical condition, the second listed diagnosis. In most cases, the disorder listed as the principal diagnosis or the reason for visit is followed by the qualifying phrase "(principal diagnosis)" or "(reason for visit)."

Provisional Diagnosis

The specifier "provisional" can be used when there is a strong presumption that the full criteria will ultimately be met for a disorder but not enough information is available to make a firm diagnosis. The clinician can indicate the diagnostic uncertainty by recording "(provisional)" following the diagnosis. For example, this diagnosis might be used when an individual who appears to have a major depressive disorder is unable to give an adequate history, and thus it cannot be established that the full criteria are met. Another use of the term *provisional* is for those situations in which differential diagnosis depends exclusively on the duration of illness. For example, a diagnosis of schizophreniform disorder requires a duration of less than 6 months but of at least 1 month and can only be given provisionally if assigned before remission has occurred.

Coding and Reporting Procedures

Each disorder is accompanied by an identifying diagnostic and statistical code, which is typically used by institutions and agencies for data collection and billing purposes. There are specific recording protocols for these diagnostic codes (identified as coding notes in the text) that were established by WHO, the U.S. Centers for Medicare and Medicaid Services (CMS), and the Centers for Disease Control and Prevention's National Center for Health Statistics to ensure consistent international recording of prevalence and mortality rates for identified health conditions. For most clinicians, the codes are used to identify the diagnosis or reason for visit for CMS and private insurance service claims. The official coding system in use in the United States as of publication of this manual is ICD-9-CM. Official adoption of ICD-10-CM is scheduled to take place on October 1, 2015, and these codes, which are shown parenthetically in this manual, should not be used until the official implementation occurs. Both ICD-9-CM and ICD-10-CM codes have been listed 1) preceding the name of the disorder in the classification and 2) accompanying the criteria set for each disorder. For some diagnoses (e.g., neurocognitive and substance/medication-induced disorders), the appropriate code depends on further specification and is listed within the criteria set for the disorder, as coding notes, and, in some cases, further clarified in a section on recording procedures. The names of some disorders are followed by alternative terms enclosed in parentheses, which, in most cases, were the DSM-IV names for the disorders.

Looking to the Future: Assessment and Monitoring Tools

The various components of DSM-5 are provided to facilitate patient assessment and to aid in developing a comprehensive case formulation. Whereas the diagnostic criteria in Section II are well-established measures that have undergone extensive review, the assessment tools, a cultural formulation interview, and conditions for further study included in Section III are those for which we determined that the scientific evidence is not yet available to support widespread clinical use. These diagnostic aids and criteria are included to highlight the evolution and direction of scientific advances in these areas and to stimulate further research.

Each of the measures in Section III is provided to aid in a comprehensive assessment of individuals that will contribute to a diagnosis and treatment plan tailored to the individual presentation and clinical context. Where cultural dynamics are particularly important for diagnostic assessment, the cultural formulation interview should be considered as a useful aid to communication with the individual. Cross-cutting symptom and diagnosis-specific severity measures provide quantitative ratings of important clinical areas that are designed to be used at the initial evaluation to establish a baseline for comparison with ratings on subsequent encounters to monitor changes and inform treatment planning.

The use of such measures will undoubtedly be facilitated by digital applications, and the measures are included in Section III to provide for further evaluation and development. As with each DSM edition, the diagnostic criteria and the DSM-5 classification of mental disorders reflect the current consensus on the evolving knowledge in our field.

Cautionary Statement for Forensic Use of DSM-5

Although the DSM-5 diagnostic criteria and text are primarily designed to assist clinicians in conducting clinical assessment, case formulation, and treatment planning, DSM-5 is also used as a reference for the courts and attorneys in assessing the forensic consequences of mental disorders. As a result, it is important to note that the definition of mental disorder included in DSM-5 was developed to meet the needs of clinicians, public health professionals, and research investigators rather than all of the technical needs of the courts and legal professionals. It is also important to note that DSM-5 does not provide treatment guidelines for any given disorder.

When used appropriately, diagnoses and diagnostic information can assist legal decision makers in their determinations. For example, when the presence of a mental disorder is the predicate for a subsequent legal determination (e.g., involuntary civil commitment), the use of an established system of diagnosis enhances the value and reliability of the determination. By providing a compendium based on a review of the pertinent clinical and research literature, DSM-5 may facilitate legal decision makers' understanding of the relevant characteristics of mental disorders. The literature related to diagnoses also serves as a check on ungrounded speculation about mental disorders and about the functioning of a particular individual. Finally, diagnostic information about longitudinal course may improve decision making when the legal issue concerns an individual's mental functioning at a past or future point in time.

However, the use of DSM-5 should be informed by an awareness of the risks and limitations of its use in forensic settings. When DSM-5 categories, criteria, and textual descriptions are employed for forensic purposes, there is a risk that diagnostic information will be misused or misunderstood. These dangers arise because of the imperfect fit between the questions of ultimate concern to the law and the information contained in a clinical diagnosis. In most situations, the clinical diagnosis of a DSM-5 mental disorder such as intellectual disability (intellectual developmental disorder), schizophrenia, major neurocognitive disorder, gambling disorder, or pedophilic disorder does not imply that an individual with such a condition meets legal criteria for the presence of a mental disorder or a specified legal standard (e.g., for competence, criminal responsibility, or disability). For the latter, additional information is usually required beyond that contained in the DSM-5 diagnosis, which might include information about the individual's functional impairments and how these impairments affect the particular abilities in question. It is precisely because impairments, abilities, and disabilities vary widely within each diagnostic category that assignment of a particular diagnosis does not imply a specific level of impairment or disability.

Use of DSM-5 to assess for the presence of a mental disorder by nonclinical, nonmedical, or otherwise insufficiently trained individuals is not advised. Nonclinical decision makers should also be cautioned that a diagnosis does not carry any necessary implications regarding the etiology or causes of the individual's mental disorder or the individual's degree of control over behaviors that may be associated with the disorder. Even when diminished control over one's behavior is a feature of the disorder, having the diagnosis in itself does not demonstrate that a particular individual is (or was) unable to control his or her behavior at a particular time.

SECTION II
Diagnostic Criteria and Codes

This section contains the diagnostic criteria approved for routine clinical use along with the ICD-9-CM codes (ICD-10 codes are shown parenthetically). For each mental disorder, the diagnostic criteria are followed by descriptive text to assist in diagnostic decision making. Where needed, specific recording procedures are presented with the diagnostic criteria to provide guidance in selecting the most appropriate code. In some cases, separate recording procedures for ICD-9-CM and ICD-10-CM are provided. Although not considered as official DSM-5 disorders, medication-induced movement disorders and other adverse effects of medication, as well as other conditions that may be a focus of clinical attention (including additional ICD-9-CM V codes and forthcoming ICD-10-CM Z codes), are provided to indicate other reasons for a clinical visit such as environmental factors and relational problems. These codes are adapted from ICD-9-CM and ICD-10-CM and were neither reviewed nor approved as official DSM-5 diagnoses, but can provide additional context for a clinical formulation and treatment plan. These three components—the criteria and their descriptive text, the medication-induced movement disorders and other adverse effects of medication, and the descriptions of other conditions that may be a focus of clinical attention—represent the key elements of the clinical diagnostic process and thus are presented together.

Neurodevelopmental Disorders

The neurodevelopmental disorders are a group of conditions with onset in the developmental period. The disorders typically manifest early in development, often before the child enters grade school, and are characterized by developmental deficits that produce impairments of personal, social, academic, or occupational functioning. The range of developmental deficits varies from very specific limitations of learning or control of executive functions to global impairments of social skills or intelligence. The neurodevelopmental disorders frequently co-occur; for example, individuals with autism spectrum disorder often have intellectual disability (intellectual developmental disorder), and many children with attention-deficit/hyperactivity disorder (ADHD) also have a specific learning disorder. For some disorders, the clinical presentation includes symptoms of excess as well as deficits and delays in achieving expected milestones. For example, autism spectrum disorder is diagnosed only when the characteristic deficits of social communication are accompanied by excessively repetitive behaviors, restricted interests, and insistence on sameness.

Intellectual disability (intellectual developmental disorder) is characterized by deficits in general mental abilities, such as reasoning, problem solving, planning, abstract thinking, judgment, academic learning, and learning from experience. The deficits result in impairments of adaptive functioning, such that the individual fails to meet standards of personal independence and social responsibility in one or more aspects of daily life, including communication, social participation, academic or occupational functioning, and personal independence at home or in community settings. Global developmental delay, as its name implies, is diagnosed when an individual fails to meet expected developmental milestones in several areas of intellectual functioning. The diagnosis is used for individuals who are unable to undergo systematic assessments of intellectual functioning, including children who are too young to participate in standardized testing. Intellectual disability may result from an acquired insult during the developmental period from, for example, a severe head injury, in which case a neurocognitive disorder also may be diagnosed.

The communication disorders include language disorder, speech sound disorder, social (pragmatic) communication disorder, and childhood-onset fluency disorder (stuttering). The first three disorders are characterized by deficits in the development and use of language, speech, and social communication, respectively. Childhood-onset fluency disorder is characterized by disturbances of the normal fluency and motor production of speech, including repetitive sounds or syllables, prolongation of consonants or vowel sounds, broken words, blocking, or words produced with an excess of physical tension. Like other neurodevelopmental disorders, communication disorders begin early in life and may produce lifelong functional impairments.

Autism spectrum disorder is characterized by persistent deficits in social communication and social interaction across multiple contexts, including deficits in social reciprocity, nonverbal communicative behaviors used for social interaction, and skills in developing, maintaining, and understanding relationships. In addition to the social communication deficits, the diagnosis of autism spectrum disorder requires the presence of restricted, repetitive patterns of behavior, interests, or activities. Because symptoms change with development and may be masked by compensatory mechanisms, the diagnostic criteria may be met based on historical information, although the current presentation must cause significant impairment.

Within the diagnosis of autism spectrum disorder, individual clinical characteristics are noted through the use of specifiers (with or without accompanying intellectual impairment; with or without accompanying structural language impairment; associated with a known medical or genetic condition or environmental factor; associated with another neurodevelopmental, mental, or behavioral disorder), as well as specifiers that describe the autistic symptoms (age at first concern; with or without loss of established skills; severity). These specifiers provide clinicians with an opportunity to individualize the diagnosis and communicate a richer clinical description of the affected individuals. For example, many individuals previously diagnosed with Asperger's disorder would now receive a diagnosis of autism spectrum disorder without language or intellectual impairment.

ADHD is a neurodevelopmental disorder defined by impairing levels of inattention, disorganization, and/or hyperactivity-impulsivity. Inattention and disorganization entail inability to stay on task, seeming not to listen, and losing materials, at levels that are inconsistent with age or developmental level. Hyperactivity-impulsivity entails overactivity, fidgeting, inability to stay seated, intruding into other people's activities, and inability to wait—symptoms that are excessive for age or developmental level. In childhood, ADHD frequently overlaps with disorders that are often considered to be "externalizing disorders," such as oppositional defiant disorder and conduct disorder. ADHD often persists into adulthood, with resultant impairments of social, academic and occupational functioning.

The neurodevelopmental motor disorders include developmental coordination disorder, stereotypic movement disorder, and tic disorders. Developmental coordination disorder is characterized by deficits in the acquisition and execution of coordinated motor skills and is manifested by clumsiness and slowness or inaccuracy of performance of motor skills that cause interference with activities of daily living. Stereotypic movement disorder is diagnosed when an individual has repetitive, seemingly driven, and apparently purposeless motor behaviors, such as hand flapping, body rocking, head banging, self-biting, or hitting. The movements interfere with social, academic, or other activities. If the behaviors cause self-injury, this should be specified as part of the diagnostic description. Tic disorders are characterized by the presence of motor or vocal tics, which are sudden, rapid, recurrent, nonrhythmic, stereotyped motor movements or vocalizations. The duration, presumed etiology, and clinical presentation define the specific tic disorder that is diagnosed: Tourette's disorder, persistent (chronic) motor or vocal tic disorder, provisional tic disorder, other specified tic disorder, and unspecified tic disorder. Tourette's disorder is diagnosed when the individual has multiple motor and vocal tics that have been present for at least 1 year and that have a waxing-waning symptom course.

Specific learning disorder, as the name implies, is diagnosed when there are specific deficits in an individual's ability to perceive or process information efficiently and accurately. This neurodevelopmental disorder first manifests during the years of formal schooling and is characterized by persistent and impairing difficulties with learning foundational academic skills in reading, writing, and/or math. The individual's performance of the affected academic skills is well below average for age, or acceptable performance levels are achieved only with extraordinary effort. Specific learning disorder may occur in individuals identified as intellectually gifted and manifest only when the learning demands or assessment procedures (e.g., timed tests) pose barriers that cannot be overcome by their innate intelligence and compensatory strategies. For all individuals, specific learning disorder can produce lifelong impairments in activities dependent on the skills, including occupational performance.

The use of specifiers for the neurodevelopmental disorder diagnoses enriches the clinical description of the individual's clinical course and current symptomatology. In addition to specifiers that describe the clinical presentation, such as age at onset or severity ratings, the neurodevelopmental disorders may include the specifier "associated with a known medical or genetic condition or environmental factor." This specifier gives clinicians an opportunity to document factors that may have played a role in the etiology of the disorder, as well as those that might affect the clinical course. Examples include genetic disorders, such as fragile X syndrome, tuberous sclerosis, and Rett syndrome; medical conditions such as epilepsy; and environmental factors, including very low birth weight and fetal alcohol exposure (even in the absence of stigmata of fetal alcohol syndrome).

Intellectual Disabilities

Intellectual Disability (Intellectual Developmental Disorder)

Diagnostic Criteria

Intellectual disability (intellectual developmental disorder) is a disorder with onset during the developmental period that includes both intellectual and adaptive functioning deficits in conceptual, social, and practical domains. The following three criteria must be met:

A. Deficits in intellectual functions, such as reasoning, problem solving, planning, abstract thinking, judgment, academic learning, and learning from experience, confirmed by both clinical assessment and individualized, standardized intelligence testing.

B. Deficits in adaptive functioning that result in failure to meet developmental and sociocultural standards for personal independence and social responsibility. Without ongoing support, the adaptive deficits limit functioning in one or more activities of daily life, such as communication, social participation, and independent living, across multiple environments, such as home, school, work, and community.

C. Onset of intellectual and adaptive deficits during the developmental period.

Note: The diagnostic term *intellectual disability* is the equivalent term for the ICD-11 diagnosis of *intellectual developmental disorders.* Although the term *intellectual disability* is used throughout this manual, both terms are used in the title to clarify relationships with other classification systems. Moreover, a federal statute in the United States (Public Law 111-256, Rosa's Law) replaces the term *mental retardation* with *intellectual disability,* and research journals use the term *intellectual disability.* Thus, *intellectual disability* is the term in common use by medical, educational, and other professions and by the lay public and advocacy groups.

Specify current severity (see Table 1):

    317 (F70)   Mild
    318.0 (F71) Moderate
    318.1 (F72) Severe
    318.2 (F73) Profound

Specifiers

The various levels of severity are defined on the basis of adaptive functioning, and not IQ scores, because it is adaptive functioning that determines the level of supports required. Moreover, IQ measures are less valid in the lower end of the IQ range.

TABLE 1   Severity levels for intellectual disability (intellectual developmental disorder)

Severity level	Conceptual domain	Social domain	Practical domain
Mild	For preschool children, there may be no obvious conceptual differences. For school-age children and adults, there are difficulties in learning academic skills involving reading, writing, arithmetic, time, or money, with support needed in one or more areas to meet age-related expectations. In adults, abstract thinking, executive function (i.e., planning, strategizing, priority setting, and cognitive flexibility), and short-term memory, as well as functional use of academic skills (e.g., reading, money management), are impaired. There is a somewhat concrete approach to problems and solutions compared with age-mates.	Compared with typically developing age-mates, the individual is immature in social interactions. For example, there may be difficulty in accurately perceiving peers' social cues. Communication, conversation, and language are more concrete or immature than expected for age. There may be difficulties regulating emotion and behavior in age-appropriate fashion; these difficulties are noticed by peers in social situations. There is limited understanding of risk in social situations; social judgment is immature for age, and the person is at risk of being manipulated by others (gullibility).	The individual may function age-appropriately in personal care. Individuals need some support with complex daily living tasks in comparison to peers. In adulthood, supports typically involve grocery shopping, transportation, home and child-care organizing, nutritious food preparation, and banking and money management. Recreational skills resemble those of age-mates, although judgment related to well-being and organization around recreation requires support. In adulthood, competitive employment is often seen in jobs that do not emphasize conceptual skills. Individuals generally need support to make health care decisions and legal decisions, and to learn to perform a skilled vocation competently. Support is typically needed to raise a family.

TABLE 1 Severity levels for intellectual disability (intellectual developmental disorder) (continued)

Severity level	Conceptual domain	Social domain	Practical domain
Moderate	All through development, the individual's conceptual skills lag markedly behind those of peers. For preschoolers, language and pre-academic skills develop slowly. For school-age children, progress in reading, writing, mathematics, and understanding of time and money occurs slowly across the school years and is markedly limited compared with that of peers. For adults, academic skill development is typically at an elementary level, and support is required for all use of academic skills in work and personal life. Ongoing assistance on a daily basis is needed to complete conceptual tasks of day-to-day life, and others may take over these responsibilities fully for the individual.	The individual shows marked differences from peers in social and communicative behavior across development. Spoken language is typically a primary tool for social communication but is much less complex than that of peers. Capacity for relationships is evident in ties to family and friends, and the individual may have successful friendships across life and sometimes romantic relations in adulthood. However, individuals may not perceive or interpret social cues accurately. Social judgment and decision-making abilities are limited, and caretakers must assist the person with life decisions. Friendships with typically developing peers are often affected by communication or social limitations. Significant social and communicative support is needed in work settings for success.	The individual can care for personal needs involving eating, dressing, elimination, and hygiene as an adult, although an extended period of teaching and time is needed for the individual to become independent in these areas, and reminders may be needed. Similarly, participation in all household tasks can be achieved by adulthood, although an extended period of teaching is needed, and ongoing supports will typically occur for adult-level performance. Independent employment in jobs that require limited conceptual and communication skills can be achieved, but considerable support from co-workers, supervisors, and others is needed to manage social expectations, job complexities, and ancillary responsibilities such as scheduling, transportation, health benefits, and money management. A variety of recreational skills can be developed. These typically require additional supports and learning opportunities over an extended period of time. Maladaptive behavior is present in a significant minority and causes social problems.

TABLE 1   Severity levels for intellectual disability (intellectual developmental disorder) *(continued)*

Severity level	Conceptual domain	Social domain	Practical domain
Severe	Attainment of conceptual skills is limited. The individual generally has little understanding of written language or of concepts involving numbers, quantity, time, and money. Caretakers provide extensive supports for problem solving throughout life.	Spoken language is quite limited in terms of vocabulary and grammar. Speech may be single words or phrases and may be supplemented through augmentative means. Speech and communication are focused on the here and now within everyday events. Language is used for social communication more than for explication. Individuals understand simple speech and gestural communication. Relationships with family members and familiar others are a source of pleasure and help.	The individual requires support for all activities of daily living, including meals, dressing, bathing, and elimination. The individual requires supervision at all times. The individual cannot make responsible decisions regarding well-being of self or others. In adulthood, participation in tasks at home, recreation, and work requires ongoing support and assistance. Skill acquisition in all domains involves long-term teaching and ongoing support. Maladaptive behavior, including self-injury, is present in a significant minority.
Profound	Conceptual skills generally involve the physical world rather than symbolic processes. The individual may use objects in goal-directed fashion for self-care, work, and recreation. Certain visuospatial skills, such as matching and sorting based on physical characteristics, may be acquired. However, co-occurring motor and sensory impairments may prevent functional use of objects.	The individual has very limited understanding of symbolic communication in speech or gesture. He or she may understand some simple instructions or gestures. The individual expresses his or her own desires and emotions largely through nonverbal, nonsymbolic communication. The individual enjoys relationships with well-known family members, caretakers, and familiar others, and initiates and responds to social interactions through gestural and emotional cues. Co-occurring sensory and physical impairments may prevent many social activities.	The individual is dependent on others for all aspects of daily physical care, health, and safety, although he or she may be able to participate in some of these activities as well. Individuals without severe physical impairments may assist with some daily work tasks at home, like carrying dishes to the table. Simple actions with objects may be the basis of participation in some vocational activities with high levels of ongoing support. Recreational activities may involve, for example, enjoyment in listening to music, watching movies, going out for walks, or participating in water activities, all with the support of others. Co-occurring physical and sensory impairments are frequent barriers to participation (beyond watching) in home, recreational, and vocational activities. Maladaptive behavior is present in a significant minority.

Diagnostic Features

The essential features of intellectual disability (intellectual developmental disorder) are deficits in general mental abilities (Criterion A) and impairment in everyday adaptive functioning, in comparison to an individual's age-, gender-, and socioculturally matched peers (Criterion B). Onset is during the developmental period (Criterion C). The diagnosis of intellectual disability is based on both clinical assessment and standardized testing of intellectual and adaptive functions.

Criterion A refers to intellectual functions that involve reasoning, problem solving, planning, abstract thinking, judgment, learning from instruction and experience, and practical understanding. Critical components include verbal comprehension, working memory, perceptual reasoning, quantitative reasoning, abstract thought, and cognitive efficacy. Intellectual functioning is typically measured with individually administered and psychometrically valid, comprehensive, culturally appropriate, psychometrically sound tests of intelligence. Individuals with intellectual disability have scores of approximately two standard deviations or more below the population mean, including a margin for measurement error (generally ±5 points). On tests with a standard deviation of 15 and a mean of 100, this involves a score of 65–75 (70 ± 5). Clinical training and judgment are required to interpret test results and assess intellectual performance.

Factors that may affect test scores include practice effects and the "Flynn effect" (i.e., overly high scores due to out-of-date test norms). Invalid scores may result from the use of brief intelligence screening tests or group tests; highly discrepant individual subtest scores may make an overall IQ score invalid. Instruments must be normed for the individual's sociocultural background and native language. Co-occurring disorders that affect communication, language, and/or motor or sensory function may affect test scores. Individual cognitive profiles based on neuropsychological testing are more useful for understanding intellectual abilities than a single IQ score. Such testing may identify areas of relative strengths and weaknesses, an assessment important for academic and vocational planning.

IQ test scores are approximations of conceptual functioning but may be insufficient to assess reasoning in real-life situations and mastery of practical tasks. For example, a person with an IQ score above 70 may have such severe adaptive behavior problems in social judgment, social understanding, and other areas of adaptive functioning that the person's actual functioning is comparable to that of individuals with a lower IQ score. Thus, clinical judgment is needed in interpreting the results of IQ tests.

Deficits in adaptive functioning (Criterion B) refer to how well a person meets community standards of personal independence and social responsibility, in comparison to others of similar age and sociocultural background. Adaptive functioning involves adaptive reasoning in three domains: conceptual, social, and practical. The *conceptual (academic) domain* involves competence in memory, language, reading, writing, math reasoning, acquisition of practical knowledge, problem solving, and judgment in novel situations, among others. The *social domain* involves awareness of others' thoughts, feelings, and experiences; empathy; interpersonal communication skills; friendship abilities; and social judgment, among others. The *practical domain* involves learning and self-management across life settings, including personal care, job responsibilities, money management, recreation, self-management of behavior, and school and work task organization, among others. Intellectual capacity, education, motivation, socialization, personality features, vocational opportunity, cultural experience, and coexisting general medical conditions or mental disorders influence adaptive functioning.

Adaptive functioning is assessed using both clinical evaluation and individualized, culturally appropriate, psychometrically sound measures. Standardized measures are used with knowledgeable informants (e.g., parent or other family member; teacher; counselor; care provider) and the individual to the extent possible. Additional sources of information include educational, developmental, medical, and mental health evaluations. Scores from standardized measures and interview sources must be interpreted using clinical judgment. When standardized testing is difficult or impossible, because of a variety of factors (e.g., sensory impairment, severe problem behavior), the individual may be diagnosed with unspecified intellectual disability. Adaptive functioning may be difficult to assess in a controlled setting (e.g., prisons, detention centers); if possible, corroborative information reflecting functioning outside those settings should be obtained.

Criterion B is met when at least one domain of adaptive functioning—conceptual, social, or practical—is sufficiently impaired that ongoing support is needed in order for the person to perform adequately in one or more life settings at school, at work, at home, or in the community. To meet diagnostic criteria for intellectual disability, the deficits in adaptive functioning must be directly related to the intellectual impairments described in Criterion A. Criterion C, onset during the developmental period, refers to recognition that intellectual and adaptive deficits are present during childhood or adolescence.

Associated Features Supporting Diagnosis

Intellectual disability is a heterogeneous condition with multiple causes. There may be associated difficulties with social judgment; assessment of risk; self-management of behavior, emotions, or interpersonal relationships; or motivation in school or work environments. Lack of communication skills may predispose to disruptive and aggressive behaviors. Gullibility is often a feature, involving naiveté in social situations and a tendency for being easily led by others. Gullibility and lack of awareness of risk may result in exploitation by others and possible victimization, fraud, unintentional criminal involvement, false confessions, and risk for physical and sexual abuse. These associated features can be important in criminal cases, including Atkins-type hearings involving the death penalty.

Individuals with a diagnosis of intellectual disability with co-occurring mental disorders are at risk for suicide. They think about suicide, make suicide attempts, and may die from them. Thus, screening for suicidal thoughts is essential in the assessment process. Because of a lack of awareness of risk and danger, accidental injury rates may be increased.

Prevalence

Intellectual disability has an overall general population prevalence of approximately 1%, and prevalence rates vary by age. Prevalence for severe intellectual disability is approximately 6 per 1,000.

Development and Course

Onset of intellectual disability is in the developmental period. The age and characteristic features at onset depend on the etiology and severity of brain dysfunction. Delayed motor, language, and social milestones may be identifiable within the first 2 years of life among those with more severe intellectual disability, while mild levels may not be identifiable until school age when difficulty with academic learning becomes apparent. All criteria (including Criterion C) must be fulfilled by history or current presentation. Some children under age 5 years whose presentation will eventually meet criteria for intellectual disability have deficits that meet criteria for global developmental delay.

When intellectual disability is associated with a genetic syndrome, there may be a characteristic physical appearance (as in, e.g., Down syndrome). Some syndromes have a *behavioral phenotype*, which refers to specific behaviors that are characteristic of particular genetic disorder (e.g., Lesch-Nyhan syndrome). In acquired forms, the onset may be abrupt following an illness such as meningitis or encephalitis or head trauma occurring during the developmental period. When intellectual disability results from a loss of previously acquired cognitive skills, as in severe traumatic brain injury, the diagnoses of intellectual disability and of a neurocognitive disorder may both be assigned.

Although intellectual disability is generally nonprogressive, in certain genetic disorders (e.g., Rett syndrome) there are periods of worsening, followed by stabilization, and in others (e.g., Sanfilippo syndrome) progressive worsening of intellectual function. After early childhood, the disorder is generally lifelong, although severity levels may change over time. The course may be influenced by underlying medical or genetic conditions and co-occurring conditions (e.g., hearing or visual impairments, epilepsy). Early and ongoing interventions may improve adaptive functioning throughout childhood and adulthood. In some cases, these result in significant improvement of intellectual functioning, such that the diagnosis of intellectual disability is no longer appropriate. Thus, it is common practice when assessing infants and young children to delay diagnosis of intellectual disability until after an appropriate course of intervention is provided. For older children and adults, the extent of support provided may allow for full participation in all activities of daily living and improved adaptive function. Diagnostic assessments must determine whether improved adaptive skills are the result of a stable, generalized new skill acquisition (in which case the diagnosis of intellectual disability may no longer be appropriate) or whether the improvement is contingent on the presence of supports and ongoing interventions (in which case the diagnosis of intellectual disability may still be appropriate).

Risk and Prognostic Factors

Genetic and physiological.   Prenatal etiologies include genetic syndromes (e.g., sequence variations or copy number variants involving one or more genes; chromosomal disorders), inborn errors of metabolism, brain malformations, maternal disease (including placental disease), and environmental influences (e.g., alcohol, other drugs, toxins, teratogens). Perinatal causes include a variety of labor and delivery-related events leading to neonatal encephalopathy. Postnatal causes include hypoxic ischemic injury, traumatic brain injury, infections, demyelinating disorders, seizure disorders (e.g., infantile spasms), severe and chronic social deprivation, and toxic metabolic syndromes and intoxications (e.g., lead, mercury).

Culture-Related Diagnostic Issues

Intellectual disability occurs in all races and cultures. Cultural sensitivity and knowledge are needed during assessment, and the individual's ethnic, cultural, and linguistic background, available experiences, and adaptive functioning within his or her community and cultural setting must be taken into account.

Gender-Related Diagnostic Issues

Overall, males are more likely than females to be diagnosed with both mild (average male:female ratio 1.6:1) and severe (average male:female ratio 1.2:1) forms of intellectual disability. However, gender ratios vary widely in reported studies. Sex-linked genetic factors and male vulnerability to brain insult may account for some of the gender differences.

Diagnostic Markers

A comprehensive evaluation includes an assessment of intellectual capacity and adaptive functioning; identification of genetic and nongenetic etiologies; evaluation for associated medical conditions (e.g., cerebral palsy, seizure disorder); and evaluation for co-occurring mental, emotional, and behavioral disorders. Components of the evaluation may include basic pre- and perinatal medical history, three-generational family pedigree, physical examination, genetic evaluation (e.g., karyotype or chromosomal microarray analysis and testing for specific genetic syndromes), and metabolic screening and neuroimaging assessment.

Differential Diagnosis

The diagnosis of intellectual disability should be made whenever Criteria A, B, and C are met. A diagnosis of intellectual disability should not be assumed because of a particular genetic or medical condition. A genetic syndrome linked to intellectual disability should be noted as a concurrent diagnosis with the intellectual disability.

Major and mild neurocognitive disorders.   Intellectual disability is categorized as a neurodevelopmental disorder and is distinct from the neurocognitive disorders, which are characterized by a loss of cognitive functioning. Major neurocognitive disorder may co-occur with intellectual disability (e.g., an individual with Down syndrome who develops Alzheimer's disease, or an individual with intellectual disability who loses further cognitive capacity following a head injury). In such cases, the diagnoses of intellectual disability and neurocognitive disorder may both be given.

Communication disorders and specific learning disorder.   These neurodevelopmental disorders are specific to the communication and learning domains and do not show deficits in intellectual and adaptive behavior. They may co-occur with intellectual disability. Both diagnoses are made if full criteria are met for intellectual disability and a communication disorder or specific learning disorder.

Autism spectrum disorder.   Intellectual disability is common among individuals with autism spectrum disorder. Assessment of intellectual ability may be complicated by social-communication and behavior deficits inherent to autism spectrum disorder, which may interfere with understanding and complying with test procedures. Appropriate assessment of intellectual functioning in autism spectrum disorder is essential, with reassessment across the developmental period, because IQ scores in autism spectrum disorder may be unstable, particularly in early childhood.

Comorbidity

Co-occurring mental, neurodevelopmental, medical, and physical conditions are frequent in intellectual disability, with rates of some conditions (e.g., mental disorders, cerebral palsy, and epilepsy) three to four times higher than in the general population. The prognosis and outcome of co-occurring diagnoses may be influenced by the presence of intellectual disability. Assessment procedures may require modifications because of associated disorders, including communication disorders, autism spectrum disorder, and motor, sensory, or other disorders. Knowledgeable informants are essential for identifying symptoms such as irritability, mood dysregulation, aggression, eating problems, and sleep problems, and for assessing adaptive functioning in various community settings.

The most common co-occurring mental and neurodevelopmental disorders are attention-deficit/hyperactivity disorder; depressive and bipolar disorders; anxiety disorders; autism spectrum disorder; stereotypic movement disorder (with or without self-injurious behavior); impulse-control disorders; and major neurocognitive disorder. Major depressive disorder may occur throughout the range of severity of intellectual disability. Self-injurious behavior requires prompt diagnostic attention and may warrant a separate diagnosis of stereotypic movement disorder. Individuals with intellectual disability, particularly those with more severe intellectual disability, may also exhibit aggression and disruptive behaviors, including harm of others or property destruction.

Relationship to Other Classifications

ICD-11 (in development at the time of this publication) uses the term *intellectual developmental disorders* to indicate that these are disorders that involve impaired brain functioning early in life. These disorders are described in ICD-11 as a metasyndrome occurring in the developmental period analogous to dementia or neurocognitive disorder in later life. There are four subtypes in ICD-11: mild, moderate, severe, and profound.

The American Association on Intellectual and Developmental Disabilities (AAIDD) also uses the term *intellectual disability* with a similar meaning to the term as used in this manual. The AAIDD's classification is multidimensional rather than categorical and is based on the disability construct. Rather than listing specifiers as is done in DSM-5, the AAIDD emphasizes a profile of supports based on severity.

Global Developmental Delay

315.8 (F88)

This diagnosis is reserved for individuals *under* the age of 5 years when the clinical severity level cannot be reliably assessed during early childhood. This category is diagnosed when an individual fails to meet expected developmental milestones in several areas of intellectual functioning, and applies to individuals who are unable to undergo systematic assessments of intellectual functioning, including children who are too young to participate in standardized testing. This category requires reassessment after a period of time.

Unspecified Intellectual Disability (Intellectual Developmental Disorder)

319 (F79)

This category is reserved for individuals *over* the age of 5 years when assessment of the degree of intellectual disability (intellectual developmental disorder) by means of locally available procedures is rendered difficult or impossible because of associated sensory or physical impairments, as in blindness or prelingual deafness; locomotor disability; or presence of severe problem behaviors or co-occurring mental disorder. This category should only be used in exceptional circumstances and requires reassessment after a period of time.

Communication Disorders

Disorders of communication include deficits in language, speech, and communication. *Speech* is the expressive production of sounds and includes an individual's articulation, fluency, voice, and resonance quality. *Language* includes the form, function, and use of a conventional system of symbols (i.e., spoken words, sign language, written words, pictures) in a rule-governed manner for communication. *Communication* includes any verbal or nonverbal behavior (whether intentional or unintentional) that influences the behavior, ideas, or attitudes of another individual. Assessments of speech, language and communication abilities must take into account the individual's cultural and language context, particularly for individuals growing up in bilingual environments. The standardized measures of language development and of nonverbal intellectual capacity must be relevant for the cultural and linguistic group (i.e., tests developed and standardized for one group may not provide appropriate norms for a different group). The diagnostic category of communication disorders includes the following: language disorder, speech sound disorder, childhood-onset fluency disorder (stuttering), social (pragmatic) communication disorder, and other specified and unspecified communication disorders.

Language Disorder

Diagnostic Criteria   **315.32 (F80.2)**

A. Persistent difficulties in the acquisition and use of language across modalities (i.e., spoken, written, sign language, or other) due to deficits in comprehension or production that include the following:

1. Reduced vocabulary (word knowledge and use).
2. Limited sentence structure (ability to put words and word endings together to form sentences based on the rules of grammar and morphology).
3. Impairments in discourse (ability to use vocabulary and connect sentences to explain or describe a topic or series of events or have a conversation).

B. Language abilities are substantially and quantifiably below those expected for age, resulting in functional limitations in effective communication, social participation, academic achievement, or occupational performance, individually or in any combination.

C. Onset of symptoms is in the early developmental period.

D. The difficulties are not attributable to hearing or other sensory impairment, motor dysfunction, or another medical or neurological condition and are not better explained by intellectual disability (intellectual developmental disorder) or global developmental delay.

Diagnostic Features

The core diagnostic features of language disorder are difficulties in the acquisition and use of language due to deficits in the comprehension or production of vocabulary, sentence structure, and discourse. The language deficits are evident in spoken communication, written communication, or sign language. Language learning and use is dependent on both receptive and expressive skills. *Expressive ability* refers to the production of vocal, gestural, or verbal signals, while *receptive ability* refers to the process of receiving and comprehending language messages. Language skills need to be assessed in both expressive and receptive modalities as these may differ in severity. For example, an individual's expressive language may be severely impaired, while his receptive language is hardly impaired at all.

Language disorder usually affects vocabulary and grammar, and these effects then limit the capacity for discourse. The child's first words and phrases are likely to be delayed in onset; vocabulary size is smaller and less varied than expected; and sentences are shorter and less complex with grammatical errors, especially in past tense. Deficits in comprehension of language are frequently underestimated, as children may be good at using context to infer meaning. There may be word-finding problems, impoverished verbal definitions, or poor understanding of synonyms, multiple meanings, or word play appropriate for age and culture. Problems with remembering new words and sentences are manifested by difficulties following instructions of increasing length, difficulties rehearsing strings of verbal information (e.g., remembering a phone number or a shopping list), and difficulties remembering novel sound sequences, a skill that may be important for learning new words. Difficulties with discourse are shown by a reduced ability to provide adequate information about the key events and to narrate a coherent story.

The language difficulty is manifest by abilities substantially and quantifiably below that expected for age and significantly interfering with academic achievement, occupational performance, effective communication, or socialization (Criterion B). A diagnosis of language disorder is made based on the synthesis of the individual's history, direct clinical observation in different contexts (i.e., home, school, or work), and scores from standardized tests of language ability that can be used to guide estimates of severity.

Associated Features Supporting Diagnosis

A positive family history of language disorders is often present. Individuals, even children, can be adept at accommodating to their limited language. They may appear to be shy or reticent to talk. Affected individuals may prefer to communicate only with family members or other familiar individuals. Although these social indicators are not diagnostic of a language disorder, if they are notable and persistent, they warrant referral for a full language assessment. Language disorder, particularly expressive deficits, may co-occur with speech sound disorder.

Development and Course

Language acquisition is marked by changes from onset in toddlerhood to the adult level of competency that appears during adolescence. Changes appear across the dimensions of language (sounds, words, grammar, narratives/expository texts, and conversational skills) in age-graded increments and synchronies. Language disorder emerges during the early developmental period; however, there is considerable variation in early vocabulary acquisition and early word combinations, and individual differences are not, as single indicators, highly predictive of later outcomes. By age 4 years, individual differences in language ability are more stable, with better measurement accuracy, and are highly predictive of later outcomes. Language disorder diagnosed from 4 years of age is likely to be stable over time and typically persists into adulthood, although the particular profile of language strengths and deficits is likely to change over the course of development.

Risk and Prognostic Factors

Children with receptive language impairments have a poorer prognosis than those with predominantly expressive impairments. They are more resistant to treatment, and difficulties with reading comprehension are frequently seen.

Genetic and physiological.   Language disorders are highly heritable, and family members are more likely to have a history of language impairment.

Differential Diagnosis

Normal variations in language.   Language disorder needs to be distinguished from normal developmental variations, and this distinction may be difficult to make before 4 years of age. Regional, social, or cultural/ethnic variations of language (e.g., dialects) must be considered when an individual is being assessed for language impairment.

Hearing or other sensory impairment.   Hearing impairment needs to be excluded as the primary cause of language difficulties. Language deficits may be associated with a hearing impairment, other sensory deficit, or a speech-motor deficit. When language deficits are in excess of those usually associated with these problems, a diagnosis of language disorder may be made.

Intellectual disability (intellectual developmental disorder).   Language delay is often the presenting feature of intellectual disability, and the definitive diagnosis may not be made until the child is able to complete standardized assessments. A separate diagnosis is not given unless the language deficits are clearly in excess of the intellectual limitations.

Neurological disorders.   Language disorder can be acquired in association with neurological disorders, including epilepsy (e.g., acquired aphasia or Landau-Kleffner syndrome).

Language regression.   Loss of speech and language in a child younger than 3 years may be a sign of autism spectrum disorder (with developmental regression) or a specific neurological condition, such as Landau-Kleffner syndrome. Among children older than 3 years, language loss may be a symptom of seizures, and a diagnostic assessment is necessary to exclude the presence of epilepsy (e.g., routine and sleep electroencephalogram).

Comorbidity

Language disorder is strongly associated with other neurodevelopmental disorders in terms of specific learning disorder (literacy and numeracy), attention-deficit/hyperactivity disorder, autism spectrum disorder, and developmental coordination disorder. It is also associated with social (pragmatic) communication disorder. A positive family history of speech or language disorders is often present.

Speech Sound Disorder

Diagnostic Criteria	315.39 (F80.0)

A. Persistent difficulty with speech sound production that interferes with speech intelligibility or prevents verbal communication of messages.
B. The disturbance causes limitations in effective communication that interfere with social participation, academic achievement, or occupational performance, individually or in any combination.
C. Onset of symptoms is in the early developmental period.
D. The difficulties are not attributable to congenital or acquired conditions, such as cerebral palsy, cleft palate, deafness or hearing loss, traumatic brain injury, or other medical or neurological conditions.

Diagnostic Features

Speech sound production describes the clear articulation of the phonemes (i.e., individual sounds) that in combination make up spoken words. Speech sound production requires both the phonological knowledge of speech sounds and the ability to coordinate the movements of the articulators (i.e., the jaw, tongue, and lips,) with breathing and vocalizing for speech. Children with speech production difficulties may experience difficulty with phonological knowledge of speech sounds or the ability to coordinate movements for speech in varying degrees. Speech sound disorder is thus heterogeneous in its underlying mechanisms and includes phonological disorder and articulation disorder. A speech sound disorder is diagnosed when speech sound production is not what would be expected based on the child's age and developmental stage and when the deficits are not the result of a physical, structural, neurological, or hearing impairment. Among typically developing children at age 4 years, overall speech should be intelligible, whereas at age 2 years, only 50% may be understandable.

Associated Features Supporting Diagnosis

Language disorder, particularly expressive deficits, may be found to co-occur with speech sound disorder. A positive family history of speech or language disorders is often present.

If the ability to rapidly coordinate the articulators is a particular aspect of difficulty, there may be a history of delay or incoordination in acquiring skills that also utilize the articulators and related facial musculature; among others, these skills include chewing, maintaining mouth closure, and blowing the nose. Other areas of motor coordination may be impaired as in developmental coordination disorder. *Verbal dyspraxia* is a term also used for speech production problems.

Speech may be differentially impaired in certain genetic conditions (e.g., Down syndrome, 22q deletion, *FoxP2* gene mutation). If present, these should also be coded.

Development and Course

Learning to produce speech sounds clearly and accurately and learning to produce connected speech fluently are developmental skills. Articulation of speech sounds follows a developmental pattern, which is reflected in the age norms of standardized tests. It is not unusual for typically developing children to use developmental processes for shortening words and syllables as they are learning to talk, but their progression in mastering speech sound production should result in mostly intelligible speech by age 3 years. Children with speech sound disorder continue to use immature phonological simplification processes past the age when most children can produce words clearly.

Most speech sounds should be produced clearly and most words should be pronounced accurately according to age and community norms by age 7 years. The most frequently mis-articulated sounds also tend to be learned later, leading them to be called the "late eight" (*l*, *r*, *s*, *z*, *th*, *ch*, *dzh*, and *zh*). Misarticulation of any of these sounds by itself could be considered within normal limits up to age 8 years. When multiple sounds are involved, it may be appropriate to target some of those sounds as part of a plan to improve intelligibility prior to the age at which almost all children can produce them accurately. Lisping (i.e., misarticulating sibilants) is particularly common and may involve frontal or lateral patterns of airstream direction. It may be associated with an abnormal tongue-thrust swallowing pattern.

Most children with speech sound disorder respond well to treatment, and speech difficulties improve over time, and thus the disorder may not be lifelong. However, when a language disorder is also present, the speech disorder has a poorer prognosis and may be associated with specific learning disorders.

Differential Diagnosis

Normal variations in speech.   Regional, social, or cultural/ethnic variations of speech should be considered before making the diagnosis.

Hearing or other sensory impairment.   Hearing impairment or deafness may result in abnormalities of speech. Deficits of speech sound production may be associated with a hearing impairment, other sensory deficit, or a speech-motor deficit. When speech deficits are in excess of those usually associated with these problems, a diagnosis of speech sound disorder may be made.

Structural deficits.   Speech impairment may be due to structural deficits (e.g., cleft palate).

Dysarthria.   Speech impairment may be attributable to a motor disorder, such as cerebral palsy. Neurological signs, as well as distinctive features of voice, differentiate dysarthria from speech sound disorder, although in young children (under 3 years) differentiation may be difficult, particularly when there is no or minimal general body motor involvement (as in, e.g., Worster-Drought syndrome).

Selective mutism.   Limited use of speech may be a sign of selective mutism, an anxiety disorder that is characterized by a lack of speech in one or more contexts or settings. Selective mutism may develop in children with a speech disorder because of embarrassment about their impairments, but many children with selective mutism exhibit normal speech in "safe" settings, such as at home or with close friends.

Childhood-Onset Fluency Disorder (Stuttering)

Diagnostic Criteria   **315.35 (F80.81)**

A. Disturbances in the normal fluency and time patterning of speech that are inappropriate for the individual's age and language skills, persist over time, and are characterized by frequent and marked occurrences of one (or more) of the following:

1. Sound and syllable repetitions.
2. Sound prolongations of consonants as well as vowels.

3. Broken words (e.g., pauses within a word).
4. Audible or silent blocking (filled or unfilled pauses in speech).
5. Circumlocutions (word substitutions to avoid problematic words).
6. Words produced with an excess of physical tension.
7. Monosyllabic whole-word repetitions (e.g., "I-I-I-I see him").

B. The disturbance causes anxiety about speaking or limitations in effective communication, social participation, or academic or occupational performance, individually or in any combination.

C. The onset of symptoms is in the early developmental period. (**Note:** Later-onset cases are diagnosed as 307.0 [F98.5] adult-onset fluency disorder.)

D. The disturbance is not attributable to a speech-motor or sensory deficit, dysfluency associated with neurological insult (e.g., stroke, tumor, trauma), or another medical condition and is not better explained by another mental disorder.

Diagnostic Features

The essential feature of childhood-onset fluency disorder (stuttering) is a disturbance in the normal fluency and time patterning of speech that is inappropriate for the individual's age. This disturbance is characterized by frequent repetitions or prolongations of sounds or syllables and by other types of speech dysfluencies, including broken words (e.g., pauses within a word), audible or silent blocking (i.e., filled or unfilled pauses in speech), circumlocutions (i.e., word substitutions to avoid problematic words), words produced with an excess of physical tension, and monosyllabic whole-word repetitions (e.g., "I-I-I-I see him"). The disturbance in fluency interferes with academic or occupational achievement or with social communication. The extent of the disturbance varies from situation to situation and often is more severe when there is special pressure to communicate (e.g., giving a report at school, interviewing for a job). Dysfluency is often absent during oral reading, singing, or talking to inanimate objects or to pets.

Associated Features Supporting Diagnosis

Fearful anticipation of the problem may develop. The speaker may attempt to avoid dysfluencies by linguistic mechanisms (e.g., altering the rate of speech, avoiding certain words or sounds) or by avoiding certain speech situations, such as telephoning or public speaking. In addition to being features of the condition, stress and anxiety have been shown to exacerbate dysfluency.

Childhood-onset fluency disorder may also be accompanied by motor movements (e.g., eye blinks, tics, tremors of the lips or face, jerking of the head, breathing movements, fist clenching). Children with fluency disorder show a range of language abilities, and the relationship between fluency disorder and language abilities is unclear.

Development and Course

Childhood-onset fluency disorder, or developmental stuttering, occurs by age 6 for 80%–90% of affected individuals, with age at onset ranging from 2 to 7 years. The onset can be insidious or more sudden. Typically, dysfluencies start gradually, with repetition of initial consonants, first words of a phrase, or long words. The child may not be aware of dysfluencies. As the disorder progresses, the dysfluencies become more frequent and interfering, occurring on the most meaningful words or phrases in the utterance. As the child becomes aware of the speech difficulty, he or she may develop mechanisms for avoiding the dysfluencies and emotional responses, including avoidance of public speaking and use of short and simple utterances. Longitudinal research shows that 65%–85% of children recover from the dysfluency, with severity of fluency disorder at age 8 years predicting recovery or persistence into adolescence and beyond.

Risk and Prognostic Factors

Genetic and physiological. The risk of stuttering among first-degree biological relatives of individuals with childhood-onset fluency disorder is more than three times the risk in the general population.

Functional Consequences of Childhood-Onset Fluency Disorder (Stuttering)

In addition to being features of the condition, stress and anxiety can exacerbate dysfluency. Impairment of social functioning may result from this anxiety.

Differential Diagnosis

Sensory deficits. Dysfluencies of speech may be associated with a hearing impairment or other sensory deficit or a speech-motor deficit. When the speech dysfluencies are in excess of those usually associated with these problems, a diagnosis of childhood-onset fluency disorder may be made.

Normal speech dysfluencies. The disorder must be distinguished from normal dysfluencies that occur frequently in young children, which include whole-word or phrase repetitions (e.g., "I want, I want ice cream"), incomplete phrases, interjections, unfilled pauses, and parenthetical remarks. If these difficulties increase in frequency or complexity as the child grows older, a diagnosis of childhood-onset fluency disorder is appropriate.

Medication side effects. Stuttering may occur as a side effect of medication and may be detected by a temporal relationship with exposure to the medication.

Adult-onset dysfluencies. If onset of dysfluencies is during or after adolescence, it is an "adult-onset dysfluency" rather than a neurodevelopmental disorder. Adult-onset dysfluencies are associated with specific neurological insults and a variety of medical conditions and mental disorders and may be specified with them, but they are not a DSM-5 diagnosis.

Tourette's disorder. Vocal tics and repetitive vocalizations of Tourette's disorder should be distinguishable from the repetitive sounds of childhood-onset fluency disorder by their nature and timing.

Social (Pragmatic) Communication Disorder

Diagnostic Criteria   315.39 (F80.82)

A. Persistent difficulties in the social use of verbal and nonverbal communication as manifested by all of the following:

1. Deficits in using communication for social purposes, such as greeting and sharing information, in a manner that is appropriate for the social context.
2. Impairment of the ability to change communication to match context or the needs of the listener, such as speaking differently in a classroom than on a playground, talking differently to a child than to an adult, and avoiding use of overly formal language.
3. Difficulties following rules for conversation and storytelling, such as taking turns in conversation, rephrasing when misunderstood, and knowing how to use verbal and nonverbal signals to regulate interaction.

4. Difficulties understanding what is not explicitly stated (e.g., making inferences) and nonliteral or ambiguous meanings of language (e.g., idioms, humor, metaphors, multiple meanings that depend on the context for interpretation).

B. The deficits result in functional limitations in effective communication, social participation, social relationships, academic achievement, or occupational performance, individually or in combination.

C. The onset of the symptoms is in the early developmental period (but deficits may not become fully manifest until social communication demands exceed limited capacities).

D. The symptoms are not attributable to another medical or neurological condition or to low abilities in the domains of word structure and grammar, and are not better explained by autism spectrum disorder, intellectual disability (intellectual developmental disorder), global developmental delay, or another mental disorder.

Diagnostic Features

Social (pragmatic) communication disorder is characterized by a primary difficulty with pragmatics, or the social use of language and communication, as manifested by deficits in understanding and following social rules of verbal and nonverbal communication in naturalistic contexts, changing language according to the needs of the listener or situation, and following rules for conversations and storytelling. The deficits in social communication result in functional limitations in effective communication, social participation, development of social relationships, academic achievement, or occupational performance. The deficits are not better explained by low abilities in the domains of structural language or cognitive ability.

Associated Features Supporting Diagnosis

The most common associated feature of social (pragmatic) communication disorder is language impairment, which is characterized by a history of delay in reaching language milestones, and historical, if not current, structural language problems (see "Language Disorder" earlier in this chapter). Individuals with social communication deficits may avoid social interactions. Attention-deficit/hyperactivity disorder (ADHD), behavioral problems, and specific learning disorders are also more common among affected individuals.

Development and Course

Because social (pragmatic) communication depends on adequate developmental progress in speech and language, diagnosis of social (pragmatic) communication disorder is rare among children younger than 4 years. By age 4 or 5 years, most children should possess adequate speech and language abilities to permit identification of specific deficits in social communication. Milder forms of the disorder may not become apparent until early adolescence, when language and social interactions become more complex.

The outcome of social (pragmatic) communication disorder is variable, with some children improving substantially over time and others continuing to have difficulties persisting into adulthood. Even among those who have significant improvements, the early deficits in pragmatics may cause lasting impairments in social relationships and behavior and also in acquisition of other related skills, such as written expression.

Risk and Prognostic Factors

Genetic and physiological. A family history of autism spectrum disorder, communication disorders, or specific learning disorder appears to increase the risk for social (pragmatic) communication disorder.

Differential Diagnosis

Autism spectrum disorder.   Autism spectrum disorder is the primary diagnostic consideration for individuals presenting with social communication deficits. The two disorders can be differentiated by the presence in autism spectrum disorder of restricted/repetitive patterns of behavior, interests, or activities and their absence in social (pragmatic) communication disorder. Individuals with autism spectrum disorder may only display the restricted/repetitive patterns of behavior, interests, and activities during the early developmental period, so a comprehensive history should be obtained. Current absence of symptoms would not preclude a diagnosis of autism spectrum disorder, if the restricted interests and repetitive behaviors were present in the past. A diagnosis of social (pragmatic) communication disorder should be considered only if the developmental history fails to reveal any evidence of restricted/repetitive patterns of behavior, interests, or activities.

Attention-deficit/hyperactivity disorder.   Primary deficits of ADHD may cause impairments in social communication and functional limitations of effective communication, social participation, or academic achievement.

Social anxiety disorder (social phobia).   The symptoms of social communication disorder overlap with those of social anxiety disorder. The differentiating feature is the timing of the onset of symptoms. In social (pragmatic) communication disorder, the individual has never had effective social communication; in social anxiety disorder, the social communication skills developed appropriately but are not utilized because of anxiety, fear, or distress about social interactions.

Intellectual disability (intellectual developmental disorder) and global developmental delay.   Social communication skills may be deficient among individuals with global developmental delay or intellectual disability, but a separate diagnosis is not given unless the social communication deficits are clearly in excess of the intellectual limitations.

Unspecified Communication Disorder

307.9 (F80.9)

This category applies to presentations in which symptoms characteristic of communication disorder that cause clinically significant distress or impairment in social, occupational, or other important areas of functioning predominate but do not meet the full criteria for communication disorder or for any of the disorders in the neurodevelopmental disorders diagnostic class. The unspecified communication disorder category is used in situations in which the clinician chooses *not* to specify the reason that the criteria are not met for communication disorder or for a specific neurodevelopmental disorder, and includes presentations in which there is insufficient information to make a more specific diagnosis.

Autism Spectrum Disorder

Autism Spectrum Disorder

Diagnostic Criteria   **299.00 (F84.0)**

A. Persistent deficits in social communication and social interaction across multiple contexts, as manifested by all of the following, currently or by history (examples are illustrative, not exhaustive; see text):

1. Deficits in social-emotional reciprocity, ranging, for example, from abnormal social approach and failure of normal back-and-forth conversation; to reduced sharing of interests, emotions, or affect; to failure to initiate or respond to social interactions.

2. Deficits in nonverbal communicative behaviors used for social interaction, ranging, for example, from poorly integrated verbal and nonverbal communication; to abnormalities in eye contact and body language or deficits in understanding and use of gestures; to a total lack of facial expressions and nonverbal communication.

3. Deficits in developing, maintaining, and understanding relationships, ranging, for example, from difficulties adjusting behavior to suit various social contexts; to difficulties in sharing imaginative play or in making friends; to absence of interest in peers.

Specify current severity:

Severity is based on social communication impairments and restricted, repetitive patterns of behavior (see Table 2).

B. Restricted, repetitive patterns of behavior, interests, or activities, as manifested by at least two of the following, currently or by history (examples are illustrative, not exhaustive; see text):

1. Stereotyped or repetitive motor movements, use of objects, or speech (e.g., simple motor stereotypies, lining up toys or flipping objects, echolalia, idiosyncratic phrases).

2. Insistence on sameness, inflexible adherence to routines, or ritualized patterns of verbal or nonverbal behavior (e.g., extreme distress at small changes, difficulties with transitions, rigid thinking patterns, greeting rituals, need to take same route or eat same food every day).

3. Highly restricted, fixated interests that are abnormal in intensity or focus (e.g., strong attachment to or preoccupation with unusual objects, excessively circumscribed or perseverative interests).

4. Hyper- or hyporeactivity to sensory input or unusual interest in sensory aspects of the environment (e.g., apparent indifference to pain/temperature, adverse response to specific sounds or textures, excessive smelling or touching of objects, visual fascination with lights or movement).

Specify current severity:

Severity is based on social communication impairments and restricted, repetitive patterns of behavior (see Table 2).

C. Symptoms must be present in the early developmental period (but may not become fully manifest until social demands exceed limited capacities, or may be masked by learned strategies in later life).

D. Symptoms cause clinically significant impairment in social, occupational, or other important areas of current functioning.

E. These disturbances are not better explained by intellectual disability (intellectual developmental disorder) or global developmental delay. Intellectual disability and autism
spectrum disorder frequently co-occur; to make comorbid diagnoses of autism spectrum disorder and intellectual disability, social communication should be below that expected for general developmental level.

Note: Individuals with a well-established DSM-IV diagnosis of autistic disorder, Asperger's
disorder, or pervasive developmental disorder not otherwise specified should be given the
diagnosis of autism spectrum disorder. Individuals who have marked deficits in social
communication, but whose symptoms do not otherwise meet criteria for autism spectrum
disorder, should be evaluated for social (pragmatic) communication disorder.

Specify if:

With or without accompanying intellectual impairment

With or without accompanying language impairment

Associated with a known medical or genetic condition or environmental factor
(**Coding note:** Use additional code to identify the associated medical or genetic condition.)

Associated with another neurodevelopmental, mental, or behavioral disorder
(**Coding note:** Use additional code[s] to identify the associated neurodevelopmental,
mental, or behavioral disorder[s].)

With catatonia (refer to the criteria for catatonia associated with another mental disorder, pp. 119–120, for definition) (**Coding note:** Use additional code 293.89 [F06.1]
catatonia associated with autism spectrum disorder to indicate the presence of the comorbid catatonia.)

Recording Procedures

For autism spectrum disorder that is associated with a known medical or genetic condition
or environmental factor, or with another neurodevelopmental, mental, or behavioral disorder, record autism spectrum disorder associated with (name of condition, disorder, or
factor) (e.g., autism spectrum disorder associated with Rett syndrome). Severity should be
recorded as level of support needed for each of the two psychopathological domains in
Table 2 (e.g., "requiring very substantial support for deficits in social communication and
requiring substantial support for restricted, repetitive behaviors"). Specification of "with
accompanying intellectual impairment" or "without accompanying intellectual impairment" should be recorded next. Language impairment specification should be recorded
thereafter. If there is accompanying language impairment, the current level of verbal functioning should be recorded (e.g., "with accompanying language impairment—no intelligible speech" or "with accompanying language impairment—phrase speech"). If catatonia is
present, record separately "catatonia associated with autism spectrum disorder."

Specifiers

The severity specifiers (see Table 2) may be used to describe succinctly the current symptomatology (which might fall below level 1), with the recognition that severity may vary by
context and fluctuate over time. Severity of social communication difficulties and restricted, repetitive behaviors should be separately rated. The descriptive severity categories
should not be used to determine eligibility for and provision of services; these can only be
developed at an individual level and through discussion of personal priorities and targets.

Regarding the specifier "with or without accompanying intellectual impairment," understanding the (often uneven) intellectual profile of a child or adult with autism spectrum
disorder is necessary for interpreting diagnostic features. Separate estimates of verbal and
nonverbal skill are necessary (e.g., using untimed nonverbal tests to assess potential
strengths in individuals with limited language).

TABLE 2 Severity levels for autism spectrum disorder

Severity level	Social communication	Restricted, repetitive behaviors
Level 3 "Requiring very substantial support"	Severe deficits in verbal and nonverbal social communication skills cause severe impairments in functioning, very limited initiation of social interactions, and minimal response to social overtures from others. For example, a person with few words of intelligible speech who rarely initiates interaction and, when he or she does, makes unusual approaches to meet needs only and responds to only very direct social approaches.	Inflexibility of behavior, extreme difficulty coping with change, or other restricted/repetitive behaviors markedly interfere with functioning in all spheres. Great distress/difficulty changing focus or action.
Level 2 "Requiring substantial support"	Marked deficits in verbal and nonverbal social communication skills; social impairments apparent even with supports in place; limited initiation of social interactions; and reduced or abnormal responses to social overtures from others. For example, a person who speaks simple sentences, whose interaction is limited to narrow special interests, and who has markedly odd nonverbal communication.	Inflexibility of behavior, difficulty coping with change, or other restricted/repetitive behaviors appear frequently enough to be obvious to the casual observer and interfere with functioning in a variety of contexts. Distress and/or difficulty changing focus or action.
Level 1 "Requiring support"	Without supports in place, deficits in social communication cause noticeable impairments. Difficulty initiating social interactions, and clear examples of atypical or unsuccessful responses to social overtures of others. May appear to have decreased interest in social interactions. For example, a person who is able to speak in full sentences and engages in communication but whose to-and-fro conversation with others fails, and whose attempts to make friends are odd and typically unsuccessful.	Inflexibility of behavior causes significant interference with functioning in one or more contexts. Difficulty switching between activities. Problems of organization and planning hamper independence.

To use the specifier "with or without accompanying language impairment," the current level of verbal functioning should be assessed and described. Examples of the specific descriptions for "with accompanying language impairment" might include no intelligible speech (nonverbal), single words only, or phrase speech. Language level in individuals "without accompanying language impairment" might be further described by speaks in full sentences or has fluent speech. Since receptive language may lag behind expressive language development in autism spectrum disorder, receptive and expressive language skills should be considered separately.

The specifier "associated with a known medical or genetic condition or environmental factor" should be used when the individual has a known genetic disorder (e.g., Rett syndrome, fragile X syndrome, Down syndrome), a medical disorder (e.g., epilepsy), or a history of environmental exposure (e.g., valproate, fetal alcohol syndrome, very low birth weight).

Additional neurodevelopmental, mental or behavioral conditions should also be noted (e.g., attention-deficit/hyperactivity disorder; developmental coordination disorder; disruptive behavior, impulse-control, or conduct disorders; anxiety, depressive, or bipolar disorders; tics or Tourette's disorder; self-injury; feeding, elimination, or sleep disorders).

Diagnostic Features

The essential features of autism spectrum disorder are persistent impairment in reciprocal social communication and social interaction (Criterion A), and restricted, repetitive patterns of behavior, interests, or activities (Criterion B). These symptoms are present from early childhood and limit or impair everyday functioning (Criteria C and D). The stage at which functional impairment becomes obvious will vary according to characteristics of the individual and his or her environment. Core diagnostic features are evident in the developmental period, but intervention, compensation, and current supports may mask difficulties in at least some contexts. Manifestations of the disorder also vary greatly depending on the severity of the autistic condition, developmental level, and chronological age; hence, the term *spectrum.* Autism spectrum disorder encompasses disorders previously referred to as early infantile autism, childhood autism, Kanner's autism, high-functioning autism, atypical autism, pervasive developmental disorder not otherwise specified, childhood disintegrative disorder, and Asperger's disorder.

The impairments in communication and social interaction specified in Criterion A are pervasive and sustained. Diagnoses are most valid and reliable when based on multiple sources of information, including clinician's observations, caregiver history, and, when possible, self-report. Verbal and nonverbal deficits in social communication have varying manifestations, depending on the individual's age, intellectual level, and language ability, as well as other factors such as treatment history and current support. Many individuals have language deficits, ranging from complete lack of speech through language delays, poor comprehension of speech, echoed speech, or stilted and overly literal language. Even when formal language skills (e.g., vocabulary, grammar) are intact, the use of language for reciprocal social communication is impaired in autism spectrum disorder.

Deficits in social-emotional reciprocity (i.e., the ability to engage with others and share thoughts and feelings) are clearly evident in young children with the disorder, who may show little or no initiation of social interaction and no sharing of emotions, along with reduced or absent imitation of others' behavior. What language exists is often one-sided, lacking in social reciprocity, and used to request or label rather than to comment, share feelings, or converse. In adults without intellectual disabilities or language delays, deficits in social-emotional reciprocity may be most apparent in difficulties processing and responding to complex social cues (e.g., when and how to join a conversation, what not to say). Adults who have developed compensation strategies for some social challenges still struggle in novel or unsupported situations and suffer from the effort and anxiety of consciously calculating what is socially intuitive for most individuals.

Deficits in nonverbal communicative behaviors used for social interaction are manifested by absent, reduced, or atypical use of eye contact (relative to cultural norms), gestures, facial expressions, body orientation, or speech intonation. An early feature of autism spectrum disorder is impaired joint attention as manifested by a lack of pointing, showing, or bringing objects to share interest with others, or failure to follow someone's pointing or eye gaze. Individuals may learn a few functional gestures, but their repertoire is smaller than that of others, and they often fail to use expressive gestures spontaneously in communication. Among adults with fluent language, the difficulty in coordinating nonverbal communication with speech may give the impression of odd, wooden, or exaggerated "body language" during interactions. Impairment may be relatively subtle within individual modes (e.g., someone may have relatively good eye contact when speaking) but noticeable in poor integration of eye contact, gesture, body posture, prosody, and facial expression for social communication.

Deficits in developing, maintaining, and understanding relationships should be judged against norms for age, gender, and culture. There may be absent, reduced, or atypical social interest, manifested by rejection of others, passivity, or inappropriate approaches that seem aggressive or disruptive. These difficulties are particularly evident in young children, in whom there is often a lack of shared social play and imagination (e.g., age-appropriate flexible pretend play) and, later, insistence on playing by very fixed rules. Older individuals may struggle to understand what behavior is considered appropriate in one situation but not another (e.g., casual behavior during a job interview), or the different ways that language may be used to communicate (e.g., irony, white lies). There may be an apparent preference for solitary activities or for interacting with much younger or older people. Frequently, there is a desire to establish friendships without a complete or realistic idea of what friendship entails (e.g., one-sided friendships or friendships based solely on shared special interests). Relationships with siblings, co-workers, and caregivers are also important to consider (in terms of reciprocity).

Autism spectrum disorder is also defined by restricted, repetitive patterns of behavior, interests, or activities (as specified in Criterion B), which show a range of manifestations according to age and ability, intervention, and current supports. Stereotyped or repetitive behaviors include simple motor stereotypies (e.g., hand flapping, finger flicking), repetitive use of objects (e.g., spinning coins, lining up toys), and repetitive speech (e.g., echolalia, the delayed or immediate parroting of heard words; use of "you" when referring to self; stereotyped use of words, phrases, or prosodic patterns). Excessive adherence to routines and restricted patterns of behavior may be manifest in resistance to change (e.g., distress at apparently small changes, such as in packaging of a favorite food; insistence on adherence to rules; rigidity of thinking) or ritualized patterns of verbal or nonverbal behavior (e.g., repetitive questioning, pacing a perimeter). Highly restricted, fixated interests in autism spectrum disorder tend to be abnormal in intensity or focus (e.g., a toddler strongly attached to a pan; a child preoccupied with vacuum cleaners; an adult spending hours writing out timetables). Some fascinations and routines may relate to apparent hyper- or hyporeactivity to sensory input, manifested through extreme responses to specific sounds or textures, excessive smelling or touching of objects, fascination with lights or spinning objects, and sometimes apparent indifference to pain, heat, or cold. Extreme reaction to or rituals involving taste, smell, texture, or appearance of food or excessive food restrictions are common and may be a presenting feature of autism spectrum disorder.

Many adults with autism spectrum disorder without intellectual or language disabilities learn to suppress repetitive behavior in public. Special interests may be a source of pleasure and motivation and provide avenues for education and employment later in life. Diagnostic criteria may be met when restricted, repetitive patterns of behavior, interests, or activities were clearly present during childhood or at some time in the past, even if symptoms are no longer present.

Criterion D requires that the features must cause clinically significant impairment in social, occupational, or other important areas of current functioning. Criterion E specifies that the social communication deficits, although sometimes accompanied by intellectual disability (intellectual developmental disorder), are not in line with the individual's developmental level; impairments exceed difficulties expected on the basis of developmental level.

Standardized behavioral diagnostic instruments with good psychometric properties, including caregiver interviews, questionnaires and clinician observation measures, are available and can improve reliability of diagnosis over time and across clinicians.

Associated Features Supporting Diagnosis

Many individuals with autism spectrum disorder also have intellectual impairment and/or language impairment (e.g., slow to talk, language comprehension behind production). Even those with average or high intelligence have an uneven profile of abilities. The gap between intellectual and adaptive functional skills is often large. Motor deficits are often present, including odd gait, clumsiness, and other abnormal motor signs (e.g., walking on tiptoes). Self-injury (e.g., head banging, biting the wrist) may occur, and disruptive/challenging behaviors are more common in children and adolescents with autism spectrum disorder than other disorders, including intellectual disability. Adolescents and adults with autism spectrum disorder are prone to anxiety and depression. Some individuals develop catatonic-like motor behavior (slowing and "freezing" mid-action), but these are typically not of the magnitude of a catatonic episode. However, it is possible for individuals with autism spectrum disorder to experience a marked deterioration in motor symptoms and display a full catatonic episode with symptoms such as mutism, posturing, grimacing and waxy flexibility. The risk period for comorbid catatonia appears to be greatest in the adolescent years.

Prevalence

In recent years, reported frequencies for autism spectrum disorder across U.S. and non-U.S. countries have approached 1% of the population, with similar estimates in child and adult samples. It remains unclear whether higher rates reflect an expansion of the diagnostic criteria of DSM-IV to include subthreshold cases, increased awareness, differences in study methodology, or a true increase in the frequency of autism spectrum disorder.

Development and Course

The age and pattern of onset also should be noted for autism spectrum disorder. Symptoms are typically recognized during the second year of life (12–24 months of age) but may be seen earlier than 12 months if developmental delays are severe, or noted later than 24 months if symptoms are more subtle. The pattern of onset description might include information about early developmental delays or any losses of social or language skills. In cases where skills have been lost, parents or caregivers may give a history of a gradual or relatively rapid deterioration in social behaviors or language skills. Typically, this would occur between 12 and 24 months of age and is distinguished from the rare instances of developmental regression occurring after at least 2 years of normal development (previously described as childhood disintegrative disorder).

The behavioral features of autism spectrum disorder first become evident in early childhood, with some cases presenting a lack of interest in social interaction in the first year of life. Some children with autism spectrum disorder experience developmental plateaus or regression, with a gradual or relatively rapid deterioration in social behaviors or use of language, often during the first 2 years of life. Such losses are rare in other disorders and may be a useful "red flag" for autism spectrum disorder. Much more unusual and warranting more extensive medical investigation are losses of skills beyond social communication (e.g., loss of self-care, toileting, motor skills) or those occurring after the second birthday (see also Rett syndrome in the section "Differential Diagnosis" for this disorder).

First symptoms of autism spectrum disorder frequently involve delayed language development, often accompanied by lack of social interest or unusual social interactions (e.g., pulling individuals by the hand without any attempt to look at them), odd play patterns (e.g., carrying toys around but never playing with them), and unusual communication patterns (e.g., knowing the alphabet but not responding to own name). Deafness may be suspected but is typically ruled out. During the second year, odd and repetitive behaviors and the absence of typical play become more apparent. Since many typically developing young children have strong preferences and enjoy repetition (e.g., eating the same foods, watching the same video multiple times), distinguishing restricted and repetitive behaviors that are diagnostic of autism spectrum disorder can be difficult in preschoolers. The clinical distinction is based on the type, frequency, and intensity of the behavior (e.g., a child who daily lines up objects for hours and is very distressed if any item is moved).

Autism spectrum disorder is not a degenerative disorder, and it is typical for learning and compensation to continue throughout life. Symptoms are often most marked in early childhood and early school years, with developmental gains typical in later childhood in at least some areas (e.g., increased interest in social interaction). A small proportion of individuals deteriorate behaviorally during adolescence, whereas most others improve. Only a minority of individuals with autism spectrum disorder live and work independently in adulthood; those who do tend to have superior language and intellectual abilities and are able to find a niche that matches their special interests and skills. In general, individuals with lower levels of impairment may be better able to function independently. However, even these individuals may remain socially naive and vulnerable, have difficulties organizing practical demands without aid, and are prone to anxiety and depression. Many adults report using compensation strategies and coping mechanisms to mask their difficulties in public but suffer from the stress and effort of maintaining a socially acceptable facade. Scarcely anything is known about old age in autism spectrum disorder.

Some individuals come for first diagnosis in adulthood, perhaps prompted by the diagnosis of autism in a child in the family or a breakdown of relations at work or home. Obtaining detailed developmental history in such cases may be difficult, and it is important to consider self-reported difficulties. Where clinical observation suggests criteria are currently met, autism spectrum disorder may be diagnosed, provided there is no evidence of good social and communication skills in childhood. For example, the report (by parents or another relative) that the individual had ordinary and sustained reciprocal friendships and good nonverbal communication skills throughout childhood would rule out a diagnosis of autism spectrum disorder; however, the absence of developmental information in itself should not do so.

Manifestations of the social and communication impairments and restricted/repetitive behaviors that define autism spectrum disorder are clear in the developmental period. In later life, intervention or compensation, as well as current supports, may mask these difficulties in at least some contexts. However, symptoms remain sufficient to cause current impairment in social, occupational, or other important areas of functioning.

Risk and Prognostic Factors

The best established prognostic factors for individual outcome within autism spectrum disorder are presence or absence of associated intellectual disability and language impairment (e.g., functional language by age 5 years is a good prognostic sign) and additional mental health problems. Epilepsy, as a comorbid diagnosis, is associated with greater intellectual disability and lower verbal ability.

Environmental.   A variety of nonspecific risk factors, such as advanced parental age, low birth weight, or fetal exposure to valproate, may contribute to risk of autism spectrum disorder.

Genetic and physiological.   Heritability estimates for autism spectrum disorder have ranged from 37% to higher than 90%, based on twin concordance rates. Currently, as many as 15% of cases of autism spectrum disorder appear to be associated with a known genetic mutation, with different de novo copy number variants or de novo mutations in specific genes associated with the disorder in different families. However, even when an autism spectrum disorder is associated with a known genetic mutation, it does not appear to be fully penetrant. Risk for the remainder of cases appears to be polygenic, with perhaps hundreds of genetic loci making relatively small contributions.

Culture-Related Diagnostic Issues

Cultural differences will exist in norms for social interaction, nonverbal communication, and relationships, but individuals with autism spectrum disorder are markedly impaired against the norms for their cultural context. Cultural and socioeconomic factors may affect age at recognition or diagnosis; for example, in the United States, late or underdiagnosis of autism spectrum disorder among African American children may occur.

Gender-Related Diagnostic Issues

Autism spectrum disorder is diagnosed four times more often in males than in females. In clinic samples, females tend to be more likely to show accompanying intellectual disability, suggesting that girls without accompanying intellectual impairments or language delays may go unrecognized, perhaps because of subtler manifestation of social and communication difficulties.

Functional Consequences of Autism Spectrum Disorder

In young children with autism spectrum disorder, lack of social and communication abilities may hamper learning, especially learning through social interaction or in settings with peers. In the home, insistence on routines and aversion to change, as well as sensory sensitivities, may interfere with eating and sleeping and make routine care (e.g., haircuts, dental work) extremely difficult. Adaptive skills are typically below measured IQ. Extreme difficulties in planning, organization, and coping with change negatively impact academic achievement, even for students with above-average intelligence. During adulthood, these individuals may have difficulties establishing independence because of continued rigidity and difficulty with novelty.

Many individuals with autism spectrum disorder, even without intellectual disability, have poor adult psychosocial functioning as indexed by measures such as independent living and gainful employment. Functional consequences in old age are unknown, but social isolation and communication problems (e.g., reduced help-seeking) are likely to have consequences for health in older adulthood.

Differential Diagnosis

Rett syndrome.   Disruption of social interaction may be observed during the regressive phase of Rett syndrome (typically between 1–4 years of age); thus, a substantial proportion of affected young girls may have a presentation that meets diagnostic criteria for autism spectrum disorder. However, after this period, most individuals with Rett syndrome improve their social communication skills, and autistic features are no longer a major area of concern. Consequently, autism spectrum disorder should be considered only when all diagnostic criteria are met.

Selective mutism.   In selective mutism, early development is not typically disturbed. The affected child usually exhibits appropriate communication skills in certain contexts and settings. Even in settings where the child is mute, social reciprocity is not impaired, nor are restricted or repetitive patterns of behavior present.

Language disorders and social (pragmatic) communication disorder.   In some forms of language disorder, there may be problems of communication and some secondary social difficulties. However, specific language disorder is not usually associated with abnormal nonverbal communication, nor with the presence of restricted, repetitive patterns of behavior, interests, or activities.

When an individual shows impairment in social communication and social interactions but does not show restricted and repetitive behavior or interests, criteria for social (pragmatic) communication disorder, instead of autism spectrum disorder, may be met. The diagnosis of autism spectrum disorder supersedes that of social (pragmatic) communication disorder whenever the criteria for autism spectrum disorder are met, and care should be taken to enquire carefully regarding past or current restricted/repetitive behavior.

Intellectual disability (intellectual developmental disorder) without autism spectrum disorder.   Intellectual disability without autism spectrum disorder may be difficult to differentiate from autism spectrum disorder in very young children. Individuals with intellectual disability who have not developed language or symbolic skills also present a challenge for differential diagnosis, since repetitive behavior often occurs in such individuals as well. A diagnosis of autism spectrum disorder in an individual with intellectual disability is appropriate when social communication and interaction are significantly impaired relative to the developmental level of the individual's nonverbal skills (e.g., fine motor skills, nonverbal problem solving). In contrast, intellectual disability is the appropriate diagnosis when there is no apparent discrepancy between the level of social-communicative skills and other intellectual skills.

Stereotypic movement disorder.   Motor stereotypies are among the diagnostic characteristics of autism spectrum disorder, so an additional diagnosis of stereotypic movement disorder is not given when such repetitive behaviors are better explained by the presence of autism spectrum disorder. However, when stereotypies cause self-injury and become a focus of treatment, both diagnoses may be appropriate.

Attention-deficit/hyperactivity disorder.   Abnormalities of attention (overly focused or easily distracted) are common in individuals with autism spectrum disorder, as is hyperactivity. A diagnosis of attention-deficit/hyperactivity disorder (ADHD) should be considered when attentional difficulties or hyperactivity exceeds that typically seen in individuals of comparable mental age.

Schizophrenia.   Schizophrenia with childhood onset usually develops after a period of normal, or near normal, development. A prodromal state has been described in which social impairment and atypical interests and beliefs occur, which could be confused with the social deficits seen in autism spectrum disorder. Hallucinations and delusions, which are defining features of schizophrenia, are not features of autism spectrum disorder. However, clinicians must take into account the potential for individuals with autism spectrum disorder to be concrete in their interpretation of questions regarding the key features of schizophrenia (e.g., "Do you hear voices when no one is there?" "Yes [on the radio]").

Comorbidity

Autism spectrum disorder is frequently associated with intellectual impairment and structural language disorder (i.e., an inability to comprehend and construct sentences with proper grammar), which should be noted under the relevant specifiers when applicable. Many individuals with autism spectrum disorder have psychiatric symptoms that do not form part of the diagnostic criteria for the disorder (about 70% of individuals with autism spectrum disorder may have one comorbid mental disorder, and 40% may have two or more comorbid mental disorders). When criteria for both ADHD and autism spectrum disorder are met, both diagnoses should be given. This same principle applies to concurrent diagnoses of autism spectrum disorder and developmental coordination disorder, anxiety disorders, depressive disorders, and other comorbid diagnoses. Among individuals who are nonverbal or have language deficits, observable signs such as changes in sleep or eating and increases in challenging behavior should trigger an evaluation for anxiety or depression. Specific learning difficulties (literacy and numeracy) are common, as is developmental coordination disorder. Medical conditions commonly associated with autism spectrum disorder should be noted under the "associated with a known medical or genetic condition or environmental factor" specifier. Such medical conditions include epilepsy, sleep problems, and constipation. Avoidant/restrictive food intake disorder is a fairly frequent presenting feature of autism spectrum disorder, and extreme and narrow food preferences may persist.

Attention-Deficit/Hyperactivity Disorder

Attention-Deficit/Hyperactivity Disorder

Diagnostic Criteria

A. A persistent pattern of inattention and/or hyperactivity-impulsivity that interferes with functioning or development, as characterized by (1) and/or (2):

1. **Inattention:** Six (or more) of the following symptoms have persisted for at least 6 months to a degree that is inconsistent with developmental level and that negatively impacts directly on social and academic/occupational activities:
   Note: The symptoms are not solely a manifestation of oppositional behavior, defiance, hostility, or failure to understand tasks or instructions. For older adolescents and adults (age 17 and older), at least five symptoms are required.

   a. Often fails to give close attention to details or makes careless mistakes in schoolwork, at work, or during other activities (e.g., overlooks or misses details, work is inaccurate).

   b. Often has difficulty sustaining attention in tasks or play activities (e.g., has difficulty remaining focused during lectures, conversations, or lengthy reading).

   c. Often does not seem to listen when spoken to directly (e.g., mind seems elsewhere, even in the absence of any obvious distraction).

   d. Often does not follow through on instructions and fails to finish schoolwork, chores, or duties in the workplace (e.g., starts tasks but quickly loses focus and is easily sidetracked).

   e. Often has difficulty organizing tasks and activities (e.g., difficulty managing sequential tasks; difficulty keeping materials and belongings in order; messy, disorganized work; has poor time management; fails to meet deadlines).

   f. Often avoids, dislikes, or is reluctant to engage in tasks that require sustained mental effort (e.g., schoolwork or homework; for older adolescents and adults, preparing reports, completing forms, reviewing lengthy papers).

   g. Often loses things necessary for tasks or activities (e.g., school materials, pencils, books, tools, wallets, keys, paperwork, eyeglasses, mobile telephones).

   h. Is often easily distracted by extraneous stimuli (for older adolescents and adults, may include unrelated thoughts).

   i. Is often forgetful in daily activities (e.g., doing chores, running errands; for older adolescents and adults, returning calls, paying bills, keeping appointments).

2. **Hyperactivity and impulsivity:** Six (or more) of the following symptoms have persisted for at least 6 months to a degree that is inconsistent with developmental level and that negatively impacts directly on social and academic/occupational activities:
    Note: The symptoms are not solely a manifestation of oppositional behavior, defiance, hostility, or a failure to understand tasks or instructions. For older adolescents and adults (age 17 and older), at least five symptoms are required.

    a. Often fidgets with or taps hands or feet or squirms in seat.
    b. Often leaves seat in situations when remaining seated is expected (e.g., leaves his or her place in the classroom, in the office or other workplace, or in other situations that require remaining in place).
    c. Often runs about or climbs in situations where it is inappropriate. (**Note:** In adolescents or adults, may be limited to feeling restless.)
    d. Often unable to play or engage in leisure activities quietly.
    e. Is often "on the go," acting as if "driven by a motor" (e.g., is unable to be or uncomfortable being still for extended time, as in restaurants, meetings; may be experienced by others as being restless or difficult to keep up with).
    f. Often talks excessively.
    g. Often blurts out an answer before a question has been completed (e.g., completes people's sentences; cannot wait for turn in conversation).
    h. Often has difficulty waiting his or her turn (e.g., while waiting in line).
    i. Often interrupts or intrudes on others (e.g., butts into conversations, games, or activities; may start using other people's things without asking or receiving permission; for adolescents and adults, may intrude into or take over what others are doing).

B. Several inattentive or hyperactive-impulsive symptoms were present prior to age 12 years.
C. Several inattentive or hyperactive-impulsive symptoms are present in two or more settings (e.g., at home, school, or work; with friends or relatives; in other activities).
D. There is clear evidence that the symptoms interfere with, or reduce the quality of, social, academic, or occupational functioning.
E. The symptoms do not occur exclusively during the course of schizophrenia or another psychotic disorder and are not better explained by another mental disorder (e.g., mood disorder, anxiety disorder, dissociative disorder, personality disorder, substance intoxication or withdrawal).

Specify whether:

314.01 (F90.2) Combined presentation: If both Criterion A1 (inattention) and Criterion A2 (hyperactivity-impulsivity) are met for the past 6 months.

314.00 (F90.0) Predominantly inattentive presentation: If Criterion A1 (inattention) is met but Criterion A2 (hyperactivity-impulsivity) is not met for the past 6 months.

314.01 (F90.1) Predominantly hyperactive/impulsive presentation: If Criterion A2 (hyperactivity-impulsivity) is met and Criterion A1 (inattention) is not met for the past 6 months.

Specify if:

In partial remission: When full criteria were previously met, fewer than the full criteria have been met for the past 6 months, and the symptoms still result in impairment in social, academic, or occupational functioning.

Specify current severity:

Mild: Few, if any, symptoms in excess of those required to make the diagnosis are present, and symptoms result in no more than minor impairments in social or occupational functioning.

Moderate: Symptoms or functional impairment between "mild" and "severe" are present.

Severe: Many symptoms in excess of those required to make the diagnosis, or several symptoms that are particularly severe, are present, or the symptoms result in marked impairment in social or occupational functioning.

Diagnostic Features

The essential feature of attention-deficit/hyperactivity disorder (ADHD) is a persistent pattern of inattention and/or hyperactivity-impulsivity that interferes with functioning or development. *Inattention* manifests behaviorally in ADHD as wandering off task, lacking persistence, having difficulty sustaining focus, and being disorganized and is not due to defiance or lack of comprehension. *Hyperactivity* refers to excessive motor activity (such as a child running about) when it is not appropriate, or excessive fidgeting, tapping, or talkativeness. In adults, hyperactivity may manifest as extreme restlessness or wearing others out with their activity. *Impulsivity* refers to hasty actions that occur in the moment without forethought and that have high potential for harm to the individual (e.g., darting into the street without looking). Impulsivity may reflect a desire for immediate rewards or an inability to delay gratification. Impulsive behaviors may manifest as social intrusiveness (e.g., interrupting others excessively) and/or as making important decisions without consideration of long-term consequences (e.g., taking a job without adequate information).

ADHD begins in childhood. The requirement that several symptoms be present before age 12 years conveys the importance of a substantial clinical presentation during childhood. At the same time, an earlier age at onset is not specified because of difficulties in establishing precise childhood onset retrospectively. Adult recall of childhood symptoms tends to be unreliable, and it is beneficial to obtain ancillary information.

Manifestations of the disorder must be present in more than one setting (e.g., home and school, work). Confirmation of substantial symptoms across settings typically cannot be done accurately without consulting informants who have seen the individual in those settings. Typically, symptoms vary depending on context within a given setting. Signs of the disorder may be minimal or absent when the individual is receiving frequent rewards for appropriate behavior, is under close supervision, is in a novel setting, is engaged in especially interesting activities, has consistent external stimulation (e.g., via electronic screens), or is interacting in one-on-one situations (e.g., the clinician's office).

Associated Features Supporting Diagnosis

Mild delays in language, motor, or social development are not specific to ADHD but often co-occur. Associated features may include low frustration tolerance, irritability, or mood lability. Even in the absence of a specific learning disorder, academic or work performance is often impaired. Inattentive behavior is associated with various underlying cognitive processes, and individuals with ADHD may exhibit cognitive problems on tests of attention, executive function, or memory, although these tests are not sufficiently sensitive or specific to serve as diagnostic indices. By early adulthood, ADHD is associated with an increased risk of suicide attempt, primarily when comorbid with mood, conduct, or substance use disorders.

No biological marker is diagnostic for ADHD. As a group, compared with peers, children with ADHD display increased slow wave electroencephalograms, reduced total brain volume on magnetic resonance imaging, and possibly a delay in posterior to anterior cortical maturation, but these findings are not diagnostic. In the uncommon cases where there is a known genetic cause (e.g., fragile X syndrome, 22q11 deletion syndrome), the ADHD presentation should still be diagnosed.

Prevalence

Population surveys suggest that ADHD occurs in most cultures in about 5% of children and about 2.5% of adults.

Development and Course

Many parents first observe excessive motor activity when the child is a toddler, but symptoms are difficult to distinguish from highly variable normative behaviors before age 4 years. ADHD is most often identified during elementary school years, and inattention becomes more prominent and impairing. The disorder is relatively stable through early adolescence, but some individuals have a worsened course with development of antisocial behaviors. In most individuals with ADHD, symptoms of motoric hyperactivity become less obvious in adolescence and adulthood, but difficulties with restlessness, inattention, poor planning, and impulsivity persist. A substantial proportion of children with ADHD remain relatively impaired into adulthood.

In preschool, the main manifestation is hyperactivity. Inattention becomes more prominent during elementary school. During adolescence, signs of hyperactivity (e.g., running and climbing) are less common and may be confined to fidgetiness or an inner feeling of jitteriness, restlessness, or impatience. In adulthood, along with inattention and restlessness, impulsivity may remain problematic even when hyperactivity has diminished.

Risk and Prognostic Factors

Temperamental.   ADHD is associated with reduced behavioral inhibition, effortful control, or constraint; negative emotionality; and/or elevated novelty seeking. These traits may predispose some children to ADHD but are not specific to the disorder.

Environmental.   Very low birth weight (less than 1,500 grams) conveys a two- to threefold risk for ADHD, but most children with low birth weight do not develop ADHD. Although ADHD is correlated with smoking during pregnancy, some of this association reflects common genetic risk. A minority of cases may be related to reactions to aspects of diet. There may be a history of child abuse, neglect, multiple foster placements, neurotoxin exposure (e.g., lead), infections (e.g., encephalitis), or alcohol exposure in utero. Exposure to environmental toxicants has been correlated with subsequent ADHD, but it is not known whether these associations are causal.

Genetic and physiological.   ADHD is elevated in the first-degree biological relatives of individuals with ADHD. The heritability of ADHD is substantial. While specific genes have been correlated with ADHD, they are neither necessary nor sufficient causal factors. Visual and hearing impairments, metabolic abnormalities, sleep disorders, nutritional deficiencies, and epilepsy should be considered as possible influences on ADHD symptoms.

ADHD is not associated with specific physical features, although rates of minor physical anomalies (e.g., hypertelorism, highly arched palate, low-set ears) may be relatively elevated. Subtle motor delays and other neurological soft signs may occur. (Note that marked co-occurring clumsiness and motor delays should be coded separately [e.g., developmental coordination disorder].)

Course modifiers.   Family interaction patterns in early childhood are unlikely to cause ADHD but may influence its course or contribute to secondary development of conduct problems.

Culture-Related Diagnostic Issues

Differences in ADHD prevalence rates across regions appear attributable mainly to different diagnostic and methodological practices. However, there also may be cultural variation in attitudes toward or interpretations of children's behaviors. Clinical identification rates in the United States for African American and Latino populations tend to be lower than for Caucasian populations. Informant symptom ratings may be influenced by cultural group of the child and the informant, suggesting that culturally appropriate practices are relevant in assessing ADHD.

Gender-Related Diagnostic Issues

ADHD is more frequent in males than in females in the general population, with a ratio of approximately 2:1 in children and 1.6:1 in adults. Females are more likely than males to present primarily with inattentive features.

Functional Consequences of Attention-Deficit/Hyperactivity Disorder

ADHD is associated with reduced school performance and academic attainment, social rejection, and, in adults, poorer occupational performance, attainment, attendance, and higher probability of unemployment as well as elevated interpersonal conflict. Children with ADHD are significantly more likely than their peers without ADHD to develop conduct disorder in adolescence and antisocial personality disorder in adulthood, consequently increasing the likelihood for substance use disorders and incarceration. The risk of subsequent substance use disorders is elevated, especially when conduct disorder or antisocial personality disorder develops. Individuals with ADHD are more likely than peers to be injured. Traffic accidents and violations are more frequent in drivers with ADHD. There may be an elevated likelihood of obesity among individuals with ADHD.

Inadequate or variable self-application to tasks that require sustained effort is often interpreted by others as laziness, irresponsibility, or failure to cooperate. Family relationships may be characterized by discord and negative interactions. Peer relationships are often disrupted by peer rejection, neglect, or teasing of the individual with ADHD. On average, individuals with ADHD obtain less schooling, have poorer vocational achievement, and have reduced intellectual scores than their peers, although there is great variability. In its severe form, the disorder is markedly impairing, affecting social, familial, and scholastic/occupational adjustment.

Academic deficits, school-related problems, and peer neglect tend to be most associated with elevated symptoms of inattention, whereas peer rejection and, to a lesser extent, accidental injury are most salient with marked symptoms of hyperactivity or impulsivity.

Differential Diagnosis

Oppositional defiant disorder. Individuals with oppositional defiant disorder may resist work or school tasks that require self-application because they resist conforming to others' demands. Their behavior is characterized by negativity, hostility, and defiance. These symptoms must be differentiated from aversion to school or mentally demanding tasks due to difficulty in sustaining mental effort, forgetting instructions, and impulsivity in individuals with ADHD. Complicating the differential diagnosis is the fact that some individuals with ADHD may develop secondary oppositional attitudes toward such tasks and devalue their importance.

Intermittent explosive disorder. ADHD and intermittent explosive disorder share high levels of impulsive behavior. However, individuals with intermittent explosive disorder show serious aggression toward others, which is not characteristic of ADHD, and they do not experience problems with sustaining attention as seen in ADHD. In addition, intermittent explosive disorder is rare in childhood. Intermittent explosive disorder may be diagnosed in the presence of ADHD.

Other neurodevelopmental disorders. The increased motoric activity that may occur in ADHD must be distinguished from the repetitive motor behavior that characterizes stereotypic movement disorder and some cases of autism spectrum disorder. In stereotypic movement disorder, the motoric behavior is generally fixed and repetitive (e.g., body rocking, self-biting), whereas the fidgetiness and restlessness in ADHD are typically generalized and not characterized by repetitive stereotypic movements. In Tourette's disorder, frequent multiple tics can be mistaken for the generalized fidgetiness of ADHD. Prolonged observation may be needed to differentiate fidgetiness from bouts of multiple tics.

Specific learning disorder.   Children with specific learning disorder may appear inattentive because of frustration, lack of interest, or limited ability. However, inattention in individuals with a specific learning disorder who do not have ADHD is not impairing outside of academic work.

Intellectual disability (intellectual developmental disorder).   Symptoms of ADHD are common among children placed in academic settings that are inappropriate to their intellectual ability. In such cases, the symptoms are not evident during non-academic tasks. A diagnosis of ADHD in intellectual disability requires that inattention or hyperactivity be excessive for mental age.

Autism spectrum disorder.   Individuals with ADHD and those with autism spectrum disorder exhibit inattention, social dysfunction, and difficult-to-manage behavior. The social dysfunction and peer rejection seen in individuals with ADHD must be distinguished from the social disengagement, isolation, and indifference to facial and tonal communication cues seen in individuals with autism spectrum disorder. Children with autism spectrum disorder may display tantrums because of an inability to tolerate a change from their expected course of events. In contrast, children with ADHD may misbehave or have a tantrum during a major transition because of impulsivity or poor self-control.

Reactive attachment disorder.   Children with reactive attachment disorder may show social disinhibition, but not the full ADHD symptom cluster, and display other features such as a lack of enduring relationships that are not characteristic of ADHD.

Anxiety disorders.   ADHD shares symptoms of inattention with anxiety disorders. Individuals with ADHD are inattentive because of their attraction to external stimuli, new activities, or preoccupation with enjoyable activities. This is distinguished from the inattention due to worry and rumination seen in anxiety disorders. Restlessness might be seen in anxiety disorders. However, in ADHD, the symptom is not associated with worry and rumination.

Depressive disorders.   Individuals with depressive disorders may present with inability to concentrate. However, poor concentration in mood disorders becomes prominent only during a depressive episode.

Bipolar disorder.   Individuals with bipolar disorder may have increased activity, poor concentration, and increased impulsivity, but these features are episodic, occurring several days at a time. In bipolar disorder, increased impulsivity or inattention is accompanied by elevated mood, grandiosity, and other specific bipolar features. Children with ADHD may show significant changes in mood within the same day; such lability is distinct from a manic episode, which must last 4 or more days to be a clinical indicator of bipolar disorder, even in children. Bipolar disorder is rare in preadolescents, even when severe irritability and anger are prominent, whereas ADHD is common among children and adolescents who display excessive anger and irritability.

Disruptive mood dysregulation disorder.   Disruptive mood dysregulation disorder is characterized by pervasive irritability, and intolerance of frustration, but impulsiveness and disorganized attention are not essential features. However, most children and adolescents with the disorder have symptoms that also meet criteria for ADHD, which is diagnosed separately.

Substance use disorders.   Differentiating ADHD from substance use disorders may be problematic if the first presentation of ADHD symptoms follows the onset of abuse or frequent use. Clear evidence of ADHD before substance misuse from informants or previous records may be essential for differential diagnosis.

Personality disorders. In adolescents and adults, it may be difficult to distinguish ADHD from borderline, narcissistic, and other personality disorders. All these disorders tend to share the features of disorganization, social intrusiveness, emotional dysregulation, and cognitive dysregulation. However, ADHD is not characterized by fear of abandonment, self-injury, extreme ambivalence, or other features of personality disorder. It may take extended clinical observation, informant interview, or detailed history to distinguish impulsive, socially intrusive, or inappropriate behavior from narcissistic, aggressive, or domineering behavior to make this differential diagnosis.

Psychotic disorders. ADHD is not diagnosed if the symptoms of inattention and hyperactivity occur exclusively during the course of a psychotic disorder.

Medication-induced symptoms of ADHD. Symptoms of inattention, hyperactivity, or impulsivity attributable to the use of medication (e.g., bronchodilators, isoniazid, neuroleptics [resulting in akathisia], thyroid replacement medication) are diagnosed as other specified or unspecified other (or unknown) substance–related disorders.

Neurocognitive disorders. Early major neurocognitive disorder (dementia) and/or mild neurocognitive disorder are not known to be associated with ADHD but may present with similar clinical features. These conditions are distinguished from ADHD by their late onset.

Comorbidity

In clinical settings, comorbid disorders are frequent in individuals whose symptoms meet criteria for ADHD. In the general population, oppositional defiant disorder co-occurs with ADHD in approximately half of children with the combined presentation and about a quarter with the predominantly inattentive presentation. Conduct disorder co-occurs in about a quarter of children or adolescents with the combined presentation, depending on age and setting. Most children and adolescents with disruptive mood dysregulation disorder have symptoms that also meet criteria for ADHD; a lesser percentage of children with ADHD have symptoms that meet criteria for disruptive mood dysregulation disorder. Specific learning disorder commonly co-occurs with ADHD. Anxiety disorders and major depressive disorder occur in a minority of individuals with ADHD but more often than in the general population. Intermittent explosive disorder occurs in a minority of adults with ADHD, but at rates above population levels. Although substance use disorders are relatively more frequent among adults with ADHD in the general population, the disorders are present in only a minority of adults with ADHD. In adults, antisocial and other personality disorders may co-occur with ADHD. Other disorders that may co-occur with ADHD include obsessive-compulsive disorder, tic disorders, and autism spectrum disorder.

Other Specified Attention-Deficit/ Hyperactivity Disorder

314.01 (F90.8)

This category applies to presentations in which symptoms characteristic of attention-deficit/hyperactivity disorder that cause clinically significant distress or impairment in social, occupational or other important areas of functioning predominate but do not meet the full criteria for attention-deficit/hyperactivity disorder or any of the disorders in the neurodevelopmental disorders diagnostic class. The other specified attention-deficit/hyperactivity disorder category is used in situations in which the clinician chooses to communicate the specific reason that the presentation does not meet the criteria for attention-deficit/ hyperactivity disorder or any specific neurodevelopmental disorder. This is done by recording "other specified attention-deficit/hyperactivity disorder" followed by the specific reason (e.g., "with insufficient inattention symptoms").

Unspecified Attention-Deficit/ Hyperactivity Disorder

314.01 (F90.9)

This category applies to presentations in which symptoms characteristic of attention-deficit/hyperactivity disorder that cause clinically significant distress or impairment in social, occupational, or other important areas of functioning predominate but do not meet the full criteria for attention-deficit/hyperactivity disorder or any of the disorders in the neurodevelopmental disorders diagnostic class. The unspecified attention-deficit/hyperactivity disorder category is used in situations in which the clinician chooses *not* to specify the reason that the criteria are not met for attention-deficit/hyperactivity disorder or for a specific neurodevelopmental disorder, and includes presentations in which there is insufficient information to make a more specific diagnosis.

Specific Learning Disorder

Specific Learning Disorder

Diagnostic Criteria

A. Difficulties learning and using academic skills, as indicated by the presence of at least one of the following symptoms that have persisted for at least 6 months, despite the provision of interventions that target those difficulties:

1. Inaccurate or slow and effortful word reading (e.g., reads single words aloud incorrectly or slowly and hesitantly, frequently guesses words, has difficulty sounding out words).
2. Difficulty understanding the meaning of what is read (e.g., may read text accurately but not understand the sequence, relationships, inferences, or deeper meanings of what is read).
3. Difficulties with spelling (e.g., may add, omit, or substitute vowels or consonants).
4. Difficulties with written expression (e.g., makes multiple grammatical or punctuation errors within sentences; employs poor paragraph organization; written expression of ideas lacks clarity).
5. Difficulties mastering number sense, number facts, or calculation (e.g., has poor understanding of numbers, their magnitude, and relationships; counts on fingers to add single-digit numbers instead of recalling the math fact as peers do; gets lost in the midst of arithmetic computation and may switch procedures).
6. Difficulties with mathematical reasoning (e.g., has severe difficulty applying mathematical concepts, facts, or procedures to solve quantitative problems).

B. The affected academic skills are substantially and quantifiably below those expected for the individual's chronological age, and cause significant interference with academic or occupational performance, or with activities of daily living, as confirmed by individually administered standardized achievement measures and comprehensive clinical assessment. For individuals age 17 years and older, a documented history of impairing learning difficulties may be substituted for the standardized assessment.

C. The learning difficulties begin during school-age years but may not become fully manifest until the demands for those affected academic skills exceed the individual's limited capacities (e.g., as in timed tests, reading or writing lengthy complex reports for a tight deadline, excessively heavy academic loads).

D. The learning difficulties are not better accounted for by intellectual disabilities, uncorrected visual or auditory acuity, other mental or neurological disorders, psychosocial adversity, lack of proficiency in the language of academic instruction, or inadequate educational instruction.

Note: The four diagnostic criteria are to be met based on a clinical synthesis of the individual's history (developmental, medical, family, educational), school reports, and psychoeducational assessment.

Coding note: Specify all academic domains and subskills that are impaired. When more than one domain is impaired, each one should be coded individually according to the following specifiers.

Specify if:

315.00 (F81.0) With impairment in reading:

Word reading accuracy

Reading rate or fluency

Reading comprehension

Note: *Dyslexia* is an alternative term used to refer to a pattern of learning difficulties characterized by problems with accurate or fluent word recognition, poor decoding, and poor spelling abilities. If dyslexia is used to specify this particular pattern of difficulties, it is important also to specify any additional difficulties that are present, such as difficulties with reading comprehension or math reasoning.

315.2 (F81.81) With impairment in written expression:

Spelling accuracy

Grammar and punctuation accuracy

Clarity or organization of written expression

315.1 (F81.2) With impairment in mathematics:

Number sense

Memorization of arithmetic facts

Accurate or fluent calculation

Accurate math reasoning

Note: *Dyscalculia* is an alternative term used to refer to a pattern of difficulties characterized by problems processing numerical information, learning arithmetic facts, and performing accurate or fluent calculations. If dyscalculia is used to specify this particular pattern of mathematic difficulties, it is important also to specify any additional difficulties that are present, such as difficulties with math reasoning or word reasoning accuracy.

Specify current severity:

Mild: Some difficulties learning skills in one or two academic domains, but of mild enough severity that the individual may be able to compensate or function well when provided with appropriate accommodations or support services, especially during the school years.

Moderate: Marked difficulties learning skills in one or more academic domains, so that the individual is unlikely to become proficient without some intervals of intensive and specialized teaching during the school years. Some accommodations or supportive services at least part of the day at school, in the workplace, or at home may be needed to complete activities accurately and efficiently.

Severe: Severe difficulties learning skills, affecting several academic domains, so that the individual is unlikely to learn those skills without ongoing intensive individualized and specialized teaching for most of the school years. Even with an array of appropriate accommodations or services at home, at school, or in the workplace, the individual may not be able to complete all activities efficiently.

Recording Procedures

Each impaired academic domain and subskill of specific learning disorder should be recorded. Because of ICD coding requirements, impairments in reading, impairments in written expression, and impairments in mathematics, with their corresponding impairments in subskills, must be coded separately. For example, impairments in reading and mathematics and impairments in the subskills of reading rate or fluency, reading comprehension, accurate or fluent calculation, and accurate math reasoning would be coded and recorded as 315.00 (F81.0) specific learning disorder with impairment in reading, with impairment in reading rate or fluency and impairment in reading comprehension; 315.1 (F81.2) specific learning disorder with impairment in mathematics, with impairment in accurate or fluent calculation and impairment in accurate math reasoning.

Diagnostic Features

Specific learning disorder is a neurodevelopmental disorder with a biological origin that is the basis for abnormalities at a cognitive level that are associated with the behavioral signs of the disorder. The biological origin includes an interaction of genetic, epigenetic, and environmental factors, which affect the brain's ability to perceive or process verbal or nonverbal information efficiently and accurately.

One essential feature of specific learning disorder is persistent difficulties learning keystone academic skills (Criterion A), with onset during the years of formal schooling (i.e., the developmental period). Key academic skills include reading of single words accurately and fluently, reading comprehension, written expression and spelling, arithmetic calculation, and mathematical reasoning (solving mathematical problems). In contrast to talking or walking, which are acquired developmental milestones that emerge with brain maturation, academic skills (e.g., reading, spelling, writing, mathematics) have to be taught and learned explicitly. Specific learning disorder disrupts the normal pattern of learning academic skills; it is not simply a consequence of lack of opportunity of learning or inadequate instruction. Difficulties mastering these key academic skills may also impede learning in other academic subjects (e.g., history, science, social studies), but those problems are attributable to difficulties learning the underlying academic skills. Difficulties learning to map letters with the sounds of one's language—to read printed words (often called *dyslexia*)—is one of the most common manifestations of specific learning disorder. The learning difficulties manifest as a range of observable, descriptive behaviors or symptoms (as listed in Criteria A1–A6). These clinical symptoms may be observed, probed by means of the clinical interview, or ascertained from school reports, rating scales, or descriptions in previous educational or psychological assessments. The learning difficulties are persistent, not transitory. In children and adolescents, *persistence* is defined as restricted progress in learning (i.e., no evidence that the individual is catching up with classmates) for at least 6 months despite the provision of extra help at home or school. For example, difficulties learning to read single words that do not fully or rapidly remit with the provision of instruction in phonological skills or word identification strategies may indicate a specific learning disorder. Evidence of persistent learning difficulties may be derived from cumulative school reports, portfolios of the child's evaluated work, curriculum-based measures, or clinical interview. In adults, persistent difficulty refers to ongoing difficulties in literacy or numeracy skills that manifest during childhood or adolescence, as indicated by cumulative evidence from school reports, evaluated portfolios of work, or previous assessments.

A second key feature is that the individual's performance of the affected academic skills is well below average for age (Criterion B). One robust clinical indicator of difficulties learning academic skills is low academic achievement for age or average achievement that is sustainable only by extraordinarily high levels of effort or support. In children, the low academic skills cause significant interference in school performance (as indicated by school reports and teacher's grades or ratings). Another clinical indicator, particularly in adults, is avoidance of activities that require the academic skills. Also in adulthood, low academic skills interfere with occupational performance or everyday activities requiring those skills (as indicated by self-report or report by others). However, this criterion also requires psychometric evidence from an individually administered, psychometrically sound and culturally appropriate test of academic achievement that is norm-referenced or criterion-referenced. Academic skills are distributed along a continuum, so there is no natural cutpoint that can be used to differentiate individuals with and without specific learning disorder. Thus, any threshold used to specify what constitutes significantly low academic achievement (e.g., academic skills well below age expectation) is to a large extent arbitrary. Low achievement scores on one or more standardized tests or subtests within an academic domain (i.e., at least 1.5 standard deviations [SD] below the population mean for age, which translates to a standard score of 78 or less, which is below the 7th percentile) are needed for the greatest diagnostic certainty. However, precise scores will vary according to the particular standardized tests that are used. On the basis of clinical judgment, a more lenient threshold may be used (e.g., 1.0–2.5 SD below the population mean for age), when learning difficulties are supported by converging evidence from clinical assessment, academic history, school reports, or test scores. Moreover, since standardized tests are not available in all languages, the diagnosis may then be based in part on clinical judgment of scores on available test measures.

A third core feature is that the learning difficulties are readily apparent in the early school years in most individuals (Criterion C). However, in others, the learning difficulties may not manifest fully until later school years, by which time learning demands have increased and exceed the individual's limited capacities.

Another key diagnostic feature is that the learning difficulties are considered "specific," for four reasons. First, they are not attributable to intellectual disabilities (intellectual disability [intellectual developmental disorder]); global developmental delay; hearing or vision disorders, or neurological or motor disorders) (Criterion D). Specific learning disorder affects learning in individuals who otherwise demonstrate normal levels of intellectual functioning (generally estimated by an IQ score of greater than about 70 [±5 points allowing for measurement error]). The phrase "unexpected academic underachievement" is often cited as the defining characteristic of specific learning disorder in that the specific learning disabilities are not part of a more general learning difficulty as manifested in intellectual disability or global developmental delay. Specific learning disorder may also occur in individuals identified as intellectually "gifted." These individuals may be able to sustain apparently adequate academic functioning by using compensatory strategies, extraordinarily high effort, or support, until the learning demands or assessment procedures (e.g., timed tests) pose barriers to their demonstrating their learning or accomplishing required tasks. Second, the learning difficulty cannot be attributed to more general external factors, such as economic or environmental disadvantage, chronic absenteeism, or lack of education as typically provided in the individual's community context. Third, the learning difficulty cannot be attributed to a neurological (e.g., pediatric stroke) or motor disorders or to vision or hearing disorders, which are often associated with problems learning academic skills but are distinguishable by presence of neurological signs.

Finally, the learning difficulty may be restricted to one academic skill or domain (e.g., reading single words, retrieving or calculating number facts).

Comprehensive assessment is required. Specific learning disorder can only be diagnosed after formal education starts but can be diagnosed at any point afterward in children, adolescents, or adults, providing there is evidence of onset during the years of formal schooling (i.e., the developmental period). No single data source is sufficient for a diagnosis of specific learning disorder. Rather, specific learning disorder is a clinical diagnosis based on a synthesis of the individual's medical, developmental, educational, and family history; the history of the learning difficulty, including its previous and current manifestation; the impact of the difficulty on academic, occupational, or social functioning; previous or current school reports; portfolios of work requiring academic skills; curriculum-based assessments; and previous or current scores from individual standardized tests of academic achievement. If an intellectual, sensory, neurological, or motor disorder is suspected, then the clinical assessment for specific learning disorder should also include methods appropriate for these disorders. Thus, comprehensive assessment will involve professionals with expertise in specific learning disorder and psychological/cognitive assessment. Since specific learning disorder typically persists into adulthood, reassessment is rarely necessary, unless indicated by marked changes in the learning difficulties (amelioration or worsening) or requested for specific purposes.

Associated Features Supporting Diagnosis

Specific learning disorder is frequently but not invariably preceded, in preschool years, by delays in attention, language, or motor skills that may persist and co-occur with specific learning disorder. An uneven profile of abilities is common, such as above-average abilities in drawing, design, and other visuospatial abilities, but slow, effortful, and inaccurate reading and poor reading comprehension and written expression. Individuals with specific learning disorder typically (but not invariably) exhibit poor performance on psychological tests of cognitive processing. However, it remains unclear whether these cognitive abnormalities are the cause, correlate, or consequence of the learning difficulties. Also, although cognitive deficits associated with difficulties learning to read words are well documented, those associated with other manifestations of specific learning disorder (e.g., reading comprehension, arithmetic computation, written expression) are underspecified or unknown. Moreover, individuals with similar behavioral symptoms or test scores are found to have a variety of cognitive deficits, and many of these processing deficits are also found in other neurodevelopmental disorders (e.g., attention-deficit/hyperactivity disorder [ADHD], autistic spectrum disorder, communication disorders, developmental coordination disorder). Thus, assessment of cognitive processing deficits is not required for diagnostic assessment. Specific learning disorder is associated with increased risk for suicidal ideation and suicide attempts in children, adolescents, and adults.

There are no known biological markers of specific learning disorder. As a group, individuals with the disorder show circumscribed alterations in cognitive processing and brain structure and function. Genetic differences are also evident at the group level. But cognitive testing, neuroimaging, or genetic testing are not useful for diagnosis at this time.

Prevalence

The prevalence of specific learning disorder across the academic domains of reading, writing, and mathematics is 5%–15% among school-age children across different languages and cultures. Prevalence in adults is unknown but appears to be approximately 4%.

Development and Course

Onset, recognition, and diagnosis of specific learning disorder usually occurs during the elementary school years when children are required to learn to read, spell, write, and learn mathematics. However, precursors such as language delays or deficits, difficulties in rhyming or counting, or difficulties with fine motor skills required for writing commonly occur in early childhood before the start of formal schooling. Manifestations may be behavioral (e.g., a reluctance to engage in learning; oppositional behavior). Specific learning disorder is lifelong, but the course and clinical expression are variable, in part depending on the interactions among the task demands of the environment, the range and severity of the individual's learning difficulties, the individual's learning abilities, comorbidity, and the available support systems and intervention. Nonetheless, problems with reading fluency and comprehension, spelling, written expression, and numeracy skills in everyday life typically persist into adulthood.

Changes in manifestation of symptoms occur with age, so that an individual may have a persistent or shifting array of learning difficulties across the lifespan.

Examples of symptoms that may be observed among preschool-age children include a lack of interest in playing games with language sounds (e.g., repetition, rhyming), and they may have trouble learning nursery rhymes. Preschool children with specific learning disorder may frequently use baby talk, mispronounce words, and have trouble remembering names of letters, numbers, or days of the week. They may fail to recognize letters in their own names and have trouble learning to count. Kindergarten-age children with specific learning disorder may be unable to recognize and write letters, may be unable to write their own names, or may use invented spelling. They may have trouble breaking down spoken words into syllables (e.g., "cowboy" into "cow" and "boy") and trouble recognizing words that rhyme (e.g., cat, bat, hat). Kindergarten-age children also may have trouble connecting letters with their sounds (e.g., letter b makes the sound /b/) and may be unable to recognize phonemes (e.g., do not know which in a set of words [e.g., dog, man, car] starts with the same sound as "cat").

Specific learning disorder in elementary school–age children typically manifests as marked difficulty learning letter-sound correspondence (particularly in English-speaking children), fluent word decoding, spelling, or math facts; reading aloud is slow, inaccurate, and effortful, and some children struggle to understand the magnitude that a spoken or written number represents. Children in primary grades (grades 1–3) may continue to have problems recognizing and manipulating phonemes, be unable to read common one-syllable words (such as mat or top), and be unable recognize common irregularly spelled words (e.g., said, two). They may commit reading errors that indicate problems in connecting sounds and letters (e.g., "big" for "got") and have difficulty sequencing numbers and letters. Children in grades 1-3 also may have difficulty remembering number facts or arithmetic procedures for adding, subtracting, and so forth, and may complain that reading or arithmetic is hard and avoid doing it. Children with specific learning disorder in the middle grades (grades 4–6) may mispronounce or skip parts of long, multisyllable words (e.g., say "conible" for "convertible," "aminal" for "animal") and confuse words that sound alike (e.g., "tornado" for "volcano"). They may have trouble remembering dates, names, and telephone numbers and may have trouble completing homework or tests on time. Children in the middle grades also may have poor comprehension with or without slow, effortful, and inaccurate reading, and they may have trouble reading small function words (e.g., that, the, an, in). They may have very poor spelling and poor written work. They may get the first part of a word correctly, then guess wildly (e.g., read "clover" as "clock"), and may express fear of reading aloud or refuse to read aloud.

By contrast, adolescents may have mastered word decoding, but reading remains slow and effortful, and they are likely to show marked problems in reading comprehension and written expression (including poor spelling) and poor mastery of math facts or mathematical problem solving. During adolescence and into adulthood, individuals with specific learning disorder may continue to make numerous spelling mistakes and read single words and connected text slowly and with much effort, with trouble pronouncing multisyllable words. They may frequently need to reread material to understand or get the main point and have trouble making inferences from written text. Adolescents and adults may avoid activities that demand reading or arithmetic (reading for pleasure, reading instructions). Adults with specific learning disorder have ongoing spelling problems, slow and effortful reading, or problems making important inferences from numerical information in work-related written documents. They may avoid both leisure and work-related activities that demand reading or writing or use alternative approaches to access print (e.g., text-to-speech/speech-to-text software, audiobooks, audiovisual media).

An alternative clinical expression is that of circumscribed learning difficulties that persist across the lifespan, such as an inability to master the basic sense of number (e.g., to know which of a pair of numbers or dots represents the larger magnitude), or lack of proficiency in word identification or spelling. Avoidance of or reluctance to engage in activities requiring academic skills is common in children, adolescents, and adults. Episodes of severe anxiety or anxiety disorders, including somatic complaints or panic attacks, are common across the lifespan and accompany both the circumscribed and the broader expression of learning difficulties.

Risk and Prognostic Factors

Environmental.   Prematurity or very low birth weight increases the risk for specific learning disorder, as does prenatal exposure to nicotine.

Genetic and physiological.   Specific learning disorder appears to aggregate in families, particularly when affecting reading, mathematics, and spelling. The relative risk of specific learning disorder in reading or mathematics is substantially higher (e.g., 4–8 times and 5–10 times higher, respectively) in first-degree relatives of individuals with these learning difficulties compared with those without them. Family history of reading difficulties (dyslexia) and parental literacy skills predict literacy problems or specific learning disorder in offspring, indicating the combined role of genetic and environmental factors.

There is high heritability for both reading ability and reading disability in alphabetic and nonalphabetic languages, including high heritability for most manifestations of learning abilities and disabilities (e.g., heritability estimate values greater than 0.6). Covariation between various manifestations of learning difficulties is high, suggesting that genes related to one presentation are highly correlated with genes related to another manifestation.

Course modifiers.   Marked problems with inattentive behavior in preschool years is predictive of later difficulties in reading and mathematics (but not necessarily specific learning disorder) and nonresponse to effective academic interventions. Delay or disorders in speech or language, or impaired cognitive processing (e.g., phonological awareness, working memory, rapid serial naming) in preschool years, predicts later specific learning disorder in reading and written expression. Comorbidity with ADHD is predictive of worse mental health outcome than that associated with specific learning disorder without ADHD. Systematic, intensive, individualized instruction, using evidence-based interventions, may improve or ameliorate the learning difficulties in some individuals or promote the use of compensatory strategies in others, thereby mitigating the otherwise poor outcomes.

Culture-Related Diagnostic Issues

Specific learning disorder occurs across languages, cultures, races, and socioeconomic conditions but may vary in its manifestation according to the nature of the spoken and written symbol systems and cultural and educational practices. For example, the cognitive processing requirements of reading and of working with numbers vary greatly across orthographies. In the English language, the observable hallmark clinical symptom of difficulties learning to read is inaccurate and slow reading of single words; in other alphabetic languages that have more direct mapping between sounds and letters (e.g., Spanish, German) and in non-alphabetic languages (e.g., Chinese, Japanese), the hallmark feature is slow but accurate reading. In English-language learners, assessment should include consideration of whether the source of reading difficulties is a limited proficiency with English or a specific learning disorder. Risk factors for specific learning disorder in English-language learners include a family history of specific learning disorder or language delay in the native language, as well as learning difficulties in English and failure to catch up with peers. If there is suspicion of cultural or language differences (e.g., as in an English-language learner), the assessment needs to take into account the individual's language proficiency in his or her first or native language as well as in the second language (in this example, English). Also, assessment should consider the linguistic and cultural context in which the individual is living, as well as his or her educational and learning history in the original culture and language.

Gender-Related Diagnostic Issues

Specific learning disorder is more common in males than in females (ratios range from about 2:1 to 3:1) and cannot be attributed to factors such as ascertainment bias, definitional or measurement variation, language, race, or socioeconomic status.

Functional Consequences of Specific Learning Disorder

Specific learning disorder can have negative functional consequences across the lifespan, including lower academic attainment, higher rates of high school dropout, lower rates of postsecondary education, high levels of psychological distress and poorer overall mental health, higher rates of unemployment and under-employment, and lower incomes. School dropout and co-occurring depressive symptoms increase the risk for poor mental health outcomes, including suicidality, whereas high levels of social or emotional support predict better mental health outcomes.

Differential Diagnosis

Normal variations in academic attainment. Specific learning disorder is distinguished from normal variations in academic attainment due to external factors (e.g., lack of educational opportunity, consistently poor instruction, learning in a second language), because the learning difficulties persist in the presence of adequate educational opportunity and exposure to the same instruction as the peer group, and competency in the language of instruction, even when it is different from one's primary spoken language.

Intellectual disability (intellectual developmental disorder). Specific learning disorder differs from general learning difficulties associated with intellectual disability, because the learning difficulties occur in the presence of normal levels of intellectual functioning (i.e., IQ score of at least 70 ± 5). If intellectual disability is present, specific learning disorder can be diagnosed only when the learning difficulties are in excess of those usually associated with the intellectual disability.

Learning difficulties due to neurological or sensory disorders. Specific learning disorder is distinguished from learning difficulties due to neurological or sensory disorders (e.g., pediatric stroke, traumatic brain injury, hearing impairment, vision impairment), because in these cases there are abnormal findings on neurological examination.

Neurocognitive disorders. Specific learning disorder is distinguished from learning problems associated with neurodegenerative cognitive disorders, because in specific learning disorder the clinical expression of specific learning difficulties occurs during the developmental period, and the difficulties do not manifest as a marked decline from a former state.

Attention-deficit/hyperactivity disorder.   Specific learning disorder is distinguished from the poor academic performance associated with ADHD, because in the latter condition the problems may not necessarily reflect specific difficulties in learning academic skills but rather may reflect difficulties in performing those skills. However, the co-occurrence of specific learning disorder and ADHD is more frequent than expected by chance. If criteria for both disorders are met, both diagnoses can be given.

Psychotic disorders.   Specific learning disorder is distinguished from the academic and cognitive-processing difficulties associated with schizophrenia or psychosis, because with these disorders there is a decline (often rapid) in these functional domains.

Comorbidity

Specific learning disorder commonly co-occurs with neurodevelopmental (e.g., ADHD, communication disorders, developmental coordination disorder, autistic spectrum disorder) or other mental disorders (e.g., anxiety disorders, depressive and bipolar disorders). These comorbidities do not necessarily exclude the diagnosis specific learning disorder but may make testing and differential diagnosis more difficult, because each of the co-occurring disorders independently interferes with the execution of activities of daily living, including learning. Thus, clinical judgment is required to attribute such impairment to learning difficulties. If there is an indication that another diagnosis could account for the difficulties learning keystone academic skills described in Criterion A, specific learning disorder should not be diagnosed.

Motor Disorders

Developmental Coordination Disorder

Diagnostic Criteria   **315.4 (F82)**

A. The acquisition and execution of coordinated motor skills is substantially below that expected given the individual's chronological age and opportunity for skill learning and use. Difficulties are manifested as clumsiness (e.g., dropping or bumping into objects) as well as slowness and inaccuracy of performance of motor skills (e.g., catching an object, using scissors or cutlery, handwriting, riding a bike, or participating in sports).
B. The motor skills deficit in Criterion A significantly and persistently interferes with activities of daily living appropriate to chronological age (e.g., self-care and self-maintenance) and impacts academic/school productivity, prevocational and vocational activities, leisure, and play.
C. Onset of symptoms is in the early developmental period.
D. The motor skills deficits are not better explained by intellectual disability (intellectual developmental disorder) or visual impairment and are not attributable to a neurological condition affecting movement (e.g., cerebral palsy, muscular dystrophy, degenerative disorder).

Diagnostic Features

The diagnosis of developmental coordination disorder is made by a clinical synthesis of the history (developmental and medical), physical examination, school or workplace report, and individual assessment using psychometrically sound and culturally appropriate standardized tests. The manifestation of impaired skills requiring motor coordination (Criterion A) varies with age. Young children may be delayed in achieving motor milestones (i.e., sitting, crawling, walking), although many achieve typical motor milestones. They also may be delayed in developing skills such as negotiating stairs, pedaling, buttoning shirts, completing puzzles, and using zippers. Even when the skill is achieved, movement execution may appear awkward, slow, or less precise than that of peers. Older children and adults may display slow speed or inaccuracy with motor aspects of activities such as assembling puzzles, building models, playing ball games (especially in teams), handwriting, typing, driving, or carrying out self-care skills.

Developmental coordination disorder is diagnosed only if the impairment in motor skills significantly interferes with the performance of, or participation in, daily activities in family, social, school, or community life (Criterion B). Examples of such activities include getting dressed, eating meals with age-appropriate utensils and without mess, engaging in physical games with others, using specific tools in class such as rulers and scissors, and participating in team exercise activities at school. Not only is ability to perform these actions impaired, but also marked slowness in execution is common. Handwriting competence is frequently affected, consequently affecting legibility and/or speed of written output and affecting academic achievement (the impact is distinguished from specific learning difficulty by the emphasis on the motoric component of written output skills). In adults, everyday skills in education and work, especially those in which speed and accuracy are required, are affected by coordination problems.

Criterion C states that the onset of symptoms of developmental coordination disorder must be in the early developmental period. However, developmental coordination disorder is typically not diagnosed before age 5 years because there is considerable variation in the age at acquisition of many motor skills or a lack of stability of measurement in early childhood (e.g., some children catch up) or because other causes of motor delay may not have fully manifested.

Criterion D specifies that the diagnosis of developmental coordination disorder is made if the coordination difficulties are not better explained by visual impairment or attributable to a neurological condition. Thus, visual function examination and neurological examination must be included in the diagnostic evaluation. If intellectual disability (intellectual developmental disorder) is present, the motor difficulties are in excess of those expected for the mental age; however, no IQ cut-off or discrepancy criterion is specified.

Developmental coordination disorder does not have discrete subtypes; however, individuals may be impaired predominantly in gross motor skills or in fine motor skills, including handwriting skills.

Other terms used to describe developmental coordination disorder include *childhood dyspraxia, specific developmental disorder of motor function,* and *clumsy child syndrome.*

Associated Features Supporting Diagnosis

Some children with developmental coordination disorder show additional (usually suppressed) motor activity, such as choreiform movements of unsupported limbs or mirror movements. These "overflow" movements are referred to as *neurodevelopmental immaturities* or *neurological soft signs* rather than neurological abnormalities. In both current literature and clinical practice, their role in diagnosis is still unclear, requiring further evaluation.

Prevalence

The prevalence of developmental coordination disorder in children ages 5–11 years is 5%–6% (in children age 7 years, 1.8% are diagnosed with severe developmental coordination disorder and 3% with probable developmental coordination disorder). Males are more often affected than females, with a male:female ratio between 2:1 and 7:1.

Development and Course

The course of developmental coordination disorder is variable but stable at least to 1 year follow-up. Although there may be improvement in the longer term, problems with coordinated movements continue through adolescence in an estimated 50%–70% of children. Onset is in early childhood. Delayed motor milestones may be the first signs, or the disorder is first recognized when the child attempts tasks such as holding a knife and fork, buttoning clothes, or playing ball games. In middle childhood, there are difficulties with motor aspects of assembling puzzles, building models, playing ball, and handwriting, as well as with organizing belongings, when motor sequencing and coordination are required. In early adulthood, there is continuing difficulty in learning new tasks involving complex/automatic motor skills, including driving and using tools. Inability to take notes and handwrite quickly may affect performance in the workplace. Co-occurrence with other disorders (see the section "Comorbidity" for this disorder) has an additional impact on presentation, course, and outcome.

Risk and Prognostic Factors

Environmental.   Developmental coordination disorder is more common following prenatal exposure to alcohol and in preterm and low-birth-weight children.

Genetic and physiological.   Impairments in underlying neurodevelopmental processes—particularly in visual-motor skills, both in visual-motor perception and spatial mentalizing—have been found and affect the ability to make rapid motoric adjustments as the complexity of the required movements increases. Cerebellar dysfunction has been proposed, but the neural basis of developmental coordination disorder remains unclear. Because of the co-occurrence of developmental coordination disorder with attention-deficit/hyperactivity disorder (ADHD), specific learning disabilities, and autism spectrum disorder, shared genetic effect has been proposed. However, consistent co-occurrence in twins appears only in severe cases.

Course modifiers.   Individuals with ADHD and with developmental coordination disorder demonstrate more impairment than individuals with ADHD without developmental coordination disorder.

Culture-Related Diagnostic Issues

Developmental coordination disorder occurs across cultures, races, and socioeconomic conditions. By definition, "activities of daily living" implies cultural differences necessitating consideration of the context in which the individual child is living as well as whether he or she has had appropriate opportunities to learn and practice such activities.

Functional Consequences of Developmental Coordination Disorder

Developmental coordination disorder leads to impaired functional performance in activities of daily living (Criterion B), and the impairment is increased with co-occurring conditions. Consequences of developmental coordination disorder include reduced participation in team play and sports; poor self-esteem and sense of self-worth; emotional or behavior problems; impaired academic achievement; poor physical fitness; and reduced physical activity and obesity.

Differential Diagnosis

Motor impairments due to another medical condition.   Problems in coordination may be associated with visual function impairment and specific neurological disorders (e.g., cerebral palsy, progressive lesions of the cerebellum, neuromuscular disorders). In such cases, there are additional findings on neurological examination.

Intellectual disability (intellectual developmental disorder).   If intellectual disability is present, motor competences may be impaired in accordance with the intellectual disability. However, if the motor difficulties are in excess of what could be accounted for by the intellectual disability, and criteria for developmental coordination disorder are met, developmental coordination disorder can be diagnosed as well.

Attention-deficit/hyperactivity disorder.   Individuals with ADHD may fall, bump into objects, or knock things over. Careful observation across different contexts is required to ascertain if lack of motor competence is attributable to distractibility and impulsiveness rather than to developmental coordination disorder. If criteria for both ADHD and developmental coordination disorder are met, both diagnoses can be given.

Autism spectrum disorder.   Individuals with autism spectrum disorder may be uninterested in participating in tasks requiring complex coordination skills, such as ball sports, which will affect test performance and function but not reflect core motor competence. Co-occurrence of developmental coordination disorder and autism spectrum disorder is common. If criteria for both disorders are met, both diagnoses can be given.

Joint hypermobility syndrome.   Individuals with syndromes causing hyperextensible joints (found on physical examination; often with a complaint of pain) may present with symptoms similar to those of developmental coordination disorder.

Comorbidity

Disorders that commonly co-occur with developmental coordination disorder include speech and language disorder; specific learning disorder (especially reading and writing); problems of inattention, including ADHD (the most frequent coexisting condition, with about 50% co-occurrence); autism spectrum disorder; disruptive and emotional behavior problems; and joint hypermobility syndrome. Different clusters of co-occurrence may be present (e.g., a cluster with severe reading disorders, fine motor problems, and handwriting problems; another cluster with impaired movement control and motor planning). Presence of other disorders does not exclude developmental coordination disorder but may make testing more difficult and may independently interfere with the execution of activities of daily living, thus requiring examiner judgment in ascribing impairment to motor skills.

Stereotypic Movement Disorder

Diagnostic Criteria   **307.3 (F98.4)**

A. Repetitive, seemingly driven, and apparently purposeless motor behavior (e.g., hand shaking or waving, body rocking, head banging, self-biting, hitting own body).
B. The repetitive motor behavior interferes with social, academic, or other activities and may result in self-injury.
C. Onset is in the early developmental period.
D. The repetitive motor behavior is not attributable to the physiological effects of a substance or neurological condition and is not better explained by another neurodevelopmental or mental disorder (e.g., trichotillomania [hair-pulling disorder], obsessive-compulsive disorder).

Specify if:
   With self-injurious behavior (or behavior that would result in an injury if preventive measures were not used)
   Without self-injurious behavior

Specify if:
   Associated with a known medical or genetic condition, neurodevelopmental disorder, or environmental factor (e.g., Lesch-Nyhan syndrome, intellectual disability [intellectual developmental disorder], intrauterine alcohol exposure)

> **Coding note:** Use additional code to identify the associated medical or genetic condition, or neurodevelopmental disorder.

Specify current severity:

    Mild: Symptoms are easily suppressed by sensory stimulus or distraction.

    Moderate: Symptoms require explicit protective measures and behavioral modification.

    Severe: Continuous monitoring and protective measures are required to prevent serious injury.

Recording Procedures

For stereotypic movement disorder that is associated with a known medical or genetic condition, neurodevelopmental disorder, or environmental factor, record stereotypic movement disorder associated with (name of condition, disorder, or factor) (e.g., stereotypic movement disorder associated with Lesch-Nyhan syndrome).

Specifiers

The severity of non-self-injurious stereotypic movements ranges from mild presentations that are easily suppressed by a sensory stimulus or distraction to continuous movements that markedly interfere with all activities of daily living. Self-injurious behaviors range in severity along various dimensions, including the frequency, impact on adaptive functioning, and severity of bodily injury (from mild bruising or erythema from hitting hand against body, to lacerations or amputation of digits, to retinal detachment from head banging).

Diagnostic Features

The essential feature of stereotypic movement disorder is repetitive, seemingly driven, and apparently purposeless motor behavior (Criterion A). These behaviors are often rhythmical movements of the head, hands, or body without obvious adaptive function. The movements may or may not respond to efforts to stop them. Among typically developing children, the repetitive movements may be stopped when attention is directed to them or when the child is distracted from performing them. Among children with neurodevelopmental disorders, the behaviors are typically less responsive to such efforts. In other cases, the individual demonstrates self-restraining behaviors (e.g., sitting on hands, wrapping arms in clothing, finding a protective device).

The repertoire of behaviors is variable; each individual presents with his or her own individually patterned, "signature" behavior. Examples of non-self-injurious stereotypic movements include, but are not limited to, body rocking, bilateral flapping or rotating hand movements, flicking or fluttering fingers in front of the face, arm waving or flapping, and head nodding. Stereotyped self-injurious behaviors include, but are not limited to, repetitive head banging, face slapping, eye poking, and biting of hands, lips, or other body parts. Eye poking is particularly concerning; it occurs more frequently among children with visual impairment. Multiple movements may be combined (e.g., cocking the head, rocking the torso, waving a small string repetitively in front of the face).

Stereotypic movements may occur many times during a day, lasting a few seconds to several minutes or longer. Frequency can vary from many occurrences in a single day to several weeks elapsing between episodes. The behaviors vary in context, occurring when the individual is engrossed in other activities, when excited, stressed, fatigued, or bored. Criterion A requires that the movements be "apparently" purposeless. However, some functions may be served by the movements. For example, stereotypic movements might reduce anxiety in response to external stressors.

Criterion B states that the stereotypic movements interfere with social, academic, or other activities and, in some children, may result in self-injury (or would if protective measures were not used). If self-injury is present, it should be coded using the specifier. Onset of stereotypic movements is in the early developmental period (Criterion C). Criterion D states that the repetitive, stereotyped behavior in stereotypic movement disorder is not attributable to the physiological effects of a substance or neurological condition and is not better explained by another neurodevelopmental or mental disorder. The presence of stereotypic movements may indicate an undetected neurodevelopmental problem, especially in children ages 1–3 years.

Prevalence

Simple stereotypic movements (e.g., rocking) are common in young typically developing children. Complex stereotypic movements are much less common (occurring in approximately 3%–4%). Between 4% and 16% of individuals with intellectual disability (intellectual developmental disorder) engage in stereotypy and self-injury. The risk is greater in individuals with severe intellectual disability. Among individuals with intellectual disability living in residential facilities, 10%–15% may have stereotypic movement disorder with self-injury.

Development and Course

Stereotypic movements typically begin within the first 3 years of life. Simple stereotypic movements are common in infancy and may be involved in acquisition of motor mastery. In children who develop complex motor stereotypies, approximately 80% exhibit symptoms before 24 months of age, 12% between 24 and 35 months, and 8% at 36 months or older. In most typically developing children, these movements resolve over time or can be suppressed. Onset of complex motor stereotypies may be in infancy or later in the developmental period. Among individuals with intellectual disability, the stereotyped, self-injurious behaviors may persist for years, even though the typography or pattern of self-injury may change.

Risk and Prognostic Factors

Environmental. Social isolation is a risk factor for self-stimulation that may progress to stereotypic movements with repetitive self-injury. Environmental stress may also trigger stereotypic behavior. Fear may alter physiological state, resulting in increased frequency of stereotypic behaviors.

Genetic and physiological. Lower cognitive functioning is linked to greater risk for stereotypic behaviors and poorer response to interventions. Stereotypic movements are more frequent among individuals with moderate-to-severe/profound intellectual disability, who by virtue of a particular syndrome (e.g., Rett syndrome) or environmental factor (e.g., an environment with relatively insufficient stimulation) seem to be at higher risk for stereotypies. Repetitive self-injurious behavior may be a behavioral phenotype in neurogenetic syndromes. For example, in Lesch-Nyhan syndrome, there are both stereotypic dystonic movements and self-mutilation of fingers, lip biting, and other forms of self-injury unless the individual is restrained, and in Rett syndrome and Cornelia de Lange syndrome, self-injury may result from the hand-to-mouth stereotypies. Stereotypic behaviors may result from a painful medical condition (e.g., middle ear infection, dental problems, gastroesophageal reflux).

Culture-Related Diagnostic Issues

Stereotypic movement disorder, with or without self-injury, occurs in all races and cultures. Cultural attitudes toward unusual behaviors may result in delayed diagnosis. Overall cultural tolerance and attitudes toward stereotypic movement vary and must be considered.

Differential Diagnosis

Normal development. Simple stereotypic movements are common in infancy and early childhood. Rocking may occur in the transition from sleep to awake, a behavior that usually resolves with age. Complex stereotypies are less common in typically developing children and can usually be suppressed by distraction or sensory stimulation. The individual's daily routine is rarely affected, and the movements generally do not cause the child distress. The diagnosis would not be appropriate in these circumstances.

Autism spectrum disorder.   Stereotypic movements may be a presenting symptom of autism spectrum disorder and should be considered when repetitive movements and behaviors are being evaluated. Deficits of social communication and reciprocity manifesting in autism spectrum disorder are generally absent in stereotypic movement disorder, and thus social interaction, social communication, and rigid repetitive behaviors and interests are distinguishing features. When autism spectrum disorder is present, stereotypic movement disorder is diagnosed only when there is self-injury or when the stereotypic behaviors are sufficiently severe to become a focus of treatment.

Tic disorders.   Typically, stereotypies have an earlier age at onset (before 3 years) than do tics, which have a mean age at onset of 5–7 years. They are consistent and fixed in their pattern or topography compared with tics, which are variable in their presentation. Stereotypies may involve arms, hands, or the entire body, while tics commonly involve eyes, face, head, and shoulders. Stereotypies are more fixed, rhythmic, and prolonged in duration than tics, which, generally, are brief, rapid, random, and fluctuating. Tics and stereotypic movements are both reduced by distraction.

Obsessive-compulsive and related disorders.   Stereotypic movement disorder is distinguished from obsessive-compulsive disorder (OCD) by the absence of obsessions, as well as by the nature of the repetitive behaviors. In OCD the individual feels driven to perform repetitive behaviors in response to an obsession or according to rules that must be applied rigidly, whereas in stereotypic movement disorder the behaviors are seemingly driven but apparently purposeless. Trichotillomania (hair-pulling disorder) and excoriation (skin-picking) disorder are characterized by body-focused repetitive behaviors (i.e., hair pulling and skin picking) that may be seemingly driven but that are not apparently purposeless, and that may not be patterned or rhythmical. Furthermore, onset in trichotillomania and excoriation disorder is not typically in the early developmental period, but rather around puberty or later.

Other neurological and medical conditions.   The diagnosis of stereotypic movements requires the exclusion of habits, mannerisms, paroxysmal dyskinesias, and benign hereditary chorea. A neurological history and examination are required to assess features suggestive of other disorders, such as myoclonus, dystonia, tics, and chorea. Involuntary movements associated with a neurological condition may be distinguished by their signs and symptoms. For example, repetitive, stereotypic movements in tardive dyskinesia can be distinguished by a history of chronic neuroleptic use and characteristic oral or facial dyskinesia or irregular trunk or limb movements. These types of movements do not result in self-injury. A diagnosis of stereotypic movement disorder is not appropriate for repetitive skin picking or scratching associated with amphetamine intoxication or abuse (e.g., patients are diagnosed with substance/medication-induced obsessive-compulsive and related disorder) and repetitive choreoathetoid movements associated with other neurological disorders.

Comorbidity

Stereotypic movement disorder may occur as a primary diagnosis or secondary to another disorder. For example, stereotypies are a common manifestation of a variety of neurogenetic disorders, such as Lesch-Nyhan syndrome, Rett syndrome, fragile X syndrome, Cornelia de Lange syndrome, and Smith-Magenis syndrome. When stereotypic movement disorder co-occurs with another medical condition, both should be coded.

Tic Disorders

Diagnostic Criteria

Note: A tic is a sudden, rapid, recurrent, nonrhythmic motor movement or vocalization.

Tourette's Disorder   307.23 (F95.2)

A. Both multiple motor and one or more vocal tics have been present at some time during the illness, although not necessarily concurrently.
B. The tics may wax and wane in frequency but have persisted for more than 1 year since first tic onset.
C. Onset is before age 18 years.
D. The disturbance is not attributable to the physiological effects of a substance (e.g., cocaine) or another medical condition (e.g., Huntington's disease, postviral encephalitis).

Persistent (Chronic) Motor or Vocal Tic Disorder   307.22 (F95.1)

A. Single or multiple motor or vocal tics have been present during the illness, but not both motor and vocal.
B. The tics may wax and wane in frequency but have persisted for more than 1 year since first tic onset.
C. Onset is before age 18 years.
D. The disturbance is not attributable to the physiological effects of a substance (e.g., cocaine) or another medical condition (e.g., Huntington's disease, postviral encephalitis).
E. Criteria have never been met for Tourette's disorder.

Specify if:
   With motor tics only
   With vocal tics only

Provisional Tic Disorder   307.21 (F95.0)

A. Single or multiple motor and/or vocal tics.
B. The tics have been present for less than 1 year since first tic onset.
C. Onset is before age 18 years.
D. The disturbance is not attributable to the physiological effects of a substance (e.g., cocaine) or another medical condition (e.g., Huntington's disease, postviral encephalitis).
E. Criteria have never been met for Tourette's disorder or persistent (chronic) motor or vocal tic disorder.

Specifiers

The "motor tics only" or "vocal tics only" specifier is only required for persistent (chronic) motor or vocal tic disorder.

Diagnostic Features

Tic disorders comprise four diagnostic categories: Tourette's disorder, persistent (chronic) motor or vocal tic disorder, provisional tic disorder, and the other specified and unspecified tic disorders. Diagnosis for any tic disorder is based on the presence of motor and/or vocal tics (Criterion A), duration of tic symptoms (Criterion B), age at onset (Criterion C), and absence of any known cause such as another medical condition or substance use (Criterion D). The tic disorders are hierarchical in order (i.e., Tourette's disorder, followed by persistent [chronic] motor or vocal tic disorder, followed by provisional tic disorder, followed by the other specified and unspecified tic disorders), such that once a tic disorder at one level of the hierarchy is diagnosed, a lower hierarchy diagnosis cannot be made (Criterion E).

Tics are sudden, rapid, recurrent, nonrhythmic motor movements or vocalizations. An individual may have various tic symptoms over time, but at any point in time, the tic repertoire recurs in a characteristic fashion. Although tics can include almost any muscle group or vocalization, certain tic symptoms, such as eye blinking or throat clearing, are common across patient populations. Tics are generally experienced as involuntary but can be voluntarily suppressed for varying lengths of time.

Tics can be either simple or complex. *Simple motor tics* are of short duration (i.e., milliseconds) and can include eye blinking, shoulder shrugging, and extension of the extremities. Simple vocal tics include throat clearing, sniffing, and grunting often caused by contraction of the diaphragm or muscles of the oropharynx. *Complex motor tics* are of longer duration (i.e., seconds) and often include a combination of simple tics such as simultaneous head turning and shoulder shrugging. Complex tics can appear purposeful, such as a tic-like sexual or obscene gesture (*copropraxia*) or a tic-like imitation of someone else's movements (*echopraxia*). Similarly, complex vocal tics include repeating one's own sounds or words (*palilalia*), repeating the last-heard word or phrase (*echolalia*), or uttering socially unacceptable words, including obscenities, or ethnic, racial, or religious slurs (*coprolalia*). Importantly, coprolalia is an abrupt, sharp bark or grunt utterance and lacks the prosody of similar inappropriate speech observed in human interactions.

The presence of motor and/or vocal tics varies across the four tic disorders (Criterion A). For Tourette's disorder, both motor and vocal tics must be present, whereas for persistent (chronic) motor or vocal tic disorder, only motor or only vocal tics are present. For provisional tic disorder, motor and/or vocal tics may be present. For other specified or unspecified tic disorders, the movement disorder symptoms are best characterized as tics but are atypical in presentation or age at onset, or have a known etiology.

The 1-year minimum duration criterion (Criterion B) assures that individuals diagnosed with either Tourette's disorder or persistent (chronic) motor or vocal tic disorder have had persistent symptoms. Tics wax and wane in severity, and some individuals may have tic-free periods of weeks to months; however, an individual who has had tic symptoms of greater than 1 year's duration since first tic onset would be considered to have persistent symptoms regardless of duration of tic-free periods. For an individual with motor and/or vocal tics of less than 1 year since first tic onset, a provisional tic disorder diagnosis can be considered. There is no duration specification for other specified and unspecified tic disorders. The onset of tics must occur prior to age 18 years (Criterion C). Tic disorders typically begin in the prepubertal period, with an average age at onset between 4 and 6 years, and with the incidence of new-onset tic disorders decreasing in the teen years. New onset of tic symptoms in adulthood is exceedingly rare and is often associated with exposures to drugs (e.g., excessive cocaine use) or is a result of a central nervous system insult (e.g., postviral encephalitis). Although tic onset is uncommon in teenagers and adults, it is not uncommon for adolescents and adults to present for an initial diagnostic assessment and, when carefully evaluated, provide a history of milder symptoms dating back to childhood. New-onset abnormal movements suggestive of tics outside of the usual age range should result in evaluation for other movement disorders or for specific etiologies.

Tic symptoms cannot be attributable to the physiological effects of a substance or another medical condition (Criterion D). When there is strong evidence from the history, physical examination, and/or laboratory results to suggest a plausible, proximal, and probable cause for a tic disorder, a diagnosis of other specified tic disorder should be used.

Having previously met diagnostic criteria for Tourette's disorder negates a possible diagnosis of persistent (chronic) motor or vocal tic disorder (Criterion E). Similarly, a previous diagnosis of persistent (chronic) motor or vocal tic disorder negates a diagnosis of provisional tic disorder or other specified or unspecified tic disorder (Criterion E).

Prevalence

Tics are common in childhood but transient in most cases. The estimated prevalence of Tourette's disorder ranges from 3 to 8 per 1,000 in school-age children. Males are more commonly affected than females, with the ratio varying from 2:1 to 4:1. A national survey in the United States estimated 3 per 1,000 for the prevalence of clinically identified cases. The frequency of identified cases was lower among African Americans and Hispanic Americans, which may be related to differences in access to care.

Development and Course

Onset of tics is typically between ages 4 and 6 years. Peak severity occurs between ages 10 and 12 years, with a decline in severity during adolescence. Many adults with tic disorders experience diminished symptoms. A small percentage of individuals will have persistently severe or worsening symptoms in adulthood.

Tic symptoms manifest similarly in all age groups and across the lifespan. Tics wax and wane in severity and change in affected muscle groups and vocalizations over time. As children get older, they begin to report their tics being associated with a premonitory urge—a somatic sensation that precedes the tic—and a feeling of tension reduction following the expression of the tic. Tics associated with a premonitory urge may be experienced as not completely "involuntary" in that the urge and the tic can be resisted. An individual may also feel the need to perform a tic in a specific way or repeat it until he or she achieves the feeling that the tic has been done "just right."

The vulnerability toward developing co-occurring conditions changes as individuals pass through the age of risk for various co-occurring conditions. For example, prepubertal children with tic disorders are more likely to experience attention-deficit/hyperactivity disorder (ADHD), obsessive-compulsive disorder (OCD), and separation anxiety disorder than are teenagers and adults, who are more likely to experience the new onset of major depressive disorder, substance use disorder, or bipolar disorder.

Risk and Prognostic Factors

Temperamental.   Tics are worsened by anxiety, excitement, and exhaustion and are better during calm, focused activities. Individuals may have fewer tics when engaged in schoolwork or tasks at work than when relaxing at home after school or in the evening. Stressful/exciting events (e.g., taking a test, participating in exciting activities) often make tics worse.

Environmental.   Observing a gesture or sound in another person may result in an individual with a tic disorder making a similar gesture or sound, which may be incorrectly perceived by others as purposeful. This can be a particular problem when the individual is interacting with authority figures (e.g., teachers, supervisors, police).

Genetic and physiological.   Genetic and environmental factors influence tic symptom expression and severity. Important risk alleles for Tourette's disorder and rare genetic variants in families with tic disorders have been identified. Obstetrical complications, older paternal age, lower birth weight, and maternal smoking during pregnancy are associated with worse tic severity.

Culture-Related Diagnostic Issues

Tic disorders do not appear to vary in clinical characteristics, course, or etiology by race, ethnicity, and culture. However, race, ethnicity, and culture may impact how tic disorders are perceived and managed in the family and community, as well as influencing patterns of help seeking, and choices of treatment.

Gender-Related Diagnostic Issues

Males are more commonly affected than females, but there are no gender differences in the kinds of tics, age at onset, or course. Women with persistent tic disorders may be more likely to experience anxiety and depression.

Functional Consequences of Tic Disorders

Many individuals with mild to moderate tic severity experience no distress or impairment in functioning and may even be unaware of their tics. Individuals with more severe symptoms generally have more impairment in daily living, but even individuals with moderate or even severe tic disorders may function well. The presence of a co-occurring condition, such as ADHD or OCD, can have greater impact on functioning. Less commonly, tics disrupt functioning in daily activities and result in social isolation, interpersonal conflict, peer victimization, inability to work or to go to school, and lower quality of life. The individual also may experience substantial psychological distress. Rare complications of Tourette's disorder include physical injury, such as eye injury (from hitting oneself in the face), and orthopedic and neurological injury (e.g., disc disease related to forceful head and neck movements).

Differential Diagnosis

Abnormal movements that may accompany other medical conditions and stereotypic movement disorder.   *Motor stereotypies* are defined as involuntary rhythmic, repetitive, predictable movements that appear purposeful but serve no obvious adaptive function or purpose and stop with distraction. Examples include repetitive hand waving/rotating, arm flapping, and finger wiggling. Motor stereotypies can be differentiated from tics based on the former's earlier age at onset (younger than 3 years), prolonged duration (seconds to minutes), constant repetitive fixed form and location, exacerbation when engrossed in activities, lack of a premonitory urge, and cessation with distraction (e.g., name called or touched). *Chorea* represents rapid, random, continual, abrupt, irregular, unpredictable, nonstereotyped actions that are usually bilateral and affect all parts of the body (i.e., face, trunk, and limbs). The timing, direction, and distribution of movements vary from moment to moment, and movements usually worsen during attempted voluntary action. *Dystonia* is the simultaneous sustained contracture of both agonist and antagonist muscles, resulting in a distorted posture or movement of parts of the body. Dystonic postures are often triggered by attempts at voluntary movements and are not seen during sleep.

Substance-induced and paroxysmal dyskinesias.   Paroxysmal dyskinesias usually occur as dystonic or choreoathetoid movements that are precipitated by voluntary movement or exertion and less commonly arise from normal background activity.

Myoclonus.   Myoclonus is characterized by a sudden unidirectional movement that is often nonrhythmic. It may be worsened by movement and occur during sleep. Myoclonus is differentiated from tics by its rapidity, lack of suppressibility, and absence of a premonitory urge.

Obsessive-compulsive and related disorders.   Differentiating obsessive-compulsive behaviors from tics may be difficult. Clues favoring an obsessive-compulsive behavior include a cognitive-based drive (e.g., fear of contamination) and the need to perform the action in a particular fashion a certain number of times, equally on both sides of the body, or until a "just right" feeling is achieved. Impulse-control problems and other repetitive behaviors, including persistent hair pulling, skin picking, and nail biting, appear more goal directed and complex than tics.

Comorbidity

Many medical and psychiatric conditions have been described as co-occurring with tic disorders, with ADHD and obsessive-compulsive and related disorders being particularly common. The obsessive-compulsive symptoms observed in tic disorder tend to be characterized by more aggressive symmetry and order symptoms and poorer response to pharmacotherapy with selective serotonin reuptake inhibitors. Children with ADHD may demonstrate disruptive behavior, social immaturity, and learning difficulties that may interfere with academic progress and interpersonal relationships and lead to greater impairment than that caused by a tic disorder. Individuals with tic disorders can also have other movement disorders and other mental disorders, such as depressive, bipolar, or substance use disorders.

Other Specified Tic Disorder

307.20 (F95.8)

This category applies to presentations in which symptoms characteristic of a tic disorder that cause clinically significant distress or impairment in social, occupational, or other important areas of functioning predominate but do not meet the full criteria for a tic disorder or any of the disorders in the neurodevelopmental disorders diagnostic class. The other specified tic disorder category is used in situations in which the clinician chooses to communicate the specific reason that the presentation does not meet the criteria for a tic disorder or any specific neurodevelopmental disorder. This is done by recording "other specified tic disorder" followed by the specific reason (e.g., "with onset after age 18 years").

Unspecified Tic Disorder

307.20 (F95.9)

This category applies to presentations in which symptoms characteristic of a tic disorder that cause clinically significant distress or impairment in social, occupational, or other important areas of functioning predominate but do not meet the full criteria for a tic disorder or for any of the disorders in the neurodevelopmental disorders diagnostic class. The unspecified tic disorder category is used in situations in which the clinician chooses *not* to specify the reason that the criteria are not met for a tic disorder or for a specific neurodevelopmental disorder, and includes presentations in which there is insufficient information to make a more specific diagnosis.

Other Neurodevelopmental Disorders

Other Specified Neurodevelopmental Disorder

315.8 (F88)

This category applies to presentations in which symptoms characteristic of a neurodevelopmental disorder that cause impairment in social, occupational, or other important areas of functioning predominate but do not meet the full criteria for any of the disorders in the neurodevelopmental disorders diagnostic class. The other specified neurodevelopmental disorder category is used in situations in which the clinician chooses to communicate the specific reason that the presentation does not meet the criteria for any specific neurodevelopmental disorder. This is done by recording "other specified neurodevelopmental disorder" followed by the specific reason (e.g., "neurodevelopmental disorder associated with prenatal alcohol exposure").

An example of a presentation that can be specified using the "other specified" designation is the following:

Neurodevelopmental disorder associated with prenatal alcohol exposure: Neurodevelopmental disorder associated with prenatal alcohol exposure is characterized by a range of developmental disabilities following exposure to alcohol in utero.

Unspecified Neurodevelopmental Disorder

315.9 (F89)

This category applies to presentations in which symptoms characteristic of a neurodevelopmental disorder that cause impairment in social, occupational, or other important areas of functioning predominate but do not meet the full criteria for any of the disorders in the neurodevelopmental disorders diagnostic class. The unspecified neurodevelopmental disorder category is used in situations in which the clinician chooses *not* to specify the reason that the criteria are not met for a specific neurodevelopmental disorder, and includes presentations in which there is insufficient information to make a more specific diagnosis (e.g., in emergency room settings).

Schizophrenia Spectrum and Other Psychotic Disorders

Schizophrenia spectrum and other psychotic disorders include schizophrenia, other psychotic disorders, and schizotypal (personality) disorder. They are defined by abnormalities in one or more of the following five domains: delusions, hallucinations, disorganized thinking (speech), grossly disorganized or abnormal motor behavior (including catatonia), and negative symptoms.

Key Features That Define the Psychotic Disorders

Delusions

Delusions are fixed beliefs that are not amenable to change in light of conflicting evidence. Their content may include a variety of themes (e.g., persecutory, referential, somatic, religious, grandiose). *Persecutory delusions* (i.e., belief that one is going to be harmed, harassed, and so forth by an individual, organization, or other group) are most common. *Referential delusions* (i.e., belief that certain gestures, comments, environmental cues, and so forth are directed at oneself) are also common. *Grandiose delusions* (i.e., when an individual believes that he or she has exceptional abilities, wealth, or fame) and *erotomanic delusions* (i.e., when an individual believes falsely that another person is in love with him or her) are also seen. *Nihilistic delusions* involve the conviction that a major catastrophe will occur, and *somatic delusions* focus on preoccupations regarding health and organ function.

Delusions are deemed *bizarre* if they are clearly implausible and not understandable to same-culture peers and do not derive from ordinary life experiences. An example of a bizarre delusion is the belief that an outside force has removed his or her internal organs and replaced them with someone else's organs without leaving any wounds or scars. An example of a nonbizarre delusion is the belief that one is under surveillance by the police, despite a lack of convincing evidence. Delusions that express a loss of control over mind or body are generally considered to be bizarre; these include the belief that one's thoughts have been "removed" by some outside force (*thought withdrawal*), that alien thoughts have been put into one's mind (*thought insertion*), or that one's body or actions are being acted on or manipulated by some outside force (*delusions of control*). The distinction between a delusion and a strongly held idea is sometimes difficult to make and depends in part on the degree of conviction with which the belief is held despite clear or reasonable contradictory evidence regarding its veracity.

Hallucinations

Hallucinations are perception-like experiences that occur without an external stimulus. They are vivid and clear, with the full force and impact of normal perceptions, and not under voluntary control. They may occur in any sensory modality, but auditory hallucinations are the most common in schizophrenia and related disorders. Auditory hallucinations are usually experienced as voices, whether familiar or unfamiliar, that are perceived as distinct from the individual's own thoughts. The hallucinations must occur in the context of a clear sensorium; those that occur while falling asleep (*hypnagogic*) or waking up (*hypnopompic*) are considered to be within the range of normal experience. Hallucinations may be a normal part of religious experience in certain cultural contexts.

Disorganized Thinking (Speech)

Disorganized thinking (formal thought disorder) is typically inferred from the individual's speech. The individual may switch from one topic to another (*derailment or loose associations*). Answers to questions may be obliquely related or completely unrelated (*tangentiality*). Rarely, speech may be so severely disorganized that it is nearly incomprehensible and resembles receptive aphasia in its linguistic disorganization (*incoherence* or "word salad"). Because mildly disorganized speech is common and nonspecific, the symptom must be severe enough to substantially impair effective communication. The severity of the impairment may be difficult to evaluate if the person making the diagnosis comes from a different linguistic background than that of the person being examined. Less severe disorganized thinking or speech may occur during the prodromal and residual periods of schizophrenia.

Grossly Disorganized or Abnormal Motor Behavior (Including Catatonia)

Grossly disorganized or abnormal motor behavior may manifest itself in a variety of ways, ranging from childlike "silliness" to unpredictable agitation. Problems may be noted in any form of goal-directed behavior, leading to difficulties in performing activities of daily living.

Catatonic behavior is a marked decrease in reactivity to the environment. This ranges from resistance to instructions (*negativism*); to maintaining a rigid, inappropriate or bizarre posture; to a complete lack of verbal and motor responses (*mutism* and *stupor*). It can also include purposeless and excessive motor activity without obvious cause (*catatonic excitement*). Other features are repeated stereotyped movements, staring, grimacing, mutism, and the echoing of speech. Although catatonia has historically been associated with schizophrenia, catatonic symptoms are nonspecific and may occur in other mental disorders (e.g., bipolar or depressive disorders with catatonia) and in medical conditions (catatonic disorder due to another medical condition).

Negative Symptoms

Negative symptoms account for a substantial portion of the morbidity associated with schizophrenia but are less prominent in other psychotic disorders. Two negative symptoms are particularly prominent in schizophrenia: diminished emotional expression and avolition. *Diminished emotional expression* includes reductions in the expression of emotions in the face, eye contact, intonation of speech (prosody), and movements of the hand, head, and face that normally give an emotional emphasis to speech. *Avolition* is a decrease in motivated self-initiated purposeful activities. The individual may sit for long periods of time and show little interest in participating in work or social activities. Other negative symptoms include alogia, anhedonia, and asociality. *Alogia* is manifested by diminished speech output. *Anhedonia* is the decreased ability to experience pleasure from positive stimuli or a degradation in the recollection of pleasure previously experienced. *Asociality* refers to the apparent lack of interest in social interactions and may be associated with avolition, but it can also be a manifestation of limited opportunities for social interactions.

Disorders in This Chapter

This chapter is organized along a gradient of psychopathology. Clinicians should first consider conditions that do not reach full criteria for a psychotic disorder or are limited to one domain of psychopathology. Then they should consider time-limited conditions. Finally, the diagnosis of a schizophrenia spectrum disorder requires the exclusion of another condition that may give rise to psychosis.

Schizotypal personality disorder is noted within this chapter as it is considered within the schizophrenia spectrum, although its full description is found in the chapter "Personality Disorders." The diagnosis schizotypal personality disorder captures a pervasive pattern of social and interpersonal deficits, including reduced capacity for close relationships; cognitive or perceptual distortions; and eccentricities of behavior, usually beginning by early adulthood but in some cases first becoming apparent in childhood and adolescence. Abnormalities of beliefs, thinking, and perception are below the threshold for the diagnosis of a psychotic disorder.

Two conditions are defined by abnormalities limited to one domain of psychosis: delusions or catatonia. Delusional disorder is characterized by at least 1 month of delusions but no other psychotic symptoms. Catatonia is described later in the chapter and further in this discussion.

Brief psychotic disorder lasts more than 1 day and remits by 1 month. Schizophreniform disorder is characterized by a symptomatic presentation equivalent to that of schizophrenia except for its duration (less than 6 months) and the absence of a requirement for a decline in functioning.

Schizophrenia lasts for at least 6 months and includes at least 1 month of active-phase symptoms. In schizoaffective disorder, a mood episode and the active-phase symptoms of schizophrenia occur together and were preceded or are followed by at least 2 weeks of delusions or hallucinations without prominent mood symptoms.

Psychotic disorders may be induced by another condition. In substance/medication-induced psychotic disorder, the psychotic symptoms are judged to be a physiological consequence of a drug of abuse, a medication, or toxin exposure and cease after removal of the agent. In psychotic disorder due to another medical condition, the psychotic symptoms are judged to be a direct physiological consequence of another medical condition.

Catatonia can occur in several disorders, including neurodevelopmental, psychotic, bipolar, depressive, and other mental disorders. This chapter also includes the diagnoses catatonia associated with another mental disorder (catatonia specifier), catatonic disorder due to another medical condition, and unspecified catatonia, and the diagnostic criteria for all three conditions are described together.

Other specified and unspecified schizophrenia spectrum and other psychotic disorders are included for classifying psychotic presentations that do not meet the criteria for any of the specific psychotic disorders, or psychotic symptomatology about which there is inadequate or contradictory information.

Clinician-Rated Assessment of Symptoms and Related Clinical Phenomena in Psychosis

Psychotic disorders are heterogeneous, and the severity of symptoms can predict important aspects of the illness, such as the degree of cognitive or neurobiological deficits. To move the field forward, a detailed framework for the assessment of severity is included in Section III "Assessment Measures," which may help with treatment planning, prognostic decision making, and research on pathophysiological mechanisms. Section III "Assessment Measures" also contains dimensional assessments of the primary symptoms of psychosis, including hallucinations, delusions, disorganized speech (except for substance/medication-induced psychotic disorder and psychotic disorder due to another medical condition), abnormal psychomotor behavior, and negative symptoms, as well as dimensional assessments of depression and mania. The severity of mood symptoms in psychosis has prognostic value and guides treatment. There is growing evidence that schizoaffective disorder is not a distinct nosological category. Thus, dimensional assessments of depression and mania for all psychotic disorders alert clinicians to mood pathology and the need to treat where appropriate. The Section III scale also includes a dimensional assessment of cognitive impairment. Many individuals with psychotic disorders have impairments in a range of cognitive domains that predict functional status. Clinical neuropsychological assessment can help guide diagnosis and treatment, but brief assessments without formal neuropsychological assessment can provide useful information that can be sufficient for diagnostic purposes. Formal neuropsychological testing, when conducted, should be administered and scored by personnel trained in the use of testing instruments. If a formal neuropsychological assessment is not conducted, the clinician should use the best available information to make a judgment. Further research on these assessments is necessary in order to determine their clinical utility; thus, the assessments available in Section III should serve as a prototype to stimulate such research.

Schizotypal (Personality) Disorder

Criteria and text for schizotypal personality disorder can be found in the chapter "Personality Disorders." Because this disorder is considered part of the schizophrenia spectrum of disorders, and is labeled in this section of ICD-9 and ICD-10 as schizotypal disorder, it is listed in this chapter and discussed in detail in the DSM-5 chapter "Personality Disorders."

Delusional Disorder

Diagnostic Criteria   297.1 (F22)

A. The presence of one (or more) delusions with a duration of 1 month or longer.
B. Criterion A for schizophrenia has never been met.
   Note: Hallucinations, if present, are not prominent and are related to the delusional theme (e.g., the sensation of being infested with insects associated with delusions of infestation).
C. Apart from the impact of the delusion(s) or its ramifications, functioning is not markedly impaired, and behavior is not obviously bizarre or odd.
D. If manic or major depressive episodes have occurred, these have been brief relative to the duration of the delusional periods.
E. The disturbance is not attributable to the physiological effects of a substance or another medical condition and is not better explained by another mental disorder, such as body dysmorphic disorder or obsessive-compulsive disorder.

Specify whether:
   Erotomanic type: This subtype applies when the central theme of the delusion is that another person is in love with the individual.
   Grandiose type: This subtype applies when the central theme of the delusion is the conviction of having some great (but unrecognized) talent or insight or having made some important discovery.
   Jealous type: This subtype applies when the central theme of the individual's delusion is that his or her spouse or lover is unfaithful.
   Persecutory type: This subtype applies when the central theme of the delusion involves the individual's belief that he or she is being conspired against, cheated, spied on, followed, poisoned or drugged, maliciously maligned, harassed, or obstructed in the pursuit of long-term goals.
   Somatic type: This subtype applies when the central theme of the delusion involves bodily functions or sensations.

Mixed type: This subtype applies when no one delusional theme predominates.

Unspecified type: This subtype applies when the dominant delusional belief cannot be clearly determined or is not described in the specific types (e.g., referential delusions without a prominent persecutory or grandiose component).

Specify if:

With bizarre content: Delusions are deemed bizarre if they are clearly implausible, not understandable, and not derived from ordinary life experiences (e.g., an individual's belief that a stranger has removed his or her internal organs and replaced them with someone else's organs without leaving any wounds or scars).

Specify if:

The following course specifiers are only to be used after a 1-year duration of the disorder:

First episode, currently in acute episode: First manifestation of the disorder meeting the defining diagnostic symptom and time criteria. An *acute episode* is a time period in which the symptom criteria are fulfilled.

First episode, currently in partial remission: *Partial remission* is a time period during which an improvement after a previous episode is maintained and in which the defining criteria of the disorder are only partially fulfilled.

First episode, currently in full remission: *Full remission* is a period of time after a previous episode during which no disorder-specific symptoms are present.

Multiple episodes, currently in acute episode

Multiple episodes, currently in partial remission

Multiple episodes, currently in full remission

Continuous: Symptoms fulfilling the diagnostic symptom criteria of the disorder are remaining for the majority of the illness course, with subthreshold symptom periods being very brief relative to the overall course.

Unspecified

Specify current severity:

Severity is rated by a quantitative assessment of the primary symptoms of psychosis, including delusions, hallucinations, disorganized speech, abnormal psychomotor behavior, and negative symptoms. Each of these symptoms may be rated for its current severity (most severe in the last 7 days) on a 5-point scale ranging from 0 (not present) to 4 (present and severe). (See Clinician-Rated Dimensions of Psychosis Symptom Severity in the chapter "Assessment Measures.")

Note: Diagnosis of delusional disorder can be made without using this severity specifier.

Subtypes

In *erotomanic type,* the central theme of the delusion is that another person is in love with the individual. The person about whom this conviction is held is usually of higher status (e.g., a famous individual or a superior at work) but can be a complete stranger. Efforts to contact the object of the delusion are common. In *grandiose type,* the central theme of the delusion is the conviction of having some great talent or insight or of having made some important discovery. Less commonly, the individual may have the delusion of having a special relationship with a prominent individual or of being a prominent person (in which case the actual individual may be regarded as an impostor). Grandiose delusions may have a religious content. In *jealous type,* the central theme of the delusion is that of an unfaithful partner. This belief is arrived at without due cause and is based on incorrect inferences supported by small bits of "evidence" (e.g., disarrayed clothing). The individual with the delusion usually confronts the spouse or lover and attempts to intervene in the imagined infidelity. In *persecutory type,* the central theme of the delusion involves the in-

most common

dividual's belief of being conspired against, cheated, spied on, followed, poisoned, maliciously maligned, harassed, or obstructed in the pursuit of long-term goals. Small slights may be exaggerated and become the focus of a delusional system. The affected individual may engage in repeated attempts to obtain satisfaction by legal or legislative action. Individuals with persecutory delusions are often resentful and angry and may resort to violence against those they believe are hurting them. In *somatic type,* the central theme of the delusion involves bodily functions or sensations. Somatic delusions can occur in several forms. Most common is the belief that the individual emits a foul odor; that there is an infestation of insects on or in the skin; that there is an internal parasite; or that parts of the body are not functioning.

Diagnostic Features

The essential feature of delusional disorder is the presence of one or more delusions that persist for at least 1 month (Criterion A). A diagnosis of delusional disorder is not given if the individual has ever had a symptom presentation that met Criterion A for schizophrenia (Criterion B). Apart from the direct impact of the delusions, impairments in psychosocial functioning may be more circumscribed than those seen in other psychotic disorders such as schizophrenia, and behavior is not obviously bizarre or odd (Criterion C). If mood episodes occur concurrently with the delusions, the total duration of these mood episodes is brief relative to the total duration of the delusional periods (Criterion D). The delusions are not attributable to the physiological effects of a substance (e.g., cocaine) or another medical condition (e.g., Alzheimer's disease) and are not better explained by another mental disorder, such as body dysmorphic disorder or obsessive-compulsive disorder (Criterion E).

In addition to the five symptom domain areas identified in the diagnostic criteria, the assessment of cognition, depression, and mania symptom domains is vital for making critically important distinctions between the various schizophrenia spectrum and other psychotic disorders.

Associated Features Supporting Diagnosis

Social, marital, or work problems can result from the delusional beliefs of delusional disorder. Individuals with delusional disorder may be able to factually describe that others view their beliefs as irrational but are unable to accept this themselves (i.e., there may be "factual insight" but no true insight). Many individuals develop irritable or dysphoric mood, which can usually be understood as a reaction to their delusional beliefs. Anger and violent behavior can occur with persecutory, jealous, and erotomanic types. The individual may engage in litigious or antagonistic behavior (e.g., sending hundreds of letters of protest to the government). Legal difficulties can occur, particularly in jealous and erotomanic types.

Prevalence

The lifetime prevalence of delusional disorder has been estimated at around 0.2%, and the most frequent subtype is persecutory. Delusional disorder, jealous type, is probably more common in males than in females, but there are no major gender differences in the overall frequency of delusional disorder.

Development and Course

On average, global function is generally better than that observed in schizophrenia. Although the diagnosis is generally stable, a proportion of individuals go on to develop schizophrenia. Delusional disorder has a significant familial relationship with both schizophrenia and schizotypal personality disorder. Although it can occur in younger age groups, the condition may be more prevalent in older individuals.

Culture-Related Diagnostic Issues

An individual's cultural and religious background must be taken into account in evaluating the possible presence of delusional disorder. The content of delusions also varies across cultural contexts.

Functional Consequences of Delusional Disorder

The functional impairment is usually more circumscribed than that seen with other psychotic disorders, although in some cases, the impairment may be substantial and include poor occupational functioning and social isolation. When poor psychosocial functioning is present, delusional beliefs themselves often play a significant role. A common characteristic of individuals with delusional disorder is the apparent normality of their behavior and appearance when their delusional ideas are not being discussed or acted on.

Differential Diagnosis

Obsessive-compulsive and related disorders.   If an individual with obsessive-compulsive disorder is completely convinced that his or her obsessive-compulsive disorder beliefs are true, then the diagnosis of obsessive-compulsive disorder, with absent insight/delusional beliefs specifier, should be given rather than a diagnosis of delusional disorder. Similarly, if an individual with body dysmorphic disorder is completely convinced that his or her body dysmorphic disorder beliefs are true, then the diagnosis of body dysmorphic disorder, with absent insight/delusional beliefs specifier, should be given rather than a diagnosis of delusional disorder.

Delirium, major neurocognitive disorder, psychotic disorder due to another medical condition, and substance/medication-induced psychotic disorder.   Individuals with these disorders may present with symptoms that suggest delusional disorder. For example, simple persecutory delusions in the context of major neurocognitive disorder would be diagnosed as major neurocognitive disorder, with behavioral disturbance. A substance/medication-induced psychotic disorder cross-sectionally may be identical in symptomatology to delusional disorder but can be distinguished by the chronological relationship of substance use to the onset and remission of the delusional beliefs.

Schizophrenia and schizophreniform disorder.   Delusional disorder can be distinguished from schizophrenia and schizophreniform disorder by the absence of the other characteristic symptoms of the active phase of schizophrenia.

Depressive and bipolar disorders and schizoaffective disorder.   These disorders may be distinguished from delusional disorder by the temporal relationship between the mood disturbance and the delusions and by the severity of the mood symptoms. If delusions occur exclusively during mood episodes, the diagnosis is depressive or bipolar disorder with psychotic features. Mood symptoms that meet full criteria for a mood episode can be superimposed on delusional disorder. Delusional disorder can be diagnosed only if the total duration of all mood episodes remains brief relative to the total duration of the delusional disturbance. If not, then a diagnosis of other specified or unspecified schizophrenia spectrum and other psychotic disorder accompanied by other specified depressive disorder, unspecified depressive disorder, other specified bipolar and related disorder, or unspecified bipolar and related disorder is appropriate.

Brief Psychotic Disorder

Diagnostic Criteria   **298.8** (F23)

A. Presence of one (or more) of the following symptoms. At least one of these must be (1), (2), or (3):

1. Delusions.
2. Hallucinations.
3. Disorganized speech (e.g., frequent derailment or incoherence).
4. Grossly disorganized or catatonic behavior.

Note: Do not include a symptom if it is a culturally sanctioned response.

B. Duration of an episode of the disturbance is at least 1 day but less than 1 month, with eventual full return to premorbid level of functioning.

C. The disturbance is not better explained by major depressive or bipolar disorder with psychotic features or another psychotic disorder such as schizophrenia or catatonia, and is not attributable to the physiological effects of a substance (e.g., a drug of abuse, a medication) or another medical condition.

Specify if:

With marked stressor(s) (brief reactive psychosis): If symptoms occur in response to events that, singly or together, would be markedly stressful to almost anyone in similar circumstances in the individual's culture.

Without marked stressor(s): If symptoms do not occur in response to events that, singly or together, would be markedly stressful to almost anyone in similar circumstances in the individual's culture.

With peripartum onset: If onset is during pregnancy or within 4 weeks postpartum.

Specify if:

With catatonia (refer to the criteria for catatonia associated with another mental disorder, pp. 119–120, for definition)

    Coding note: Use additional code 293.89 (F06.1) catatonia associated with brief psychotic disorder to indicate the presence of the comorbid catatonia.

Specify current severity:

Severity is rated by a quantitative assessment of the primary symptoms of psychosis, including delusions, hallucinations, disorganized speech, abnormal psychomotor behavior, and negative symptoms. Each of these symptoms may be rated for its current severity (most severe in the last 7 days) on a 5-point scale ranging from 0 (not present) to 4 (present and severe). (See Clinician-Rated Dimensions of Psychosis Symptom Severity in the chapter "Assessment Measures.")

Note: Diagnosis of brief psychotic disorder can be made without using this severity specifier.

Diagnostic Features

The essential feature of brief psychotic disorder is a disturbance that involves the sudden onset of at least one of the following positive psychotic symptoms: delusions, hallucinations, disorganized speech (e.g., frequent derailment or incoherence), or grossly abnormal psychomotor behavior, including catatonia (Criterion A). *Sudden onset* is defined as change from a nonpsychotic state to a clearly psychotic state within 2 weeks, usually without a prodrome. An episode of the disturbance lasts at least 1 day but less than 1 month, and the individual eventually has a full return to the premorbid level of functioning (Criterion B). The disturbance is not better explained by a depressive or bipolar disorder with psychotic features, by schizoaffective disorder, or by schizophrenia and is not attributable to the physiological effects of a substance (e.g., a hallucinogen) or another medical condition (e.g., subdural hematoma) (Criterion C).

In addition to the five symptom domain areas identified in the diagnostic criteria, the assessment of cognition, depression, and mania symptom domains is vital for making critically important distinctions between the various schizophrenia spectrum and other psychotic disorders.

Associated Features Supporting Diagnosis

Individuals with brief psychotic disorder typically experience emotional turmoil or overwhelming confusion. They may have rapid shifts from one intense affect to another. Although the disturbance is brief, the level of impairment may be severe, and supervision may be required to ensure that nutritional and hygienic needs are met and that the individual is protected from the consequences of poor judgment, cognitive impairment, or acting on the basis of delusions. There appears to be an increased risk of suicidal behavior, particularly during the acute episode.

Prevalence

In the United States, brief psychotic disorder may account for 9% of cases of first-onset psychosis. Psychotic disturbances that meet Criteria A and C, but not Criterion B, for brief psychotic disorder (i.e., duration of active symptoms is 1–6 months as opposed to remission within 1 month) are more common in developing countries than in developed countries. Brief psychotic disorder is twofold more common in females than in males.

Development and Course

Brief psychotic disorder may appear in adolescence or early adulthood, and onset can occur across the lifespan, with the average age at onset being the mid 30s. By definition, a diagnosis of brief psychotic disorder requires a full remission of all symptoms and an eventual full return to the premorbid level of functioning within 1 month of the onset of the disturbance. In some individuals, the duration of psychotic symptoms may be quite brief (e.g., a few days).

Risk and Prognostic Factors

Temperamental.   Preexisting personality disorders and traits (e.g., schizotypal personality disorder; borderline personality disorder; or traits in the psychoticism domain, such as perceptual dysregulation, and the negative affectivity domain, such as suspiciousness) may predispose the individual to the development of the disorder.

Culture-Related Diagnostic Issues

It is important to distinguish symptoms of brief psychotic disorder from culturally sanctioned response patterns. For example, in some religious ceremonies, an individual may report hearing voices, but these do not generally persist and are not perceived as abnormal by most members of the individual's community. In addition, cultural and religious background must be taken into account when considering whether beliefs are delusional.

Functional Consequences of Brief Psychotic Disorder

Despite high rates of relapse, for most individuals, outcome is excellent in terms of social functioning and symptomatology.

Differential Diagnosis

Other medical conditions. A variety of medical disorders can manifest with psychotic symptoms of short duration. Psychotic disorder due to another medical condition or a delirium is diagnosed when there is evidence from the history, physical examination, or laboratory tests that the delusions or hallucinations are the direct physiological consequence of a specific medical condition (e.g., Cushing's syndrome, brain tumor) (see "Psychotic Disorder Due to Another Medical Condition" later in this chapter).

Substance-related disorders. Substance/medication-induced psychotic disorder, substance-induced delirium, and substance intoxication are distinguished from brief psychotic disorder by the fact that a substance (e.g., a drug of abuse, a medication, exposure to a toxin) is judged to be etiologically related to the psychotic symptoms (see "Substance/Medication-Induced Psychotic Disorder" later in this chapter). Laboratory tests, such as a urine drug screen or a blood alcohol level, may be helpful in making this determination, as may a careful history of substance use with attention to temporal relationships between substance intake and onset of the symptoms and to the nature of the substance being used.

Depressive and bipolar disorders. The diagnosis of brief psychotic disorder cannot be made if the psychotic symptoms are better explained by a mood episode (i.e., the psychotic symptoms occur exclusively during a full major depressive, manic, or mixed episode).

Other psychotic disorders. If the psychotic symptoms persist for 1 month or longer, the diagnosis is either schizophreniform disorder, delusional disorder, depressive disorder with psychotic features, bipolar disorder with psychotic features, or other specified or unspecified schizophrenia spectrum and other psychotic disorder, depending on the other symptoms in the presentation. The differential diagnosis between brief psychotic disorder and schizophreniform disorder is difficult when the psychotic symptoms have remitted before 1 month in response to successful treatment with medication. Careful attention should be given to the possibility that a recurrent disorder (e.g., bipolar disorder, recurrent acute exacerbations of schizophrenia) may be responsible for any recurring psychotic episodes.

Malingering and factitious disorders. An episode of factitious disorder, with predominantly psychological signs and symptoms, may have the appearance of brief psychotic disorder, but in such cases there is evidence that the symptoms are intentionally produced. When malingering involves apparently psychotic symptoms, there is usually evidence that the illness is being feigned for an understandable goal.

Personality disorders. In certain individuals with personality disorders, psychosocial stressors may precipitate brief periods of psychotic symptoms. These symptoms are usually transient and do not warrant a separate diagnosis. If psychotic symptoms persist for at least 1 day, an additional diagnosis of brief psychotic disorder may be appropriate.

Schizophreniform Disorder

Diagnostic Criteria   **295.40 (F20.81)**

A. Two (or more) of the following, each present for a significant portion of time during a 1-month period (or less if successfully treated). At least one of these must be (1), (2), or (3):

   1. Delusions.
   2. Hallucinations.
   3. Disorganized speech (e.g., frequent derailment or incoherence).
   4. Grossly disorganized or catatonic behavior.
   5. Negative symptoms (i.e., diminished emotional expression or avolition).

B. An episode of the disorder lasts at least 1 month but less than 6 months. When the diagnosis must be made without waiting for recovery, it should be qualified as "provisional."

C. Schizoaffective disorder and depressive or bipolar disorder with psychotic features have been ruled out because either 1) no major depressive or manic episodes have occurred concurrently with the active-phase symptoms, or 2) if mood episodes have occurred during active-phase symptoms, they have been present for a minority of the total duration of the active and residual periods of the illness.

D. The disturbance is not attributable to the physiological effects of a substance (e.g., a drug of abuse, a medication) or another medical condition.

Specify if:

With good prognostic features: This specifier requires the presence of at least two of the following features: onset of prominent psychotic symptoms within 4 weeks of the first noticeable change in usual behavior or functioning; confusion or perplexity; good premorbid social and occupational functioning; and absence of blunted or flat affect.

Without good prognostic features: This specifier is applied if two or more of the above features have not been present.

Specify if:

With catatonia (refer to the criteria for catatonia associated with another mental disorder, pp. 119–120, for definition).

Coding note: Use additional code 293.89 (F06.1) catatonia associated with schizophreniform disorder to indicate the presence of the comorbid catatonia.

Specify current severity:

Severity is rated by a quantitative assessment of the primary symptoms of psychosis, including delusions, hallucinations, disorganized speech, abnormal psychomotor behavior, and negative symptoms. Each of these symptoms may be rated for its current severity (most severe in the last 7 days) on a 5-point scale ranging from 0 (not present) to 4 (present and severe). (See Clinician-Rated Dimensions of Psychosis Symptom Severity in the chapter "Assessment Measures.")

Note: Diagnosis of schizophreniform disorder can be made without using this severity specifier.

Note: For additional information on Associated Features Supporting Diagnosis, Development and Course (age-related factors), Culture-Related Diagnostic Issues, Gender-Related Diagnostic Issues, Differential Diagnosis, and Comorbidity, see the corresponding sections in schizophrenia.

Diagnostic Features

The characteristic symptoms of schizophreniform disorder are identical to those of schizophrenia (Criterion A). Schizophreniform disorder is distinguished by its difference in duration: the total duration of the illness, including prodromal, active, and residual phases, is at least 1 month but less than 6 months (Criterion B). The duration requirement for schizophreniform disorder is intermediate between that for brief psychotic disorder, which lasts more than 1 day and remits by 1 month, and schizophrenia, which lasts for at least 6 months. The diagnosis of schizophreniform disorder is made under two conditions: 1) when an episode of illness lasts between 1 and 6 months and the individual has already recovered, and 2) when an individual is symptomatic for less than the 6 months' duration required for the diagnosis of schizophrenia but has not yet recovered. In this case, the diagnosis should be noted as "schizophreniform disorder (provisional)" because it is uncertain if the individual will recover from the disturbance within the 6-month period. If the disturbance persists beyond 6 months, the diagnosis should be changed to schizophrenia.

Another distinguishing feature of schizophreniform disorder is the lack of a criterion requiring impaired social and occupational functioning. While such impairments may potentially be present, they are not necessary for a diagnosis of schizophreniform disorder.

In addition to the five symptom domain areas identified in the diagnostic criteria, the assessment of cognition, depression, and mania symptom domains is vital for making critically important distinctions between the various schizophrenia spectrum and other psychotic disorders.

Associated Features Supporting Diagnosis

As with schizophrenia, currently there are no laboratory or psychometric tests for schizophreniform disorder. There are multiple brain regions where neuroimaging, neuropathological, and neurophysiological research has indicated abnormalities, but none are diagnostic.

Prevalence

Incidence of schizophreniform disorder across sociocultural settings is likely similar to that observed in schizophrenia. In the United States and other developed countries, the incidence is low, possibly fivefold less than that of schizophrenia. In developing countries, the incidence may be higher, especially for the specifier "with good prognostic features"; in some of these settings schizophreniform disorder may be as common as schizophrenia.

Development and Course

The development of schizophreniform disorder is similar to that of schizophrenia. About one-third of individuals with an initial diagnosis of schizophreniform disorder (provisional) recover within the 6-month period and schizophreniform disorder is their final diagnosis. The majority of the remaining two-thirds of individuals will eventually receive a diagnosis of schizophrenia or schizoaffective disorder.

Risk and Prognostic Factors

Genetic and physiological.   Relatives of individuals with schizophreniform disorder have an increased risk for schizophrenia.

Functional Consequences of Schizophreniform Disorder

For the majority of individuals with schizophreniform disorder who eventually receive a diagnosis of schizophrenia or schizoaffective disorder, the functional consequences are similar to the consequences of those disorders. Most individuals experience dysfunction in several areas of daily functioning, such as school or work, interpersonal relationships, and self-care. Individuals who recover from schizophreniform disorder have better functional outcomes.

Differential Diagnosis

Other mental disorders and medical conditions.   A wide variety of mental and medical conditions can manifest with psychotic symptoms that must be considered in the differential diagnosis of schizophreniform disorder. These include psychotic disorder due to another medical condition or its treatment; delirium or major neurocognitive disorder; substance/medication-induced psychotic disorder or delirium; depressive or bipolar disorder with psychotic features; schizoaffective disorder; other specified or unspecified bipolar and related disorder; depressive or bipolar disorder with catatonic features; schizophrenia; brief psychotic disorder; delusional disorder; other specified or unspecified schizo-phrenia spectrum and other psychotic disorder; schizotypal, schizoid, or paranoid personality disorders; autism spectrum disorder; disorders presenting in childhood with disorganized speech; attention-deficit/hyperactivity disorder; obsessive-compulsive disorder; posttraumatic stress disorder; and traumatic brain injury.

Since the diagnostic criteria for schizophreniform disorder and schizophrenia differ primarily in duration of illness, the discussion of the differential diagnosis of schizophrenia also applies to schizophreniform disorder.

Brief psychotic disorder.   Schizophreniform disorder differs in duration from brief psychotic disorder, which has a duration of less than 1 month.

Schizophrenia

Diagnostic Criteria	295.90 (F20.9)

A. Two (or more) of the following, each present for a significant portion of time during a 1-month period (or less if successfully treated). At least one of these must be (1), (2), or (3):

   1. Delusions.
   2. Hallucinations.
   3. Disorganized speech (e.g., frequent derailment or incoherence).
   4. Grossly disorganized or catatonic behavior.
   5. Negative symptoms (i.e., diminished emotional expression or avolition).

B. For a significant portion of the time since the onset of the disturbance, level of functioning in one or more major areas, such as work, interpersonal relations, or self-care, is markedly below the level achieved prior to the onset (or when the onset is in childhood or adolescence, there is failure to achieve expected level of interpersonal, academic, or occupational functioning).

C. Continuous signs of the disturbance persist for at least 6 months. This 6-month period must include at least 1 month of symptoms (or less if successfully treated) that meet Criterion A (i.e., active-phase symptoms) and may include periods of prodromal or residual symptoms. During these prodromal or residual periods, the signs of the disturbance may be manifested by only negative symptoms or by two or more symptoms listed in Criterion A present in an attenuated form (e.g., odd beliefs, unusual perceptual experiences).

D. Schizoaffective disorder and depressive or bipolar disorder with psychotic features have been ruled out because either 1) no major depressive or manic episodes have occurred concurrently with the active-phase symptoms, or 2) if mood episodes have occurred during active-phase symptoms, they have been present for a minority of the total duration of the active and residual periods of the illness.

E. The disturbance is not attributable to the physiological effects of a substance (e.g., a drug of abuse, a medication) or another medical condition.

F. If there is a history of autism spectrum disorder or a communication disorder of childhood onset, the additional diagnosis of schizophrenia is made only if prominent delusions or hallucinations, in addition to the other required symptoms of schizophrenia, are also present for at least 1 month (or less if successfully treated).

Specify if:
The following course specifiers are only to be used after a 1-year duration of the disorder and if they are not in contradiction to the diagnostic course criteria.

   First episode, currently in acute episode: First manifestation of the disorder meeting the defining diagnostic symptom and time criteria. An *acute episode* is a time period in which the symptom criteria are fulfilled.

First episode, currently in partial remission: *Partial remission* is a period of time during which an improvement after a previous episode is maintained and in which the defining criteria of the disorder are only partially fulfilled.

First episode, currently in full remission: *Full remission* is a period of time after a previous episode during which no disorder-specific symptoms are present.

Multiple episodes, currently in acute episode: Multiple episodes may be determined after a minimum of two episodes (i.e., after a first episode, a remission and a minimum of one relapse).

Multiple episodes, currently in partial remission

Multiple episodes, currently in full remission

Continuous: Symptoms fulfilling the diagnostic symptom criteria of the disorder are remaining for the majority of the illness course, with subthreshold symptom periods being very brief relative to the overall course.

Unspecified

Specify if:

With catatonia (refer to the criteria for catatonia associated with another mental disorder, pp. 119–120, for definition).

> **Coding note:** Use additional code 293.89 (F06.1) catatonia associated with schizophrenia to indicate the presence of the comorbid catatonia.

Specify current severity:

Severity is rated by a quantitative assessment of the primary symptoms of psychosis, including delusions, hallucinations, disorganized speech, abnormal psychomotor behavior, and negative symptoms. Each of these symptoms may be rated for its current severity (most severe in the last 7 days) on a 5-point scale ranging from 0 (not present) to 4 (present and severe). (See Clinician-Rated Dimensions of Psychosis Symptom Severity in the chapter "Assessment Measures.")

Note: Diagnosis of schizophrenia can be made without using this severity specifier.

Diagnostic Features

The characteristic symptoms of schizophrenia involve a range of cognitive, behavioral, and emotional dysfunctions, but no single symptom is pathognomonic of the disorder. The diagnosis involves the recognition of a constellation of signs and symptoms associated with impaired occupational or social functioning. Individuals with the disorder will vary substantially on most features, as schizophrenia is a heterogeneous clinical syndrome.

At least two Criterion A symptoms must be present for a significant portion of time during a 1-month period or longer. At least one of these symptoms must be the clear presence of delusions (Criterion A1), hallucinations (Criterion A2), or disorganized speech (Criterion A3). Grossly disorganized or catatonic behavior (Criterion A4) and negative symptoms (Criterion A5) may also be present. In those situations in which the active-phase symptoms remit within a month in response to treatment, Criterion A is still met if the clinician estimates that they would have persisted in the absence of treatment.

Schizophrenia involves impairment in one or more major areas of functioning (Criterion B). If the disturbance begins in childhood or adolescence, the expected level of function is not attained. Comparing the individual with unaffected siblings may be helpful. The dysfunction persists for a substantial period during the course of the disorder and does not appear to be a direct result of any single feature. Avolition (i.e., reduced drive to pursue goal-directed behavior; Criterion A5) is linked to the social dysfunction described under Criterion B. There is also strong evidence for a relationship between cognitive impairment (see the section "Associated Features Supporting Diagnosis" for this disorder) and functional impairment in individuals with schizophrenia.

Some signs of the disturbance must persist for a continuous period of at least 6 months (Criterion C). Prodromal symptoms often precede the active phase, and residual symptoms may follow it, characterized by mild or subthreshold forms of hallucinations or delusions. Individuals may express a variety of unusual or odd beliefs that are not of delusional proportions (e.g., ideas of reference or magical thinking); they may have unusual perceptual experiences (e.g., sensing the presence of an unseen person); their speech may be generally understandable but vague; and their behavior may be unusual but not grossly disorganized (e.g., mumbling in public). Negative symptoms are common in the prodromal and residual phases and can be severe. Individuals who had been socially active may become withdrawn from previous routines. Such behaviors are often the first sign of a disorder.

Mood symptoms and full mood episodes are common in schizophrenia and may be concurrent with active-phase symptomatology. However, as distinct from a psychotic mood disorder, a schizophrenia diagnosis requires the presence of delusions or hallucinations in the absence of mood episodes. In addition, mood episodes, taken in total, should be present for only a minority of the total duration of the active and residual periods of the illness.

In addition to the five symptom domain areas identified in the diagnostic criteria, the assessment of cognition, depression, and mania symptom domains is vital for making critically important distinctions between the various schizophrenia spectrum and other psychotic disorders.

Associated Features Supporting Diagnosis

Individuals with schizophrenia may display inappropriate affect (e.g., laughing in the absence of an appropriate stimulus); a dysphoric mood that can take the form of depression, anxiety, or anger; a disturbed sleep pattern (e.g., daytime sleeping and nighttime activity); and a lack of interest in eating or food refusal. Depersonalization, derealization, and somatic concerns may occur and sometimes reach delusional proportions. Anxiety and phobias are common. Cognitive deficits in schizophrenia are common and are strongly linked to vocational and functional impairments. These deficits can include decrements in declarative memory, working memory, language function, and other executive functions, as well as slower processing speed. Abnormalities in sensory processing and inhibitory capacity, as well as reductions in attention, are also found. Some individuals with schizophrenia show social cognition deficits, including deficits in the ability to infer the intentions of other people (theory of mind), and may attend to and then interpret irrelevant events or stimuli as meaningful, perhaps leading to the generation of explanatory delusions. These impairments frequently persist during symptomatic remission.

Some individuals with psychosis may lack insight or awareness of their disorder (i.e., anosognosia). This lack of "insight" includes unawareness of symptoms of schizophrenia and may be present throughout the entire course of the illness. Unawareness of illness is typically a symptom of schizophrenia itself rather than a coping strategy. It is comparable to the lack of awareness of neurological deficits following brain damage, termed *anosognosia*. This symptom is the most common predictor of non-adherence to treatment, and it predicts higher relapse rates, increased number of involuntary treatments, poorer psychosocial functioning, aggression, and a poorer course of illness.

Hostility and aggression can be associated with schizophrenia, although spontaneous or random assault is uncommon. Aggression is more frequent for younger males and for individuals with a past history of violence, non-adherence with treatment, substance abuse, and impulsivity. It should be noted that the vast majority of persons with schizophrenia are not aggressive and are more frequently victimized than are individuals in the general population.

Currently, there are no radiological, laboratory, or psychometric tests for the disorder. Differences are evident in multiple brain regions between groups of healthy individuals and persons with schizophrenia, including evidence from neuroimaging, neuropathological, and neurophysiological studies. Differences are also evident in cellular architecture, white matter connectivity, and gray matter volume in a variety of regions such as the prefrontal and temporal cortices. Reduced overall brain volume has been observed, as well as increased brain volume reduction with age. Brain volume reductions with age are more pronounced in individuals with schizophrenia than in healthy individuals. Finally, individuals with schizophrenia appear to differ from individuals without the disorder in eye-tracking and electrophysiological indices.

Neurological soft signs common in individuals with schizophrenia include impairments in motor coordination, sensory integration, and motor sequencing of complex movements; left-right confusion; and disinhibition of associated movements. In addition, minor physical anomalies of the face and limbs may occur.

Prevalence

The lifetime prevalence of schizophrenia appears to be approximately 0.3%–0.7%, although there is reported variation by race/ethnicity, across countries, and by geographic origin for immigrants and children of immigrants. The sex ratio differs across samples and populations: for example, an emphasis on negative symptoms and longer duration of disorder (associated with poorer outcome) shows higher incidence rates for males, whereas definitions allowing for the inclusion of more mood symptoms and brief presentations (associated with better outcome) show equivalent risks for both sexes.

Development and Course

The psychotic features of schizophrenia typically emerge between the late teens and the mid-30s; onset prior to adolescence is rare. The peak age at onset for the first psychotic episode is in the early- to mid-20s for males and in the late-20s for females. The onset may be abrupt or insidious, but the majority of individuals manifest a slow and gradual development of a variety of clinically significant signs and symptoms. Half of these individuals complain of depressive symptoms. Earlier age at onset has traditionally been seen as a predictor of worse prognosis. However, the effect of age at onset is likely related to gender, with males having worse premorbid adjustment, lower educational achievement, more prominent negative symptoms and cognitive impairment, and in general a worse outcome. Impaired cognition is common, and alterations in cognition are present during development and precede the emergence of psychosis, taking the form of stable cognitive impairments during adulthood. Cognitive impairments may persist when other symptoms are in remission and contribute to the disability of the disease.

The predictors of course and outcome are largely unexplained, and course and outcome may not be reliably predicted. The course appears to be favorable in about 20% of those with schizophrenia, and a small number of individuals are reported to recover completely. However, most individuals with schizophrenia still require formal or informal daily living supports, and many remain chronically ill, with exacerbations and remissions of active symptoms, while others have a course of progressive deterioration.

Psychotic symptoms tend to diminish over the life course, perhaps in association with normal age-related declines in dopamine activity. Negative symptoms are more closely related to prognosis than are positive symptoms and tend to be the most persistent. Furthermore, cognitive deficits associated with the illness may not improve over the course of the illness.

The essential features of schizophrenia are the same in childhood, but it is more difficult to make the diagnosis. In children, delusions and hallucinations may be less elaborate than in adults, and visual hallucinations are more common and should be distinguished from normal fantasy play. Disorganized speech occurs in many disorders with childhood onset (e.g., autism spectrum disorder), as does disorganized behavior (e.g., attention-deficit/

hyperactivity disorder). These symptoms should not be attributed to schizophrenia without due consideration of the more common disorders of childhood. Childhood-onset cases tend to resemble poor-outcome adult cases, with gradual onset and prominent negative symptoms. Children who later receive the diagnosis of schizophrenia are more likely to have experienced nonspecific emotional-behavioral disturbances and psychopathology, intellectual and language alterations, and subtle motor delays.

Late-onset cases (i.e., onset after age 40 years) are overrepresented by females, who may have married. Often, the course is characterized by a predominance of psychotic symptoms with preservation of affect and social functioning. Such late-onset cases can still meet the diagnostic criteria for schizophrenia, but it is not yet clear whether this is the same condition as schizophrenia diagnosed prior to mid-life (e.g., prior to age 55 years).

Risk and Prognostic Factors

Environmental.   Season of birth has been linked to the incidence of schizophrenia, including late winter/early spring in some locations and summer for the deficit form of the disease. The incidence of schizophrenia and related disorders is higher for children growing up in an urban environment and for some minority ethnic groups.

Genetic and physiological.   There is a strong contribution for genetic factors in determining risk for schizophrenia, although most individuals who have been diagnosed with schizophrenia have no family history of psychosis. Liability is conferred by a spectrum of risk alleles, common and rare, with each allele contributing only a small fraction to the total population variance. The risk alleles identified to date are also associated with other mental disorders, including bipolar disorder, depression, and autism spectrum disorder.

Pregnancy and birth complications with hypoxia and greater paternal age are associated with a higher risk of schizophrenia for the developing fetus. In addition, other prenatal and perinatal adversities, including stress, infection, malnutrition, maternal diabetes, and other medical conditions, have been linked with schizophrenia. However, the vast majority of offspring with these risk factors do not develop schizophrenia.

Culture-Related Diagnostic Issues

Cultural and socioeconomic factors must be considered, particularly when the individual and the clinician do not share the same cultural and socioeconomic background. Ideas that appear to be delusional in one culture (e.g., witchcraft) may be commonly held in another. In some cultures, visual or auditory hallucinations with a religious content (e.g., hearing God's voice) are a normal part of religious experience. In addition, the assessment of disorganized speech may be made difficult by linguistic variation in narrative styles across cultures. The assessment of affect requires sensitivity to differences in styles of emotional expression, eye contact, and body language, which vary across cultures. If the assessment is conducted in a language that is different from the individual's primary language, care must be taken to ensure that alogia is not related to linguistic barriers. In certain cultures, distress may take the form of hallucinations or pseudo-hallucinations and overvalued ideas that may present clinically similar to true psychosis but are normative to the patient's subgroup.

Gender-Related Diagnostic Issues

A number of features distinguish the clinical expression of schizophrenia in females and males. The general incidence of schizophrenia tends to be slightly lower in females, particularly among treated cases. The age at onset is later in females, with a second mid-life peak as described earlier (see the section "Development and Course" for this disorder). Symptoms tend to be more affect-laden among females, and there are more psychotic symptoms, as well as a greater propensity for psychotic symptoms to worsen in later life.

Other symptom differences include less frequent negative symptoms and disorganization. Finally, social functioning tends to remain better preserved in females. There are, however, frequent exceptions to these general caveats.

Suicide Risk

Approximately 5%–6% of individuals with schizophrenia die by suicide, about 20% attempt suicide on one or more occasions, and many more have significant suicidal ideation. Suicidal behavior is sometimes in response to command hallucinations to harm oneself or others. Suicide risk remains high over the whole lifespan for males and females, although it may be especially high for younger males with comorbid substance use. Other risk factors include having depressive symptoms or feelings of hopelessness and being unemployed, and the risk is higher, also, in the period after a psychotic episode or hospital discharge.

Functional Consequences of Schizophrenia

Schizophrenia is associated with significant social and occupational dysfunction. Making educational progress and maintaining employment are frequently impaired by avolition or other disorder manifestations, even when the cognitive skills are sufficient for the tasks at hand. Most individuals are employed at a lower level than their parents, and most, particularly men, do not marry or have limited social contacts outside of their family.

Differential Diagnosis

Major depressive or bipolar disorder with psychotic or catatonic features.   The distinction between schizophrenia and major depressive or bipolar disorder with psychotic features or with catatonia depends on the temporal relationship between the mood disturbance and the psychosis, and on the severity of the depressive or manic symptoms. If delusions or hallucinations occur exclusively during a major depressive or manic episode, the diagnosis is depressive or bipolar disorder with psychotic features.

Schizoaffective disorder.   A diagnosis of schizoaffective disorder requires that a major depressive or manic episode occur concurrently with the active-phase symptoms and that the mood symptoms be present for a majority of the total duration of the active periods.

Schizophreniform disorder and brief psychotic disorder.   These disorders are of shorter duration than schizophrenia as specified in Criterion C, which requires 6 months of symptoms. In schizophreniform disorder, the disturbance is present less than 6 months, and in brief psychotic disorder, symptoms are present at least 1 day but less than 1 month.

Delusional disorder.   Delusional disorder can be distinguished from schizophrenia by the absence of the other symptoms characteristic of schizophrenia (e.g., delusions, prominent auditory or visual hallucinations, disorganized speech, grossly disorganized or catatonic behavior, negative symptoms).

Schizotypal personality disorder.   Schizotypal personality disorder may be distinguished from schizophrenia by subthreshold symptoms that are associated with persistent personality features.

Obsessive-compulsive disorder and body dysmorphic disorder.   Individuals with obsessive-compulsive disorder and body dysmorphic disorder may present with poor or absent insight, and the preoccupations may reach delusional proportions. But these disorders are distinguished from schizophrenia by their prominent obsessions, compulsions, preoccupations with appearance or body odor, hoarding, or body-focused repetitive behaviors.

Posttraumatic stress disorder.   Posttraumatic stress disorder may include flashbacks that have a hallucinatory quality, and hypervigilance may reach paranoid proportions. But a traumatic event and characteristic symptom features relating to reliving or reacting to the event are required to make the diagnosis.

Autism spectrum disorder or communication disorders.   These disorders may also have symptoms resembling a psychotic episode but are distinguished by their respective deficits in social interaction with repetitive and restricted behaviors and other cognitive and communication deficits. An individual with autism spectrum disorder or communication disorder must have symptoms that meet full criteria for schizophrenia, with prominent hallucinations or delusions for at least 1 month, in order to be diagnosed with schizophrenia as a comorbid condition.

Other mental disorders associated with a psychotic episode.   The diagnosis of schizophrenia is made only when the psychotic episode is persistent and not attributable to the physiological effects of a substance or another medical condition. Individuals with a delirium or major or minor neurocognitive disorder may present with psychotic symptoms, but these would have a temporal relationship to the onset of cognitive changes consistent with those disorders. Individuals with substance/medication-induced psychotic disorder may present with symptoms characteristic of Criterion A for schizophrenia, but the substance/medication-induced psychotic disorder can usually be distinguished by the chronological relationship of substance use to the onset and remission of the psychosis in the absence of substance use.

Comorbidity

Rates of comorbidity with substance-related disorders are high in schizophrenia. Over half of individuals with schizophrenia have tobacco use disorder and smoke cigarettes regularly. Comorbidity with anxiety disorders is increasingly recognized in schizophrenia. Rates of obsessive-compulsive disorder and panic disorder are elevated in individuals with schizophrenia compared with the general population. Schizotypal or paranoid personality disorder may sometimes precede the onset of schizophrenia.

Life expectancy is reduced in individuals with schizophrenia because of associated medical conditions. Weight gain, diabetes, metabolic syndrome, and cardiovascular and pulmonary disease are more common in schizophrenia than in the general population. Poor engagement in health maintenance behaviors (e.g., cancer screening, exercise) increases the risk of chronic disease, but other disorder factors, including medications, lifestyle, cigarette smoking, and diet, may also play a role. A shared vulnerability for psychosis and medical disorders may explain some of the medical comorbidity of schizophrenia.

Schizoaffective Disorder

Diagnostic Criteria

A. An uninterrupted period of illness during which there is a major mood episode (major depressive or manic) concurrent with Criterion A of schizophrenia.
   Note: The major depressive episode must include Criterion A1: Depressed mood.
B. Delusions or hallucinations for 2 or more weeks in the absence of a major mood episode (depressive or manic) during the lifetime duration of the illness.
C. Symptoms that meet criteria for a major mood episode are present for the majority of the total duration of the active and residual portions of the illness.
D. The disturbance is not attributable to the effects of a substance (e.g., a drug of abuse, a medication) or another medical condition.

Specify whether:

295.70 (F25.0) Bipolar type: This subtype applies if a manic episode is part of the presentation. Major depressive episodes may also occur.

295.70 (F25.1) Depressive type: This subtype applies if only major depressive episodes are part of the presentation.

Specify if:

With catatonia (refer to the criteria for catatonia associated with another mental disorder, pp. 119–120, for definition).

> **Coding note:** Use additional code 293.89 (F06.1) catatonia associated with schizoaffective disorder to indicate the presence of the comorbid catatonia.

Specify if:

The following course specifiers are only to be used after a 1-year duration of the disorder and if they are not in contradiction to the diagnostic course criteria.

First episode, currently in acute episode: First manifestation of the disorder meeting the defining diagnostic symptom and time criteria. An *acute episode* is a time period in which the symptom criteria are fulfilled.

First episode, currently in partial remission: *Partial remission* is a time period during which an improvement after a previous episode is maintained and in which the defining criteria of the disorder are only partially fulfilled.

First episode, currently in full remission: *Full remission* is a period of time after a previous episode during which no disorder-specific symptoms are present.

Multiple episodes, currently in acute episode: Multiple episodes may be determined after a minimum of two episodes (i.e., after a first episode, a remission and a minimum of one relapse).

Multiple episodes, currently in partial remission

Multiple episodes, currently in full remission

Continuous: Symptoms fulfilling the diagnostic symptom criteria of the disorder are remaining for the majority of the illness course, with subthreshold symptom periods being very brief relative to the overall course.

Unspecified

Specify current severity:

Severity is rated by a quantitative assessment of the primary symptoms of psychosis, including delusions, hallucinations, disorganized speech, abnormal psychomotor behavior, and negative symptoms. Each of these symptoms may be rated for its current severity (most severe in the last 7 days) on a 5-point scale ranging from 0 (not present) to 4 (present and severe). (See Clinician-Rated Dimensions of Psychosis Symptom Severity in the chapter "Assessment Measures.")

Note: Diagnosis of schizoaffective disorder can be made without using this severity specifier.

Note: For additional information on Development and Course (age-related factors), Risk and Prognostic Factors (environmental risk factors), Culture-Related Diagnostic Issues, and Gender-Related Diagnostic Issues, see the corresponding sections in schizophrenia, bipolar I and II disorders, and major depressive disorder in their respective chapters.

Diagnostic Features

The diagnosis of schizoaffective disorder is based on the assessment of an uninterrupted period of illness during which the individual continues to display active or residual symptoms of psychotic illness. The diagnosis is usually, but not necessarily, made during the period of psychotic illness. At some time during the period, Criterion A for schizophrenia has to be met. Criteria B (social dysfunction) and F (exclusion of autism spectrum disorder or other communication disorder of childhood onset) for schizophrenia do not have to be met. In addition to meeting Criterion A for schizophrenia, there is a major mood episode (major depressive or manic) (Criterion A for schizoaffective disorder). Because loss of interest or pleasure is common in schizophrenia, to meet Criterion A for schizoaffective disorder, the major depressive episode must include pervasive depressed mood (i.e., the presence of markedly diminished interest or pleasure is not sufficient). Episodes of depression or mania are present for the majority of the total duration of the illness (i.e., after Criterion A has been met) (Criterion C for schizoaffective disorder). To separate schizoaffective disorder from a depressive or bipolar disorder with psychotic features, delusions or hallucinations must be present for at least 2 weeks in the absence of a major mood episode (depressive or manic) at some point during the lifetime duration of the illness (Criterion B for schizoaffective disorder). The symptoms must not be attributable to the effects of a substance or another medical condition (Criterion D for schizoaffective disorder).

Criterion C for schizoaffective disorder specifies that mood symptoms meeting criteria for a major mood episode must be present for the majority of the total duration of the active and residual portion of the illness. Criterion C requires the assessment of mood symptoms for the entire course of a psychotic illness, which differs from the criterion in DSM-IV, which required only an assessment of the current period of illness. If the mood symptoms are present for only a relatively brief period, the diagnosis is schizophrenia, not schizoaffective disorder. When deciding whether an individual's presentation meets Criterion C, the clinician should review the total duration of psychotic illness (i.e., both active and residual symptoms) and determine when significant mood symptoms (untreated or in need of treatment with antidepressant and/or mood-stabilizing medication) accompanied the psychotic symptoms. This determination requires sufficient historical information and clinical judgment. For example, an individual with a 4-year history of active and residual symptoms of schizophrenia develops depressive and manic episodes that, taken together, do not occupy more than 1 year during the 4-year history of psychotic illness. This presentation would not meet Criterion C.

In addition to the five symptom domain areas identified in the diagnostic criteria, the assessment of cognition, depression, and mania symptom domains is vital for making critically important distinctions between the various schizophrenia spectrum and other psychotic disorders.

Associated Features Supporting Diagnosis

Occupational functioning is frequently impaired, but this is not a defining criterion (in contrast to schizophrenia). Restricted social contact and difficulties with self-care are associated with schizoaffective disorder, but negative symptoms may be less severe and less persistent than those seen in schizophrenia. Anosognosia (i.e., poor insight) is also common in schizoaffective disorder, but the deficits in insight may be less severe and pervasive than those in schizophrenia. Individuals with schizoaffective disorder may be at increased risk for later developing episodes of major depressive disorder or bipolar disorder if mood symptoms continue following the remission of symptoms meeting Criterion A for schizophrenia. There may be associated alcohol and other substance-related disorders.

There are no tests or biological measures that can assist in making the diagnosis of schizoaffective disorder. Whether schizoaffective disorder differs from schizophrenia with regard to associated features such as structural or functional brain abnormalities, cognitive deficits, or genetic risk factors is not clear.

Prevalence

Schizoaffective disorder appears to be about one-third as common as schizophrenia. Lifetime prevalence of schizoaffective disorder is estimated to be 0.3%. The incidence of schizoaffective disorder is higher in females than in males, mainly due to an increased incidence of the depressive type among females.

Development and Course

The typical age at onset of schizoaffective disorder is early adulthood, although onset can occur anywhere from adolescence to late in life. A significant number of individuals diagnosed with another psychotic illness initially will receive the diagnosis schizoaffective disorder later when the pattern of mood episodes has become more apparent. With the current diagnostic Criterion C, it is expected that the diagnosis for some individuals will convert from schizoaffective disorder to another disorder as mood symptoms become less prominent. The prognosis for schizoaffective disorder is somewhat better than the prognosis for schizophrenia but worse than the prognosis for mood disorders.

Schizoaffective disorder may occur in a variety of temporal patterns. The following is a typical pattern: An individual may have pronounced auditory hallucinations and persecutory delusions for 2 months before the onset of a prominent major depressive episode. The psychotic symptoms and the full major depressive episode are then present for 3 months. Then, the individual recovers completely from the major depressive episode, but the psychotic symptoms persist for another month before they too disappear. During this period of illness, the individual's symptoms concurrently met criteria for a major depressive episode and Criterion A for schizophrenia, and during this same period of illness, auditory hallucinations and delusions were present both before and after the depressive phase. The total period of illness lasted for about 6 months, with psychotic symptoms alone present during the initial 2 months, both depressive and psychotic symptoms present during the next 3 months, and psychotic symptoms alone present during the last month. In this instance, the duration of the depressive episode was not brief relative to the total duration of the psychotic disturbance, and thus the presentation qualifies for a diagnosis of schizoaffective disorder.

The expression of psychotic symptoms across the lifespan is variable. Depressive or manic symptoms can occur before the onset of psychosis, during acute psychotic episodes, during residual periods, and after cessation of psychosis. For example, an individual might present with prominent mood symptoms during the prodromal stage of schizophrenia. This pattern is not necessarily indicative of schizoaffective disorder, since it is the co-occurrence of psychotic and mood symptoms that is diagnostic. For an individual with symptoms that clearly meet the criteria for schizoaffective disorder but who on further follow-up only presents with residual psychotic symptoms (such as subthreshold psychosis and/or prominent negative symptoms), the diagnosis may be changed to schizophrenia, as the total proportion of psychotic illness compared with mood symptoms becomes more prominent. Schizoaffective disorder, bipolar type, may be more common in young adults, whereas schizoaffective disorder, depressive type, may be more common in older adults.

Risk and Prognostic Factors

Genetic and physiological.   Among individuals with schizophrenia, there may be an increased risk for schizoaffective disorder in first-degree relatives. The risk for schizoaffective disorder may be increased among individuals who have a first-degree relative with schizophrenia, bipolar disorder, or schizoaffective disorder.

Culture-Related Diagnostic Issues

Cultural and socioeconomic factors must be considered, particularly when the individual and the clinician do not share the same cultural and economic background. Ideas that appear to be delusional in one culture (e.g., witchcraft) may be commonly held in another. There is also some evidence in the literature for the overdiagnosis of schizophrenia compared with schizoaffective disorder in African American and Hispanic populations, so care must be taken to ensure a culturally appropriate evaluation that includes both psychotic and affective symptoms.

Suicide Risk

The lifetime risk of suicide for schizophrenia and schizoaffective disorder is 5%, and the presence of depressive symptoms is correlated with a higher risk for suicide. There is evidence that suicide rates are higher in North American populations than in European, Eastern European, South American, and Indian populations of individuals with schizophrenia or schizoaffective disorder.

Functional Consequences of Schizoaffective Disorder

Schizoaffective disorder is associated with social and occupational dysfunction, but dysfunction is not a diagnostic criterion (as it is for schizophrenia), and there is substantial variability between individuals diagnosed with schizoaffective disorder.

Differential Diagnosis

Other mental disorders and medical conditions.   A wide variety of psychiatric and medical conditions can manifest with psychotic and mood symptoms that must be considered in the differential diagnosis of schizoaffective disorder. These include psychotic disorder due to another medical condition; delirium; major neurocognitive disorder; substance/medication-induced psychotic disorder or neurocognitive disorder; bipolar disorders with psychotic features; major depressive disorder with psychotic features; depressive or bipolar disorders with catatonic features; schizotypal, schizoid, or paranoid personality disorder; brief psychotic disorder; schizophreniform disorder; schizophrenia; delusional disorder; and other specified and unspecified schizophrenia spectrum and other psychotic disorders. Medical conditions and substance use can present with a combination of psychotic and mood symptoms, and thus psychotic disorder due to another medical condition needs to be excluded. Distinguishing schizoaffective disorder from schizophrenia and from depressive and bipolar disorders with psychotic features is often difficult. Criterion C is designed to separate schizoaffective disorder from schizophrenia, and Criterion B is designed to distinguish schizoaffective disorder from a depressive or bipolar disorder with psychotic features. More specifically, schizoaffective disorder can be distinguished from a depressive or bipolar disorder with psychotic features due to the presence of prominent delusions and/or hallucinations for at least 2 weeks in the absence of a major mood episode. In contrast, in depressive or bipolar disorders with psychotic features, the psychotic features primarily occur during the mood episode(s). Because the relative proportion of mood to psychotic symptoms may change over time, the appropriate diagnosis may change from and to schizoaffective disorder (e.g., a diagnosis of schizoaffective disorder for a severe and prominent major depressive episode lasting 3 months during the first 6 months of a persistent psychotic illness would be changed to schizophrenia if active psychotic or prominent residual symptoms persist over several years without a recurrence of another mood episode).

Psychotic disorder due to another medical condition.   Other medical conditions and substance use can manifest with a combination of psychotic and mood symptoms, and thus psychotic disorder due to another medical condition needs to be excluded.

Schizophrenia, bipolar, and depressive disorders.   Distinguishing schizoaffective disorder from schizophrenia and from depressive and bipolar disorders with psychotic features is often difficult. Criterion C is designed to separate schizoaffective disorder from schizophrenia, and Criterion B is designed to distinguish schizoaffective disorder from a depressive or bipolar disorder with psychotic features. More specifically, schizoaffective disorder can be distinguished from a depressive or bipolar disorder with psychotic features based on the presence of prominent delusions and/or hallucinations for at least 2 weeks in the absence of a major mood episode. In contrast, in depressive or bipolar disorder with psychotic features, the psychotic features primarily occur during the mood episode(s). Because the relative proportion of mood to psychotic symptoms may change over time, the appropriate diagnosis may change from and to schizoaffective disorder. (For example, a diagnosis of schizoaffective disorder for a severe and prominent major depressive episode lasting 3 months during the first 6 months of a chronic psychotic illness would be changed to schizophrenia if active psychotic or prominent residual symptoms persist over several years without a recurrence of another mood episode.)

Comorbidity

Many individuals diagnosed with schizoaffective disorder are also diagnosed with other mental disorders, especially substance use disorders and anxiety disorders. Similarly, the incidence of medical conditions is increased above base rate for the general population and leads to decreased life expectancy.

Substance/Medication-Induced Psychotic Disorder

Diagnostic Criteria

A. Presence of one or both of the following symptoms:

1. Delusions.
2. Hallucinations.

B. There is evidence from the history, physical examination, or laboratory findings of both (1) and (2):

1. The symptoms in Criterion A developed during or soon after substance intoxication or withdrawal or after exposure to a medication.
2. The involved substance/medication is capable of producing the symptoms in Criterion A.

C. The disturbance is not better explained by a psychotic disorder that is not substance/medication-induced. Such evidence of an independent psychotic disorder could include the following:

> The symptoms preceded the onset of the substance/medication use; the symptoms persist for a substantial period of time (e.g., about 1 month) after the cessation of acute withdrawal or severe intoxication; or there is other evidence of an independent non-substance/medication-induced psychotic disorder (e.g., a history of recurrent non-substance/medication-related episodes).

D. The disturbance does not occur exclusively during the course of a delirium.

E. The disturbance causes clinically significant distress or impairment in social, occupational, or other important areas of functioning.

Note: This diagnosis should be made instead of a diagnosis of substance intoxication or substance withdrawal only when the symptoms in Criterion A predominate in the clinical picture and when they are sufficiently severe to warrant clinical attention.

Coding note: The ICD-9-CM and ICD-10-CM codes for the [specific substance/medication]-induced psychotic disorders are indicated in the table below. Note that the ICD-10-CM code depends on whether or not there is a comorbid substance use disorder present for the same class of substance. If a mild substance use disorder is comorbid with the substance-induced psychotic disorder, the 4th position character is "1," and the clinician should record "mild [substance] use disorder" before the substance-induced psychotic disorder (e.g., "mild cocaine use disorder with cocaine-induced psychotic disorder"). If a moderate or severe substance use disorder is comorbid with the substance-induced psychotic disorder, the 4th position character is "2," and the clinician should record "moderate [substance] use disorder" or "severe [substance] use disorder," depending on the severity of the comorbid substance use disorder. If there is no comorbid substance use disorder (e.g., after a one-time heavy use of the substance), then the 4th position character is "9," and the clinician should record only the substance-induced psychotic disorder.

		ICD-10-CM		
	ICD-9-CM	With use disorder, mild	With use disorder, moderate or severe	Without use disorder
Alcohol	291.9	F10.159	F10.259	F10.959
Cannabis	292.9	F12.159	F12.259	F12.959
Phencyclidine	292.9	F16.159	F16.259	F16.959
Other hallucinogen	292.9	F16.159	F16.259	F16.959
Inhalant	292.9	F18.159	F18.259	F18.959
Sedative, hypnotic, or anxiolytic	292.9	F13.159	F13.259	F13.959
Amphetamine (or other stimulant)	292.9	F15.159	F15.259	F15.959
Cocaine	292.9	F14.159	F14.259	F14.959
Other (or unknown) substance	292.9	F19.159	F19.259	F19.959

Specify if (see Table 1 in the chapter "Substance-Related and Addictive Disorders" for diagnoses associated with substance class):

With onset during intoxication: If the criteria are met for intoxication with the substance and the symptoms develop during intoxication.

With onset during withdrawal: If the criteria are met for withdrawal from the substance and the symptoms develop during, or shortly after, withdrawal.

Specify current severity:

Severity is rated by a quantitative assessment of the primary symptoms of psychosis, including delusions, hallucinations, abnormal psychomotor behavior, and negative symptoms. Each of these symptoms may be rated for its current severity (most severe in the last 7 days) on a 5-point scale ranging from 0 (not present) to 4 (present and severe). (See Clinician-Rated Dimensions of Psychosis Symptom Severity in the chapter "Assessment Measures.")

Note: Diagnosis of substance/medication-induced psychotic disorder can be made without using this severity specifier.

Recording Procedures

ICD-9-CM.   The name of the substance/medication-induced psychotic disorder begins with the specific substance (e.g., cocaine, dexamethasone) that is presumed to be causing the delusions or hallucinations. The diagnostic code is selected from the table included in the criteria set, which is based on the drug class. For substances that do not fit into any of the classes (e.g., dexamethasone), the code for "other substance" should be used; and in cases in which a substance is judged to be an etiological factor but the specific class of substance is unknown, the category "unknown substance" should be used.

The name of the disorder is followed by the specification of onset (i.e., onset during intoxication, onset during withdrawal). Unlike the recording procedures for ICD-10-CM, which combine the substance-induced disorder and substance use disorder into a single code, for ICD-9-CM a separate diagnostic code is given for the substance use disorder. For example, in the case of delusions occurring during intoxication in a man with a severe cocaine use disorder, the diagnosis is 292.9 cocaine-induced psychotic disorder, with onset during intoxication. An additional diagnosis of 304.20 severe cocaine use disorder is also given. When more than one substance is judged to play a significant role in the development of psychotic symptoms, each should be listed separately (e.g., 292.9 cannabis-induced psychotic disorder with onset during intoxication, with severe cannabis use disorder; 292.9 phencyclidine-induced psychotic disorder, with onset during intoxication, with mild phencyclidine use disorder).

ICD-10-CM.   The name of the substance/medication-induced psychotic disorder begins with the specific substance (e.g., cocaine, dexamethasone) that is presumed to be causing the delusions or hallucinations. The diagnostic code is selected from the table included in the criteria set, which is based on the drug class and presence or absence of a comorbid substance use disorder. For substances that do not fit into any of the classes (e.g., dexamethasone), the code for "other substance" with no comorbid substance use should be used; and in cases in which a substance is judged to be an etiological factor but the specific class of substance is unknown, the category "unknown substance" with no comorbid substance use should be used.

When recording the name of the disorder, the comorbid substance use disorder (if any) is listed first, followed by the word "with," followed by the name of the substance-induced psychotic disorder, followed by the specification of onset (i.e., onset during intoxication, onset during withdrawal). For example, in the case of delusions occurring during intoxication in a man with a severe cocaine use disorder, the diagnosis is F14.259 severe cocaine use disorder with cocaine-induced psychotic disorder, with onset during intoxication. A separate diagnosis of the comorbid severe cocaine use disorder is not given. If the substance-induced psychotic disorder occurs without a comorbid substance use disorder (e.g., after a one-time heavy use of the substance), no accompanying substance use disorder is noted (e.g., F16.959 phencyclidine-induced psychotic disorder, with onset during intoxication). When more than one substance is judged to play a significant role in the development of psychotic symptoms, each should be listed separately (e.g., F12.259 severe cannabis use disorder with cannabis-induced psychotic disorder, with onset during intoxication; F16.159 mild phencyclidine use disorder with phencyclidine-induced psychotic disorder, with onset during intoxication).

Diagnostic Features

The essential features of substance/medication-induced psychotic disorder are prominent delusions and/or hallucinations (Criterion A) that are judged to be due to the physiological effects of a substance/medication (i.e., a drug of abuse, a medication, or a toxin exposure) (Criterion B). Hallucinations that the individual realizes are substance/medication-induced are not included here and instead would be diagnosed as substance intoxication or substance withdrawal with the accompanying specifier "with perceptual disturbances" (applies to alcohol withdrawal; cannabis intoxication; sedative, hypnotic, or anxiolytic withdrawal; and stimulant intoxication).

A substance/medication-induced psychotic disorder is distinguished from a primary psychotic disorder by considering the onset, course, and other factors. For drugs of abuse, there must be evidence from the history, physical examination, or laboratory findings of substance use, intoxication, or withdrawal. Substance/medication-induced psychotic disorders arise during or soon after exposure to a medication or after substance intoxication or withdrawal but can persist for weeks, whereas primary psychotic disorders may precede the onset of substance/medication use or may occur during times of sustained abstinence. Once initiated, the psychotic symptoms may continue as long as the substance/medication use continues. Another consideration is the presence of features that are atypical of a primary psychotic disorder (e.g., atypical age at onset or course). For example, the appearance of delusions de novo in a person older than 35 years without a known history of a primary psychotic disorder should suggest the possibility of a substance/medication-induced psychotic disorder. Even a prior history of a primary psychotic disorder does not rule out the possibility of a substance/medication-induced psychotic disorder. In contrast, factors that suggest that the psychotic symptoms are better accounted for by a primary psychotic disorder include persistence of psychotic symptoms for a substantial period of time (i.e., a month or more) after the end of substance intoxication or acute substance withdrawal or after cessation of medication use; or a history of prior recurrent primary psychotic disorders. Other causes of psychotic symptoms must be considered even in an individual with substance intoxication or withdrawal, because substance use problems are not uncommon among individuals with non-substance/medication-induced psychotic disorders.

In addition to the four symptom domain areas identified in the diagnostic criteria, the assessment of cognition, depression, and mania symptom domains is vital for making critically important distinctions between the various schizophrenia spectrum and other psychotic disorders.

Associated Features Supporting Diagnosis

Psychotic disorders can occur in association with intoxication with the following classes of substances: alcohol; cannabis; hallucinogens, including phencyclidine and related substances; inhalants; sedatives, hypnotics, and anxiolytics; stimulants (including cocaine); and other (or unknown) substances. Psychotic disorders can occur in association with withdrawal from the following classes of substances: alcohol; sedatives, hypnotics, and anxiolytics; and other (or unknown) substances.

Some of the medications reported to evoke psychotic symptoms include anesthetics and analgesics, anticholinergic agents, anticonvulsants, antihistamines, antihypertensive and cardiovascular medications, antimicrobial medications, antiparkinsonian medications, chemotherapeutic agents (e.g., cyclosporine, procarbazine), corticosteroids, gastrointestinal medications, muscle relaxants, nonsteroidal anti-inflammatory medications, other over-the-counter medications (e.g., phenylephrine, pseudoephedrine), antidepressant medication, and disulfiram. Toxins reported to induce psychotic symptoms include anticholinesterase, organophosphate insecticides, sarin and other nerve gases, carbon monoxide, carbon dioxide, and volatile substances such as fuel or paint.

Prevalence

Prevalence of substance/medication-induced psychotic disorder in the general population is unknown. Between 7% and 25% of individuals presenting with a first episode of psychosis in different settings are reported to have substance/medication-induced psychotic disorder.

Development and Course

The initiation of the disorder may vary considerably with the substance. For example, smoking a high dose of cocaine may produce psychosis within minutes, whereas days or weeks of high-dose alcohol or sedative use may be required to produce psychosis. Alcohol-induced psychotic disorder, with hallucinations, usually occurs only after prolonged, heavy ingestion of alcohol in individuals who have moderate to severe alcohol use disorder, and the hallucinations are generally auditory in nature.

Psychotic disorders induced by amphetamine and cocaine share similar clinical features. Persecutory delusions may rapidly develop shortly after use of amphetamine or a similarly acting sympathomimetic. The hallucination of bugs or vermin crawling in or under the skin (formication) can lead to scratching and extensive skin excoriations. Cannabis-induced psychotic disorder may develop shortly after high-dose cannabis use and usually involves persecutory delusions, marked anxiety, emotional lability, and depersonalization. The disorder usually remits within a day but in some cases may persist for a few days.

Substance/medication-induced psychotic disorder may at times persist when the offending agent is removed, such that it may be difficult initially to distinguish it from an independent psychotic disorder. Agents such as amphetamines, phencyclidine, and cocaine have been reported to evoke temporary psychotic states that can sometimes persist for weeks or longer despite removal of the agent and treatment with neuroleptic medication. In later life, polypharmacy for medical conditions and exposure to medications for parkinsonism, cardiovascular disease, and other medical disorders may be associated with a greater likelihood of psychosis induced by prescription medications as opposed to substances of abuse.

Diagnostic Markers

With substances for which relevant blood levels are available (e.g., blood alcohol level, other quantifiable blood levels such as digoxin), the presence of a level consistent with toxicity may increase diagnostic certainty.

Functional Consequences of Substance/Medication-Induced Psychotic Disorder

Substance/medication-induced psychotic disorder is typically severely disabling and consequently is observed most frequently in emergency rooms, as individuals are often brought to the acute-care setting when it occurs. However, the disability is typically self-limited and resolves upon removal of the offending agent.

Differential Diagnosis

Substance intoxication or substance withdrawal.   Individuals intoxicated with stimulants, cannabis, the opioid meperidine, or phencyclidine, or those withdrawing from alcohol or sedatives, may experience altered perceptions that they recognize as drug effects. If reality testing for these experiences remains intact (i.e., the individual recognizes that the perception is substance induced and neither believes in nor acts on it), the diagnosis is not substance/medication-induced psychotic disorder. Instead, substance intoxication or substance withdrawal, with perceptual disturbances, is diagnosed (e.g., cocaine intoxication, with perceptual disturbances). "Flashback" hallucinations that can occur long after the use of hallucinogens has stopped are diagnosed as hallucinogen persisting perception disorder. If substance/medication-induced psychotic symptoms occur exclusively during the course of a delirium, as in severe forms of alcohol withdrawal, the psychotic symptoms are considered to be an associated feature of the delirium and are not diagnosed separately. Delusions in the context of a major or mild neurocognitive disorder would be diagnosed as major or mild neurocognitive disorder, with behavioral disturbance.

Primary psychotic disorder.   A substance/medication-induced psychotic disorder is distinguished from a primary psychotic disorder, such as schizophrenia, schizoaffective disorder, delusional disorder, brief psychotic disorder, other specified schizophrenia spectrum and other psychotic disorder, or unspecified schizophrenia spectrum and other psychotic disorder, by the fact that a substance is judged to be etiologically related to the symptoms.

Psychotic disorder due to another medical condition.   A substance/medication-induced psychotic disorder due to a prescribed treatment for a mental or medical condition must have its onset while the individual is receiving the medication (or during withdrawal, if there is a withdrawal syndrome associated with the medication). Because individuals with medical conditions often take medications for those conditions, the clinician must consider the possibility that the psychotic symptoms are caused by the physiological consequences of the medical condition rather than the medication, in which case psychotic disorder due to another medical condition is diagnosed. The history often provides the primary basis for such a judgment. At times, a change in the treatment for the medical condition (e.g., medication substitution or discontinuation) may be needed to determine empirically for that individual whether the medication is the causative agent. If the clinician has ascertained that the disturbance is attributable to both a medical condition and substance/medication use, both diagnoses (i.e., psychotic disorder due to another medical condition and substance/medication-induced psychotic disorder) may be given.

Psychotic Disorder
Due to Another Medical Condition

Diagnostic Criteria

A. Prominent hallucinations or delusions.
B. There is evidence from the history, physical examination, or laboratory findings that the disturbance is the direct pathophysiological consequence of another medical condition.
C. The disturbance is not better explained by another mental disorder.
D. The disturbance does not occur exclusively during the course of a delirium.
E. The disturbance causes clinically significant distress or impairment in social, occupational, or other important areas of functioning.

Specify whether:
Code based on predominant symptom:
   293.81 (F06.2) With delusions: If delusions are the predominant symptom.
   293.82 (F06.0) With hallucinations: If hallucinations are the predominant symptom.

Coding note: Include the name of the other medical condition in the name of the mental disorder (e.g., 293.81 [F06.2] psychotic disorder due to malignant lung neoplasm, with delusions). The other medical condition should be coded and listed separately immediately before the psychotic disorder due to the medical condition (e.g., 162.9 [C34.90] malignant lung neoplasm; 293.81 [F06.2] psychotic disorder due to malignant lung neoplasm, with delusions).

Specify current severity:
   Severity is rated by a quantitative assessment of the primary symptoms of psychosis, including delusions, hallucinations, abnormal psychomotor behavior, and negative symptoms. Each of these symptoms may be rated for its current severity (most severe in the last 7 days) on a 5-point scale ranging from 0 (not present) to 4 (present and

severe). (See Clinician-Rated Dimensions of Psychosis Symptom Severity in the chapter "Assessment Measures.")

Note: Diagnosis of psychotic disorder due to another medical condition can be made without using this severity specifier.

Specifiers

In addition to the symptom domain areas identified in the diagnostic criteria, the assessment of cognition, depression, and mania symptom domains is vital for making critically important distinctions between the various schizophrenia spectrum and other psychotic disorders.

Diagnostic Features

The essential features of psychotic disorder due to another medical condition are prominent delusions or hallucinations that are judged to be attributable to the physiological effects of another medical condition and are not better explained by another mental disorder (e.g., the symptoms are not a psychologically mediated response to a severe medical condition, in which case a diagnosis of brief psychotic disorder, with marked stressor, would be appropriate).

Hallucinations can occur in any sensory modality (i.e., visual, olfactory, gustatory, tactile, or auditory), but certain etiological factors are likely to evoke specific hallucinatory phenomena. Olfactory hallucinations are suggestive of temporal lobe epilepsy. Hallucinations may vary from simple and unformed to highly complex and organized, depending on etiological and environmental factors. Psychotic disorder due to another medical condition is generally not diagnosed if the individual maintains reality testing for the hallucinations and appreciates that they result from the medical condition. Delusions may have a variety of themes, including somatic, grandiose, religious, and, most commonly, persecutory. On the whole, however, associations between delusions and particular medical conditions appear to be less specific than is the case for hallucinations.

In determining whether the psychotic disturbance is attributable to another medical condition, the presence of a medical condition must be identified and considered to be the etiology of the psychosis through a physiological mechanism. Although there are no infallible guidelines for determining whether the relationship between the psychotic disturbance and the medical condition is etiological, several considerations provide some guidance. One consideration is the presence of a temporal association between the onset, exacerbation, or remission of the medical condition and that of the psychotic disturbance. A second consideration is the presence of features that are atypical for a psychotic disorder (e.g., atypical age at onset or presence of visual or olfactory hallucinations). The disturbance must also be distinguished from a substance/medication-induced psychotic disorder or another mental disorder (e.g., an adjustment disorder).

Associated Features Supporting Diagnosis

The temporal association of the onset or exacerbation of the medical condition offers the greatest diagnostic certainty that the delusions or hallucinations are attributable to a medical condition. Additional factors may include concomitant treatments for the underlying medical condition that confer a risk for psychosis independently, such as steroid treatment for autoimmune disorders.

Prevalence

Prevalence rates for psychotic disorder due to another medical condition are difficult to estimate given the wide variety of underlying medical etiologies. Lifetime prevalence has been estimated to range from 0.21% to 0.54%. When the prevalence findings are stratified by age group, individuals older than 65 years have a significantly greater prevalence of 0.74% compared with those in younger age groups. Rates of psychosis also vary according to the underlying medical condition; conditions most commonly associated with psychosis include untreated endocrine and metabolic disorders, autoimmune disorders (e.g., systemic lupus erythematosus, N-methyl-D-aspartate (NMDA) receptor autoimmune encephalitis), or temporal lobe epilepsy. Psychosis due to epilepsy has been further differentiated into ictal, postictal, and interictal psychosis. The most common of these is postictal psychosis, observed in 2%–7.8% of epilepsy patients. Among older individuals, there may be a higher prevalence of the disorder in females, although additional gender-related features are not clear and vary considerably with the gender distributions of the underlying medical conditions.

Development and Course

Psychotic disorder due to another medical condition may be a single transient state or it may be recurrent, cycling with exacerbations and remissions of the underlying medical condition. Although treatment of the underlying medical condition often results in a resolution of the psychosis, this is not always the case, and psychotic symptoms may persist long after the medical event (e.g., psychotic disorder due to focal brain injury). In the context of chronic conditions such as multiple sclerosis or chronic interictal psychosis of epilepsy, the psychosis may assume a long-term course.

The expression of psychotic disorder due to another medical condition does not differ substantially in phenomenology depending on age at occurrence. However, older age groups have a higher prevalence of the disorder, which is most likely due to the increasing medical burden associated with advanced age and the cumulative effects of deleterious exposures and age-related processes (e.g., atherosclerosis). The nature of the underlying medical conditions is likely to change across the lifespan, with younger age groups more affected by epilepsy, head trauma, autoimmune, and neoplastic diseases of early to midlife, and older age groups more affected by stroke disease, anoxic events, and multiple system comorbidities. Underlying factors with increasing age, such as preexisting cognitive impairment as well as vision and hearing impairments, may incur a greater risk for psychosis, possibly by serving to lower the threshold for experiencing psychosis.

Risk and Prognostic Factors

Course modifiers. Identification and treatment of the underlying medical condition has the greatest impact on course, although preexisting central nervous system injury may confer a worse course outcome (e.g., head trauma, cerebrovascular disease).

Diagnostic Markers

The diagnosis of psychotic disorder due to another medical condition depends on the clinical condition of each individual, and the diagnostic tests will vary according to that condition. A variety of medical conditions may cause psychotic symptoms. These include neurological conditions (e.g., neoplasms, cerebrovascular disease, Huntington's disease, multiple sclerosis, epilepsy, auditory or visual nerve injury or impairment, deafness, migraine, central nervous system infections), endocrine conditions (e.g., hyper- and hypothyroidism, hyper- and hypoparathyroidism, hyper- and hypoadrenocorticism), metabolic conditions (e.g., hypoxia, hypercarbia, hypoglycemia), fluid or electrolyte imbalances, hepatic or renal diseases, and autoimmune disorders with central nervous system involvement (e.g., systemic lupus erythematosus). The associated physical examination findings, laboratory findings, and patterns of prevalence or onset reflect the etiological medical condition.

Suicide Risk

Suicide risk in the context of psychotic disorder due to another medical condition is not clearly delineated, although certain conditions such as epilepsy and multiple sclerosis are associated with increased rates of suicide, which may be further increased in the presence of psychosis.

Functional Consequences of Psychotic Disorder Due to Another Medical Condition

Functional disability is typically severe in the context of psychotic disorder due to another medical condition but will vary considerably by the type of condition and likely improve with successful resolution of the condition.

Differential Diagnosis

Delirium.   Hallucinations and delusions commonly occur in the context of a delirium; however, a separate diagnosis of psychotic disorder due to another medical condition is not given if the disturbance occurs exclusively during the course of a delirium. Delusions in the context of a major or mild neurocognitive disorder would be diagnosed as major or mild neurocognitive disorder, with behavioral disturbance.

Substance/medication-induced psychotic disorder.   If there is evidence of recent or prolonged substance use (including medications with psychoactive effects), withdrawal from a substance, or exposure to a toxin (e.g., LSD [lysergic acid diethylamide] intoxication, alcohol withdrawal), a substance/medication-induced psychotic disorder should be considered. Symptoms that occur during or shortly after (i.e., within 4 weeks) of substance intoxication or withdrawal or after medication use may be especially indicative of a substance-induced psychotic disorder, depending on the character, duration, or amount of the substance used. If the clinician has ascertained that the disturbance is due to both a medical condition and substance use, both diagnoses (i.e., psychotic disorder due to another medical condition and substance/medication-induced psychotic disorder) can be given.

Psychotic disorder.   Psychotic disorder due to another medical condition must be distinguished from a psychotic disorder (e.g., schizophrenia, delusional disorder, schizoaffective disorder) or a depressive or bipolar disorder, with psychotic features. In psychotic disorders and in depressive or bipolar disorders, with psychotic features, no specific and direct causative physiological mechanisms associated with a medical condition can be demonstrated. Late age at onset and the absence of a personal or family history of schizophrenia or delusional disorder suggest the need for a thorough assessment to rule out the diagnosis of psychotic disorder due to another medical condition. Auditory hallucinations that involve voices speaking complex sentences are more characteristic of schizophrenia than of psychotic disorder due to a medical condition. Other types of hallucinations (e.g., visual, olfactory) commonly signal a psychotic disorder due to another medical condition or a substance/medication-induced psychotic disorder.

Comorbidity

Psychotic disorder due to another medical condition in individuals older than 80 years is associated with concurrent major neurocognitive disorder (dementia).

Catatonia

Catatonia can occur in the context of several disorders, including neurodevelopmental, psychotic, bipolar, depressive disorders, and other medical conditions (e.g., cerebral folate deficiency, rare autoimmune and paraneoplastic disorders). The manual does not treat catatonia as an independent class but recognizes a) catatonia associated with another mental disorder (i.e., a neurodevelopmental, psychotic disorder, a bipolar disorder, a depressive disorder, or other mental disorder), b) catatonic disorder due to another medical condition, and c) unspecified catatonia.

Catatonia is defined by the presence of three or more of 12 psychomotor features in the diagnostic criteria for catatonia associated with another mental disorder and catatonic disorder due to another medical condition. The essential feature of catatonia is a marked psychomotor disturbance that may involve decreased motor activity, decreased engagement during interview or physical examination, or excessive and peculiar motor activity. The clinical presentation of catatonia can be puzzling, as the psychomotor disturbance may range from marked unresponsiveness to marked agitation. Motoric immobility may be severe (stupor) or moderate (catalepsy and waxy flexibility). Similarly, decreased engagement may be severe (mutism) or moderate (negativism). Excessive and peculiar motor behaviors can be complex (e.g., stereotypy) or simple (agitation) and may include echolalia and echopraxia. In extreme cases, the same individual may wax and wane between decreased and excessive motor activity. The seemingly opposing clinical features and variable manifestations of the diagnosis contribute to a lack of awareness and decreased recognition of catatonia. During severe stages of catatonia, the individual may need careful supervision to avoid self-harm or harming others. There are potential risks from malnutrition, exhaustion, hyperpyrexia and self-inflicted injury.

Catatonia Associated With Another Mental Disorder (Catatonia Specifier)

293.89 (F06.1)

A. The clinical picture is dominated by three (or more) of the following symptoms:
1. Stupor (i.e., no psychomotor activity; not actively relating to environment).
2. Catalepsy (i.e., passive induction of a posture held against gravity).
3. Waxy flexibility (i.e., slight, even resistance to positioning by examiner).
4. Mutism (i.e., no, or very little, verbal response [exclude if known aphasia]).
5. Negativism (i.e., opposition or no response to instructions or external stimuli).
6. Posturing (i.e., spontaneous and active maintenance of a posture against gravity).
7. Mannerism (i.e., odd, circumstantial caricature of normal actions).
8. Stereotypy (i.e., repetitive, abnormally frequent, non-goal-directed movements).
9. Agitation, not influenced by external stimuli.
10. Grimacing.
11. Echolalia (i.e., mimicking another's speech).
12. Echopraxia (i.e., mimicking another's movements).

Coding note: Indicate the name of the associated mental disorder when recording the name of the condition (i.e., 293.89 [F06.1] catatonia associated with major depressive disorder). Code first the associated mental disorder (e.g., neurodevelopmental disorder, brief psychotic disorder, schizophreniform disorder, schizophrenia, schizoaffective disorder, bipolar disorder, major depressive disorder, or other mental disorder) (e.g., 295.70 [F25.1] schizoaffective disorder, depressive type; 293.89 [F06.1] catatonia associated with schizoaffective disorder).

Diagnostic Features

Catatonia associated with another mental disorder (catatonia specifier) may be used when criteria are met for catatonia during the course of a neurodevelopmental, psychotic, bipolar, depressive, or other mental disorder. The catatonia specifier is appropriate when the clinical picture is characterized by marked psychomotor disturbance and involves at least three of the 12 diagnostic features listed in Criterion A. Catatonia is typically diagnosed in an inpatient setting and occurs in up to 35% of individuals with schizophrenia, but the majority of catatonia cases involve individuals with depressive or bipolar disorders. Before the catatonia specifier is used in neurodevelopmental, psychotic, bipolar, depressive, or other mental disorders, a wide variety of other medical conditions need to be ruled out; these conditions include, but are not limited to, medical conditions due to infectious, metabolic, or neurological conditions (see "Catatonic Disorder Due to Another Medical Condition"). Catatonia can also be a side effect of a medication (see the chapter "Medication-Induced Movement Disorders and Other Adverse Effects of Medication"). Because of the seriousness of the complications, particular attention should be paid to the possibility that the catatonia is attributable to 333.92 (G21.0) neuroleptic malignant syndrome.

Catatonic Disorder Due to Another Medical Condition

Diagnostic Criteria   **293.89 (F06.1)**

A. The clinical picture is dominated by three (or more) of the following symptoms:
   1. Stupor (i.e., no psychomotor activity; not actively relating to environment).
   2. Catalepsy (i.e., passive induction of a posture held against gravity).
   3. Waxy flexibility (i.e., slight, even resistance to positioning by examiner).
   4. Mutism (i.e., no, or very little, verbal response [**Note:** not applicable if there is an established aphasia]).
   5. Negativism (i.e., opposition or no response to instructions or external stimuli).
   6. Posturing (i.e., spontaneous and active maintenance of a posture against gravity).
   7. Mannerism (i.e., odd, circumstantial caricature of normal actions).
   8. Stereotypy (i.e., repetitive, abnormally frequent, non-goal-directed movements).
   9. Agitation, not influenced by external stimuli.
   10. Grimacing.
   11. Echolalia (i.e., mimicking another's speech).
   12. Echopraxia (i.e., mimicking another's movements).
B. There is evidence from the history, physical examination, or laboratory findings that the disturbance is the direct pathophysiological consequence of another medical condition.
C. The disturbance is not better explained by another mental disorder (e.g., a manic episode).
D. The disturbance does not occur exclusively during the course of a delirium.
E. The disturbance causes clinically significant distress or impairment in social, occupational, or other important areas of functioning.

Coding note: Include the name of the medical condition in the name of the mental disorder (e.g., 293.89 [F06.1]) catatonic disorder due to hepatic encephalopathy). The other medical condition should be coded and listed separately immediately before the catatonic disorder due to the medical condition (e.g., 572.2 [K71.90] hepatic encephalopathy; 293.89 [F06.1] catatonic disorder due to hepatic encephalopathy).

Diagnostic Features

The essential feature of catatonic disorder due to another medical condition is the presence of catatonia that is judged to be attributed to the physiological effects of another medical condition. Catatonia can be diagnosed by the presence of at least three of the 12 clinical features in Criterion A. There must be evidence from the history, physical examination, or laboratory findings that the catatonia is attributable to another medical condition (Criterion B). The diagnosis is not given if the catatonia is better explained by another mental disorder (e.g., manic episode) (Criterion C) or if it occurs exclusively during the course of a delirium (Criterion D).

Associated Features Supporting Diagnosis

A variety of medical conditions may cause catatonia, especially neurological conditions (e.g., neoplasms, head trauma, cerebrovascular disease, encephalitis) and metabolic conditions (e.g., hypercalcemia, hepatic encephalopathy, homocystinuria, diabetic ketoacidosis). The associated physical examination findings, laboratory findings, and patterns of prevalence and onset reflect those of the etiological medical condition.

Differential Diagnosis

A separate diagnosis of catatonic disorder due to another medical condition is not given if the catatonia occurs exclusively during the course of a delirium or neuroleptic malignant syndrome. If the individual is currently taking neuroleptic medication, consideration should be given to medication-induced movement disorders (e.g., abnormal positioning may be due to neuroleptic-induced acute dystonia) or neuroleptic malignant syndrome (e.g., catatonic-like features may be present, along with associated vital sign and/or laboratory abnormalities). Catatonic symptoms may be present in any of the following five psychotic disorders: brief psychotic disorder, schizophreniform disorder, schizophrenia, schizoaffective disorder, and substance/medication-induced psychotic disorder. It may also be present in some of the neurodevelopmental disorders, in all of the bipolar and depressive disorders, and in other mental disorders.

Unspecified Catatonia

This category applies to presentations in which symptoms characteristic of catatonia cause clinically significant distress or impairment in social, occupational, or other important areas of functioning but either the nature of the underlying mental disorder or other medical condition is unclear, full criteria for catatonia are not met, or there is insufficient information to make a more specific diagnosis (e.g., in emergency room settings).

Coding note: Code first **781.99 (R29.818)** other symptoms involving nervous and musculoskeletal systems, followed by **293.89 (F06.1)** unspecified catatonia.

Other Specified Schizophrenia Spectrum and Other Psychotic Disorder

298.8 (F28)

This category applies to presentations in which symptoms characteristic of a schizophrenia spectrum and other psychotic disorder that cause clinically significant distress or impairment in social, occupational, or other important areas of functioning predominate but do not meet the full criteria for any of the disorders in the schizophrenia spectrum and other psychotic disorders diagnostic class. The other specified schizophrenia spectrum and other psychotic disorder category is used in situations in which the clinician chooses to communicate the specific reason that the presentation does not meet the criteria for any specific schizophrenia spectrum and other psychotic disorder. This is done by recording "other specified schizophrenia spectrum and other psychotic disorder" followed by the specific reason (e.g., "persistent auditory hallucinations").

Examples of presentations that can be specified using the "other specified" designation include the following:

1. **Persistent auditory hallucinations** occurring in the absence of any other features.
2. **Delusions with significant overlapping mood episodes:** This includes persistent delusions with periods of overlapping mood episodes that are present for a substantial portion of the delusional disturbance (such that the criterion stipulating only brief mood disturbance in delusional disorder is not met).
3. **Attenuated psychosis syndrome:** This syndrome is characterized by psychotic-like symptoms that are below a threshold for full psychosis (e.g., the symptoms are less severe and more transient, and insight is relatively maintained).
4. **Delusional symptoms in partner of individual with delusional disorder:** In the context of a relationship, the delusional material from the dominant partner provides content for delusional belief by the individual who may not otherwise entirely meet criteria for delusional disorder.

Unspecified Schizophrenia Spectrum and Other Psychotic Disorder

298.9 (F29)

This category applies to presentations in which symptoms characteristic of a schizophrenia spectrum and other psychotic disorder that cause clinically significant distress or impairment in social, occupational, or other important areas of functioning predominate but do not meet the full criteria for any of the disorders in the schizophrenia spectrum and other psychotic disorders diagnostic class. The unspecified schizophrenia spectrum and other psychotic disorder category is used in situations in which the clinician chooses *not* to specify the reason that the criteria are not met for a specific schizophrenia spectrum and other psychotic disorder, and includes presentations in which there is insufficient information to make a more specific diagnosis (e.g., in emergency room settings).

Bipolar and Related Disorders

Bipolar and related disorders are separated from the depressive disorders in DSM-5 and placed between the chapters on schizophrenia spectrum and other psychotic disorders and depressive disorders in recognition of their place as a bridge between the two diagnostic classes in terms of symptomatology, family history, and genetics. The diagnoses included in this chapter are bipolar I disorder, bipolar II disorder, cyclothymic disorder, substance/medication-induced bipolar and related disorder, bipolar and related disorder due to another medical condition, other specified bipolar and related disorder, and unspecified bipolar and related disorder.

The bipolar I disorder criteria represent the modern understanding of the classic manic-depressive disorder or affective psychosis described in the nineteenth century, differing from that classic description only to the extent that neither psychosis nor the lifetime experience of a major depressive episode is a requirement. However, the vast majority of individuals whose symptoms meet the criteria for a fully syndromal manic episode also experience major depressive episodes during the course of their lives.

Bipolar II disorder, requiring the lifetime experience of at least one episode of major depression and at least one hypomanic episode, is no longer thought to be a "milder" condition than bipolar I disorder, largely because of the amount of time individuals with this condition spend in depression and because the instability of mood experienced by individuals with bipolar II disorder is typically accompanied by serious impairment in work and social functioning.

The diagnosis of cyclothymic disorder is given to adults who experience at least 2 years (for children, a full year) of both hypomanic and depressive periods without ever fulfilling the criteria for an episode of mania, hypomania, or major depression.

A large number of substances of abuse, some prescribed medications, and several medical conditions can be associated with manic-like phenomena. This fact is recognized in the diagnoses of substance/medication-induced bipolar and related disorder and bipolar and related disorder due to another medical condition.

The recognition that many individuals, particularly children and, to a lesser extent, adolescents, experience bipolar-like phenomena that do not meet the criteria for bipolar I, bipolar II, or cyclothymic disorder is reflected in the availability of the other specified bipolar and related disorder category. Indeed, specific criteria for a disorder involving short-duration hypomania are provided in Section III in the hope of encouraging further study of this disorder.

Bipolar I Disorder

Diagnostic Criteria

For a diagnosis of bipolar I disorder, it is necessary to meet the following criteria for a manic episode. The manic episode may have been preceded by and may be followed by hypomanic or major depressive episodes.

Manic Episode

A. A distinct period of abnormally and persistently elevated, expansive, or irritable mood and abnormally and persistently increased activity or energy, lasting at least 1 week and present most of the day, nearly every day (or any duration if hospitalization is necessary).

B. During the period of mood disturbance and increased energy or activity, three (or more) of the following symptoms (four if the mood is only irritable) are present to a significant degree and represent a noticeable change from usual behavior:

1. Inflated self-esteem or grandiosity.
2. Decreased need for sleep (e.g., feels rested after only 3 hours of sleep).
3. More talkative than usual or pressure to keep talking.
4. Flight of ideas or subjective experience that thoughts are racing.
5. Distractibility (i.e., attention too easily drawn to unimportant or irrelevant external stimuli), as reported or observed.
6. Increase in goal-directed activity (either socially, at work or school, or sexually) or psychomotor agitation (i.e., purposeless non-goal-directed activity).
7. Excessive involvement in activities that have a high potential for painful consequences (e.g., engaging in unrestrained buying sprees, sexual indiscretions, or foolish business investments).

C. The mood disturbance is sufficiently severe to cause marked impairment in social or occupational functioning or to necessitate hospitalization to prevent harm to self or others, or there are psychotic features.

D. The episode is not attributable to the physiological effects of a substance (e.g., a drug of abuse, a medication, other treatment) or another medical condition.

Note: A full manic episode that emerges during antidepressant treatment (e.g., medication, electroconvulsive therapy) but persists at a fully syndromal level beyond the physiological effect of that treatment is sufficient evidence for a manic episode and, therefore, a bipolar I diagnosis.

Note: Criteria A–D constitute a manic episode. At least one lifetime manic episode is required for the diagnosis of bipolar I disorder.

Hypomanic Episode

A. A distinct period of abnormally and persistently elevated, expansive, or irritable mood and abnormally and persistently increased activity or energy, lasting at least 4 consecutive days and present most of the day, nearly every day.

B. During the period of mood disturbance and increased energy and activity, three (or more) of the following symptoms (four if the mood is only irritable) have persisted, represent a noticeable change from usual behavior, and have been present to a significant degree:

1. Inflated self-esteem or grandiosity.
2. Decreased need for sleep (e.g., feels rested after only 3 hours of sleep).
3. More talkative than usual or pressure to keep talking.
4. Flight of ideas or subjective experience that thoughts are racing.
5. Distractibility (i.e., attention too easily drawn to unimportant or irrelevant external stimuli), as reported or observed.
6. Increase in goal-directed activity (either socially, at work or school, or sexually) or psychomotor agitation.
7. Excessive involvement in activities that have a high potential for painful consequences (e.g., engaging in unrestrained buying sprees, sexual indiscretions, or foolish business investments).

C. The episode is associated with an unequivocal change in functioning that is uncharacteristic of the individual when not symptomatic.

D. The disturbance in mood and the change in functioning are observable by others.

E. The episode is not severe enough to cause marked impairment in social or occupational functioning or to necessitate hospitalization. If there are psychotic features, the episode is, by definition, manic.

F. The episode is not attributable to the physiological effects of a substance (e.g., a drug of abuse, a medication, other treatment) or another medical condition.

Note: A full hypomanic episode that emerges during antidepressant treatment (e.g., medication, electroconvulsive therapy) but persists at a fully syndromal level beyond the physiological effect of that treatment is sufficient evidence for a hypomanic episode diagnosis. However, caution is indicated so that one or two symptoms (particularly increased irritability, edginess, or agitation following antidepressant use) are not taken as sufficient for diagnosis of a hypomanic episode, nor necessarily indicative of a bipolar diathesis.

Note: Criteria A–F constitute a hypomanic episode. Hypomanic episodes are common in bipolar I disorder but are not required for the diagnosis of bipolar I disorder.

Major Depressive Episode

A. Five (or more) of the following symptoms have been present during the same 2-week period and represent a change from previous functioning; at least one of the symptoms is either (1) depressed mood or (2) loss of interest or pleasure.

Note: Do not include symptoms that are clearly attributable to another medical condition.

1. Depressed mood most of the day, nearly every day, as indicated by either subjective report (e.g., feels sad, empty, or hopeless) or observation made by others (e.g., appears tearful). (**Note:** In children and adolescents, can be irritable mood.)

2. Markedly diminished interest or pleasure in all, or almost all, activities most of the day, nearly every day (as indicated by either subjective account or observation).

3. Significant weight loss when not dieting or weight gain (e.g., a change of more than 5% of body weight in a month), or decrease or increase in appetite nearly every day. (**Note:** In children, consider failure to make expected weight gain.)

4. Insomnia or hypersomnia nearly every day.

5. Psychomotor agitation or retardation nearly every day (observable by others; not merely subjective feelings of restlessness or being slowed down).

6. Fatigue or loss of energy nearly every day.

7. Feelings of worthlessness or excessive or inappropriate guilt (which may be delusional) nearly every day (not merely self-reproach or guilt about being sick).

8. Diminished ability to think or concentrate, or indecisiveness, nearly every day (either by subjective account or as observed by others).

9. Recurrent thoughts of death (not just fear of dying), recurrent suicidal ideation without a specific plan, or a suicide attempt or a specific plan for committing suicide.

B. The symptoms cause clinically significant distress or impairment in social, occupational, or other important areas of functioning.

C. The episode is not attributable to the physiological effects of a substance or another medical condition.

Note: Criteria A–C constitute a major depressive episode. Major depressive episodes are common in bipolar I disorder but are not required for the diagnosis of bipolar I disorder.

Note: Responses to a significant loss (e.g., bereavement, financial ruin, losses from a natural disaster, a serious medical illness or disability) may include the feelings of intense sadness, rumination about the loss, insomnia, poor appetite, and weight loss noted in Criterion A, which may resemble a depressive episode. Although such symptoms may be understandable or considered appropriate to the loss, the presence of a major depressive episode in addition to the normal response to a significant loss should also be carefully considered. This decision inevitably requires the exercise of clinical judgment based on the individual's history and the cultural norms for the expression of distress in the context of loss.[1]

Bipolar I Disorder

A. Criteria have been met for at least one manic episode (Criteria A–D under "Manic Episode" above).

B. The occurrence of the manic and major depressive episode(s) is not better explained by schizoaffective disorder, schizophrenia, schizophreniform disorder, delusional disorder, or other specified or unspecified schizophrenia spectrum and other psychotic disorder.

Coding and Recording Procedures

The diagnostic code for bipolar I disorder is based on type of current or most recent episode and its status with respect to current severity, presence of psychotic features, and remission status. Current severity and psychotic features are only indicated if full criteria are currently met for a manic or major depressive episode. Remission specifiers are only indicated if the full criteria are not currently met for a manic, hypomanic, or major depressive episode. Codes are as follows:

Bipolar I disorder	Current or most recent episode manic	Current or most recent episode hypomanic*	Current or most recent episode depressed	Current or most recent episode unspecified**
Mild (p. 154)	296.41 (F31.11)	NA	296.51 (F31.31)	NA
Moderate (p. 154)	296.42 (F31.12)	NA	296.52 (F31.32)	NA
Severe (p. 154)	296.43 (F31.13)	NA	296.53 (F31.4)	NA

---

[1] In distinguishing grief from a major depressive episode (MDE), it is useful to consider that in grief the predominant affect is feelings of emptiness and loss, while in an MDE it is persistent depressed mood and the inability to anticipate happiness or pleasure. The dysphoria in grief is likely to decrease in intensity over days to weeks and occurs in waves, the so-called pangs of grief. These waves tend to be associated with thoughts or reminders of the deceased. The depressed mood of an MDE is more persistent and not tied to specific thoughts or preoccupations. The pain of grief may be accompanied by positive emotions and humor that are uncharacteristic of the pervasive unhappiness and misery characteristic of an MDE. The thought content associated with grief generally features a preoccupation with thoughts and memories of the deceased, rather than the self-critical or pessimistic ruminations seen in an MDE. In grief, self-esteem is generally preserved, whereas in an MDE, feelings of worthlessness and self-loathing are common. If self-derogatory ideation is present in grief, it typically involves perceived failings vis-à-vis the deceased (e.g., not visiting frequently enough, not telling the deceased how much he or she was loved). If a bereaved individual thinks about death and dying, such thoughts are generally focused on the deceased and possibly about "joining" the deceased, whereas in an MDE such thoughts are focused on ending one's own life because of feeling worthless, undeserving of life, or unable to cope with the pain of depression.

Bipolar I disorder	Current or most recent episode manic	Current or most recent episode hypomanic*	Current or most recent episode depressed	Current or most recent episode unspecified**
With psychotic features*** (p. 152)	296.44 (F31.2)	NA	296.54 (F31.5)	NA
In partial remission (p. 154)	296.45 (F31.73)	296.45 (F31.71)	296.55 (F31.75)	NA
In full remission (p. 154)	296.46 (F31.74)	296.46 (F31.72)	296.56 (F31.76)	NA
Unspecified	296.40 (F31.9)	296.40 (F31.9)	296.50 (F31.9)	NA

*Severity and psychotic specifiers do not apply; code 296.40 (F31.0) for cases not in remission.
**Severity, psychotic, and remission specifiers do not apply. Code 296.7 (F31.9).
***If psychotic features are present, code the "with psychotic features" specifier irrespective of episode severity.

In recording the name of a diagnosis, terms should be listed in the following order: bipolar I disorder, type of current or most recent episode, severity/psychotic/remission specifiers, followed by as many specifiers without codes as apply to the current or most recent episode.

Specify:
   With anxious distress (p. 149)
   With mixed features (pp. 149–150)
   With rapid cycling (pp. 150–151)
   With melancholic features (p. 151)
   With atypical features (pp. 151–152)
   With mood-congruent psychotic features (p. 152)
   With mood-incongruent psychotic features (p. 152)
   With catatonia (p. 152). **Coding note:** Use additional code 293.89 (F06.1).
   With peripartum onset (pp. 152–153)
   With seasonal pattern (pp. 153–154)

Diagnostic Features

The essential feature of a manic episode is a distinct period during which there is an abnormally, persistently elevated, expansive, or irritable mood and persistently increased activity or energy that is present for most of the day, nearly every day, for a period of at least 1 week (or any duration if hospitalization is necessary), accompanied by at least three additional symptoms from Criterion B. If the mood is irritable rather than elevated or expansive, at least four Criterion B symptoms must be present.

Mood in a manic episode is often described as euphoric, excessively cheerful, high, or "feeling on top of the world." In some cases, the mood is of such a highly infectious quality that it is easily recognized as excessive and may be characterized by unlimited and haphazard enthusiasm for interpersonal, sexual, or occupational interactions. For example, the individual may spontaneously start extensive conversations with strangers in public. Often the predominant mood is irritable rather than elevated, particularly when the individual's wishes are denied or if the individual has been using substances. Rapid shifts in mood over brief periods of time may occur and are referred to as lability (i.e., the alternation among euphoria, dysphoria, and irritability). In children, happiness, silliness and "goofiness" are normal in the context of special occasions; however, if these symptoms are recurrent, inappropriate to the context, and beyond what is expected for the developmental level of the child, they may meet Criterion A. If the happiness is unusual for a child (i.e., distinct from baseline), and the mood change occurs at the same time as symptoms that meet Criterion B for mania, diagnostic certainty is increased; however, the mood change must be accompanied by persistently increased activity or energy levels that are obvious to those who know the child well.

During the manic episode, the individual may engage in multiple overlapping new projects. The projects are often initiated with little knowledge of the topic, and nothing seems out of the individual's reach. The increased activity levels may manifest at unusual hours of the day.

Inflated self-esteem is typically present, ranging from uncritical self-confidence to marked grandiosity, and may reach delusional proportions (Criterion B1). Despite lack of any particular experience or talent, the individual may embark on complex tasks such as writing a novel or seeking publicity for some impractical invention. Grandiose delusions (e.g., of having a special relationship to a famous person) are common. In children, overestimation of abilities and belief that, for example, they are the best at a sport or the smartest in the class is normal; however, when such beliefs are present despite clear evidence to the contrary or the child attempts feats that are clearly dangerous and, most important, represent a change from the child's normal behavior, the grandiosity criterion should be considered satisfied.

One of the most common features is a decreased need for sleep (Criterion B2) and is distinct from insomnia in which the individual wants to sleep or feels the need to sleep but is unable. The individual may sleep little, if at all, or may awaken several hours earlier than usual, feeling rested and full of energy. When the sleep disturbance is severe, the individual may go for days without sleep, yet not feel tired. Often a decreased need for sleep heralds the onset of a manic episode.

Speech can be rapid, pressured, loud, and difficult to interrupt (Criterion B3). Individuals may talk continuously and without regard for others' wishes to communicate, often in an intrusive manner or without concern for the relevance of what is said. Speech is sometimes characterized by jokes, puns, amusing irrelevancies, and theatricality, with dramatic mannerisms, singing, and excessive gesturing. Loudness and forcefulness of speech often become more important than what is conveyed. If the individual's mood is more irritable than expansive, speech may be marked by complaints, hostile comments, or angry tirades, particularly if attempts are made to interrupt the individual. Both Criterion A and Criterion B symptoms may be accompanied by symptoms of the opposite (i.e., depressive) pole (see "with mixed features" specifier, pp. 149–150).

Often the individual's thoughts race at a rate faster than they can be expressed through speech (Criterion B4). Frequently there is flight of ideas evidenced by a nearly continuous flow of accelerated speech, with abrupt shifts from one topic to another. When flight of ideas is severe, speech may become disorganized, incoherent, and particularly distressful to the individual. Sometimes thoughts are experienced as so crowded that it is very difficult to speak.

Distractibility (Criterion B5) is evidenced by an inability to censor immaterial external stimuli (e.g., the interviewer's attire, background noises or conversations, furnishings in the room) and often prevents individuals experiencing mania from holding a rational conversation or attending to instructions.

The increase in goal-directed activity often consists of excessive planning and participation in multiple activities, including sexual, occupational, political, or religious activities. Increased sexual drive, fantasies, and behavior are often present. Individuals in a manic episode usually show increased sociability (e.g., renewing old acquaintances or calling or contacting friends or even strangers), without regard to the intrusive, domineering, and demanding nature of these interactions. They often display psychomotor agitation or restlessness (i.e., purposeless activity) by pacing or by holding multiple conversations simultaneously. Some individuals write excessive letters, e-mails, text messages, and so forth, on many different topics to friends, public figures, or the media.

The increased activity criterion can be difficult to ascertain in children; however, when the child takes on many tasks simultaneously, starts devising elaborate and unrealistic plans for projects, develops previously absent and developmentally inappropriate sexual preoccupations (not accounted for by sexual abuse or exposure to sexually explicit material), then Criterion B might be met based on clinical judgment. It is essential to determine whether the behavior represents a change from the child's baseline behavior; occurs most of the day, nearly every day for the requisite time period; and occurs in temporal association with other symptoms of mania.

The expansive mood, excessive optimism, grandiosity, and poor judgment often lead to reckless involvement in activities such as spending sprees, giving away possessions, reckless driving, foolish business investments, and sexual promiscuity that is unusual for the individual, even though these activities are likely to have catastrophic consequences (Criterion B7). The individual may purchase many unneeded items without the money to pay for them and, in some cases, give them away. Sexual behavior may include infidelity or indiscriminate sexual encounters with strangers, often disregarding the risk of sexually transmitted diseases or interpersonal consequences.

The manic episode must result in marked impairment in social or occupational functioning or require hospitalization to prevent harm to self or others (e.g., financial losses, illegal activities, loss of employment, self-injurious behavior). By definition, the presence of psychotic features during a manic episode also satisfies Criterion C.

Manic symptoms or syndromes that are attributable to the physiological effects of a drug of abuse (e.g., in the context of cocaine or amphetamine intoxication), the side effects of medications or treatments (e.g., steroids, L-dopa, antidepressants, stimulants), or another medical condition do not count toward the diagnosis of bipolar I disorder. However, a fully syndromal manic episode that arises during treatment (e.g., with medications, electroconvulsive therapy, light therapy) or drug use and persists beyond the physiological effect of the inducing agent (i.e., after a medication is fully out of the individual's system or the effects of electroconvulsive therapy would be expected to have dissipated completely) is sufficient evidence for a manic episode diagnosis (Criterion D). Caution is indicated so that one or two symptoms (particularly increased irritability, edginess, or agitation following antidepressant use) are not taken as sufficient for diagnosis of a manic or hypomanic episode, nor necessarily an indication of a bipolar disorder diathesis. It is necessary to meet criteria for a manic episode to make a diagnosis of bipolar I disorder, but it is not required to have hypomanic or major depressive episodes. However, they may precede or follow a manic episode. Full descriptions of the diagnostic features of a hypomanic episode may be found within the text for bipolar II disorder, and the features of a major depressive episode are described within the text for major depressive disorder.

Associated Features Supporting Diagnosis

During a manic episode, individuals often do not perceive that they are ill or in need of treatment and vehemently resist efforts to be treated. Individuals may change their dress, makeup, or personal appearance to a more sexually suggestive or flamboyant style. Some perceive a sharper sense of smell, hearing, or vision. Gambling and antisocial behaviors may accompany the manic episode. Some individuals may become hostile and physically threatening to others and, when delusional, may become physically assaultive or suicidal. Catastrophic consequences of a manic episode (e.g., involuntary hospitalization, difficulties with the law, serious financial difficulties) often result from poor judgment, loss of insight, and hyperactivity.

Mood may shift very rapidly to anger or depression. Depressive symptoms may occur during a manic episode and, if present, may last moments, hours, or, more rarely, days (see "with mixed features" specifier, pp. 149–150).

Prevalence

The 12-month prevalence estimate in the continental United States was 0.6% for bipolar I disorder as defined in DSM-IV. Twelve-month prevalence of bipolar I disorder across 11 countries ranged from 0.0% to 0.6%. The lifetime male-to-female prevalence ratio is approximately 1.1:1.

Development and Course

Mean age at onset of the first manic, hypomanic, or major depressive episode is approximately 18 years for bipolar I disorder. Special considerations are necessary to detect the diagnosis in children. Since children of the same chronological age may be at different developmental stages, it is difficult to define with precision what is "normal" or "expected" at any given point. Therefore, each child should be judged according to his or her own baseline. Onset occurs throughout the life cycle, including first onsets in the 60s or 70s. Onset of manic symptoms (e.g., sexual or social disinhibition) in late mid-life or late-life should prompt consideration of medical conditions (e.g., frontotemporal neurocognitive disorder) and of substance ingestion or withdrawal.

More than 90% of individuals who have a single manic episode go on to have recurrent mood episodes. Approximately 60% of manic episodes occur immediately before a major depressive episode. Individuals with bipolar I disorder who have multiple (four or more) mood episodes (major depressive, manic, or hypomanic) within 1 year receive the specifier "with rapid cycling."

Risk and Prognostic Factors

Environmental. Bipolar disorder is more common in high-income than in low-income countries (1.4% vs. 0.7%). Separated, divorced, or widowed individuals have higher rates of bipolar I disorder than do individuals who are married or have never been married, but the direction of the association is unclear.

Genetic and physiological. A family history of bipolar disorder is one of the strongest and most consistent risk factors for bipolar disorders. There is an average 10-fold increased risk among adult relatives of individuals with bipolar I and bipolar II disorders. Magnitude of risk increases with degree of kinship. Schizophrenia and bipolar disorder likely share a genetic origin, reflected in familial co-aggregation of schizophrenia and bipolar disorder.

Course modifiers. After an individual has a manic episode with psychotic features, subsequent manic episodes are more likely to include psychotic features. Incomplete interepisode recovery is more common when the current episode is accompanied by mood-incongruent psychotic features.

Culture-Related Diagnostic Issues

Little information exists on specific cultural differences in the expression of bipolar I disorder. One possible explanation for this may be that diagnostic instruments are often translated and applied in different cultures with no transcultural validation. In one U.S. study, 12-month prevalence of bipolar I disorder was significantly lower for Afro-Caribbeans than for African Americans or whites.

Gender-Related Diagnostic Issues

Females are more likely to experience rapid cycling and mixed states, and to have patterns of comorbidity that differ from those of males, including higher rates of lifetime eating disorders. Females with bipolar I or II disorder are more likely to experience depressive symptoms than males. They also have a higher lifetime risk of alcohol use disorder than do males and a much greater likelihood of alcohol use disorder than do females in the general population.

Suicide Risk

The lifetime risk of suicide in individuals with bipolar disorder is estimated to be at least 15 times that of the general population. In fact, bipolar disorder may account for one-quarter of all completed suicides. A past history of suicide attempt and percent days spent depressed in the past year are associated with greater risk of suicide attempts or completions.

Functional Consequences of Bipolar I Disorder

Although many individuals with bipolar disorder return to a fully functional level between episodes, approximately 30% show severe impairment in work role function. Functional recovery lags substantially behind recovery from symptoms, especially with respect to occupational recovery, resulting in lower socioeconomic status despite equivalent levels of education when compared with the general population. Individuals with bipolar I disorder perform more poorly than healthy individuals on cognitive tests. Cognitive impairments may contribute to vocational and interpersonal difficulties and persist through the lifespan, even during euthymic periods.

Differential Diagnosis

Major depressive disorder.   Major depressive disorder may also be accompanied by hypomanic or manic symptoms (i.e., fewer symptoms or for a shorter duration than required for mania or hypomania). When the individual presents in an episode of major depression, one must depend on corroborating history regarding past episodes of mania or hypomania. Symptoms of irritability may be associated with either major depressive disorder or bipolar disorder, adding to diagnostic complexity.

Other bipolar disorders.   Diagnosis of bipolar I disorder is differentiated from bipolar II disorder by determining whether there have been any past episodes of mania. Other specified and unspecified bipolar and related disorders should be differentiated from bipolar I and II disorders by considering whether either the episodes involving manic or hypomanic symptoms or the episodes of depressive symptoms fail to meet the full criteria for those conditions.

Bipolar disorder due to another medical condition may be distinguished from bipolar I and II disorders by identifying, based on best clinical evidence, a causally related medical condition.

Generalized anxiety disorder, panic disorder, posttraumatic stress disorder, or other anxiety disorders.   These disorders need to be considered in the differential diagnosis as either the primary disorder or, in some cases, a comorbid disorder. A careful history of symptoms is needed to differentiate generalized anxiety disorder from bipolar disorder, as anxious ruminations may be mistaken for racing thoughts, and efforts to minimize anxious feelings may be taken as impulsive behavior. Similarly, symptoms of posttraumatic stress disorder need to be differentiated from bipolar disorder. It is helpful to assess the episodic nature of the symptoms described, as well as to consider symptom triggers, in making this differential diagnosis.

Substance/medication-induced bipolar disorder.   Substance use disorders may manifest with substance/medication-induced manic symptoms that must be distinguished from bipolar I disorder; response to mood stabilizers during a substance/medication-induced mania may not necessarily be diagnostic for bipolar disorder. There may be substantial overlap in view of the tendency for individuals with bipolar I disorder to overuse substances during an episode. A primary diagnosis of bipolar disorder must be established based on symptoms that remain once substances are no longer being used.

Attention-deficit/hyperactivity disorder.   This disorder may be misdiagnosed as bipolar disorder, especially in adolescents and children. Many symptoms overlap with the symptoms of mania, such as rapid speech, racing thoughts, distractibility, and less need for sleep. The "double counting" of symptoms toward both ADHD and bipolar disorder can be avoided if the clinician clarifies whether the symptom(s) represents a distinct episode.

Personality disorders.   Personality disorders such as borderline personality disorder may have substantial symptomatic overlap with bipolar disorders, since mood lability and impulsivity are common in both conditions. Symptoms must represent a distinct episode, and the noticeable increase over baseline required for the diagnosis of bipolar disorder must be present. A diagnosis of a personality disorder should not be made during an untreated mood episode.

Disorders with prominent irritability.   In individuals with severe irritability, particularly children and adolescents, care must be taken to apply the diagnosis of bipolar disorder only to those who have had a clear episode of mania or hypomania—that is, a distinct time period, of the required duration, during which the irritability was clearly different from the individual's baseline and was accompanied by the onset of Criterion B symptoms. When a child's irritability is persistent and particularly severe, the diagnosis of disruptive mood dysregulation disorder would be more appropriate. Indeed, when any child is being assessed for mania, it is essential that the symptoms represent a clear change from the child's typical behavior.

Comorbidity

Co-occurring mental disorders are common, with the most frequent disorders being any anxiety disorder (e.g., panic attacks, social anxiety disorder [social phobia], specific phobia), occurring in approximately three-fourths of individuals; ADHD, any disruptive, impulse-control, or conduct disorder (e.g., intermittent explosive disorder, oppositional defiant disorder, conduct disorder), and any substance use disorder (e.g., alcohol use disorder) occur in over half of individuals with bipolar I disorder. Adults with bipolar I disorder have high rates of serious and/or untreated co-occurring medical conditions. Metabolic syndrome and migraine are more common among individuals with bipolar disorder than in the general population. More than half of individuals whose symptoms meet criteria for bipolar disorder have an alcohol use disorder, and those with both disorders are at greater risk for suicide attempt.

Bipolar II Disorder

Diagnostic Criteria   **296.89** (F31.81)

For a diagnosis of bipolar II disorder, it is necessary to meet the following criteria for a current or past hypomanic episode *and* the following criteria for a current or past major depressive episode:

Hypomanic Episode

A. A distinct period of abnormally and persistently elevated, expansive, or irritable mood and abnormally and persistently increased activity or energy, lasting at least 4 consecutive days and present most of the day, nearly every day.

B. During the period of mood disturbance and increased energy and activity, three (or more) of the following symptoms have persisted (four if the mood is only irritable), represent a noticeable change from usual behavior, and have been present to a significant degree:

1. Inflated self-esteem or grandiosity.
2. Decreased need for sleep (e.g., feels rested after only 3 hours of sleep).
3. More talkative than usual or pressure to keep talking.

4. Flight of ideas or subjective experience that thoughts are racing.
5. Distractibility (i.e., attention too easily drawn to unimportant or irrelevant external stimuli), as reported or observed.
6. Increase in goal-directed activity (either socially, at work or school, or sexually) or psychomotor agitation.
7. Excessive involvement in activities that have a high potential for painful consequences (e.g., engaging in unrestrained buying sprees, sexual indiscretions, or foolish business investments).

C. The episode is associated with an unequivocal change in functioning that is uncharacteristic of the individual when not symptomatic.
D. The disturbance in mood and the change in functioning are observable by others.
E. The episode is not severe enough to cause marked impairment in social or occupational functioning or to necessitate hospitalization. If there are psychotic features, the episode is, by definition, manic.
F. The episode is not attributable to the physiological effects of a substance (e.g., a drug of abuse, a medication, other treatment) or another medical condition.
   Note: A full hypomanic episode that emerges during antidepressant treatment (e.g., medication, electroconvulsive therapy) but persists at a fully syndromal level beyond the physiological effect of that treatment is sufficient evidence for a hypomanic episode diagnosis. However, caution is indicated so that one or two symptoms (particularly increased irritability, edginess, or agitation following antidepressant use) are not taken as sufficient for diagnosis of a hypomanic episode, nor necessarily indicative of a bipolar diathesis.

Major Depressive Episode
A. Five (or more) of the following symptoms have been present during the same 2-week period and represent a change from previous functioning; at least one of the symptoms is either (1) depressed mood or (2) loss of interest or pleasure.
   Note: Do not include symptoms that are clearly attributable to a medical condition.

   1. Depressed mood most of the day, nearly every day, as indicated by either subjective report (e.g., feels sad, empty, or hopeless) or observation made by others (e.g., appears tearful). (**Note:** In children and adolescents, can be irritable mood.)
   2. Markedly diminished interest or pleasure in all, or almost all, activities most of the day, nearly every day (as indicated by either subjective account or observation).
   3. Significant weight loss when not dieting or weight gain (e.g., a change of more than 5% of body weight in a month), or decrease or increase in appetite nearly every day. (**Note:** In children, consider failure to make expected weight gain.)
   4. Insomnia or hypersomnia nearly every day.
   5. Psychomotor agitation or retardation nearly every day (observable by others; not merely subjective feelings of restlessness or being slowed down).
   6. Fatigue or loss of energy nearly every day.
   7. Feelings of worthlessness or excessive or inappropriate guilt (which may be delusional) nearly every day (not merely self-reproach or guilt about being sick).
   8. Diminished ability to think or concentrate, or indecisiveness, nearly every day (either by subjective account or as observed by others).
   9. Recurrent thoughts of death (not just fear of dying), recurrent suicidal ideation without a specific plan, a suicide attempt, or a specific plan for committing suicide.

B. The symptoms cause clinically significant distress or impairment in social, occupational, or other important areas of functioning.
C. The episode is not attributable to the physiological effects of a substance or another medical condition.

Note: Criteria A–C above constitute a major depressive episode.

Note: Responses to a significant loss (e.g., bereavement, financial ruin, losses from a natural disaster, a serious medical illness or disability) may include the feelings of intense sadness, rumination about the loss, insomnia, poor appetite, and weight loss noted in Criterion A, which may resemble a depressive episode. Although such symptoms may be understandable or considered appropriate to the loss, the presence of a major depressive episode in addition to the normal response to a significant loss should be carefully considered. This decision inevitably requires the exercise of clinical judgment based on the individual's history and the cultural norms for the expression of distress in the context of loss.[1]

Bipolar II Disorder

A. Criteria have been met for at least one hypomanic episode (Criteria A–F under "Hypomanic Episode" above) and at least one major depressive episode (Criteria A–C under "Major Depressive Episode" above).

B. There has never been a manic episode.

C. The occurrence of the hypomanic episode(s) and major depressive episode(s) is not better explained by schizoaffective disorder, schizophrenia, schizophreniform disorder, delusional disorder, or other specified or unspecified schizophrenia spectrum and other psychotic disorder.

D. The symptoms of depression or the unpredictability caused by frequent alternation between periods of depression and hypomania causes clinically significant distress or impairment in social, occupational, or other important areas of functioning.

Coding and Recording Procedures

Bipolar II disorder has one diagnostic code: 296.89 (F31.81). Its status with respect to current severity, presence of psychotic features, course, and other specifiers cannot be coded but should be indicated in writing (e.g., 296.89 [F31.81] bipolar II disorder, current episode depressed, moderate severity, with mixed features; 296.89 [F31.81] bipolar II disorder, most recent episode depressed, in partial remission).

Specify current or most recent episode:
Hypomanic
Depressed

Specify if:
With anxious distress (p. 149)
With mixed features (pp. 149–150)

---

[1] In distinguishing grief from a major depressive episode (MDE), it is useful to consider that in grief the predominant affect is feelings of emptiness and loss, while in an MDE it is persistent depressed mood and the inability to anticipate happiness or pleasure. The dysphoria in grief is likely to decrease in intensity over days to weeks and occurs in waves, the so-called pangs of grief. These waves tend to be associated with thoughts or reminders of the deceased. The depressed mood of an MDE is more persistent and not tied to specific thoughts or preoccupations. The pain of grief may be accompanied by positive emotions and humor that are uncharacteristic of the pervasive unhappiness and misery characteristic of an MDE. The thought content associated with grief generally features a preoccupation with thoughts and memories of the deceased, rather than the self-critical or pessimistic ruminations seen in an MDE. In grief, self-esteem is generally preserved, whereas in an MDE feelings of worthlessness and self-loathing are common. If self-derogatory ideation is present in grief, it typically involves perceived failings vis-à-vis the deceased (e.g., not visiting frequently enough, not telling the deceased how much he or she was loved). If a bereaved individual thinks about death and dying, such thoughts are generally focused on the deceased and possibly about "joining" the deceased, whereas in an MDE such thoughts are focused on ending one's own life because of feeling worthless, undeserving of life, or unable to cope with the pain of depression.

With rapid cycling (pp. 150–151)
With melancholic features (p. 151)
With atypical features (pp. 151–152)
With mood-congruent psychotic features (p. 152)
With mood-incongruent psychotic features (p. 152)
With catatonia (p. 152). **Coding note:** Use additional code 293.89 (F06.1).
With peripartum onset (pp. 152–153)
With seasonal pattern (pp. 153–154)

Specify course if full criteria for a mood episode are not currently met:
In partial remission (p. 154)
In full remission (p. 154)

Specify severity if full criteria for a major depressive episode are currently met:
Mild (p. 154)
Moderate (p. 154)
Severe (p. 154)

Diagnostic Features

Bipolar II disorder is characterized by a clinical course of recurring mood episodes consisting of one or more major depressive episodes (Criteria A–C under "Major Depressive Episode") and at least one hypomanic episode (Criteria A–F under "Hypomanic Episode"). The major depressive episode must last at least 2 weeks, and the hypomanic episode must last at least 4 days, to meet the diagnostic criteria. During the mood episode(s), the requisite number of symptoms must be present most of the day, nearly every day, and represent a noticeable change from usual behavior and functioning. The presence of a manic episode during the course of illness precludes the diagnosis of bipolar II disorder (Criterion B under "Bipolar II Disorder"). Episodes of substance/medication-induced depressive disorder or substance/medication-induced bipolar and related disorder (representing the physiological effects of a medication, other somatic treatments for depression, drugs of abuse, or toxin exposure) or of depressive and related disorder due to another medical condition or bipolar and related disorder due to another medical condition do not count toward a diagnosis of bipolar II disorder unless they persist beyond the physiological effects of the treatment or substance and then meet duration criteria for an episode. In addition, the episodes must not be better accounted for by schizoaffective disorder and are not superimposed on schizophrenia, schizophreniform disorder, delusional disorder, or other specified or unspecified schizophrenia spectrum or other psychotic disorders (Criterion C under "Bipolar II Disorder"). The depressive episodes or hypomanic fluctuations must cause clinically significant distress or impairment in social, occupational, or other important areas of functioning (Criterion D under "Bipolar II Disorder"); however, for hypomanic episodes, this requirement does not have to be met. A hypomanic episode that causes significant impairment would likely qualify for the diagnosis of manic episode and, therefore, for a lifetime diagnosis of bipolar I disorder. The recurrent major depressive episodes are often more frequent and lengthier than those occurring in bipolar I disorder.

Individuals with bipolar II disorder typically present to a clinician during a major depressive episode and are unlikely to complain initially of hypomania. Typically, the hypomanic episodes themselves do not cause impairment. Instead, the impairment results from the major depressive episodes or from a persistent pattern of unpredictable mood changes and fluctuating, unreliable interpersonal or occupational functioning. Individuals with bipolar II disorder may not view the hypomanic episodes as pathological or disadvantageous, although others may be troubled by the individual's erratic behavior. Clinical information from other informants, such as close friends or relatives, is often useful in establishing the diagnosis of bipolar II disorder.

A hypomanic episode should not be confused with the several days of euthymia and restored energy or activity that may follow remission of a major depressive episode. Despite the substantial differences in duration and severity between a manic and hypomanic episode, bipolar II disorder is not a "milder form" of bipolar I disorder. Compared with individuals with bipolar I disorder, individuals with bipolar II disorder have greater chronicity of illness and spend, on average, more time in the depressive phase of their illness, which can be severe and/or disabling. Depressive symptoms co-occurring with a hypomanic episode or hypomanic symptoms co-occurring with a depressive episode are common in individuals with bipolar II disorder and are overrepresented in females, particularly hypomania with mixed features. Individuals experiencing hypomania with mixed features may not label their symptoms as hypomania, but instead experience them as depression with increased energy or irritability.

Associated Features Supporting Diagnosis

A common feature of bipolar II disorder is impulsivity, which can contribute to suicide attempts and substance use disorders. Impulsivity may also stem from a concurrent personality disorder, substance use disorder, anxiety disorder, another mental disorder, or a medical condition. There may be heightened levels of creativity in some individuals with a bipolar disorder. However, that relationship may be nonlinear; that is, greater lifetime creative accomplishments have been associated with milder forms of bipolar disorder, and higher creativity has been found in unaffected family members. The individual's attachment to heightened creativity during hypomanic episodes may contribute to ambivalence about seeking treatment or undermine adherence to treatment.

Prevalence

The 12-month prevalence of bipolar II disorder, internationally, is 0.3%. In the United States, 12-month prevalence is 0.8%. The prevalence rate of pediatric bipolar II disorder is difficult to establish. DSM-IV bipolar I, bipolar II, and bipolar disorder not otherwise specified yield a combined prevalence rate of 1.8% in U.S. and non-U.S. community samples, with higher rates (2.7% inclusive) in youths age 12 years or older.

Development and Course

Although bipolar II disorder can begin in late adolescence and throughout adulthood, average age at onset is the mid-20s, which is slightly later than for bipolar I disorder but earlier than for major depressive disorder. The illness most often begins with a depressive episode and is not recognized as bipolar II disorder until a hypomanic episode occurs; this happens in about 12% of individuals with the initial diagnosis of major depressive disorder. Anxiety, substance use, or eating disorders may also precede the diagnosis, complicating its detection. Many individuals experience several episodes of major depression prior to the first recognized hypomanic episode.

The number of lifetime episodes (both hypomanic and major depressive episodes) tends to be higher for bipolar II disorder than for major depressive disorder or bipolar I disorder. However, individuals with bipolar I disorder are actually more likely to experience hypomanic symptoms than are individuals with bipolar II disorder. The interval between mood episodes in the course of bipolar II disorder tends to decrease as the individual ages. While the hypomanic episode is the feature that defines bipolar II disorder, depressive episodes are more enduring and disabling over time. Despite the predominance of depression, once a hypomanic episode has occurred, the diagnosis becomes bipolar II disorder and never reverts to major depressive disorder.

Approximately 5%–15% of individuals with bipolar II disorder have multiple (four or more) mood episodes (hypomanic or major depressive) within the previous 12 months. If this pattern is present, it is noted by the specifier "with rapid cycling." By definition, psychotic symptoms do not occur in hypomanic episodes, and they appear to be less frequent in the major depressive episodes in bipolar II disorder than in those of bipolar I disorder.

Switching from a depressive episode to a manic or hypomanic episode (with or without mixed features) may occur, both spontaneously and during treatment for depression. About 5%–15% of individuals with bipolar II disorder will ultimately develop a manic episode, which changes the diagnosis to bipolar I disorder, regardless of subsequent course.

Making the diagnosis in children is often a challenge, especially in those with irritability and hyperarousal that is *nonepisodic* (i.e., lacks the well-demarcated periods of altered mood). Nonepisodic irritability in youth is associated with an elevated risk for anxiety disorders and major depressive disorder, but not bipolar disorder, in adulthood. Persistently irritable youths have lower familial rates of bipolar disorder than do youths who have bipolar disorder. For a hypomanic episode to be diagnosed, the child's symptoms must exceed what is expected in a given environment and culture for the child's developmental stage. Compared with adult onset of bipolar II disorder, childhood or adolescent onset of the disorder may be associated with a more severe lifetime course. The 3-year incidence rate of first-onset bipolar II disorder in adults older than 60 years is 0.34%. However, distinguishing individuals older than 60 years with bipolar II disorder by late versus early age at onset does not appear to have any clinical utility.

Risk and Prognostic Factors

Genetic and physiological.   The risk of bipolar II disorder tends to be highest among relatives of individuals with bipolar II disorder, as opposed to individuals with bipolar I disorder or major depressive disorder. There may be genetic factors influencing the age at onset for bipolar disorders.

Course modifiers.   A rapid-cycling pattern is associated with a poorer prognosis. Return to previous level of social function for individuals with bipolar II disorder is more likely for individuals of younger age and with less severe depression, suggesting adverse effects of prolonged illness on recovery. More education, fewer years of illness, and being married are independently associated with functional recovery in individuals with bipolar disorder, even after diagnostic type (I vs. II), current depressive symptoms, and presence of psychiatric comorbidity are taken into account.

Gender-Related Diagnostic Issues

Whereas the gender ratio for bipolar I disorder is equal, findings on gender differences in bipolar II disorder are mixed, differing by type of sample (i.e., registry, community, or clinical) and country of origin. There is little to no evidence of bipolar gender differences, whereas some, but not all, clinical samples suggest that bipolar II disorder is more common in females than in males, which may reflect gender differences in treatment seeking or other factors.

Patterns of illness and comorbidity, however, seem to differ by gender, with females being more likely than males to report hypomania with mixed depressive features and a rapid-cycling course. Childbirth may be a specific trigger for a hypomanic episode, which can occur in 10%–20% of females in nonclinical populations and most typically in the early postpartum period. Distinguishing hypomania from the elated mood and reduced sleep that normally accompany the birth of a child may be challenging. Postpartum hypomania may foreshadow the onset of a depression that occurs in about half of females who experience postpartum "highs." Accurate detection of bipolar II disorder may help in establishing appropriate treatment of the depression, which may reduce the risk of suicide and infanticide.

Suicide Risk

Suicide risk is high in bipolar II disorder. Approximately one-third of individuals with bipolar II disorder report a lifetime history of suicide attempt. The prevalence rates of lifetime attempted suicide in bipolar II and bipolar I disorder appear to be similar (32.4% and 36.3%, respectively). However, the lethality of attempts, as defined by a lower ratio of attempts to completed suicides, may be higher in individuals with bipolar II disorder compared with individuals with bipolar I disorder. There may be an association between genetic markers and increased risk for suicidal behavior in individuals with bipolar disorder, including a 6.5-fold higher risk of suicide among first-degree relatives of bipolar II probands compared with those with bipolar I disorder.

Functional Consequences of Bipolar II Disorder

Although many individuals with bipolar II disorder return to a fully functional level between mood episodes, at least 15% continue to have some inter-episode dysfunction, and 20% transition directly into another mood episode without inter-episode recovery. Functional recovery lags substantially behind recovery from symptoms of bipolar II disorder, especially in regard to occupational recovery, resulting in lower socioeconomic status despite equivalent levels of education with the general population. Individuals with bipolar II disorder perform more poorly than healthy individuals on cognitive tests and, with the exception of memory and semantic fluency, have similar cognitive impairment as do individuals with bipolar I disorder. Cognitive impairments associated with bipolar II disorder may contribute to vocational difficulties. Prolonged unemployment in individuals with bipolar disorder is associated with more episodes of depression, older age, increased rates of current panic disorder, and lifetime history of alcohol use disorder.

Differential Diagnosis

Major depressive disorder.   Perhaps the most challenging differential diagnosis to consider is major depressive disorder, which may be accompanied by hypomanic or manic symptoms that do not meet full criteria (i.e., either fewer symptoms or a shorter duration than required for a hypomanic episode). This is especially true in evaluating individuals with symptoms of irritability, which may be associated with either major depressive disorder or bipolar II disorder.

Cyclothymic disorder.   In cyclothymic disorder, there are numerous periods of hypomanic symptoms and numerous periods of depressive symptoms that do not meet symptom or duration criteria for a major depressive episode. Bipolar II disorder is distinguished from cyclothymic disorder by the presence of one or more major depressive episodes. If a major depressive episode occurs after the first 2 years of cyclothymic disorder, the additional diagnosis of bipolar II disorder is given.

Schizophrenia spectrum and other related psychotic disorders.   Bipolar II disorder must be distinguished from psychotic disorders (e.g., schizoaffective disorder, schizophrenia, and delusional disorder). Schizophrenia, schizoaffective disorder, and delusional disorder are all characterized by periods of psychotic symptoms that occur in the absence of prominent mood symptoms. Other helpful considerations include the accompanying symptoms, previous course, and family history.

Panic disorder or other anxiety disorders.   Anxiety disorders need to be considered in the differential diagnosis and may frequently be present as co-occurring disorders.

Substance use disorders.   Substance use disorders are included in the differential diagnosis.

Attention-deficit/hyperactivity disorder.   Attention-deficit/hyperactivity disorder (ADHD) may be misdiagnosed as bipolar II disorder, especially in adolescents and children. Many symptoms of ADHD, such as rapid speech, racing thoughts, distractibility, and less need for sleep, overlap with the symptoms of hypomania. The double counting of symptoms toward both ADHD and bipolar II disorder can be avoided if the clinician clarifies whether the symptoms represent a distinct episode and if the noticeable increase over baseline required for the diagnosis of bipolar II disorder is present.

Personality disorders.   The same convention as applies for ADHD also applies when evaluating an individual for a personality disorder such as borderline personality disorder, since mood lability and impulsivity are common in both personality disorders and bipolar II disorder. Symptoms must represent a distinct episode, and the noticeable increase over baseline required for the diagnosis of bipolar II disorder must be present. A diagnosis of a personality disorder should not be made during an untreated mood episode unless the lifetime history supports the presence of a personality disorder.

Other bipolar disorders.   Diagnosis of bipolar II disorder should be differentiated from bipolar I disorder by carefully considering whether there have been any past episodes of mania and from other specified and unspecified bipolar and related disorders by confirming the presence of fully syndromal hypomania and depression.

Comorbidity

Bipolar II disorder is more often than not associated with one or more co-occurring mental disorders, with anxiety disorders being the most common. Approximately 60% of individuals with bipolar II disorder have three or more co-occurring mental disorders; 75% have an anxiety disorder; and 37% have a substance use disorder. Children and adolescents with bipolar II disorder have a higher rate of co-occurring anxiety disorders compared with those with bipolar I disorder, and the anxiety disorder most often predates the bipolar disorder. Anxiety and substance use disorders occur in individuals with bipolar II disorder at a higher rate than in the general population. Approximately 14% of individuals with bipolar II disorder have at least one lifetime eating disorder, with binge-eating disorder being more common than bulimia nervosa and anorexia nervosa.

These commonly co-occurring disorders do not seem to follow a course of illness that is truly independent from that of the bipolar disorder, but rather have strong associations with mood states. For example, anxiety and eating disorders tend to associate most with depressive symptoms, and substance use disorders are moderately associated with manic symptoms.

Cyclothymic Disorder

Diagnostic Criteria   **301.13** (F34.0)

A. For at least 2 years (at least 1 year in children and adolescents) there have been numerous periods with hypomanic symptoms that do not meet criteria for a hypomanic episode and numerous periods with depressive symptoms that do not meet criteria for a major depressive episode.
B. During the above 2-year period (1 year in children and adolescents), the hypomanic and depressive periods have been present for at least half the time and the individual has not been without the symptoms for more than 2 months at a time.
C. Criteria for a major depressive, manic, or hypomanic episode have never been met.
D. The symptoms in Criterion A are not better explained by schizoaffective disorder, schizophrenia, schizophreniform disorder, delusional disorder, or other specified or unspecified schizophrenia spectrum and other psychotic disorder.
E. The symptoms are not attributable to the physiological effects of a substance (e.g., a drug of abuse, a medication) or another medical condition (e.g., hyperthyroidism).

F. The symptoms cause clinically significant distress or impairment in social, occupational, or other important areas of functioning.

Specify if:
   With anxious distress (see p. 149)

Diagnostic Features

The essential feature of cyclothymic disorder is a chronic, fluctuating mood disturbance involving numerous periods of hypomanic symptoms and periods of depressive symptoms that are distinct from each other (Criterion A). The hypomanic symptoms are of insufficient number, severity, pervasiveness, or duration to meet full criteria for a hypomanic episode, and the depressive symptoms are of insufficient number, severity, pervasiveness, or duration to meet full criteria for a major depressive episode. During the initial 2-year period (1 year for children or adolescents), the symptoms must be persistent (present more days than not), and any symptom-free intervals last no longer than 2 months (Criterion B). The diagnosis of cyclothymic disorder is made only if the criteria for a major depressive, manic, or hypomanic episode have never been met (Criterion C).

If an individual with cyclothymic disorder subsequently (i.e., after the initial 2 years in adults or 1 year in children or adolescents) experiences a major depressive, manic, or hypomanic episode, the diagnosis changes to major depressive disorder, bipolar I disorder, or other specified or unspecified bipolar and related disorder (subclassified as hypomanic episode without prior major depressive episode), respectively, and the cyclothymic disorder diagnosis is dropped.

The cyclothymic disorder diagnosis is not made if the pattern of mood swings is better explained by schizoaffective disorder, schizophrenia, schizophreniform disorder, delusional disorder, or other specified and unspecified schizophrenia spectrum and other psychotic disorders (Criterion D), in which case the mood symptoms are considered associated features of the psychotic disorder. The mood disturbance must also not be attributable to the physiological effects of a substance (e.g., a drug of abuse, a medication) or another medical condition (e.g., hyperthyroidism) (Criterion E). Although some individuals may function particularly well during some of the periods of hypomania, over the prolonged course of the disorder, there must be clinically significant distress or impairment in social, occupational, or other important areas of functioning as a result of the mood disturbance (Criterion F). The impairment may develop as a result of prolonged periods of cyclical, often unpredictable mood changes (e.g., the individual may be regarded as temperamental, moody, unpredictable, inconsistent, or unreliable).

Prevalence

The lifetime prevalence of cyclothymic disorder is approximately 0.4%–1%. Prevalence in mood disorders clinics may range from 3% to 5%. In the general population, cyclothymic disorder is apparently equally common in males and females. In clinical settings, females with cyclothymic disorder may be more likely to present for treatment than males.

Development and Course

Cyclothymic disorder usually begins in adolescence or early adult life and is sometimes considered to reflect a temperamental predisposition to other disorders in this chapter. Cyclothymic disorder usually has an insidious onset and a persistent course. There is a 15%–50% risk that an individual with cyclothymic disorder will subsequently develop bipolar I disorder or bipolar II disorder. Onset of persistent, fluctuating hypomanic and depressive symptoms late in adult life needs to be clearly differentiated from bipolar and related disorder due to another medical condition and depressive disorder due to another medical condition (e.g., multiple sclerosis) before the cyclothymic disorder diagnosis is assigned. Among children with cyclothymic disorder, the mean age at onset of symptoms is 6.5 years of age.

Risk and Prognostic Factors

Genetic and physiological.   Major depressive disorder, bipolar I disorder, and bipolar II disorder are more common among first-degree biological relatives of individuals with cyclothymic disorder than in the general population. There may also be an increased familial risk of substance-related disorders. Cyclothymic disorder may be more common in the first-degree biological relatives of individuals with bipolar I disorder than in the general population.

Differential Diagnosis

Bipolar and related disorder due to another medical condition and depressive disorder due to another medical condition.   The diagnosis of bipolar and related disorder due to another medical condition or depressive disorder due to another medical condition is made when the mood disturbance is judged to be attributable to the physiological effect of a specific, usually chronic medical condition (e.g., hyperthyroidism). This determination is based on the history, physical examination, or laboratory findings. If it is judged that the hypomanic and depressive symptoms are not the physiological consequence of the medical condition, then the primary mental disorder (i.e., cyclothymic disorder) and the medical condition are coded. For example, this would be the case if the mood symptoms are considered to be the psychological (not the physiological) consequence of having a chronic medical condition, or if there is no etiological relationship between the hypomanic and depressive symptoms and the medical condition.

Substance/medication-induced bipolar and related disorder and substance/medication-induced depressive disorder.   Substance/medication-induced bipolar and related disorder and substance/medication-induced depressive disorder are distinguished from cyclothymic disorder by the judgment that a substance/medication (especially stimulants) is etiologically related to the mood disturbance. The frequent mood swings in these disorders that are suggestive of cyclothymic disorder usually resolve following cessation of substance/medication use.

Bipolar I disorder, with rapid cycling, and bipolar II disorder, with rapid cycling. Both disorders may resemble cyclothymic disorder by virtue of the frequent marked shifts in mood. By definition, in cyclothymic disorder the criteria for a major depressive, manic, or hypomanic episode has never been met, whereas the bipolar I disorder and bipolar II disorder specifier "with rapid cycling" requires that full mood episodes be present.

Borderline personality disorder.   Borderline personality disorder is associated with marked shifts in mood that may suggest cyclothymic disorder. If the criteria are met for both disorders, both borderline personality disorder and cyclothymic disorder may be diagnosed.

Comorbidity

Substance-related disorders and sleep disorders (i.e., difficulties in initiating and maintaining sleep) may be present in individuals with cyclothymic disorder. Most children with cyclothymic disorder treated in outpatient psychiatric settings have comorbid mental conditions; they are more likely than other pediatric patients with mental disorders to have comorbid attention-deficit/hyperactivity disorder.

Substance/Medication-Induced Bipolar and Related Disorder

Diagnostic Criteria

A. A prominent and persistent disturbance in mood that predominates in the clinical picture and is characterized by elevated, expansive, or irritable mood, with or without depressed mood, or markedly diminished interest or pleasure in all, or almost all, activities.

B. There is evidence from the history, physical examination, or laboratory findings of both (1) and (2):

1. The symptoms in Criterion A developed during or soon after substance intoxication or withdrawal or after exposure to a medication.
2. The involved substance/medication is capable of producing the symptoms in Criterion A.

C. The disturbance is not better explained by a bipolar or related disorder that is not substance/medication-induced. Such evidence of an independent bipolar or related disorder could include the following:

The symptoms precede the onset of the substance/medication use; the symptoms persist for a substantial period of time (e.g., about 1 month) after the cessation of acute withdrawal or severe intoxication; or there is other evidence suggesting the existence of an independent non-substance/medication-induced bipolar and related disorder (e.g., a history of recurrent non-substance/medication-related episodes).

D. The disturbance does not occur exclusively during the course of a delirium.

E. The disturbance causes clinically significant distress or impairment in social, occupational, or other important areas of functioning.

Coding note: The ICD-9-CM and ICD-10-CM codes for the [specific substance/medication]-induced bipolar and related disorders are indicated in the table below. Note that the ICD-10-CM code depends on whether or not there is a comorbid substance use disorder present for the same class of substance. If a mild substance use disorder is comorbid with the substance-induced bipolar and related disorder, the 4th position character is "1," and the clinician should record "mild [substance] use disorder" before the substance-induced bipolar and related disorder (e.g., "mild cocaine use disorder with cocaine-induced bipolar and related disorder"). If a moderate or severe substance use disorder is comorbid with the substance-induced bipolar and related disorder, the 4th position character is "2," and the clinician should record "moderate [substance] use disorder" or "severe [substance] use disorder," depending on the severity of the comorbid substance use disorder. If there is no comorbid substance use disorder (e.g., after a one-time heavy use of the substance), then the 4th position character is "9," and the clinician should record only the substance-induced bipolar and related disorder.

| | | ICD-10-CM | | |
	ICD-9-CM	With use disorder, mild	With use disorder, moderate or severe	Without use disorder
Alcohol	291.89	F10.14	F10.24	F10.94
Phencyclidine	292.84	F16.14	F16.24	F16.94
Other hallucinogen	292.84	F16.14	F16.24	F16.94

	ICD-9-CM	ICD-10-CM		
		With use disorder, mild	With use disorder, moderate or severe	Without use disorder
Sedative, hypnotic, or anxiolytic	292.84	F13.14	F13.24	F13.94
Amphetamine (or other stimulant)	292.84	F15.14	F15.24	F15.94
Cocaine	292.84	F14.14	F14.24	F14.94
Other (or unknown) substance	292.84	F19.14	F19.24	F19.94

Specify if (see Table 1 in the chapter "Substance-Related and Addictive Disorders" for diagnoses associated with substance class):

With onset during intoxication: If the criteria are met for intoxication with the substance and the symptoms develop during intoxication.

With onset during withdrawal: If criteria are met for withdrawal from the substance and the symptoms develop during, or shortly after, withdrawal.

Recording Procedures

ICD-9-CM. The name of the substance/medication-induced bipolar and related disorder begins with the specific substance (e.g., cocaine, dexamethasone) that is presumed to be causing the bipolar mood symptoms. The diagnostic code is selected from the table included in the criteria set, which is based on the drug class. For substances that do not fit into any of the classes (e.g., dexamethasone), the code for "other substance" should be used; and in cases in which a substance is judged to be an etiological factor but the specific class of substance is unknown, the category "unknown substance" should be used.

The name of the disorder is followed by the specification of onset (i.e., onset during intoxication, onset during withdrawal). Unlike the recording procedures for ICD-10-CM, which combine the substance-induced disorder and substance use disorder into a single code, for ICD-9-CM a separate diagnostic code is given for the substance use disorder. For example, in the case of irritable symptoms occurring during intoxication in a man with a severe cocaine use disorder, the diagnosis is 292.84 cocaine-induced bipolar and related disorder, with onset during intoxication. An additional diagnosis of 304.20 severe cocaine use disorder is also given. When more than one substance is judged to play a significant role in the development of bipolar mood symptoms, each should be listed separately (e.g., 292.84 methylphenidate-induced bipolar and related disorder, with onset during intoxication; 292.84 dexamethasone-induced bipolar and related disorder, with onset during intoxication).

ICD-10-CM. The name of the substance/medication-induced bipolar and related disorder begins with the specific substance (e.g., cocaine, dexamethasone) that is presumed to be causing the bipolar mood symptoms. The diagnostic code is selected from the table included in the criteria set, which is based on the drug class and presence or absence of a comorbid substance use disorder. For substances that do not fit into any of the classes (e.g., dexamethasone), the code for "other substance" should be used; and in cases in which a substance is judged to be an etiological factor but the specific class of substance is unknown, the category "unknown substance" should be used.

When recording the name of the disorder, the comorbid substance use disorder (if any) is listed first, followed by the word "with," followed by the name of the substance-induced bipolar and related disorder, followed by the specification of onset (i.e., onset during in-toxication, onset during withdrawal). For example, in the case of irritable symptoms oc-curring during intoxication in a man with a severe cocaine use disorder, the diagnosis is F14.24 severe cocaine use disorder with cocaine-induced bipolar and related disorder, with onset during intoxication. A separate diagnosis of the comorbid severe cocaine use disorder is not given. If the substance-induced bipolar and related disorder occurs without a comorbid substance use disorder (e.g., after a one-time heavy use of the substance), no accompanying substance use disorder is noted (e.g., F15.94 amphetamine-induced bipolar and related disorder, with onset during intoxication). When more than one substance is judged to play a significant role in the development of bipolar mood symptoms, each should be listed separately (e.g., F15.24 severe methylphenidate use disorder with meth-ylphenidate-induced bipolar and related disorder, with onset during intoxication; F19.94 dexamethasone-induced bipolar and related disorder, with onset during intoxication).

Diagnostic Features

The diagnostic features of substance/medication-induced bipolar and related disorder are es-sentially the same as those for mania, hypomania, or depression. A key exception to the diag-nosis of substance/medication-induced bipolar and related disorder is the case of hypomania or mania that occurs after antidepressant medication use or other treatments and persists be-yond the physiological effects of the medication. This condition is considered an indicator of true bipolar disorder, not substance/medication-induced bipolar and related disorder. Simi-larly, individuals with apparent electroconvulsive therapy–induced manic or hypomanic ep-isodes that persist beyond the physiological effects of the treatment are diagnosed with bipolar disorder, not substance/medication-induced bipolar and related disorder.

Side effects of some antidepressants and other psychotropic drugs (e.g., edginess, ag-itation) may resemble the primary symptoms of a manic syndrome, but they are funda-mentally distinct from bipolar symptoms and are insufficient for the diagnosis. That is, the criterion symptoms of mania/hypomania have specificity (simple agitation is not the same as excess involvement in purposeful activities), and a sufficient number of symptoms must be present (not just one or two symptoms) to make these diagnoses. In particular, the appearance of one or two nonspecific symptoms—irritability, edginess, or agitation during antidepressant treatment—in the absence of a full manic or hypomanic syndrome should not be taken to support a diagnosis of a bipolar disorder.

Associated Features Supporting Diagnosis

Etiology (causally related to the use of psychotropic medications or substances of abuse based on best clinical evidence) is the key variable in this etiologically specified form of bi-polar disorder. Substances/medications that are typically considered to be associated with substance/medication-induced bipolar and related disorder include the stimulant class of drugs, as well as phencyclidine and steroids; however, a number of potential sub-stances continue to emerge as new compounds are synthesized (e.g., so-called bath salts). A history of such substance use may help increase diagnostic certainty.

Prevalence

There are no epidemiological studies of substance/medication-induced mania or bipolar disorder. Each etiological substance may have its own individual risk of inducing a bipo-lar (manic/hypomanic) disorder.

Development and Course

In phencyclidine-induced mania, the initial presentation may be one of a delirium with af-fective features, which then becomes an atypically appearing manic or mixed manic state.

This condition follows the ingestion or inhalation quickly, usually within hours or, at the most, a few days. In stimulant-induced manic or hypomanic states, the response is in minutes to 1 hour after one or several ingestions or injections. The episode is very brief and typically resolves over 1–2 days. With corticosteroids and some immunosuppressant medications, the mania (or mixed or depressed state) usually follows several days of ingestion, and the higher doses appear to have a much greater likelihood of producing bipolar symptoms.

Diagnostic Markers

Determination of the substance of use can be made through markers in the blood or urine to corroborate diagnosis.

Differential Diagnosis

Substance/medication-induced bipolar and related disorder should be differentiated from other bipolar disorders, substance intoxication or substance-induced delirium, and medication side effects (as noted earlier). A full manic episode that emerges during antidepressant treatment (e.g., medication, electroconvulsive therapy) but persists at a fully syndromal level beyond the physiological effect of that treatment is sufficient evidence for a bipolar I diagnosis. A full hypomanic episode that emerges during antidepressant treatment (e.g., medication, electroconvulsive therapy) but persists at a fully syndromal level beyond the physiological effect of that treatment is sufficient evidence for a bipolar II diagnosis only if preceded by a major depressive episode.

Comorbidity

Comorbidities are those associated with the use of illicit substances (in the case of illegal stimulants or phencyclidine) or diversion of prescribed stimulants. Comorbidities related to steroid or immunosuppressant medications are those medical indications for these preparations. Delirium can occur before or along with manic symptoms in individuals ingesting phencyclidine or those who are prescribed steroid medications or other immunosuppressant medications.

Bipolar and Related Disorder Due to Another Medical Condition

Diagnostic Criteria

A. A prominent and persistent period of abnormally elevated, expansive, or irritable mood and abnormally increased activity or energy that predominates in the clinical picture.
B. There is evidence from the history, physical examination, or laboratory findings that the disturbance is the direct pathophysiological consequence of another medical condition.
C. The disturbance is not better explained by another mental disorder.
D. The disturbance does not occur exclusively during the course of a delirium.
E. The disturbance causes clinically significant distress or impairment in social, occupational, or other important areas of functioning, or necessitates hospitalization to prevent harm to self or others, or there are psychotic features.

Coding note: The ICD-9-CM code for bipolar and related disorder due to another medical condition is **293.83,** which is assigned regardless of the specifier. The ICD-10-CM code depends on the specifier (see below).

Specify if:

(F06.33) With manic features: Full criteria are not met for a manic or hypomanic episode.

(F06.33) With manic- or hypomanic-like episode: Full criteria are met except Criterion D for a manic episode or except Criterion F for a hypomanic episode.

(F06.34) With mixed features: Symptoms of depression are also present but do not predominate in the clinical picture.

Coding note: Include the name of the other medical condition in the name of the mental disorder (e.g., 293.83 [F06.33] bipolar disorder due to hyperthyroidism, with manic features). The other medical condition should also be coded and listed separately immediately before the bipolar and related disorder due to the medical condition (e.g., 242.90 [E05.90] hyperthyroidism; 293.83 [F06.33] bipolar disorder due to hyperthyroidism, with manic features).

Diagnostic Features

The essential features of bipolar and related disorder due to another medical condition are presence of a prominent and persistent period of abnormally elevated, expansive, or irritable mood and abnormally increased activity or energy predominating in the clinical picture that is attributable to another medical condition (Criterion B). In most cases the manic or hypomanic picture may appear during the initial presentation of the medical condition (i.e., within 1 month); however, there are exceptions, especially in chronic medical conditions that might worsen or relapse and herald the appearance of the manic or hypomanic picture. Bipolar and related disorder due to another medical condition would not be diagnosed when the manic or hypomanic episodes definitely preceded the medical condition, since the proper diagnosis would be bipolar disorder (except in the unusual circumstance in which all preceding manic or hypomanic episodes—or, when only one such episode has occurred, the preceding manic or hypomanic episode—were associated with ingestion of a substance/medication). The diagnosis of bipolar and related disorder due to another medical condition should not be made during the course of a delirium (Criterion D). The manic or hypomanic episode in bipolar and related disorder due to another medical condition must cause clinically significant distress or impairment in social, occupational, or other important areas of functioning to qualify for this diagnosis (Criterion E).

Associated Features Supporting Diagnosis

Etiology (i.e., a causal relationship to another medical condition based on best clinical evidence) is the key variable in this etiologically specified form of bipolar disorder. The listing of medical conditions that are said to be able to induce mania is never complete, and the clinician's best judgment is the essence of this diagnosis. Among the best known of the medical conditions that can cause a bipolar manic or hypomanic condition are Cushing's disease and multiple sclerosis, as well as stroke and traumatic brain injuries.

Development and Course

Bipolar and related disorder due to another medical condition usually has its onset acutely or subacutely within the first weeks or month of the onset of the associated medical condition. However, this is not always the case, as a worsening or later relapse of the associated medical condition may precede the onset of the manic or hypomanic syndrome. The clinician must make a clinical judgment in these situations about whether the medical condition is causative, based on temporal sequence as well as plausibility of a causal relationship. Finally, the condition may remit before or just after the medical condition remits, particularly when treatment of the manic/hypomanic symptoms is effective.

Culture-Related Diagnostic Issues

Culture-related differences, to the extent that there is any evidence, pertain to those associated with the medical condition (e.g., rates of multiple sclerosis and stroke vary around the world based on dietary, genetic factors, and other environmental factors).

Gender-Related Diagnostic Issues

Gender differences pertain to those associated with the medical condition (e.g., systemic lupus erythematosus is more common in females; stroke is somewhat more common in middle-age males compared with females).

Diagnostic Markers

Diagnostic markers pertain to those associated with the medical condition (e.g., steroid levels in blood or urine to help corroborate the diagnosis of Cushing's disease, which can be associated with manic or depressive syndromes; laboratory tests confirming the diagnosis of multiple sclerosis).

Functional Consequences of Bipolar and Related Disorder Due to Another Medical Condition

Functional consequences of the bipolar symptoms may exacerbate impairments associated with the medical condition and may incur worse outcomes due to interference with medical treatment. In general, it is believed, but not established, that the illness, when induced by Cushing's disease, will not recur if the Cushing's disease is cured or arrested. However, it is also suggested, but not established, that mood syndromes, including depressive and manic/hypomanic ones, may be episodic (i.e., recurring) with static brain injuries and other central nervous system diseases.

Differential Diagnosis

Symptoms of delirium, catatonia, and acute anxiety.   It is important to differentiate symptoms of mania from excited or hypervigilant delirious symptoms; from excited catatonic symptoms; and from agitation related to acute anxiety states.

Medication-induced depressive or manic symptoms.   An important differential diagnostic observation is that the other medical condition may be treated with medications (e.g., steroids or alpha-interferon) that can induce depressive or manic symptoms. In these cases, clinical judgment using all of the evidence in hand is the best way to try to separate the most likely and/or the most important of two etiological factors (i.e., association with the medical condition vs. a substance/medication-induced syndrome). The differential diagnosis of the associated medical conditions is relevant but largely beyond the scope of the present manual.

Comorbidity

Conditions comorbid with bipolar and related disorder due to another medical condition are those associated with the medical conditions of etiological relevance. Delirium can occur before or along with manic symptoms in individuals with Cushing's disease.

Other Specified Bipolar and Related Disorder

296.89 (F31.89)

This category applies to presentations in which symptoms characteristic of a bipolar and related disorder that cause clinically significant distress or impairment in social, occupational, or other important areas of functioning predominate but do not meet the full criteria for any of the disorders in the bipolar and related disorders diagnostic class. The other specified bipolar and related disorder category is used in situations in which the clinician chooses to communicate the specific reason that the presentation does not meet the criteria for any specific bipolar and related disorder. This is done by recording "other specified bipolar and related disorder" followed by the specific reason (e.g., "short-duration cyclothymia").

Examples of presentations that can be specified using the "other specified" designation include the following:

1. **Short-duration hypomanic episodes (2–3 days) and major depressive episodes:** A lifetime history of one or more major depressive episodes in individuals whose presentation has never met full criteria for a manic or hypomanic episode but who have experienced two or more episodes of short-duration hypomania that meet the full symptomatic criteria for a hypomanic episode but that only last for 2–3 days. The episodes of hypomanic symptoms do not overlap in time with the major depressive episodes, so the disturbance does not meet criteria for major depressive episode, with mixed features.

2. **Hypomanic episodes with insufficient symptoms and major depressive episodes:** A lifetime history of one or more major depressive episodes in individuals whose presentation has never met full criteria for a manic or hypomanic episode but who have experienced one or more episodes of hypomania that do not meet full symptomatic criteria (i.e., at least 4 consecutive days of elevated mood and one or two of the other symptoms of a hypomanic episode, or irritable mood and two or three of the other symptoms of a hypomanic episode). The episodes of hypomanic symptoms do not overlap in time with the major depressive episodes, so the disturbance does not meet criteria for major depressive episode, with mixed features.

3. **Hypomanic episode without prior major depressive episode:** One or more hypomanic episodes in an individual whose presentation has never met full criteria for a major depressive episode or a manic episode. If this occurs in an individual with an established diagnosis of persistent depressive disorder (dysthymia), both diagnoses can be concurrently applied during the periods when the full criteria for a hypomanic episode are met.

4. **Short-duration cyclothymia (less than 24 months):** Multiple episodes of hypomanic symptoms that do not meet criteria for a hypomanic episode and multiple episodes of depressive symptoms that do not meet criteria for a major depressive episode that persist over a period of less than 24 months (less than 12 months for children or adolescents) in an individual whose presentation has never met full criteria for a major depressive, manic, or hypomanic episode and does not meet criteria for any psychotic disorder. During the course of the disorder, the hypomanic or depressive symptoms are present for more days than not, the individual has not been without symptoms for more than 2 months at a time, and the symptoms cause clinically significant distress or impairment.

Unspecified Bipolar and Related Disorder

296.80 (F31.9)

This category applies to presentations in which symptoms characteristic of a bipolar and related disorder that cause clinically significant distress or impairment in social, occupational, or other important areas of functioning predominate but do not meet the full criteria for any of the disorders in the bipolar and related disorders diagnostic class. The unspecified bipolar and related disorder category is used in situations in which the clinician chooses *not* to specify the reason that the criteria are not met for a specific bipolar and related disorder, and includes presentations in which there is insufficient information to make a more specific diagnosis (e.g., in emergency room settings).

Specifiers for Bipolar and Related Disorders

Specify if:

With anxious distress: The presence of at least two of the following symptoms during the majority of days of the current or most recent episode of mania, hypomania, or depression:

1. Feeling keyed up or tense.
2. Feeling unusually restless.
3. Difficulty concentrating because of worry.
4. Fear that something awful may happen.
5. Feeling that the individual might lose control of himself or herself.

> *Specify* current severity:
> **Mild:** Two symptoms.
> **Moderate:** Three symptoms.
> **Moderate-severe:** Four or five symptoms.
> **Severe:** Four or five symptoms with motor agitation.

Note: Anxious distress has been noted as a prominent feature of both bipolar and major depressive disorder in both primary care and specialty mental health settings. High levels of anxiety have been associated with higher suicide risk, longer duration of illness, and greater likelihood of treatment nonresponse. As a result, it is clinically useful to specify accurately the presence and severity levels of anxious distress for treatment planning and monitoring of response to treatment.

With mixed features: The mixed features specifier can apply to the current manic, hypomanic, or depressive episode in bipolar I or bipolar II disorder:

Manic or hypomanic episode, with mixed features:

A. Full criteria are met for a manic episode or hypomanic episode, and at least three of the following symptoms are present during the majority of days of the current or most recent episode of mania or hypomania:

1. Prominent dysphoria or depressed mood as indicated by either subjective report (e.g., feels sad or empty) or observation made by others (e.g., appears tearful).
2. Diminished interest or pleasure in all, or almost all, activities (as indicated by either subjective account or observation made by others).
3. Psychomotor retardation nearly every day (observable by others; not merely subjective feelings of being slowed down).

4. Fatigue or loss of energy.
5. Feelings of worthlessness or excessive or inappropriate guilt (not merely self-reproach or guilt about being sick).
6. Recurrent thoughts of death (not just fear of dying), recurrent suicidal ideation without a specific plan, or a suicide attempt or a specific plan for committing suicide.

B. Mixed symptoms are observable by others and represent a change from the person's usual behavior.
C. For individuals whose symptoms meet full episode criteria for both mania and depression simultaneously, the diagnosis should be manic episode, with mixed features, due to the marked impairment and clinical severity of full mania.
D. The mixed symptoms are not attributable to the physiological effects of a substance (e.g., a drug of abuse, a medication, other treatment).

Depressive episode, with mixed features:

A. Full criteria are met for a major depressive episode, and at least three of the following manic/hypomanic symptoms are present during the majority of days of the current or most recent episode of depression:

1. Elevated, expansive mood.
2. Inflated self-esteem or grandiosity.
3. More talkative than usual or pressure to keep talking.
4. Flight of ideas or subjective experience that thoughts are racing.
5. Increase in energy or goal-directed activity (either socially, at work or school, or sexually).
6. Increased or excessive involvement in activities that have a high potential for painful consequences (e.g., engaging in unrestrained buying sprees, sexual indiscretions, or foolish business investments).
7. Decreased need for sleep (feeling rested despite sleeping less than usual; to be contrasted with insomnia).

B. Mixed symptoms are observable by others and represent a change from the person's usual behavior.
C. For individuals whose symptoms meet full episode criteria for both mania and depression simultaneously, the diagnosis should be manic episode, with mixed features.
D. The mixed symptoms are not attributable to the physiological effects of a substance (e.g., a drug of abuse, a medication, other treatment).

Note: Mixed features associated with a major depressive episode have been found to be a significant risk factor for the development of bipolar I or bipolar II disorder. As a result, it is clinically useful to note the presence of this specifier for treatment planning and monitoring of response to treatment.

With rapid cycling (can be applied to bipolar I or bipolar II disorder): Presence of at least four mood episodes in the previous 12 months that meet the criteria for manic, hypomanic, or major depressive episode.

Note: Episodes are demarcated by either partial or full remissions of at least 2 months or a switch to an episode of the opposite polarity (e.g., major depressive episode to manic episode).

Note: The essential feature of a rapid-cycling bipolar disorder is the occurrence of at least four mood episodes during the previous 12 months. These episodes can occur in any combination and order. The episodes must meet both the duration and symptom number criteria for a major depressive, manic, or hypomanic episode and must be demarcated by either a period of full remission or a switch to an episode of the opposite polarity. Manic and hypomanic episodes are counted as being on the same pole. Except for the fact that they occur more frequently, the episodes that occur in a rapid-cycling pattern are no different from those that occur in a non-rapid-cycling pattern. Mood episodes that count toward defining a rapid-cycling pattern exclude those episodes directly caused by a substance (e.g., cocaine, corticosteroids) or another medical condition.

With melancholic features:

A. One of the following is present during the most severe period of the current episode:

1. Loss of pleasure in all, or almost all, activities.
2. Lack of reactivity to usually pleasurable stimuli (does not feel much better, even temporarily, when something good happens).

B. Three (or more) of the following:

1. A distinct quality of depressed mood characterized by profound despondency, despair, and/or moroseness or by so-called empty mood.
2. Depression that is regularly worse in the morning.
3. Early-morning awakening (i.e., at least 2 hours before usual awakening).
4. Marked psychomotor agitation or retardation.
5. Significant anorexia or weight loss.
6. Excessive or inappropriate guilt.

Note: The specifier "with melancholic features" is applied if these features are present at the most severe stage of the episode. There is a near-complete absence of the capacity for pleasure, not merely a diminution. A guideline for evaluating the lack of reactivity of mood is that even highly desired events are not associated with marked brightening of mood. Either mood does not brighten at all, or it brightens only partially (e.g., up to 20%–40% of normal for only minutes at a time). The "distinct quality" of mood that is characteristic of the "with melancholic features" specifier is experienced as qualitatively different from that during a nonmelancholic depressive episode. A depressed mood that is described as merely more severe, longer lasting, or present without a reason is not considered distinct in quality. Psychomotor changes are nearly always present and are observable by others.

Melancholic features exhibit only a modest tendency to repeat across episodes in the same individual. They are more frequent in inpatients, as opposed to outpatients; are less likely to occur in milder than in more severe major depressive episodes; and are more likely to occur in those with psychotic features.

With atypical features: This specifier can be applied when these features predominate during the majority of days of the current or most recent major depressive episode.

A. Mood reactivity (i.e., mood brightens in response to actual or potential positive events).

B. Two (or more) of the following features:

1. Significant weight gain or increase in appetite.
2. Hypersomnia.
3. Leaden paralysis (i.e., heavy, leaden feelings in arms or legs).
4. A long-standing pattern of interpersonal rejection sensitivity (not limited to episodes of mood disturbance) that results in significant social or occupational impairment.

C. Criteria are not met for "with melancholic features" or "with catatonia" during the same episode.

Note: "Atypical depression" has historical significance (i.e., atypical in contradistinction to the more classical agitated, "endogenous" presentations of depression that were the norm when depression was rarely diagnosed in outpatients and almost never in adolescents or younger adults) and today does not connote an uncommon or unusual clinical presentation as the term might imply.

Mood reactivity is the capacity to be cheered up when presented with positive events (e.g., a visit from children, compliments from others). Mood may become euthymic (not sad) even for extended periods of time if the external circumstances remain favorable. Increased appetite may be manifested by an obvious increase in food intake or by weight gain. Hypersomnia may include either an extended period of nighttime sleep or daytime napping that totals at least 10 hours of sleep per day (or at least 2 hours more than when not depressed). Leaden paralysis is defined as feeling heavy, leaden, or weighted down, usually in the arms or legs. This sensation is generally present for at least an hour a day but often lasts for many hours at a time. Unlike the other atypical features, pathological sensitivity to perceived interpersonal rejection is a trait that has an early onset and persists throughout most of adult life. Rejection sensitivity occurs both when the person is and is not depressed, though it may be exacerbated during depressive periods.

With psychotic features: Delusions or hallucinations are present at any time in the episode. If psychotic features are present, specify if mood-congruent or mood-incongruent:

With mood-congruent psychotic features: During manic episodes, the content of all delusions and hallucinations is consistent with the typical manic themes of grandiosity, invulnerability, etc., but may also include themes of suspiciousness or paranoia, especially with respect to others' doubts about the individual's capacities, accomplishments, and so forth.

With mood-incongruent psychotic features: The content of delusions and hallucinations is inconsistent with the episode polarity themes as described above, or the content is a mixture of mood-incongruent and mood-congruent themes.

With catatonia: This specifier can apply to an episode of mania or depression if catatonic features are present during most of the episode. See criteria for catatonia associated with a mental disorder in the chapter "Schizophrenia Spectrum and Other Psychotic Disorders."

With peripartum onset: This specifier can be applied to the current or, if the full criteria are not currently met for a mood episode, most recent episode of mania, hypomania, or major depression in bipolar I or bipolar II disorder if onset of mood symptoms occurs during pregnancy or in the 4 weeks following delivery.

Note: Mood episodes can have their onset either during pregnancy or postpartum. Although the estimates differ according to the period of follow-up after delivery, between 3% and 6% of women will experience the onset of a major depressive episode during pregnancy or in the weeks or months following delivery. Fifty percent of "postpartum" major depressive episodes actually begin prior to delivery. Thus, these episodes are referred to collectively as *peripartum* episodes. Women with peripartum major depressive episodes often have severe anxiety and even panic attacks. Prospective studies have demonstrated that mood and anxiety symptoms during pregnancy, as well as the "baby blues," increase the risk for a postpartum major depressive episode.

Peripartum-onset mood episodes can present either with or without psychotic features. Infanticide is most often associated with postpartum psychotic episodes that are characterized by command hallucinations to kill the infant or delusions that the infant is possessed, but psychotic symptoms can also occur in severe postpartum mood episodes without such specific delusions or hallucinations.

Postpartum mood (major depressive or manic) episodes with psychotic features appear to occur in from 1 in 500 to 1 in 1,000 deliveries and may be more common in primiparous women. The risk of postpartum episodes with psychotic features is particularly increased for women with prior postpartum mood episodes but is also elevated for those with a prior history of a depressive or bipolar disorder (especially bipolar I disorder) and those with a family history of bipolar disorders.

Once a woman has had a postpartum episode with psychotic features, the risk of recurrence with each subsequent delivery is between 30% and 50%. Postpartum episodes must be differentiated from delirium occurring in the postpartum period, which is distinguished by a fluctuating level of awareness or attention. The postpartum period is unique with respect to the degree of neuroendocrine alterations and psychosocial adjustments, the potential impact of breast-feeding on treatment planning, and the long-term implications of a history of postpartum mood disorder on subsequent family planning.

With seasonal pattern: This specifier applies to the lifetime pattern of mood episodes. The essential feature is a regular seasonal pattern of at least one type of episode (i.e., mania, hypomania, or depression). The other types of episodes may not follow this pattern. For example, an individual may have seasonal manias, but his or her depressions do not regularly occur at a specific time of year.

A. There has been a regular temporal relationship between the onset of manic, hypomanic, or major depressive episodes and a particular time of the year (e.g., in the fall or winter) in bipolar I or bipolar II disorder.

Note: Do not include cases in which there is an obvious effect of seasonally related psychosocial stressors (e.g., regularly being unemployed every winter).

B. Full remissions (or a change from major depression to mania or hypomania or vice versa) also occur at a characteristic time of the year (e.g., depression disappears in the spring).

C. In the last 2 years, the individual's manic, hypomanic, or major depressive episodes have demonstrated a temporal seasonal relationship, as defined above, and no non-seasonal episodes of that polarity have occurred during that 2-year period.

D. Seasonal manias, hypomanias, or depressions (as described above) substantially outnumber any nonseasonal manias, hypomanias, or depressions that may have occurred over the individual's lifetime.

Note: This specifier can be applied to the pattern of major depressive episodes in bipolar I disorder, bipolar II disorder, or major depressive disorder, recurrent. The essential feature is the onset and remission of major depressive episodes at characteristic times of the year. In most cases, the episodes begin in fall or winter and remit in spring. Less commonly, there may be recurrent summer depressive episodes. This pattern of onset and remission of episodes must have occurred during at least a 2-year period, without any nonseasonal episodes occurring during this period. In addition, the seasonal depressive episodes must substantially outnumber any nonseasonal depressive episodes over the individual's lifetime.

This specifier does not apply to those situations in which the pattern is better explained by seasonally linked psychosocial stressors (e.g., seasonal unemployment or school schedule). Major depressive episodes that occur in a seasonal pattern are often characterized by loss of energy, hypersomnia, overeating, weight gain, and a craving for carbohydrates. It is unclear whether a seasonal pattern is more likely in recurrent major depressive disorder or in bipolar disorders. However, within the bipolar disorders group, a seasonal pattern appears to be more likely in bipolar II disorder than in bipolar I disorder. In some individuals, the onset of manic or hypomanic episodes may also be linked to a particular season.

The prevalence of winter-type seasonal pattern appears to vary with latitude, age, and sex. Prevalence increases with higher latitudes. Age is also a strong predictor of seasonality, with younger persons at higher risk for winter depressive episodes.

Specify if:

In partial remission: Symptoms of the immediately previous manic, hypomanic, or major depressive episode are present but full criteria are not met, or there is a period lasting less than 2 months without any significant symptoms of a manic, hypomanic, or major depressive episode following the end of such an episode.

In full remission: During the past 2 months, no significant signs or symptoms of the disturbance were present.

Specify current severity of manic episode:

Severity is based on the number of criterion symptoms, the severity of those symptoms, and the degree of functional disability.

Mild: Minimum symptom criteria are met for a manic episode.

Moderate: Extreme increase in activity or impairment in judgment.

Severe: Almost continual supervision is required in order to prevent physical harm to self or others.

Specify current severity of major depressive episode:

Severity is based on the number of criterion symptoms, the severity of those symptoms, and the degree of functional disability.

Mild: Few, if any, symptoms in excess of those required to meet the diagnostic criteria are present, the intensity of the symptoms is distressing but manageable, and the symptoms result in minor impairment in social or occupational functioning.

Moderate: The number of symptoms, intensity of symptoms, and/or functional impairment are between those specified for "mild" and "severe."

Severe: The number of symptoms is substantially in excess of those required to make the diagnosis, the intensity of the symptoms is seriously distressing and unmanageable, and the symptoms markedly interfere with social and occupational functioning.

Depressive Disorders

Depressive disorders include disruptive mood dysregulation disorder, major depressive disorder (including major depressive episode), persistent depressive disorder (dysthymia), premenstrual dysphoric disorder, substance/medication-induced depressive disorder, depressive disorder due to another medical condition, other specified depressive disorder, and unspecified depressive disorder. Unlike in DSM-IV, this chapter "Depressive Disorders" has been separated from the previous chapter "Bipolar and Related Disorders." The common feature of all of these disorders is the presence of sad, empty, or irritable mood, accompanied by somatic and cognitive changes that significantly affect the individual's capacity to function. What differs among them are issues of duration, timing, or presumed etiology.

In order to address concerns about the potential for the overdiagnosis of and treatment for bipolar disorder in children, a new diagnosis, disruptive mood dysregulation disorder, referring to the presentation of children with persistent irritability and frequent episodes of extreme behavioral dyscontrol, is added to the depressive disorders for children up to 12 years of age. Its placement in this chapter reflects the finding that children with this symptom pattern typically develop unipolar depressive disorders or anxiety disorders, rather than bipolar disorders, as they mature into adolescence and adulthood.

Major depressive disorder represents the classic condition in this group of disorders. It is characterized by discrete episodes of at least 2 weeks' duration (although most episodes last considerably longer) involving clear-cut changes in affect, cognition, and neurovegetative functions and inter-episode remissions. A diagnosis based on a single episode is possible, although the disorder is a recurrent one in the majority of cases. Careful consideration is given to the delineation of normal sadness and grief from a major depressive episode. Bereavement may induce great suffering, but it does not typically induce an episode of major depressive disorder. When they do occur together, the depressive symptoms and functional impairment tend to be more severe and the prognosis is worse compared with bereavement that is not accompanied by major depressive disorder. Bereavement-related depression tends to occur in persons with other vulnerabilities to depressive disorders, and recovery may be facilitated by antidepressant treatment.

A more chronic form of depression, persistent depressive disorder (dysthymia), can be diagnosed when the mood disturbance continues for at least 2 years in adults or 1 year in children. This diagnosis, new in DSM-5, includes both the DSM-IV diagnostic categories of chronic major depression and dysthymia.

After careful scientific review of the evidence, premenstrual dysphoric disorder has been moved from an appendix of DSM-IV ("Criteria Sets and Axes Provided for Further Study") to Section II of DSM-5. Almost 20 years of additional research on this condition has confirmed a specific and treatment-responsive form of depressive disorder that begins sometime following ovulation and remits within a few days of menses and has a marked impact on functioning.

A large number of substances of abuse, some prescribed medications, and several medical conditions can be associated with depression-like phenomena. This fact is recognized in the diagnoses of substance/medication-induced depressive disorder and depressive disorder due to another medical condition.

Disruptive Mood Dysregulation Disorder

Diagnostic Criteria   **296.99** (F34.81)

A. Severe recurrent temper outbursts manifested verbally (e.g., verbal rages) and/or be-
   haviorally (e.g., physical aggression toward people or property) that are grossly out of
   proportion in intensity or duration to the situation or provocation.
B. The temper outbursts are inconsistent with developmental level.
C. The temper outbursts occur, on average, three or more times per week.
D. The mood between temper outbursts is persistently irritable or angry most of the day,
   nearly every day, and is observable by others (e.g., parents, teachers, peers).
E. Criteria A–D have been present for 12 or more months. Throughout that time, the indi-
   vidual has not had a period lasting 3 or more consecutive months without all of the
   symptoms in Criteria A–D.
F. Criteria A and D are present in at least two of three settings (i.e., at home, at school,
   with peers) and are severe in at least one of these.
G. The diagnosis should not be made for the first time before age 6 years or after age 18
   years.
H. By history or observation, the age at onset of Criteria A–E is before 10 years.
I. There has never been a distinct period lasting more than 1 day during which the full
   symptom criteria, except duration, for a manic or hypomanic episode have been met.
   Note: Developmentally appropriate mood elevation, such as occurs in the context of a
   highly positive event or its anticipation, should not be considered as a symptom of mania or hypomania.
J. The behaviors do not occur exclusively during an episode of major depressive disorder
   and are not better explained by another mental disorder (e.g., autism spectrum disorder, posttraumatic stress disorder, separation anxiety disorder, persistent depressive
   disorder [dysthymia]).
   Note: This diagnosis cannot coexist with oppositional defiant disorder, intermittent explosive disorder, or bipolar disorder, though it can coexist with others, including major
   depressive disorder, attention-deficit/hyperactivity disorder, conduct disorder, and
   substance use disorders. Individuals whose symptoms meet criteria for both disruptive
   mood dysregulation disorder and oppositional defiant disorder should only be given the
   diagnosis of disruptive mood dysregulation disorder. If an individual has ever experienced a manic or hypomanic episode, the diagnosis of disruptive mood dysregulation
   disorder should not be assigned.
K. The symptoms are not attributable to the physiological effects of a substance or another medical or neurological condition.

Diagnostic Features

The core feature of disruptive mood dysregulation disorder is chronic, severe persistent irritability. This severe irritability has two prominent clinical manifestations, the first of
which is frequent temper outbursts. These outbursts typically occur in response to frustration and can be verbal or behavioral (the latter in the form of aggression against property, self, or others). They must occur frequently (i.e., on average, three or more times per
week) (Criterion C) over at least 1 year in at least two settings (Criteria E and F), such as in
the home and at school, and they must be developmentally inappropriate (Criterion B).
The second manifestation of severe irritability consists of chronic, persistently irritable or
angry mood that is present between the severe temper outbursts. This irritable or angry
mood must be characteristic of the child, being present most of the day, nearly every day,
and noticeable by others in the child's environment (Criterion D).

The clinical presentation of disruptive mood dysregulation disorder must be carefully distinguished from presentations of other, related conditions, particularly pediatric bipolar disorder. In fact, disruptive mood dysregulation disorder was added to DSM-5 to address the considerable concern about the appropriate classification and treatment of children who present with chronic, persistent irritability relative to children who present with classic (i.e., episodic) bipolar disorder.

Some researchers view severe, non-episodic irritability as characteristic of bipolar disorder in children, although both DSM-IV and DSM-5 require that both children and adults have distinct episodes of mania or hypomania to qualify for the diagnosis of bipolar I disorder. During the latter decades of the 20th century, this contention by researchers that severe, nonepisodic irritability is a manifestation of pediatric mania coincided with an upsurge in the rates at which clinicians assigned the diagnosis of bipolar disorder to their pediatric patients. This sharp increase in rates appears to be attributable to clinicians combining at least two clinical presentations into a single category. That is, both classic, episodic presentations of mania and non-episodic presentations of severe irritability have been labeled as bipolar disorder in children. In DSM-5, the term *bipolar disorder* is explicitly reserved for episodic presentations of bipolar symptoms. DSM-IV did not include a diagnosis designed to capture youths whose hallmark symptoms consisted of very severe, nonepisodic irritability, whereas DSM-5, with the inclusion of disruptive mood dysregulation disorder, provides a distinct category for such presentations.

Prevalence

Disruptive mood dysregulation disorder is common among children presenting to pediatric mental health clinics. Prevalence estimates of the disorder in the community are unclear. Based on rates of chronic and severe persistent irritability, which is the core feature of the disorder, the overall 6-month to 1-year period-prevalence of disruptive mood dysregulation disorder among children and adolescents probably falls in the 2%–5% range. However, rates are expected to be higher in males and school-age children than in females and adolescents.

Development and Course

The onset of disruptive mood dysregulation disorder must be before age 10 years, and the diagnosis should not be applied to children with a developmental age of less than 6 years. It is unknown whether the condition presents only in this age-delimited fashion. Because the symptoms of disruptive mood dysregulation disorder are likely to change as children mature, use of the diagnosis should be restricted to age groups similar to those in which validity has been established (6–18 years). Approximately half of children with severe, chronic irritability will have a presentation that continues to meet criteria for the condition 1 year later. Rates of conversion from severe, nonepisodic irritability to bipolar disorder are very low. Instead, children with chronic irritability are at risk to develop unipolar depressive and/or anxiety disorders in adulthood.

Age-related variations also differentiate classic bipolar disorder and disruptive mood dysregulation disorder. Rates of bipolar disorder generally are very low prior to adolescence (<1%), with a steady increase into early adulthood (1%–2% prevalence). Disruptive mood dysregulation disorder is more common than bipolar disorder prior to adolescence, and symptoms of the condition generally become less common as children transition into adulthood.

Risk and Prognostic Factors

Temperamental.   Children with chronic irritability typically exhibit complicated psychiatric histories. In such children, a relatively extensive history of chronic irritability is common, typically manifesting before full criteria for the syndrome are met. Such prediagnostic presentations may have qualified for a diagnosis of oppositional defiant disorder. Many children with disruptive mood dysregulation disorder have symptoms that also meet criteria for attention-deficit/hyperactivity disorder (ADHD) and for an anxiety disorder, with such diagnoses often being present from a relatively early age. For some children, the criteria for major depressive disorder may also be met.

Genetic and physiological.   In terms of familial aggregation and genetics, it has been suggested that children presenting with chronic, non-episodic irritability can be differentiated from children with bipolar disorder in their family-based risk. However, these two groups do not differ in familial rates of anxiety disorders, unipolar depressive disorders, or substance abuse. Compared with children with pediatric bipolar disorder or other mental illnesses, those with disruptive mood dysregulation disorder exhibit both commonalities and differences in information-processing deficits. For example, face-emotion labeling deficits, as well as perturbed decision making and cognitive control, are present in children with bipolar disorder and chronically irritable children, as well as in children with some other psychiatric conditions. There is also evidence for disorder-specific dysfunction, such as during tasks assessing attention deployment in response to emotional stimuli, which has demonstrated unique signs of dysfunction in children with chronic irritability.

Gender-Related Diagnostic Issues

Children presenting to clinics with features of disruptive mood dysregulation disorder are predominantly male. Among community samples, a male preponderance appears to be supported. This difference in prevalence between males and females differentiates disruptive mood dysregulation disorder from bipolar disorder, in which there is an equal gender prevalence.

Suicide Risk

In general, evidence documenting suicidal behavior and aggression, as well as other severe functional consequences, in disruptive mood dysregulation disorder should be noted when evaluating children with chronic irritability.

Functional Consequences of Disruptive Mood Dysregulation Disorder

Chronic, severe irritability, such as is seen in disruptive mood dysregulation disorder, is associated with marked disruption in a child's family and peer relationships, as well as in school performance. Because of their extremely low frustration tolerance, such children generally have difficulty succeeding in school; they are often unable to participate in the activities typically enjoyed by healthy children; their family life is severely disrupted by their outbursts and irritability; and they have trouble initiating or sustaining friendships. Levels of dysfunction in children with bipolar disorder and disruptive mood dysregulation disorder are generally comparable. Both conditions cause severe disruption in the lives of the affected individual and their families. In both disruptive mood dysregulation disorder and pediatric bipolar disorder, dangerous behavior, suicidal ideation or suicide attempts, severe aggression, and psychiatric hospitalization are common.

Differential Diagnosis

Because chronically irritable children and adolescents typically present with complex histories, the diagnosis of disruptive mood dysregulation disorder must be made while considering the presence or absence of multiple other conditions. Despite the need to consider many other syndromes, differentiation of disruptive mood dysregulation disorder from bipolar disorder and oppositional defiant disorder requires particularly careful assessment.

Bipolar disorders.   The central feature differentiating disruptive mood dysregulation disorder and bipolar disorders in children involves the longitudinal course of the core symptoms. In children, as in adults, bipolar I disorder and bipolar II disorder manifest as an episodic illness with discrete episodes of mood perturbation that can be differentiated from the child's typical presentation. The mood perturbation that occurs during a manic episode is distinctly different from the child's usual mood. In addition, during a manic episode, the change in mood must be accompanied by the onset, or worsening, of associated cognitive, behavioral, and physical symptoms (e.g., distractibility, increased goal-directed activity), which are also present to a degree that is distinctly different from the child's usual baseline. Thus, in the case of a manic episode, parents (and, depending on developmental level, children) should be able to identify a distinct time period during which the child's mood and behavior were markedly different from usual. In contrast, the irritability of disruptive mood dysregulation disorder is persistent and is present over many months; while it may wax and wane to a certain degree, severe irritability is characteristic of the child with disruptive mood dysregulation disorder. Thus, while bipolar disorders are episodic conditions, disruptive mood dysregulation disorder is not. In fact, the diagnosis of disruptive mood dysregulation disorder cannot be assigned to a child who has ever experienced a full-duration hypomanic or manic episode (irritable or euphoric) or who has ever had a manic or hypomanic episode lasting more than 1 day. Another central differentiating feature between bipolar disorders and disruptive mood dysregulation disorder is the presence of elevated or expansive mood and grandiosity. These symptoms are common features of mania but are not characteristic of disruptive mood dysregulation disorder.

Oppositional defiant disorder.   While symptoms of oppositional defiant disorder typically do occur in children with disruptive mood dysregulation disorder, mood symptoms of disruptive mood dysregulation disorder are relatively rare in children with oppositional defiant disorder. The key features that warrant the diagnosis of disruptive mood dysregulation disorder in children whose symptoms also meet criteria for oppositional defiant disorder are the presence of severe and frequently recurrent outbursts and a persistent disruption in mood between outbursts. In addition, the diagnosis of disruptive mood dysregulation disorder requires severe impairment in at least one setting (i.e., home, school, or among peers) and mild to moderate impairment in a second setting. For this reason, while most children whose symptoms meet criteria for disruptive mood dysregulation disorder will also have a presentation that meets criteria for oppositional defiant disorder, the reverse is not the case. That is, in only approximately 15% of individuals with oppositional defiant disorder would criteria for disruptive mood dysregulation disorder be met. Moreover, even for children in whom criteria for both disorders are met, only the diagnosis of disruptive mood dysregulation disorder should be made. Finally, both the prominent mood symptoms in disruptive mood dysregulation disorder and the high risk for depressive and anxiety disorders in follow-up studies justify placement of disruptive mood dysregulation disorder among the depressive disorders in DSM-5. (Oppositional defiant disorder is included in the chapter "Disruptive, Impulse-Control, and Conduct Disorders.") This reflects the more prominent mood component among individuals with disruptive mood dysregulation disorder, as compared with individuals with oppositional defiant disorder. Nevertheless, it also should be noted that disruptive mood dysregulation disorder appears to carry a high risk for behavioral problems as well as mood problems.

Attention-deficit/hyperactivity disorder, major depressive disorder, anxiety disorders, and autism spectrum disorder.   Unlike children diagnosed with bipolar disorder or oppositional defiant disorder, a child whose symptoms meet criteria for disruptive mood dysregulation disorder also can receive a comorbid diagnosis of ADHD, major depressive disorder, and/or anxiety disorder. However, children whose irritability is present only in the context of a major depressive episode or persistent depressive disorder (dysthymia) should receive one of those diagnoses rather than disruptive mood dysregulation disorder. Children with disruptive mood dysregulation disorder may have symptoms that also meet criteria for an anxiety disorder and can receive both diagnoses, but children whose irritability is manifest only in the context of exacerbation of an anxiety disorder should receive the relevant anxiety disorder diagnosis rather than disruptive mood dysregulation disorder. In addition, children with autism spectrum disorders frequently present with temper outbursts when, for example, their routines are disturbed. In that instance, the temper outbursts would be considered secondary to the autism spectrum disorder, and the child should not receive the diagnosis of disruptive mood dysregulation disorder.

Intermittent explosive disorder.   Children with symptoms suggestive of intermittent explosive disorder present with instances of severe temper outbursts, much like children with disruptive mood dysregulation disorder. However, unlike disruptive mood dysregulation disorder, intermittent explosive disorder does not require persistent disruption in mood between outbursts. In addition, intermittent explosive disorder requires only 3 months of active symptoms, in contrast to the 12-month requirement for disruptive mood dysregulation disorder. Thus, these two diagnoses should not be made in the same child. For children with outbursts and intercurrent, persistent irritability, only the diagnosis of disruptive mood dysregulation disorder should be made.

Comorbidity

Rates of comorbidity in disruptive mood dysregulation disorder are extremely high. It is rare to find individuals whose symptoms meet criteria for disruptive mood dysregulation disorder alone. Comorbidity between disruptive mood dysregulation disorder and other DSM-defined syndromes appears higher than for many other pediatric mental illnesses; the strongest overlap is with oppositional defiant disorder. Not only is the overall rate of comorbidity high in disruptive mood dysregulation disorder, but also the range of comorbid illnesses appears particularly diverse. These children typically present to the clinic with a wide range of disruptive behavior, mood, anxiety, and even autism spectrum symptoms and diagnoses. However, children with disruptive mood dysregulation disorder should not have symptoms that meet criteria for bipolar disorder, as in that context, only the bipolar disorder diagnosis should be made. If children have symptoms that meet criteria for oppositional defiant disorder or intermittent explosive disorder *and* disruptive mood dysregulation disorder, only the diagnosis of disruptive mood dysregulation disorder should be assigned. Also, as noted earlier, the diagnosis of disruptive mood dysregulation disorder should not be assigned if the symptoms occur only in an anxiety-provoking context, when the routines of a child with autism spectrum disorder or obsessive-compulsive disorder are disturbed, or in the context of a major depressive episode.

Major Depressive Disorder

Diagnostic Criteria

A. Five (or more) of the following symptoms have been present during the same 2-week period and represent a change from previous functioning; at least one of the symptoms is either (1) depressed mood or (2) loss of interest or pleasure.
   Note: Do not include symptoms that are clearly attributable to another medical condition.

   1. Depressed mood most of the day, nearly every day, as indicated by either subjective report (e.g., feels sad, empty, hopeless) or observation made by others (e.g., appears tearful). (**Note:** In children and adolescents, can be irritable mood.)
   2. Markedly diminished interest or pleasure in all, or almost all, activities most of the day, nearly every day (as indicated by either subjective account or observation).

3. Significant weight loss when not dieting or weight gain (e.g., a change of more than 5% of body weight in a month), or decrease or increase in appetite nearly every day. (**Note:** In children, consider failure to make expected weight gain.)
4. Insomnia or hypersomnia nearly every day.
5. Psychomotor agitation or retardation nearly every day (observable by others, not merely subjective feelings of restlessness or being slowed down).
6. Fatigue or loss of energy nearly every day.
7. Feelings of worthlessness or excessive or inappropriate guilt (which may be delusional) nearly every day (not merely self-reproach or guilt about being sick).
8. Diminished ability to think or concentrate, or indecisiveness, nearly every day (either by subjective account or as observed by others).
9. Recurrent thoughts of death (not just fear of dying), recurrent suicidal ideation without a specific plan, or a suicide attempt or a specific plan for committing suicide.

B. The symptoms cause clinically significant distress or impairment in social, occupational, or other important areas of functioning.
C. The episode is not attributable to the physiological effects of a substance or another medical condition.

Note: Criteria A–C represent a major depressive episode.

Note: Responses to a significant loss (e.g., bereavement, financial ruin, losses from a natural disaster, a serious medical illness or disability) may include the feelings of intense sadness, rumination about the loss, insomnia, poor appetite, and weight loss noted in Criterion A, which may resemble a depressive episode. Although such symptoms may be understandable or considered appropriate to the loss, the presence of a major depressive episode in addition to the normal response to a significant loss should also be carefully considered. This decision inevitably requires the exercise of clinical judgment based on the individual's history and the cultural norms for the expression of distress in the context of loss.[1]

D. The occurrence of the major depressive episode is not better explained by schizoaffective disorder, schizophrenia, schizophreniform disorder, delusional disorder, or other specified and unspecified schizophrenia spectrum and other psychotic disorders.
E. There has never been a manic episode or a hypomanic episode.
   Note: This exclusion does not apply if all of the manic-like or hypomanic-like episodes are substance-induced or are attributable to the physiological effects of another medical condition.

---

[1] In distinguishing grief from a major depressive episode (MDE), it is useful to consider that in grief the predominant affect is feelings of emptiness and loss, while in an MDE it is persistent depressed mood and the inability to anticipate happiness or pleasure. The dysphoria in grief is likely to decrease in intensity over days to weeks and occurs in waves, the so-called pangs of grief. These waves tend to be associated with thoughts or reminders of the deceased. The depressed mood of an MDE is more persistent and not tied to specific thoughts or preoccupations. The pain of grief may be accompanied by positive emotions and humor that are uncharacteristic of the pervasive unhappiness and misery characteristic of an MDE. The thought content associated with grief generally features a preoccupation with thoughts and memories of the deceased, rather than the self-critical or pessimistic ruminations seen in an MDE. In grief, self-esteem is generally preserved, whereas in an MDE feelings of worthlessness and self-loathing are common. If self-derogatory ideation is present in grief, it typically involves perceived failings vis-à-vis the deceased (e.g., not visiting frequently enough, not telling the deceased how much he or she was loved). If a bereaved individual thinks about death and dying, such thoughts are generally focused on the deceased and possibly about "joining" the deceased, whereas in an MDE such thoughts are focused on ending one's own life because of feeling worthless, undeserving of life, or unable to cope with the pain of depression.

Coding and Recording Procedures

The diagnostic code for major depressive disorder is based on whether this is a single or recurrent episode, current severity, presence of psychotic features, and remission status. Current severity and psychotic features are only indicated if full criteria are currently met for a major depressive episode. Remission specifiers are only indicated if the full criteria are not currently met for a major depressive episode. Codes are as follows:

Severity/course specifier	Single episode	Recurrent episode*
Mild (p. 188)	296.21 (F32.0)	296.31 (F33.0)
Moderate (p. 188)	296.22 (F32.1)	296.32 (F33.1)
Severe (p. 188)	296.23 (F32.2)	296.33 (F33.2)
With psychotic features** (p. 186)	296.24 (F32.3)	296.34 (F33.3)
In partial remission (p. 188)	296.25 (F32.4)	296.35 (F33.41)
In full remission (p. 188)	296.26 (F32.5)	296.36 (F33.42)
Unspecified	296.20 (F32.9)	296.30 (F33.9)

*For an episode to be considered recurrent, there must be an interval of at least 2 consecutive months between separate episodes in which criteria are not met for a major depressive episode. The definitions of specifiers are found on the indicated pages.

**If psychotic features are present, code the "with psychotic features" specifier irrespective of episode severity.

In recording the name of a diagnosis, terms should be listed in the following order: major depressive disorder, single or recurrent episode, severity/psychotic/remission specifiers, followed by as many of the following specifiers without codes that apply to the current episode.

Specify:
>   **With anxious distress** (p. 184)
>   **With mixed features** (pp. 184–185)
>   **With melancholic features** (p. 185)
>   **With atypical features** (pp. 185–186)
>   **With mood-congruent psychotic features** (p. 186)
>   **With mood-incongruent psychotic features** (p. 186)
>   **With catatonia** (p. 186). **Coding note:** Use additional code 293.89 (F06.1).
>   **With peripartum onset** (pp. 186–187)
>   **With seasonal pattern** (recurrent episode only) (pp. 187–188)

Diagnostic Features

The criterion symptoms for major depressive disorder must be present nearly every day to be considered present, with the exception of weight change and suicidal ideation. Depressed mood must be present for most of the day, in addition to being present nearly every day. Often insomnia or fatigue is the presenting complaint, and failure to probe for accompanying depressive symptoms will result in underdiagnosis. Sadness may be denied at first but may be elicited through interview or inferred from facial expression and demeanor. With individuals who focus on a somatic complaint, clinicians should determine whether the distress from that complaint is associated with specific depressive symptoms. Fatigue and sleep disturbance are present in a high proportion of cases; psychomotor disturbances are much less common but are indicative of greater overall severity, as is the presence of delusional or near-delusional guilt.

The essential feature of a major depressive episode is a period of at least 2 weeks during which there is either depressed mood or the loss of interest or pleasure in nearly all activities (Criterion A). In children and adolescents, the mood may be irritable rather than sad. The individual must also experience at least four additional symptoms drawn from a list that includes changes in appetite or weight, sleep, and psychomotor activity; decreased energy; feelings of worthlessness or guilt; difficulty thinking, concentrating, or making decisions; or recurrent thoughts of death or suicidal ideation or suicide plans or attempts. To count toward a major depressive episode, a symptom must either be newly present or must have clearly worsened compared with the person's pre-episode status. The symptoms must persist for most of the day, nearly every day, for at least 2 consecutive weeks. The episode must be accompanied by clinically significant distress or impairment in social, occupational, or other important areas of functioning. For some individuals with milder episodes, functioning may appear to be normal but requires markedly increased effort.

The mood in a major depressive episode is often described by the person as depressed, sad, hopeless, discouraged, or "down in the dumps" (Criterion A1). In some cases, sadness may be denied at first but may subsequently be elicited by interview (e.g., by pointing out that the individual looks as if he or she is about to cry). In some individuals who complain of feeling "blah," having no feelings, or feeling anxious, the presence of a depressed mood can be inferred from the person's facial expression and demeanor. Some individuals emphasize somatic complaints (e.g., bodily aches and pains) rather than reporting feelings of sadness. Many individuals report or exhibit increased irritability (e.g., persistent anger, a tendency to respond to events with angry outbursts or blaming others, an exaggerated sense of frustration over minor matters). In children and adolescents, an irritable or cranky mood may develop rather than a sad or dejected mood. This presentation should be differentiated from a pattern of irritability when frustrated.

Loss of interest or pleasure is nearly always present, at least to some degree. Individuals may report feeling less interested in hobbies, "not caring anymore," or not feeling any enjoyment in activities that were previously considered pleasurable (Criterion A2). Family members often notice social withdrawal or neglect of pleasurable avocations (e.g., a formerly avid golfer no longer plays, a child who used to enjoy soccer finds excuses not to practice). In some individuals, there is a significant reduction from previous levels of sexual interest or desire.

Appetite change may involve either a reduction or increase. Some depressed individuals report that they have to force themselves to eat. Others may eat more and may crave specific foods (e.g., sweets or other carbohydrates). When appetite changes are severe (in either direction), there may be a significant loss or gain in weight, or, in children, a failure to make expected weight gains may be noted (Criterion A3).

Sleep disturbance may take the form of either difficulty sleeping or sleeping excessively (Criterion A4). When insomnia is present, it typically takes the form of middle insomnia (i.e., waking up during the night and then having difficulty returning to sleep) or terminal insomnia (i.e., waking too early and being unable to return to sleep). Initial insomnia (i.e., difficulty falling asleep) may also occur. Individuals who present with oversleeping (hypersomnia) may experience prolonged sleep episodes at night or increased daytime sleep. Sometimes the reason that the individual seeks treatment is for the disturbed sleep.

Psychomotor changes include agitation (e.g., the inability to sit still, pacing, handwringing; or pulling or rubbing of the skin, clothing, or other objects) or retardation (e.g., slowed speech, thinking, and body movements; increased pauses before answering; speech that is decreased in volume, inflection, amount, or variety of content, or muteness) (Criterion A5). The psychomotor agitation or retardation must be severe enough to be observable by others and not represent merely subjective feelings.

Decreased energy, tiredness, and fatigue are common (Criterion A6). A person may report sustained fatigue without physical exertion. Even the smallest tasks seem to require substantial effort. The efficiency with which tasks are accomplished may be reduced. For example, an individual may complain that washing and dressing in the morning are exhausting and take twice as long as usual.

The sense of worthlessness or guilt associated with a major depressive episode may include unrealistic negative evaluations of one's worth or guilty preoccupations or ruminations over minor past failings (Criterion A7). Such individuals often misinterpret neutral or trivial day-to-day events as evidence of personal defects and have an exaggerated sense of responsibility for untoward events. The sense of worthlessness or guilt may be of delusional proportions (e.g., an individual who is convinced that he or she is personally responsible for world poverty). Blaming oneself for being sick and for failing to meet occupational or interpersonal responsibilities as a result of the depression is very common and, unless delusional, is not considered sufficient to meet this criterion.

Many individuals report impaired ability to think, concentrate, or make even minor decisions (Criterion A8). They may appear easily distracted or complain of memory difficulties. Those engaged in cognitively demanding pursuits are often unable to function. In children, a precipitous drop in grades may reflect poor concentration. In elderly individuals, memory difficulties may be the chief complaint and may be mistaken for early signs of a dementia ("pseudodementia"). When the major depressive episode is successfully treated, the memory problems often fully abate. However, in some individuals, particularly elderly persons, a major depressive episode may sometimes be the initial presentation of an irreversible dementia.

Thoughts of death, suicidal ideation, or suicide attempts (Criterion A9) are common. They may range from a passive wish not to awaken in the morning or a belief that others would be better off if the individual were dead, to transient but recurrent thoughts of committing suicide, to a specific suicide plan. More severely suicidal individuals may have put their affairs in order (e.g., updated wills, settled debts), acquired needed materials (e.g., a rope or a gun), and chosen a location and time to accomplish the suicide. Motivations for suicide may include a desire to give up in the face of perceived insurmountable obstacles, an intense wish to end what is perceived as an unending and excruciatingly painful emotional state, an inability to foresee any enjoyment in life, or the wish to not be a burden to others. The resolution of such thinking may be a more meaningful measure of diminished suicide risk than denial of further plans for suicide.

The evaluation of the symptoms of a major depressive episode is especially difficult when they occur in an individual who also has a general medical condition (e.g., cancer, stroke, myocardial infarction, diabetes, pregnancy). Some of the criterion signs and symptoms of a major depressive episode are identical to those of general medical conditions (e.g., weight loss with untreated diabetes; fatigue with cancer; hypersomnia early in pregnancy; insomnia later in pregnancy or the postpartum). Such symptoms count toward a major depressive diagnosis except when they are clearly and fully attributable to a general medical condition. Nonvegetative symptoms of dysphoria, anhedonia, guilt or worthlessness, impaired concentration or indecision, and suicidal thoughts should be assessed with particular care in such cases. Definitions of major depressive episodes that have been modified to include only these nonvegetative symptoms appear to identify nearly the same individuals as do the full criteria.

Associated Features Supporting Diagnosis

Major depressive disorder is associated with high mortality, much of which is accounted for by suicide; however, it is not the only cause. For example, depressed individuals admitted to nursing homes have a markedly increased likelihood of death in the first year. Individuals frequently present with tearfulness, irritability, brooding, obsessive rumination, anxiety, phobias, excessive worry over physical health, and complaints of pain (e.g., headaches; joint, abdominal, or other pains). In children, separation anxiety may occur.

Although an extensive literature exists describing neuroanatomical, neuroendocrinological, and neurophysiological correlates of major depressive disorder, no laboratory test has yielded results of sufficient sensitivity and specificity to be used as a diagnostic tool for this disorder. Until recently, hypothalamic-pituitary-adrenal axis hyperactivity had been the most extensively investigated abnormality associated with major depressive episodes, and it appears to be associated with melancholia, psychotic features, and risks for eventual suicide. Molecular studies have also implicated peripheral factors, including genetic variants in neurotrophic factors and pro-inflammatory cytokines. Additionally, functional magnetic resonance imaging studies provide evidence for functional abnormalities in specific neural systems supporting emotion processing, reward seeking, and emotion regulation in adults with major depression.

Prevalence

Twelve-month prevalence of major depressive disorder in the United States is approximately 7%, with marked differences by age group such that the prevalence in 18- to 29-year-old individuals is threefold higher than the prevalence in individuals age 60 years or older. Females experience 1.5- to 3-fold higher rates than males beginning in early adolescence.

Development and Course

Major depressive disorder may first appear at any age, but the likelihood of onset increases markedly with puberty. In the United States, incidence appears to peak in the 20s; however, first onset in late life is not uncommon.

The course of major depressive disorder is quite variable, such that some individuals rarely, if ever, experience remission (a period of 2 or more months with no symptoms, or only one or two symptoms to no more than a mild degree), while others experience many years with few or no symptoms between discrete episodes. It is important to distinguish individuals who present for treatment during an exacerbation of a chronic depressive illness from those whose symptoms developed recently. Chronicity of depressive symptoms substantially increases the likelihood of underlying personality, anxiety, and substance use disorders and decreases the likelihood that treatment will be followed by full symptom resolution. It is therefore useful to ask individuals presenting with depressive symptoms to identify the last period of at least 2 months during which they were entirely free of depressive symptoms.

Recovery typically begins within 3 months of onset for two in five individuals with major depression and within 1 year for four in five individuals. Recency of onset is a strong determinant of the likelihood of near-term recovery, and many individuals who have been depressed only for several months can be expected to recover spontaneously. Features associated with lower recovery rates, other than current episode duration, include psychotic features, prominent anxiety, personality disorders, and symptom severity.

The risk of recurrence becomes progressively lower over time as the duration of remission increases. The risk is higher in individuals whose preceding episode was severe, in younger individuals, and in individuals who have already experienced multiple episodes. The persistence of even mild depressive symptoms during remission is a powerful predictor of recurrence.

Many bipolar illnesses begin with one or more depressive episodes, and a substantial proportion of individuals who initially appear to have major depressive disorder will prove, in time, to instead have a bipolar disorder. This is more likely in individuals with onset of the illness in adolescence, those with psychotic features, and those with a family history of bipolar illness. The presence of a "with mixed features" specifier also increases the risk for future manic or hypomanic diagnosis. Major depressive disorder, particularly with psychotic features, may also transition into schizophrenia, a change that is much more frequent than the reverse.

Despite consistent differences between genders in prevalence rates for depressive disorders, there appear to be no clear differences by gender in phenomenology, course, or treatment response. Similarly, there are no clear effects of current age on the course or treatment response of major depressive disorder. Some symptom differences exist, though, such that hypersomnia and hyperphagia are more likely in younger individuals, and melancholic symptoms, particularly psychomotor disturbances, are more common in older individuals. The likelihood of suicide attempts lessens in middle and late life, although the risk of completed suicide does not. Depressions with earlier ages at onset are more familial and more likely to involve personality disturbances. The course of major depressive disorder within individuals does not generally change with aging. Mean times to recovery appear to be stable over long periods, and the likelihood of being in an episode does not generally increase or decrease with time.

Risk and Prognostic Factors

Temperamental.   Neuroticism (negative affectivity) is a well-established risk factor for the onset of major depressive disorder, and high levels appear to render individuals more likely to develop depressive episodes in response to stressful life events.

Environmental.   Adverse childhood experiences, particularly when there are multiple experiences of diverse types, constitute a set of potent risk factors for major depressive disorder. Stressful life events are well recognized as precipitants of major depressive episodes, but the presence or absence of adverse life events near the onset of episodes does not appear to provide a useful guide to prognosis or treatment selection.

Genetic and physiological.   First-degree family members of individuals with major depressive disorder have a risk for major depressive disorder two- to fourfold higher than that of the general population. Relative risks appear to be higher for early-onset and recurrent forms. Heritability is approximately 40%, and the personality trait neuroticism accounts for a substantial portion of this genetic liability.

Course modifiers.   Essentially all major nonmood disorders increase the risk of an individual developing depression. Major depressive episodes that develop against the background of another disorder often follow a more refractory course. Substance use, anxiety, and borderline personality disorders are among the most common of these, and the presenting depressive symptoms may obscure and delay their recognition. However, sustained clinical improvement in depressive symptoms may depend on the appropriate treatment of underlying illnesses. Chronic or disabling medical conditions also increase risks for major depressive episodes. Such prevalent illnesses as diabetes, morbid obesity, and cardiovascular disease are often complicated by depressive episodes, and these episodes are more likely to become chronic than are depressive episodes in medically healthy individuals.

Culture-Related Diagnostic Issues

Surveys of major depressive disorder across diverse cultures have shown sevenfold differences in 12-month prevalence rates but much more consistency in female-to-male ratio, mean ages at onset, and the degree to which presence of the disorder raises the likelihood of comorbid substance abuse. While these findings suggest substantial cultural differences in the expression of major depressive disorder, they do not permit simple linkages between particular cultures and the likelihood of specific symptoms. Rather, clinicians should be aware that in most countries the majority of cases of depression go unrecognized in primary care settings and that in many cultures, somatic symptoms are very likely to constitute the presenting complaint. Among the Criterion A symptoms, insomnia and loss of energy are the most uniformly reported.

Gender-Related Diagnostic Issues

Although the most reproducible finding in the epidemiology of major depressive disorder has been a higher prevalence in females, there are no clear differences between genders in symptoms, course, treatment response, or functional consequences. In women, the risk for suicide attempts is higher, and the risk for suicide completion is lower. The disparity in suicide rate by gender is not as great among those with depressive disorders as it is in the population as a whole.

Suicide Risk

The possibility of suicidal behavior exists at all times during major depressive episodes. The most consistently described risk factor is a past history of suicide attempts or threats, but it should be remembered that most completed suicides are not preceded by unsuccessful attempts. Other features associated with an increased risk for completed suicide include male sex, being single or living alone, and having prominent feelings of hopelessness. The presence of borderline personality disorder markedly increases risk for future suicide attempts.

Functional Consequences of Major Depressive Disorder

Many of the functional consequences of major depressive disorder derive from individual symptoms. Impairment can be very mild, such that many of those who interact with the affected individual are unaware of depressive symptoms. Impairment may, however, range to complete incapacity such that the depressed individual is unable to attend to basic self-care needs or is mute or catatonic. Among individuals seen in general medical settings, those with major depressive disorder have more pain and physical illness and greater decreases in physical, social, and role functioning.

Differential Diagnosis

Manic episodes with irritable mood or mixed episodes.   Major depressive episodes with prominent irritable mood may be difficult to distinguish from manic episodes with irritable mood or from mixed episodes. This distinction requires a careful clinical evaluation of the presence of manic symptoms.

Mood disorder due to another medical condition.   A major depressive episode is the appropriate diagnosis if the mood disturbance is not judged, based on individual history, physical examination, and laboratory findings, to be the direct pathophysiological consequence of a specific medical condition (e.g., multiple sclerosis, stroke, hypothyroidism).

Substance/medication-induced depressive or bipolar disorder.   This disorder is distinguished from major depressive disorder by the fact that a substance (e.g., a drug of abuse, a medication, a toxin) appears to be etiologically related to the mood disturbance. For example, depressed mood that occurs only in the context of withdrawal from cocaine would be diagnosed as cocaine-induced depressive disorder.

Attention-deficit/hyperactivity disorder.   Distractibility and low frustration tolerance can occur in both attention-deficit/ hyperactivity disorder and a major depressive episode; if the criteria are met for both, attention-deficit/hyperactivity disorder may be diagnosed in addition to the mood disorder. However, the clinician must be cautious not to overdiagnose a major depressive episode in children with attention-deficit/hyperactivity disorder whose disturbance in mood is characterized by irritability rather than by sadness or loss of interest.

Adjustment disorder with depressed mood.   A major depressive episode that occurs in response to a psychosocial stressor is distinguished from adjustment disorder with depressed mood by the fact that the full criteria for a major depressive episode are not met in adjustment disorder.

Sadness.   Finally, periods of sadness are inherent aspects of the human experience. These periods should not be diagnosed as a major depressive episode unless criteria are met for severity (i.e., five out of nine symptoms), duration (i.e., most of the day, nearly every day for at least 2 weeks), and clinically significant distress or impairment. The diagnosis other specified depressive disorder may be appropriate for presentations of depressed mood with clinically significant impairment that do not meet criteria for duration or severity.

Comorbidity

Other disorders with which major depressive disorder frequently co-occurs are substance-related disorders, panic disorder, obsessive-compulsive disorder, anorexia nervosa, bulimia nervosa, and borderline personality disorder.

Persistent Depressive Disorder (Dysthymia)

Diagnostic Criteria   **300.4 (F34.1)**

This disorder represents a consolidation of DSM-IV-defined chronic major depressive disorder and dysthymic disorder.

A. Depressed mood for most of the day, for more days than not, as indicated by either subjective account or observation by others, for at least 2 years.

   Note: In children and adolescents, mood can be irritable and duration must be at least 1 year.

B. Presence, while depressed, of two (or more) of the following:

   1. Poor appetite or overeating.
   2. Insomnia or hypersomnia.
   3. Low energy or fatigue.
   4. Low self-esteem.
   5. Poor concentration or difficulty making decisions.
   6. Feelings of hopelessness.

C. During the 2-year period (1 year for children or adolescents) of the disturbance, the individual has never been without the symptoms in Criteria A and B for more than 2 months at a time.

D. Criteria for a major depressive disorder may be continuously present for 2 years.

E. There has never been a manic episode or a hypomanic episode, and criteria have never been met for cyclothymic disorder.

F. The disturbance is not better explained by a persistent schizoaffective disorder, schizophrenia, delusional disorder, or other specified or unspecified schizophrenia spectrum and other psychotic disorder.

G. The symptoms are not attributable to the physiological effects of a substance (e.g., a drug of abuse, a medication) or another medical condition (e.g., hypothyroidism).

H. The symptoms cause clinically significant distress or impairment in social, occupational, or other important areas of functioning.

Note: Because the criteria for a major depressive episode include four symptoms that are absent from the symptom list for persistent depressive disorder (dysthymia), a very limited number of individuals will have depressive symptoms that have persisted longer than 2 years but will not meet criteria for persistent depressive disorder. If full criteria for a major depressive episode have been met at some point during the current episode of illness, they should be given a diagnosis of major depressive disorder. Otherwise, a diagnosis of other specified depressive disorder or unspecified depressive disorder is warranted.

Specify if:

With anxious distress (p. 184)
With mixed features (pp. 184–185)
With melancholic features (p. 185)
With atypical features (pp. 185–186)
With mood-congruent psychotic features (p. 186)
With mood-incongruent psychotic features (p. 186)
With peripartum onset (pp. 186–187)

Specify if:

In partial remission (p. 188)
In full remission (p. 188)

Specify if:

Early onset: If onset is before age 21 years.
Late onset: If onset is at age 21 years or older.

Specify if (for most recent 2 years of persistent depressive disorder):

With pure dysthymic syndrome: Full criteria for a major depressive episode have not been met in at least the preceding 2 years.
With persistent major depressive episode: Full criteria for a major depressive episode have been met throughout the preceding 2-year period.
With intermittent major depressive episodes, with current episode: Full criteria for a major depressive episode are currently met, but there have been periods of at least 8 weeks in at least the preceding 2 years with symptoms below the threshold for a full major depressive episode.
With intermittent major depressive episodes, without current episode: Full criteria for a major depressive episode are not currently met, but there has been one or more major depressive episodes in at least the preceding 2 years.

Specify current severity:

Mild (p. 188)
Moderate (p. 188)
Severe (p. 188)

Diagnostic Features

The essential feature of persistent depressive disorder (dysthymia) is a depressed mood that occurs for most of the day, for more days than not, for at least 2 years, or at least 1 year for children and adolescents (Criterion A). This disorder represents a consolidation of DSM-IV-defined chronic major depressive disorder and dysthymic disorder. Major depression may precede persistent depressive disorder, and major depressive episodes may occur during persistent depressive disorder. Individuals whose symptoms meet major depressive disorder criteria for 2 years should be given a diagnosis of persistent depressive disorder as well as major depressive disorder.

Individuals with persistent depressive disorder describe their mood as sad or "down in the dumps." During periods of depressed mood, at least two of the six symptoms from Criterion B are present. Because these symptoms have become a part of the individual's day-to-day experience, particularly in the case of early onset (e.g., "I've always been this way"), they may not be reported unless the individual is directly prompted. During the 2-year period (1 year for children or adolescents), any symptom-free intervals last no longer than 2 months (Criterion C).

Prevalence

Persistent depressive disorder is effectively an amalgam of DSM-IV dysthymic disorder and chronic major depressive episode. The 12-month prevalence in the United States is approximately 0.5% for persistent depressive disorder and 1.5% for chronic major depressive disorder.

Development and Course

Persistent depressive disorder often has an early and insidious onset (i.e., in childhood, adolescence, or early adult life) and, by definition, a chronic course. Among individuals with both persistent depressive disorder and borderline personality disorder, the covariance of the corresponding features over time suggests the operation of a common mechanism. Early onset (i.e., before age 21 years) is associated with a higher likelihood of comorbid personality disorders and substance use disorders.

When symptoms rise to the level of a major depressive episode, they are likely to subsequently revert to a lower level. However, depressive symptoms are much less likely to resolve in a given period of time in the context of persistent depressive disorder than they are in a major depressive episode.

Risk and Prognostic Factors

Temperamental. Factors predictive of poorer long-term outcome include higher levels of neuroticism (negative affectivity), greater symptom severity, poorer global functioning, and presence of anxiety disorders or conduct disorder.

Environmental. Childhood risk factors include parental loss or separation.

Genetic and physiological. There are no clear differences in illness development, course, or family history between DSM-IV dysthymic disorder and chronic major depressive disorder. Earlier findings pertaining to either disorder are therefore likely to apply to persistent depressive disorder. It is thus likely that individuals with persistent depressive disorder will have a higher proportion of first-degree relatives with persistent depressive disorder than do individuals with major depressive disorder, and more depressive disorders in general.

A number of brain regions (e.g., prefrontal cortex, anterior cingulate, amygdala, hippocampus) have been implicated in persistent depressive disorder. Possible polysomnographic abnormalities exist as well.

Functional Consequences of Persistent Depressive Disorder

The degree to which persistent depressive disorder impacts social and occupational functioning is likely to vary widely, but effects can be as great as or greater than those of major depressive disorder.

Differential Diagnosis

Major depressive disorder. If there is a depressed mood plus two or more symptoms meeting criteria for a persistent depressive episode for 2 years or more, then the diagnosis of persistent depressive disorder is made. The diagnosis depends on the 2-year duration, which distinguishes it from episodes of depression that do not last 2 years. If the symptom criteria are sufficient for a diagnosis of a major depressive episode at any time during this period, then the diagnosis of major depression should be made and also noted as a specifier with the diagnosis of persistent depressive disorder. If the individual's symptoms currently meet full criteria for a major depressive episode, then the specifier of "with intermittent major depressive episodes, with current episode" would be made. If the major depressive episode has persisted for at least a 2-year duration and remains present, then the specifier "with persistent major depressive episode" is used. When full major depressive episode criteria are not currently met but there has been at least one previous episode of major depression in the context of at least 2 years of persistent depressive symptoms, then the specifier of "with intermittent major depressive episodes, without current episode" is used. If the individual has not experienced an episode of major depression in the last 2 years, then the specifier "with pure dysthymic syndrome" is used.

Psychotic disorders.   Depressive symptoms are a common associated feature of chronic psychotic disorders (e.g., schizoaffective disorder, schizophrenia, delusional disorder). A separate diagnosis of persistent depressive disorder is not made if the symptoms occur only during the course of the psychotic disorder (including residual phases).

Depressive or bipolar and related disorder due to another medical condition.   Persistent depressive disorder must be distinguished from a depressive or bipolar and related disorder due to another medical condition. The diagnosis is depressive or bipolar and related disorder due to another medical condition if the mood disturbance is judged, based on history, physical examination, or laboratory findings, to be attributable to the direct pathophysiological effects of a specific, usually chronic, medical condition (e.g., multiple sclerosis). If it is judged that the depressive symptoms are not attributable to the physiological effects of another medical condition, then the primary mental disorder (e.g., persistent depressive disorder) is recorded, and the medical condition is noted as a concomitant medical condition (e.g., diabetes mellitus).

Substance/medication-induced depressive or bipolar disorder.   A substance/medication-induced depressive or bipolar and related disorder is distinguished from persistent depressive disorder when a substance (e.g., a drug of abuse, a medication, a toxin) is judged to be etiologically related to the mood disturbance.

Personality disorders.   Often, there is evidence of a coexisting personality disturbance. When an individual's presentation meets the criteria for both persistent depressive disorder and a personality disorder, both diagnoses are given.

Comorbidity

In comparison to individuals with major depressive disorder, those with persistent depressive disorder are at higher risk for psychiatric comorbidity in general, and for anxiety disorders and substance use disorders in particular. Early-onset persistent depressive disorder is strongly associated with DSM-IV Cluster B and C personality disorders.

Premenstrual Dysphoric Disorder

Diagnostic Criteria	625.4 (F32.81)

A. In the majority of menstrual cycles, at least five symptoms must be present in the final week before the onset of menses, start to *improve* within a few days after the onset of menses, and become *minimal* or absent in the week postmenses.

B. One (or more) of the following symptoms must be present:

   1. Marked affective lability (e.g., mood swings; feeling suddenly sad or tearful, or increased sensitivity to rejection).

   2. Marked irritability or anger or increased interpersonal conflicts.
   3. Marked depressed mood, feelings of hopelessness, or self-deprecating thoughts.
   4. Marked anxiety, tension, and/or feelings of being keyed up or on edge.
C. One (or more) of the following symptoms must additionally be present, to reach a total of *five* symptoms when combined with symptoms from Criterion B above.
   1. Decreased interest in usual activities (e.g., work, school, friends, hobbies).
   2. Subjective difficulty in concentration.
   3. Lethargy, easy fatigability, or marked lack of energy.
   4. Marked change in appetite; overeating; or specific food cravings.
   5. Hypersomnia or insomnia.
   6. A sense of being overwhelmed or out of control.
   7. Physical symptoms such as breast tenderness or swelling, joint or muscle pain, a sensation of "bloating," or weight gain.

Note: The symptoms in Criteria A–C must have been met for most menstrual cycles that occurred in the preceding year.

D. The symptoms are associated with clinically significant distress or interference with work, school, usual social activities, or relationships with others (e.g., avoidance of social activities; decreased productivity and efficiency at work, school, or home).
E. The disturbance is not merely an exacerbation of the symptoms of another disorder, such as major depressive disorder, panic disorder, persistent depressive disorder (dysthymia), or a personality disorder (although it may co-occur with any of these disorders).
F. Criterion A should be confirmed by prospective daily ratings during at least two symptomatic cycles. (**Note:** The diagnosis may be made provisionally prior to this confirmation.)
G. The symptoms are not attributable to the physiological effects of a substance (e.g., a drug of abuse, a medication, other treatment) or another medical condition (e.g., hyperthyroidism).

Recording Procedures

If symptoms have not been confirmed by prospective daily ratings of at least two symptomatic cycles, "provisional" should be noted after the name of the diagnosis (i.e., "premenstrual dysphoric disorder, provisional").

Diagnostic Features

The essential features of premenstrual dysphoric disorder are the expression of mood lability, irritability, dysphoria, and anxiety symptoms that occur repeatedly during the premenstrual phase of the cycle and remit around the onset of menses or shortly thereafter. These symptoms may be accompanied by behavioral and physical symptoms. Symptoms must have occurred in most of the menstrual cycles during the past year and must have an adverse effect on work or social functioning. The intensity and/or expressivity of the accompanying symptoms may be closely related to social and cultural background characteristics of the affected female, family perspectives, and more specific factors such as religious beliefs, social tolerance, and female gender role issues.

Typically, symptoms peak around the time of the onset of menses. Although it is not uncommon for symptoms to linger into the first few days of menses, the individual must have a symptom-free period in the follicular phase after the menstrual period begins. While the core symptoms include mood and anxiety symptoms, behavioral and somatic symptoms commonly also occur. However, the presence of physical and/or behavioral symptoms in the absence of mood and/or anxious symptoms is not sufficient for a diagnosis. Symptoms are of comparable severity (but not duration) to those of another mental disorder, such as a major depressive episode or generalized anxiety disorder. In order to confirm a provisional diagnosis, daily prospective symptom ratings are required for at least two symptomatic cycles.

Associated Features Supporting Diagnosis

Delusions and hallucinations have been described in the late luteal phase of the menstrual cycle but are rare. The premenstrual phase has been considered by some to be a risk period for suicide.

Prevalence

Twelve-month prevalence of premenstrual dysphoric disorder is between 1.8% and 5.8% of menstruating women. Estimates are substantially inflated if they are based on retrospective reports rather than prospective daily ratings. However, estimated prevalence based on a daily record of symptoms for 1–2 months may be less representative, as individuals with the most severe symptoms may be unable to sustain the rating process. The most rigorous estimate of premenstrual dysphoric disorder is 1.8% for women whose symptoms meet the full criteria without functional impairment and 1.3% for women whose symptoms meet the current criteria with functional impairment and without co-occurring symptoms from another mental disorder.

Development and Course

Onset of premenstrual dysphoric disorder can occur at any point after menarche. Incidence of new cases over a 40-month follow-up period is 2.5% (95% confidence interval = 1.7–3.7). Anecdotally, many individuals, as they approach menopause, report that symptoms worsen. Symptoms cease after menopause, although cyclical hormone replacement can trigger the re-expression of symptoms.

Risk and Prognostic Factors

Environmental. Environmental factors associated with the expression of premenstrual dysphoric disorder include stress, history of interpersonal trauma, seasonal changes, and sociocultural aspects of female sexual behavior in general, and female gender role in particular.

Genetic and physiological. Heritability of premenstrual dysphoric disorder is unknown. However, for premenstrual symptoms, estimates for heritability range between 30% and 80%, with the most stable component of premenstrual symptoms estimated to be about 50% heritable.

Course modifiers. Women who use oral contraceptives may have fewer premenstrual complaints than do women who do not use oral contraceptives.

Culture-Related Diagnostic Issues

Premenstrual dysphoric disorder is not a culture-bound syndrome and has been observed in individuals in the United States, Europe, India, and Asia. It is unclear as to whether rates differ by race. Nevertheless, frequency, intensity, and expressivity of symptoms and help-seeking patterns may be significantly influenced by cultural factors.

Diagnostic Markers

As indicated earlier, the diagnosis of premenstrual dysphoric disorder is appropriately confirmed by 2 months of prospective symptom ratings. A number of scales, including the

Daily Rating of Severity of Problems and the Visual Analogue Scales for Premenstrual Mood Symptoms, have undergone validation and are commonly used in clinical trials for premenstrual dysphoric disorder. The Premenstrual Tension Syndrome Rating Scale has a self-report and an observer version, both of which have been validated and used widely to measure illness severity in women who have premenstrual dysphoric disorder.

Functional Consequences of Premenstrual Dysphoric Disorder

Symptoms must be associated with clinically meaningful distress and/or an obvious and marked impairment in the ability to function socially or occupationally in the week prior to menses. Impairment in social functioning may be manifested by marital discord and problems with children, other family members, or friends. Chronic marital or job problems should not be confused with dysfunction that occurs only in association with premenstrual dysphoric disorder.

Differential Diagnosis

Premenstrual syndrome.   Premenstrual syndrome differs from premenstrual dysphoric disorder in that a minimum of five symptoms is not required, and there is no stipulation of affective symptoms for individuals who have premenstrual syndrome. This condition may be more common than premenstrual dysphoric disorder, although the estimated prevalence of premenstrual syndrome varies. While premenstrual syndrome shares the feature of symptom expression during the premenstrual phase of the menstrual cycle, it is generally considered to be less severe than premenstrual dysphoric disorder. The presence of physical or behavioral symptoms in the premenstruum, without the required affective symptoms, likely meets criteria for premenstrual syndrome and not for premenstrual dysphoric disorder.

Dysmenorrhea.   Dysmenorrhea is a syndrome of painful menses, but this is distinct from a syndrome characterized by affective changes. Moreover, symptoms of dysmenorrhea begin with the onset of menses, whereas symptoms of premenstrual dysphoric disorder, by definition, begin before the onset of menses, even if they linger into the first few days of menses.

Bipolar disorder, major depressive disorder, and persistent depressive disorder (dysthymia).   Many women with (either naturally occurring or substance/medication-induced) bipolar or major depressive disorder or persistent depressive disorder believe that they have premenstrual dysphoric disorder. However, when they chart symptoms, they realize that the symptoms do not follow a premenstrual pattern. Women with another mental disorder may experience chronic symptoms or intermittent symptoms that are unrelated to menstrual cycle phase. However, because the onset of menses constitutes a memorable event, they may report that symptoms occur only during the premenstruum or that symptoms worsen premenstrually. This is one of the rationales for the requirement that symptoms be confirmed by daily prospective ratings. The process of differential diagnosis, particularly if the clinician relies on retrospective symptoms only, is made more difficult because of the overlap between symptoms of premenstrual dysphoric disorder and some other diagnoses. The overlap of symptoms is particularly salient for differentiating premenstrual dysphoric disorder from major depressive episodes, persistent depressive disorder, bipolar disorders, and borderline personality disorder. However, the rate of personality disorders is no higher in individuals with premenstrual dysphoric disorder than in those without the disorder.

Use of hormonal treatments.   Some women who present with moderate to severe premenstrual symptoms may be using hormonal treatments, including hormonal contraceptives. If such symptoms occur after initiation of exogenous hormone use, the symptoms may be due to the use of hormones rather than to the underlying condition of premenstrual dysphoric disorder. If the woman stops hormones and the symptoms disappear, this is consistent with substance/medication-induced depressive disorder.

Comorbidity

A major depressive episode is the most frequently reported previous disorder in individuals presenting with premenstrual dysphoric disorder. A wide range of medical (e.g., migraine, asthma, allergies, seizure disorders) or other mental disorders (e.g., depressive and bipolar disorders, anxiety disorders, bulimia nervosa, substance use disorders) may worsen in the premenstrual phase; however, the absence of a symptom-free period during the postmenstrual interval obviates a diagnosis of premenstrual dysphoric disorder. These conditions are better considered premenstrual exacerbation of a current mental or medical disorder. Although the diagnosis of premenstrual dysphoric disorder should not be assigned in situations in which an individual only experiences a premenstrual exacerbation of another mental or physical disorder, it can be considered in addition to the diagnosis of another mental or physical disorder if the individual experiences symptoms and changes in level of functioning that are characteristic of premenstrual dysphoric disorder and markedly different from the symptoms experienced as part of the ongoing disorder.

Substance/Medication-Induced Depressive Disorder

Diagnostic Criteria

A. A prominent and persistent disturbance in mood that predominates in the clinical picture and is characterized by depressed mood or markedly diminished interest or pleasure in all, or almost all, activities.

B. There is evidence from the history, physical examination, or laboratory findings of both (1) and (2):

1. The symptoms in Criterion A developed during or soon after substance intoxication or withdrawal or after exposure to a medication.
2. The involved substance/medication is capable of producing the symptoms in Criterion A.

C. The disturbance is not better explained by a depressive disorder that is not substance/medication-induced. Such evidence of an independent depressive disorder could include the following:

The symptoms preceded the onset of the substance/medication use; the symptoms persist for a substantial period of time (e.g., about 1 month) after the cessation of acute withdrawal or severe intoxication; or there is other evidence suggesting the existence of an independent non-substance/medication-induced depressive disorder (e.g., a history of recurrent non-substance/medication-related episodes).

D. The disturbance does not occur exclusively during the course of a delirium.

E. The disturbance causes clinically significant distress or impairment in social, occupational, or other important areas of functioning.

Note: This diagnosis should be made instead of a diagnosis of substance intoxication or substance withdrawal only when the symptoms in Criterion A predominate in the clinical picture and when they are sufficiently severe to warrant clinical attention.

Coding note: The ICD-9-CM and ICD-10-CM codes for the [specific substance/medication]-induced depressive disorders are indicated in the table below. Note that the ICD-10-

CM code depends on whether or not there is a comorbid substance use disorder present for the same class of substance. If a mild substance use disorder is comorbid with the substance-induced depressive disorder, the 4th position character is "1," and the clinician should record "mild [substance] use disorder" before the substance-induced depressive disorder (e.g., "mild cocaine use disorder with cocaine-induced depressive disorder"). If a moderate or severe substance use disorder is comorbid with the substance-induced depressive disorder, the 4th position character is "2," and the clinician should record "moderate [substance] use disorder" or "severe [substance] use disorder," depending on the severity of the comorbid substance use disorder. If there is no comorbid substance use disorder (e.g., after a one-time heavy use of the substance), then the 4th position character is "9," and the clinician should record only the substance-induced depressive disorder.

		ICD-10-CM		
	ICD-9-CM	With use disorder, mild	With use disorder, moderate or severe	Without use disorder
Alcohol	291.89	F10.14	F10.24	F10.94
Phencyclidine	292.84	F16.14	F16.24	F16.94
Other hallucinogen	292.84	F16.14	F16.24	F16.94
Inhalant	292.84	F18.14	F18.24	F18.94
Opioid	292.84	F11.14	F11.24	F11.94
Sedative, hypnotic, or anxiolytic	292.84	F13.14	F13.24	F13.94
Amphetamine (or other stimulant)	292.84	F15.14	F15.24	F15.94
Cocaine	292.84	F14.14	F14.24	F14.94
Other (or unknown) substance	292.84	F19.14	F19.24	F19.94

Specify if (see Table 1 in the chapter "Substance-Related and Addictive Disorders" for diagnoses associated with substance class):
   With onset during intoxication: If criteria are met for intoxication with the substance and the symptoms develop during intoxication.
   With onset during withdrawal: If criteria are met for withdrawal from the substance and the symptoms develop during, or shortly after, withdrawal.

Recording Procedures

ICD-9-CM.   The name of the substance/medication-induced depressive disorder begins with the specific substance (e.g., cocaine, dexamethasone) that is presumed to be causing the depressive symptoms. The diagnostic code is selected from the table included in the criteria set, which is based on the drug class. For substances that do not fit into any of the classes (e.g., dexamethasone), the code for "other substance" should be used; and in cases in which a substance is judged to be an etiological factor but the specific class of substance is unknown, the category "unknown substance" should be used.

The name of the disorder is followed by the specification of onset (i.e., onset during intoxication, onset during withdrawal). Unlike the recording procedures for ICD-10-CM, which combine the substance-induced disorder and substance use disorder into a single code, for ICD-9-CM a separate diagnostic code is given for the substance use disorder. For example, in the case of depressive symptoms occurring during withdrawal in a man with a severe cocaine use disorder, the diagnosis is 292.84 cocaine-induced depressive disorder, with onset during withdrawal. An additional diagnosis of 304.20 severe cocaine use disorder is also given. When more than one substance is judged to play a significant role in the development of depressive mood symptoms, each should be listed separately (e.g., 292.84 methylphenidate-induced depressive disorder, with onset during withdrawal; 292.84 dexamethasone-induced depressive disorder, with onset during intoxication).

ICD-10-CM. The name of the substance/medication-induced depressive disorder begins with the specific substance (e.g., cocaine, dexamethasone) that is presumed to be causing the depressive symptoms. The diagnostic code is selected from the table included in the criteria set, which is based on the drug class and presence or absence of a comorbid substance use disorder. For substances that do not fit into any of the classes (e.g., dexamethasone), the code for "other substance" should be used; and in cases in which a substance is judged to be an etiological factor but the specific class of substance is unknown, the category "unknown substance" should be used.

When recording the name of the disorder, the comorbid substance use disorder (if any) is listed first, followed by the word "with," followed by the name of the substance-induced depressive disorder, followed by the specification of onset (i.e., onset during intoxication, onset during withdrawal). For example, in the case of depressive symptoms occurring during withdrawal in a man with a severe cocaine use disorder, the diagnosis is F14.24 severe cocaine use disorder with cocaine-induced depressive disorder, with onset during withdrawal. A separate diagnosis of the comorbid severe cocaine use disorder is not given. If the substance-induced depressive disorder occurs without a comorbid substance use disorder (e.g., after a one-time heavy use of the substance), no accompanying substance use disorder is noted (e.g., F16.94 phencyclidine-induced depressive disorder, with onset during intoxication). When more than one substance is judged to play a significant role in the development of depressive mood symptoms, each should be listed separately (e.g., F15.24 severe methylphenidate use disorder with methylphenidate-induced depressive disorder, with onset during withdrawal; F19.94 dexamethasone-induced depressive disorder, with onset during intoxication).

Diagnostic Features

The diagnostic features of substance/medication-induced depressive disorder include the symptoms of a depressive disorder, such as major depressive disorder; however, the depressive symptoms are associated with the ingestion, injection, or inhalation of a substance (e.g., drug of abuse, toxin, psychotropic medication, other medication), and the depressive symptoms persist beyond the expected length of physiological effects, intoxication, or withdrawal period. As evidenced by clinical history, physical examination, or laboratory findings, the relevant depressive disorder should have developed during or within 1 month after use of a substance that is capable of producing the depressive disorder (Criterion B1). In addition, the diagnosis is not better explained by an independent depressive disorder. Evidence of an independent depressive disorder includes the depressive disorder preceded the onset of ingestion or withdrawal from the substance; the depressive disorder persists beyond a substantial period of time after the cessation of substance use; or other evidence suggests the existence of an independent non-substance/medication-induced depressive disorder (Criterion C). This diagnosis should not be made when symptoms occur exclusively during the course of a delirium (Criterion D). The depressive disorder associated with the substance use, intoxication, or withdrawal must cause clinically significant distress or impairment in social, occupational, or other important areas of functioning to qualify for this diagnosis (Criterion E).

Some medications (e.g., stimulants, steroids, L-dopa, antibiotics, central nervous system drugs, dermatological agents, chemotherapeutic drugs, immunological agents) can induce depressive mood disturbances. Clinical judgment is essential to determine whether the medication is truly associated with inducing the depressive disorder or whether a primary depressive disorder happened to have its onset while the person was receiving the treatment. For example, a depressive episode that developed within the first several weeks of beginning alpha-methyldopa (an antihypertensive agent) in an individual with no history of major depressive disorder would qualify for the diagnosis of medication-induced depressive disorder. In some cases, a previously established condition (e.g., major depressive disorder, recurrent) can recur while the individual is coincidentally taking a medication that has the capacity to cause depressive symptoms (e.g., L-dopa, oral contraceptives). In such cases, the clinician must make a judgment as to whether the medication is causative in this particular situation.

A substance/medication-induced depressive disorder is distinguished from a primary depressive disorder by considering the onset, course, and other factors associated with the substance use. There must be evidence from the history, physical examination, or laboratory findings of substance use, abuse, intoxication, or withdrawal prior to the onset of the depressive disorder. The withdrawal state for some substances can be relatively protracted, and thus intense depressive symptoms can last for a long period after the cessation of substance use.

Prevalence

In a nationally representative U.S. adult population, the lifetime prevalence of substance/medication-induced depressive disorder is 0.26%.

Development and Course

A depressive disorder associated with the use of substance (i.e., alcohol, illicit drugs, or a prescribed treatment for a mental disorder or another medical condition) must have its onset while the individual is using the substance or during withdrawal, if there is a withdrawal syndrome associated with the substance. Most often, the depressive disorder has its onset within the first few weeks or 1 month of use of the substance. Once the substance is discontinued, the depressive symptoms usually remit within days to several weeks, depending on the half-life of the substance/medication and the presence of a withdrawal syndrome. If symptoms persist 4 weeks beyond the expected time course of withdrawal of a particular substance/medication, other causes for the depressive mood symptoms should be considered.

Although there are a few prospective controlled trials examining the association of depressive symptoms with use of a medication, most reports are from postmarketing surveillance studies, retrospective observational studies, or case reports, making evidence of causality difficult to determine. Substances implicated in medication-induced depressive disorder, with varying degrees of evidence, include antiviral agents (efavirenz), cardiovascular agents (clonidine, guanethidine, methyldopa, reserpine), retinoic acid derivatives (isotretinoin), antidepressants, anticonvulsants, anti-migraine agents (triptans), antipsychotics, hormonal agents (corticosteroids, oral contraceptives, gonadotropin-releasing hormone agonists, tamoxifen), smoking cessation agents (varenicline), and immunological agents (interferon). However, other potential substances continue to emerge as new compounds are synthesized. A history of such substance use may help increase diagnostic certainty.

Risk and Prognostic Factors

Temperamental.   Factors that appear to increase the risk of substance/medication-induced depressive disorder can be conceptualized as pertaining to the specific type of drug or to a group of individuals with underlying alcohol or drug use disorders. Risk factors common to all drugs include history of major depressive disorder, history of drug-induced depression, and psychosocial stressors.

Environmental.   There are also risk factors pertaining to a specific type of medication (e.g., increased immune activation prior to treatment for hepatitis C associated with inter-feron-alfa-induced depression); high doses (greater than 80 mg/day prednisone-equivalents) of corticosteroids or high plasma concentrations of efavirenz; and high estrogen/progesterone content in oral contraceptives.

Course modifiers.   In a representative U.S. adult population, compared with individuals with major depressive disorder who did not have a substance use disorder, individuals with substance-induced depressive disorder were more likely to be male, to be black, to have at most a high school diploma, to lack insurance, and to have lower family income. They were also more likely to report higher family history of substance use disorders and antisocial behavior, higher 12-month history of stressful life events, and a greater number of DSM-IV major depressive disorder criteria. They were more likely to report feelings of worthlessness, insomnia/hypersomnia, and thoughts of death and suicide attempts, but less likely to report depressed mood and parental loss by death before age 18 years.

Diagnostic Markers

Determination of the substance of use can sometimes be made through laboratory assays of the suspected substance in the blood or urine to corroborate the diagnosis.

Suicide Risk

Drug-induced or treatment-emergent suicidality represents a marked change in thoughts and behavior from the person's baseline, is usually temporally associated with initiation of a substance, and must be distinguished from the underlying primary mental disorders.

In regard to the treatment-emergent suicidality associated with antidepressants, a U.S. Food and Drug Administration (FDA) advisory committee considered meta-analyses of 99,839 participants enrolled in 372 randomized clinical trials of antidepressants in trials for mental disorders. The analyses showed that when the data were pooled across all adult age groups, there was no perceptible increased risk of suicidal behavior or ideation. However, in age-stratified analyses, the risk for patients ages 18–24 years was elevated, albeit not significantly (odds ratio [OR] = 1.55; 95% confidence interval [CI] = 0.91–2.70). The FDA meta-analyses reveal an absolute risk of suicide in patients taking investigational antidepressants of 0.01%. In conclusion, suicide is clearly an extremely rare treatment-emergent phenomenon, but the outcome of suicide was serious enough to prompt the FDA to issue an expanded black-box warning in 2007 regarding the importance of careful monitoring of treatment-emergent suicidal ideation in patients receiving antidepressants.

Differential Diagnosis

Substance intoxication and withdrawal.   Depressive symptoms occur commonly in substance intoxication and substance withdrawal, and the diagnosis of the substance-specific intoxication or withdrawal will usually suffice to categorize the symptom presentation. A diagnosis of substance-induced depressive disorder should be made instead of a diagnosis of substance intoxication or substance withdrawal when the mood symptoms are sufficiently severe to warrant independent clinical attention. For example, dysphoric mood is a characteristic feature of cocaine withdrawal. Substance/medication-induced depressive disorder should be diagnosed instead of cocaine withdrawal only if the mood disturbance is substantially more intense or longer lasting than what is usually encountered with cocaine withdrawal and is sufficiently severe to be a separate focus of attention and treatment.

Primary depressive disorder.   A substance/medication-induced depressive disorder is distinguished from a primary depressive disorder by the fact that a substance is judged to be etiologically related to the symptoms, as described earlier (see section "Development and Course" for this disorder).

Depressive disorder due to another medical condition.   Because individuals with other medical conditions often take medications for those conditions, the clinician must consider the possibility that the mood symptoms are caused by the physiological consequences of the medical condition rather than the medication, in which case depressive disorder due to another medical condition is diagnosed. The history often provides the primary basis for such a judgment. At times, a change in the treatment for the other medical condition (e.g., medication substitution or discontinuation) may be needed to determine empirically whether the medication is the causative agent. If the clinician has ascertained that the disturbance is a function of both another medical condition and substance use or withdrawal, both diagnoses (i.e., depressive disorder due to another medical condition and substance/medication-induced depressive disorder) may be given. When there is insufficient evidence to determine whether the depressive symptoms are associated with substance (including a medication) ingestion or withdrawal or with another medical condition or are primary (i.e., not a function of either a substance or another medical condition), a diagnosis of other specified depressive disorder or unspecified depressive disorder would be indicated.

Comorbidity

Compared with individuals with major depressive disorder and no comorbid substance use disorder, those with substance/medication-induced depressive disorder have higher rates of comorbidity with any DSM-IV mental disorder; are more likely to have specific DSM-IV disorders of pathological gambling and paranoid, histrionic, and antisocial personality disorders; and are less likely to have persistent depressive disorder (dysthymia). Compared with individuals with major depressive disorder and a comorbid substance use disorder, individuals with substance/medication-induced depressive disorder are more likely to have alcohol use disorder, any other substance use disorder, and histrionic personality disorder; however, they are less likely to have persistent depressive disorder.

Depressive Disorder
Due to Another Medical Condition

Diagnostic Criteria

A. A prominent and persistent period of depressed mood or markedly diminished interest or pleasure in all, or almost all, activities that predominates in the clinical picture.

B. There is evidence from the history, physical examination, or laboratory findings that the disturbance is the direct pathophysiological consequence of another medical condition.

C. The disturbance is not better explained by another mental disorder (e.g., adjustment disorder, with depressed mood, in which the stressor is a serious medical condition).

D. The disturbance does not occur exclusively during the course of a delirium.

E. The disturbance causes clinically significant distress or impairment in social, occupational, or other important areas of functioning.

Coding note: The ICD-9-CM code for depressive disorder due to another medical condition is **293.83,** which is assigned regardless of the specifier. The ICD-10-CM code depends on the specifier (see below).

Specify if:
  (F06.31) With depressive features: Full criteria are not met for a major depressive episode.
  (F06.32) With major depressive–like episode: Full criteria are met (except Criterion C) for a major depressive episode.
  (F06.34) With mixed features: Symptoms of mania or hypomania are also present but do not predominate in the clinical picture.

Coding note: Include the name of the other medical condition in the name of the mental disorder (e.g., 293.83 [F06.31] depressive disorder due to hypothyroidism, with depressive features). The other medical condition should also be coded and listed separately immediately before the depressive disorder due to the medical condition (e.g., 244.9 [E03.9] hypothyroidism; 293.83 [F06.31] depressive disorder due to hypothyroidism, with depressive features).

Diagnostic Features

The essential feature of depressive disorder due to another medical condition is a prominent and persistent period of depressed mood or markedly diminished interest or pleasure in all, or almost all, activities that predominates in the clinical picture (Criterion A) and that is thought to be related to the direct physiological effects of another medical condition (Criterion B). In determining whether the mood disturbance is due to a general medical condition, the clinician must first establish the presence of a general medical condition. Further, the clinician must establish that the mood disturbance is etiologically related to the general medical condition through a physiological mechanism. A careful and comprehensive assessment of multiple factors is necessary to make this judgment. Although there are no infallible guidelines for determining whether the relationship between the mood disturbance and the general medical condition is etiological, several considerations provide some guidance in this area. One consideration is the presence of a temporal association between the onset, exacerbation, or remission of the general medical condition and that of the mood disturbance. A second consideration is the presence of features that are atypical of primary Mood Disorders (e.g., atypical age at onset or course or absence of family history). Evidence from the literature that suggests that there can be a direct association between the general medical condition in question and the development of mood symptoms can provide a useful context in the assessment of a particular situation.

Associated Features Supporting Diagnosis

Etiology (i.e., a causal relationship to another medical condition based on best clinical evidence) is the key variable in depressive disorder due to another medical condition. The listing of the medical conditions that are said to be able to induce major depression is never complete, and the clinician's best judgment is the essence of this diagnosis.

There are clear associations, as well as some neuroanatomical correlates, of depression with stroke, Huntington's disease, Parkinson's disease, and traumatic brain injury. Among the neuroendocrine conditions most closely associated with depression are Cushing's disease and hypothyroidism. There are numerous other conditions thought to be associated with depression, such as multiple sclerosis. However, the literature's support for a causal association is greater with some conditions, such as Parkinson's disease and Huntington's disease, than with others, for which the differential diagnosis may be adjustment disorder, with depressed mood.

Development and Course

Following stroke, the onset of depression appears to be very acute, occurring within 1 day or a few days of the cerebrovascular accident (CVA) in the largest case series. However, in some cases, onset of the depression is weeks to months following the CVA. In the largest series, the duration of the major depressive episode following stroke was 9–11 months on average. Similarly, in Huntington's disease the depressive state comes quite early in the course of the illness. With Parkinson's disease and Huntington's disease, it often precedes the major motor impairments and cognitive impairments associated with each condition. This is more prominently the case for Huntington's disease, in which depression is considered to be the first neuropsychiatric symptom. There is some observational evidence that depression is less common as the dementia of Huntington's disease progresses.

Risk and Prognostic Factors

The risk of acute onset of a major depressive disorder following a CVA (within 1 day to a week of the event) appears to be strongly correlated with lesion location, with greatest risk associated with left frontal strokes and least risk apparently associated with right frontal lesions in those individuals who present within days of the stroke. The association with frontal regions and laterality is not observed in depressive states that occur in the 2–6 months following stroke.

Gender-Related Diagnostic Issues

Gender differences pertain to those associated with the medical condition (e.g., systemic lupus erythematosus is more common in females; stroke is somewhat more common in middle-age males compared with females).

Diagnostic Markers

Diagnostic markers pertain to those associated with the medical condition (e.g., steroid levels in blood or urine to help corroborate the diagnosis of Cushing's disease, which can be associated with manic or depressive syndromes).

Suicide Risk

There are no epidemiological studies that provide evidence to differentiate the risk of suicide from a major depressive episode due to another medical condition compared with the risk from a major depressive episode in general. There are case reports of suicides in association with major depressive episodes associated with another medical condition. There is a clear association between serious medical illnesses and suicide, particularly shortly after onset or diagnosis of the illness. Thus, it would be prudent to assume that the risk of suicide for major depressive episodes associated with medical conditions is not less than that for other forms of major depressive episode, and might even be greater.

Functional Consequences of Depressive Disorder Due to Another Medical Condition

Functional consequences pertain to those associated with the medical condition. In general, it is believed, but not established, that a major depressive episode induced by Cushing's disease will not recur if the Cushing's disease is cured or arrested. However, it is also suggested, but not established, that mood syndromes, including depressive and manic/hypomanic ones, may be episodic (i.e., recurring) in some individuals with static brain injuries and other central nervous system diseases.

Differential Diagnosis

Depressive disorders not due to another medical condition.   Determination of whether a medical condition accompanying a depressive disorder is causing the disorder depends on a) the absence of an episode(s) of depressive episodes prior to the onset of the medical condition, b) the probability that the associated medical condition has a potential to promote or cause a depressive disorder, and c) a course of the depressive symptoms shortly after the onset or worsening of the medical condition, especially if the depressive symptoms remit near the time that the medical disorder is effectively treated or remits.

Medication-induced depressive disorder.   An important caveat is that some medical conditions are treated with medications (e.g., steroids or alpha-interferon) that can induce depressive or manic symptoms. In these cases, clinical judgment, based on all the evidence in hand, is the best way to try to separate the most likely and/or the most important of two etiological factors (i.e., association with the medical condition vs. a substance-induced syndrome).

Adjustment disorders.   It is important to differentiate a depressive episode from an adjustment disorder, as the onset of the medical condition is in itself a life stressor that could bring on either an adjustment disorder or an episode of major depression. The major differentiating elements are the pervasiveness the depressive picture and the number and quality of the depressive symptoms that the patient reports or demonstrates on the mental status examination. The differential diagnosis of the associated medical conditions is relevant but largely beyond the scope of the present manual.

Comorbidity

Conditions comorbid with depressive disorder due to another medical condition are those associated with the medical conditions of etiological relevance. It has been noted that delirium can occur before or along with depressive symptoms in individuals with a variety of medical conditions, such as Cushing's disease. The association of anxiety symptoms, usually generalized symptoms, is common in depressive disorders, regardless of cause.

Other Specified Depressive Disorder

311 (F32.89)

This category applies to presentations in which symptoms characteristic of a depressive disorder that cause clinically significant distress or impairment in social, occupational, or other important areas of functioning predominate but do not meet the full criteria for any of the disorders in the depressive disorders diagnostic class. The other specified depressive disorder category is used in situations in which the clinician chooses to communicate the specific reason that the presentation does not meet the criteria for any specific depressive disorder. This is done by recording "other specified depressive disorder" followed by the specific reason (e.g., "short-duration depressive episode").

Examples of presentations that can be specified using the "other specified" designation include the following:

1. **Recurrent brief depression:** Concurrent presence of depressed mood and at least four other symptoms of depression for 2–13 days at least once per month (not associated with the menstrual cycle) for at least 12 consecutive months in an individual whose presentation has never met criteria for any other depressive or bipolar disorder and does not currently meet active or residual criteria for any psychotic disorder.

2. **Short-duration depressive episode (4–13 days):** Depressed affect and at least four of the other eight symptoms of a major depressive episode associated with clinically significant distress or impairment that persists for more than 4 days, but less than 14 days, in an individual whose presentation has never met criteria for any other depressive or bipolar disorder, does not currently meet active or residual criteria for any psychotic disorder, and does not meet criteria for recurrent brief depression.

3. **Depressive episode with insufficient symptoms:** Depressed affect and at least one of the other eight symptoms of a major depressive episode associated with clinically

significant distress or impairment that persist for at least 2 weeks in an individual whose presentation has never met criteria for any other depressive or bipolar disorder, does not currently meet active or residual criteria for any psychotic disorder, and does not meet criteria for mixed anxiety and depressive disorder symptoms.

Unspecified Depressive Disorder

311 (F32.9)

This category applies to presentations in which symptoms characteristic of a depressive disorder that cause clinically significant distress or impairment in social, occupational, or other important areas of functioning predominate but do not meet the full criteria for any of the disorders in the depressive disorders diagnostic class. The unspecified depressive disorder category is used in situations in which the clinician chooses *not* to specify the reason that the criteria are not met for a specific depressive disorder, and includes presentations for which there is insufficient information to make a more specific diagnosis (e.g., in emergency room settings).

Specifiers for Depressive Disorders

Specify if:

With anxious distress: Anxious distress is defined as the presence of at least two of the following symptoms during the majority of days of a major depressive episode or persistent depressive disorder (dysthymia):

1. Feeling keyed up or tense.
2. Feeling unusually restless.
3. Difficulty concentrating because of worry.
4. Fear that something awful may happen.
5. Feeling that the individual might lose control of himself or herself.

Specify current severity:

Mild: Two symptoms.
Moderate: Three symptoms.
Moderate-severe: Four or five symptoms.
Severe: Four or five symptoms and with motor agitation.

Note: Anxious distress has been noted as a prominent feature of both bipolar and major depressive disorder in both primary care and specialty mental health settings. High levels of anxiety have been associated with higher suicide risk, longer duration of illness, and greater likelihood of treatment nonresponse. As a result, it is clinically useful to specify accurately the presence and severity levels of anxious distress for treatment planning and monitoring of response to treatment.

With mixed features:

A. At least three of the following manic/hypomanic symptoms are present during the majority of days of a major depressive episode:

   1. Elevated, expansive mood.
   2. Inflated self-esteem or grandiosity.
   3. More talkative than usual or pressure to keep talking.
   4. Flight of ideas or subjective experience that thoughts are racing.
   5. Increase in energy or goal-directed activity (either socially, at work or school, or sexually).

6. Increased or excessive involvement in activities that have a high potential for painful consequences (e.g., engaging in unrestrained buying sprees, sexual indiscretions, foolish business investments).

7. Decreased need for sleep (feeling rested despite sleeping less than usual; to be contrasted with insomnia).

B. Mixed symptoms are observable by others and represent a change from the person's usual behavior.

C. For individuals whose symptoms meet full criteria for either mania or hypomania, the diagnosis should be bipolar I or bipolar II disorder.

D. The mixed symptoms are not attributable to the physiological effects of a substance (e.g., a drug of abuse, a medication or other treatment).

Note: Mixed features associated with a major depressive episode have been found to be a significant risk factor for the development of bipolar I or bipolar II disorder. As a result, it is clinically useful to note the presence of this specifier for treatment planning and monitoring of response to treatment.

With melancholic features:

A. One of the following is present during the most severe period of the current episode:

1. Loss of pleasure in all, or almost all, activities.

2. Lack of reactivity to usually pleasurable stimuli (does not feel much better, even temporarily, when something good happens).

B. Three (or more) of the following:

1. A distinct quality of depressed mood characterized by profound despondency, despair, and/or moroseness or by so-called empty mood.

2. Depression that is regularly worse in the morning.

3. Early-morning awakening (i.e., at least 2 hours before usual awakening).

4. Marked psychomotor agitation or retardation.

5. Significant anorexia or weight loss.

6. Excessive or inappropriate guilt.

Note: The specifier "with melancholic features" is applied if these features are present at the most severe stage of the episode. There is a near-complete absence of the capacity for pleasure, not merely a diminution. A guideline for evaluating the lack of reactivity of mood is that even highly desired events are not associated with marked brightening of mood. Either mood does not brighten at all, or it brightens only partially (e.g., up to 20%–40% of normal for only minutes at a time). The "distinct quality" of mood that is characteristic of the "with melancholic features" specifier is experienced as qualitatively different from that during a nonmelancholic depressive episode. A depressed mood that is described as merely more severe, longer lasting, or present without a reason is not considered distinct in quality. Psychomotor changes are nearly always present and are observable by others.

Melancholic features exhibit only a modest tendency to repeat across episodes in the same individual. They are more frequent in inpatients, as opposed to outpatients; are less likely to occur in milder than in more severe major depressive episodes; and are more likely to occur in those with psychotic features.

With atypical features: This specifier can be applied when these features predominate during the majority of days of the current or most recent major depressive episode or persistent depressive disorder.

A. Mood reactivity (i.e., mood brightens in response to actual or potential positive events).

B. Two (or more) of the following:

1. Significant weight gain or increase in appetite.
2. Hypersomnia.
3. Leaden paralysis (i.e., heavy, leaden feelings in arms or legs).
4. A long-standing pattern of interpersonal rejection sensitivity (not limited to episodes of mood disturbance) that results in significant social or occupational impairment.

C. Criteria are not met for "with melancholic features" or "with catatonia" during the same episode.

Note: "Atypical depression" has historical significance (i.e., atypical in contradistinction to the more classical agitated, "endogenous" presentations of depression that were the norm when depression was rarely diagnosed in outpatients and almost never in adolescents or younger adults) and today does not connote an uncommon or unusual clinical presentation as the term might imply.

Mood reactivity is the capacity to be cheered up when presented with positive events (e.g., a visit from children, compliments from others). Mood may become euthymic (not sad) even for extended periods of time if the external circumstances remain favorable. Increased appetite may be manifested by an obvious increase in food intake or by weight gain. Hypersomnia may include either an extended period of nighttime sleep or daytime napping that totals at least 10 hours of sleep per day (or at least 2 hours more than when not depressed). Leaden paralysis is defined as feeling heavy, leaden, or weighted down, usually in the arms or legs. This sensation is generally present for at least an hour a day but often lasts for many hours at a time. Unlike the other atypical features, pathological sensitivity to perceived interpersonal rejection is a trait that has an early onset and persists throughout most of adult life. Rejection sensitivity occurs both when the person is and is not depressed, though it may be exacerbated during depressive periods.

With psychotic features: Delusions and/or hallucinations are present.

With mood-congruent psychotic features: The content of all delusions and hallucinations is consistent with the typical depressive themes of personal inadequacy, guilt, disease, death, nihilism, or deserved punishment.

With mood-incongruent psychotic features: The content of the delusions or hallucinations does not involve typical depressive themes of personal inadequacy, guilt, disease, death, nihilism, or deserved punishment, or the content is a mixture of mood-incongruent and mood-congruent themes.

With catatonia: The catatonia specifier can apply to an episode of depression if catatonic features are present during most of the episode. See criteria for catatonia associated with a mental disorder (for a description of catatonia, see the chapter "Schizophrenia Spectrum and Other Psychotic Disorders").

With peripartum onset: This specifier can be applied to the current or, if full criteria are not currently met for a major depressive episode, most recent episode of major depression if onset of mood symptoms occurs during pregnancy or in the 4 weeks following delivery.

Note: Mood episodes can have their onset either during pregnancy or postpartum. Although the estimates differ according to the period of follow-up after delivery, between 3% and 6% of women will experience the onset of a major depressive episode during pregnancy or in the weeks or months following delivery. Fifty percent of "postpartum" major depressive episodes actually begin prior to delivery. Thus, these episodes are referred to collectively as *peripartum* episodes. Women with peripartum major depressive episodes often have severe anxiety and even panic attacks. Prospective studies have demonstrated that mood and anxiety symptoms during pregnancy, as well as the "baby blues," increase the risk for a postpartum major depressive episode.

Peripartum-onset mood episodes can present either with or without psychotic features. Infanticide is most often associated with postpartum psychotic episodes that are characterized by command hallucinations to kill the infant or delusions that the infant is possessed, but psychotic symptoms can also occur in severe postpartum mood episodes without such specific delusions or hallucinations.

Postpartum mood (major depressive or manic) episodes with psychotic features appear to occur in from 1 in 500 to 1 in 1,000 deliveries and may be more common in primiparous women. The risk of postpartum episodes with psychotic features is particularly increased for women with prior postpartum mood episodes but is also elevated for those with a prior history of a depressive or bipolar disorder (especially bipolar I disorder) and those with a family history of bipolar disorders.

Once a woman has had a postpartum episode with psychotic features, the risk of recurrence with each subsequent delivery is between 30% and 50%. Postpartum episodes must be differentiated from delirium occurring in the postpartum period, which is distinguished by a fluctuating level of awareness or attention. The postpartum period is unique with respect to the degree of neuroendocrine alterations and psychosocial adjustments, the potential impact of breast-feeding on treatment planning, and the long-term implications of a history of postpartum mood disorder on subsequent family planning.

With seasonal pattern: This specifier applies to recurrent major depressive disorder.

A. There has been a regular temporal relationship between the onset of major depressive episodes in major depressive disorder and a particular time of the year (e.g., in the fall or winter).

Note: Do not include cases in which there is an obvious effect of seasonally related psychosocial stressors (e.g., regularly being unemployed every winter).

B. Full remissions (or a change from major depression to mania or hypomania) also occur at a characteristic time of the year (e.g., depression disappears in the spring).

C. In the last 2 years, two major depressive episodes have occurred that demonstrate the temporal seasonal relationships defined above and no nonseasonal major depressive episodes have occurred during that same period.

D. Seasonal major depressive episodes (as described above) substantially outnumber the nonseasonal major depressive episodes that may have occurred over the individual's lifetime.

Note: The specifier "with seasonal pattern" can be applied to the pattern of major depressive episodes in major depressive disorder, recurrent. The essential feature is the onset and remission of major depressive episodes at characteristic times of the year. In most cases, the episodes begin in fall or winter and remit in spring. Less commonly, there may be recurrent summer depressive episodes. This pattern of onset and remission of episodes must have occurred during at least a 2-year period, without any nonseasonal episodes occurring during this period. In addition, the seasonal depressive episodes must substantially outnumber any nonseasonal depressive episodes over the individual's lifetime.

This specifier does not apply to those situations in which the pattern is better explained by seasonally linked psychosocial stressors (e.g., seasonal unemployment or school schedule). Major depressive episodes that occur in a seasonal pattern are often characterized by loss of energy, hypersomnia, overeating, weight gain, and a craving for carbohydrates. It is unclear whether a seasonal pattern is more likely in recurrent major depressive disorder or in bipolar disorders. However, within the bipolar disorders group, a seasonal pattern appears to be more likely in bipolar II disorder than in bipolar I disorder. In some individuals, the onset of manic or hypomanic episodes may also be linked to a particular season.

The prevalence of winter-type seasonal pattern appears to vary with latitude, age, and sex. Prevalence increases with higher latitudes. Age is also a strong predictor of seasonality, with younger persons at higher risk for winter depressive episodes.

Specify if:

In partial remission: Symptoms of the immediately previous major depressive episode are present but full criteria are not met, or there is a period lasting less than 2 months without any significant symptoms of a major depressive episode following the end of such an episode.

In full remission: During the past 2 months, no significant signs or symptoms of the disturbance were present.

Specify current severity:

Severity is based on the number of criterion symptoms, the severity of those symptoms, and the degree of functional disability.

Mild: Few, if any, symptoms in excess of those required to make the diagnosis are present, the intensity of the symptoms is distressing but manageable, and the symptoms result in minor impairment in social or occupational functioning.

Moderate: The number of symptoms, intensity of symptoms, and/or functional impairment are between those specified for "mild" and "severe."

Severe: The number of symptoms is substantially in excess of that required to make the diagnosis, the intensity of the symptoms is seriously distressing and unmanageable, and the symptoms markedly interfere with social and occupational functioning.

Anxiety Disorders

Anxiety disorders include disorders that share features of excessive fear and anxiety and related behavioral disturbances. *Fear* is the emotional response to real or perceived imminent threat, whereas *anxiety* is anticipation of future threat. Obviously, these two states overlap, but they also differ, with fear more often associated with surges of autonomic arousal necessary for fight or flight, thoughts of immediate danger, and escape behaviors, and anxiety more often associated with muscle tension and vigilance in preparation for future danger and cautious or avoidant behaviors. Sometimes the level of fear or anxiety is reduced by pervasive avoidance behaviors. *Panic attacks* feature prominently within the anxiety disorders as a particular type of fear response. Panic attacks are not limited to anxiety disorders but rather can be seen in other mental disorders as well.

The anxiety disorders differ from one another in the types of objects or situations that induce fear, anxiety, or avoidance behavior, and the associated cognitive ideation. Thus, while the anxiety disorders tend to be highly comorbid with each other, they can be differentiated by close examination of the types of situations that are feared or avoided and the content of the associated thoughts or beliefs.

Anxiety disorders differ from developmentally normative fear or anxiety by being excessive or persisting beyond developmentally appropriate periods. They differ from transient fear or anxiety, often stress-induced, by being persistent (e.g., typically lasting 6 months or more), although the criterion for duration is intended as a general guide with allowance for some degree of flexibility and is sometimes of shorter duration in children (as in separation anxiety disorder and selective mutism). Since individuals with anxiety disorders typically overestimate the danger in situations they fear or avoid, the primary determination of whether the fear or anxiety is excessive or out of proportion is made by the clinician, taking cultural contextual factors into account. Many of the anxiety disorders develop in childhood and tend to persist if not treated. Most occur more frequently in females than in males (approximately 2:1 ratio). Each anxiety disorder is diagnosed only when the symptoms are not attributable to the physiological effects of a substance/medication or to another medical condition or are not better explained by another mental disorder.

The chapter is arranged developmentally, with disorders sequenced according to the typical age at onset. The individual with separation anxiety disorder is fearful or anxious about separation from attachment figures to a degree that is developmentally inappropriate. There is persistent fear or anxiety about harm coming to attachment figures and events that could lead to loss of or separation from attachment figures and reluctance to go away from attachment figures, as well as nightmares and physical symptoms of distress. Although the symptoms often develop in childhood, they can be expressed throughout adulthood as well.

Selective mutism is characterized by a consistent failure to speak in social situations in which there is an expectation to speak (e.g., school) even though the individual speaks in other situations. The failure to speak has significant consequences on achievement in academic or occupational settings or otherwise interferes with normal social communication.

Individuals with specific phobia are fearful or anxious about or avoidant of circumscribed objects or situations. A specific cognitive ideation is not featured in this disorder, as it is in other anxiety disorders. The fear, anxiety, or avoidance is almost always immediately induced by the phobic situation, to a degree that is persistent and out of proportion to the actual risk posed. There are various types of specific phobias: animal; natural environment; blood-injection-injury; situational; and other situations.

In social anxiety disorder (social phobia), the individual is fearful or anxious about or avoidant of social interactions and situations that involve the possibility of being scrutinized. These include social interactions such as meeting unfamiliar people, situations in which the individual may be observed eating or drinking, and situations in which the individual performs in front of others. The cognitive ideation is of being negatively evaluated by others, by being embarrassed, humiliated, or rejected, or offending others.

In panic disorder, the individual experiences recurrent unexpected panic attacks and is persistently concerned or worried about having more panic attacks or changes his or her behavior in maladaptive ways because of the panic attacks (e.g., avoidance of exercise or of unfamiliar locations). Panic attacks are abrupt surges of intense fear or intense discomfort that reach a peak within minutes, accompanied by physical and/or cognitive symptoms. Limited-symptom panic attacks include fewer than four symptoms. Panic attacks may be *expected*, such as in response to a typically feared object or situation, or *unexpected*, meaning that the panic attack occurs for no apparent reason. Panic attacks function as a marker and prognostic factor for severity of diagnosis, course, and comorbidity across an array of disorders, including, but not limited to, the anxiety disorders (e.g., substance use, depressive and psychotic disorders). Panic attack may therefore be used as a descriptive specifier for any anxiety disorder as well as other mental disorders.

Individuals with agoraphobia are fearful and anxious about two or more of the following situations: using public transportation; being in open spaces; being in enclosed places; standing in line or being in a crowd; or being outside of the home alone in other situations. The individual fears these situations because of thoughts that escape might be difficult or help might not be available in the event of developing panic-like symptoms or other incapacitating or embarrassing symptoms. These situations almost always induce fear or anxiety and are often avoided or require the presence of a companion.

The key features of generalized anxiety disorder are persistent and excessive anxiety and worry about various domains, including work and school performance, that the individual finds difficult to control. In addition, the individual experiences physical symptoms, including restlessness or feeling keyed up or on edge; being easily fatigued; difficulty concentrating or mind going blank; irritability; muscle tension; and sleep disturbance.

Substance/medication-induced anxiety disorder involves anxiety due to substance intoxication or withdrawal or to a medication treatment. In anxiety disorder due to another medical condition, anxiety symptoms are the physiological consequence of another medical condition.

Disorder-specific scales are available to better characterize the severity of each anxiety disorder and to capture change in severity over time. For ease of use, particularly for individuals with more than one anxiety disorder, these scales have been developed to have the same format (but different focus) across the anxiety disorders, with ratings of behavioral symptoms, cognitive ideation symptoms, and physical symptoms relevant to each disorder.

Separation Anxiety Disorder

Diagnostic Criteria	309.21 (F93.0)

A. Developmentally inappropriate and excessive fear or anxiety concerning separation from those to whom the individual is attached, as evidenced by at least three of the following:

   1. Recurrent excessive distress when anticipating or experiencing separation from home or from major attachment figures.

2. Persistent and excessive worry about losing major attachment figures or about possible harm to them, such as illness, injury, disasters, or death.
3. Persistent and excessive worry about experiencing an untoward event (e.g., getting lost, being kidnapped, having an accident, becoming ill) that causes separation from a major attachment figure.
4. Persistent reluctance or refusal to go out, away from home, to school, to work, or elsewhere because of fear of separation.
5. Persistent and excessive fear of or reluctance about being alone or without major attachment figures at home or in other settings.
6. Persistent reluctance or refusal to sleep away from home or to go to sleep without being near a major attachment figure.
7. Repeated nightmares involving the theme of separation.
8. Repeated complaints of physical symptoms (e.g., headaches, stomachaches, nausea, vomiting) when separation from major attachment figures occurs or is anticipated.

B. The fear, anxiety, or avoidance is persistent, lasting at least 4 weeks in children and adolescents and typically 6 months or more in adults.

C. The disturbance causes clinically significant distress or impairment in social, academic, occupational, or other important areas of functioning.

D. The disturbance is not better explained by another mental disorder, such as refusing to leave home because of excessive resistance to change in autism spectrum disorder; delusions or hallucinations concerning separation in psychotic disorders; refusal to go outside without a trusted companion in agoraphobia; worries about ill health or other harm befalling significant others in generalized anxiety disorder; or concerns about having an illness in illness anxiety disorder.

Diagnostic Features

The essential feature of separation anxiety disorder is excessive fear or anxiety concerning separation from home or attachment figures. The anxiety exceeds what may be expected given the person's developmental level (Criterion A). Individuals with separation anxiety disorder have symptoms that meet at least three of the following criteria: They experience recurrent excessive distress when separation from home or major attachment figures is anticipated or occurs (Criterion A1). They worry about the well-being or death of attachment figures, particularly when separated from them, and they need to know the whereabouts of their attachment figures and want to stay in touch with them (Criterion A2). They also worry about untoward events to themselves, such as getting lost, being kidnapped, or having an accident, that would keep them from ever being reunited with their major attachment figure (Criterion A3). Individuals with separation anxiety disorder are reluctant or refuse to go out by themselves because of separation fears (Criterion A4). They have persistent and excessive fear or reluctance about being alone or without major attachment figures at home or in other settings. Children with separation anxiety disorder may be unable to stay or go in a room by themselves and may display "clinging" behavior, staying close to or "shadowing" the parent around the house, or requiring someone to be with them when going to another room in the house (Criterion A5). They have persistent reluctance or refusal to go to sleep without being near a major attachment figure or to sleep away from home (Criterion A6). Children with this disorder often have difficulty at bedtime and may insist that someone stay with them until they fall asleep. During the night, they may make their way to their parents' bed (or that of a significant other, such as a sibling). Children may be reluctant or refuse to attend camp, to sleep at friends' homes, or to go on errands. Adults may be uncomfortable when traveling independently (e.g., sleeping in a hotel room). There may be repeated nightmares in which the content expresses the individual's separation anxiety (e.g., destruction of the family through fire, murder, or other catastrophe) (Criterion A7). Physical symptoms (e.g., headaches, abdominal complaints, nausea, vomiting) are common in children when separation from major attachment figures occurs or is anticipated (Criterion A8). Cardiovascular symptoms such as palpitations, dizziness, and feeling faint are rare in younger children but may occur in adolescents and adults.

The disturbance must last for a period of at least 4 weeks in children and adolescents younger than 18 years and is typically 6 months or longer in adults (Criterion B). However, the duration criterion for adults should be used as a general guide, with allowance for some degree of flexibility. The disturbance must cause clinically significant distress or impairment in social, academic, occupational, or other important areas of functioning (Criterion C).

Associated Features Supporting Diagnosis

When separated from major attachment figures, children with separation anxiety disorder may exhibit social withdrawal, apathy, sadness, or difficulty concentrating on work or play. Depending on their age, individuals may have fears of animals, monsters, the dark, muggers, burglars, kidnappers, car accidents, plane travel, and other situations that are perceived as presenting danger to the family or themselves. Some individuals become homesick and uncomfortable to the point of misery when away from home. Separation anxiety disorder in children may lead to school refusal, which in turn may lead to academic difficulties and social isolation. When extremely upset at the prospect of separation, children may show anger or occasionally aggression toward someone who is forcing separation. When alone, especially in the evening or the dark, young children may report unusual perceptual experiences (e.g., seeing people peering into their room, frightening creatures reaching for them, feeling eyes staring at them). Children with this disorder may be described as demanding, intrusive, and in need of constant attention, and, as adults, may appear dependent and overprotective. The individual's excessive demands often become a source of frustration for family members, leading to resentment and conflict in the family.

Prevalence

The 12-month prevalence of separation anxiety disorder among adults in the United States is 0.9%–1.9%. In children, 6- to 12-month prevalence is estimated to be approximately 4%. In adolescents in the United States, the 12-month prevalence is 1.6%. Separation anxiety disorder decreases in prevalence from childhood through adolescence and adulthood and is the most prevalent anxiety disorder in children younger than 12 years. In clinical samples of children, the disorder is equally common in males and females. In the community, the disorder is more frequent in females.

Development and Course

Periods of heightened separation anxiety from attachment figures are part of normal early development and may indicate the development of secure attachment relationships (e.g., around 1 year of age, when infants may suffer from stranger anxiety). Onset of separation anxiety disorder may be as early as preschool age and may occur at any time during childhood and more rarely in adolescence. Typically there are periods of exacerbation and remission. In some cases, both the anxiety about possible separation and the avoidance of situations involving separation from the home or nuclear family (e.g., going away to college, moving away from attachment figures) may persist through adulthood. However, the majority of children with separation anxiety disorder are free of impairing anxiety disorders over their lifetimes. Many adults with separation anxiety disorder do not recall a childhood onset of separation anxiety disorder, although they may recall symptoms.

The manifestations of separation anxiety disorder vary with age. Younger children are more reluctant to go to school or may avoid school altogether. Younger children may not express worries or specific fears of definite threats to parents, home, or themselves, and the anxiety is manifested only when separation is experienced. As children age, worries emerge; these are often worries about specific dangers (e.g., accidents, kidnapping, mugging, death) or vague concerns about not being reunited with attachment figures. In adults, separation anxiety disorder may limit their ability to cope with changes in circumstances (e.g., moving, getting married). Adults with the disorder are typically overconcerned about their offspring and spouses and experience marked discomfort when separated from them. They may also experience significant disruption in work or social experiences because of needing to continuously check on the whereabouts of a significant other.

Risk and Prognostic Factors

Environmental. Separation anxiety disorder often develops after life stress, especially a loss (e.g., the death of a relative or pet; an illness of the individual or a relative; a change of schools; parental divorce; a move to a new neighborhood; immigration; a disaster that involved periods of separation from attachment figures). In young adults, other examples of life stress include leaving the parental home, entering into a romantic relationship, and becoming a parent. Parental overprotection and intrusiveness may be associated with separation anxiety disorder.

Genetic and physiological. Separation anxiety disorder in children may be heritable. Heritability was estimated at 73% in a community sample of 6-year-old twins, with higher rates in girls. Children with separation anxiety disorder display particularly enhanced sensitivity to respiratory stimulation using CO_2-enriched air.

Culture-Related Diagnostic Issues

There are cultural variations in the degree to which it is considered desirable to tolerate separation, so that demands and opportunities for separation between parents and children are avoided in some cultures. For example, there is wide variation across countries and cultures with respect to the age at which it is expected that offspring should leave the parental home. It is important to differentiate separation anxiety disorder from the high value some cultures place on strong interdependence among family members.

Gender-Related Diagnostic Issues

Girls manifest greater reluctance to attend or avoidance of school than boys. Indirect expression of fear of separation may be more common in males than in females, for example, by limited independent activity, reluctance to be away from home alone, or distress when spouse or offspring do things independently or when contact with spouse or offspring is not possible.

Suicide Risk

Separation anxiety disorder in children may be associated with an increased risk for suicide. In a community sample, the presence of mood disorders, anxiety disorders, or substance use has been associated with suicidal ideation and attempts. However, this association is not specific to separation anxiety disorder and is found in several anxiety disorders.

Functional Consequences of Separation Anxiety Disorder

Individuals with separation anxiety disorder often limit independent activities away from home or attachment figures (e.g., in children, avoiding school, not going to camp, having difficulty sleeping alone; in adolescents, not going away to college; in adults, not leaving the parental home, not traveling, not working outside the home).

Differential Diagnosis

Generalized anxiety disorder.   Separation anxiety disorder is distinguished from generalized anxiety disorder in that the anxiety predominantly concerns separation from attachment figures, and if other worries occur, they do not predominate the clinical picture.

Panic disorder.   Threats of separation may lead to extreme anxiety and even a panic attack. In separation anxiety disorder, in contrast to panic disorder, the anxiety concerns the possibility of being away from attachment figures and worry about untoward events befalling them, rather than being incapacitated by an unexpected panic attack.

Agoraphobia.   Unlike individuals with agoraphobia, those with separation anxiety disorder are not anxious about being trapped or incapacitated in situations from which escape is perceived as difficult in the event of panic-like symptoms or other incapacitating symptoms.

Conduct disorder.   School avoidance (truancy) is common in conduct disorder, but anxiety about separation is not responsible for school absences, and the child or adolescent usually stays away from, rather than returns to, the home.

Social anxiety disorder.   School refusal may be due to social anxiety disorder (social phobia). In such instances, the school avoidance is due to fear of being judged negatively by others rather than to worries about being separated from the attachment figures.

Posttraumatic stress disorder.   Fear of separation from loved ones is common after traumatic events such as a disasters, particularly when periods of separation from loved ones were experienced during the traumatic event. In posttraumatic stress disorder (PTSD), the central symptoms concern intrusions about, and avoidance of, memories associated with the traumatic event itself, whereas in separation anxiety disorder, the worries and avoidance concern the well-being of attachment figures and separation from them.

Illness anxiety disorder.   Individuals with illness anxiety disorder worry about specific illnesses they may have, but the main concern is about the medical diagnosis itself, not about being separated from attachment figures.

Bereavement.   Intense yearning or longing for the deceased, intense sorrow and emotional pain, and preoccupation with the deceased or the circumstances of the death are expected responses occurring in bereavement, whereas fear of separation from other attachment figures is central in separation anxiety disorder.

Depressive and bipolar disorders.   These disorders may be associated with reluctance to leave home, but the main concern is not worry or fear of untoward events befalling attachment figures, but rather low motivation for engaging with the outside world. However, individuals with separation anxiety disorder may become depressed while being separated or in anticipation of separation.

Oppositional defiant disorder.   Children and adolescents with separation anxiety disorder may be oppositional in the context of being forced to separate from attachment figures. Oppositional defiant disorder should be considered only when there is persistent oppositional behavior unrelated to the anticipation or occurrence of separation from attachment figures.

Psychotic disorders.   Unlike the hallucinations in psychotic disorders, the unusual perceptual experiences that may occur in separation anxiety disorder are usually based on a misperception of an actual stimulus, occur only in certain situations (e.g., nighttime), and are reversed by the presence of an attachment figure.

Personality disorders.   Dependent personality disorder is characterized by an indiscriminate tendency to rely on others, whereas separation anxiety disorder involves concern about the proximity and safety of main attachment figures. Borderline personality disorder is characterized by fear of abandonment by loved ones, but problems in identity, self-direction, interpersonal functioning, and impulsivity are additionally central to that disorder, whereas they are not central to separation anxiety disorder.

Comorbidity

In children, separation anxiety disorder is highly comorbid with generalized anxiety disorder and specific phobia. In adults, common comorbidities include specific phobia, PTSD, panic disorder, generalized anxiety disorder, social anxiety disorder, agoraphobia, obsessive-compulsive disorder, and personality disorders. Depressive and bipolar disorders are also comorbid with separation anxiety disorder in adults.

Selective Mutism

Diagnostic Criteria   **313.23** (F94.0)

A. Consistent failure to speak in specific social situations in which there is an expectation for speaking (e.g., at school) despite speaking in other situations.

B. The disturbance interferes with educational or occupational achievement or with social communication.

C. The duration of the disturbance is at least 1 month (not limited to the first month of school).

D. The failure to speak is not attributable to a lack of knowledge of, or comfort with, the spoken language required in the social situation.

E. The disturbance is not better explained by a communication disorder (e.g., childhood-onset fluency disorder) and does not occur exclusively during the course of autism spectrum disorder, schizophrenia, or another psychotic disorder.

Diagnostic Features

When encountering other individuals in social interactions, children with selective mutism do not initiate speech or reciprocally respond when spoken to by others. Lack of speech occurs in social interactions with children or adults. Children with selective mutism will speak in their home in the presence of immediate family members but often not even in front of close friends or second-degree relatives, such as grandparents or cousins. The disturbance is often marked by high social anxiety. Children with selective mutism often refuse to speak at school, leading to academic or educational impairment, as teachers often find it difficult to assess skills such as reading. The lack of speech may interfere with social communication, although children with this disorder sometimes use nonspoken or nonverbal means (e.g., grunting, pointing, writing) to communicate and may be willing or eager to perform or engage in social encounters when speech is not required (e.g., nonverbal parts in school plays).

Associated Features Supporting Diagnosis

Associated features of selective mutism may include excessive shyness, fear of social embarrassment, social isolation and withdrawal, clinging, compulsive traits, negativism, temper tantrums, or mild oppositional behavior. Although children with this disorder generally have normal language skills, there may occasionally be an associated communication disorder, although no particular association with a specific communication disorder has been identified. Even when these disorders are present, anxiety is present as well. In clinical settings, children with selective mutism are almost always given an additional diagnosis of another anxiety disorder—most commonly, social anxiety disorder (social phobia).

Prevalence

Selective mutism is a relatively rare disorder and has not been included as a diagnostic category in epidemiological studies of prevalence of childhood disorders. Point prevalence using various clinic or school samples ranges between 0.03% and 1% depending on the setting (e.g., clinic vs. school vs. general population) and ages of the individuals in the sample. The prevalence of the disorder does not seem to vary by sex or race/ethnicity. The disorder is more likely to manifest in young children than in adolescents and adults.

Development and Course

The onset of selective mutism is usually before age 5 years, but the disturbance may not come to clinical attention until entry into school, where there is an increase in social interaction and performance tasks, such as reading aloud. The persistence of the disorder is variable. Although clinical reports suggest that many individuals "outgrow" selective mutism, the longitudinal course of the disorder is unknown. In some cases, particularly in individuals with social anxiety disorder, selective mutism may disappear, but symptoms of social anxiety disorder remain.

Risk and Prognostic Factors

Temperamental.   Temperamental risk factors for selective mutism are not well identified. Negative affectivity (neuroticism) or behavioral inhibition may play a role, as may parental history of shyness, social isolation, and social anxiety. Children with selective mutism may have subtle receptive language difficulties compared with their peers, although receptive language is still within the normal range.

Environmental.   Social inhibition on the part of parents may serve as a model for social reticence and selective mutism in children. Furthermore, parents of children with selective mutism have been described as overprotective or more controlling than parents of children with other anxiety disorders or no disorder.

Genetic and physiological factors.   Because of the significant overlap between selective mutism and social anxiety disorder, there may be shared genetic factors between these conditions.

Culture-Related Diagnostic Issues

Children in families who have immigrated to a country where a different language is spoken may refuse to speak the new language because of lack of knowledge of the language. If comprehension of the new language is adequate but refusal to speak persists, a diagnosis of selective mutism may be warranted.

Functional Consequences of Selective Mutism

Selective mutism may result in social impairment, as children may be too anxious to engage in reciprocal social interaction with other children. As children with selective mutism mature, they may face increasing social isolation. In school settings, these children may suffer academic impairment, because often they do not communicate with teachers regarding their academic or personal needs (e.g., not understanding a class assignment, not asking to use the restroom). Severe impairment in school and social functioning, including that resulting from teasing by peers, is common. In certain instances, selective mutism may serve as a compensatory strategy to decrease anxious arousal in social encounters.

Differential Diagnosis

Communication disorders.   Selective mutism should be distinguished from speech disturbances that are better explained by a communication disorder, such as language disorder, speech sound disorder (previously phonological disorder), childhood-onset fluency disorder (stuttering), or pragmatic (social) communication disorder. Unlike selective mutism, the speech disturbance in these conditions is not restricted to a specific social situation.

Neurodevelopmental disorders and schizophrenia and other psychotic disorders. Individuals with an autism spectrum disorder, schizophrenia or another psychotic disorder, or severe intellectual disability may have problems in social communication and be unable to speak appropriately in social situations. In contrast, selective mutism should be diagnosed only when a child has an established capacity to speak in some social situations (e.g., typically at home).

Social anxiety disorder (social phobia).   The social anxiety and social avoidance in social anxiety disorder may be associated with selective mutism. In such cases, both diagnoses may be given.

Comorbidity

The most common comorbid conditions are other anxiety disorders, most commonly social anxiety disorder, followed by separation anxiety disorder and specific phobia. Oppositional behaviors have been noted to occur in children with selective mutism, although oppositional behavior may be limited to situations requiring speech. Communication delays or disorders also may appear in some children with selective mutism.

Specific Phobia

Diagnostic Criteria

A. Marked fear or anxiety about a specific object or situation (e.g., flying, heights, animals, receiving an injection, seeing blood).

   Note: In children, the fear or anxiety may be expressed by crying, tantrums, freezing, or clinging.

B. The phobic object or situation almost always provokes immediate fear or anxiety.

C. The phobic object or situation is actively avoided or endured with intense fear or anxiety.

D. The fear or anxiety is out of proportion to the actual danger posed by the specific object or situation and to the sociocultural context.

E. The fear, anxiety, or avoidance is persistent, typically lasting for 6 months or more.

F. The fear, anxiety, or avoidance causes clinically significant distress or impairment in social, occupational, or other important areas of functioning.

G. The disturbance is not better explained by the symptoms of another mental disorder, including fear, anxiety, and avoidance of situations associated with panic-like symptoms or other incapacitating symptoms (as in agoraphobia); objects or situations related to obsessions (as in obsessive-compulsive disorder); reminders of traumatic events (as in posttraumatic stress disorder); separation from home or attachment figures (as in separation anxiety disorder); or social situations (as in social anxiety disorder).

Specify if:

Code based on the phobic stimulus:

300.29 (F40.218) Animal (e.g., spiders, insects, dogs).

300.29 (F40.228) Natural environment (e.g., heights, storms, water).

300.29 (F40.23x) Blood-injection-injury (e.g., needles, invasive medical procedures).

> **Coding note:** Select specific ICD-10-CM code as follows: **F40.230** fear of blood; **F40.231** fear of injections and transfusions; **F40.232** fear of other medical care; or **F40.233** fear of injury.

300.29 (F40.248) Situational (e.g., airplanes, elevators, enclosed places).

300.29 (F40.298) Other (e.g., situations that may lead to choking or vomiting; in children, e.g., loud sounds or costumed characters).

Coding note: When more than one phobic stimulus is present, code all ICD-10-CM codes that apply (e.g., for fear of snakes and flying, F40.218 specific phobia, animal, and F40.248 specific phobia, situational).

Specifiers

It is common for individuals to have multiple specific phobias. The average individual with specific phobia fears three objects or situations, and approximately 75% of individuals with specific phobia fear more than one situation or object. In such cases, multiple specific phobia diagnoses, each with its own diagnostic code reflecting the phobic stimulus, would need to be given. For example, if an individual fears thunderstorms and flying, then two diagnoses would be given: specific phobia, natural environment, and specific phobia, situational.

Diagnostic Features

A key feature of this disorder is that the fear or anxiety is circumscribed to the presence of a particular situation or object (Criterion A), which may be termed the *phobic stimulus*. The categories of feared situations or objects are provided as specifiers. Many individuals fear objects or situations from more than one category, or phobic stimulus. For the diagnosis of specific phobia, the response must differ from normal, transient fears that commonly occur in the population. To meet the criteria for a diagnosis, the fear or anxiety must be intense or severe (i.e., "marked") (Criterion A). The amount of fear experienced may vary with proximity to the feared object or situation and may occur in anticipation of or in the actual presence of the object or situation. Also, the fear or anxiety may take the form of a full or limited symptom panic attack (i.e., expected panic attack). Another characteristic of specific phobias is that fear or anxiety is evoked nearly every time the individual comes into contact with the phobic stimulus (Criterion B). Thus, an individual who becomes anxious only occasionally upon being confronted with the situation or object (e.g., becomes anxious when flying only on one out of every five airplane flights) would not be diagnosed with specific phobia. However, the degree of fear or anxiety expressed may vary (from anticipatory anxiety to a full panic attack) across different occasions of encountering the phobic object or situation because of various contextual factors such as the presence of others, duration of exposure, and other threatening elements such as turbulence on a flight for individuals who fear flying. Fear and anxiety are often expressed differently between children and adults. Also, the fear or anxiety occurs as soon as the phobic object or situation is encountered (i.e., immediately rather than being delayed).

The individual actively avoids the situation, or if he or she either is unable or decides not to avoid it, the situation or object evokes intense fear or anxiety (Criterion C). *Active avoidance* means the individual intentionally behaves in ways that are designed to prevent or minimize contact with phobic objects or situations (e.g., takes tunnels instead of bridges on daily commute to work for fear of heights; avoids entering a dark room for fear of spiders; avoids accepting a job in a locale where a phobic stimulus is more common). Avoidance behaviors are often obvious (e.g., an individual who fears blood refusing to go to the doctor) but are sometimes less obvious (e.g., an individual who fears snakes refusing to look at pictures that resemble the form or shape of snakes). Many individuals with specific phobias have suffered over many years and have changed their living circumstances in ways designed to avoid the phobic object or situation as much as possible (e.g., an individual diagnosed with specific phobia, animal, who moves to reside in an area devoid of the particular feared animal). Therefore, they no longer experience fear or anxiety in their daily life. In such instances, avoidance behaviors or ongoing refusal to engage in activities that would involve exposure to the phobic object or situation (e.g., repeated refusal to accept offers for work-related travel because of fear of flying) may be helpful in confirming the diagnosis in the absence of overt anxiety or panic.

The fear or anxiety is out of proportion to the actual danger that the object or situation poses, or more intense than is deemed necessary (Criterion D). Although individuals with specific phobia often recognize their reactions as disproportionate, they tend to overestimate the danger in their feared situations, and thus the judgment of being out of proportion is made by the clinician. The individual's sociocultural context should also be taken into account. For example, fears of the dark may be reasonable in a context of ongoing violence, and fear of insects may be more disproportionate in settings where insects are consumed in the diet. The fear, anxiety, or avoidance is persistent, typically lasting for 6 months or more (Criterion E), which helps distinguish the disorder from transient fears that are common in the population, particularly among children. However, the duration criterion should be used as a general guide, with allowance for some degree of flexibility. The specific phobia must cause clinically significant distress or impairment in social, occupational, or other important areas of functioning in order for the disorder to be diagnosed (Criterion F).

Associated Features Supporting Diagnosis

Individuals with specific phobia typically experience an increase in physiological arousal in anticipation of or during exposure to a phobic object or situation. However, the physiological response to the feared situation or object varies. Whereas individuals with situational, natural environment, and animal specific phobias are likely to show sympathetic nervous system arousal, individuals with blood-injection-injury specific phobia often demonstrate a vasovagal fainting or near-fainting response that is marked by initial brief acceleration of heart rate and elevation of blood pressure followed by a deceleration of heart rate and a drop in blood pressure. Current neural systems models for specific phobia emphasize the amygdala and related structures, much as in other anxiety disorders.

Prevalence

In the United States, the 12-month community prevalence estimate for specific phobia is approximately 7%–9%. Prevalence rates in European countries are largely similar to those in the United States (e.g., about 6%), but rates are generally lower in Asian, African, and Latin American countries (2%–4%). Prevalence rates are approximately 5% in children and are approximately 16% in 13- to 17-year-olds. Prevalence rates are lower in older individuals (about 3%–5%), possibly reflecting diminishing severity to subclinical levels. Females are more frequently affected than males, at a rate of approximately 2:1, although rates vary across different phobic stimuli. That is, animal, natural environment, and situational specific phobias are predominantly experienced by females, whereas blood-injection-injury phobia is experienced nearly equally by both genders.

Development and Course

Specific phobia sometimes develops following a traumatic event (e.g., being attacked by an animal or stuck in an elevator), observation of others going through a traumatic event (e.g., watching someone drown), an unexpected panic attack in the to be feared situation (e.g., an unexpected panic attack while on the subway), or informational transmission (e.g., extensive media coverage of a plane crash). However, many individuals with specific phobia are unable to recall the specific reason for the onset of their phobias. Specific phobia usually develops in early childhood, with the majority of cases developing prior to age 10 years. The median age at onset is between 7 and 11 years, with the mean at about 10 years. Situational specific phobias tend to have a later age at onset than natural environment, animal, or blood-injection-injury specific phobias. Specific phobias that develop in childhood and adolescence are likely to wax and wane during that period. However, phobias that do persist into adulthood are unlikely to remit for the majority of individuals.

When specific phobia is being diagnosed in children, two issues should be considered. First, young children may express their fear and anxiety by crying, tantrums, freezing, or clinging. Second, young children typically are not able to understand the concept of avoidance. Therefore, the clinician should assemble additional information from parents, teachers, or others who know the child well. Excessive fears are quite common in young children but are usually transitory and only mildly impairing and thus considered developmentally appropriate. In such cases a diagnosis of specific phobia would not be made. When the diagnosis of specific phobia is being considered in a child, it is important to assess the degree of impairment and the duration of the fear, anxiety, or avoidance, and whether it is typical for the child's particular developmental stage.

Although the prevalence of specific phobia is lower in older populations, it remains one of the more commonly experienced disorders in late life. Several issues should be considered when diagnosing specific phobia in older populations. First, older individuals may be more likely to endorse natural environment specific phobias, as well as phobias of falling. Second, specific phobia (like all anxiety disorders) tends to co-occur with medical concerns in older individuals, including coronary heart disease and chronic obstructive pulmonary disease. Third, older individuals may be more likely to attribute the symptoms of anxiety to medical conditions. Fourth, older individuals may be more likely to manifest anxiety in an atypical manner (e.g., involving symptoms of both anxiety and depression) and thus be more likely to warrant a diagnosis of unspecified anxiety disorder. Additionally, the presence of specific phobia in older adults is associated with decreased quality of life and may serve as a risk factor for major neurocognitive disorder.

Although most specific phobias develop in childhood and adolescence, it is possible for a specific phobia to develop at any age, often as the result of experiences that are traumatic. For example, phobias of choking almost always follow a near-choking event at any age.

Risk and Prognostic Factors

Temperamental.   Temperamental risk factors for specific phobia, such as negative affectivity (neuroticism) or behavioral inhibition, are risk factors for other anxiety disorders as well.

Environmental.   Environmental risk factors for specific phobias, such as parental overprotectiveness, parental loss and separation, and physical and sexual abuse, tend to predict other anxiety disorders as well. As noted earlier, negative or traumatic encounters with the feared object or situation sometimes (but not always) precede the development of specific phobia.

Genetic and physiological.   There may be a genetic susceptibility to a certain category of specific phobia (e.g., an individual with a first-degree relative with a specific phobia of animals is significantly more likely to have the same specific phobia than any other category of phobia). Individuals with blood-injection-injury phobia show a unique propensity to vasovagal syncope (fainting) in the presence of the phobic stimulus.

Culture-Related Diagnostic Issues

In the United States, Asians and Latinos report significantly lower rates of specific phobia than non-Latino whites, African Americans, and Native Americans. In addition to having lower prevalence rates of specific phobia, some countries outside of the United States, particularly Asian and African countries, show differing phobia content, age at onset, and gender ratios.

Suicide Risk

Individuals with specific phobia are up to 60% more likely to make a suicide attempt than are individuals without the diagnosis. However, it is likely that these elevated rates are primarily due to comorbidity with personality disorders and other anxiety disorders.

Functional Consequences of Specific Phobia

Individuals with specific phobia show similar patterns of impairment in psychosocial functioning and decreased quality of life as individuals with other anxiety disorders and alcohol and substance use disorders, including impairments in occupational and interpersonal functioning. In older adults, impairment may be seen in caregiving duties and volunteer activities. Also, fear of falling in older adults can lead to reduced mobility and reduced physical and social functioning, and may lead to receiving formal or informal home support. The distress and impairment caused by specific phobias tend to increase with the number of feared objects and situations. Thus, an individual who fears four objects or situations is likely to have more impairment in his or her occupational and social roles and a lower quality of life than an individual who fears only one object or situation. Individuals with blood-injection-injury specific phobia are often reluctant to obtain medical care even when a medical concern is present. Additionally, fear of vomiting and choking may substantially reduce dietary intake.

Differential Diagnosis

Agoraphobia. Situational specific phobia may resemble agoraphobia in its clinical presentation, given the overlap in feared situations (e.g., flying, enclosed places, elevators). If an individual fears only one of the agoraphobia situations, then specific phobia, situational, may be diagnosed. If two or more agoraphobic situations are feared, a diagnosis of agoraphobia is likely warranted. For example, an individual who fears airplanes and elevators (which overlap with the "public transportation" agoraphobic situation) but does not fear other agoraphobic situations would be diagnosed with specific phobia, situational, whereas an individual who fears airplanes, elevators, and crowds (which overlap with two agoraphobic situations, "using public transportation" and "standing in line and or being in a crowd") would be diagnosed with agoraphobia. Criterion B of agoraphobia (the situations are feared or avoided "because of thoughts that escape might be difficult or help might not be available in the event of developing panic-like symptoms or other incapacitating or embarrassing symptoms") can also be useful in differentiating agoraphobia from specific phobia. If the situations are feared for other reasons, such as fear of being harmed directly by the object or situations (e.g., fear of the plane crashing, fear of the animal biting), a specific phobia diagnosis may be more appropriate.

Social anxiety disorder. If the situations are feared because of negative evaluation, social anxiety disorder should be diagnosed instead of specific phobia.

Separation anxiety disorder. If the situations are feared because of separation from a primary caregiver or attachment figure, separation anxiety disorder should be diagnosed instead of specific phobia.

Panic disorder. Individuals with specific phobia may experience panic attacks when confronted with their feared situation or object. A diagnosis of specific phobia would be given if the panic attacks only occurred in response to the specific object or situation, whereas a diagnosis of panic disorder would be given if the individual also experienced panic attacks that were unexpected (i.e., not in response to the specific phobia object or situation).

Obsessive-compulsive disorder. If an individual's primary fear or anxiety is of an object or situation as a result of obsessions (e.g., fear of blood due to obsessive thoughts about contamination from blood-borne pathogens [i.e., HIV]; fear of driving due to obsessive images of harming others), and if other diagnostic criteria for obsessive-compulsive disorder are met, then obsessive-compulsive disorder should be diagnosed.

Trauma- and stressor-related disorders. If the phobia develops following a traumatic event, posttraumatic stress disorder (PTSD) should be considered as a diagnosis. However, traumatic events can precede the onset of PTSD and specific phobia. In this case, a diagnosis of specific phobia would be assigned only if all of the criteria for PTSD are not met.

Eating disorders. A diagnosis of specific phobia is not given if the avoidance behavior is exclusively limited to avoidance of food and food-related cues, in which case a diagnosis of anorexia nervosa or bulimia nervosa should be considered.

Schizophrenia spectrum and other psychotic disorders. When the fear and avoidance are due to delusional thinking (as in schizophrenia or other schizophrenia spectrum and other psychotic disorders), a diagnosis of specific phobia is not warranted.

Comorbidity

Specific phobia is rarely seen in medical-clinical settings in the absence of other psychopathology and is more frequently seen in nonmedical mental health settings. Specific phobia is frequently associated with a range of other disorders, especially depression in older adults. Because of early onset, specific phobia is typically the temporally primary disorder. Individuals with specific phobia are at increased risk for the development of other disorders, including other anxiety disorders, depressive and bipolar disorders, substance-related disorders, somatic symptom and related disorders, and personality disorders (particularly dependent personality disorder).

Social Anxiety Disorder (Social Phobia)

Diagnostic Criteria   **300.23** (F40.10)

A. Marked fear or anxiety about one or more social situations in which the individual is exposed to possible scrutiny by others. Examples include social interactions (e.g., having a conversation, meeting unfamiliar people), being observed (e.g., eating or drinking), and performing in front of others (e.g., giving a speech).

   Note: In children, the anxiety must occur in peer settings and not just during interactions with adults.

B. The individual fears that he or she will act in a way or show anxiety symptoms that will be negatively evaluated (i.e., will be humiliating or embarrassing; will lead to rejection or offend others).

C. The social situations almost always provoke fear or anxiety.

   Note: In children, the fear or anxiety may be expressed by crying, tantrums, freezing, clinging, shrinking, or failing to speak in social situations.

D. The social situations are avoided or endured with intense fear or anxiety.

E. The fear or anxiety is out of proportion to the actual threat posed by the social situation and to the sociocultural context.

F. The fear, anxiety, or avoidance is persistent, typically lasting for 6 months or more.

G. The fear, anxiety, or avoidance causes clinically significant distress or impairment in social, occupational, or other important areas of functioning.

H. The fear, anxiety, or avoidance is not attributable to the physiological effects of a substance (e.g., a drug of abuse, a medication) or another medical condition.

I. The fear, anxiety, or avoidance is not better explained by the symptoms of another mental disorder, such as panic disorder, body dysmorphic disorder, or autism spectrum disorder.

J. If another medical condition (e.g., Parkinson's disease, obesity, disfigurement from burns or injury) is present, the fear, anxiety, or avoidance is clearly unrelated or is excessive.

Specify if:
Performance only: If the fear is restricted to speaking or performing in public.

Specifiers

Individuals with the performance only type of social anxiety disorder have performance fears that are typically most impairing in their professional lives (e.g., musicians, dancers, performers, athletes) or in roles that require regular public speaking. Performance fears may also manifest in work, school, or academic settings in which regular public presentations are required. Individuals with performance only social anxiety disorder do not fear or avoid nonperformance social situations.

Diagnostic Features

The essential feature of social anxiety disorder is a marked, or intense, fear or anxiety of social situations in which the individual may be scrutinized by others. In children the fear or anxiety must occur in peer settings and not just during interactions with adults (Criterion A). When exposed to such social situations, the individual fears that he or she will be negatively evaluated. The individual is concerned that he or she will be judged as anxious, weak, crazy, stupid, boring, intimidating, dirty, or unlikable. The individual fears that he or she will act or appear in a certain way or show anxiety symptoms, such as blushing, trembling, sweating, stumbling over one's words, or staring, that will be negatively evaluated by others (Criterion B). Some individuals fear offending others or being rejected as a result. Fear of offending others—for example, by a gaze or by showing anxiety symptoms—may be the predominant fear in individuals from cultures with strong collectivistic orientations. An individual with fear of trembling of the hands may avoid drinking, eating, writing, or pointing in public; an individual with fear of sweating may avoid shaking hands or eating spicy foods; and an individual with fear of blushing may avoid public performance, bright lights, or discussion about intimate topics. Some individuals fear and avoid urinating in public restrooms when other individuals are present (i.e., paruresis, or "shy bladder syndrome").

The social situations almost always provoke fear or anxiety (Criterion C). Thus, an individual who becomes anxious only occasionally in the social situation(s) would not be diagnosed with social anxiety disorder. However, the degree and type of fear and anxiety may vary (e.g., anticipatory anxiety, a panic attack) across different occasions. The anticipatory anxiety may occur sometimes far in advance of upcoming situations (e.g., worrying every day for weeks before attending a social event, repeating a speech for days in advance). In children, the fear or anxiety may be expressed by crying, tantrums, freezing, clinging, or shrinking in social situations. The individual will often avoid the feared social situations. Alternatively, the situations are endured with intense fear or anxiety (Criterion D). Avoidance can be extensive (e.g., not going to parties, refusing school) or subtle (e.g., overpreparing the text of a speech, diverting attention to others, limiting eye contact).

The fear or anxiety is judged to be out of proportion to the actual risk of being negatively evaluated or to the consequences of such negative evaluation (Criterion E). Sometimes, the anxiety may not be judged to be excessive, because it is related to an actual danger (e.g., being bullied or tormented by others). However, individuals with social anxiety disorder often overestimate the negative consequences of social situations, and thus the judgment of being out of proportion is made by the clinician. The individual's sociocultural context needs to be taken into account when this judgment is being made. For example, in certain cultures, behavior that might otherwise appear socially anxious may be considered appropriate in social situations (e.g., might be seen as a sign of respect).

The duration of the disturbance is typically at least 6 months (Criterion F). This duration threshold helps distinguish the disorder from transient social fears that are common, particularly among children and in the community. However, the duration criterion should be used as a general guide, with allowance for some degree of flexibility. The fear, anxiety, and avoidance must interfere significantly with the individual's normal routine, occupational or academic functioning, or social activities or relationships, or must cause clinically significant distress or impairment in social, occupational, or other important areas of functioning (Criterion G). For example, an individual who is afraid to speak in public would not receive a diagnosis of social anxiety disorder if this activity is not routinely encountered on the job or in classroom work, and if the individual is not significantly distressed about it. However, if the individual avoids, or is passed over for, the job or education he or she really wants because of social anxiety symptoms, Criterion G is met.

Associated Features Supporting Diagnosis

Individuals with social anxiety disorder may be inadequately assertive or excessively submissive or, less commonly, highly controlling of the conversation. They may show overly rigid body posture or inadequate eye contact, or speak with an overly soft voice. These individuals may be shy or withdrawn, and they may be less open in conversations and disclose little about themselves. They may seek employment in jobs that do not require social contact, although this is not the case for individuals with social anxiety disorder, performance only. They may live at home longer. Men may be delayed in marrying and having a family, whereas women who would want to work outside the home may live a life as homemaker and mother. Self-medication with substances is common (e.g., drinking before going to a party). Social anxiety among older adults may also include exacerbation of symptoms of medical illnesses, such as increased tremor or tachycardia. Blushing is a hallmark physical response of social anxiety disorder.

Prevalence

The 12-month prevalence estimate of social anxiety disorder for the United States is approximately 7%. Lower 12-month prevalence estimates are seen in much of the world using the same diagnostic instrument, clustering around 0.5%–2.0%; median prevalence in Europe is 2.3%. The 12-month prevalence rates in children and adolescents are comparable to those in adults. Prevalence rates decrease with age. The 12-month prevalence for older adults ranges from 2% to 5%. In general, higher rates of social anxiety disorder are found in females than in males in the general population (with odds ratios ranging from 1.5 to 2.2), and the gender difference in prevalence is more pronounced in adolescents and young adults. Gender rates are equivalent or slightly higher for males in clinical samples, and it is assumed that gender roles and social expectations play a significant role in explaining the heightened help-seeking behavior in male patients. Prevalence in the United States is higher in American Indians and lower in persons of Asian, Latino, African American, and Afro-Caribbean descent compared with non-Hispanic whites.

Development and Course

Median age at onset of social anxiety disorder in the United States is 13 years, and 75% of individuals have an age at onset between 8 and 15 years. The disorder sometimes emerges out of a childhood history of social inhibition or shyness in U.S. and European studies. Onset can also occur in early childhood. Onset of social anxiety disorder may follow a stressful or humiliating experience (e.g., being bullied, vomiting during a public speech), or it may be insidious, developing slowly. First onset in adulthood is relatively rare and is more likely to occur after a stressful or humiliating event or after life changes that require new social roles (e.g., marrying someone from a different social class, receiving a job promotion). Social anxiety disorder may diminish after an individual with fear of dating marries and may reemerge after divorce. Among individuals presenting to clinical care, the disorder tends to be particularly persistent.

Adolescents endorse a broader pattern of fear and avoidance, including of dating, compared with younger children. Older adults express social anxiety at lower levels but across a broader range of situations, whereas younger adults express higher levels of social anxiety for specific situations. In older adults, social anxiety may concern disability due to declining sensory functioning (hearing, vision) or embarrassment about one's appearance (e.g., tremor as a symptom of Parkinson's disease) or functioning due to medical conditions, incontinence, or cognitive impairment (e.g., forgetting people's names). In the community approximately 30% of individuals with social anxiety disorder experience remission of symptoms within 1 year, and about 50% experience remission within a few years. For approximately 60% of individuals without a specific treatment for social anxiety disorder, the course takes several years or longer.

Detection of social anxiety disorder in older adults may be challenging because of several factors, including a focus on somatic symptoms, comorbid medical illness, limited insight, changes to social environment or roles that may obscure impairment in social functioning, or reticence about describing psychological distress.

Risk and Prognostic Factors

Temperamental. Underlying traits that predispose individuals to social anxiety disorder include behavioral inhibition and fear of negative evaluation.

Environmental. There is no causative role of increased rates of childhood maltreatment or other early-onset psychosocial adversity in the development of social anxiety disorder. However, childhood maltreatment and adversity are risk factors for social anxiety disorder.

Genetic and physiological. Traits predisposing individuals to social anxiety disorder, such as behavioral inhibition, are strongly genetically influenced. The genetic influence is subject to gene-environment interaction; that is, children with high behavioral inhibition are more susceptible to environmental influences, such as socially anxious modeling by parents. Also, social anxiety disorder is heritable (but performance-only anxiety less so). First-degree relatives have a two to six times greater chance of having social anxiety disorder, and liability to the disorder involves the interplay of disorder-specific (e.g., fear of negative evaluation) and nonspecific (e.g., neuroticism) genetic factors.

Culture-Related Diagnostic Issues

The syndrome of *taijin kyofusho* (e.g., in Japan and Korea) is often characterized by social-evaluative concerns, fulfilling criteria for social anxiety disorder, that are associated with the fear that the individual makes *other* people uncomfortable (e.g., "My gaze upsets people so they look away and avoid me"), a fear that is at times experienced with delusional intensity. This symptom may also be found in non-Asian settings. Other presentations of *taijin kyofusho* may fulfill criteria for body dysmorphic disorder or delusional disorder.

Immigrant status is associated with significantly lower rates of social anxiety disorder in both Latino and non-Latino white groups. Prevalence rates of social anxiety disorder may not be in line with self-reported social anxiety levels in the same culture—that is, societies with strong collectivistic orientations may report high levels of social anxiety but low prevalence of social anxiety disorder.

Gender-Related Diagnostic Issues

Females with social anxiety disorder report a greater number of social fears and comorbid depressive, bipolar, and anxiety disorders, whereas males are more likely to fear dating, have oppositional defiant disorder or conduct disorder, and use alcohol and illicit drugs to relieve symptoms of the disorder. Paruresis is more common in males.

Functional Consequences of Social Anxiety Disorder

Social anxiety disorder is associated with elevated rates of school dropout and with decreased well-being, employment, workplace productivity, socioeconomic status, and quality of life. Social anxiety disorder is also associated with being single, unmarried, or divorced and with not having children, particularly among men. In older adults, there may be impairment in caregiving duties and volunteer activities. Social anxiety disorder also impedes leisure activities. Despite the extent of distress and social impairment associated with social anxiety disorder, only about half of individuals with the disorder in Western societies ever seek treatment, and they tend to do so only after 15–20 years of experiencing symptoms. Not being employed is a strong predictor for the persistence of social anxiety disorder.

Differential Diagnosis

Normative shyness.   Shyness (i.e., social reticence) is a common personality trait and is not by itself pathological. In some societies, shyness is even evaluated positively. However, when there is a significant adverse impact on social, occupational, and other important areas of functioning, a diagnosis of social anxiety disorder should be considered, and when full diagnostic criteria for social anxiety disorder are met, the disorder should be diagnosed. Only a minority (12%) of self-identified shy individuals in the United States have symptoms that meet diagnostic criteria for social anxiety disorder.

Agoraphobia.   Individuals with agoraphobia may fear and avoid social situations (e.g., going to a movie) because escape might be difficult or help might not be available in the event of incapacitation or panic-like symptoms, whereas individuals with social anxiety disorder are most fearful of scrutiny by others. Moreover, individuals with social anxiety disorder are likely to be calm when left entirely alone, which is often not the case in agoraphobia.

Panic disorder.   Individuals with social anxiety disorder may have panic attacks, but the concern is about fear of negative evaluation, whereas in panic disorder the concern is about the panic attacks themselves.

Generalized anxiety disorder.   Social worries are common in generalized anxiety disorder, but the focus is more on the nature of ongoing relationships rather than on fear of negative evaluation. Individuals with generalized anxiety disorder, particularly children, may have excessive worries about the quality of their social performance, but these worries also pertain to nonsocial performance and when the individual is not being evaluated by others. In social anxiety disorder, the worries focus on social performance and others' evaluation.

Separation anxiety disorder.   Individuals with separation anxiety disorder may avoid social settings (including school refusal) because of concerns about being separated from attachment figures or, in children, about requiring the presence of a parent when it is not developmentally appropriate. Individuals with separation anxiety disorder are usually comfortable in social settings when their attachment figure is present or when they are at home, whereas those with social anxiety disorder may be uncomfortable when social situations occur at home or in the presence of attachment figures.

Specific phobias.   Individuals with specific phobias may fear embarrassment or humiliation (e.g., embarrassment about fainting when they have their blood drawn), but they do not generally fear negative evaluation in other social situations.

Selective mutism.   Individuals with selective mutism may fail to speak because of fear of negative evaluation, but they do not fear negative evaluation in social situations where no speaking is required (e.g., nonverbal play).

Major depressive disorder.   Individuals with major depressive disorder may be concerned about being negatively evaluated by others because they feel they are bad or not worthy of being liked. In contrast, individuals with social anxiety disorder are worried about being negatively evaluated because of certain social behaviors or physical symptoms.

Body dysmorphic disorder.   Individuals with body dysmorphic disorder are preoccupied with one or more perceived defects or flaws in their physical appearance that are not observable or appear slight to others; this preoccupation often causes social anxiety and avoidance. If their social fears and avoidance are caused only by their beliefs about their appearance, a separate diagnosis of social anxiety disorder is not warranted.

Delusional disorder.   Individuals with delusional disorder may have nonbizarre delusions and/or hallucinations related to the delusional theme that focus on being rejected by or offending others. Although extent of insight into beliefs about social situations may vary, many individuals with social anxiety disorder have good insight that their beliefs are out of proportion to the actual threat posed by the social situation.

Autism spectrum disorder.   Social anxiety and social communication deficits are hallmarks of autism spectrum disorder. Individuals with social anxiety disorder typically have adequate age-appropriate social relationships and social communication capacity, although they may appear to have impairment in these areas when first interacting with unfamiliar peers or adults.

Personality disorders.   Given its frequent onset in childhood and its persistence into and through adulthood, social anxiety disorder may resemble a personality disorder. The most apparent overlap is with avoidant personality disorder. Individuals with avoidant personality disorder have a broader avoidance pattern than those with social anxiety disorder. Nonetheless, social anxiety disorder is typically more comorbid with avoidant personality disorder than with other personality disorders, and avoidant personality disorder is more comorbid with social anxiety disorder than with other anxiety disorders.

Other mental disorders.   Social fears and discomfort can occur as part of schizophrenia, but other evidence for psychotic symptoms is usually present. In individuals with an eating disorder, it is important to determine that fear of negative evaluation about eating disorder symptoms or behaviors (e.g., purging and vomiting) is not the sole source of social anxiety before applying a diagnosis of social anxiety disorder. Similarly, obsessive-compulsive disorder may be associated with social anxiety, but the additional diagnosis of social anxiety disorder is used only when social fears and avoidance are independent of the foci of the obsessions and compulsions.

Other medical conditions.   Medical conditions may produce symptoms that may be embarrassing (e.g., trembling in Parkinson's disease). When the fear of negative evaluation due to other medical conditions is excessive, a diagnosis of social anxiety disorder should be considered.

Oppositional defiant disorder.   Refusal to speak due to opposition to authority figures should be differentiated from failure to speak due to fear of negative evaluation.

Comorbidity

Social anxiety disorder is often comorbid with other anxiety disorders, major depressive disorder, and substance use disorders, and the onset of social anxiety disorder generally precedes that of the other disorders, except for specific phobia and separation anxiety disorder. Chronic social isolation in the course of a social anxiety disorder may result in major depressive disorder. Comorbidity with depression is high also in older adults. Substances may be used as self-medication for social fears, but the symptoms of substance intoxication or withdrawal, such as trembling, may also be a source of (further) social fear. Social anxiety disorder is frequently comorbid with bipolar disorder or body dysmorphic disorder; for example, an individual has body dysmorphic disorder concerning a preoccupation with a slight irregularity of her nose, as well as social anxiety disorder because of a severe fear of sounding unintelligent. The more generalized form of social anxiety disorder, but not social anxiety disorder, performance only, is often comorbid with avoidant personality disorder. In children, comorbidities with high-functioning autism and selective mutism are common.

Panic Disorder

Diagnostic Criteria   **300.01 (F41.0)**

A. Recurrent unexpected panic attacks. A panic attack is an abrupt surge of intense fear or intense discomfort that reaches a peak within minutes, and during which time four (or more) of the following symptoms occur:

Note: The abrupt surge can occur from a calm state or an anxious state.

1. Palpitations, pounding heart, or accelerated heart rate.
2. Sweating.
3. Trembling or shaking.
4. Sensations of shortness of breath or smothering.
5. Feelings of choking.
6. Chest pain or discomfort.
7. Nausea or abdominal distress.
8. Feeling dizzy, unsteady, light-headed, or faint.
9. Chills or heat sensations.
10. Paresthesias (numbness or tingling sensations).
11. Derealization (feelings of unreality) or depersonalization (being detached from oneself).
12. Fear of losing control or "going crazy."
13. Fear of dying.

Note: Culture-specific symptoms (e.g., tinnitus, neck soreness, headache, uncontrollable screaming or crying) may be seen. Such symptoms should not count as one of the four required symptoms.

B. At least one of the attacks has been followed by 1 month (or more) of one or both of the following:

1. Persistent concern or worry about additional panic attacks or their consequences (e.g., losing control, having a heart attack, "going crazy").
2. A significant maladaptive change in behavior related to the attacks (e.g., behaviors designed to avoid having panic attacks, such as avoidance of exercise or unfamiliar situations).

C. The disturbance is not attributable to the physiological effects of a substance (e.g., a drug of abuse, a medication) or another medical condition (e.g., hyperthyroidism, cardiopulmonary disorders).

D. The disturbance is not better explained by another mental disorder (e.g., the panic attacks do not occur only in response to feared social situations, as in social anxiety disorder; in response to circumscribed phobic objects or situations, as in specific phobia; in response to obsessions, as in obsessive-compulsive disorder; in response to reminders of traumatic events, as in posttraumatic stress disorder; or in response to separation from attachment figures, as in separation anxiety disorder).

Diagnostic Features

Panic disorder refers to recurrent unexpected panic attacks (Criterion A). A panic attack is an abrupt surge of intense fear or intense discomfort that reaches a peak within minutes, and during which time four or more of a list of 13 physical and cognitive symptoms occur. The term *recurrent* literally means more than one unexpected panic attack. The term *unexpected* refers to a panic attack for which there is no obvious cue or trigger at the time of occurrence—that is, the attack appears to occur from out of the blue, such as when the individual is relaxing or emerging from sleep (nocturnal panic attack). In contrast, *expected* panic attacks are attacks for which there is an obvious cue or trigger, such as a situation in which panic attacks typically occur. The determination of whether panic attacks are expected or unexpected is made by the clinician, who makes this judgment based on a combination of careful questioning as to the sequence of events preceding or leading up to the attack and the individual's own judgment of whether or not the attack seemed to occur for no apparent reason. Cultural interpretations may influence the assignment of panic attacks as expected or unexpected (see section "Culture-Related Diagnostic Issues" for this disorder). In the United States and Europe, approximately one-half of individuals with panic disorder have expected panic attacks as well as unexpected panic attacks. Thus, the presence of expected panic attacks does not rule out the diagnosis of panic disorder. For more details regarding expected versus unexpected panic attacks, see the text accompanying panic attacks (pp. 214–217).

The frequency and severity of panic attacks vary widely. In terms of frequency, there may be moderately frequent attacks (e.g., one per week) for months at a time, or short bursts of more frequent attacks (e.g., daily) separated by weeks or months without any attacks or with less frequent attacks (e.g., two per month) over many years. Persons who have infrequent panic attacks resemble persons with more frequent panic attacks in terms of panic attack symptoms, demographic characteristics, comorbidity with other disorders, family history, and biological data. In terms of severity, individuals with panic disorder may have both full-symptom (four or more symptoms) and limited-symptom (fewer than four symptoms) attacks, and the number and type of panic attack symptoms frequently differ from one panic attack to the next. However, more than one unexpected full-symptom panic attack is required for the diagnosis of panic disorder.

The worries about panic attacks or their consequences usually pertain to physical concerns, such as worry that panic attacks reflect the presence of life-threatening illnesses (e.g., cardiac disease, seizure disorder); social concerns, such as embarrassment or fear of being judged negatively by others because of visible panic symptoms; and concerns about mental functioning, such as "going crazy" or losing control (Criterion B). The maladaptive changes in behavior represent attempts to minimize or avoid panic attacks or their consequences. Examples include avoiding physical exertion, reorganizing daily life to ensure that help is available in the event of a panic attack, restricting usual daily activities, and avoiding agoraphobia-type situations, such as leaving home, using public transportation, or shopping. If agoraphobia is present, a separate diagnosis of agoraphobia is given.

Associated Features Supporting Diagnosis

One type of unexpected panic attack is a *nocturnal* panic attack (i.e., waking from sleep in a state of panic, which differs from panicking after fully waking from sleep). In the United States, this type of panic attack has been estimated to occur at least one time in roughly one-quarter to one-third of individuals with panic disorder, of whom the majority also have daytime panic attacks. In addition to worry about panic attacks and their consequences, many individuals with panic disorder report constant or intermittent feelings of anxiety that are more broadly related to health and mental health concerns. For example, individuals with panic disorder often anticipate a catastrophic outcome from a mild physical symptom or medication side effect (e.g., thinking that they may have heart disease or that a headache means presence of a brain tumor). Such individuals often are relatively intolerant of medication side effects. In addition, there may be pervasive concerns about abilities to complete daily tasks or withstand daily stressors, excessive use of drugs (e.g., alcohol, prescribed medications or illicit drugs) to control panic attacks, or extreme behaviors aimed at controlling panic attacks (e.g., severe restrictions on food intake or avoidance of specific foods or medications because of concerns about physical symptoms that provoke panic attacks).

Prevalence

In the general population, the 12-month prevalence estimate for panic disorder across the United States and several European countries is about 2%–3% in adults and adolescents. In the United States, significantly lower rates of panic disorder are reported among Latinos, African Americans, Caribbean blacks, and Asian Americans, compared with non-Latino whites; American Indians, by contrast, have significantly higher rates. Lower estimates have been reported for Asian, African, and Latin American countries, ranging from 0.1% to 0.8%. Females are more frequently affected than males, at a rate of approximately 2:1. The gender differentiation occurs in adolescence and is already observable before age 14 years. Although panic attacks occur in children, the overall prevalence of panic disorder is low before age 14 years (<0.4%). The rates of panic disorder show a gradual increase during adolescence, particularly in females, and possibly following the onset of puberty, and peak during adulthood. The prevalence rates decline in older individuals (i.e., 0.7% in adults over the age of 64), possibly reflecting diminishing severity to subclinical levels.

Development and Course

The median age at onset for panic disorder in the United States is 20–24 years. A small number of cases begin in childhood, and onset after age 45 years is unusual but can occur. The usual course, if the disorder is untreated, is chronic but waxing and waning. Some individuals may have episodic outbreaks with years of remission in between, and others may have continuous severe symptomatology. Only a minority of individuals have full remission without subsequent relapse within a few years. The course of panic disorder typically is complicated by a range of other disorders, in particular other anxiety disorders, depressive disorders, and substance use disorders (see section "Comorbidity" for this disorder).

Although panic disorder is very rare in childhood, first occurrence of "fearful spells" is often dated retrospectively back to childhood. As in adults, panic disorder in adolescents tends to have a chronic course and is frequently comorbid with other anxiety, depressive, and bipolar disorders. To date, no differences in the clinical presentation between adolescents and adults have been found. However, adolescents may be less worried about additional panic attacks than are young adults. Lower prevalence of panic disorder in older adults appears to be attributable to age-related "dampening" of the autonomic nervous system response. Many older individuals with "panicky feelings" are observed to have a "hybrid" of limited-symptom panic attacks and generalized anxiety. Also, older adults tend to attribute their panic attacks to certain stressful situations, such as a medical procedure or social setting. Older individuals may retrospectively endorse explanations for the panic attack (which would preclude the diagnosis of panic disorder), even if an attack might actually have been unexpected in the moment (and thus qualify as the basis for a panic disorder diagnosis). This may result in under-endorsement of unexpected panic attacks in older individuals. Thus, careful questioning of older adults is required to assess whether panic attacks were expected before entering the situation, so that unexpected panic attacks and the diagnosis of panic disorder are not overlooked.

While the low rate of panic disorder in children could relate to difficulties in symptom reporting, this seems unlikely given that children are capable of reporting intense fear or panic in relation to separation and to phobic objects or phobic situations. Adolescents might be less willing than adults to openly discuss panic attacks. Therefore, clinicians should be aware that unexpected panic attacks do occur in adolescents, much as they do in adults, and be attuned to this possibility when encountering adolescents presenting with episodes of intense fear or distress.

Risk and Prognostic Factors

Temperamental.   Negative affectivity (neuroticism) (i.e., proneness to experiencing negative emotions) and anxiety sensitivity (i.e., the disposition to believe that symptoms of anxiety are harmful) are risk factors for the onset of panic attacks and, separately, for worry about panic, although their risk status for the diagnosis of panic disorder is unknown. History of "fearful spells" (i.e., limited-symptom attacks that do not meet full criteria for a panic attack) may be a risk factor for later panic attacks and panic disorder. Although separation anxiety in childhood, especially when severe, may precede the later development of panic disorder, it is not a consistent risk factor.

Environmental.   Reports of childhood experiences of sexual and physical abuse are more common in panic disorder than in certain other anxiety disorders. Smoking is a risk factor for panic attacks and panic disorder. Most individuals report identifiable stressors in the months before their first panic attack (e.g., interpersonal stressors and stressors related to physical well-being, such as negative experiences with illicit or prescription drugs, disease, or death in the family).

Genetic and physiological.   It is believed that multiple genes confer vulnerability to panic disorder. However, the exact genes, gene products, or functions related to the genetic regions implicated remain unknown. Current neural systems models for panic disorder emphasize the amygdala and related structures, much as in other anxiety disorders. There is an increased risk for panic disorder among offspring of parents with anxiety, depressive, and bipolar disorders. Respiratory disturbance, such as asthma, is associated with panic disorder, in terms of past history, comorbidity, and family history.

Culture-Related Diagnostic Issues

The rate of fears about mental and somatic symptoms of anxiety appears to vary across cultures and may influence the rate of panic attacks and panic disorder. Also, cultural expectations may influence the classification of panic attacks as expected or unexpected. For example, a Vietnamese individual who has a panic attack after walking out into a windy environment (*trúng gió;* "hit by the wind") may attribute the panic attack to exposure to wind as a result of the cultural syndrome that links these two experiences, resulting in classification of the panic attack as expected. Various other cultural syndromes are associated with panic disorder, including *ataque de nervios* ("attack of nerves") among Latin Americans and *khyâl* attacks and "soul loss" among Cambodians. *Ataque de nervios* may involve trembling, uncontrollable screaming or crying, aggressive or suicidal behavior, and depersonalization or derealization, which may be experienced longer than the few minutes typical of panic attacks. Some clinical presentations of *ataque de nervios* fulfill criteria for conditions other than panic attack (e.g., other specified dissociative disorder). These syndromes impact the symptoms and frequency of panic disorder, including the individual's attribution of unexpectedness, as cultural syndromes may create fear of certain situations, ranging from interpersonal arguments (associated with *ataque de nervios*), to types of exertion (associated with *khyâl* attacks), to atmospheric wind (associated with *trúng gió* attacks). Clarification of the details of cultural attributions may aid in distinguishing expected and unexpected panic attacks. For more information regarding cultural syndromes, refer to the "Glossary of Cultural Concepts of Distress" in the Appendix.

The specific worries about panic attacks or their consequences are likely to vary from one culture to another (and across different age groups and gender). For panic disorder, U.S. community samples of non-Latino whites have significantly less functional impairment than African Americans. There are also higher rates of objectively defined severity in non-Latino Caribbean blacks with panic disorder, and lower rates of panic disorder overall in both African American and Afro-Caribbean groups, suggesting that among individuals of African descent, the criteria for panic disorder may be met only when there is substantial severity and impairment.

Gender-Related Diagnostic Issues

The clinical features of panic disorder do not appear to differ between males and females. There is some evidence for sexual dimorphism, with an association between panic disorder and the catechol-O-methyltransferase (COMT) gene in females only.

Diagnostic Markers

Agents with disparate mechanisms of action, such as sodium lactate, caffeine, isoproterenol, yohimbine, carbon dioxide, and cholecystokinin, provoke panic attacks in individuals with panic disorder to a much greater extent than in healthy control subjects (and in some cases, than in individuals with other anxiety, depressive, or bipolar disorders without panic attacks). Also, for a proportion of individuals with panic disorder, panic attacks are related to hypersensitive medullary carbon dioxide detectors, resulting in hypocapnia and other respiratory irregularities. However, none of these laboratory findings are considered diagnostic of panic disorder.

Suicide Risk

Panic attacks and a diagnosis of panic disorder in the past 12 months are related to a higher rate of suicide attempts and suicidal ideation in the past 12 months even when comorbidity and a history of childhood abuse and other suicide risk factors are taken into account.

Functional Consequences of Panic Disorder

Panic disorder is associated with high levels of social, occupational, and physical disability; considerable economic costs; and the highest number of medical visits among the anxiety disorders, although the effects are strongest with the presence of agoraphobia. Individuals with panic disorder may be frequently absent from work or school for doctor and emergency room visits, which can lead to unemployment or dropping out of school. In older adults, impairment may be seen in caregiving duties or volunteer activities. Full-symptom panic attacks typically are associated with greater morbidity (e.g., greater health care utilization, more disability, poorer quality of life) than limited-symptom attacks.

Differential Diagnosis

Other specified anxiety disorder or unspecified anxiety disorder. Panic disorder should not be diagnosed if full-symptom (unexpected) panic attacks have never been experienced. In the case of only limited-symptom unexpected panic attacks, an other specified anxiety disorder or unspecified anxiety disorder diagnosis should be considered.

Anxiety disorder due to another medical condition.   Panic disorder is not diagnosed if the panic attacks are judged to be a direct physiological consequence of another medical condition. Examples of medical conditions that can cause panic attacks include hyperthyroidism, hyperparathyroidism, pheochromocytoma, vestibular dysfunctions, seizure disorders, and cardiopulmonary conditions (e.g., arrhythmias, supraventricular tachycardia, asthma, chronic obstructive pulmonary disease [COPD]). Appropriate laboratory tests (e.g., serum calcium levels for hyperparathyroidism; Holter monitor for arrhythmias) or physical examinations (e.g., for cardiac conditions) may be helpful in determining the etiological role of another medical condition.

Substance/medication-induced anxiety disorder.   Panic disorder is not diagnosed if the panic attacks are judged to be a direct physiological consequence of a substance. Intoxication with central nervous system stimulants (e.g., cocaine, amphetamines, caffeine) or cannabis and withdrawal from central nervous system depressants (e.g., alcohol, barbiturates) can precipitate a panic attack. However, if panic attacks continue to occur outside of the context of substance use (e.g., long after the effects of intoxication or withdrawal have ended), a diagnosis of panic disorder should be considered. In addition, because panic disorder may precede substance use in some individuals and may be associated with increased substance use, especially for purposes of self-medication, a detailed history should be taken to determine if the individual had panic attacks prior to excessive substance use. If this is the case, a diagnosis of panic disorder should be considered in addition to a diagnosis of substance use disorder. Features such as onset after age 45 years or the presence of atypical symptoms during a panic attack (e.g., vertigo, loss of consciousness, loss of bladder or bowel control, slurred speech, amnesia) suggest the possibility that another medical condition or a substance may be causing the panic attack symptoms.

Other mental disorders with panic attacks as an associated feature (e.g., other anxiety disorders and psychotic disorders).   Panic attacks that occur as a symptom of other anxiety disorders are expected (e.g., triggered by social situations in social anxiety disorder, by phobic objects or situations in specific phobia or agoraphobia, by worry in generalized anxiety disorder, by separation from home or attachment figures in separation anxiety disorder) and thus would not meet criteria for panic disorder. (**Note:** Sometimes an unexpected panic attack is associated with the onset of another anxiety disorder, but then the attacks become expected, whereas panic disorder is characterized by recurrent unexpected panic attacks.) If the panic attacks occur only in response to specific triggers, then only the relevant anxiety disorder is assigned. However, if the individual experiences unexpected panic attacks as well and shows persistent concern and worry or behavioral change because of the attacks, then an additional diagnosis of panic disorder should be considered.

Comorbidity

Panic disorder infrequently occurs in clinical settings in the absence of other psychopathology. The prevalence of panic disorder is elevated in individuals with other disorders, particularly other anxiety disorders (and especially agoraphobia), major depression, bipolar disorder, and possibly mild alcohol use disorder. While panic disorder often has an earlier age at onset than the comorbid disorder(s), onset sometimes occurs after the comorbid disorder and may be seen as a severity marker of the comorbid illness.

Reported lifetime rates of comorbidity between major depressive disorder and panic disorder vary widely, ranging from 10% to 65% in individuals with panic disorder. In approximately one-third of individuals with both disorders, the depression precedes the onset of panic disorder. In the remaining two-thirds, depression occurs coincident with or following the onset of panic disorder. A subset of individuals with panic disorder develop a substance-related disorder, which for some represents an attempt to treat their anxiety with alcohol or medications. Comorbidity with other anxiety disorders and illness anxiety disorder is also common.

Panic disorder is significantly comorbid with numerous general medical symptoms and conditions, including, but not limited to, dizziness, cardiac arrhythmias, hyperthyroidism, asthma, COPD, and irritable bowel syndrome. However, the nature of the association (e.g., cause and effect) between panic disorder and these conditions remains unclear. Although mitral valve prolapse and thyroid disease are more common among individuals with panic disorder than in the general population, the differences in prevalence are not consistent.

Panic Attack Specifier

Note: Symptoms are presented for the purpose of identifying a panic attack; however, panic attack is not a mental disorder and cannot be coded. Panic attacks can occur in the context of any anxiety disorder as well as other mental disorders (e.g., depressive disorders, posttraumatic stress disorder, substance use disorders) and some medical conditions (e.g., cardiac, respiratory, vestibular, gastrointestinal). When the presence of a panic attack is identified, it should be noted as a specifier (e.g., "posttraumatic stress disorder with panic attacks"). For panic disorder, the presence of panic attack is contained within the criteria for the disorder and panic attack is not used as a specifier.

An abrupt surge of intense fear or intense discomfort that reaches a peak within minutes, and during which time four (or more) of the following symptoms occur:

Note: The abrupt surge can occur from a calm state or an anxious state.

1. Palpitations, pounding heart, or accelerated heart rate.
2. Sweating.
3. Trembling or shaking.
4. Sensations of shortness of breath or smothering.
5. Feelings of choking.
6. Chest pain or discomfort.
7. Nausea or abdominal distress.
8. Feeling dizzy, unsteady, light-headed, or faint.
9. Chills or heat sensations.
10. Paresthesias (numbness or tingling sensations).
11. Derealization (feelings of unreality) or depersonalization (being detached from oneself).
12. Fear of losing control or "going crazy."
13. Fear of dying.

Note: Culture-specific symptoms (e.g., tinnitus, neck soreness, headache, uncontrollable screaming or crying) may be seen. Such symptoms should not count as one of the four required symptoms.

Features

The essential feature of a panic attack is an abrupt surge of intense fear or intense discomfort that reaches a peak within minutes and during which time four or more of 13 physical and cognitive symptoms occur. Eleven of these 13 symptoms are physical (e.g., palpitations, sweating), while two are cognitive (i.e., fear of losing control or going crazy, fear of dying). "Fear of going crazy" is a colloquialism often used by individuals with panic attacks and is not intended as a pejorative or diagnostic term. The term *within minutes* means that the time to peak intensity is literally only a few minutes. A panic attack can arise from either a calm state or an anxious state, and time to peak intensity should be assessed independently of any preceding anxiety. That is, the start of the panic attack is the point at which there is an abrupt increase in discomfort rather than the point at which anxiety first developed. Likewise, a panic attack can return to either an anxious state or a calm state and possibly peak again. A panic attack is distinguished from ongoing anxiety by its time to peak intensity, which occurs within minutes; its discrete nature; and its typically greater severity. Attacks that meet all other criteria but have fewer than four physical and/or cognitive symptoms are referred to as *limited-symptom attacks.*

There are two characteristic types of panic attacks: expected and unexpected. *Expected panic attacks* are attacks for which there is an obvious cue or trigger, such as situations in which panic attacks have typically occurred. *Unexpected panic attacks* are those for which there is no obvious cue or trigger at the time of occurrence (e.g., when relaxing or out of sleep [nocturnal panic attack]). The determination of whether panic attacks are expected or unexpected is made by the clinician, who makes this judgment based on a combination of careful questioning as to the sequence of events preceding or leading up to the attack and the individual's own judgment of whether or not the attack seemed to occur for no apparent reason. Cultural interpretations may influence their determination as expected or unexpected. Culture-specific symptoms (e.g., tinnitus, neck soreness, headache, uncontrollable screaming or crying) may be seen; however, such symptoms should not count as one of the four required symptoms. Panic attacks can occur in the context of any mental disorder (e.g., anxiety disorders, depressive disorders, bipolar disorders, eating disorders, obsessive-compulsive and related disorders, personality disorders, psychotic disorders, substance use disorders) and some medical conditions (e.g., cardiac, respiratory, vestibular, gastrointestinal), with the majority never meeting criteria for panic disorder. Recurrent unexpected panic attacks are required for a diagnosis of panic disorder.

Associated Features

One type of unexpected panic attack is a *nocturnal panic attack* (i.e., waking from sleep in a state of panic), which differs from panicking after fully waking from sleep. Panic attacks are related to a higher rate of suicide attempts and suicidal ideation even when comorbidity and other suicide risk factors are taken into account.

Prevalence

In the general population, 12-month prevalence estimates for panic attacks in the United States is 11.2% in adults. Twelve-month prevalence estimates do not appear to differ significantly among African Americans, Asian Americans, and Latinos. Lower 12-month prevalence estimates for European countries appear to range from 2.7% to 3.3%. Females are more frequently affected than males, although this gender difference is more pronounced for panic disorder. Panic attacks can occur in children but are relatively rare until the age of puberty, when the prevalence rates increase. The prevalence rates decline in older individuals, possibly reflecting diminishing severity to subclinical levels.

Development and Course

The mean age at onset for panic attacks in the United States is approximately 22–23 years among adults. However, the course of panic attacks is likely influenced by the course of any co-occurring mental disorder(s) and stressful life events. Panic attacks are uncommon, and unexpected panic attacks are rare, in preadolescent children. Adolescents might be less willing than adults to openly discuss panic attacks, even though they present with episodes of intense fear or discomfort. Lower prevalence of panic attacks in older individuals may be related to a weaker autonomic response to emotional states relative to younger individuals. Older individuals may be less inclined to use the word "fear" and more inclined to use the word "discomfort" to describe panic attacks. Older individuals with "panicky feelings" may have a hybrid of limited-symptom attacks and generalized anxiety. In addition, older individuals tend to attribute panic attacks to certain situations that are stressful (e.g., medical procedures, social settings) and may retrospectively endorse explanations for the panic attack even if it was unexpected in the moment. This may result in under-endorsement of unexpected panic attacks in older individuals.

Risk and Prognostic Factors

Temperamental.   Negative affectivity (neuroticism) (i.e., proneness to experiencing negative emotions) and anxiety sensitivity (i.e., the disposition to believe that symptoms of anxiety are harmful) are risk factors for the onset of panic attacks. History of "fearful spells" (i.e., limited-symptom attacks that do not meet full criteria for a panic attack) may be a risk factor for later panic attacks.

Environmental.   Smoking is a risk factor for panic attacks. Most individuals report identifiable stressors in the months before their first panic attack (e.g., interpersonal stressors and stressors related to physical well-being, such as negative experiences with illicit or prescription drugs, disease, or death in the family).

Culture-Related Diagnostic Issues

Cultural interpretations may influence the determination of panic attacks as expected or unexpected. Culture-specific symptoms (e.g., tinnitus, neck soreness, headache, and uncontrollable screaming or crying) may be seen; however, such symptoms should not count as one of the four required symptoms. Frequency of each of the 13 symptoms varies cross-culturally (e.g., higher rates of paresthesias in African Americans and of dizziness in several Asian groups). Cultural syndromes also influence the cross-cultural presentation of panic attacks, resulting in different symptom profiles across different cultural groups. Examples include *khyâl* (wind) attacks, a Cambodian cultural syndrome involving dizziness, tinnitus, and neck soreness; and *trúng gió* (wind-related) attacks, a Vietnamese cultural syndrome associated with headaches. *Ataque de nervios* (attack of nerves) is a cultural syndrome among Latin Americans that may involve trembling, uncontrollable screaming or crying, aggressive or suicidal behavior, and depersonalization or derealization, and which may be experienced for longer than only a few minutes. Some clinical presentations of *ataque de nervios* fulfill criteria for conditions other than panic attack (e.g., other specified dissociative disorder). Also, cultural expectations may influence the classification of panic attacks as expected or unexpected, as cultural syndromes may create fear of certain situations, ranging from interpersonal arguments (associated with *ataque de nervios*), to types of exertion (associated with *khyâl* attacks), to atmospheric wind (associated with *trúng gió* attacks). Clarification of the details of cultural attributions may aid in distinguishing expected and unexpected panic attacks. For more information about cultural syndromes, see "Glossary of Cultural Concepts of Distress" in the Appendix to this manual.

Gender-Related Diagnostic Issues

Panic attacks are more common in females than in males, but clinical features or symptoms of panic attacks do not differ between males and females.

Diagnostic Markers

Physiological recordings of naturally occurring panic attacks in individuals with panic disorder indicate abrupt surges of arousal, usually of heart rate, that reach a peak within minutes and subside within minutes, and for a proportion of these individuals the panic attack may be preceded by cardiorespiratory instabilities.

Functional Consequences of Panic Attacks

In the context of co-occurring mental disorders, including anxiety disorders, depressive disorders, bipolar disorder, substance use disorders, psychotic disorders, and personality disorders, panic attacks are associated with increased symptom severity, higher rates of comorbidity and suicidality, and poorer treatment response. Also, full-symptom panic attacks typically are associated with greater morbidity (e.g., greater health care utilization, more disability, poorer quality of life) than limited-symptom attacks.

Differential Diagnosis

Other paroxysmal episodes (e.g., "anger attacks"). Panic attacks should not be diagnosed if the episodes do not involve the essential feature of an abrupt surge of intense fear or intense discomfort, but rather other emotional states (e.g., anger, grief).

Anxiety disorder due to another medical condition. Medical conditions that can cause or be misdiagnosed as panic attacks include hyperthyroidism, hyperparathyroidism, pheochromocytoma, vestibular dysfunctions, seizure disorders, and cardiopulmonary conditions (e.g., arrhythmias, supraventricular tachycardia, asthma, chronic obstructive pulmonary disease). Appropriate laboratory tests (e.g., serum calcium levels for hyperparathyroidism; Holter monitor for arrhythmias) or physical examinations (e.g., for cardiac conditions) may be helpful in determining the etiological role of another medical condition.

Substance/medication-induced anxiety disorder. Intoxication with central nervous system stimulants (e.g., cocaine, amphetamines, caffeine) or cannabis and withdrawal from central nervous system depressants (e.g., alcohol, barbiturates) can precipitate a panic attack. A detailed history should be taken to determine if the individual had panic attacks prior to excessive substance use. Features such as onset after age 45 years or the presence of atypical symptoms during a panic attack (e.g., vertigo, loss of consciousness, loss of bladder or bowel control, slurred speech, or amnesia) suggest the possibility that a medical condition or a substance may be causing the panic attack symptoms.

Panic disorder. Repeated unexpected panic attacks are required but are not sufficient for the diagnosis of panic disorder (i.e., full diagnostic criteria for panic disorder must be met).

Comorbidity

Panic attacks are associated with increased likelihood of various comorbid mental disorders, including anxiety disorders, depressive disorders, bipolar disorders, impulse-control disorders, and substance use disorders. Panic attacks are associated with increased likelihood of later developing anxiety disorders, depressive disorders, bipolar disorders, and possibly other disorders.

Agoraphobia

Diagnostic Criteria	**300.22 (F40.00)**

A. Marked fear or anxiety about two (or more) of the following five situations:

  1. Using public transportation (e.g., automobiles, buses, trains, ships, planes).
  2. Being in open spaces (e.g., parking lots, marketplaces, bridges).
  3. Being in enclosed places (e.g., shops, theaters, cinemas).
  4. Standing in line or being in a crowd.
  5. Being outside of the home alone.

B. The individual fears or avoids these situations because of thoughts that escape might be difficult or help might not be available in the event of developing panic-like symptoms or other incapacitating or embarrassing symptoms (e.g., fear of falling in the elderly; fear of incontinence).

C. The agoraphobic situations almost always provoke fear or anxiety.

D. The agoraphobic situations are actively avoided, require the presence of a companion, or are endured with intense fear or anxiety.

E. The fear or anxiety is out of proportion to the actual danger posed by the agoraphobic situations and to the sociocultural context.

F. The fear, anxiety, or avoidance is persistent, typically lasting for 6 months or more.

G. The fear, anxiety, or avoidance causes clinically significant distress or impairment in social, occupational, or other important areas of functioning.

H. If another medical condition (e.g., inflammatory bowel disease, Parkinson's disease) is present, the fear, anxiety, or avoidance is clearly excessive.

I. The fear, anxiety, or avoidance is not better explained by the symptoms of another mental disorder—for example, the symptoms are not confined to specific phobia, situational type; do not involve only social situations (as in social anxiety disorder); and are not related exclusively to obsessions (as in obsessive-compulsive disorder), perceived defects or flaws in physical appearance (as in body dysmorphic disorder), reminders of traumatic events (as in posttraumatic stress disorder), or fear of separation (as in separation anxiety disorder).

Note: Agoraphobia is diagnosed irrespective of the presence of panic disorder. If an individual's presentation meets criteria for panic disorder and agoraphobia, both diagnoses should be assigned.

Diagnostic Features

The essential feature of agoraphobia is marked, or intense, fear or anxiety triggered by the real or anticipated exposure to a wide range of situations (Criterion A). The diagnosis requires endorsement of symptoms occurring in at least two of the following five situations: 1) using public transportation, such as automobiles, buses, trains, ships, or planes; 2) being in open spaces, such as parking lots, marketplaces, or bridges; 3) being in enclosed spaces, such as shops, theaters, or cinemas; 4) standing in line or being in a crowd; or 5) being outside of the home alone. The examples for each situation are not exhaustive; other situations may be feared. When experiencing fear and anxiety cued by such situations, individuals typically experience thoughts that something terrible might happen (Criterion B). Individuals frequently believe that escape from such situations might be difficult (e.g., "can't get out of here") or that help might be unavailable (e.g., "there is nobody to help me") when panic-like symptoms or other incapacitating or embarrassing symptoms occur. "Panic-like symptoms" refer to any of the 13 symptoms included in the criteria for panic attack, such as dizziness, faintness, and fear of dying. "Other incapacitating or embarrassing symptoms" include symptoms such as vomiting and inflammatory bowel symptoms, as well as, in older adults, a fear of falling or, in children, a sense of disorientation and getting lost.

The amount of fear experienced may vary with proximity to the feared situation and may occur in anticipation of or in the actual presence of the agoraphobic situation. Also, the fear or anxiety may take the form of a full- or limited-symptom panic attack (i.e., an expected panic attack). Fear or anxiety is evoked nearly every time the individual comes into contact with the feared situation (Criterion C). Thus, an individual who becomes anxious only occasionally in an agoraphobic situation (e.g., becomes anxious when standing in line on only one out of every five occasions) would not be diagnosed with agoraphobia. The individual actively avoids the situation or, if he or she either is unable or decides not to avoid it, the situation evokes intense fear or anxiety (Criterion D). *Active avoidance* means the individual is currently behaving in ways that are intentionally designed to prevent or minimize contact with agoraphobic situations. Avoidance can be behavioral (e.g., changing daily routines, choosing a job nearby to avoid using public transportation, arranging for food delivery to avoid entering shops and supermarkets) as well as cognitive (e.g., using distraction to get through agoraphobic situations) in nature. The avoidance can become so severe that the person is completely homebound. Often, an individual is better able to confront a feared situation when accompanied by a companion, such as a partner, friend, or health professional.

The fear, anxiety, or avoidance must be out of proportion to the actual danger posed by the agoraphobic situations and to the sociocultural context (Criterion E). Differentiating clinically significant agoraphobic fears from reasonable fears (e.g., leaving the house during a bad storm) or from situations that are deemed dangerous (e.g., walking in a parking lot or using public transportation in a high-crime area) is important for a number of reasons. First, what constitutes avoidance may be difficult to judge across cultures and sociocultural contexts (e.g., it is socioculturally appropriate for orthodox Muslim women in certain parts of the world to avoid leaving the house alone, and thus such avoidance would not be considered indicative of agoraphobia). Second, older adults are likely to overattribute their fears to age-related constraints and are less likely to judge their fears as being out of proportion to the actual risk. Third, individuals with agoraphobia are likely to overestimate danger in relation to panic-like or other bodily symptoms. Agoraphobia should be diagnosed only if the fear, anxiety, or avoidance persists (Criterion F) and if it causes clinically significant distress or impairment in social, occupational, or other important areas of functioning (Criterion G). The duration of "typically lasting for 6 months or more" is meant to exclude individuals with short-lived, transient problems. However, the duration criterion should be used as a general guide, with allowance for some degree of flexibility.

Associated Features Supporting Diagnosis

In its most severe forms, agoraphobia can cause individuals to become completely homebound, unable to leave their home and dependent on others for services or assistance to provide even for basic needs. Demoralization and depressive symptoms, as well as abuse of alcohol and sedative medication as inappropriate self-medication strategies, are common.

Prevalence

Every year approximately 1.7% of adolescents and adults have a diagnosis of agoraphobia. Females are twice as likely as males to experience agoraphobia. Agoraphobia may occur in childhood, but incidence peaks in late adolescence and early adulthood. Twelve-month prevalence in individuals older than 65 years is 0.4%. Prevalence rates do not appear to vary systematically across cultural/racial groups.

Development and Course

The percentage of individuals with agoraphobia reporting panic attacks or panic disorder preceding the onset of agoraphobia ranges from 30% in community samples to more than 50% in clinic samples. The majority of individuals with panic disorder show signs of anxiety and agoraphobia before the onset of panic disorder.

In two-thirds of all cases of agoraphobia, initial onset is before age 35 years. There is a substantial incidence risk in late adolescence and early adulthood, with indications for a second high incidence risk phase after age 40 years. First onset in childhood is rare. The overall mean age at onset for agoraphobia is 17 years, although the age at onset without preceding panic attacks or panic disorder is 25–29 years.

The course of agoraphobia is typically persistent and chronic. Complete remission is rare (10%), unless the agoraphobia is treated. With more severe agoraphobia, rates of full remission decrease, whereas rates of relapse and chronicity increase. A range of other disorders, in particular other anxiety disorders, depressive disorders, substance use disorders, and personality disorders, may complicate the course of agoraphobia. The long-term course and outcome of agoraphobia are associated with substantially elevated risk of secondary major depressive disorder, persistent depressive disorder (dysthymia), and substance use disorders.

The clinical features of agoraphobia are relatively consistent across the lifespan, although the type of agoraphobic situations triggering fear, anxiety, or avoidance, as well as the type of cognitions, may vary. For example, in children, being outside of the home alone is the most frequent situation feared, whereas in older adults, being in shops, standing in line, and being in open spaces are most often feared. Also, cognitions often pertain to becoming lost (in children), to experiencing panic-like symptoms (in adults), to falling (in older adults).

The low prevalence of agoraphobia in children could reflect difficulties in symptom reporting, and thus assessments in young children may require solicitation of information from multiple sources, including parents or teachers. Adolescents, particularly males, may be less willing than adults to openly discuss agoraphobic fears and avoidance; however, agoraphobia can occur prior to adulthood and should be assessed in children and adolescents. In older adults, comorbid somatic symptom disorders, as well as motor disturbances (e.g., sense of falling or having medical complications), are frequently mentioned by individuals as the reason for their fear and avoidance. In these instances, care is to be taken in evaluating whether the fear and avoidance are out of proportion to the real danger involved.

Risk and Prognostic Factors

Temperamental.   Behavioral inhibition and neurotic disposition (i.e., negative affectivity [neuroticism] and anxiety sensitivity) are closely associated with agoraphobia but are relevant to most anxiety disorders (phobic disorders, panic disorder, generalized anxiety disorder). Anxiety sensitivity (the disposition to believe that symptoms of anxiety are harmful) is also characteristic of individuals with agoraphobia.

Environmental.   Negative events in childhood (e.g., separation, death of parent) and other stressful events, such as being attacked or mugged, are associated with the onset of agoraphobia. Furthermore, individuals with agoraphobia describe the family climate and child-rearing behavior as being characterized by reduced warmth and increased overprotection.

Genetic and physiological.   Heritability for agoraphobia is 61%. Of the various phobias, agoraphobia has the strongest and most specific association with the genetic factor that represents proneness to phobias.

Gender-Related Diagnostic Issues

Females have different patterns of comorbid disorders than males. Consistent with gender differences in the prevalence of mental disorders, males have higher rates of comorbid substance use disorders.

Functional Consequences of Agoraphobia

Agoraphobia is associated with considerable impairment and disability in terms of role functioning, work productivity, and disability days. Agoraphobia severity is a strong determinant of the degree of disability, irrespective of the presence of comorbid panic disorder, panic attacks, and other comorbid conditions. More than one-third of individuals with agoraphobia are completely homebound and unable to work.

Differential Diagnosis

When diagnostic criteria for agoraphobia and another disorder are fully met, both diagnoses should be assigned, unless the fear, anxiety, or avoidance of agoraphobia is attributable to the other disorder. Weighting of criteria and clinical judgment may be helpful in some cases.

Specific phobia, situational type. Differentiating agoraphobia from situational specific phobia can be challenging in some cases, because these conditions share several symptom characteristics and criteria. Specific phobia, situational type, should be diagnosed versus agoraphobia if the fear, anxiety, or avoidance is limited to one of the agoraphobic situations. Requiring fears from two or more of the agoraphobic situations is a robust means for differentiating agoraphobia from specific phobias, particularly the situational subtype. Additional differentiating features include the cognitive ideation. Thus, if the situation is feared for reasons other than panic-like symptoms or other incapacitating or embarrassing symptoms (e.g., fears of being directly harmed by the situation itself, such as fear of the plane crashing for individuals who fear flying), then a diagnosis of specific phobia may be more appropriate.

Separation anxiety disorder. Separation anxiety disorder can be best differentiated from agoraphobia by examining cognitive ideation. In separation anxiety disorder, the thoughts are about detachment from significant others and the home environment (i.e., parents or other attachment figures), whereas in agoraphobia the focus is on panic-like symptoms or other incapacitating or embarrassing symptoms in the feared situations.

Social anxiety disorder (social phobia). Agoraphobia should be differentiated from social anxiety disorder based primarily on the situational clusters that trigger fear, anxiety, or avoidance and the cognitive ideation. In social anxiety disorder, the focus is on fear of being negatively evaluated.

Panic disorder. When criteria for panic disorder are met, agoraphobia should not be diagnosed if the avoidance behaviors associated with the panic attacks do not extend to avoidance of two or more agoraphobic situations.

Acute stress disorder and posttraumatic stress disorder. Acute stress disorder and posttraumatic stress disorder (PTSD) can be differentiated from agoraphobia by examining whether the fear, anxiety, or avoidance is related only to situations that remind the individual of a traumatic event. If the fear, anxiety, or avoidance is restricted to trauma reminders, and if the avoidance behavior does not extend to two or more agoraphobic situations, then a diagnosis of agoraphobia is not warranted.

Major depressive disorder. In major depressive disorder, the individual may avoid leaving home because of apathy, loss of energy, low self-esteem, and anhedonia. If the avoidance is unrelated to fears of panic-like or other incapacitating or embarrassing symptoms, then agoraphobia should not be diagnosed.

Other medical conditions. Agoraphobia is not diagnosed if the avoidance of situations is judged to be a physiological consequence of a medical condition. This determination is based on history, laboratory findings, and a physical examination. Other relevant medical conditions may include neurodegenerative disorders with associated motor disturbances (e.g., Parkinson's disease, multiple sclerosis), as well as cardiovascular disorders. Individuals with certain medical conditions may avoid situations because of realistic concerns about being incapacitated (e.g., fainting in an individual with transient ischemic attacks) or being embarrassed (e.g., diarrhea in an individual with Crohn's disease). The diagnosis of agoraphobia should be given only when the fear or avoidance is clearly in excess of that usually associated with these medical conditions.

Comorbidity

The majority of individuals with agoraphobia also have other mental disorders. The most frequent additional diagnoses are other anxiety disorders (e.g., specific phobias, panic disorder, social anxiety disorder), depressive disorders (major depressive disorder), PTSD, and alcohol use disorder. Whereas other anxiety disorders (e.g., separation anxiety disorder, specific phobias, panic disorder) frequently precede onset of agoraphobia, depressive disorders and substance use disorders typically occur secondary to agoraphobia.

Generalized Anxiety Disorder

Diagnostic Criteria   **300.02 (F41.1)**

A. Excessive anxiety and worry (apprehensive expectation), occurring more days than not for at least 6 months, about a number of events or activities (such as work or school performance).

B. The individual finds it difficult to control the worry.

C. The anxiety and worry are associated with three (or more) of the following six symptoms (with at least some symptoms having been present for more days than not for the past 6 months):

Note: Only one item is required in children.

1. Restlessness or feeling keyed up or on edge.
2. Being easily fatigued.
3. Difficulty concentrating or mind going blank.
4. Irritability.
5. Muscle tension.
6. Sleep disturbance (difficulty falling or staying asleep, or restless, unsatisfying sleep).

D. The anxiety, worry, or physical symptoms cause clinically significant distress or impairment in social, occupational, or other important areas of functioning.

E. The disturbance is not attributable to the physiological effects of a substance (e.g., a drug of abuse, a medication) or another medical condition (e.g., hyperthyroidism).

F. The disturbance is not better explained by another mental disorder (e.g., anxiety or worry about having panic attacks in panic disorder, negative evaluation in social anxiety disorder [social phobia], contamination or other obsessions in obsessive-compulsive disorder, separation from attachment figures in separation anxiety disorder, reminders of traumatic events in posttraumatic stress disorder, gaining weight in anorexia nervosa, physical complaints in somatic symptom disorder, perceived appearance flaws in body dysmorphic disorder, having a serious illness in illness anxiety disorder, or the content of delusional beliefs in schizophrenia or delusional disorder).

Diagnostic Features

The essential feature of generalized anxiety disorder is excessive anxiety and worry (apprehensive expectation) about a number of events or activities. The intensity, duration, or frequency of the anxiety and worry is out of proportion to the actual likelihood or impact of the anticipated event. The individual finds it difficult to control the worry and to keep worrisome thoughts from interfering with attention to tasks at hand. Adults with generalized anxiety disorder often worry about everyday, routine life circumstances, such as possible job responsibilities, health and finances, the health of family members, misfortune to their children, or minor matters (e.g., doing household chores or being late for appointments). Children with generalized anxiety disorder tend to worry excessively about their competence or the quality of their performance. During the course of the disorder, the focus of worry may shift from one concern to another.

Several features distinguish generalized anxiety disorder from nonpathological anxiety. First, the worries associated with generalized anxiety disorder are excessive and typically interfere significantly with psychosocial functioning, whereas the worries of everyday life are not excessive and are perceived as more manageable and may be put off when more pressing matters arise. Second, the worries associated with generalized anxiety disorder are more pervasive, pronounced, and distressing; have longer duration; and frequently occur without precipitants. The greater the range of life circumstances about which a person worries (e.g., finances, children's safety, job performance), the more likely his or her symptoms are to meet criteria for generalized anxiety disorder. Third, everyday worries are much less likely to be accompanied by physical symptoms (e.g., restlessness or feeling keyed up or on edge). Individuals with generalized anxiety disorder report subjective distress due to constant worry and related impairment in social, occupational, or other important areas of functioning.

The anxiety and worry are accompanied by at least three of the following additional symptoms: restlessness or feeling keyed up or on edge, being easily fatigued, difficulty concentrating or mind going blank, irritability, muscle tension, and disturbed sleep, although only one additional symptom is required in children.

Associated Features Supporting Diagnosis

Associated with muscle tension, there may be trembling, twitching, feeling shaky, and muscle aches or soreness. Many individuals with generalized anxiety disorder also experience somatic symptoms (e.g., sweating, nausea, diarrhea) and an exaggerated startle response. Symptoms of autonomic hyperarousal (e.g., accelerated heart rate, shortness of breath, dizziness) are less prominent in generalized anxiety disorder than in other anxiety disorders, such as panic disorder. Other conditions that may be associated with stress (e.g., irritable bowel syndrome, headaches) frequently accompany generalized anxiety disorder.

Prevalence

The 12-month prevalence of generalized anxiety disorder is 0.9% among adolescents and 2.9% among adults in the general community of the United States. The 12-month prevalence for the disorder in other countries ranges from 0.4% to 3.6%. The lifetime morbid risk is 9.0%. Females are twice as likely as males to experience generalized anxiety disorder. The prevalence of the diagnosis peaks in middle age and declines across the later years of life.

Individuals of European descent tend to experience generalized anxiety disorder more frequently than do individuals of non-European descent (i.e., Asian, African, Native American and Pacific Islander). Furthermore, individuals from developed countries are more likely than individuals from nondeveloped countries to report that they have experienced symptoms that meet criteria for generalized anxiety disorder in their lifetime.

Development and Course

Many individuals with generalized anxiety disorder report that they have felt anxious and nervous all of their lives. The median age at onset for generalized anxiety disorder is 30 years; however, age at onset is spread over a very broad range. The median age at onset is later than that for the other anxiety disorders. The symptoms of excessive worry and anxiety may occur early in life but are then manifested as an anxious temperament. Onset of the disorder rarely occurs prior to adolescence. The symptoms of generalized anxiety disorder tend to be chronic and wax and wane across the lifespan, fluctuating between syndromal and subsyndromal forms of the disorder. Rates of full remission are very low.

The clinical expression of generalized anxiety disorder is relatively consistent across the lifespan. The primary difference across age groups is in the content of the individual's worry. Children and adolescents tend to worry more about school and sporting performance, whereas older adults report greater concern about the well-being of family or their own physical heath. Thus, the content of an individual's worry tends to be age appropriate. Younger adults experience greater severity of symptoms than do older adults.

The earlier in life individuals have symptoms that meet criteria for generalized anxiety disorder, the more comorbidity they tend to have and the more impaired they are likely to be. The advent of chronic physical disease can be a potent issue for excessive worry in the elderly. In the frail elderly, worries about safety—and especially about falling—may limit activities. In those with early cognitive impairment, what appears to be excessive worry about, for example, the whereabouts of things is probably better regarded as realistic given the cognitive impairment.

In children and adolescents with generalized anxiety disorder, the anxieties and worries often concern the quality of their performance or competence at school or in sporting events, even when their performance is not being evaluated by others. There may be excessive concerns about punctuality. They may also worry about catastrophic events, such as earthquakes or nuclear war. Children with the disorder may be overly conforming, perfectionist, and unsure of themselves and tend to redo tasks because of excessive dissatisfaction with less-than-perfect performance. They are typically overzealous in seeking reassurance and approval and require excessive reassurance about their performance and other things they are worried about.

Generalized anxiety disorder may be overdiagnosed in children. When this diagnosis is being considered in children, a thorough evaluation for the presence of other childhood anxiety disorders and other mental disorders should be done to determine whether the worries may be better explained by one of these disorders. Separation anxiety disorder, social anxiety disorder (social phobia), and obsessive-compulsive disorder are often accompanied by worries that may mimic those described in generalized anxiety disorder. For example, a child with social anxiety disorder may be concerned about school performance because of fear of humiliation. Worries about illness may also be better explained by separation anxiety disorder or obsessive-compulsive disorder.

Risk and Prognostic Factors

Temperamental.   Behavioral inhibition, negative affectivity (neuroticism), and harm avoidance have been associated with generalized anxiety disorder.

Environmental.   Although childhood adversities and parental overprotection have been associated with generalized anxiety disorder, no environmental factors have been identified as specific to generalized anxiety disorder or necessary or sufficient for making the diagnosis.

Genetic and physiological.   One-third of the risk of experiencing generalized anxiety disorder is genetic, and these genetic factors overlap with the risk of neuroticism and are shared with other anxiety and mood disorders, particularly major depressive disorder.

Culture-Related Diagnostic Issues

There is considerable cultural variation in the expression of generalized anxiety disorder. For example, in some cultures, somatic symptoms predominate in the expression of the disorder, whereas in other cultures cognitive symptoms tend to predominate. This difference may be more evident on initial presentation than subsequently, as more symptoms are reported over time. There is no information as to whether the propensity for excessive worrying is related to culture, although the topic being worried about can be culture specific. It is important to consider the social and cultural context when evaluating whether worries about certain situations are excessive.

Gender-Related Diagnostic Issues

In clinical settings, generalized anxiety disorder is diagnosed somewhat more frequently in females than in males (about 55%–60% of those presenting with the disorder are female). In epidemiological studies, approximately two-thirds are female. Females and males who experience generalized anxiety disorder appear to have similar symptoms but demonstrate different patterns of comorbidity consistent with gender differences in the prevalence of disorders. In females, comorbidity is largely confined to the anxiety disorders and unipolar depression, whereas in males, comorbidity is more likely to extend to the substance use disorders as well.

Functional Consequences of Generalized Anxiety Disorder

Excessive worrying impairs the individual's capacity to do things quickly and efficiently, whether at home or at work. The worrying takes time and energy; the associated symptoms of muscle tension and feeling keyed up or on edge, tiredness, difficulty concentrating, and disturbed sleep contribute to the impairment. Importantly the excessive worrying may impair the ability of individuals with generalized anxiety disorder to encourage confidence in their children.

Generalized anxiety disorder is associated with significant disability and distress that is independent of comorbid disorders, and most non-institutionalized adults with the disorder are moderately to seriously disabled. Generalized anxiety disorder accounts for 110 million disability days per annum in the U.S. population.

Differential Diagnosis

Anxiety disorder due to another medical condition.   The diagnosis of anxiety disorder associated with another medical condition should be assigned if the individual's anxiety and worry are judged, based on history, laboratory findings, or physical examination, to be a physiological effect of another specific medical condition (e.g., pheochromocytoma, hyperthyroidism).

Substance/medication-induced anxiety disorder.   A substance/medication-induced anxiety disorder is distinguished from generalized anxiety disorder by the fact that a substance or medication (e.g., a drug of abuse, exposure to a toxin) is judged to be etiologically related to the anxiety. For example, severe anxiety that occurs only in the context of heavy coffee consumption would be diagnosed as caffeine-induced anxiety disorder.

Social anxiety disorder.   Individuals with social anxiety disorder often have anticipatory anxiety that is focused on upcoming social situations in which they must perform or be evaluated by others, whereas individuals with generalized anxiety disorder worry, whether or not they are being evaluated.

Obsessive-compulsive disorder.   Several features distinguish the excessive worry of generalized anxiety disorder from the obsessional thoughts of obsessive-compulsive disorder. In generalized anxiety disorder the focus of the worry is about forthcoming problems, and it is the excessiveness of the worry about future events that is abnormal. In obsessive-compulsive disorder, the obsessions are inappropriate ideas that take the form of intrusive and unwanted thoughts, urges, or images.

Posttraumatic stress disorder and adjustment disorders.   Anxiety is invariably present in posttraumatic stress disorder. Generalized anxiety disorder is not diagnosed if the anxiety and worry are better explained by symptoms of posttraumatic stress disorder. Anxiety may also be present in adjustment disorder, but this residual category should be used only when the criteria are not met for any other disorder (including generalized anxiety disorder). Moreover, in adjustment disorders, the anxiety occurs in response to an identifiable stressor within 3 months of the onset of the stressor and does not persist for more than 6 months after the termination of the stressor or its consequences.

Depressive, bipolar, and psychotic disorders.   Although generalized anxiety/worry is a common associated feature of depressive, bipolar, and psychotic disorders, generalized anxiety disorder may be diagnosed comorbidly if the anxiety/worry is sufficiently severe to warrant clinical attention.

Comorbidity

Individuals whose presentation meets criteria for generalized anxiety disorder are likely to have met, or currently meet, criteria for other anxiety and unipolar depressive disorders. The neuroticism or emotional liability that underpins this pattern of comorbidity is associated with temperamental antecedents and genetic and environmental risk factors shared between these disorders, although independent pathways are also possible. Comorbidity with substance use, conduct, psychotic, neurodevelopmental, and neurocognitive disorders is less common.

Substance/Medication-Induced Anxiety Disorder

Diagnostic Criteria

A. Panic attacks or anxiety is predominant in the clinical picture.
B. There is evidence from the history, physical examination, or laboratory findings of both (1) and (2):
   1. The symptoms in Criterion A developed during or soon after substance intoxication or withdrawal or after exposure to a medication.
   2. The involved substance/medication is capable of producing the symptoms in Criterion A.
C. The disturbance is not better explained by an anxiety disorder that is not substance/medication-induced. Such evidence of an independent anxiety disorder could include the following:

   The symptoms precede the onset of the substance/medication use; the symptoms persist for a substantial period of time (e.g., about 1 month) after the cessation of acute withdrawal or severe intoxication; or there is other evidence suggesting the existence of an independent non-substance/medication-induced anxiety disorder (e.g., a history of recurrent non-substance/medication-related episodes).
D. The disturbance does not occur exclusively during the course of a delirium.
E. The disturbance causes clinically significant distress or impairment in social, occupational, or other important areas of functioning.

Note: This diagnosis should be made instead of a diagnosis of substance intoxication or substance withdrawal only when the symptoms in Criterion A predominate in the clinical picture and they are sufficiently severe to warrant clinical attention.

Coding note: The ICD-9-CM and ICD-10-CM codes for the [specific substance/medication]-induced anxiety disorders are indicated in the table below. Note that the ICD-10-CM code depends on whether or not there is a comorbid substance use disorder present for the same class of substance. If a mild substance use disorder is comorbid with the substance-induced anxiety disorder, the 4th position character is "1," and the clinician should record "mild [substance] use disorder" before the substance-induced anxiety disorder (e.g., "mild cocaine use disorder with cocaine-induced anxiety disorder"). If a moderate or severe substance use disorder is comorbid with the substance-induced anxiety disorder, the 4th position character is "2," and the clinician should record "moderate [substance] use disorder" or "severe [substance] use disorder," depending on the severity of the comorbid substance use disorder. If there is no comorbid substance use disorder (e.g., after a one-time heavy use of the substance), then the 4th position character is "9," and the clinician should record only the substance-induced anxiety disorder.

	ICD-9-CM	ICD-10-CM		
		With use disorder, mild	With use disorder, moderate or severe	Without use disorder
Alcohol	291.89	F10.180	F10.280	F10.980
Caffeine	292.89	F15.180	F15.280	F15.980
Cannabis	292.89	F12.180	F12.280	F12.980
Phencyclidine	292.89	F16.180	F16.280	F16.980
Other hallucinogen	292.89	F16.180	F16.280	F16.980
Inhalant	292.89	F18.180	F18.280	F18.980
Opioid	292.89	F11.188	F11.288	F11.988
Sedative, hypnotic, or anxiolytic	292.89	F13.180	F13.280	F13.980
Amphetamine (or other stimulant)	292.89	F15.180	F15.280	F15.980
Cocaine	292.89	F14.180	F14.280	F14.980
Other (or unknown) substance	292.89	F19.180	F19.280	F19.980

Specify if (see Table 1 in the chapter "Substance-Related and Addictive Disorders" for diagnoses associated with substance class):

With onset during intoxication: This specifier applies if criteria are met for intoxication with the substance and the symptoms develop during intoxication.

With onset during withdrawal: This specifier applies if criteria are met for withdrawal from the substance and the symptoms develop during, or shortly after, withdrawal.

With onset after medication use: Symptoms may appear either at initiation of medication or after a modification or change in use.

Recording Procedures

ICD-9-CM.   The name of the substance/medication-induced anxiety disorder begins with the specific substance (e.g., cocaine, salbutamol) that is presumed to be causing the anxiety symptoms. The diagnostic code is selected from the table included in the criteria set, which is based on the drug class. For substances that do not fit into any of the classes (e.g., salbutamol), the code for "other substance" should be used; and in cases in which a substance is judged to be an etiological factor but the specific class of substance is unknown, the category "unknown substance" should be used.

The name of the disorder is followed by the specification of onset (i.e., onset during intoxication, onset during withdrawal, with onset during medication use). Unlike the recording procedures for ICD-10-CM, which combine the substance-induced disorder and substance use disorder into a single code, for ICD-9-CM a separate diagnostic code is given for the substance use disorder. For example, in the case of anxiety symptoms occurring during withdrawal in a man with a severe lorazepam use disorder, the diagnosis is 292.89 lorazepam-induced anxiety disorder, with onset during withdrawal. An additional diagnosis of 304.10 severe lorazepam use disorder is also given. When more than one substance is judged to play a significant role in the development of anxiety symptoms, each should be listed separately (e.g., 292.89 methylphenidate-induced anxiety disorder, with onset during intoxication; 292.89 salbutamol-induced anxiety disorder, with onset after medication use).

ICD-10-CM.   The name of the substance/medication-induced anxiety disorder begins with the specific substance (e.g., cocaine, salbutamol) that is presumed to be causing the anxiety symptoms. The diagnostic code is selected from the table included in the criteria set, which is based on the drug class and presence or absence of a comorbid substance use disorder. For substances that do not fit into any of the classes (e.g., salbutamol), the code for "other substance" should be used; and in cases in which a substance is judged to be an etiological factor but the specific class of substance is unknown, the category "unknown substance" should be used.

When recording the name of the disorder, the comorbid substance use disorder (if any) is listed first, followed by the word "with," followed by the name of the substance-induced anxiety disorder, followed by the specification of onset (i.e., onset during intoxication, onset during withdrawal, with onset during medication use). For example, in the case of anxiety symptoms occurring during withdrawal in a man with a severe lorazepam use disorder, the diagnosis is F13.280 severe lorazepam use disorder with lorazepam-induced anxiety disorder, with onset during withdrawal. A separate diagnosis of the comorbid severe lorazepam use disorder is not given. If the substance-induced anxiety disorder occurs without a comorbid substance use disorder (e.g., after a one-time heavy use of the substance), no accompanying substance use disorder is noted (e.g., F16.980 psilocybin-induced anxiety disorder, with onset during intoxication). When more than one substance is judged to play a significant role in the development of anxiety symptoms, each should be listed separately (e.g., F15.280 severe methylphenidate use disorder with methylphenidate-induced anxiety disorder, with onset during intoxication; F19.980 salbutamol-induced anxiety disorder, with onset after medication use).

Diagnostic Features

The essential features of substance/medication-induced anxiety disorder are prominent symptoms of panic or anxiety (Criterion A) that are judged to be due to the effects of a substance (e.g., a drug of abuse, a medication, or a toxin exposure). The panic or anxiety symptoms must have developed during or soon after substance intoxication or withdrawal or after exposure to a medication, and the substances or medications must be capable of producing the symptoms (Criterion B2). Substance/medication-induced anxiety disorder due to a prescribed treatment for a mental disorder or another medical condition must have its onset while the individual is receiving the medication (or during withdrawal, if a withdrawal is associated with the medication). Once the treatment is discontinued, the panic or anxiety symptoms will usually improve or remit within days to several weeks to a month (depending on the half-life of the substance/medication and the presence of withdrawal). The diagnosis of substance/medication-induced anxiety disorder should not be given if the onset of the panic or anxiety symptoms precedes the substance/medication intoxication or withdrawal, or if the symptoms persist for a substantial period of time (i.e., usually longer than 1 month) from the time of severe intoxication or withdrawal. If the panic or anxiety symptoms persist for substantial periods of time, other causes for the symptoms should be considered.

The substance/medication-induced anxiety disorder diagnosis should be made instead of a diagnosis of substance intoxication or substance withdrawal only when the symptoms in Criterion A are predominant in the clinical picture and are sufficiently severe to warrant independent clinical attention.

Associated Features Supporting Diagnosis

Panic or anxiety can occur in association with intoxication with the following classes of substances: alcohol, caffeine, cannabis, phencyclidine, other hallucinogens, inhalants, stimulants (including cocaine), and other (or unknown) substances. Panic or anxiety can occur in association with withdrawal from the following classes of substances: alcohol; opioids; sedatives, hypnotics, and anxiolytics; stimulants (including cocaine); and other (or unknown) substances. Some medications that evoke anxiety symptoms include anesthetics and analgesics, sympathomimetics or other bronchodilators, anticholinergics, insulin, thyroid preparations, oral contraceptives, antihistamines, antiparkinsonian medications, corticosteroids, antihypertensive and cardiovascular medications, anticonvulsants, lithium carbonate, antipsychotic medications, and antidepressant medications. Heavy metals and toxins (e.g., organophosphate insecticide, nerve gases, carbon monoxide, carbon dioxide, volatile substances such as gasoline and paint) may also cause panic or anxiety symptoms.

Prevalence

The prevalence of substance/medication-induced anxiety disorder is not clear. General population data suggest that it may be rare, with a 12-month prevalence of approximately 0.002%. However, in clinical populations, the prevalence is likely to be higher.

Diagnostic Markers

Laboratory assessments (e.g., urine toxicology) may be useful to measure substance intoxication as part of an assessment for substance/medication-induced anxiety disorder.

Differential Diagnosis

Substance intoxication and substance withdrawal.   Anxiety symptoms commonly occur in substance intoxication and substance withdrawal. The diagnosis of the substance-specific intoxication or substance-specific withdrawal will usually suffice to categorize the symptom presentation. A diagnosis of substance/medication-induced anxiety disorder should be made in addition to substance intoxication or substance withdrawal when the panic or anxiety symptoms are predominant in the clinical picture and are sufficiently severe to warrant independent clinical attention. For example, panic or anxiety symptoms are characteristic of alcohol withdrawal.

Anxiety disorder (i.e., not induced by a substance/medication).   Substance/medication-induced anxiety disorder is judged to be etiologically related to the substance/medication. Substance/medication-induced anxiety disorder is distinguished from a primary anxiety disorder based on the onset, course, and other factors with respect to substances/medications. For drugs of abuse, there must be evidence from the history, physical examination, or laboratory findings for use, intoxication, or withdrawal. Substance/medication-induced anxiety disorders arise only in association with intoxication or withdrawal states, whereas primary anxiety disorders may precede the onset of substance/medication use. The presence of features that are atypical of a primary anxiety disorder, such as atypical age at onset (e.g., onset of panic disorder after age 45 years) or symptoms (e.g., atypical panic attack symptoms such as true vertigo, loss of balance, loss of consciousness, loss of bladder control, headaches, slurred speech) may suggest a substance/medication-induced etiology. A primary anxiety disorder diagnosis is warranted if the panic or anxiety symptoms persist for a substantial period of time (about 1 month or longer) after the end of the substance intoxication or acute withdrawal or there is a history of an anxiety disorder.

Delirium.   If panic or anxiety symptoms occur exclusively during the course of delirium, they are considered to be an associated feature of the delirium and are not diagnosed separately.

Anxiety disorder due to another medical condition.   If the panic or anxiety symptoms are attributed to the physiological consequences of another medical condition (i.e., rather than to the medication taken for the medical condition), anxiety disorder due to another medical condition should be diagnosed. The history often provides the basis for such a judgment. At times, a change in the treatment for the other medical condition (e.g., medication substitution or discontinuation) may be needed to determine whether the medication is the causative agent (in which case the symptoms may be better explained by substance/medication-induced anxiety disorder). If the disturbance is attributable to both another medical condition and substance use, both diagnoses (i.e., anxiety disorder due to another medical condition and substance/medication-induced anxiety disorder) may be given. When there is insufficient evidence to determine whether the panic or anxiety symptoms are attributable to a substance/medication or to another medical condition or are primary (i.e., not attributable to either a substance or another medical condition), a diagnosis of other specified or unspecified anxiety disorder would be indicated.

Anxiety Disorder Due to Another Medical Condition

Diagnostic Criteria   293.84 (F06.4)

A. Panic attacks or anxiety is predominant in the clinical picture.
B. There is evidence from the history, physical examination, or laboratory findings that the disturbance is the direct pathophysiological consequence of another medical condition.
C. The disturbance is not better explained by another mental disorder.
D. The disturbance does not occur exclusively during the course of a delirium.
E. The disturbance causes clinically significant distress or impairment in social, occupational, or other important areas of functioning.

Coding note: Include the name of the other medical condition within the name of the mental disorder (e.g., 293.84 [F06.4] anxiety disorder due to pheochromocytoma). The other medical condition should be coded and listed separately immediately before the anxiety disorder due to the medical condition (e.g., 227.0 [D35.00] pheochromocytoma; 293.84 [F06.4] anxiety disorder due to pheochromocytoma).

Diagnostic Features

The essential feature of anxiety disorder due to another medical condition is clinically significant anxiety that is judged to be best explained as a physiological effect of another medical condition. Symptoms can include prominent anxiety symptoms or panic attacks (Criterion A). The judgment that the symptoms are best explained by the associated physical condition must be based on evidence from the history, physical examination, or laboratory findings (Criterion B). Additionally, it must be judged that the symptoms are not better accounted for by another mental disorder, in particular, adjustment disorder, with anxiety, in which the stressor is the medical condition (Criterion C). In this case, an individual with adjustment disorder is especially distressed about the meaning or the consequences of the associated medical condition. By contrast, there is often a prominent physical component to the anxiety (e.g., shortness of breath) when the anxiety is due to another medical condition. The diagnosis is not made if the anxiety symptoms occur only during the course of a delirium (Criterion D). The anxiety symptoms must cause clinically significant distress or impairment in social, occupational, or other important areas of functioning (Criterion E).

In determining whether the anxiety symptoms are attributable to another medical condition, the clinician must first establish the presence of the medical condition. Furthermore, it must be established that anxiety symptoms can be etiologically related to the medical condition through a physiological mechanism before making a judgment that this is the best explanation for the symptoms in a specific individual. A careful and comprehensive assessment of multiple factors is necessary to make this judgment. Several aspects of the clinical presentation should be considered: 1) the presence of a clear temporal association between the onset, exacerbation, or remission of the medical condition and the anxiety symptoms; 2) the presence of features that are atypical of a primary anxiety disorder (e.g., atypical age at onset or course); and 3) evidence in the literature that a known physiological mechanism (e.g., hyperthyroidism) causes anxiety. In addition, the disturbance must not be better explained by a primary anxiety disorder, a substance/medication-induced anxiety disorder, or another primary mental disorder (e.g., adjustment disorder).

Associated Features Supporting Diagnosis

A number of medical conditions are known to include anxiety as a symptomatic manifestation. Examples include endocrine disease (e.g., hyperthyroidism, pheochromocytoma, hypoglycemia, hyperadrenocortisolism), cardiovascular disorders (e.g., congestive heart failure, pulmonary embolism, arrhythmia such as atrial fibrillation), respiratory illness (e.g., chronic obstructive pulmonary disease, asthma, pneumonia), metabolic disturbances (e.g., vitamin B_{12} deficiency, porphyria), and neurological illness (e.g., neoplasms, vestibular dysfunction, encephalitis, seizure disorders). Anxiety due to another medical condition is diagnosed when the medical condition is known to induce anxiety and when the medical condition preceded the onset of the anxiety.

Prevalence

The prevalence of anxiety disorder due to another medical condition is unclear. There appears to be an elevated prevalence of anxiety disorders among individuals with a variety of medical conditions, including asthma, hypertension, ulcers, and arthritis. However, this increased prevalence may be due to reasons other than the anxiety disorder directly causing the medical condition.

Development and Course

The development and course of anxiety disorder due to another medical condition generally follows the course of the underlying illness. This diagnosis is not meant to include primary anxiety disorders that arise in the context of chronic medical illness. This is important to consider with older adults, who may experience chronic medical illness and then develop independent anxiety disorders secondary to the chronic medical illness.

Diagnostic Markers

Laboratory assessments and/or medical examinations are necessary to confirm the diagnosis of the associated medical condition.

Differential Diagnosis

Delirium.   A separate diagnosis of anxiety disorder due to another medical condition is not given if the anxiety disturbance occurs exclusively during the course of a delirium. However, a diagnosis of anxiety disorder due to another medical condition may be given in addition to a diagnosis of major neurocognitive disorder (dementia) if the etiology of anxiety is judged to be a physiological consequence of the pathological process causing the neurocognitive disorder and if anxiety is a prominent part of the clinical presentation.

Mixed presentation of symptoms (e.g., mood and anxiety).   If the presentation includes a mix of different types of symptoms, the specific mental disorder due to another medical condition depends on which symptoms predominate in the clinical picture.

Substance/medication-induced anxiety disorder.   If there is evidence of recent or prolonged substance use (including medications with psychoactive effects), withdrawal from a substance, or exposure to a toxin, a substance/medication-induced anxiety disorder should be considered. Certain medications are known to increase anxiety (e.g., corticosteroids, estrogens, metoclopramide), and when this is the case, the medication may be the most likely etiology, although it may be difficult to distinguish whether the anxiety is attributable to the medications or to the medical illness itself. When a diagnosis of substance-induced anxiety is being made in relation to recreational or nonprescribed drugs, it may be useful to obtain a urine or blood drug screen or other appropriate laboratory evaluation. Symptoms that occur during or shortly after (i.e., within 4 weeks of) substance intoxication or withdrawal or after medication use may be especially indicative of a substance/medication-induced anxiety disorder, depending on the type, duration, or amount of the substance used. If the disturbance is associated with both another medical condition and substance use, both diagnoses (i.e., anxiety disorder due to another medical condition and substance/medication-induced anxiety disorder) can be given. Features such as onset after age 45 years or the presence of atypical symptoms during a panic attack (e.g., vertigo, loss of consciousness, loss of bladder or bowel control, slurred speech, amnesia) suggest the possibility that another medical condition or a substance may be causing the panic attack symptoms.

Anxiety disorder (not due to a known medical condition).   Anxiety disorder due to another medical condition should be distinguished from other anxiety disorders (especially panic disorder and generalized anxiety disorder). In other anxiety disorders, no specific and direct causative physiological mechanisms associated with another medical condition can be demonstrated. Late age at onset, atypical symptoms, and the absence of a personal or family history of anxiety disorders suggest the need for a thorough assessment to rule out the diagnosis of anxiety disorder due to another medical condition. Anxiety disorders can exacerbate or pose increased risk for medical conditions such as cardiovascular events and myocardial infarction and should not be diagnosed as anxiety disorder due to another medical condition in these cases.

Illness anxiety disorder.   Anxiety disorder due to another medical condition should be distinguished from illness anxiety disorder. Illness anxiety disorder is characterized by worry about illness, concern about pain, and bodily preoccupations. In the case of illness anxiety disorder, individuals may or may not have diagnosed medical conditions. Although an individual with illness anxiety disorder and a diagnosed medical condition is likely to experience anxiety about the medical condition, the medical condition is not physiologically related to the anxiety symptoms.

Adjustment disorders.   Anxiety disorder due to another medical condition should be distinguished from adjustment disorders, with anxiety, or with anxiety and depressed mood. Adjustment disorder is warranted when individuals experience a maladaptive response to the stress of having another medical condition. The reaction to stress usually concerns the meaning or consequences of the stress, as compared with the experience of anxiety or mood symptoms that occur as a physiological consequence of the other medical condition. In adjustment disorder, the anxiety symptoms are typically related to coping with the stress of having a general medical condition, whereas in anxiety disorder due to another medical condition, individuals are more likely to have prominent physical symptoms and to be focused on issues other than the stress of the illness itself.

Associated feature of another mental disorder.   Anxiety symptoms may be an associated feature of another mental disorder (e.g., schizophrenia, anorexia nervosa).

Other specified or unspecified anxiety disorder.   This diagnosis is given if it cannot be determined whether the anxiety symptoms are primary, substance-induced, or associated with another medical condition.

Other Specified Anxiety Disorder

300.09 (F41.8)

This category applies to presentations in which symptoms characteristic of an anxiety disorder that cause clinically significant distress or impairment in social, occupational, or other important areas of functioning predominate but do not meet the full criteria for any of the disorders in the anxiety disorders diagnostic class. The other specified anxiety disorder category is used in situations in which the clinician chooses to communicate the specific reason that the presentation does not meet the criteria for any specific anxiety disorder. This is done by recording "other specified anxiety disorder" followed by the specific reason (e.g., "generalized anxiety not occurring more days than not").

Examples of presentations that can be specified using the "other specified" designation include the following:

1. **Limited-symptom attacks.**
2. **Generalized anxiety not occurring more days than not.**
3. *Khyâl cap* **(wind attacks):** See "Glossary of Cultural Concepts of Distress" in the Appendix.
4. *Ataque de nervios* **(attack of nerves):** See "Glossary of Cultural Concepts of Distress" in the Appendix.

Unspecified Anxiety Disorder

300.00 (F41.9)

This category applies to presentations in which symptoms characteristic of an anxiety disorder that cause clinically significant distress or impairment in social, occupational, or other important areas of functioning predominate but do not meet the full criteria for any of the disorders in the anxiety disorders diagnostic class. The unspecified anxiety disorder category is used in situations in which the clinician chooses *not* to specify the reason that the criteria are not met for a specific anxiety disorder, and includes presentations in which there is insufficient information to make a more specific diagnosis (e.g., in emergency room settings).

Obsessive-Compulsive and Related Disorders

Obsessive-compulsive and related disorders include obsessive-compulsive disorder (OCD), body dysmorphic disorder, hoarding disorder, trichotillomania (hair-pulling disorder), excoriation (skin-picking) disorder, substance/medication-induced obsessive-compulsive and related disorder, obsessive-compulsive and related disorder due to another medical condition, and other specified obsessive-compulsive and related disorder and unspecified obsessive-compulsive and related disorder (e.g., body-focused repetitive behavior disorder, obsessional jealousy).

OCD is characterized by the presence of obsessions and/or compulsions. *Obsessions* are recurrent and persistent thoughts, urges, or images that are experienced as intrusive and unwanted, whereas *compulsions* are repetitive behaviors or mental acts that an individual feels driven to perform in response to an obsession or according to rules that must be applied rigidly. Some other obsessive-compulsive and related disorders are also characterized by preoccupations and by repetitive behaviors or mental acts in response to the preoccupations. Other obsessive-compulsive and related disorders are characterized primarily by recurrent body-focused repetitive behaviors (e.g., hair pulling, skin picking) and repeated attempts to decrease or stop the behaviors.

The inclusion of a chapter on obsessive-compulsive and related disorders in DSM-5 reflects the increasing evidence of these disorders' relatedness to one another in terms of a range of diagnostic validators as well as the clinical utility of grouping these disorders in the same chapter. Clinicians are encouraged to screen for these conditions in individuals who present with one of them and be aware of overlaps between these conditions. At the same time, there are important differences in diagnostic validators and treatment approaches across these disorders. Moreover, there are close relationships between the anxiety disorders and some of the obsessive-compulsive and related disorders (e.g., OCD), which is reflected in the sequence of DSM-5 chapters, with obsessive-compulsive and related disorders following anxiety disorders.

The obsessive-compulsive and related disorders differ from developmentally normative preoccupations and rituals by being excessive or persisting beyond developmentally appropriate periods. The distinction between the presence of subclinical symptoms and a clinical disorder requires assessment of a number of factors, including the individual's level of distress and impairment in functioning.

The chapter begins with OCD. It then covers body dysmorphic disorder and hoarding disorder, which are characterized by cognitive symptoms such as perceived defects or flaws in physical appearance or the perceived need to save possessions, respectively. The chapter then covers trichotillomania (hair-pulling disorder) and excoriation (skin-picking) disorder, which are characterized by recurrent body-focused repetitive behaviors. Finally, it covers substance/medication-induced obsessive-compulsive and related disorder, obsessive-compulsive and related disorder due to another medical condition, and other specified obsessive-compulsive and related disorder and unspecified obsessive-compulsive and related disorder.

While the specific content of obsessions and compulsions varies among individuals, certain symptom dimensions are common in OCD, including those of cleaning (contamination obsessions and cleaning compulsions); symmetry (symmetry obsessions and repeating, ordering, and counting compulsions); forbidden or taboo thoughts (e.g., aggressive, sexual, and religious obsessions and related compulsions); and harm (e.g., fears of harm to oneself or others and related checking compulsions). The tic-related specifier of OCD is used when an individual has a current or past history of a tic disorder.

Body dysmorphic disorder is characterized by preoccupation with one or more perceived defects or flaws in physical appearance that are not observable or appear only slight to others, and by repetitive behaviors (e.g., mirror checking, excessive grooming, skin picking, or reassurance seeking) or mental acts (e.g., comparing one's appearance with that of other people) in response to the appearance concerns. The appearance preoccupations are not better explained by concerns with body fat or weight in an individual with an eating disorder. Muscle dysmorphia is a form of body dysmorphic disorder that is characterized by the belief that one's body build is too small or is insufficiently muscular.

Hoarding disorder is characterized by persistent difficulty discarding or parting with possessions, regardless of their actual value, as a result of a strong perceived need to save the items and to distress associated with discarding them. Hoarding disorder differs from normal collecting. For example, symptoms of hoarding disorder result in the accumulation of a large number of possessions that congest and clutter active living areas to the extent that their intended use is substantially compromised. The excessive acquisition form of hoarding disorder, which characterizes most but not all individuals with hoarding disorder, consists of excessive collecting, buying, or stealing of items that are not needed or for which there is no available space.

Trichotillomania (hair-pulling disorder) is characterized by recurrent pulling out of one's hair resulting in hair loss, and repeated attempts to decrease or stop hair pulling. Excoriation (skin-picking) disorder is characterized by recurrent picking of one's skin resulting in skin lesions and repeated attempts to decrease or stop skin picking. The body-focused repetitive behaviors that characterize these two disorders are not triggered by obsessions or preoccupations; however, they may be preceded or accompanied by various emotional states, such as feelings of anxiety or boredom. They may also be preceded by an increasing sense of tension or may lead to gratification, pleasure, or a sense of relief when the hair is pulled out or the skin is picked. Individuals with these disorders may have varying degrees of conscious awareness of the behavior while engaging in it, with some individuals displaying more focused attention on the behavior (with preceding tension and subsequent relief) and other individuals displaying more automatic behavior (with the behaviors seeming to occur without full awareness).

Substance/medication-induced obsessive-compulsive and related disorder consists of symptoms that are due to substance intoxication or withdrawal or to a medication. Obsessive-compulsive and related disorder due to another medical condition involves symptoms characteristic of obsessive-compulsive and related disorders that are the direct pathophysiological consequence of a medical disorder. Other specified obsessive-compulsive and related disorder and unspecified obsessive-compulsive and related disorder consist of symptoms that do not meet criteria for a specific obsessive-compulsive and related disorder because of atypical presentation or uncertain etiology; these categories are also used for other specific syndromes that are not listed in Section II and when insufficient information is available to diagnose the presentation as another obsessive-compulsive and related disorder. Examples of specific syndromes not listed in Section II, and therefore diagnosed as other specified obsessive-compulsive and related disorder or as unspecified obsessive-compulsive and related disorder include body-focused repetitive behavior disorder and obsessional jealousy.

Obsessive-compulsive and related disorders that have a cognitive component have insight as the basis for specifiers; in each of these disorders, insight ranges from "good or fair insight" to "poor insight" to "absent insight/delusional beliefs" with respect to disorder-related beliefs. For individuals whose obsessive-compulsive and related disorder symptoms warrant the "with absent insight/delusional beliefs" specifier, these symptoms should not be diagnosed as a psychotic disorder.

Obsessive-Compulsive Disorder

Diagnostic Criteria	**300.3** (F42.2)

A. Presence of obsessions, compulsions, or both:

Obsessions are defined by (1) and (2):

1. Recurrent and persistent thoughts, urges, or images that are experienced, at some time during the disturbance, as intrusive and unwanted, and that in most individuals cause marked anxiety or distress.
2. The individual attempts to ignore or suppress such thoughts, urges, or images, or to neutralize them with some other thought or action (i.e., by performing a compulsion).

Compulsions are defined by (1) and (2):

1. Repetitive behaviors (e.g., hand washing, ordering, checking) or mental acts (e.g., praying, counting, repeating words silently) that the individual feels driven to per- form in response to an obsession or according to rules that must be applied rigidly.
2. The behaviors or mental acts are aimed at preventing or reducing anxiety or dis- tress, or preventing some dreaded event or situation; however, these behaviors or mental acts are not connected in a realistic way with what they are designed to neu- tralize or prevent, or are clearly excessive.
   Note: Young children may not be able to articulate the aims of these behaviors or mental acts.

B. The obsessions or compulsions are time-consuming (e.g., take more than 1 hour per day) or cause clinically significant distress or impairment in social, occupational, or other important areas of functioning.

C. The obsessive-compulsive symptoms are not attributable to the physiological effects of a substance (e.g., a drug of abuse, a medication) or another medical condition.

D. The disturbance is not better explained by the symptoms of another mental disorder (e.g., excessive worries, as in generalized anxiety disorder; preoccupation with ap- pearance, as in body dysmorphic disorder; difficulty discarding or parting with posses- sions, as in hoarding disorder; hair pulling, as in trichotillomania [hair-pulling disorder]; skin picking, as in excoriation [skin-picking] disorder; stereotypies, as in stereotypic movement disorder; ritualized eating behavior, as in eating disorders; preoccupation with substances or gambling, as in substance-related and addictive disorders; preoc- cupation with having an illness, as in illness anxiety disorder; sexual urges or fantasies, as in paraphilic disorders; impulses, as in disruptive, impulse-control, and conduct dis- orders; guilty ruminations, as in major depressive disorder; thought insertion or delu- sional preoccupations, as in schizophrenia spectrum and other psychotic disorders; or repetitive patterns of behavior, as in autism spectrum disorder).

Specify if:
   With good or fair insight: The individual recognizes that obsessive-compulsive dis- order beliefs are definitely or probably not true or that they may or may not be true.
   With poor insight: The individual thinks obsessive-compulsive disorder beliefs are probably true.
   With absent insight/delusional beliefs: The individual is completely convinced that obsessive-compulsive disorder beliefs are true.

Specify if:
   Tic-related: The individual has a current or past history of a tic disorder.

Specifiers

Many individuals with obsessive-compulsive disorder (OCD) have dysfunctional beliefs. These beliefs can include an inflated sense of responsibility and the tendency to overestimate threat; perfectionism and intolerance of uncertainty; and over-importance of thoughts (e.g., believing that having a forbidden thought is as bad as acting on it) and the need to control thoughts.

Individuals with OCD vary in the degree of insight they have about the accuracy of the beliefs that underlie their obsessive-compulsive symptoms. Many individuals have *good or fair insight* (e.g., the individual believes that the house definitely will not, probably will not, or may or may not burn down if the stove is not checked 30 times). Some have *poor insight* (e.g., the individual believes that the house will probably burn down if the stove is not checked 30 times), and a few (4% or less) have *absent insight/delusional beliefs* (e.g., the individual is convinced that the house will burn down if the stove is not checked 30 times). Insight can vary within an individual over the course of the illness. Poorer insight has been linked to worse long-term outcome.

Up to 30% of individuals with OCD have a lifetime tic disorder. This is most common in males with onset of OCD in childhood. These individuals tend to differ from those without a history of tic disorders in the themes of their OCD symptoms, comorbidity, course, and pattern of familial transmission.

Diagnostic Features

The characteristic symptoms of OCD are the presence of obsessions and compulsions (Criterion A). *Obsessions* are repetitive and persistent thoughts (e.g., of contamination), images (e.g., of violent or horrific scenes), or urges (e.g., to stab someone). Importantly, obsessions are not pleasurable or experienced as voluntary: they are intrusive and unwanted and cause marked distress or anxiety in most individuals. The individual attempts to ignore or suppress these obsessions (e.g., avoiding triggers or using thought suppression) or to neutralize them with another thought or action (e.g., performing a compulsion). *Compulsions* (or rituals) are repetitive behaviors (e.g., washing, checking) or mental acts (e.g., counting, repeating words silently) that the individual feels driven to perform in response to an obsession or according to rules that must be applied rigidly. Most individuals with OCD have both obsessions and compulsions. Compulsions are typically performed in response to an obsession (e.g., thoughts of contamination leading to washing rituals or that something is incorrect leading to repeating rituals until it feels "just right"). The aim is to reduce the distress triggered by obsessions or to prevent a feared event (e.g., becoming ill). However, these compulsions either are not connected in a realistic way to the feared event (e.g., arranging items symmetrically to prevent harm to a loved one) or are clearly excessive (e.g., showering for hours each day). Compulsions are not done for pleasure, although some individuals experience relief from anxiety or distress.

Criterion B emphasizes that obsessions and compulsions must be time-consuming (e.g., more than 1 hour per day) or cause clinically significant distress or impairment to warrant a diagnosis of OCD. This criterion helps to distinguish the disorder from the occasional intrusive thoughts or repetitive behaviors that are common in the general population (e.g., double-checking that a door is locked). The frequency and severity of obsessions and compulsions vary across individuals with OCD (e.g., some have mild to moderate symptoms, spending 1–3 hours per day obsessing or doing compulsions, whereas others have nearly constant intrusive thoughts or compulsions that can be incapacitating).

Associated Features Supporting Diagnosis

The specific content of obsessions and compulsions varies between individuals. However, certain themes, or dimensions, are common, including those of cleaning (contamination obsessions and cleaning compulsions); symmetry (symmetry obsessions and repeating, ordering, and counting compulsions); forbidden or taboo thoughts (e.g., aggressive, sexual, or religious obsessions and related compulsions); and harm (e.g., fears of harm to oneself or others and checking compulsions). Some individuals also have difficulties discarding and accumulate (hoard) objects as a consequence of typical obsessions and compulsions, such as fears of harming others. These themes occur across different cultures, are relatively consistent over time in adults with the disorder, and may be associated with different neural substrates. Importantly, individuals often have symptoms in more than one dimension.

Individuals with OCD experience a range of affective responses when confronted with situations that trigger obsessions and compulsions. For example, many individuals experience marked anxiety that can include recurrent panic attacks. Others report strong feelings of disgust. While performing compulsions, some individuals report a distressing sense of "incompleteness" or uneasiness until things look, feel, or sound "just right."

It is common for individuals with the disorder to avoid people, places, and things that trigger obsessions and compulsions. For example, individuals with contamination concerns might avoid public situations (e.g., restaurants, public restrooms) to reduce exposure to feared contaminants; individuals with intrusive thoughts about causing harm might avoid social interactions.

Prevalence

The 12-month prevalence of OCD in the United States is 1.2%, with a similar prevalence internationally (1.1%–1.8%). Females are affected at a slightly higher rate than males in adulthood, although males are more commonly affected in childhood.

Development and Course

In the United States, the mean age at onset of OCD is 19.5 years, and 25% of cases start by age 14 years. Onset after age 35 years is unusual but does occur. Males have an earlier age at onset than females: nearly 25% of males have onset before age 10 years. The onset of symptoms is typically gradual; however, acute onset has also been reported.

If OCD is untreated, the course is usually chronic, often with waxing and waning symptoms. Some individuals have an episodic course, and a minority have a deteriorating course. Without treatment, remission rates in adults are low (e.g., 20% for those reevaluated 40 years later). Onset in childhood or adolescence can lead to a lifetime of OCD. However, 40% of individuals with onset of OCD in childhood or adolescence may experience remission by early adulthood. The course of OCD is often complicated by the co-occurrence of other disorders (see section "Comorbidity" for this disorder).

Compulsions are more easily diagnosed in children than obsessions are because compulsions are observable. However, most children have both obsessions and compulsions (as do most adults). The pattern of symptoms in adults can be stable over time, but it is more variable in children. Some differences in the content of obsessions and compulsions have been reported when children and adolescent samples have been compared with adult samples. These differences likely reflect content appropriate to different developmental stages (e.g., higher rates of sexual and religious obsessions in adolescents than in children; higher rates of harm obsessions [e.g., fears of catastrophic events, such as death or illness to self or loved ones] in children and adolescents than in adults).

Risk and Prognostic Factors

Temperamental.   Greater internalizing symptoms, higher negative emotionality, and behavioral inhibition in childhood are possible temperamental risk factors.

Environmental.   Physical and sexual abuse in childhood and other stressful or traumatic events have been associated with an increased risk for developing OCD. Some children may develop the sudden onset of obsessive-compulsive symptoms, which has been associated with different environmental factors, including various infectious agents and a post-infectious autoimmune syndrome.

Genetic and physiological.   The rate of OCD among first-degree relatives of adults with OCD is approximately two times that among first-degree relatives of those without the disorder; however, among first-degree relatives of individuals with onset of OCD in childhood or adolescence, the rate is increased 10-fold. Familial transmission is due in part to genetic factors (e.g., a concordance rate of 0.57 for monozygotic vs. 0.22 for dizygotic twins). Dysfunction in the orbitofrontal cortex, anterior cingulate cortex, and striatum have been most strongly implicated.

Culture-Related Diagnostic Issues

OCD occurs across the world. There is substantial similarity across cultures in the gender distribution, age at onset, and comorbidity of OCD. Moreover, around the globe, there is a similar symptom structure involving cleaning, symmetry, hoarding, taboo thoughts, or fear of harm. However, regional variation in symptom expression exists, and cultural factors may shape the content of obsessions and compulsions.

Gender-Related Diagnostic Issues

Males have an earlier age at onset of OCD than females and are more likely to have comorbid tic disorders. Gender differences in the pattern of symptom dimensions have been reported, with, for example, females more likely to have symptoms in the cleaning dimension and males more likely to have symptoms in the forbidden thoughts and symmetry dimensions. Onset or exacerbation of OCD, as well as symptoms that can interfere with the mother-infant relationship (e.g., aggressive obsessions leading to avoidance of the infant), have been reported in the peripartum period.

Suicide Risk

Suicidal thoughts occur at some point in as many as about half of individuals with OCD. Suicide attempts are also reported in up to one-quarter of individuals with OCD; the presence of comorbid major depressive disorder increases the risk.

Functional Consequences of Obsessive-Compulsive Disorder

OCD is associated with reduced quality of life as well as high levels of social and occupational impairment. Impairment occurs across many different domains of life and is associated with symptom severity. Impairment can be caused by the time spent obsessing and doing compulsions. Avoidance of situations that can trigger obsessions or compulsions can also severely restrict functioning. In addition, specific symptoms can create specific obstacles. For example, obsessions about harm can make relationships with family and friends feel hazardous; the result can be avoidance of these relationships. Obsessions about symmetry can derail the timely completion of school or work projects because the project never feels "just right," potentially resulting in school failure or job loss. Health consequences can also occur. For example, individuals with contamination concerns may avoid doctors' offices and hospitals (e.g., because of fears of exposure to germs) or develop dermatological problems (e.g., skin lesions due to excessive washing). Sometimes the symptoms of the disorder interfere with its own treatment (e.g., when medications are considered contaminated). When the disorder starts in childhood or adolescence, individuals may experience developmental difficulties. For example, adolescents may avoid socializing with peers; young adults may struggle when they leave home to live independently.

The result can be few significant relationships outside the family and a lack of autonomy and financial independence from their family of origin. In addition, some individuals with OCD try to impose rules and prohibitions on family members because of their disorder (e.g., no one in the family can have visitors to the house for fear of contamination), and this can lead to family dysfunction.

Differential Diagnosis

Anxiety disorders.   Recurrent thoughts, avoidant behaviors, and repetitive requests for reassurance can also occur in anxiety disorders. However, the recurrent thoughts that are present in generalized anxiety disorder (i.e., worries) are usually about real-life concerns, whereas the obsessions of OCD usually do not involve real-life concerns and can include content that is odd, irrational, or of a seemingly magical nature; moreover, compulsions are often present and usually linked to the obsessions. Like individuals with OCD, individuals with specific phobia can have a fear reaction to specific objects or situations; however, in specific phobia the feared object is usually much more circumscribed, and rituals are not present. In social anxiety disorder (social phobia), the feared objects or situations are limited to social interactions, and avoidance or reassurance seeking is focused on reducing this social fear.

Major depressive disorder.   OCD can be distinguished from the rumination of major depressive disorder, in which thoughts are usually mood-congruent and not necessarily experienced as intrusive or distressing; moreover, ruminations are not linked to compulsions, as is typical in OCD.

Other obsessive-compulsive and related disorders.   In body dysmorphic disorder, the obsessions and compulsions are limited to concerns about physical appearance; and in trichotillomania (hair-pulling disorder), the compulsive behavior is limited to hair pulling in the absence of obsessions. Hoarding disorder symptoms focus exclusively on the persistent difficulty discarding or parting with possessions, marked distress associated with discarding items, and excessive accumulation of objects. However, if an individual has obsessions that are typical of OCD (e.g., concerns about incompleteness or harm), and these obsessions lead to compulsive hoarding behaviors (e.g., acquiring all objects in a set to attain a sense of completeness or not discarding old newspapers because they may contain information that could prevent harm), a diagnosis of OCD should be given instead.

Eating disorders.   OCD can be distinguished from anorexia nervosa in that in OCD the obsessions and compulsions are not limited to concerns about weight and food.

Tics (in tic disorder) and stereotyped movements.   A *tic* is a sudden, rapid, recurrent, nonrhythmic motor movement or vocalization (e.g., eye blinking, throat clearing). A *stereotyped movement* is a repetitive, seemingly driven, nonfunctional motor behavior (e.g., head banging, body rocking, self-biting). Tics and stereotyped movements are typically less complex than compulsions and are not aimed at neutralizing obsessions. However, distinguishing between complex tics and compulsions can be difficult. Whereas compulsions are usually preceded by obsessions, tics are often preceded by premonitory sensory urges. Some individuals have symptoms of both OCD and a tic disorder, in which case both diagnoses may be warranted.

Psychotic disorders.   Some individuals with OCD have poor insight or even delusional OCD beliefs. However, they have obsessions and compulsions (distinguishing their condition from delusional disorder) and do not have other features of schizophrenia or schizoaffective disorder (e.g., hallucinations or formal thought disorder).

Other compulsive-like behaviors.   Certain behaviors are sometimes described as "compulsive," including sexual behavior (in the case of paraphilias), gambling (i.e., gambling disorder), and substance use (e.g., alcohol use disorder). However, these behaviors differ from the compulsions of OCD in that the person usually derives pleasure from the activity and may wish to resist it only because of its deleterious consequences.

Obsessive-compulsive personality disorder.   Although obsessive-compulsive personality disorder and OCD have similar names, the clinical manifestations of these disorders are quite different. Obsessive-compulsive personality disorder is not characterized by intrusive thoughts, images, or urges or by repetitive behaviors that are performed in response to these intrusions; instead, it involves an enduring and pervasive maladaptive pattern of excessive perfectionism and rigid control. If an individual manifests symptoms of both OCD and obsessive-compulsive personality disorder, both diagnoses can be given.

Comorbidity

Individuals with OCD often have other psychopathology. Many adults with the disorder have a lifetime diagnosis of an anxiety disorder (76%; e.g., panic disorder, social anxiety disorder, generalized anxiety disorder, specific phobia) or a depressive or bipolar disorder (63% for any depressive or bipolar disorder, with the most common being major depressive disorder [41%]). Onset of OCD is usually later than for most comorbid anxiety disorders (with the exception of separation anxiety disorder) and PTSD but often precedes that of depressive disorders. Comorbid obsessive-compulsive personality disorder is also common in individuals with OCD (e.g., ranging from 23% to 32%).

Up to 30% of individuals with OCD also have a lifetime tic disorder. A comorbid tic disorder is most common in males with onset of OCD in childhood. These individuals tend to differ from those without a history of tic disorders in the themes of their OCD symptoms, comorbidity, course, and pattern of familial transmission. A triad of OCD, tic disorder, and attention-deficit/hyperactivity disorder can also be seen in children.

Disorders that occur more frequently in individuals with OCD than in those without the disorder include several obsessive-compulsive and related disorders such as body dysmorphic disorder, trichotillomania (hair-pulling disorder), and excoriation (skin-picking) disorder. Finally, an association between OCD and some disorders characterized by impulsivity, such as oppositional defiant disorder, has been reported.

OCD is also much more common in individuals with certain other disorders than would be expected based on its prevalence in the general population; when one of those other disorders is diagnosed, the individual should be assessed for OCD as well. For example, in individuals with schizophrenia or schizoaffective disorder, the prevalence of OCD is approximately 12%. Rates of OCD are also elevated in bipolar disorder; eating disorders, such as anorexia nervosa and bulimia nervosa; and Tourette's disorder.

Body Dysmorphic Disorder

Diagnostic Criteria   **300.7** (F45.22)

A. Preoccupation with one or more perceived defects or flaws in physical appearance that are not observable or appear slight to others.
B. At some point during the course of the disorder, the individual has performed repetitive behaviors (e.g., mirror checking, excessive grooming, skin picking, reassurance seeking) or mental acts (e.g., comparing his or her appearance with that of others) in response to the appearance concerns.
C. The preoccupation causes clinically significant distress or impairment in social, occupational, or other important areas of functioning.
D. The appearance preoccupation is not better explained by concerns with body fat or weight in an individual whose symptoms meet diagnostic criteria for an eating disorder.

Specify if:

> **With muscle dysmorphia:** The individual is preoccupied with the idea that his or her body build is too small or insufficiently muscular. This specifier is used even if the individual is preoccupied with other body areas, which is often the case.

Specify if:

Indicate degree of insight regarding body dysmorphic disorder beliefs (e.g., "I look ugly" or "I look deformed").

> **With good or fair insight:** The individual recognizes that the body dysmorphic disorder beliefs are definitely or probably not true or that they may or may not be true.
>
> **With poor insight:** The individual thinks that the body dysmorphic disorder beliefs are probably true.
>
> **With absent insight/delusional beliefs:** The individual is completely convinced that the body dysmorphic disorder beliefs are true.

Diagnostic Features

Individuals with body dysmorphic disorder (formerly known as *dysmorphophobia*) are preoccupied with one or more perceived defects or flaws in their physical appearance, which they believe look ugly, unattractive, abnormal, or deformed (Criterion A). The perceived flaws are not observable or appear only slight to other individuals. Concerns range from looking "unattractive" or "not right" to looking "hideous" or "like a monster." Preoccupations can focus on one or many body areas, most commonly the skin (e.g., perceived acne, scars, lines, wrinkles, paleness), hair (e.g., "thinning" hair or "excessive" body or facial hair), or nose (e.g., size or shape). However, any body area can be the focus of concern (e.g., eyes, teeth, weight, stomach, breasts, legs, face size or shape, lips, chin, eyebrows, genitals). Some individuals are concerned about perceived asymmetry of body areas. The preoccupations are intrusive, unwanted, time-consuming (occurring, on average, 3–8 hours per day), and usually difficult to resist or control.

Excessive repetitive behaviors or mental acts (e.g., comparing) are performed in response to the preoccupation (Criterion B). The individual feels driven to perform these behaviors, which are not pleasurable and may increase anxiety and dysphoria. They are typically time-consuming and difficult to resist or control. Common behaviors are comparing one's appearance with that of other individuals; repeatedly checking perceived defects in mirrors or other reflecting surfaces or examining them directly; excessively grooming (e.g., combing, styling, shaving, plucking, or pulling hair); camouflaging (e.g., repeatedly applying makeup or covering disliked areas with such things as a hat, clothing, makeup, or hair); seeking reassurance about how the perceived flaws look; touching disliked areas to check them; excessively exercising or weight lifting; and seeking cosmetic procedures. Some individuals excessively tan (e.g., to darken "pale" skin or diminish perceived acne), repeatedly change their clothes (e.g., to camouflage perceived defects), or compulsively shop (e.g., for beauty products). Compulsive skin picking intended to improve perceived skin defects is common and can cause skin damage, infections, or ruptured blood vessels. The preoccupation must cause clinically significant distress or impairment in social, occupational, or other important areas of functioning (Criterion C); usually both are present. Body dysmorphic disorder must be differentiated from an eating disorder.

Muscle dysmorphia, a form of body dysmorphic disorder occurring almost exclusively in males, consists of preoccupation with the idea that one's body is too small or insufficiently lean or muscular. Individuals with this form of the disorder actually have a normal-looking body or are even very muscular. They may also be preoccupied with other body areas, such as skin or hair. A majority (but not all) diet, exercise, and/or lift weights excessively, sometimes causing bodily damage. Some use potentially dangerous anabolic-androgenic steroids and other substances to try to make their body bigger and more muscular. Body dysmorphic disorder by proxy is a form of body dysmorphic disorder in which individuals are preoccupied with defects they perceive in another person's appearance.

Insight regarding body dysmorphic disorder beliefs can range from good to absent/ delusional (i.e., delusional beliefs consisting of complete conviction that the individual's view of their appearance is accurate and undistorted). On average, insight is poor; one-third or more of individuals currently have delusional body dysmorphic disorder beliefs. Individuals with delusional body dysmorphic disorder tend to have greater morbidity in some areas (e.g., suicidality), but this appears accounted for by their tendency to have more severe body dysmorphic disorder symptoms.

Associated Features Supporting Diagnosis

Many individuals with body dysmorphic disorder have ideas or delusions of reference, believing that other people take special notice of them or mock them because of how they look. Body dysmorphic disorder is associated with high levels of anxiety, social anxiety, social avoidance, depressed mood, neuroticism, and perfectionism as well as low extroversion and low self-esteem. Many individuals are ashamed of their appearance and their excessive focus on how they look, and are reluctant to reveal their concerns to others. A majority of individuals receive cosmetic treatment to try to improve their perceived defects. Dermatological treatment and surgery are most common, but any type (e.g., dental, electrolysis) may be received. Occasionally, individuals may perform surgery on themselves. Body dysmorphic disorder appears to respond poorly to such treatments and sometimes becomes worse. Some individuals take legal action or are violent toward the clinician because they are dissatisfied with the cosmetic outcome.

Body dysmorphic disorder has been associated with executive dysfunction and visual processing abnormalities, with a bias for analyzing and encoding details rather than holistic or configural aspects of visual stimuli. Individuals with this disorder tend to have a bias for negative and threatening interpretations of facial expressions and ambiguous scenarios.

Prevalence

The point prevalence among U.S. adults is 2.4% (2.5% in females and 2.2% in males). Outside the United States (i.e., Germany), current prevalence is approximately 1.7%–1.8%, with a gender distribution similar to that in the United States. The current prevalence is 9%–15% among dermatology patients, 7%–8% among U.S. cosmetic surgery patients, 3%–16% among international cosmetic surgery patients (most studies), 8% among adult orthodontia patients, and 10% among patients presenting for oral or maxillofacial surgery.

Development and Course

The mean age at disorder onset is 16–17 years, the median age at onset is 15 years, and the most common age at onset is 12–13 years. Two-thirds of individuals have disorder onset before age 18. Subclinical body dysmorphic disorder symptoms begin, on average, at age 12 or 13 years. Subclinical concerns usually evolve gradually to the full disorder, although some individuals experience abrupt onset of body dysmorphic disorder. The disorder appears to usually be chronic, although improvement is likely when evidence-based treatment is received. The disorder's clinical features appear largely similar in children/ adolescents and adults. Body dysmorphic disorder occurs in the elderly, but little is known about the disorder in this age group. Individuals with disorder onset before age 18 years are more likely to attempt suicide, have more comorbidity, and have gradual (rather than acute) disorder onset than those with adult-onset body dysmorphic disorder.

Risk and Prognostic Factors

Environmental.   Body dysmorphic disorder has been associated with high rates of childhood neglect and abuse.

Genetic and physiological.   The prevalence of body dysmorphic disorder is elevated in first-degree relatives of individuals with obsessive-compulsive disorder (OCD).

Culture-Related Diagnostic Issues

Body dysmorphic disorder has been reported internationally. It appears that the disorder may have more similarities than differences across races and cultures but that cultural values and preferences may influence symptom content to some degree. *Taijin kyofusho,* included in the traditional Japanese diagnostic system, has a subtype similar to body dysmorphic disorder: *shubo-kyofu* ("the phobia of a deformed body").

Gender-Related Diagnostic Issues

Females and males appear to have more similarities than differences in terms of most clinical features— for example, disliked body areas, types of repetitive behaviors, symptom severity, suicidality, comorbidity, illness course, and receipt of cosmetic procedures for body dysmorphic disorder. However, males are more likely to have genital preoccupations, and females are more likely to have a comorbid eating disorder. Muscle dysmorphia occurs almost exclusively in males.

Suicide Risk

Rates of suicidal ideation and suicide attempts are high in both adults and children/adolescents with body dysmorphic disorder. Furthermore, risk for suicide appears high in adolescents. A substantial proportion of individuals attribute suicidal ideation or suicide attempts primarily to their appearance concerns. Individuals with body dysmorphic disorder have many risk factors for completed suicide, such as high rates of suicidal ideation and suicide attempts, demographic characteristics associated with suicide, and high rates of comorbid major depressive disorder.

Functional Consequences of Body Dysmorphic Disorder

Nearly all individuals with body dysmorphic disorder experience impaired psychosocial functioning because of their appearance concerns. Impairment can range from moderate (e.g., avoidance of some social situations) to extreme and incapacitating (e.g., being completely housebound). On average, psychosocial functioning and quality of life are markedly poor. More severe body dysmorphic disorder symptoms are associated with poorer functioning and quality of life. Most individuals experience impairment in their job, academic, or role functioning (e.g., as a parent or caregiver), which is often severe (e.g., performing poorly, missing school or work, not working). About 20% of youths with body dysmorphic disorder report dropping out of school primarily because of their body dysmorphic disorder symptoms. Impairment in social functioning (e.g., social activities, relationships, intimacy), including avoidance, is common. Individuals may be housebound because of their body dysmorphic disorder symptoms, sometimes for years. A high proportion of adults and adolescents have been psychiatrically hospitalized.

Differential Diagnosis

Normal appearance concerns and clearly noticeable physical defects.   Body dysmorphic disorder differs from normal appearance concerns in being characterized by excessive appearance-related preoccupations and repetitive behaviors that are time-consuming, are usually difficult to resist or control, and cause clinically significant distress or impairment in functioning. Physical defects that are clearly noticeable (i.e., not slight) are not diagnosed as body dysmorphic disorder. However, skin picking as a symptom of body dysmorphic disorder can cause noticeable skin lesions and scarring; in such cases, body dysmorphic disorder should be diagnosed.

Eating disorders.   In an individual with an eating disorder, concerns about being fat are considered a symptom of the eating disorder rather than body dysmorphic disorder. However, weight concerns may occur in body dysmorphic disorder. Eating disorders and body dysmorphic disorder can be comorbid, in which case both should be diagnosed.

Other obsessive-compulsive and related disorders.   The preoccupations and repetitive behaviors of body dysmorphic disorder differ from obsessions and compulsions in OCD in that the former focus only on appearance. These disorders have other differences, such as poorer insight in body dysmorphic disorder. When skin picking is intended to improve the appearance of perceived skin defects, body dysmorphic disorder, rather than excoriation (skin-picking) disorder, is diagnosed. When hair removal (plucking, pulling, or other types of removal) is intended to improve perceived defects in the appearance of facial or body hair, body dysmorphic disorder is diagnosed rather than trichotillomania (hair-pulling disorder).

Illness anxiety disorder.   Individuals with body dysmorphic disorder are not preoccupied with having or acquiring a serious illness and do not have particularly elevated levels of somatization.

Major depressive disorder.   The prominent preoccupation with appearance and excessive repetitive behaviors in body dysmorphic disorder differentiate it from major depressive disorder. However, major depressive disorder and depressive symptoms are common in individuals with body dysmorphic disorder, often appearing to be secondary to the distress and impairment that body dysmorphic disorder causes. Body dysmorphic disorder should be diagnosed in depressed individuals if diagnostic criteria for body dysmorphic disorder are met.

Anxiety disorders.   Social anxiety and avoidance are common in body dysmorphic disorder. However, unlike social anxiety disorder (social phobia), agoraphobia, and avoidant personality disorder, body dysmorphic disorder includes prominent appearance-related preoccupation, which may be delusional, and repetitive behaviors, and the social anxiety and avoidance are due to concerns about perceived appearance defects and the belief or fear that other people will consider these individuals ugly, ridicule them, or reject them because of their physical features. Unlike generalized anxiety disorder, anxiety and worry in body dysmorphic disorder focus on perceived appearance flaws.

Psychotic disorders.   Many individuals with body dysmorphic disorder have delusional appearance beliefs (i.e., complete conviction that their view of their perceived defects is accurate), which is diagnosed as body dysmorphic disorder, with absent insight/delusional beliefs, not as delusional disorder. Appearance-related ideas or delusions of reference are common in body dysmorphic disorder; however, unlike schizophrenia or schizoaffective disorder, body dysmorphic disorder involves prominent appearance preoccupations and related repetitive behaviors, and disorganized behavior and other psychotic symptoms are absent (except for appearance beliefs, which may be delusional).

Other disorders and symptoms.   Body dysmorphic disorder should not be diagnosed if the preoccupation is limited to discomfort with or a desire to be rid of one's primary and/or secondary sex characteristics in an individual with gender dysphoria or if the preoccupation focuses on the belief that one emits a foul or offensive body odor as in olfactory reference syndrome (which is not a DSM-5 disorder). Body identity integrity disorder (apotemnophilia) (which is not a DSM-5 disorder) involves a desire to have a limb amputated to correct an experience of mismatch between a person's sense of body identity and his or her actual anatomy. However, the concern does not focus on the limb's appearance, as it would in body dysmorphic disorder. *Koro,* a culturally related disorder that usually occurs in epidemics in Southeastern Asia, consists of a fear that the penis (labia, nipples, or breasts in females) is shrinking or retracting and will disappear into the abdomen, often accompanied by a belief that death will result. Koro differs from body dysmorphic disorder in several ways, including a focus on death rather than preoccupation with perceived ugliness. *Dysmorphic concern* (which is not a DSM-5 disorder) is a much broader construct than, and is not equivalent to, body dysmorphic disorder. It involves symptoms reflecting an overconcern with slight or imagined flaws in appearance.

Comorbidity

Major depressive disorder is the most common comorbid disorder, with onset usually after that of body dysmorphic disorder. Comorbid social anxiety disorder (social phobia), OCD, and substance-related disorders are also common.

Hoarding Disorder

Diagnostic Criteria	300.3 (F42.3)

A. Persistent difficulty discarding or parting with possessions, regardless of their actual value.
B. This difficulty is due to a perceived need to save the items and to distress associated with discarding them.
C. The difficulty discarding possessions results in the accumulation of possessions that congest and clutter active living areas and substantially compromises their intended use. If living areas are uncluttered, it is only because of the interventions of third parties (e.g., family members, cleaners, authorities).
D. The hoarding causes clinically significant distress or impairment in social, occupational, or other important areas of functioning (including maintaining a safe environment for self and others).
E. The hoarding is not attributable to another medical condition (e.g., brain injury, cerebrovascular disease, Prader-Willi syndrome).
F. The hoarding is not better explained by the symptoms of another mental disorder (e.g., obsessions in obsessive-compulsive disorder, decreased energy in major depressive disorder, delusions in schizophrenia or another psychotic disorder, cognitive deficits in major neurocognitive disorder, restricted interests in autism spectrum disorder).

Specify if:
With excessive acquisition: If difficulty discarding possessions is accompanied by excessive acquisition of items that are not needed or for which there is no available space.

Specify if:
With good or fair insight: The individual recognizes that hoarding-related beliefs and behaviors (pertaining to difficulty discarding items, clutter, or excessive acquisition) are problematic.
With poor insight: The individual is mostly convinced that hoarding-related beliefs and behaviors (pertaining to difficulty discarding items, clutter, or excessive acquisition) are not problematic despite evidence to the contrary.
With absent insight/delusional beliefs: The individual is completely convinced that hoarding-related beliefs and behaviors (pertaining to difficulty discarding items, clutter, or excessive acquisition) are not problematic despite evidence to the contrary.

Specifiers

With excessive acquisition.   Approximately 80%–90% of individuals with hoarding disorder display excessive acquisition. The most frequent form of acquisition is excessive buying, followed by acquisition of free items (e.g., leaflets, items discarded by others). Stealing is less common. Some individuals may deny excessive acquisition when first assessed, yet it may appear later during the course of treatment. Individuals with hoarding disorder typically experience distress if they are unable to or are prevented from acquiring items.

Diagnostic Features

The essential feature of hoarding disorder is persistent difficulties discarding or parting with possessions, regardless of their actual value (Criterion A). The term *persistent* indicates a long-standing difficulty rather than more transient life circumstances that may lead to excessive clutter, such as inheriting property. The difficulty in discarding possessions noted in Criterion A refers to any form of discarding, including throwing away, selling, giving away, or recycling. The main reasons given for these difficulties are the perceived utility or aesthetic value of the items or strong sentimental attachment to the possessions. Some individuals feel responsible for the fate of their possessions and often go to great lengths to avoid being wasteful. Fears of losing important information are also common. The most commonly saved items are newspapers, magazines, old clothing, bags, books, mail, and paperwork, but virtually any item can be saved. The nature of items is not limited to possessions that most other people would define as useless or of limited value. Many individuals collect and save large numbers of valuable things as well, which are often found in piles mixed with other less valuable items.

Individuals with hoarding disorder purposefully save possessions and experience distress when facing the prospect of discarding them (Criterion B). This criterion emphasizes that the saving of possessions is intentional, which discriminates hoarding disorder from other forms of psychopathology that are characterized by the passive accumulation of items or the absence of distress when possessions are removed.

Individuals accumulate large numbers of items that fill up and clutter active living areas to the extent that their intended use is no longer possible (Criterion C). For example, the individual may not be able to cook in the kitchen, sleep in his or her bed, or sit in a chair. If the space can be used, it is only with great difficulty. *Clutter* is defined as a large group of usually unrelated or marginally related objects piled together in a disorganized fashion in spaces designed for other purposes (e.g., tabletops, floor, hallway). Criterion C emphasizes the "active" living areas of the home, rather than more peripheral areas, such as garages, attics, or basements, that are sometimes cluttered in homes of individuals without hoarding disorder. However, individuals with hoarding disorder often have possessions that spill beyond the active living areas and can occupy and impair the use of other spaces, such as vehicles, yards, the workplace, and friends' and relatives' houses. In some cases, living areas may be uncluttered because of the intervention of third parties (e.g., family members, cleaners, local authorities). Individuals who have been forced to clear their homes still have a symptom picture that meets criteria for hoarding disorder because the lack of clutter is due to a third-party intervention. Hoarding disorder contrasts with normative collecting behavior, which is organized and systematic, even if in some cases the actual amount of possessions may be similar to the amount accumulated by an individual with hoarding disorder. Normative collecting does not produce the clutter, distress, or impairment typical of hoarding disorder.

Symptoms (i.e., difficulties discarding and/or clutter) must cause clinically significant distress or impairment in social, occupational, or other important areas of functioning, including maintaining a safe environment for self and others (Criterion D). In some cases, particularly when there is poor insight, the individual may not report distress, and the impairment may be apparent only to those around the individual. However, any attempts to discard or clear the possessions by third parties result in high levels of distress.

Associated Features Supporting Diagnosis

Other common features of hoarding disorder include indecisiveness, perfectionism, avoidance, procrastination, difficulty planning and organizing tasks, and distractibility. Some individuals with hoarding disorder live in unsanitary conditions that may be a logical consequence of severely cluttered spaces and/or that are related to planning and organizing difficulties. *Animal hoarding* can be defined as the accumulation of a large number of animals and a failure to provide minimal standards of nutrition, sanitation, and veterinary care and to act on the deteriorating condition of the animals (including disease, starvation, or death) and the environment (e.g., severe overcrowding, extremely unsanitary conditions). Animal hoarding may be a special manifestation of hoarding disorder. Most individuals who hoard animals also hoard inanimate objects. The most prominent differences between animal and object hoarding are the extent of unsanitary conditions and the poorer insight in animal hoarding.

Prevalence

Nationally representative prevalence studies of hoarding disorder are not available. Community surveys estimate the point prevalence of clinically significant hoarding in the United States and Europe to be approximately 2%–6%. Hoarding disorder affects both males and females, but some epidemiological studies have reported a significantly greater prevalence among males. This contrasts with clinical samples, which are predominantly female. Hoarding symptoms appear to be almost three times more prevalent in older adults (ages 55–94 years) compared with younger adults (ages 34–44 years).

Development and Course

Hoarding appears to begin early in life and spans well into the late stages. Hoarding symptoms may first emerge around ages 11–15 years, start interfering with the individual's everyday functioning by the mid-20s, and cause clinically significant impairment by the mid-30s. Participants in clinical research studies are usually in their 50s. Thus, the severity of hoarding increases with each decade of life. Once symptoms begin, the course of hoarding is often chronic, with few individuals reporting a waxing and waning course.

Pathological hoarding in children appears to be easily distinguished from developmentally adaptive saving and collecting behaviors. Because children and adolescents typically do not control their living environment and discarding behaviors, the possible intervention of third parties (e.g., parents keeping the spaces usable and thus reducing interference) should be considered when making the diagnosis.

Risk and Prognostic Factors

Temperamental. Indecisiveness is a prominent feature of individuals with hoarding disorder and their first-degree relatives.

Environmental. Individuals with hoarding disorder often retrospectively report stressful and traumatic life events preceding the onset of the disorder or causing an exacerbation.

Genetic and physiological. Hoarding behavior is familial, with about 50% of individuals who hoard reporting having a relative who also hoards. Twin studies indicate that approximately 50% of the variability in hoarding behavior is attributable to additive genetic factors.

Culture-Related Diagnostic Issues

While most of the research has been done in Western, industrialized countries and urban communities, the available data from non-Western and developing countries suggest that hoarding is a universal phenomenon with consistent clinical features.

Gender-Related Diagnostic Issues

The key features of hoarding disorder (i.e., difficulties discarding, excessive amount of clutter) are generally comparable in males and females, but females tend to display more excessive acquisition, particularly excessive buying, than do males.

Functional Consequences of Hoarding Disorder

Clutter impairs basic activities, such as moving through the house, cooking, cleaning, personal hygiene, and even sleeping. Appliances may be broken, and utilities such as water and electricity may be disconnected, as access for repair work may be difficult. Quality of life is often considerably impaired. In severe cases, hoarding can put individuals at risk for fire, falling (especially elderly individuals), poor sanitation, and other health risks. Hoarding disorder is associated with occupational impairment, poor physical health, and high social service utilization. Family relationships are frequently under great strain. Conflict with neighbors and local authorities is common, and a substantial proportion of individuals with severe hoarding disorder have been involved in legal eviction proceedings, and some have a history of eviction.

Differential Diagnosis

Other medical conditions.   Hoarding disorder is not diagnosed if the symptoms are judged to be a direct consequence of another medical condition (Criterion E), such as traumatic brain injury, surgical resection for treatment of a tumor or seizure control, cerebrovascular disease, infections of the central nervous system (e.g., herpes simplex encephalitis), or neurogenetic conditions such as Prader-Willi syndrome. Damage to the anterior ventromedial prefrontal and cingulate cortices has been particularly associated with the excessive accumulation of objects. In these individuals, the hoarding behavior is not present prior to the onset of the brain damage and appears shortly after the brain damage occurs. Some of these individuals appear to have little interest in the accumulated items and are able to discard them easily or do not care if others discard them, whereas others appear to be very reluctant to discard anything.

Neurodevelopmental disorders.   Hoarding disorder is not diagnosed if the accumulation of objects is judged to be a direct consequence of a neurodevelopmental disorder, such as autism spectrum disorder or intellectual disability (intellectual developmental disorder).

Schizophrenia spectrum and other psychotic disorders.   Hoarding disorder is not diagnosed if the accumulation of objects is judged to be a direct consequence of delusions or negative symptoms in schizophrenia spectrum and other psychotic disorders.

Major depressive episode.   Hoarding disorder is not diagnosed if the accumulation of objects is judged to be a direct consequence of psychomotor retardation, fatigue, or loss of energy during a major depressive episode.

Obsessive-compulsive disorder.   Hoarding disorder is not diagnosed if the symptoms are judged to be a direct consequence of typical obsessions or compulsions, such as fears of contamination, harm, or feelings of incompleteness in obsessive-compulsive disorder (OCD). Feelings of incompleteness (e.g., losing one's identity, or having to document and preserve all life experiences) are the most frequent OCD symptoms associated with this form of hoarding. The accumulation of objects can also be the result of persistently avoiding onerous rituals (e.g., not discarding objects in order to avoid endless washing or checking rituals).

In OCD, the behavior is generally unwanted and highly distressing, and the individual experiences no pleasure or reward from it. Excessive acquisition is usually not present; if excessive acquisition is present, items are acquired because of a specific obsession (e.g., the need to buy items that have been accidentally touched in order to avoid contaminating other people), not because of a genuine desire to possess the items. Individuals who hoard in the context of OCD are also more likely to accumulate bizarre items, such as trash, feces, urine, nails, hair, used diapers, or rotten food. Accumulation of such items is very unusual in hoarding disorder.

When severe hoarding appears concurrently with other typical symptoms of OCD but is judged to be independent from these symptoms, both hoarding disorder and OCD may be diagnosed.

Neurocognitive disorders.   Hoarding disorder is not diagnosed if the accumulation of objects is judged to be a direct consequence of a degenerative disorder, such as neurocognitive disorder associated with frontotemporal lobar degeneration or Alzheimer's disease. Typically, onset of the accumulating behavior is gradual and follows onset of the neurocognitive disorder. The accumulating behavior may be accompanied by self-neglect and severe domestic squalor, alongside other neuropsychiatric symptoms, such as disinhibition, gambling, rituals/stereotypies, tics, and self-injurious behaviors.

Comorbidity

Approximately 75% of individuals with hoarding disorder have a comorbid mood or anxiety disorder. The most common comorbid conditions are major depressive disorder (up to 50% of cases), social anxiety disorder (social phobia), and generalized anxiety disorder. Approximately 20% of individuals with hoarding disorder also have symptoms that meet diagnostic criteria for OCD. These comorbidities may often be the main reason for consultation, because individuals are unlikely to spontaneously report hoarding symptoms, and these symptoms are often not asked about in routine clinical interviews.

Trichotillomania (Hair-Pulling Disorder)

Diagnostic Criteria   **312.39** (F63.3)

A. Recurrent pulling out of one's hair, resulting in hair loss.
B. Repeated attempts to decrease or stop hair pulling.
C. The hair pulling causes clinically significant distress or impairment in social, occupational, or other important areas of functioning.
D. The hair pulling or hair loss is not attributable to another medical condition (e.g., a dermatological condition).
E. The hair pulling is not better explained by the symptoms of another mental disorder (e.g., attempts to improve a perceived defect or flaw in appearance in body dysmorphic disorder).

Diagnostic Features

The essential feature of trichotillomania (hair-pulling disorder) is the recurrent pulling out of one's own hair (Criterion A). Hair pulling may occur from any region of the body in which hair grows; the most common sites are the scalp, eyebrows, and eyelids, while less common sites are axillary, facial, pubic, and peri-rectal regions. Hair-pulling sites may vary over time. Hair pulling may occur in brief episodes scattered throughout the day or during less frequent but more sustained periods that can continue for hours, and such hair pulling may endure for months or years. Criterion A requires that hair pulling lead to hair loss, although individuals with this disorder may pull hair in a widely distributed pattern (i.e., pulling single hairs from all over a site) such that hair loss may not be clearly visible. Alternatively, individuals may attempt to conceal or camouflage hair loss (e.g., by using makeup, scarves, or wigs). Individuals with trichotillomania have made repeated attempts to decrease or stop hair pulling (Criterion B). Criterion C indicates that hair pulling causes clinically significant distress or impairment in social, occupational, or other important areas of functioning. The term *distress* includes negative affects that may be experienced by individuals with hair pulling, such as feeling a loss of control, embarrassment, and shame. Significant impairment may occur in several different areas of functioning (e.g., social, occupational, academic, and leisure), in part because of avoidance of work, school, or other public situations.

Associated Features Supporting Diagnosis

Hair pulling may be accompanied by a range of behaviors or rituals involving hair. Thus, individuals may search for a particular kind of hair to pull (e.g., hairs with a specific texture or color), may try to pull out hair in a specific way (e.g., so that the root comes out intact), or may visually examine or tactilely or orally manipulate the hair after it has been pulled (e.g., rolling the hair between the fingers, pulling the strand between the teeth, biting the hair into pieces, or swallowing the hair).

Hair pulling may also be preceded or accompanied by various emotional states; it may be triggered by feelings of anxiety or boredom, may be preceded by an increasing sense of tension (either immediately before pulling out the hair or when attempting to resist the urge to pull), or may lead to gratification, pleasure, or a sense of relief when the hair is pulled out. Hair-pulling behavior may involve varying degrees of conscious awareness, with some individuals displaying more focused attention on the hair pulling (with preceding tension and subsequent relief), and other individuals displaying more automatic behavior (in which the hair pulling seems to occur without full awareness). Many individuals report a mix of both behavioral styles. Some individuals experience an "itch-like" or tingling sensation in the scalp that is alleviated by the act of pulling hair. Pain does not usually accompany hair pulling.

Patterns of hair loss are highly variable. Areas of complete alopecia, as well as areas of thinned hair density, are common. When the scalp is involved, there may be a predilection for pulling out hair in the crown or parietal regions. There may be a pattern of nearly complete baldness except for a narrow perimeter around the outer margins of the scalp, particularly at the nape of the neck ("tonsure trichotillomania"). Eyebrows and eyelashes may be completely absent.

Hair pulling does not usually occur in the presence of other individuals, except immediate family members. Some individuals have urges to pull hair from other individuals and may sometimes try to find opportunities to do so surreptitiously. Some individuals may pull hairs from pets, dolls, and other fibrous materials (e.g., sweaters or carpets). Some individuals may deny their hair pulling to others. The majority of individuals with trichotillomania also have one or more other body-focused repetitive behaviors, including skin picking, nail biting, and lip chewing.

Prevalence

In the general population, the 12-month prevalence estimate for trichotillomania in adults and adolescents is 1%–2%. Females are more frequently affected than males, at a ratio of approximately 10:1. This estimate likely reflects the true gender ratio of the condition, although it may also reflect differential treatment seeking based on gender or cultural attitudes regarding appearance (e.g., acceptance of normative hair loss among males). Among children with trichotillomania, males and females are more equally represented.

Development and Course

Hair pulling may be seen in infants, and this behavior typically resolves during early development. Onset of hair pulling in trichotillomania most commonly coincides with, or follows the onset of, puberty. Sites of hair pulling may vary over time. The usual course of trichotillomania is chronic, with some waxing and waning if the disorder is untreated. Symptoms may possibly worsen in females accompanying hormonal changes (e.g., menstruation, perimenopause). For some individuals, the disorder may come and go for weeks, months, or years at a time. A minority of individuals remit without subsequent relapse within a few years of onset.

Risk and Prognostic Factors

Genetic and physiological.　There is evidence for a genetic vulnerability to trichotillomania. The disorder is more common in individuals with obsessive-compulsive disorder (OCD) and their first-degree relatives than in the general population.

Culture-Related Diagnostic Issues

Trichotillomania appears to manifest similarly across cultures, although there is a paucity of data from non-Western regions.

Diagnostic Markers

Most individuals with trichotillomania admit to hair pulling; thus, dermatopathological diagnosis is rarely required. Skin biopsy and dermoscopy (or trichoscopy) of trichotillomania are able to differentiate the disorder from other causes of alopecia. In trichotillomania, dermoscopy shows a range of characteristic features, including decreased hair density, short vellus hair, and broken hairs with different shaft lengths.

Functional Consequences of Trichotillomania (Hair-Pulling Disorder)

Trichotillomania is associated with distress as well as with social and occupational impairment. There may be irreversible damage to hair growth and hair quality. Infrequent medical consequences of trichotillomania include digit purpura, musculoskeletal injury (e.g., carpal tunnel syndrome; back, shoulder and neck pain), blepharitis, and dental damage (e.g., worn or broken teeth due to hair biting). Swallowing of hair (trichophagia) may lead to trichobezoars, with subsequent anemia, abdominal pain, hematemesis, nausea and vomiting, bowel obstruction, and even perforation.

Differential Diagnosis

Normative hair removal/manipulation.　Trichotillomania should not be diagnosed when hair removal is performed solely for cosmetic reasons (i.e., to improve one's physical appearance). Many individuals twist and play with their hair, but this behavior does not usually qualify for a diagnosis of trichotillomania. Some individuals may bite rather than pull hair; again, this does not qualify for a diagnosis of trichotillomania.

Other obsessive-compulsive and related disorders.　Individuals with OCD and symmetry concerns may pull out hairs as part of their symmetry rituals, and individuals with body dysmorphic disorder may remove body hair that they perceive as ugly, asymmetrical, or abnormal; in such cases a diagnosis of trichotillomania is not given. The description of body-focused repetitive behavior disorder in other specified obsessive-compulsive and related disorder excludes individuals who meet diagnostic criteria for trichotillomania.

Neurodevelopmental disorders.   In neurodevelopmental disorders, hair pulling may meet the definition of stereotypies (e.g., in stereotypic movement disorder). Tics (in tic disorders) rarely lead to hair pulling.

Psychotic disorder.   Individuals with a psychotic disorder may remove hair in response to a delusion or hallucination. Trichotillomania is not diagnosed in such cases.

Another medical condition.   Trichotillomania is not diagnosed if the hair pulling or hair loss is attributable to another medical condition (e.g., inflammation of the skin or other dermatological conditions). Other causes of scarring alopecia (e.g., alopecia areata, androgenic alopecia, telogen effluvium) or nonscarring alopecia (e.g., chronic discoid lupus erythematosus, lichen planopilaris, central centrifugal cicatricial alopecia, pseudopelade, folliculitis decalvans, dissecting folliculitis, acne keloidalis nuchae) should be considered in individuals with hair loss who deny hair pulling. Skin biopsy or dermoscopy can be used to differentiate individuals with trichotillomania from those with dermatological disorders.

Substance-related disorders.   Hair-pulling symptoms may be exacerbated by certain substances—for example, stimulants—but it is less likely that substances are the primary cause of persistent hair pulling.

Comorbidity

Trichotillomania is often accompanied by other mental disorders, most commonly major depressive disorder and excoriation (skin-picking) disorder. Repetitive body-focused symptoms other than hair pulling or skin picking (e.g., nail biting) occur in the majority of individuals with trichotillomania and may deserve an additional diagnosis of other specified obsessive-compulsive and related disorder (i.e., body-focused repetitive behavior disorder).

Excoriation (Skin-Picking) Disorder

Diagnostic Criteria   **698.4** (F42.4)

A. Recurrent skin picking resulting in skin lesions.
B. Repeated attempts to decrease or stop skin picking.
C. The skin picking causes clinically significant distress or impairment in social, occupational, or other important areas of functioning.
D. The skin picking is not attributable to the physiological effects of a substance (e.g., cocaine) or another medical condition (e.g., scabies).
E. The skin picking is not better explained by symptoms of another mental disorder (e.g., delusions or tactile hallucinations in a psychotic disorder, attempts to improve a perceived defect or flaw in appearance in body dysmorphic disorder, stereotypies in stereotypic movement disorder, or intention to harm oneself in nonsuicidal self-injury).

Diagnostic Features

The essential feature of excoriation (skin-picking) disorder is recurrent picking at one's own skin (Criterion A). The most commonly picked sites are the face, arms, and hands, but many individuals pick from multiple body sites. Individuals may pick at healthy skin, at minor skin irregularities, at lesions such as pimples or calluses, or at scabs from previous picking. Most individuals pick with their fingernails, although many use tweezers, pins, or other objects. In addition to skin picking, there may be skin rubbing, squeezing, lancing, and biting. Individuals with excoriation disorder often spend significant amounts of time on their picking behavior, sometimes several hours per day, and such skin picking may endure for months or years. Criterion A requires that skin picking lead to skin lesions, although individuals with this disorder often attempt to conceal or camouflage such lesions (e.g., with makeup or clothing). Individuals with excoriation disorder have made repeated attempts to decrease or stop skin picking (Criterion B).

Criterion C indicates that skin picking causes clinically significant distress or impairment in social, occupational, or other important areas of functioning. The term *distress* includes negative affects that may be experienced by individuals with skin picking, such as feeling a loss of control, embarrassment, and shame. Significant impairment may occur in several different areas of functioning (e.g., social, occupational, academic, and leisure), in part because of avoidance of social situations.

Associated Features Supporting Diagnosis

Skin picking may be accompanied by a range of behaviors or rituals involving skin or scabs. Thus, individuals may search for a particular kind of scab to pull, and they may examine, play with, or mouth or swallow the skin after it has been pulled. Skin picking may also be preceded or accompanied by various emotional states. Skin picking may be triggered by feelings of anxiety or boredom, may be preceded by an increasing sense of tension (either immediately before picking the skin or when attempting to resist the urge to pick), and may lead to gratification, pleasure, or a sense of relief when the skin or scab has been picked. Some individuals report picking in response to a minor skin irregularity or to relieve an uncomfortable bodily sensation. Pain is not routinely reported to accompany skin picking. Some individuals engage in skin picking that is more focused (i.e., with preceding tension and subsequent relief), whereas others engage in more automatic picking (i.e., when skin picking occurs without preceding tension and without full awareness), and many have a mix of both behavioral styles. Skin picking does not usually occur in the presence of other individuals, except immediate family members. Some individuals report picking the skin of others.

Prevalence

In the general population, the lifetime prevalence for excoriation disorder in adults is 1.4% or somewhat higher. Three-quarters or more of individuals with the disorder are female. This likely reflects the true gender ratio of the condition, although it may also reflect differential treatment seeking based on gender or cultural attitudes regarding appearance.

Development and Course

Although individuals with excoriation disorder may present at various ages, the skin picking most often has onset during adolescence, commonly coinciding with or following the onset of puberty. The disorder frequently begins with a dermatological condition, such as acne. Sites of skin picking may vary over time. The usual course is chronic, with some waxing and waning if untreated. For some individuals, the disorder may come and go for weeks, months, or years at a time.

Risk and Prognostic Factors

Genetic and physiological.   Excoriation disorder is more common in individuals with obsessive-compulsive disorder (OCD) and their first-degree family members than in the general population.

Diagnostic Markers

Most individuals with excoriation disorder admit to skin picking; therefore, dermatopathological diagnosis is rarely required. However, the disorder may have characteristic features on histopathology.

Functional Consequences of Excoriation (Skin-Picking) Disorder

Excoriation disorder is associated with distress as well as with social and occupational impairment. The majority of individuals with this condition spend at least 1 hour per day picking, thinking about picking, and resisting urges to pick. Many individuals report avoiding social or entertainment events as well as going out in public. A majority of individuals with the disorder also report experiencing work interference from skin picking on at least a daily or weekly basis. A significant proportion of students with excoriation disorder report having missed school, having experienced difficulties managing responsibilities at school, or having had difficulties studying because of skin picking. Medical complications of skin picking include tissue damage, scarring, and infection and can be life-threatening. Rarely, synovitis of the wrists due to chronic picking has been reported. Skin picking often results in significant tissue damage and scarring. It frequently requires antibiotic treatment for infection, and on occasion it may require surgery.

Differential Diagnosis

Psychotic disorder.   Skin picking may occur in response to a delusion (i.e., parasitosis) or tactile hallucination (i.e., formication) in a psychotic disorder. In such cases, excoriation disorder should not be diagnosed.

Other obsessive-compulsive and related disorders.   Excessive washing compulsions in response to contamination obsessions in individuals with OCD may lead to skin lesions, and skin picking may occur in individuals with body dysmorphic disorder who pick their skin solely because of appearance concerns; in such cases, excoriation disorder should not be diagnosed. The description of body-focused repetitive behavior disorder in other specified obsessive-compulsive and related disorder excludes individuals whose symptoms meet diagnostic criteria for excoriation disorder.

Neurodevelopmental disorders.   While stereotypic movement disorder may be characterized by repetitive self-injurious behavior, onset is in the early developmental period. For example, individuals with the neurogenetic condition Prader-Willi syndrome may have early onset of skin picking, and their symptoms may meet criteria for stereotypic movement disorder. While tics in individuals with Tourette's disorder may lead to self-injury, the behavior is not tic-like in excoriation disorder.

Somatic symptom and related disorders.   Excoriation disorder is not diagnosed if the skin lesion is primarily attributable to deceptive behaviors in factitious disorder.

Other disorders.   Excoriation disorder is not diagnosed if the skin picking is primarily attributable to the intention to harm oneself that is characteristic of nonsuicidal self-injury.

Other medical conditions.   Excoriation disorder is not diagnosed if the skin picking is primarily attributable to another medical condition. For example, scabies is a dermatological condition invariably associated with severe itching and scratching. However, excoriation disorder may be precipitated or exacerbated by an underlying dermatological condition. For example, acne may lead to some scratching and picking, which may also be associated with comorbid excoriation disorder. The differentiation between these two clinical situations (acne with some scratching and picking vs. acne with comorbid excoriation disorder) requires an assessment of the extent to which the individual's skin picking has become independent of the underlying dermatological condition.

Substance/medication-induced disorders.   Skin-picking symptoms may also be induced by certain substances (e.g., cocaine), in which case excoriation disorder should not be diagnosed. If such skin picking is clinically significant, then a diagnosis of substance/medication-induced obsessive-compulsive and related disorder should be considered.

Comorbidity

Excoriation disorder is often accompanied by other mental disorders. Such disorders include OCD and trichotillomania (hair-pulling disorder), as well as major depressive disorder. Repetitive body-focused symptoms other than skin picking and hair pulling (e.g., nail biting) occur in many individuals with excoriation disorder and may deserve an additional diagnosis of other specified obsessive-compulsive and related disorder (i.e., body-focused repetitive behavior disorder).

Substance/Medication-Induced Obsessive-Compulsive and Related Disorder

Diagnostic Criteria

A. Obsessions, compulsions, skin picking, hair pulling, other body-focused repetitive behaviors, or other symptoms characteristic of the obsessive-compulsive and related disorders predominate in the clinical picture.

B. There is evidence from the history, physical examination, or laboratory findings of both (1) and (2):

   1. The symptoms in Criterion A developed during or soon after substance intoxication or withdrawal or after exposure to a medication.
   2. The involved substance/medication is capable of producing the symptoms in Criterion A.

C. The disturbance is not better explained by an obsessive-compulsive and related disorder that is not substance/medication-induced. Such evidence of an independent obsessive-compulsive and related disorder could include the following:

   The symptoms precede the onset of the substance/medication use; the symptoms persist for a substantial period of time (e.g., about 1 month) after the cessation of acute withdrawal or severe intoxication; or there is other evidence suggesting the existence of an independent non-substance/medication-induced obsessive-compulsive and related disorder (e.g., a history of recurrent non-substance/medication-related episodes).

D. The disturbance does not occur exclusively during the course of a delirium.

E. The disturbance causes clinically significant distress or impairment in social, occupational, or other important areas of functioning.

Note: This diagnosis should be made in addition to a diagnosis of substance intoxication or substance withdrawal only when the symptoms in Criterion A predominate in the clinical picture and are sufficiently severe to warrant clinical attention.

Coding note: The ICD-9-CM and ICD-10-CM codes for the [specific substance/medication]-induced obsessive-compulsive and related disorders are indicated in the table below. Note that the ICD-10-CM code depends on whether or not there is a comorbid substance use disorder present for the same class of substance. If a mild substance use disorder is comorbid with the substance-induced obsessive-compulsive and related disorder, the 4th position character is "1," and the clinician should record "mild [substance] use disorder" before the substance-induced obsessive-compulsive and related disorder (e.g., "mild cocaine use disorder with cocaine-induced obsessive-compulsive and related disorder"). If a moderate or severe substance use disorder is comorbid with the substance-induced obsessive-compulsive and related disorder, the 4th position character is "2," and the clinician should record "moderate [substance] use disorder" or "severe [substance] use disorder," depending on the severity of the comorbid substance use disorder. If there is no comorbid substance use disorder (e.g., after a one-time heavy use of the substance), then the 4th position character is "9," and the clinician should record only the substance-induced obsessive-compulsive and related disorder.

		ICD-10-CM		
	ICD-9-CM	With use disorder, mild	With use disorder, moderate or severe	Without use disorder
Amphetamine (or other stimulant)	292.89	F15.188	F15.288	F15.988
Cocaine	292.89	F14.188	F14.288	F14.988
Other (or unknown) substance	292.89	F19.188	F19.288	F19.988

Specify if (see Table 1 in the chapter "Substance-Related and Addictive Disorders" for diagnoses associated with substance class):

With onset during intoxication: If the criteria are met for intoxication with the substance and the symptoms develop during intoxication.

With onset during withdrawal: If criteria are met for withdrawal from the substance and the symptoms develop during, or shortly after, withdrawal.

With onset after medication use: Symptoms may appear either at initiation of medication or after a modification or change in use.

Recording Procedures

ICD-9-CM. The name of the substance/medication-induced obsessive-compulsive and related disorder begins with the specific substance (e.g., cocaine) that is presumed to be causing the obsessive-compulsive and related symptoms. The diagnostic code is selected from the table included in the criteria set, which is based on the drug class. For substances that do not fit into any of the classes, the code for "other substance" should be used; and in cases in which a substance is judged to be an etiological factor but the specific class of substance is unknown, the category "unknown substance" should be used.

The name of the disorder is followed by the specification of onset (i.e., onset during intoxication, onset during withdrawal, with onset after medication use). Unlike the recording procedures for ICD-10-CM, which combine the substance-induced disorder and substance use disorder into a single code, for ICD-9-CM a separate diagnostic code is given for the substance use disorder. For example, in the case of repetitive behaviors occurring during intoxication in a man with a severe cocaine use disorder, the diagnosis is 292.89 cocaine-induced obsessive-compulsive and related disorder, with onset during intoxication. An additional diagnosis of 304.20 severe cocaine use disorder is also given. When more than one substance is judged to play a significant role in the development of the obsessive-compulsive and related disorder, each should be listed separately.

ICD-10-CM. The name of the substance/medication-induced obsessive-compulsive and related disorder begins with the specific substance (e.g., cocaine) that is presumed to be causing the obsessive-compulsive and related symptoms. The diagnostic code is selected from the table included in the criteria set, which is based on the drug class and presence or absence of a comorbid substance use disorder. For substances that do not fit into any of the classes, the code for "other substance" with no comorbid substance use should be used; and in cases in which a substance is judged to be an etiological factor but the specific class of substance is unknown, the category "unknown substance" with no comorbid substance use should be used.

When recording the name of the disorder, the comorbid substance use disorder (if any) is listed first, followed by the word "with," followed by the name of the substance-induced obsessive-compulsive and related disorder, followed by the specification of onset (i.e., onset during intoxication, onset during withdrawal, with onset after medication use). For example, in the case of repetitive behaviors occurring during intoxication in a man with a severe cocaine use disorder, the diagnosis is F14.288 severe cocaine use disorder with cocaine-induced obsessive-compulsive and related disorder, with onset during intoxication. A separate diagnosis of the comorbid severe cocaine use disorder is not given. If the substance-induced obsessive-compulsive and related disorder occurs without a comorbid substance use disorder (e.g., after a one-time heavy use of the substance), no accompanying substance use disorder is noted (e.g., F15.988 amphetamine-induced obsessive-compulsive and related disorder, with onset during intoxication). When more than one substance is judged to play a significant role in the development of the obsessive-compulsive and related disorder, each should be listed separately.

Diagnostic Features

The essential features of substance/medication-induced obsessive-compulsive and related disorder are prominent symptoms of an obsessive-compulsive and related disorder (Criterion A) that are judged to be attributable to the effects of a substance (e.g., drug of abuse, medication). The obsessive-compulsive and related disorder symptoms must have developed during or soon after substance intoxication or withdrawal or after exposure to a medication or toxin, and the substance/medication must be capable of producing the symptoms (Criterion B). Substance/medication-induced obsessive-compulsive and related disorder due to a prescribed treatment for a mental disorder or general medical condition must have its onset while the individual is receiving the medication. Once the treatment is discontinued, the obsessive-compulsive and related disorder symptoms will usually improve or remit within days to several weeks to 1 month (depending on the half-life of the substance/medication). The diagnosis of substance/medication-induced obsessive-compulsive and related disorder should not be given if onset of the obsessive-compulsive and related disorder symptoms precedes the substance intoxication or medication use, or if the symptoms persist for a substantial period of time, usually longer than 1 month, from the time of severe intoxication or withdrawal. If the obsessive-compulsive and related disorder symptoms persist for a substantial period of time, other causes for the symptoms should be considered. The substance/medication-induced obsessive-compulsive and related disorder diagnosis should be made in addition to a diagnosis of substance intoxication only when the symptoms in Criterion A predominate in the clinical picture and are sufficiently severe to warrant independent clinical attention

Associated Features Supporting Diagnosis

Obsessions, compulsions, hair pulling, skin picking, or other body-focused repetitive behaviors can occur in association with intoxication with the following classes of substances: stimulants (including cocaine) and other (or unknown) substances. Heavy metals and toxins may also cause obsessive-compulsive and related disorder symptoms. Laboratory assessments (e.g., urine toxicology) may be useful to measure substance intoxication as part of an assessment for obsessive-compulsive and related disorders.

Prevalence

In the general population, the very limited data that are available indicate that substance-induced obsessive-compulsive and related disorder is very rare.

Differential Diagnosis

Substance intoxication.   Obsessive-compulsive and related disorder symptoms may occur in substance intoxication. The diagnosis of the substance-specific intoxication will usually suffice to categorize the symptom presentation. A diagnosis of an obsessive-compulsive and related disorder should be made in addition to substance intoxication when the symptoms are judged to be in excess of those usually associated with intoxication and are sufficiently severe to warrant independent clinical attention.

Obsessive-compulsive and related disorder (i.e., not induced by a substance).   Substance/medication-induced obsessive-compulsive and related disorder is judged to be etiologically related to the substance/medication. Substance/medication-induced obsessive-compulsive and related disorder is distinguished from a primary obsessive-compulsive and related disorder by considering the onset, course, and other factors with respect to substances/medications. For drugs of abuse, there must be evidence from the history, physical examination, or laboratory findings for use or intoxication. Substance/medication-induced obsessive-compulsive and related disorder arises only in association with intoxication, whereas a primary obsessive-compulsive and related disorder may precede the onset of substance/medication use. The presence of features that are atypical of a primary obsessive-compulsive and related disorder, such as atypical age at onset of symptoms, may suggest a substance-induced etiology. A primary obsessive-compulsive and related disorder diagnosis is warranted if the symptoms persist for a substantial period of time (about 1 month or longer) after the end of the substance intoxication or the individual has a history of an obsessive-compulsive and related disorder.

Obsessive-compulsive and related disorder due to another medical condition.   If the obsessive-compulsive and related disorder symptoms are attributable to another medical condition (i.e., rather than to the medication taken for the other medical condition), obsessive-compulsive and related disorder due to another medical condition should be diagnosed. The history often provides the basis for judgment. At times, a change in the treatment for the other medical condition (e.g., medication substitution or discontinuation) may be needed to determine whether or not the medication is the causative agent (in which case the symptoms may be better explained by substance/medication-induced obsessive-compulsive and related disorder). If the disturbance is attributable to both another medical condition and substance use, both diagnoses (i.e., obsessive-compulsive and related disorder due to another medical condition and substance/medication-induced obsessive-compulsive and related disorder) may be given. When there is insufficient evidence to determine whether the symptoms are attributable to either a substance/medication or another medical condition or are primary (i.e., attributable to neither a substance/medication nor another medical condition), a diagnosis of other specified or unspecified obsessive-compulsive and related disorder would be indicated.

Delirium.   If obsessive-compulsive and related disorder symptoms occur exclusively during the course of delirium, they are considered to be an associated feature of the delirium and are not diagnosed separately.

Obsessive-Compulsive and Related Disorder Due to Another Medical Condition

Diagnostic Criteria   **294.8 (F06.8)**

A. Obsessions, compulsions, preoccupations with appearance, hoarding, skin picking, hair pulling, other body-focused repetitive behaviors, or other symptoms characteristic of obsessive-compulsive and related disorder predominate in the clinical picture.

B. There is evidence from the history, physical examination, or laboratory findings that the disturbance is the direct pathophysiological consequence of another medical condition.

C. The disturbance is not better explained by another mental disorder.

D. The disturbance does not occur exclusively during the course of a delirium.

E. The disturbance causes clinically significant distress or impairment in social, occupational, or other important areas of functioning.

Specify if:

With obsessive-compulsive disorder–like symptoms: If obsessive-compulsive disorder–like symptoms predominate in the clinical presentation.

With appearance preoccupations: If preoccupation with perceived appearance defects or flaws predominates in the clinical presentation.

With hoarding symptoms: If hoarding predominates in the clinical presentation.

With hair-pulling symptoms: If hair pulling predominates in the clinical presentation.

With skin-picking symptoms: If skin picking predominates in the clinical presentation.

Coding note: Include the name of the other medical condition in the name of the mental disorder (e.g., 294.8 [F06.8] obsessive-compulsive and related disorder due to cerebral infarction). The other medical condition should be coded and listed separately immediately before the obsessive-compulsive and related disorder due to the medical condition (e.g., 438.89 [I69.398] cerebral infarction; 294.8 [F06.8] obsessive-compulsive and related disorder due to cerebral infarction).

Diagnostic Features

The essential feature of obsessive-compulsive and related disorder due to another medical condition is clinically significant obsessive-compulsive and related symptoms that are judged to be best explained as the direct pathophysiological consequence of another medical condition. Symptoms can include prominent obsessions, compulsions, preoccupations with appearance, hoarding, hair pulling, skin picking, or other body-focused repetitive behaviors (Criterion A). The judgment that the symptoms are best explained by the associated medical condition must be based on evidence from the history, physical examination, or laboratory findings (Criterion B). Additionally, it must be judged that the symptoms are not better explained by another mental disorder (Criterion C). The diagnosis is not made if the obsessive-compulsive and related symptoms occur only during the course of a delirium (Criterion D). The obsessive-compulsive and related symptoms must cause clinically significant distress or impairment in social, occupational, or other important areas of functioning (Criterion E).

In determining whether the obsessive-compulsive and related symptoms are attributable to another medical condition, a relevant medical condition must be present. Furthermore, it must be established that obsessive-compulsive and related symptoms can be etiologically related to the medical condition through a pathophysiological mechanism and that this best explains the symptoms in the individual. Although there are no infallible guidelines for determining whether the relationship between the obsessive-compulsive and related symptoms and the medical condition is etiological, considerations that may provide some guidance in making this diagnosis include the presence of a clear temporal association between the onset, exacerbation, or remission of the medical condition and the obsessive-compulsive and related symptoms; the presence of features that are atypical of a primary obsessive-compulsive and related disorder (e.g., atypical age at onset or course); and evidence in the literature that a known physiological mechanism (e.g., striatal damage) causes obsessive-compulsive and related symptoms. In addition, the disturbance cannot be better explained by a primary obsessive-compulsive and related disorder, a substance/medication-induced obsessive-compulsive and related disorder, or another mental disorder.

There is some controversy about whether obsessive-compulsive and related disorders can be attributed to Group A streptococcal infection. Sydenham's chorea is the neurological manifestation of rheumatic fever, which is in turn due to Group A streptococcal infection. Sydenham's chorea is characterized by a combination of motor and nonmotor features. Nonmotor features include obsessions, compulsions, attention deficit, and emotional lability. Although individuals with Sydenham's chorea may present with non-neuropsychiatric features of acute rheumatic fever, such as carditis and arthritis, they may present with obsessive-compulsive disorder–like symptoms; such individuals should be diagnosed with obsessive-compulsive and related disorder due to another medical condition.

Pediatric autoimmune neuropsychiatric disorders associated with streptococcal infections (PANDAS) has been identified as another post-infectious autoimmune disorder characterized by the sudden onset of obsessions, compulsions, and/or tics accompanied by a variety of acute neuropsychiatric symptoms in the absence of chorea, carditis, or arthritis, after Group A streptococcal infection. Although there is a body of evidence that supports the existence of PANDAS, it remains a controversial diagnosis. Given this ongoing controversy, the description of PANDAS has been modified to eliminate etiological factors and to designate an expanded clinical entity: pediatric acute-onset neuropsychiatric syndrome (PANS) or idiopathic childhood acute neuropsychiatric symptoms (CANS), which deserves further study.

Associated Features Supporting Diagnosis

A number of other medical disorders are known to include obsessive-compulsive and related symptoms as a manifestation. Examples include disorders leading to striatal damage, such as cerebral infarction.

Development and Course

The development and course of obsessive-compulsive and related disorder due to another medical condition generally follows the course of the underlying illness.

Diagnostic Markers

Laboratory assessments and/or medical examinations are necessary to confirm the diagnosis of another medical condition.

Differential Diagnosis

Delirium.   A separate diagnosis of obsessive-compulsive and related disorder due to another medical condition is not given if the disturbance occurs exclusively during the course of a delirium. However, a diagnosis of obsessive-compulsive and related disorder due to another medical condition may be given in addition to a diagnosis of major neurocognitive disorder (dementia) if the etiology of the obsessive-compulsive symptoms is judged to be a physiological consequence of the pathological process causing the dementia and if obsessive-compulsive symptoms are a prominent part of the clinical presentation.

Mixed presentation of symptoms (e.g., mood and obsessive-compulsive and related disorder symptoms).   If the presentation includes a mix of different types of symptoms, the specific mental disorder due to another medical condition depends on which symptoms predominate in the clinical picture.

Substance/medication-induced obsessive-compulsive and related disorders.   If there is evidence of recent or prolonged substance use (including medications with psychoactive effects), withdrawal from a substance, or exposure to a toxin, a substance/medication-induced obsessive-compulsive and related disorder should be considered. When a substance/medication-induced obsessive-compulsive and related disorder is being diagnosed in relation to drugs of abuse, it may be useful to obtain a urine or blood drug screen or other appropriate laboratory evaluation. Symptoms that occur during or shortly after (i.e., within 4 weeks of) substance intoxication or withdrawal or after medication use may be especially indicative of a substance/medication-induced obsessive-compulsive and related disorder, depending on the type, duration, or amount of the substance used.

Obsessive-compulsive and related disorders (primary).   Obsessive-compulsive and related disorder due to another medical condition should be distinguished from a primary obsessive-compulsive and related disorder. In primary mental disorders, no specific and direct causative physiological mechanisms associated with a medical condition can be demonstrated. Late age at onset or atypical symptoms suggest the need for a thorough assessment to rule out the diagnosis of obsessive-compulsive and related disorder due to another medical condition.

Illness anxiety disorder.   Illness anxiety disorder is characterized by a preoccupation with having or acquiring a serious illness. In the case of illness anxiety disorder, individuals may or may not have diagnosed medical conditions.

Associated feature of another mental disorder.   Obsessive-compulsive and related symptoms may be an associated feature of another mental disorder (e.g., schizophrenia, anorexia nervosa).

Other specified obsessive-compulsive and related disorder or unspecified obsessive-compulsive and related disorder.   These diagnoses are given if it is unclear whether the obsessive-compulsive and related symptoms are primary, substance-induced, or due to another medical condition.

Other Specified Obsessive-Compulsive and Related Disorder

300.3 (F42.8)

This category applies to presentations in which symptoms characteristic of an obsessive-compulsive and related disorder that cause clinically significant distress or impairment in social, occupational, or other important areas of functioning predominate but do not meet the full criteria for any of the disorders in the obsessive-compulsive and related disorders diagnostic class. The other specified obsessive-compulsive and related disorder category is used in situations in which the clinician chooses to communicate the specific reason that the presentation does not meet the criteria for any specific obsessive-compulsive and related disorder. This is done by recording "other specified obsessive-compulsive and related disorder" followed by the specific reason (e.g., "body-focused repetitive behavior disorder").

Examples of presentations that can be specified using the "other specified" designation include the following:

1. **Body dysmorphic–like disorder with actual flaws:** This is similar to body dysmorphic disorder except that the defects or flaws in physical appearance are clearly observable by others (i.e., they are more noticeable than "slight"). In such cases, the preoccupation with these flaws is clearly excessive and causes significant impairment or distress.
2. **Body dysmorphic–like disorder without repetitive behaviors:** Presentations that meet body dysmorphic disorder except that the individual has not performed repetitive behaviors or mental acts in response to the appearance concerns.
3. **Body-focused repetitive behavior disorder:** This is characterized by recurrent body-focused repetitive behaviors (e.g., nail biting, lip biting, cheek chewing) and repeated attempts to decrease or stop the behaviors. These symptoms cause clinically significant

distress or impairment in social, occupational, or other important areas of functioning and are not better explained by trichotillomania (hair-pulling disorder), excoriation (skin-picking) disorder, stereotypic movement disorder, or nonsuicidal self-injury.

4. **Obsessional jealousy:** This is characterized by nondelusional preoccupation with a partner's perceived infidelity. The preoccupations may lead to repetitive behaviors or mental acts in response to the infidelity concerns; they cause clinically significant distress or impairment in social, occupational, or other important areas of functioning; and they are not better explained by another mental disorder such as delusional disorder, jealous type, or paranoid personality disorder.

5. ***Shubo-kyofu:*** A variant of *taijin kyofusho* (see "Glossary of Cultural Concepts of Distress" in the Appendix) that is similar to body dysmorphic disorder and is characterized by excessive fear of having a bodily deformity.

6. ***Koro:*** Related to *dhat syndrome* (see "Glossary of Cultural Concepts of Distress" in the Appendix), an episode of sudden and intense anxiety that the penis (or the vulva and nipples in females) will recede into the body, possibly leading to death.

7. ***Jikoshu-kyofu:*** A variant of *taijin kyofusho* (see "Glossary of Cultural Concepts of Distress" in the Appendix) characterized by fear of having an offensive body odor (also termed *olfactory reference syndrome*).

Unspecified Obsessive-Compulsive and Related Disorder

300.3 (F42.9)

This category applies to presentations in which symptoms characteristic of an obsessive-compulsive and related disorder that cause clinically significant distress or impairment in social, occupational, or other important areas of functioning predominate but do not meet the full criteria for any of the disorders in the obsessive-compulsive and related disorders diagnostic class. The unspecified obsessive-compulsive and related disorder category is used in situations in which the clinician chooses *not* to specify the reason that the criteria are not met for a specific obsessive-compulsive and related disorder, and includes presentations in which there is insufficient information to make a more specific diagnosis (e.g., in emergency room settings).

Trauma- and Stressor-Related Disorders

Trauma- and stressor-related disorders include disorders in which exposure to a traumatic or stressful event is listed explicitly as a diagnostic criterion. These include reactive attachment disorder, disinhibited social engagement disorder, posttraumatic stress disorder (PTSD), acute stress disorder, and adjustment disorders. Placement of this chapter reflects the close relationship between these diagnoses and disorders in the surrounding chapters on anxiety disorders, obsessive-compulsive and related disorders, and dissociative disorders.

Psychological distress following exposure to a traumatic or stressful event is quite variable. In some cases, symptoms can be well understood within an anxiety- or fear-based context. It is clear, however, that many individuals who have been exposed to a traumatic or stressful event exhibit a phenotype in which, rather than anxiety- or fear-based symptoms, the most prominent clinical characteristics are anhedonic and dysphoric symptoms, externalizing angry and aggressive symptoms, or dissociative symptoms. Because of these variable expressions of clinical distress following exposure to catastrophic or aversive events, the aforementioned disorders have been grouped under a separate category: *trauma- and stressor-related disorders*. Furthermore, it is not uncommon for the clinical picture to include some combination of the above symptoms (with or without anxiety- or fear-based symptoms). Such a heterogeneous picture has long been recognized in adjustment disorders, as well. Social neglect—that is, the absence of adequate caregiving during childhood—is a diagnostic requirement of both reactive attachment disorder and disinhibited social engagement disorder. Although the two disorders share a common etiology, the former is expressed as an internalizing disorder with depressive symptoms and withdrawn behavior, while the latter is marked by disinhibition and externalizing behavior.

Reactive Attachment Disorder

Diagnostic Criteria   313.89 (F94.1)

A. A consistent pattern of inhibited, emotionally withdrawn behavior toward adult caregivers, manifested by both of the following:

   1. The child rarely or minimally seeks comfort when distressed.
   2. The child rarely or minimally responds to comfort when distressed.

B. A persistent social and emotional disturbance characterized by at least two of the following:

   1. Minimal social and emotional responsiveness to others.
   2. Limited positive affect.
   3. Episodes of unexplained irritability, sadness, or fearfulness that are evident even during nonthreatening interactions with adult caregivers.

C. The child has experienced a pattern of extremes of insufficient care as evidenced by at least one of the following:

   1. Social neglect or deprivation in the form of persistent lack of having basic emotional needs for comfort, stimulation, and affection met by caregiving adults.

2. Repeated changes of primary caregivers that limit opportunities to form stable attachments (e.g., frequent changes in foster care).
3. Rearing in unusual settings that severely limit opportunities to form selective attachments (e.g., institutions with high child-to-caregiver ratios).

D. The care in Criterion C is presumed to be responsible for the disturbed behavior in Criterion A (e.g., the disturbances in Criterion A began following the lack of adequate care in Criterion C).
E. The criteria are not met for autism spectrum disorder.
F. The disturbance is evident before age 5 years.
G. The child has a developmental age of at least 9 months.

Specify if:

Persistent: The disorder has been present for more than 12 months.

Specify current severity:

Reactive attachment disorder is specified as **severe** when a child exhibits all symptoms of the disorder, with each symptom manifesting at relatively high levels.

Diagnostic Features

Reactive attachment disorder is characterized by a pattern of markedly disturbed and developmentally inappropriate attachment behaviors, in which a child rarely or minimally turns preferentially to an attachment figure for comfort, support, protection, and nurturance. The essential feature is absent or grossly underdeveloped attachment between the child and putative caregiving adults. Children with reactive attachment disorder are believed to have the capacity to form selective attachments. However, because of limited opportunities during early development, they fail to show the behavioral manifestations of selective attachments. That is, when distressed, they show no consistent effort to obtain comfort, support, nurturance, or protection from caregivers. Furthermore, when distressed, children with this disorder do not respond more than minimally to comforting efforts of caregivers. Thus, the disorder is associated with the absence of expected comfort seeking and response to comforting behaviors. As such, children with reactive attachment disorder show diminished or absent expression of positive emotions during routine interactions with caregivers. In addition, their emotion regulation capacity is compromised, and they display episodes of negative emotions of fear, sadness, or irritability that are not readily explained. A diagnosis of reactive attachment disorder should not be made in children who are developmentally unable to form selective attachments. For this reason, the child must have a developmental age of at least 9 months.

Associated Features Supporting Diagnosis

Because of the shared etiological association with social neglect, reactive attachment disorder often co-occurs with developmental delays, especially in delays in cognition and language. Other associated features include stereotypies and other signs of severe neglect (e.g., malnutrition or signs of poor care).

Prevalence

The prevalence of reactive attachment disorder is unknown, but the disorder is seen relatively rarely in clinical settings. The disorder has been found in young children exposed to severe neglect before being placed in foster care or raised in institutions. However, even in populations of severely neglected children, the disorder is uncommon, occurring in less than 10% of such children.

Development and Course

Conditions of social neglect are often present in the first months of life in children diagnosed with reactive attachment disorder, even before the disorder is diagnosed. The clinical features of the disorder manifest in a similar fashion between the ages of 9 months and 5 years. That is, signs of absent-to-minimal attachment behaviors and associated emotionally aberrant behaviors are evident in children throughout this age range, although differing cognitive and motor abilities may affect how these behaviors are expressed. Without remediation and recovery through normative caregiving environments, it appears that signs of the disorder may persist, at least for several years.

It is unclear whether reactive attachment disorder occurs in older children and, if so, how it differs from its presentation in young children. Because of this, the diagnosis should be made with caution in children older than 5 years.

Risk and Prognostic Factors

Environmental. Serious social neglect is a diagnostic requirement for reactive attachment disorder and is also the only known risk factor for the disorder. However, the majority of severely neglected children do not develop the disorder. Prognosis appears to depend on the quality of the caregiving environment following serious neglect.

Culture-Related Diagnostic Issues

Similar attachment behaviors have been described in young children in many different cultures around the world. However, caution should be exercised in making the diagnosis of reactive attachment disorder in cultures in which attachment has not been studied.

Functional Consequences of Reactive Attachment Disorder

Reactive attachment disorder significantly impairs young children's abilities to relate interpersonally to adults or peers and is associated with functional impairment across many domains of early childhood.

Differential Diagnosis

Autism spectrum disorder. Aberrant social behaviors manifest in young children with reactive attachment disorder, but they also are key features of autism spectrum disorder. Specifically, young children with either condition can manifest dampened expression of positive emotions, cognitive and language delays, and impairments in social reciprocity. As a result, reactive attachment disorder must be differentiated from autism spectrum disorder. These two disorders can be distinguished based on differential histories of neglect and on the presence of restricted interests or ritualized behaviors, specific deficit in social communication, and selective attachment behaviors. Children with reactive attachment disorder have experienced a history of severe social neglect, although it is not always possible to obtain detailed histories about the precise nature of their experiences, especially in initial evaluations. Children with autistic spectrum disorder will only rarely have a history of social neglect. The restricted interests and repetitive behaviors characteristic of autism spectrum disorder are not a feature of reactive attachment disorder. These clinical features manifest as excessive adherence to rituals and routines; restricted, fixated interests; and unusual sensory reactions. However, it is important to note that children with either condition can exhibit stereotypic behaviors such as rocking or flapping. Children with either disorder also may exhibit a range of intellectual functioning, but only children with autistic spectrum disorder exhibit selective impairments in social communicative behaviors, such as intentional communication (i.e., impairment in communication that is deliberate, goal-directed, and aimed at influencing the behavior of the recipient). Children with reactive attachment disorder show social communicative functioning comparable to their overall level of intellectual functioning. Finally, children with autistic spectrum disorder regularly show attachment behavior typical for their developmental level. In contrast, children with reactive attachment disorder do so only rarely or inconsistently, if at all.

Intellectual disability (intellectual developmental disorder).   Developmental delays often accompany reactive attachment disorder, but they should not be confused with the disorder. Children with intellectual disability should exhibit social and emotional skills comparable to their cognitive skills and do not demonstrate the profound reduction in positive affect and emotion regulation difficulties evident in children with reactive attachment disorder. In addition, developmentally delayed children who have reached a cognitive age of 7–9 months should demonstrate selective attachments regardless of their chronological age. In contrast, children with reactive attachment disorder show lack of preferred attachment despite having attained a developmental age of at least 9 months.

Depressive disorders.   Depression in young children is also associated with reductions in positive affect. There is limited evidence, however, to suggest that children with depressive disorders have impairments in attachment. That is, young children who have been diagnosed with depressive disorders still should seek and respond to comforting efforts by caregivers.

Comorbidity

Conditions associated with neglect, including cognitive delays, language delays, and stereotypies, often co-occur with reactive attachment disorder. Medical conditions, such as severe malnutrition, may accompany signs of the disorder. Depressive symptoms also may co-occur with reactive attachment disorder.

Disinhibited Social Engagement Disorder

Diagnostic Criteria   **313.89** (F94.2)

A. A pattern of behavior in which a child actively approaches and interacts with unfamiliar adults and exhibits at least two of the following:
   1. Reduced or absent reticence in approaching and interacting with unfamiliar adults.
   2. Overly familiar verbal or physical behavior (that is not consistent with culturally sanctioned and with age-appropriate social boundaries).
   3. Diminished or absent checking back with adult caregiver after venturing away, even in unfamiliar settings.
   4. Willingness to go off with an unfamiliar adult with minimal or no hesitation.
B. The behaviors in Criterion A are not limited to impulsivity (as in attention-deficit/hyperactivity disorder) but include socially disinhibited behavior.
C. The child has experienced a pattern of extremes of insufficient care as evidenced by at least one of the following:
   1. Social neglect or deprivation in the form of persistent lack of having basic emotional needs for comfort, stimulation, and affection met by caregiving adults.
   2. Repeated changes of primary caregivers that limit opportunities to form stable attachments (e.g., frequent changes in foster care).
   3. Rearing in unusual settings that severely limit opportunities to form selective attachments (e.g., institutions with high child-to-caregiver ratios).

D. The care in Criterion C is presumed to be responsible for the disturbed behavior in Criterion A (e.g., the disturbances in Criterion A began following the pathogenic care in Criterion C).

E. The child has a developmental age of at least 9 months.

Specify if:

Persistent: The disorder has been present for more than 12 months.

Specify current severity:

Disinhibited social engagement disorder is specified as **severe** when the child exhibits all symptoms of the disorder, with each symptom manifesting at relatively high levels.

Diagnostic Features

The essential feature of disinhibited social engagement disorder is a pattern of behavior that involves culturally inappropriate, overly familiar behavior with relative strangers (Criterion A). This overly familiar behavior violates the social boundaries of the culture. A diagnosis of disinhibited social engagement disorder should not be made before children are developmentally able to form selective attachments. For this reason, the child must have a developmental age of at least 9 months.

Associated Features Supporting Diagnosis

Because of the shared etiological association with social neglect, disinhibited social engagement disorder may co-occur with developmental delays, especially cognitive and language delays, stereotypies, and other signs of severe neglect, such as malnutrition or poor care. However, signs of the disorder often persist even after these other signs of neglect are no longer present. Therefore, it is not uncommon for children with the disorder to present with no current signs of neglect. Moreover, the condition can present in children who show no signs of disordered attachment. Thus, disinhibited social engagement disorder may be seen in children with a history of neglect who lack attachments or whose attachments to their caregivers range from disturbed to secure.

Prevalence

The prevalence of disinhibited social attachment disorder is unknown. Nevertheless, the disorder appears to be rare, occurring in a minority of children, even those who have been severely neglected and subsequently placed in foster care or raised in institutions. In such high-risk populations, the condition occurs in only about 20% of children. The condition is seen rarely in other clinical settings.

Development and Course

Conditions of social neglect are often present in the first months of life in children diagnosed with disinhibited social engagement disorder, even before the disorder is diagnosed. However, there is no evidence that neglect beginning after age 2 years is associated with manifestations of the disorder. If neglect occurs early and signs of the disorder appear, clinical features of the disorder are moderately stable over time, particularly if conditions of neglect persist. Indiscriminate social behavior and lack of reticence with unfamiliar adults in toddlerhood are accompanied by attention-seeking behaviors in preschoolers. When the disorder persists into middle childhood, clinical features manifest as verbal and physical overfamiliarity as well as inauthentic expression of emotions. These signs appear particularly apparent when the child interacts with adults. Peer relationships are most affected in adolescence, with both indiscriminate behavior and conflicts apparent. The disorder has not been described in adults.

Disinhibited social engagement disorder has been described from the second year of life through adolescence. There are some differences in manifestations of the disorder from early childhood through adolescence. At the youngest ages, across many cultures, children show reticence when interacting with strangers. Young children with the disorder fail to show reticence to approach, engage with, and even accompany adults. In preschool children, verbal and social intrusiveness appear most prominent, often accompanied by attention-seeking behavior. Verbal and physical overfamiliarity continue through middle childhood, accompanied by inauthentic expressions of emotion. In adolescence, indiscriminate behavior extends to peers. Relative to healthy adolescents, adolescents with the disorder have more "superficial" peer relationships and more peer conflicts. Adult manifestations of the disorder are unknown.

Risk and Prognostic Factors

Environmental.   Serious social neglect is a diagnostic requirement for disinhibited social engagement disorder and is also the only known risk factor for the disorder. However, the majority of severely neglected children do not develop the disorder. Neurobiological vulnerability may differentiate neglected children who do and do not develop the disorder. However, no clear link with any specific neurobiological factors has been established. The disorder has not been identified in children who experience social neglect only after age 2 years. Prognosis is only modestly associated with quality of the caregiving environment following serious neglect. In many cases, the disorder persists, even in children whose caregiving environment becomes markedly improved.

Course modifiers.   Caregiving quality seems to moderate the course of disinhibited social engagement disorder. Nevertheless, even after placement in normative caregiving environments, some children show persistent signs of the disorder, at least through adolescence.

Functional Consequences of Disinhibited Social Engagement Disorder

Disinhibited social engagement disorder significantly impairs young children's abilities to relate interpersonally to adults and peers.

Differential Diagnosis

Attention-deficit/hyperactivity disorder.   Because of social impulsivity that sometimes accompanies attention-deficit/hyperactivity disorder (ADHD), it is necessary to differentiate the two disorders. Children with disinhibited social engagement disorder may be distinguished from those with ADHD because the former do not show difficulties with attention or hyperactivity.

Comorbidity

Limited research has examined the issue of disorders comorbid with disinhibited social engagement disorder. Conditions associated with neglect, including cognitive delays, language delays, and stereotypies, may co-occur with disinhibited social engagement disorder. In addition, children may be diagnosed with ADHD and disinhibited social engagement disorder concurrently.

Posttraumatic Stress Disorder

Diagnostic Criteria	**309.81 (F43.10)**

Posttraumatic Stress Disorder

Note: The following criteria apply to adults, adolescents, and children older than 6 years. For children 6 years and younger, see corresponding criteria below.

A. Exposure to actual or threatened death, serious injury, or sexual violence in one (or more) of the following ways:

   1. Directly experiencing the traumatic event(s).
   2. Witnessing, in person, the event(s) as it occurred to others.
   3. Learning that the traumatic event(s) occurred to a close family member or close friend. In cases of actual or threatened death of a family member or friend, the event(s) must have been violent or accidental.
   4. Experiencing repeated or extreme exposure to aversive details of the traumatic event(s) (e.g., first responders collecting human remains; police officers repeatedly exposed to details of child abuse).

   Note: Criterion A4 does not apply to exposure through electronic media, television, movies, or pictures, unless this exposure is work related.

B. Presence of one (or more) of the following intrusion symptoms associated with the traumatic event(s), beginning after the traumatic event(s) occurred:

   1. Recurrent, involuntary, and intrusive distressing memories of the traumatic event(s).

   Note: In children older than 6 years, repetitive play may occur in which themes or aspects of the traumatic event(s) are expressed.

   2. Recurrent distressing dreams in which the content and/or affect of the dream are related to the traumatic event(s).

   Note: In children, there may be frightening dreams without recognizable content.

   3. Dissociative reactions (e.g., flashbacks) in which the individual feels or acts as if the traumatic event(s) were recurring. (Such reactions may occur on a continuum, with the most extreme expression being a complete loss of awareness of present surroundings.)

   Note: In children, trauma-specific reenactment may occur in play.

   4. Intense or prolonged psychological distress at exposure to internal or external cues that symbolize or resemble an aspect of the traumatic event(s).
   5. Marked physiological reactions to internal or external cues that symbolize or resemble an aspect of the traumatic event(s).

C. Persistent avoidance of stimuli associated with the traumatic event(s), beginning after the traumatic event(s) occurred, as evidenced by one or both of the following:

   1. Avoidance of or efforts to avoid distressing memories, thoughts, or feelings about or closely associated with the traumatic event(s).
   2. Avoidance of or efforts to avoid external reminders (people, places, conversations, activities, objects, situations) that arouse distressing memories, thoughts, or feelings about or closely associated with the traumatic event(s).

D. Negative alterations in cognitions and mood associated with the traumatic event(s), beginning or worsening after the traumatic event(s) occurred, as evidenced by two (or more) of the following:

   1. Inability to remember an important aspect of the traumatic event(s) (typically due to dissociative amnesia and not to other factors such as head injury, alcohol, or drugs).

2. Persistent and exaggerated negative beliefs or expectations about oneself, others, or the world (e.g., "I am bad," "No one can be trusted," "The world is completely dangerous," "My whole nervous system is permanently ruined").

3. Persistent, distorted cognitions about the cause or consequences of the traumatic event(s) that lead the individual to blame himself/herself or others.

4. Persistent negative emotional state (e.g., fear, horror, anger, guilt, or shame).

5. Markedly diminished interest or participation in significant activities.

6. Feelings of detachment or estrangement from others.

7. Persistent inability to experience positive emotions (e.g., inability to experience happiness, satisfaction, or loving feelings).

E. Marked alterations in arousal and reactivity associated with the traumatic event(s), beginning or worsening after the traumatic event(s) occurred, as evidenced by two (or more) of the following:

1. Irritable behavior and angry outbursts (with little or no provocation) typically expressed as verbal or physical aggression toward people or objects.

2. Reckless or self-destructive behavior.

3. Hypervigilance.

4. Exaggerated startle response.

5. Problems with concentration.

6. Sleep disturbance (e.g., difficulty falling or staying asleep or restless sleep).

F. Duration of the disturbance (Criteria B, C, D, and E) is more than 1 month.

G. The disturbance causes clinically significant distress or impairment in social, occupational, or other important areas of functioning.

H. The disturbance is not attributable to the physiological effects of a substance (e.g., medication, alcohol) or another medical condition.

Specify whether:

With dissociative symptoms: The individual's symptoms meet the criteria for posttraumatic stress disorder, and in addition, in response to the stressor, the individual experiences persistent or recurrent symptoms of either of the following:

1. **Depersonalization:** Persistent or recurrent experiences of feeling detached from, and as if one were an outside observer of, one's mental processes or body (e.g., feeling as though one were in a dream; feeling a sense of unreality of self or body or of time moving slowly).

2. **Derealization:** Persistent or recurrent experiences of unreality of surroundings (e.g., the world around the individual is experienced as unreal, dreamlike, distant, or distorted).

Note: To use this subtype, the dissociative symptoms must not be attributable to the physiological effects of a substance (e.g., blackouts, behavior during alcohol intoxication) or another medical condition (e.g., complex partial seizures).

Specify if:

With delayed expression: If the full diagnostic criteria are not met until at least 6 months after the event (although the onset and expression of some symptoms may be immediate).

Posttraumatic Stress Disorder for Children 6 Years and Younger

A. In children 6 years and younger, exposure to actual or threatened death, serious injury, or sexual violence in one (or more) of the following ways:

1. Directly experiencing the traumatic event(s).

2. Witnessing, in person, the event(s) as it occurred to others, especially primary caregivers.

Note: Witnessing does not include events that are witnessed only in electronic media, television, movies, or pictures.

3. Learning that the traumatic event(s) occurred to a parent or caregiving figure.

B. Presence of one (or more) of the following intrusion symptoms associated with the traumatic event(s), beginning after the traumatic event(s) occurred:

1. Recurrent, involuntary, and intrusive distressing memories of the traumatic event(s).

   Note: Spontaneous and intrusive memories may not necessarily appear distressing and may be expressed as play reenactment.

2. Recurrent distressing dreams in which the content and/or affect of the dream are related to the traumatic event(s).

   Note: It may not be possible to ascertain that the frightening content is related to the traumatic event.

3. Dissociative reactions (e.g., flashbacks) in which the child feels or acts as if the traumatic event(s) were recurring. (Such reactions may occur on a continuum, with the most extreme expression being a complete loss of awareness of present surroundings.) Such trauma-specific reenactment may occur in play.

4. Intense or prolonged psychological distress at exposure to internal or external cues that symbolize or resemble an aspect of the traumatic event(s).

5. Marked physiological reactions to reminders of the traumatic event(s).

C. One (or more) of the following symptoms, representing either persistent avoidance of stimuli associated with the traumatic event(s) or negative alterations in cognitions and mood associated with the traumatic event(s), must be present, beginning after the event(s) or worsening after the event(s):

Persistent Avoidance of Stimuli

1. Avoidance of or efforts to avoid activities, places, or physical reminders that arouse recollections of the traumatic event(s).

2. Avoidance of or efforts to avoid people, conversations, or interpersonal situations that arouse recollections of the traumatic event(s).

Negative Alterations in Cognitions

3. Substantially increased frequency of negative emotional states (e.g., fear, guilt, sadness, shame, confusion).

4. Markedly diminished interest or participation in significant activities, including constriction of play.

5. Socially withdrawn behavior.

6. Persistent reduction in expression of positive emotions.

D. Alterations in arousal and reactivity associated with the traumatic event(s), beginning or worsening after the traumatic event(s) occurred, as evidenced by two (or more) of the following:

1. Irritable behavior and angry outbursts (with little or no provocation) typically expressed as verbal or physical aggression toward people or objects (including extreme temper tantrums).

2. Hypervigilance.

3. Exaggerated startle response.

4. Problems with concentration.

5. Sleep disturbance (e.g., difficulty falling or staying asleep or restless sleep).

E. The duration of the disturbance is more than 1 month.

F. The disturbance causes clinically significant distress or impairment in relationships with parents, siblings, peers, or other caregivers or with school behavior.

G. The disturbance is not attributable to the physiological effects of a substance (e.g., medication or alcohol) or another medical condition.

Specify whether:

With dissociative symptoms: The individual's symptoms meet the criteria for post-traumatic stress disorder, and the individual experiences persistent or recurrent symptoms of either of the following:

1. **Depersonalization:** Persistent or recurrent experiences of feeling detached from, and as if one were an outside observer of, one's mental processes or body (e.g., feeling as though one were in a dream; feeling a sense of unreality of self or body or of time moving slowly).

2. **Derealization:** Persistent or recurrent experiences of unreality of surroundings (e.g., the world around the individual is experienced as unreal, dreamlike, distant, or distorted).

Note: To use this subtype, the dissociative symptoms must not be attributable to the physiological effects of a substance (e.g., blackouts) or another medical condition (e.g., complex partial seizures).

Specify if:

With delayed expression: If the full diagnostic criteria are not met until at least 6 months after the event (although the onset and expression of some symptoms may be immediate).

Diagnostic Features

The essential feature of posttraumatic stress disorder (PTSD) is the development of characteristic symptoms following exposure to one or more traumatic events. Emotional reactions to the traumatic event (e.g., fear, helplessness, horror) are no longer a part of Criterion A. The clinical presentation of PTSD varies. In some individuals, fear-based re-experiencing, emotional, and behavioral symptoms may predominate. In others, anhedonic or dysphoric mood states and negative cognitions may be most distressing. In some other individuals, arousal and reactive-externalizing symptoms are prominent, while in others, dissociative symptoms predominate. Finally, some individuals exhibit combinations of these symptom patterns.

The directly experienced traumatic events in Criterion A include, but are not limited to, exposure to war as a combatant or civilian, threatened or actual physical assault (e.g., physical attack, robbery, mugging, childhood physical abuse), threatened or actual sexual violence (e.g., forced sexual penetration, alcohol/drug-facilitated sexual penetration, abusive sexual contact, noncontact sexual abuse, sexual trafficking), being kidnapped, being taken hostage, terrorist attack, torture, incarceration as a prisoner of war, natural or human-made disasters, and severe motor vehicle accidents. For children, sexually violent events may include developmentally inappropriate sexual experiences without physical violence or injury. A life-threatening illness or debilitating medical condition is not necessarily considered a traumatic event. Medical incidents that qualify as traumatic events involve sudden, catastrophic events (e.g., waking during surgery, anaphylactic shock). Witnessed events include, but are not limited to, observing threatened or serious injury, unnatural death, physical or sexual abuse of another person due to violent assault, domestic violence, accident, war or disaster, or a medical catastrophe in one's child (e.g., a life-threatening hemorrhage). Indirect exposure through learning about an event is limited to experiences affecting close relatives or friends and experiences that are violent or accidental (e.g., death due to natural causes does not qualify). Such events include violent personal assault, suicide, serious accident, and serious injury. The disorder may be especially severe or long-lasting when the stressor is interpersonal and intentional (e.g., torture, sexual violence).

The traumatic event can be reexperienced in various ways. Commonly, the individual has recurrent, involuntary, and intrusive recollections of the event (Criterion B1). Intrusive recollections in PTSD are distinguished from depressive rumination in that they apply only to involuntary and intrusive distressing memories. The emphasis is on recurrent memories of the event that usually include sensory, emotional, or physiological behavioral components. A common reexperiencing symptom is distressing dreams that replay the event itself or that are representative or thematically related to the major threats involved in the traumatic event (Criterion B2). The individual may experience dissociative states that last from a few seconds to several hours or even days, during which components of the event are relived and the individual behaves as if the event were occurring at that moment (Criterion B3). Such events occur on a continuum from brief visual or other sensory intrusions about part of the traumatic event without loss of reality orientation, to complete loss of awareness of present surroundings. These episodes, often referred to as "flashbacks," are typically brief but can be associated with prolonged distress and heightened arousal. For young children, reenactment of events related to trauma may appear in play or in dissociative states. Intense psychological distress (Criterion B4) or physiological reactivity (Criterion B5) often occurs when the individual is exposed to triggering events that resemble or symbolize an aspect of the traumatic event (e.g., windy days after a hurricane; seeing someone who resembles one's perpetrator). The triggering cue could be a physical sensation (e.g., dizziness for survivors of head trauma; rapid heartbeat for a previously traumatized child), particularly for individuals with highly somatic presentations.

Stimuli associated with the trauma are persistently (e.g., always or almost always) avoided. The individual commonly makes deliberate efforts to avoid thoughts, memories, feelings, or talking about the traumatic event (e.g., utilizing distraction techniques to avoid internal reminders) (Criterion C1) and to avoid activities, objects, situations, or people who arouse recollections of it (Criterion C2).

Negative alterations in cognitions or mood associated with the event begin or worsen after exposure to the event. These negative alterations can take various forms, including an inability to remember an important aspect of the traumatic event; such amnesia is typically due to dissociative amnesia and is not due to head injury, alcohol, or drugs (Criterion D1). Another form is persistent (i.e., always or almost always) and exaggerated negative expectations regarding important aspects of life applied to oneself, others, or the future (e.g., "I have always had bad judgment"; "People in authority can't be trusted") that may manifest as a negative change in perceived identity since the trauma (e.g., "I can't trust anyone ever again"; Criterion D2). Individuals with PTSD may have persistent erroneous cognitions about the causes of the traumatic event that lead them to blame themselves or others (e.g., "It's all my fault that my uncle abused me") (Criterion D3). A persistent negative mood state (e.g., fear, horror, anger, guilt, shame) either began or worsened after exposure to the event (Criterion D4). The individual may experience markedly diminished interest or participation in previously enjoyed activities (Criterion D5), feeling detached or estranged from other people (Criterion D6), or a persistent inability to feel positive emotions (especially happiness, joy, satisfaction, or emotions associated with intimacy, tenderness, and sexuality) (Criterion D7).

Individuals with PTSD may be quick tempered and may even engage in aggressive verbal and/or physical behavior with little or no provocation (e.g., yelling at people, getting into fights, destroying objects) (Criterion E1). They may also engage in reckless or self-destructive behavior such as dangerous driving, excessive alcohol or drug use, or self-injurious or suicidal behavior (Criterion E2). PTSD is often characterized by a heightened sensitivity to potential threats, including those that are related to the traumatic experience (e.g., following a motor vehicle accident, being especially sensitive to the threat potentially caused by cars or trucks) and those not related to the traumatic event (e.g., being fearful of suffering a heart attack) (Criterion E3). Individuals with PTSD may be very reactive to unexpected stimuli, displaying a heightened startle response, or jumpiness, to loud noises or unexpected movements (e.g., jumping markedly in response to a telephone ringing) (Criterion E4). Concentration difficulties, including difficulty remembering daily events (e.g., forgetting one's telephone number) or attending to focused tasks (e.g., following a conversation for a sustained period of time), are commonly reported (Criterion E5). Problems with sleep onset and maintenance are common and may be associated with nightmares and safety concerns or with generalized elevated arousal that interferes with adequate sleep (Criterion E6). Some individuals also experience persistent dissociative symptoms of detachment from their bodies (depersonalization) or the world around them (derealization); this is reflected in the "with dissociative symptoms" specifier.

Associated Features Supporting Diagnosis

Developmental regression, such as loss of language in young children, may occur. Auditory pseudo-hallucinations, such as having the sensory experience of hearing one's thoughts spoken in one or more different voices, as well as paranoid ideation, can be present. Following prolonged, repeated, and severe traumatic events (e.g., childhood abuse, torture), the individual may additionally experience difficulties in regulating emotions or maintaining stable interpersonal relationships, or dissociative symptoms. When the traumatic event produces violent death, symptoms of both problematic bereavement and PTSD may be present.

Prevalence

In the United States, projected lifetime risk for PTSD using DSM-IV criteria at age 75 years is 8.7%. Twelve-month prevalence among U.S. adults is about 3.5%. Lower estimates are seen in Europe and most Asian, African, and Latin American countries, clustering around 0.5%–1.0%. Although different groups have different levels of exposure to traumatic events, the conditional probability of developing PTSD following a similar level of exposure may also vary across cultural groups. Rates of PTSD are higher among veterans and others whose vocation increases the risk of traumatic exposure (e.g., police, firefighters, emergency medical personnel). Highest rates (ranging from one-third to more than one-half of those exposed) are found among survivors of rape, military combat and captivity, and ethnically or politically motivated internment and genocide. The prevalence of PTSD may vary across development; children and adolescents, including preschool children, generally have displayed lower prevalence following exposure to serious traumatic events; however, this may be because previous criteria were insufficiently developmentally informed. The prevalence of full-threshold PTSD also appears to be lower among older adults compared with the general population; there is evidence that subthreshold presentations are more common than full PTSD in later life and that these symptoms are associated with substantial clinical impairment. Compared with U.S. non-Latino whites, higher rates of PTSD have been reported among U.S. Latinos, African Americans, and American Indians, and lower rates have been reported among Asian Americans, after adjustment for traumatic exposure and demographic variables.

Development and Course

PTSD can occur at any age, beginning after the first year of life. Symptoms usually begin within the first 3 months after the trauma, although there may be a delay of months, or even years, before criteria for the diagnosis are met. There is abundant evidence for what DSM-IV called "delayed onset" but is now called "delayed expression," with the recognition that some symptoms typically appear immediately and that the delay is in meeting full criteria.

Frequently, an individual's reaction to a trauma initially meets criteria for acute stress disorder in the immediate aftermath of the trauma. The symptoms of PTSD and the relative predominance of different symptoms may vary over time. Duration of the symptoms also varies, with complete recovery within 3 months occurring in approximately one-half of adults, while some individuals remain symptomatic for longer than 12 months and sometimes for more than 50 years. Symptom recurrence and intensification may occur in response to reminders of the original trauma, ongoing life stressors, or newly experienced traumatic events. For older individuals, declining health, worsening cognitive functioning, and social isolation may exacerbate PTSD symptoms.

The clinical expression of reexperiencing can vary across development. Young children may report new onset of frightening dreams without content specific to the traumatic event. Before age 6 years (see criteria for preschool subtype), young children are more likely to express reexperiencing symptoms through play that refers directly or symbolically to the trauma. They may not manifest fearful reactions at the time of the exposure or during reexperiencing. Parents may report a wide range of emotional or behavioral changes in young children. Children may focus on imagined interventions in their play or storytelling. In addition to avoidance, children may become preoccupied with reminders. Because of young children's limitations in expressing thoughts or labeling emotions, negative alterations in mood or cognition tend to involve primarily mood changes. Children may experience co-occurring traumas (e.g., physical abuse, witnessing domestic violence) and in chronic circumstances may not be able to identify onset of symptomatology. Avoidant behavior may be associated with restricted play or exploratory behavior in young children; reduced participation in new activities in school-age children; or reluctance to pursue developmental opportunities in adolescents (e.g., dating, driving). Older children and adolescents may judge themselves as cowardly. Adolescents may harbor beliefs of being changed in ways that make them socially undesirable and estrange them from peers (e.g., "Now I'll never fit in") and lose aspirations for the future. Irritable or aggressive behavior in children and adolescents can interfere with peer relationships and school behavior. Reckless behavior may lead to accidental injury to self or others, thrill-seeking, or high-risk behaviors. Individuals who continue to experience PTSD into older adulthood may express fewer symptoms of hyperarousal, avoidance, and negative cognitions and mood compared with younger adults with PTSD, although adults exposed to traumatic events during later life may display more avoidance, hyperarousal, sleep problems, and crying spells than do younger adults exposed to the same traumatic events. In older individuals, the disorder is associated with negative health perceptions, primary care utilization, and suicidal ideation.

Risk and Prognostic Factors

Risk (and protective) factors are generally divided into pretraumatic, peritraumatic, and posttraumatic factors.

Pretraumatic factors

Temperamental. These include childhood emotional problems by age 6 years (e.g., prior traumatic exposure, externalizing or anxiety problems) and prior mental disorders (e.g., panic disorder, depressive disorder, PTSD, or obsessive-compulsive disorder [OCD]).

Environmental. These include lower socioeconomic status; lower education; exposure to prior trauma (especially during childhood); childhood adversity (e.g., economic deprivation, family dysfunction, parental separation or death); cultural characteristics (e.g., fatalistic or self-blaming coping strategies); lower intelligence; minority racial/ethnic status; and a family psychiatric history. Social support prior to event exposure is protective.

Genetic and physiological. These include female gender and younger age at the time of trauma exposure (for adults). Certain genotypes may either be protective or increase risk of PTSD after exposure to traumatic events.

Peritraumatic factors

Environmental. These include severity (dose) of the trauma (the greater the magnitude of trauma, the greater the likelihood of PTSD), perceived life threat, personal injury, interpersonal violence (particularly trauma perpetrated by a caregiver or involving a witnessed threat to a caregiver in children), and, for military personnel, being a perpetrator, witnessing atrocities, or killing the enemy. Finally, dissociation that occurs during the trauma and persists afterward is a risk factor.

Posttraumatic factors

Temperamental. These include negative appraisals, inappropriate coping strategies, and development of acute stress disorder.

Environmental. These include subsequent exposure to repeated upsetting reminders, subsequent adverse life events, and financial or other trauma-related losses. Social support (including family stability, for children) is a protective factor that moderates outcome after trauma.

Culture-Related Diagnostic Issues

The risk of onset and severity of PTSD may differ across cultural groups as a result of variation in the type of traumatic exposure (e.g., genocide), the impact on disorder severity of the meaning attributed to the traumatic event (e.g., inability to perform funerary rites after a mass killing), the ongoing sociocultural context (e.g., residing among unpunished perpetrators in postconflict settings), and other cultural factors (e.g., acculturative stress in immigrants). The relative risk for PTSD of particular exposures (e.g., religious persecution) may vary across cultural groups. The clinical expression of the symptoms or symptom clusters of PTSD may vary culturally, particularly with respect to avoidance and numbing symptoms, distressing dreams, and somatic symptoms (e.g., dizziness, shortness of breath, heat sensations).

Cultural syndromes and idioms of distress influence the expression of PTSD and the range of comorbid disorders in different cultures by providing behavioral and cognitive templates that link traumatic exposures to specific symptoms. For example, panic attack symptoms may be salient in PTSD among Cambodians and Latin Americans because of the association of traumatic exposure with panic-like *khyâl* attacks and *ataque de nervios*. Comprehensive evaluation of local expressions of PTSD should include assessment of cultural concepts of distress (see the chapter "Cultural Formulation" in Section III).

Gender-Related Diagnostic Issues

PTSD is more prevalent among females than among males across the lifespan. Females in the general population experience PTSD for a longer duration than do males. At least some of the increased risk for PTSD in females appears to be attributable to a greater likelihood of exposure to traumatic events, such as rape, and other forms of interpersonal violence. Within populations exposed specifically to such stressors, gender differences in risk for PTSD are attenuated or nonsignificant.

Suicide Risk

Traumatic events such as childhood abuse increase a person's suicide risk. PTSD is associated with suicidal ideation and suicide attempts, and presence of the disorder may indicate which individuals with ideation eventually make a suicide plan or actually attempt suicide.

Functional Consequences of Posttraumatic Stress Disorder

PTSD is associated with high levels of social, occupational, and physical disability, as well as considerable economic costs and high levels of medical utilization. Impaired functioning is exhibited across social, interpersonal, developmental, educational, physical health, and occupational domains. In community and veteran samples, PTSD is associated with poor social and family relationships, absenteeism from work, lower income, and lower educational and occupational success.

Differential Diagnosis

Adjustment disorders.   In adjustment disorders, the stressor can be of any severity or type rather than that required by PTSD Criterion A. The diagnosis of an adjustment disorder is used when the response to a stressor that meets PTSD Criterion A does not meet all other PTSD criteria (or criteria for another mental disorder). An adjustment disorder is also diagnosed when the symptom pattern of PTSD occurs in response to a stressor that does not meet PTSD Criterion A (e.g., spouse leaving, being fired).

Other posttraumatic disorders and conditions.   Not all psychopathology that occurs in individuals exposed to an extreme stressor should necessarily be attributed to PTSD. The diagnosis requires that trauma exposure precede the onset or exacerbation of pertinent symptoms. Moreover, if the symptom response pattern to the extreme stressor meets criteria for another mental disorder, these diagnoses should be given instead of, or in addition to, PTSD. Other diagnoses and conditions are excluded if they are better explained by PTSD (e.g., symptoms of panic disorder that occur only after exposure to traumatic reminders). If severe, symptom response patterns to the extreme stressor may warrant a separate diagnosis (e.g., dissociative amnesia).

Acute stress disorder.   Acute stress disorder is distinguished from PTSD because the symptom pattern in acute stress disorder is restricted to a duration of 3 days to 1 month following exposure to the traumatic event.

Anxiety disorders and obsessive-compulsive disorder.   In OCD, there are recurrent intrusive thoughts, but these meet the definition of an obsession. In addition, the intrusive thoughts are not related to an experienced traumatic event, compulsions are usually present, and other symptoms of PTSD or acute stress disorder are typically absent. Neither the arousal and dissociative symptoms of panic disorder nor the avoidance, irritability, and anxiety of generalized anxiety disorder are associated with a specific traumatic event. The symptoms of separation anxiety disorder are clearly related to separation from home or family, rather than to a traumatic event.

Major depressive disorder.   Major depression may or may not be preceded by a traumatic event and should be diagnosed if other PTSD symptoms are absent. Specifically, major depressive disorder does not include any PTSD Criterion B or C symptoms. Nor does it include a number of symptoms from PTSD Criterion D or E.

Personality disorders.   Interpersonal difficulties that had their onset, or were greatly exacerbated, after exposure to a traumatic event may be an indication of PTSD, rather than a personality disorder, in which such difficulties would be expected independently of any traumatic exposure.

Dissociative disorders.   Dissociative amnesia, dissociative identity disorder, and depersonalization-derealization disorder may or may not be preceded by exposure to a traumatic event or may or may not have co-occurring PTSD symptoms. When full PTSD criteria are also met, however, the PTSD "with dissociative symptoms" subtype should be considered.

Conversion disorder (functional neurological symptom disorder).   New onset of somatic symptoms within the context of posttraumatic distress might be an indication of PTSD rather than conversion disorder (functional neurological symptom disorder).

Psychotic disorders.   Flashbacks in PTSD must be distinguished from illusions, hallucinations, and other perceptual disturbances that may occur in schizophrenia, brief psychotic disorder, and other psychotic disorders; depressive and bipolar disorders with psychotic features; delirium; substance/medication-induced disorders; and psychotic disorders due to another medical condition.

Traumatic brain injury.   When a brain injury occurs in the context of a traumatic event (e.g., traumatic accident, bomb blast, acceleration/deceleration trauma), symptoms of PTSD may appear. An event causing head trauma may also constitute a psychological traumatic event, and traumatic brain injury (TBI)–related neurocognitive symptoms are not mutually exclusive and may occur concurrently. Symptoms previously termed *postconcussive* (e.g., headaches, dizziness, sensitivity to light or sound, irritability, concentration deficits) can occur in brain-injured and non-brain-injured populations, including individuals with PTSD. Because symptoms of PTSD and TBI-related neurocognitive symptoms can overlap, a differential diagnosis between PTSD and neurocognitive disorder symptoms attributable to TBI may be possible based on the presence of symptoms that are distinctive to each presentation. Whereas reexperiencing and avoidance are characteristic of PTSD and not the effects of TBI, persistent disorientation and confusion are more specific to TBI (neurocognitive effects) than to PTSD.

Comorbidity

Individuals with PTSD are 80% more likely than those without PTSD to have symptoms that meet diagnostic criteria for at least one other mental disorder (e.g., depressive, bipolar, anxiety, or substance use disorders). Comorbid substance use disorder and conduct disorder are more common among males than among females. Among U.S. military personnel and combat veterans who have been deployed to recent wars in Afghanistan and Iraq, co-occurrence of PTSD and mild TBI is 48%. Although most young children with PTSD also have at least one other diagnosis, the patterns of comorbidity are different than in adults, with oppositional defiant disorder and separation anxiety disorder predominating. Finally, there is considerable comorbidity between PTSD and major neurocognitive disorder and some overlapping symptoms between these disorders.

Acute Stress Disorder

Diagnostic Criteria   **308.3 (F43.0)**

A. Exposure to actual or threatened death, serious injury, or sexual violation in one (or more) of the following ways:

   1. Directly experiencing the traumatic event(s).
   2. Witnessing, in person, the event(s) as it occurred to others.
   3. Learning that the event(s) occurred to a close family member or close friend. **Note:** In cases of actual or threatened death of a family member or friend, the event(s) must have been violent or accidental.
   4. Experiencing repeated or extreme exposure to aversive details of the traumatic event(s) (e.g., first responders collecting human remains, police officers repeatedly exposed to details of child abuse).

   Note: This does not apply to exposure through electronic media, television, movies, or pictures, unless this exposure is work related.

B. Presence of nine (or more) of the following symptoms from any of the five categories of intrusion, negative mood, dissociation, avoidance, and arousal, beginning or worsening after the traumatic event(s) occurred:

   Intrusion Symptoms

   1. Recurrent, involuntary, and intrusive distressing memories of the traumatic event(s). **Note:** In children, repetitive play may occur in which themes or aspects of the traumatic event(s) are expressed.

2. Recurrent distressing dreams in which the content and/or affect of the dream are related to the event(s). **Note:** In children, there may be frightening dreams without recognizable content.
3. Dissociative reactions (e.g., flashbacks) in which the individual feels or acts as if the traumatic event(s) were recurring. (Such reactions may occur on a continuum, with the most extreme expression being a complete loss of awareness of present surroundings.) **Note:** In children, trauma-specific reenactment may occur in play.
4. Intense or prolonged psychological distress or marked physiological reactions in response to internal or external cues that symbolize or resemble an aspect of the traumatic event(s).

Negative Mood

5. Persistent inability to experience positive emotions (e.g., inability to experience happiness, satisfaction, or loving feelings).

Dissociative Symptoms

6. An altered sense of the reality of one's surroundings or oneself (e.g., seeing oneself from another's perspective, being in a daze, time slowing).
7. Inability to remember an important aspect of the traumatic event(s) (typically due to dissociative amnesia and not to other factors such as head injury, alcohol, or drugs).

Avoidance Symptoms

8. Efforts to avoid distressing memories, thoughts, or feelings about or closely associated with the traumatic event(s).
9. Efforts to avoid external reminders (people, places, conversations, activities, objects, situations) that arouse distressing memories, thoughts, or feelings about or closely associated with the traumatic event(s).

Arousal Symptoms

10. Sleep disturbance (e.g., difficulty falling or staying asleep, restless sleep).
11. Irritable behavior and angry outbursts (with little or no provocation), typically expressed as verbal or physical aggression toward people or objects.
12. Hypervigilance.
13. Problems with concentration.
14. Exaggerated startle response.

C. Duration of the disturbance (symptoms in Criterion B) is 3 days to 1 month after trauma exposure.

   Note: Symptoms typically begin immediately after the trauma, but persistence for at least 3 days and up to a month is needed to meet disorder criteria.

D. The disturbance causes clinically significant distress or impairment in social, occupational, or other important areas of functioning.

E. The disturbance is not attributable to the physiological effects of a substance (e.g., medication or alcohol) or another medical condition (e.g., mild traumatic brain injury) and is not better explained by brief psychotic disorder.

Diagnostic Features

The essential feature of acute stress disorder is the development of characteristic symptoms lasting from 3 days to 1 month following exposure to one or more traumatic events. Traumatic events that are experienced directly include, but are not limited to, exposure to war as a combatant or civilian, threatened or actual violent personal assault (e.g., sexual violence, physical attack, active combat, mugging, childhood physical and/or sexual violence, being kidnapped, being taken hostage, terrorist attack, torture), natural or human-made disasters (e.g., earthquake, hurricane, airplane crash), and severe accident (e.g., severe motor vehicle, industrial accident). For children, sexually traumatic events may include inappropriate sexual experiences without violence or injury. A life-threatening illness or debilitating medical condition is not necessarily considered a traumatic event. Medical incidents that qualify as traumatic events involve sudden, catastrophic events (e.g., waking during surgery, anaphylactic shock). Stressful events that do not possess the severe and traumatic components of events encompassed by Criterion A may lead to an adjustment disorder but not to acute stress disorder.

The clinical presentation of acute stress disorder may vary by individual but typically involves an anxiety response that includes some form of reexperiencing of or reactivity to the traumatic event. In some individuals, a dissociative or detached presentation can predominate, although these individuals typically will also display strong emotional or physiological reactivity in response to trauma reminders. In other individuals, there can be a strong anger response in which reactivity is characterized by irritable or possibly aggressive responses. The full symptom picture must be present for at least 3 days after the traumatic event and can be diagnosed only up to 1 month after the event. Symptoms that occur immediately after the event but resolve in less than 3 days would not meet criteria for acute stress disorder.

Witnessed events include, but are not limited to, observing threatened or serious injury, unnatural death, physical or sexual violence inflicted on another individual as a result of violent assault, severe domestic violence, severe accident, war, and disaster; it may also include witnessing a medical catastrophe (e.g., a life-threatening hemorrhage) involving one's child. Events experienced indirectly through learning about the event are limited to close relatives or close friends. Such events must have been violent or accidental—death due to natural causes does not qualify—and include violent personal assault, suicide, serious accident, or serious injury. The disorder may be especially severe when the stressor is interpersonal and intentional (e.g., torture, rape). The likelihood of developing this disorder may increase as the intensity of and physical proximity to the stressor increase.

The traumatic event can be reexperienced in various ways. Commonly, the individual has recurrent and intrusive recollections of the event (Criterion B1). The recollections are spontaneous or triggered recurrent memories of the event that usually occur in response to a stimulus that is reminiscent of the traumatic experience (e.g., the sound of a backfiring car triggering memories of gunshots). These intrusive memories often include sensory (e.g., sensing the intense heat that was perceived in a house fire), emotional (e.g., experiencing the fear of believing that one was about to be stabbed), or physiological (e.g., experiencing the shortness of breath that one suffered during a near-drowning) components.

Distressing dreams may contain themes that are representative of or thematically related to the major threats involved in the traumatic event. (For example, in the case of a motor vehicle accident survivor, the distressing dreams may involve crashing cars generally; in the case of a combat soldier, the distressing dreams may involve being harmed in ways other than combat.)

Dissociative states may last from a few seconds to several hours, or even days, during which components of the event are relived and the individual behaves as though experiencing the event at that moment. While dissociative responses are common during a traumatic event, only dissociative responses that persist beyond 3 days after trauma exposure are considered for the diagnosis of acute stress disorder. For young children, reenactment of events related to trauma may appear in play and may include dissociative moments (e.g., a child who survives a motor vehicle accident may repeatedly crash toy cars during play in a focused and distressing manner). These episodes, often referred to as *flashbacks*, are typically brief but involve a sense that the traumatic event is occurring in the present rather than being remembered in the past and are associated with significant distress.

Some individuals with the disorder do not have intrusive memories of the event itself, but instead experience intense psychological distress or physiological reactivity when they are exposed to triggering events that resemble or symbolize an aspect of the traumatic event (e.g., windy days for children after a hurricane, entering an elevator for a male or female who was raped in an elevator, seeing someone who resembles one's perpetrator). The triggering cue could be a physical sensation (e.g., a sense of heat for a burn victim, dizziness for survivors of head trauma), particularly for individuals with highly somatic presentations. The individual may have a persistent inability to feel positive emotions (e.g., happiness, joy, satisfaction, or emotions associated with intimacy, tenderness, or sexuality) but can experience negative emotions such as fear, sadness, anger, guilt, or shame.

Alterations in awareness can include *depersonalization,* a detached sense of oneself (e.g., seeing oneself from the other side of the room), or *derealization,* having a distorted view of one's surroundings (e.g., perceiving that things are moving in slow motion, seeing things in a daze, not being aware of events that one would normally encode). Some individuals also report an inability to remember an important aspect of the traumatic event that was presumably encoded. This symptom is attributable to dissociative amnesia and is not attributable to head injury, alcohol, or drugs.

Stimuli associated with the trauma are persistently avoided. The individual may refuse to discuss the traumatic experience or may engage in avoidance strategies to minimize awareness of emotional reactions (e.g., excessive alcohol use when reminded of the experience). This behavioral avoidance may include avoiding watching news coverage of the traumatic experience, refusing to return to a workplace where the trauma occurred, or avoiding interacting with others who shared the same traumatic experience.

It is very common for individuals with acute stress disorder to experience problems with sleep onset and maintenance, which may be associated with nightmares or with generalized elevated arousal that prevents adequate sleep. Individuals with acute stress disorder may be quick tempered and may even engage in aggressive verbal and/or physical behavior with little provocation. Acute stress disorder is often characterized by a heightened sensitivity to potential threats, including those that are related to the traumatic experience (e.g., a motor vehicle accident victim may be especially sensitive to the threat potentially caused by any cars or trucks) or those not related to the traumatic event (e.g., fear of having a heart attack). Concentration difficulties, including difficulty remembering daily events (e.g., forgetting one's telephone number) or attending to focused tasks (e.g., following a conversation for a sustained period of time), are commonly reported. Individuals with acute stress disorder may be very reactive to unexpected stimuli, displaying a heightened startle response or jumpiness to loud noises or unexpected movements (e.g., the individual may jump markedly in the response to a telephone ringing).

Associated Features Supporting Diagnosis

Individuals with acute stress disorder commonly engage in catastrophic or extremely negative thoughts about their role in the traumatic event, their response to the traumatic experience, or the likelihood of future harm. For example, an individual with acute stress disorder may feel excessively guilty about not having prevented the traumatic event or about not adapting to the experience more successfully. Individuals with acute stress disorder may also interpret their symptoms in a catastrophic manner, such that flashback memories or emotional numbing may be interpreted as a sign of diminished mental capacity. It is common for individuals with acute stress disorder to experience panic attacks in the initial month after trauma exposure that may be triggered by trauma reminders or may apparently occur spontaneously. Additionally, individuals with acute stress disorder may display chaotic or impulsive behavior. For example, individuals may drive recklessly, make irrational decisions, or gamble excessively. In children, there may be significant separation anxiety, possibly manifested by excessive needs for attention from caregivers. In the case of bereavement following a death that occurred in traumatic circumstances, the symptoms of acute stress disorder can involve acute grief reactions. In such cases, reexperiencing, dissociative, and arousal symptoms may involve reactions to the loss, such as intrusive memories of the circumstances of the individual's death, disbelief that the individual has died, and anger about the death. Postconcussive symptoms (e.g., headaches, dizziness, sensitivity to light or sound, irritability, concentration deficits), which occur frequently following mild traumatic brain injury, are also frequently seen in individuals with acute stress disorder. Postconcussive symptoms are equally common in brain-injured and non–brain-injured populations, and the frequent occurrence of postconcussive symptoms could be attributable to acute stress disorder symptoms.

Prevalence

The prevalence of acute stress disorder in recently trauma-exposed populations (i.e., within 1 month of trauma exposure) varies according to the nature of the event and the context in which it is assessed. In both U.S. and non-U.S. populations, acute stress disorder tends to be identified in less than 20% of cases following traumatic events that do not involve interpersonal assault; 13%–21% of motor vehicle accidents, 14% of mild traumatic brain injury, 19% of assault, 10% of severe burns, and 6%–12% of industrial accidents. Higher rates (i.e., 20%–50%) are reported following interpersonal traumatic events, including assault, rape, and witnessing a mass shooting.

Development and Course

Acute stress disorder cannot be diagnosed until 3 days after a traumatic event. Although acute stress disorder may progress to posttraumatic stress disorder (PTSD) after 1 month, it may also be a transient stress response that remits within 1 month of trauma exposure and does not result in PTSD. Approximately half of individuals who eventually develop PTSD initially present with acute stress disorder. Symptom worsening during the initial month can occur, often as a result of ongoing life stressors or further traumatic events.

The forms of reexperiencing can vary across development. Unlike adults or adolescents, young children may report frightening dreams without content that clearly reflects aspects of the trauma (e.g., waking in fright in the aftermath of the trauma but being unable to relate the content of the dream to the traumatic event). Children age 6 years and younger are more likely than older children to express reexperiencing symptoms through play that refers directly or symbolically to the trauma. For example, a very young child who survived a fire may draw pictures of flames. Young children also do not necessarily manifest fearful reactions at the time of the exposure or even during reexperiencing. Parents typically report a range of emotional expressions, such as anger, shame, or withdrawal, and even excessively bright positive affect, in young children who are traumatized. Although children may avoid reminders of the trauma, they sometimes become preoccupied with reminders (e.g., a young child bitten by a dog may talk about dogs constantly yet avoid going outside because of fear of coming into contact with a dog).

Risk and Prognostic Factors

Temperamental.   Risk factors include prior mental disorder, high levels of negative affectivity (neuroticism), greater perceived severity of the traumatic event, and an avoidant coping style. Catastrophic appraisals of the traumatic experience, often characterized by exaggerated appraisals of future harm, guilt, or hopelessness, are strongly predictive of acute stress disorder.

Environmental.   First and foremost, an individual must be exposed to a traumatic event to be at risk for acute stress disorder. Risk factors for the disorder include a history of prior trauma.

Genetic and physiological. Females are at greater risk for developing acute stress disorder.

Elevated reactivity, as reflected by acoustic startle response, prior to trauma exposure increases the risk for developing acute stress disorder.

Culture-Related Diagnostic Issues

The profile of symptoms of acute stress disorder may vary cross-culturally, particularly with respect to dissociative symptoms, nightmares, avoidance, and somatic symptoms (e.g., dizziness, shortness of breath, heat sensations). Cultural syndromes and idioms of distress shape the local symptom profiles of acute stress disorder. Some cultural groups may display variants of dissociative responses, such as possession or trancelike behaviors in the initial month after trauma exposure. Panic symptoms may be salient in acute stress disorder among Cambodians because of the association of traumatic exposure with panic-like *khyâl* attacks, and *ataque de nervios* among Latin Americans may also follow a traumatic exposure.

Gender-Related Diagnostic Issues

Acute stress disorder is more prevalent among females than among males. Sex-linked neurobiological differences in stress response may contribute to females' increased risk for acute stress disorder. The increased risk for the disorder in females may be attributable in part to a greater likelihood of exposure to the types of traumatic events with a high conditional risk for acute stress disorder, such as rape and other interpersonal violence.

Functional Consequences of Acute Stress Disorder

Impaired functioning in social, interpersonal, or occupational domains has been shown across survivors of accidents, assault, and rape who develop acute stress disorder. The extreme levels of anxiety that may be associated with acute stress disorder may interfere with sleep, energy levels, and capacity to attend to tasks. Avoidance in acute stress disorder can result in generalized withdrawal from many situations that are perceived as potentially threatening, which can lead to nonattendance of medical appointments, avoidance of driving to important appointments, and absenteeism from work.

Differential Diagnosis

Adjustment disorders. In adjustment disorders, the stressor can be of any severity rather than of the severity and type required by Criterion A of acute stress disorder. The diagnosis of an adjustment disorder is used when the response to a Criterion A event does not meet the criteria for acute stress disorder (or another specific mental disorder) and when the symptom pattern of acute stress disorder occurs in response to a stressor that does not meet Criterion A for exposure to actual or threatened death, serious injury, or sexual violence (e.g., spouse leaving, being fired). For example, severe stress reactions to life-threatening illnesses that may include some acute stress disorder symptoms may be more appropriately described as an adjustment disorder. Some forms of acute stress response do not include acute stress disorder symptoms and may be characterized by anger, depression, or guilt. These responses are more appropriately described as primarily an adjustment disorder. Depressive or anger responses in an adjustment disorder may involve rumination about the traumatic event, as opposed to involuntary and intrusive distressing memories in acute stress disorder.

Panic disorder. Spontaneous panic attacks are very common in acute stress disorder. However, panic disorder is diagnosed only if panic attacks are unexpected and there is anxiety about future attacks or maladaptive changes in behavior associated with fear of dire consequences of the attacks.

Dissociative disorders.   Severe dissociative responses (in the absence of characteristic acute stress disorder symptoms) may be diagnosed as derealization/depersonalization disorder. If severe amnesia of the trauma persists in the absence of characteristic acute stress disorder symptoms, the diagnosis of dissociative amnesia may be indicated.

Posttraumatic stress disorder.   Acute stress disorder is distinguished from PTSD because the symptom pattern in acute stress disorder must occur within 1 month of the traumatic event and resolve within that 1-month period. If the symptoms persist for more than 1 month and meet criteria for PTSD, the diagnosis is changed from acute stress disorder to PTSD.

Obsessive-compulsive disorder.   In obsessive-compulsive disorder, there are recurrent intrusive thoughts, but these meet the definition of an obsession. In addition, the intrusive thoughts are not related to an experienced traumatic event, compulsions are usually present, and other symptoms of acute stress disorder are typically absent.

Psychotic disorders.   Flashbacks in acute stress disorder must be distinguished from illusions, hallucinations, and other perceptual disturbances that may occur in schizophrenia, other psychotic disorders, depressive or bipolar disorder with psychotic features, a delirium, substance/medication-induced disorders, and psychotic disorders due to another medical condition. Acute stress disorder flashbacks are distinguished from these other perceptual disturbances by being directly related to the traumatic experience and by occurring in the absence of other psychotic or substance-induced features.

Traumatic brain injury.   When a brain injury occurs in the context of a traumatic event (e.g., traumatic accident, bomb blast, acceleration/deceleration trauma), symptoms of acute stress disorder may appear. An event causing head trauma may also constitute a psychological traumatic event, and traumatic brain injury (TBI)–related neurocognitive symptoms are not mutually exclusive and may occur concurrently. Symptoms previously termed *postconcussive* (e.g., headaches, dizziness, sensitivity to light or sound, irritability, concentration deficits) can occur in brain-injured and non–brain injured populations, including individuals with acute stress disorder. Because symptoms of acute stress disorder and TBI-related neurocognitive symptoms can overlap, a differential diagnosis between acute stress disorder and neurocognitive disorder symptoms attributable to TBI may be possible based on the presence of symptoms that are distinctive to each presentation. Whereas reexperiencing and avoidance are characteristic of acute stress disorder and not the effects of TBI, persistent disorientation and confusion are more specific to TBI (neurocognitive effects) than to acute stress disorder. Furthermore, differential is aided by the fact that symptoms of acute stress disorder persist for up to only 1 month following trauma exposure.

Adjustment Disorders

Diagnostic Criteria

A. The development of emotional or behavioral symptoms in response to an identifiable stressor(s) occurring within 3 months of the onset of the stressor(s).

B. These symptoms or behaviors are clinically significant, as evidenced by one or both of the following:

1. Marked distress that is out of proportion to the severity or intensity of the stressor, taking into account the external context and the cultural factors that might influence symptom severity and presentation.

2. Significant impairment in social, occupational, or other important areas of functioning.

C. The stress-related disturbance does not meet the criteria for another mental disorder and is not merely an exacerbation of a preexisting mental disorder.

D. The symptoms do not represent normal bereavement.

E. Once the stressor or its consequences have terminated, the symptoms do not persist for more than an additional 6 months.

Specify whether:

309.0 (F43.21) With depressed mood: Low mood, tearfulness, or feelings of hopelessness are predominant.

309.24 (F43.22) With anxiety: Nervousness, worry, jitteriness, or separation anxiety is predominant.

309.28 (F43.23) With mixed anxiety and depressed mood: A combination of depression and anxiety is predominant.

309.3 (F43.24) With disturbance of conduct: Disturbance of conduct is predominant.

309.4 (F43.25) With mixed disturbance of emotions and conduct: Both emotional symptoms (e.g., depression, anxiety) and a disturbance of conduct are predominant.

309.9 (F43.20) Unspecified: For maladaptive reactions that are not classifiable as one of the specific subtypes of adjustment disorder.

Diagnostic Features

The presence of emotional or behavioral symptoms in response to an identifiable stressor is the essential feature of adjustment disorders (Criterion A). The stressor may be a single event (e.g., a termination of a romantic relationship), or there may be multiple stressors (e.g., marked business difficulties and marital problems). Stressors may be recurrent (e.g., associated with seasonal business crises, unfulfilling sexual relationships) or continuous (e.g., a persistent painful illness with increasing disability, living in a crime-ridden neighborhood). Stressors may affect a single individual, an entire family, or a larger group or community (e.g., a natural disaster). Some stressors may accompany specific developmental events (e.g., going to school, leaving a parental home, reentering a parental home, getting married, becoming a parent, failing to attain occupational goals, retirement).

Adjustment disorders may be diagnosed following the death of a loved one when the intensity, quality, or persistence of grief reactions exceeds what normally might be expected, when cultural, religious, or age-appropriate norms are taken into account. A more specific set of bereavement-related symptoms has been designated *persistent complex bereavement disorder.*

Adjustment disorders are associated with an increased risk of suicide attempts and completed suicide.

Prevalence

Adjustment disorders are common, although prevalence may vary widely as a function of the population studied and the assessment methods used. The percentage of individuals in outpatient mental health treatment with a principal diagnosis of an adjustment disorder ranges from approximately 5% to 20%. In a hospital psychiatric consultation setting, it is often the most common diagnosis, frequently reaching 50%.

Development and Course

By definition, the disturbance in adjustment disorders begins within 3 months of onset of a stressor and lasts no longer than 6 months after the stressor or its consequences have ceased. If the stressor is an acute event (e.g., being fired from a job), the onset of the disturbance is usually immediate (i.e., within a few days) and the duration is relatively brief (i.e., no more than a few months). If the stressor or its consequences persist, the adjustment disorder may also continue to be present and become the persistent form.

Risk and Prognostic Factors

Environmental.   Individuals from disadvantaged life circumstances experience a high rate of stressors and may be at increased risk for adjustment disorders.

Culture-Related Diagnostic Issues

The context of the individual's cultural setting should be taken into account in making the clinical judgment of whether the individual's response to the stressor is maladaptive or whether the associated distress is in excess of what would be expected. The nature, meaning, and experience of the stressors and the evaluation of the response to the stressors may vary across cultures.

Functional Consequences of Adjustment Disorders

The subjective distress or impairment in functioning associated with adjustment disorders is frequently manifested as decreased performance at work or school and temporary changes in social relationships. An adjustment disorder may complicate the course of illness in individuals who have a general medical condition (e.g., decreased compliance with the recommended medical regimen; increased length of hospital stay).

Differential Diagnosis

Major depressive disorder.   If an individual has symptoms that meet criteria for a major depressive disorder in response to a stressor, the diagnosis of an adjustment disorder is not applicable. The symptom profile of major depressive disorder differentiates it from adjustment disorders.

Posttraumatic stress disorder and acute stress disorder.   In adjustment disorders, the stressor can be of any severity rather than of the severity and type required by Criterion A of acute stress disorder and posttraumatic stress disorder (PTSD). In distinguishing adjustment disorders from these two posttraumatic diagnoses, there are both timing and symptom profile considerations. Adjustment disorders can be diagnosed immediately and persist up to 6 months after exposure to the traumatic event, whereas acute stress disorder can only occur between 3 days and 1 month of exposure to the stressor, and PTSD cannot be diagnosed until at least 1 month has passed since the occurrence of the traumatic stressor. The required symptom profile for PTSD and acute stress disorder differentiates them from the adjustment disorders. With regard to symptom profiles, an adjustment disorder may be diagnosed following a traumatic event when an individual exhibits symptoms of either acute stress disorder or PTSD that do not meet or exceed the diagnostic threshold for either disorder. An adjustment disorder should also be diagnosed for individuals who have not been exposed to a traumatic event but who otherwise exhibit the full symptom profile of either acute stress disorder or PTSD.

Personality disorders.   With regard to personality disorders, some personality features may be associated with a vulnerability to situational distress that may resemble an adjustment disorder. The lifetime history of personality functioning will help inform the interpretation of distressed behaviors to aid in distinguishing a long-standing personality disorder from an adjustment disorder. In addition to some personality disorders incurring vulnerability to distress, stressors may also exacerbate personality disorder symptoms. In the presence of a personality disorder, if the symptom criteria for an adjustment disorder are met, and the stress-related disturbance exceeds what may be attributable to maladaptive personality disorder symptoms (i.e., Criterion C is met), then the diagnosis of an adjustment disorder should be made.

Psychological factors affecting other medical conditions. In psychological factors affecting other medical conditions, specific psychological entities (e.g., psychological symptoms, behaviors, other factors) exacerbate a medical condition. These psychological factors can precipitate, exacerbate, or put an individual at risk for medical illness, or they can worsen an existing condition. In contrast, an adjustment disorder is a reaction to the stressor (e.g., having a medical illness).

Normative stress reactions. When bad things happen, most people get upset. This is not an adjustment disorder. The diagnosis should only be made when the magnitude of the distress (e.g., alterations in mood, anxiety, or conduct) exceeds what would normally be expected (which may vary in different cultures) or when the adverse event precipitates functional impairment.

Comorbidity

Adjustment disorders can accompany most mental disorders and any medical disorder. Adjustment disorders can be diagnosed in addition to another mental disorder only if the latter does not explain the particular symptoms that occur in reaction to the stressor. For example, an individual may develop an adjustment disorder, with depressed mood, after losing a job and at the same time have a diagnosis of obsessive-compulsive disorder. Or, an individual may have a depressive or bipolar disorder and an adjustment disorder as long as the criteria for both are met. Adjustment disorders are common accompaniments of medical illness and may be the major psychological response to a medical disorder.

Other Specified Trauma- and Stressor-Related Disorder

309.89 (F43.8)

This category applies to presentations in which symptoms characteristic of a trauma- and stressor-related disorder that cause clinically significant distress or impairment in social, occupational, or other important areas of functioning predominate but do not meet the full criteria for any of the disorders in the trauma- and stressor-related disorders diagnostic class. The other specified trauma- and stressor-related disorder category is used in situations in which the clinician chooses to communicate the specific reason that the presentation does not meet the criteria for any specific trauma- and stressor-related disorder. This is done by recording "other specified trauma- and stressor-related disorder" followed by the specific reason (e.g., "persistent complex bereavement disorder").

Examples of presentations that can be specified using the "other specified" designation include the following:

1. **Adjustment-like disorders with delayed onset of symptoms that occur more than 3 months after the stressor.**
2. **Adjustment-like disorders with prolonged duration of more than 6 months without prolonged duration of stressor.**
3. *Ataque de nervios:* See "Glossary of Cultural Concepts of Distress" in the Appendix.
4. **Other cultural syndromes:** See "Glossary of Cultural Concepts of Distress" in the Appendix.
5. **Persistent complex bereavement disorder:** This disorder is characterized by severe and persistent grief and mourning reactions (see the chapter "Conditions for Further Study").

Unspecified Trauma- and Stressor-Related Disorder

309.9 (F43.9)

This category applies to presentations in which symptoms characteristic of a trauma- and stressor-related disorder that cause clinically significant distress or impairment in social, occupational, or other important areas of functioning predominate but do not meet the full criteria for any of the disorders in the trauma- and stressor-related disorders diagnostic class. The unspecified trauma- and stressor-related disorder category is used in situations in which the clinician chooses *not* to specify the reason that the criteria are not met for a specific trauma- and stressor-related disorder, and includes presentations in which there is insufficient information to make a more specific diagnosis (e.g., in emergency room settings).

Dissociative Disorders

Dissociative disorders are characterized by a disruption of and/or discontinuity in the normal integration of consciousness, memory, identity, emotion, perception, body representation, motor control, and behavior. Dissociative symptoms can potentially disrupt every area of psychological functioning. This chapter includes dissociative identity disorder, dissociative amnesia, depersonalization/derealization disorder, other specified dissociative disorder, and unspecified dissociative disorder.

Dissociative symptoms are experienced as a) unbidden intrusions into awareness and behavior, with accompanying losses of continuity in subjective experience (i.e., "positive" dissociative symptoms such as fragmentation of identity, depersonalization, and derealization) and/or b) inability to access information or to control mental functions that normally are readily amenable to access or control (i.e., "negative" dissociative symptoms such as amnesia).

The dissociative disorders are frequently found in the aftermath of trauma, and many of the symptoms, including embarrassment and confusion about the symptoms or a desire to hide them, are influenced by the proximity to trauma. In DSM-5, the dissociative disorders are placed next to, but are not part of, the trauma- and stressor-related disorders, reflecting the close relationship between these diagnostic classes. Both acute stress disorder and posttraumatic stress disorder contain dissociative symptoms, such as amnesia, flashbacks, numbing, and depersonalization/derealization.

Depersonalization/derealization disorder is characterized by clinically significant persistent or recurrent depersonalization (i.e., experiences of unreality or detachment from one's mind, self, or body) and/or derealization (i.e., experiences of unreality or detachment from one's surroundings). These alterations of experience are accompanied by intact reality testing. There is no evidence of any distinction between individuals with predominantly depersonalization versus derealization symptoms. Therefore, individuals with this disorder can have depersonalization, derealization, or both.

Dissociative amnesia is characterized by an inability to recall autobiographical information. This amnesia may be localized (i.e., an event or period of time), selective (i.e., a specific aspect of an event), or generalized (i.e., identity and life history). Dissociative amnesia is fundamentally an inability to recall autobiographical information that is inconsistent with normal forgetting. It may or may not involve purposeful travel or bewildered wandering (i.e., fugue). Although some individuals with amnesia promptly notice that they have "lost time" or that they have a gap in their memory, most individuals with dissociative disorders are initially unaware of their amnesias. For them, awareness of amnesia occurs only when personal identity is lost or when circumstances make these individuals aware that autobiographical information is missing (e.g., when they discover evidence of events they cannot recall or when others tell them or ask them about events they cannot recall). Until and unless this happens, these individuals have "amnesia for their amnesia." Amnesia is experienced as an essential feature of dissociative amnesia; individuals may experience localized or selective amnesia most commonly, or generalized amnesia rarely. Dissociative fugue is rare in persons with dissociative amnesia but common in dissociative identity disorder.

Dissociative identity disorder is characterized by a) the presence of two or more distinct personality states or an experience of possession and b) recurrent episodes of amnesia. The fragmentation of identity may vary with culture (e.g., possession-form presentations) and circumstance. Thus, individuals may experience discontinuities in identity and memory that may not be immediately evident to others or are obscured by attempts to hide dysfunction. Individuals with dissociative identity disorder experience a) recurrent, inexplicable intrusions into their conscious functioning and sense of self (e.g., voices; dissociated actions and speech; intrusive thoughts, emotions, and impulses), b) alterations of sense of self (e.g., attitudes, preferences, and feeling like one's body or actions are not one's own), c) odd changes of perception (e.g., depersonalization or derealization, such as feeling detached from one's body while cutting), and d) intermittent functional neurological symptoms. Stress often produces transient exacerbation of dissociative symptoms that makes them more evident.

The residual category of other specified dissociative disorder has seven examples: chronic or recurrent mixed dissociative symptoms that approach, but fall short of, the diagnostic criteria for dissociative identity disorder; dissociative states secondary to brainwashing or thought reform; two acute presentations, of less than 1 month's duration, of mixed dissociative symptoms, one of which is also marked by the presence of psychotic symptoms; and three single-symptom dissociative presentations—dissociative trance, dissociative stupor or coma, and Ganser's syndrome (the giving of approximate and vague answers).

Dissociative Identity Disorder

Diagnostic Criteria   300.14 (F44.81)

A. Disruption of identity characterized by two or more distinct personality states, which may be described in some cultures as an experience of possession. The disruption in identity involves marked discontinuity in sense of self and sense of agency, accompanied by related alterations in affect, behavior, consciousness, memory, perception, cognition, and/or sensory-motor functioning. These signs and symptoms may be observed by others or reported by the individual.

B. Recurrent gaps in the recall of everyday events, important personal information, and/or traumatic events that are inconsistent with ordinary forgetting.

C. The symptoms cause clinically significant distress or impairment in social, occupational, or other important areas of functioning.

D. The disturbance is not a normal part of a broadly accepted cultural or religious practice.
Note: In children, the symptoms are not better explained by imaginary playmates or other fantasy play.

E. The symptoms are not attributable to the physiological effects of a substance (e.g., blackouts or chaotic behavior during alcohol intoxication) or another medical condition (e.g., complex partial seizures).

Diagnostic Features

The defining feature of dissociative identity disorder is the presence of two or more distinct personality states or an experience of possession (Criterion A). The overtness or covertness of these personality states, however, varies as a function of psychological motivation, current level of stress, culture, internal conflicts and dynamics, and emotional resilience. Sustained periods of identity disruption may occur when psychosocial pressures are severe and/or prolonged. In many possession-form cases of dissociative identity disorder, and in a small proportion of non-possession-form cases, manifestations of alternate identities are highly overt. Most individuals with non-possession-form dissociative identity disorder do not overtly display their discontinuity of identity for long periods of time; only a small minority present to clinical attention with observable alternation of identities. When alternate personality states are not directly observed, the disorder can be identified by two clusters of symptoms: 1) sudden alterations or discontinuities in sense of self and sense of agency (Criterion A), and 2) recurrent dissociative amnesias (Criterion B).

Criterion A symptoms are related to discontinuities of experience that can affect any aspect of an individual's functioning. Individuals with dissociative identity disorder may report the feeling that they have suddenly become depersonalized observers of their "own" speech and actions, which they may feel powerless to stop (sense of self). Such individuals may also report perceptions of voices (e.g., a child's voice; crying; the voice of a spiritual being). In some cases, voices are experienced as multiple, perplexing, independent thought streams over which the individual experiences no control. Strong emotions, impulses, and even speech or other actions may suddenly emerge, without a sense of personal ownership or control (sense of agency). These emotions and impulses are frequently reported as ego-dystonic and puzzling. Attitudes, outlooks, and personal preferences (e.g., about food, activities, dress) may suddenly shift and then shift back. Individuals may report that their bodies feel different (e.g., like a small child, like the opposite gender, huge and muscular). Alterations in sense of self and loss of personal agency may be accompanied by a feeling that these attitudes, emotions, and behaviors—even one's body—are "not mine" and/or are "not under my control." Although most Criterion A symptoms are subjective, many of these sudden discontinuities in speech, affect, and behavior can be witnessed by family, friends, or the clinician. Non-epileptic seizures and other conversion symptoms are prominent in some presentations of dissociative identity disorder, especially in some non-Western settings.

The dissociative amnesia of individuals with dissociative identity disorder manifests in three primary ways: as 1) gaps in remote memory of personal life events (e.g., periods of childhood or adolescence; some important life events, such as the death of a grandparent, getting married, giving birth); 2) lapses in dependable memory (e.g., of what happened today, of well-learned skills such as how to do their job, use a computer, read, drive); and 3) discovery of evidence of their everyday actions and tasks that they do not recollect doing (e.g., finding unexplained objects in their shopping bags or among their possessions; finding perplexing writings or drawings that they must have created; discovering injuries; "coming to" in the midst of doing something). Dissociative fugues, wherein the person discovers dissociated travel, are common. Thus, individuals with dissociative identity disorder may report that they have suddenly found themselves at the beach, at work, in a nightclub, or somewhere at home (e.g., in the closet, on a bed or sofa, in the corner) with no memory of how they came to be there. Amnesia in individuals with dissociative identity disorder is not limited to stressful or traumatic events; these individuals often cannot recall everyday events as well.

Individuals with dissociative identity disorder vary in their awareness and attitude toward their amnesias. It is common for these individuals to minimize their amnestic symptoms. Some of their amnestic behaviors may be apparent to others—as when these persons do not recall something they were witnessed to have done or said, when they cannot remember their own name, or when they do not recognize their spouse, children, or close friends.

Possession-form identities in dissociative identity disorder typically manifest as behaviors that appear as if a "spirit," supernatural being, or outside person has taken control, such that the individual begins speaking or acting in a distinctly different manner. For example, an individual's behavior may give the appearance that her identity has been replaced by the "ghost" of a girl who committed suicide in the same community years before, speaking and acting as though she were still alive. Or an individual may be "taken over" by a demon or deity, resulting in profound impairment, and demanding that the individual or a relative be punished for a past act, followed by more subtle periods of identity alteration. However, the majority of possession states around the world are normal, usually part of spiritual practice, and do not meet criteria for dissociative identity disorder. The identities that arise during possession-form dissociative identity disorder present recurrently, are unwanted and involuntary, cause clinically significant distress or impairment (Criterion C), and are not a normal part of a broadly accepted cultural or religious practice (Criterion D).

Associated Features Supporting Diagnosis

Individuals with dissociative identity disorder typically present with comorbid depression, anxiety, substance abuse, self-injury, non-epileptic seizures, or another common symptom. They often conceal, or are not fully aware of, disruptions in consciousness, amnesia, or other dissociative symptoms. Many individuals with dissociative identity disorder report dissociative flashbacks during which they undergo a sensory reliving of a previous event as though it were occurring in the present, often with a change of identity, a partial or complete loss of contact with or disorientation to current reality during the flashback, and a subsequent amnesia for the content of the flashback. Individuals with the disorder typically report multiple types of interpersonal maltreatment during childhood and adulthood. Nonmaltreatment forms of overwhelming early life events, such as multiple long, painful, early-life medical procedures, also may be reported. Self-mutilation and suicidal behavior are frequent. On standardized measures, these individuals report higher levels of hypnotizability and dissociativity compared with other clinical groups and healthy control subjects. Some individuals experience transient psychotic phenomena or episodes. Several brain regions have been implicated in the pathophysiology of dissociative identity disorder, including the orbitofrontal cortex, hippocampus, parahippocampal gyrus, and amygdala.

Prevalence

The 12-month prevalence of dissociative identity disorder among adults in a small U.S. community study was 1.5%. The prevalence across genders in that study was 1.6% for males and 1.4% for females.

Development and Course

Dissociative identity disorder is associated with overwhelming experiences, traumatic events, and/or abuse occurring in childhood. The full disorder may first manifest at almost any age (from earliest childhood to late life). Dissociation in children may generate problems with memory, concentration, attachment, and traumatic play. Nevertheless, children usually do not present with identity changes; instead they present primarily with overlap and interference among mental states (Criterion A phenomena), with symptoms related to discontinuities of experience. Sudden changes in identity during adolescence may appear to be just adolescent turmoil or the early stages of another mental disorder. Older individuals may present to treatment with what appear to be late-life mood disorders, obsessive-compulsive disorder, paranoia, psychotic mood disorders, or even cognitive disorders due to dissociative amnesia. In some cases, disruptive affects and memories may increasingly intrude into awareness with advancing age.

Psychological decompensation and overt changes in identity may be triggered by 1) removal from the traumatizing situation (e.g., through leaving home); 2) the individual's children reaching the same age at which the individual was originally abused or traumatized; 3) later traumatic experiences, even seemingly inconsequential ones, like a minor motor vehicle accident; or 4) the death of, or the onset of a fatal illness in, their abuser(s).

Risk and Prognostic Factors

Environmental.   Interpersonal physical and sexual abuse is associated with an increased risk of dissociative identity disorder. Prevalence of childhood abuse and neglect in the

United States, Canada, and Europe among those with the disorder is about 90%. Other forms of traumatizing experiences, including childhood medical and surgical procedures, war, childhood prostitution, and terrorism, have been reported.

Course modifiers. Ongoing abuse, later-life retraumatization, comorbidity with mental disorders, severe medical illness, and delay in appropriate treatment are associated with poorer prognosis.

Culture-Related Diagnostic Issues

Many features of dissociative identity disorder can be influenced by the individual's cultural background. Individuals with this disorder may present with prominent medically unexplained neurological symptoms, such as non-epileptic seizures, paralyses, or sensory loss, in cultural settings where such symptoms are common. Similarly, in settings where normative possession is common (e.g., rural areas in the developing world, among certain religious groups in the United States and Europe), the fragmented identities may take the form of possessing spirits, deities, demons, animals, or mythical figures. Acculturation or prolonged intercultural contact may shape the characteristics of the other identities (e.g., identities in India may speak English exclusively and wear Western clothes). Possession-form dissociative identity disorder can be distinguished from culturally accepted possession states in that the former is involuntary, distressing, uncontrollable, and often recurrent or persistent; involves conflict between the individual and his or her surrounding family, social, or work milieu; and is manifested at times and in places that violate the norms of the culture or religion.

Gender-Related Diagnostic Issues

Females with dissociative identity disorder predominate in adult clinical settings but not in child clinical settings. Adult males with dissociative identity disorder may deny their symptoms and trauma histories, and this can lead to elevated rates of false negative diagnosis. Females with dissociative identity disorder present more frequently with acute dissociative states (e.g., flashbacks, amnesia, fugue, functional neurological [conversion] symptoms, hallucinations, self-mutilation). Males commonly exhibit more criminal or violent behavior than females; among males, common triggers of acute dissociative states include combat, prison conditions, and physical or sexual assaults.

Suicide Risk

Over 70% of outpatients with dissociative identity disorder have attempted suicide; multiple attempts are common, and other self-injurious behavior is frequent. Assessment of suicide risk may be complicated when there is amnesia for past suicidal behavior or when the presenting identity does not feel suicidal and is unaware that other dissociated identities do.

Functional Consequences of Dissociative Identity Disorder

Impairment varies widely, from apparently minimal (e.g., in high-functioning professionals) to profound. Regardless of level of disability, individuals with dissociative identity disorder commonly minimize the impact of their dissociative and posttraumatic symptoms. The symptoms of higher-functioning individuals may impair their relational, marital, family, and parenting functions more than their occupational and professional life (although the latter also may be affected). With appropriate treatment, many impaired individuals show marked improvement in occupational and personal functioning. However, some remain highly impaired in most activities of living. These individuals may only respond to treatment very slowly, with gradual reduction in or improved tolerance of their dissociative and posttraumatic symptoms. Long-term supportive treatment may slowly increase these individuals' ability to manage their symptoms and decrease use of more restrictive levels of care.

Differential Diagnosis

Other specified dissociative disorder.   The core of dissociative identity disorder is the division of identity, with recurrent disruption of conscious functioning and sense of self. This central feature is shared with one form of other specified dissociative disorder, which may be distinguished from dissociative identity disorder by the presence of chronic or recurrent mixed dissociative symptoms that do not meet Criterion A for dissociative identity disorder or are not accompanied by recurrent amnesia.

Major depressive disorder.   Individuals with dissociative identity disorder are often depressed, and their symptoms may appear to meet the criteria for a major depressive episode. Rigorous assessment indicates that this depression in some cases does not meet full criteria for major depressive disorder. Other specified depressive disorder in individuals with dissociative identity disorder often has an important feature: the depressed mood and cognitions *fluctuate* because they are experienced in some identity states but not others.

Bipolar disorders.   Individuals with dissociative identity disorder are often misdiagnosed with a bipolar disorder, most often bipolar II disorder. The relatively rapid shifts in mood in individuals with this disorder—typically within minutes or hours, in contrast to the slower mood changes typically seen in individuals with bipolar disorders—are due to the rapid, subjective shifts in mood commonly reported across dissociative states, sometimes accompanied by fluctuation in levels of activation. Furthermore, in dissociative identity disorder, elevated or depressed mood may be displayed in conjunction with overt identities, so one or the other mood may predominate for a relatively long period of time (often for days) or may shift within minutes.

Posttraumatic stress disorder.   Some traumatized individuals have both posttraumatic stress disorder (PTSD) and dissociative identity disorder. Accordingly, it is crucial to distinguish between individuals with PTSD only and individuals who have both PTSD and dissociative identity disorder. This differential diagnosis requires that the clinician establish the presence or absence of dissociative symptoms that are not characteristic of acute stress disorder or PTSD. Some individuals with PTSD manifest dissociative symptoms that also occur in dissociative identity disorder: 1) amnesia for some aspects of trauma, 2) dissociative flashbacks (i.e., reliving of the trauma, with reduced awareness of one's current orientation), and 3) symptoms of intrusion and avoidance, negative alterations in cognition and mood, and hyperarousal that are focused around the traumatic event. On the other hand, individuals with dissociative identity disorder manifest dissociative symptoms that are not a manifestation of PTSD: 1) amnesias for many everyday (i.e., nontraumatic) events, 2) dissociative flashbacks that may be followed by amnesia for the content of the flashback, 3) disruptive intrusions (unrelated to traumatic material) by dissociated identity states into the individual's sense of self and agency, and 4) infrequent, full-blown changes among different identity states.

Psychotic disorders.   Dissociative identity disorder may be confused with schizophrenia or other psychotic disorders. The personified, internally communicative inner voices of dissociative identity disorder, especially of a child (e.g., "I hear a little girl crying in a closet and an angry man yelling at her"), may be mistaken for psychotic hallucinations. Dissociative experiences of identity fragmentation or possession, and of perceived loss of control over thoughts, feelings, impulses, and acts, may be confused with signs of formal thought disorder, such as thought insertion or withdrawal. Individuals with dissociative identity disorder may also report visual, tactile, olfactory, gustatory, and somatic hallucinations, which are usually related to posttraumatic and dissociative factors, such as partial flashbacks. Individuals with dissociative identity disorder experience these symptoms as caused by alternate identities, do not have delusional explanations for the phenomena, and often describe the symptoms in a personified way (e.g., "I feel like someone else wants to cry with my eyes"). Persecutory and derogatory internal voices in dissociative identity disorder associated with depressive symptoms may be misdiagnosed as major depression with psychotic features. Chaotic identity change and acute intrusions that disrupt thought processes may be distinguished from brief psychotic disorder by the predominance of dissociative symptoms and amnesia for the episode, and diagnostic evaluation after cessation of the crisis can help confirm the diagnosis.

Substance/medication-induced disorders.   Symptoms associated with the physiological effects of a substance can be distinguished from dissociative identity disorder if the substance in question is judged to be etiologically related to the disturbance.

Personality disorders.   Individuals with dissociative identity disorder often present identities that appear to encapsulate a variety of severe personality disorder features, suggesting a differential diagnosis of personality disorder, especially of the borderline type. Importantly, however, the individual's longitudinal variability in personality style (due to inconsistency among identities) differs from the pervasive and persistent dysfunction in affect management and interpersonal relationships typical of those with personality disorders.

Conversion disorder (functional neurological symptom disorder).   This disorder may be distinguished from dissociative identity disorder by the absence of an identity disruption characterized by two or more distinct personality states or an experience of possession. Dissociative amnesia in conversion disorder is more limited and circumscribed (e.g., amnesia for a non-epileptic seizure).

Seizure disorders.   Individuals with dissociative identity disorder may present with seizurelike symptoms and behaviors that resemble complex partial seizures with temporal lobe foci. These include déjà vu, jamais vu, depersonalization, derealization, out-of-body experiences, amnesia, disruptions of consciousness, hallucinations, and other intrusion phenomena of sensation, affect, and thought. Normal electroencephalographic findings, including telemetry, differentiate non-epileptic seizures from the seizurelike symptoms of dissociative identity disorder. Also, individuals with dissociative identity disorder obtain very high dissociation scores, whereas individuals with complex partial seizures do not.

Factitious disorder and malingering.   Individuals who feign dissociative identity disorder do not report the subtle symptoms of intrusion characteristic of the disorder; instead they tend to overreport well-publicized symptoms of the disorder, such as dissociative amnesia, while underreporting less-publicized comorbid symptoms, such as depression. Individuals who feign dissociative identity disorder tend to be relatively undisturbed by or may even seem to enjoy "having" the disorder. In contrast, individuals with genuine dissociative identity disorder tend to be ashamed of and overwhelmed by their symptoms and to underreport their symptoms or deny their condition. Sequential observation, corroborating history, and intensive psychometric and psychological assessment may be helpful in assessment.

Individuals who malinger dissociative identity disorder usually create limited, stereotyped alternate identities, with feigned amnesia, related to the events for which gain is sought. For example, they may present an "all-good" identity and an "all-bad" identity in hopes of gaining exculpation for a crime.

Comorbidity

Many individuals with dissociative identity disorder present with a comorbid disorder. If not assessed and treated specifically for the dissociative disorder, these individuals often receive prolonged treatment for the comorbid diagnosis only, with limited overall treatment response and resultant demoralization, and disability.

Individuals with dissociative identity disorder usually exhibit a large number of co-morbid disorders. In particular, most develop PTSD. Other disorders that are highly co-morbid with dissociative identity disorder include depressive disorders, trauma- and stressor-related disorders, personality disorders (especially avoidant and borderline personality disorders), conversion disorder (functional neurological symptom disorder), somatic symptom disorder, eating disorders, substance-related disorders, obsessive-compulsive disorder, and sleep disorders. Dissociative alterations in identity, memory, and consciousness may affect the symptom presentation of comorbid disorders.

Dissociative Amnesia

Diagnostic Criteria   **300.12** (F44.0)

A. An inability to recall important autobiographical information, usually of a traumatic or stressful nature, that is inconsistent with ordinary forgetting.
   Note: Dissociative amnesia most often consists of localized or selective amnesia for a specific event or events; or generalized amnesia for identity and life history.
B. The symptoms cause clinically significant distress or impairment in social, occupational, or other important areas of functioning.
C. The disturbance is not attributable to the physiological effects of a substance (e.g., alcohol or other drug of abuse, a medication) or a neurological or other medical condition (e.g., partial complex seizures, transient global amnesia, sequelae of a closed head injury/traumatic brain injury, other neurological condition).
D. The disturbance is not better explained by dissociative identity disorder, posttraumatic stress disorder, acute stress disorder, somatic symptom disorder, or major or mild neurocognitive disorder.

Coding note: The code for dissociative amnesia without dissociative fugue is **300.12 (F44.0).** The code for dissociative amnesia with dissociative fugue is **300.13 (F44.1).**

Specify if:
   300.13 (F44.1) With dissociative fugue: Apparently purposeful travel or bewildered wandering that is associated with amnesia for identity or for other important autobiographical information.

Diagnostic Features

The defining characteristic of dissociative amnesia is an inability to recall important autobiographical information that 1) should be successfully stored in memory and 2) ordinarily would be readily remembered (Criterion A). Dissociative amnesia differs from the permanent amnesias due to neurobiological damage or toxicity that prevent memory storage or retrieval in that it is always potentially reversible because the memory has been successfully stored.

Localized amnesia, a failure to recall events during a circumscribed period of time, is the most common form of dissociative amnesia. Localized amnesia may be broader than amnesia for a single traumatic event (e.g., months or years associated with child abuse or intense combat). In *selective amnesia,* the individual can recall some, but not all, of the events during a circumscribed period of time. Thus, the individual may remember part of a traumatic event but not other parts. Some individuals report both localized and selective amnesias.

Generalized amnesia, a complete loss of memory for one's life history, is rare. Individuals with generalized amnesia may forget personal identity. Some lose previous knowledge about the world (i.e., semantic knowledge) and can no longer access well-learned skills (i.e., procedural knowledge). Generalized amnesia has an acute onset; the perplexity, disorientation, and purposeless wandering of individuals with generalized amnesia usually bring them to the attention of the police or psychiatric emergency services. Generalized amnesia may be more common among combat veterans, sexual assault victims, and individuals experiencing extreme emotional stress or conflict.

Individuals with dissociative amnesia are frequently unaware (or only partially aware) of their memory problems. Many, especially those with localized amnesia, minimize the importance of their memory loss and may become uncomfortable when prompted to address it. In *systematized amnesia*, the individual loses memory for a specific category of information (e.g., all memories relating to one's family, a particular person, or childhood sexual abuse). In *continuous amnesia*, an individual forgets each new event as it occurs.

Associated Features Supporting Diagnosis

Many individuals with dissociative amnesia are chronically impaired in their ability to form and sustain satisfactory relationships. Histories of trauma, child abuse, and victimization are common. Some individuals with dissociative amnesia report dissociative flashbacks (i.e., behavioral reexperiencing of traumatic events). Many have a history of self-mutilation, suicide attempts, and other high-risk behaviors. Depressive and functional neurological symptoms are common, as are depersonalization, auto-hypnotic symptoms, and high hypnotizability. Sexual dysfunctions are common. Mild traumatic brain injury may precede dissociative amnesia.

Prevalence

The 12-month prevalence for dissociative amnesia among adults in a small U.S. community study was 1.8% (1.0% for males; 2.6% for females).

Development and Course

Onset of generalized amnesia is usually sudden. Less is known about the onset of localized and selective amnesias because these amnesias are seldom evident, even to the individual. Although overwhelming or intolerable events typically precede localized amnesia, its onset may be delayed for hours, days, or longer.

Individuals may report multiple episodes of dissociative amnesia. A single episode may predispose to future episodes. In between episodes of amnesia, the individual may or may not appear to be acutely symptomatic. The duration of the forgotten events can range from minutes to decades. Some episodes of dissociative amnesia resolve rapidly (e.g., when the person is removed from combat or some other stressful situation), whereas other episodes persist for long periods of time. Some individuals may gradually recall the dissociated memories years later. Dissociative capacities may decline with age, but not always. As the amnesia remits, there may be considerable distress, suicidal behavior, and symptoms of posttraumatic stress disorder (PTSD).

Dissociative amnesia has been observed in young children, adolescents, and adults. Children may be the most difficult to evaluate because they often have difficulty understanding questions about amnesia, and interviewers may find it difficult to formulate child-friendly questions about memory and amnesia. Observations of apparent dissociative amnesia are often difficult to differentiate from inattention, absorption, anxiety, oppositional behavior, and learning disorders. Reports from several different sources (e.g., teacher, therapist, case worker) may be needed to diagnose amnesia in children.

Risk and Prognostic Factors

Environmental. Single or repeated traumatic experiences (e.g., war, childhood maltreatment, natural disaster, internment in concentration camps, genocide) are common antecedents. Dissociative amnesia is more likely to occur with 1) a greater number of adverse childhood experiences, particularly physical and/or sexual abuse, 2) interpersonal violence; and 3) increased severity, frequency, and violence of the trauma.

Genetic and physiological.   There are no genetic studies of dissociative amnesia. Studies of dissociation report significant genetic and environmental factors in both clinical and nonclinical samples.

Course modifiers.   Removal from the traumatic circumstances underlying the dissociative amnesia (e.g., combat) may bring about a rapid return of memory. The memory loss of individuals with dissociative fugue may be particularly refractory. Onset of PTSD symptoms may decrease localized, selective, or systematized amnesia. The returning memory, however, may be experienced as flashbacks that alternate with amnesia for the content of the flashbacks.

Culture-Related Diagnostic Issues

In Asia, the Middle East, and Latin America, non-epileptic seizures and other functional neurological symptoms may accompany dissociative amnesia. In cultures with highly restrictive social traditions, the precipitants of dissociative amnesia often do not involve frank trauma. Instead, the amnesia is preceded by severe psychological stresses or conflicts (e.g., marital conflict, other family disturbances, attachment problems, conflicts due to restriction or oppression).

Suicide Risk

Suicidal and other self-destructive behaviors are common in individuals with dissociative amnesia. Suicidal behavior may be a particular risk when the amnesia remits suddenly and overwhelms the individual with intolerable memories.

Functional Consequences of Dissociative Amnesia

The impairment of individuals with localized, selective, or systematized dissociative amnesia ranges from limited to severe. Individuals with chronic generalized dissociative amnesia usually have impairment in all aspects of functioning. Even when these individuals "re-learn" aspects of their life history, autobiographical memory remains very impaired. Most become vocationally and interpersonally disabled.

Differential Diagnosis

Dissociative identity disorder.   Individuals with dissociative amnesia may report depersonalization and auto-hypnotic symptoms. Individuals with dissociative identity disorder report pervasive discontinuities in sense of self and agency, accompanied by many other dissociative symptoms. The amnesias of individuals with localized, selective, and/or systematized dissociative amnesias are relatively stable. Amnesias in dissociative identity disorder include amnesia for everyday events, finding of unexplained possessions, sudden fluctuations in skills and knowledge, major gaps in recall of life history, and brief amnesic gaps in interpersonal interactions.

Posttraumatic stress disorder.   Some individuals with PTSD cannot recall part or all of a specific traumatic event (e.g., a rape victim with depersonalization and/or derealization symptoms who cannot recall most events for the entire day of the rape). When that amnesia extends beyond the immediate time of the trauma, a comorbid diagnosis of dissociative amnesia is warranted.

Neurocognitive disorders.   In neurocognitive disorders, memory loss for personal information is usually embedded in cognitive, linguistic, affective, attentional, and behavioral disturbances. In dissociative amnesia, memory deficits are primarily for autobiographical information; intellectual and cognitive abilities are preserved.

Substance-related disorders.   In the context of repeated intoxication with alcohol or other substances/medications, there may be episodes of "black outs" or periods for which the individual has no memory. To aid in distinguishing these episodes from dissociative amnesia, a longitudinal history noting that the amnestic episodes occur only in the context of intoxication and do not occur in other situations would help identify the source as substance-induced; however the distinction may be difficult when the individual with dissociative amnesia may also misuse alcohol or other substances in the context of stressful situations that may also exacerbate dissociative symptoms. Some individuals with comorbid dissociative amnesia and substance use disorders will attribute their memory problems solely to the substance use. Prolonged use of alcohol or other substances may result in a substance-induced neurocognitive disorder that may be associated with impaired cognitive function, but in this context the protracted history of substance use and the persistent deficits associated with the neurocognitive disorder would serve to distinguish it from dissociative amnesia, where there is typically no evidence of persistent impairment in intellectual functioning.

Posttraumatic amnesia due to brain injury.   Amnesia may occur in the context of a traumatic brain injury (TBI) when there has been an impact to the head or other mechanisms of rapid movement or displacement of the brain within the skull TBI. Other characteristics of TBI include loss of consciousness, disorientation and confusion, or, in more severe cases, neurological signs (e.g., abnormalities on neuroimaging, a new onset of seizures or a marked worsening of a preexisting seizure disorder, visual field cuts, anosmia). A neurocognitive disorder attributable to TBI must present either immediately after brain injury occurs or immediately after the individual recovers consciousness after the injury, and persist past the acute post-injury period. The cognitive presentation of a neurocognitive disorder following TBI is variable and includes difficulties in the domains of complex attention, executive function, learning and memory as well as slowed speed of information processing and disturbances in social cognition. These additional features help distinguish it from dissociative amnesia.

Seizure disorders.   Individuals with seizure disorders may exhibit complex behavior during seizures or post-ictally with subsequent amnesia. Some individuals with a seizure disorder engage in nonpurposive wandering that is limited to the period of seizure activity. Conversely, behavior during a dissociative fugue is usually purposeful, complex, and goal-directed and may last for days, weeks, or longer. Occasionally, individuals with a seizure disorder will report that earlier autobiographical memories have been "wiped out" as the seizure disorder progresses. Such memory loss is not associated with traumatic circumstances and appears to occur randomly. Serial electroencephalograms usually show abnormalities. Telemetric electroencephalographic monitoring usually shows an association between the episodes of amnesia and seizure activity. Dissociative and epileptic amnesias may coexist.

Catatonic stupor.   Mutism in catatonic stupor may suggest dissociative amnesia, but failure of recall is absent. Other catatonic symptoms (e.g., rigidity, posturing, negativism) are usually present.

Factitious disorder and malingering.   There is no test, battery of tests, or set of procedures that invariably distinguishes dissociative amnesia from feigned amnesia. Individuals with factitious disorder or malingering have been noted to continue their deception even during hypnotic or barbiturate-facilitated interviews. Feigned amnesia is more common in individuals with 1) acute, florid dissociative amnesia; 2) financial, sexual, or legal problems; or 3) a wish to escape stressful circumstances. True amnesia can be associated with those same circumstances. Many individuals who malinger confess spontaneously or when confronted.

Normal and age-related changes in memory.   Memory decrements in major and mild neurocognitive disorders differ from those of dissociative amnesia, which are usually associated with stressful events and are more specific, extensive, and/or complex.

Comorbidity

As dissociative amnesia begins to remit, a wide variety of affective phenomena may surface: dysphoria, grief, rage, shame, guilt, psychological conflict and turmoil, and suicidal and homicidal ideation, impulses, and acts. These individuals may have symptoms that then meet diagnostic criteria for persistent depressive disorder (dysthymia); major depressive disorder; other specified or unspecified depressive disorder; adjustment disorder, with depressed mood; or adjustment disorder, with mixed disturbance of emotions and conduct. Many individuals with dissociative amnesia develop PTSD at some point during their life, especially when the traumatic antecedents of their amnesia are brought into conscious awareness.

Many individuals with dissociative amnesia have symptoms that meet diagnostic criteria for a comorbid somatic symptom or related disorder (and vice versa), including somatic symptom disorder and conversion disorder (functional neurological symptom disorder). Many individuals with dissociative amnesia have symptoms that meet diagnostic criteria for a personality disorder, especially dependent, avoidant, and borderline.

Depersonalization/Derealization Disorder

Diagnostic Criteria   300.6 (F48.1)

A. The presence of persistent or recurrent experiences of depersonalization, derealization, or both:

1. **Depersonalization:** Experiences of unreality, detachment, or being an outside observer with respect to one's thoughts, feelings, sensations, body, or actions (e.g., perceptual alterations, distorted sense of time, unreal or absent self, emotional and/or physical numbing).

2. **Derealization:** Experiences of unreality or detachment with respect to surroundings (e.g., individuals or objects are experienced as unreal, dreamlike, foggy, lifeless, or visually distorted).

B. During the depersonalization or derealization experiences, reality testing remains intact.

C. The symptoms cause clinically significant distress or impairment in social, occupational, or other important areas of functioning.

D. The disturbance is not attributable to the physiological effects of a substance (e.g., a drug of abuse, medication) or another medical condition (e.g., seizures).

E. The disturbance is not better explained by another mental disorder, such as schizophrenia, panic disorder, major depressive disorder, acute stress disorder, posttraumatic stress disorder, or another dissociative disorder.

Diagnostic Features

The essential features of depersonalization/derealization disorder are persistent or recurrent episodes of depersonalization, derealization, or both. Episodes of depersonalization are characterized by a feeling of unreality or detachment from, or unfamiliarity with, one's whole self or from aspects of the self (Criterion A1). The individual may feel detached from his or her entire being (e.g., "I am no one," "I have no self"). He or she may also feel subjectively detached from aspects of the self, including feelings (e.g., hypoemotionality:

"I know I have feelings but I don't feel them"), thoughts (e.g., "My thoughts don't feel like my own," "head filled with cotton"), whole body or body parts, or sensations (e.g., touch, proprioception, hunger, thirst, libido). There may also be a diminished sense of agency (e.g., feeling robotic, like an automaton; lacking control of one's speech or movements). The depersonalization experience can sometimes be one of a split self, with one part observing and one participating, known as an "out-of-body experience" in its most extreme form. The unitary symptom of "depersonalization" consists of several symptom factors: anomalous body experiences (i.e., unreality of the self and perceptual alterations); emotional or physical numbing; and temporal distortions with anomalous subjective recall.

Episodes of derealization are characterized by a feeling of unreality or detachment from, or unfamiliarity with, the world, be it individuals, inanimate objects, or all surroundings (Criterion A2). The individual may feel as if he or she were in a fog, dream, or bubble, or as if there were a veil or a glass wall between the individual and world around. Surroundings may be experienced as artificial, colorless, or lifeless. Derealization is commonly accompanied by subjective visual distortions, such as blurriness, heightened acuity, widened or narrowed visual field, two-dimensionality or flatness, exaggerated three-dimensionality, or altered distance or size of objects (i.e., macropsia or micropsia). Auditory distortions can also occur, whereby voices or sounds are muted or heightened. In addition, Criterion C requires the presence of clinically significant distress or impairment in social, occupational, or other important areas of functioning, and Criteria D and E describe exclusionary diagnoses.

Associated Features Supporting Diagnosis

Individuals with depersonalization/derealization disorder may have difficulty describing their symptoms and may think they are "crazy" or "going crazy". Another common experience is the fear of irreversible brain damage. A commonly associated symptom is a subjectively altered sense of time (i.e., too fast or too slow), as well as a subjective difficulty in vividly recalling past memories and owning them as personal and emotional. Vague somatic symptoms, such as head fullness, tingling, or lightheadedness, are not uncommon. Individuals may suffer extreme rumination or obsessional preoccupation (e.g., constantly obsessing about whether they really exist, or checking their perceptions to determine whether they appear real). Varying degrees of anxiety and depression are also common associated features. Individuals with the disorder have been found to have physiological hyporeactivity to emotional stimuli. Neural substrates of interest include the hypothalamic-pituitary-adrenocortical axis, inferior parietal lobule, and prefrontal cortical-limbic circuits.

Prevalence

Transient depersonalization/derealization symptoms lasting hours to days are common in the general population. The 12-month prevalence of depersonalization/derealization disorder is thought to be markedly less than for transient symptoms, although precise estimates for the disorder are unavailable. In general, approximately one-half of all adults have experienced at least one lifetime episode of depersonalization/derealization. However, symptomatology that meets full criteria for depersonalization/derealization disorder is markedly less common than transient symptoms. Lifetime prevalence in U.S. and non-U.S. countries is approximately 2% (range of 0.8% to 2.8%). The gender ratio for the disorder is 1:1.

Development and Course

The mean age at onset of depersonalization/derealization disorder is 16 years, although the disorder can start in early or middle childhood; a minority cannot recall ever not having had the symptoms. Less than 20% of individuals experience onset after age 20 years and only 5% after age 25 years. Onset in the fourth decade of life or later is highly unusual. Onset can range from extremely sudden to gradual. Duration of depersonalization/derealization disorder episodes can vary greatly, from brief (hours or days) to prolonged (weeks, months, or years). Given the rarity of disorder onset after age 40 years, in such cases the individual should be examined more closely for underlying medical conditions (e.g., brain lesions, seizure disorders, sleep apnea). The course of the disorder is often persistent. About one-third of cases involve discrete episodes; another third, continuous symptoms from the start; and still another third, an initially episodic course that eventually becomes continuous.

While in some individuals the intensity of symptoms can wax and wane considerably, others report an unwavering level of intensity that in extreme cases can be constantly present for years or decades. Internal and external factors that affect symptom intensity vary between individuals, yet some typical patterns are reported. Exacerbations can be triggered by stress, worsening mood or anxiety symptoms, novel or overstimulating settings, and physical factors such as lighting or lack of sleep.

Risk and Prognostic Factors

Temperamental.   Individuals with depersonalization/derealization disorder are characterized by harm-avoidant temperament, immature defenses, and both disconnection and overconnection schemata. Immature defenses such as idealization/devaluation, projection and acting out result in denial of reality and poor adaptation. *Cognitive disconnection schemata* reflect defectiveness and emotional inhibition and subsume themes of abuse, neglect, and deprivation. *Overconnection schemata* involve impaired autonomy with themes of dependency, vulnerability, and incompetence.

Environmental.   There is a clear association between the disorder and childhood interpersonal traumas in a substantial portion of individuals, although this association is not as prevalent or as extreme in the nature of the traumas as in other dissociative disorders, such as dissociative identity disorder. In particular, emotional abuse and emotional neglect have been most strongly and consistently associated with the disorder. Other stressors can include physical abuse; witnessing domestic violence; growing up with a seriously impaired, mentally ill parent; or unexpected death or suicide of a family member or close friend. Sexual abuse is a much less common antecedent but can be encountered. The most common proximal precipitants of the disorder are severe stress (interpersonal, financial, occupational), depression, anxiety (particularly panic attacks), and illicit drug use. Symptoms may be specifically induced by substances such as tetrahydrocannabinol, hallucinogens, ketamine, MDMA (3,4-methylene-dioxymethamphetamine; "ecstasy") and salvia. Marijuana use may precipitate new-onset panic attacks and depersonalization/derealization symptoms simultaneously.

Culture-Related Diagnostic Issues

Volitionally induced experiences of depersonalization/derealization can be a part of meditative practices that are prevalent in many religions and cultures and should not be diagnosed as a disorder. However, there are individuals who initially induce these states intentionally but over time lose control over them and may develop a fear and aversion for related practices.

Functional Consequences of Depersonalization/Derealization Disorder

Symptoms of depersonalization/derealization disorder are highly distressing and are associated with major morbidity. The affectively flattened and robotic demeanor that these individuals often demonstrate may appear incongruent with the extreme emotional pain reported by those with the disorder. Impairment is often experienced in both interpersonal and occupational spheres, largely due to the hypoemotionality with others, subjective difficulty in focusing and retaining information, and a general sense of disconnectedness from life.

Differential Diagnosis

Illness anxiety disorder. Although individuals with depersonalization/derealization disorder can present with vague somatic complaints as well as fears of permanent brain damage, the diagnosis of depersonalization/derealization disorder is characterized by the presence of a constellation of typical depersonalization/derealization symptoms and the absence of other manifestations of illness anxiety disorder.

Major depressive disorder. Feelings of numbness, deadness, apathy, and being in a dream are not uncommon in major depressive episodes. However, in depersonalization/derealization disorder, such symptoms are associated with further symptoms of the disorder. If the depersonalization/derealization clearly precedes the onset of a major depressive episode or clearly continues after its resolution, the diagnosis of depersonalization/derealization disorder applies.

Obsessive-compulsive disorder. Some individuals with depersonalization/derealization disorder can become obsessively preoccupied with their subjective experience or develop rituals checking on the status of their symptoms. However, other symptoms of obsessive-compulsive disorder unrelated to depersonalization/derealization are not present.

Other dissociative disorders. In order to diagnose depersonalization/derealization disorder, the symptoms should not occur in the context of another dissociative disorder, such as dissociative identity disorder. Differentiation from dissociative amnesia and conversion disorder (functional neurological symptom disorder) is simpler, as the symptoms of these disorders do not overlap with those of depersonalization/derealization disorder.

Anxiety disorders. Depersonalization/derealization is one of the symptoms of panic attacks, increasingly common as panic attack severity increases. Therefore, depersonalization/derealization disorder should not be diagnosed when the symptoms occur only during panic attacks that are part of panic disorder, social anxiety disorder, or specific phobia. In addition, it is not uncommon for depersonalization/derealization symptoms to first begin in the context of new-onset panic attacks or as panic disorder progresses and worsens. In such presentations, the diagnosis of depersonalization/derealization disorder can be made if 1) the depersonalization/derealization component of the presentation is very prominent from the start, clearly exceeding in duration and intensity the occurrence of actual panic attacks; or 2) the depersonalization/derealization continues after panic disorder has remitted or has been successfully treated.

Psychotic disorders. The presence of intact reality testing specifically regarding the depersonalization/derealization symptoms is essential to differentiating depersonalization/derealization disorder from psychotic disorders. Rarely, positive-symptom schizophrenia can pose a diagnostic challenge when nihilistic delusions are present. For example, an individual may complain that he or she is dead or the world is not real; this could be either a subjective experience that the individual knows is not true or a delusional conviction.

Substance/medication-induced disorders. Depersonalization/derealization associated with the physiological effects of substances during acute intoxication or withdrawal is not diagnosed as depersonalization/derealization disorder. The most common precipitating substances are the illicit drugs marijuana, hallucinogens, ketamine, ecstasy, and salvia. In about 15% of all cases of depersonalization/derealization disorder, the symptoms are precipitated by ingestion of such substances. If the symptoms persist for some time in the absence of any further substance or medication use, the diagnosis of depersonalization/derealization disorder applies. This diagnosis is usually easy to establish since the vast majority of individuals with this presentation become highly phobic and aversive to the triggering substance and do not use it again.

Mental disorders due to another medical condition.   Features such as onset after age 40 years or the presence of atypical symptoms and course in any individual suggest the possibility of an underlying medical condition. In such cases, it is essential to conduct a thorough medical and neurological evaluation, which may include standard laboratory studies, viral titers, an electroencephalogram, vestibular testing, visual testing, sleep studies, and/or brain imaging. When the suspicion of an underlying seizure disorder proves difficult to confirm, an ambulatory electroencephalogram may be indicated; although temporal lobe epilepsy is most commonly implicated, parietal and frontal lobe epilepsy may also be associated.

Comorbidity

In a convenience sample of adults recruited for a number of depersonalization research studies, lifetime comorbidities were high for unipolar depressive disorder and for any anxiety disorder, with a significant proportion of the sample having both disorders. Comorbidity with posttraumatic stress disorder was low. The three most commonly co-occurring personality disorders were avoidant, borderline, and obsessive-compulsive.

Other Specified Dissociative Disorder

300.15 (F44.89)

This category applies to presentations in which symptoms characteristic of a dissociative disorder that cause clinically significant distress or impairment in social, occupational, or other important areas of functioning predominate but do not meet the full criteria for any of the disorders in the dissociative disorders diagnostic class. The other specified dissociative disorder category is used in situations in which the clinician chooses to communicate the specific reason that the presentation does not meet the criteria for any specific dissociative disorder. This is done by recording "other specified dissociative disorder" followed by the specific reason (e.g., "dissociative trance").

Examples of presentations that can be specified using the "other specified" designation include the following:

1. **Chronic and recurrent syndromes of mixed dissociative symptoms:** This category includes identity disturbance associated with less-than-marked discontinuities in sense of self and agency, or alterations of identity or episodes of possession in an individual who reports no dissociative amnesia.

2. **Identity disturbance due to prolonged and intense coercive persuasion:** Individuals who have been subjected to intense coercive persuasion (e.g., brainwashing, thought reform, indoctrination while captive, torture, long-term political imprisonment, recruitment by sects/cults or by terror organizations) may present with prolonged changes in, or conscious questioning of, their identity.

3. **Acute dissociative reactions to stressful events:** This category is for acute, transient conditions that typically last less than 1 month, and sometimes only a few hours or days. These conditions are characterized by constriction of consciousness; depersonalization; derealization; perceptual disturbances (e.g., time slowing, macropsia);

micro-amnesias; transient stupor; and/or alterations in sensory-motor functioning (e.g., analgesia, paralysis).

4. **Dissociative trance:** This condition is characterized by an acute narrowing or complete loss of awareness of immediate surroundings that manifests as profound unresponsiveness or insensitivity to environmental stimuli. The unresponsiveness may be accompanied by minor stereotyped behaviors (e.g., finger movements) of which the individual is unaware and/or that he or she cannot control, as well as transient paralysis or loss of consciousness. The dissociative trance is not a normal part of a broadly accepted collective cultural or religious practice.

Unspecified Dissociative Disorder

300.15 (F44.9)

This category applies to presentations in which symptoms characteristic of a dissociative disorder that cause clinically significant distress or impairment in social, occupational, or other important areas of functioning predominate but do not meet the full criteria for any of the disorders in the dissociative disorders diagnostic class. The unspecified dissociative disorder category is used in situations in which the clinician chooses *not* to specify the reason that the criteria are not met for a specific dissociative disorder, and includes presentations for which there is insufficient information to make a more specific diagnosis (e.g., in emergency room settings).

Somatic Symptom and Related Disorders

Somatic symptom disorder and other disorders with prominent somatic symptoms constitute a new category in DSM-5 called *somatic symptom and related disorders*. This chapter includes the diagnoses of somatic symptom disorder, illness anxiety disorder, conversion disorder (functional neurological symptom disorder), psychological factors affecting other medical conditions, factitious disorder, other specified somatic symptom and related disorder, and unspecified somatic symptom and related disorder. All of the disorders in this chapter share a common feature: the prominence of somatic symptoms associated with significant distress and impairment. Individuals with disorders with prominent somatic symptoms are commonly encountered in primary care and other medical settings but are less commonly encountered in psychiatric and other mental health settings. These reconceptualized diagnoses, based on a reorganization of DSM-IV somatoform disorder diagnoses, are more useful for primary care and other medical (nonpsychiatric) clinicians.

The major diagnosis in this diagnostic class, somatic symptom disorder, emphasizes diagnosis made on the basis of positive symptoms and signs (distressing somatic symptoms plus abnormal thoughts, feelings, and behaviors in response to these symptoms) rather than the absence of a medical explanation for somatic symptoms. A distinctive characteristic of many individuals with somatic symptom disorder is not the somatic symptoms per se, but instead the way they present and interpret them. Incorporating affective, cognitive, and behavioral components into the criteria for somatic symptom disorder provides a more comprehensive and accurate reflection of the true clinical picture than can be achieved by assessing the somatic complaints alone.

The principles behind the changes in the somatic symptom and related diagnoses from DSM-IV are crucial in understanding the DSM-5 diagnoses. The DSM-IV term *somatoform disorders* was confusing and is replaced by *somatic symptom and related disorders*. In DSM-IV there was a great deal of overlap across the somatoform disorders and a lack of clarity about the boundaries of diagnoses. Although individuals with these disorders primarily present in medical rather than mental health settings, nonpsychiatric physicians found the DSM-IV somatoform diagnoses difficult to understand and use. The current DSM-5 classification recognizes this overlap by reducing the total number of disorders as well as their subcategories.

The previous criteria overemphasized the centrality of medically unexplained symptoms. Such symptoms are present to various degrees, particularly in conversion disorder, but somatic symptom disorders can also accompany diagnosed medical disorders. The reliability of determining that a somatic symptom is medically unexplained is limited, and grounding a diagnosis on the absence of an explanation is problematic and reinforces mind-body dualism. It is not appropriate to give an individual a mental disorder diagnosis solely because a medical cause cannot be demonstrated. Furthermore, the presence of a medical diagnosis does not exclude the possibility of a comorbid mental disorder, including a somatic symptom and related disorder. Perhaps because of the predominant focus on lack of medical explanation, individuals regarded these diagnoses as pejorative and demeaning, implying that their physical symptoms were not "real." The new classification defines the major diagnosis, somatic symptom disorder, on the basis of positive symptoms (distressing somatic symptoms plus abnormal thoughts, feelings, and behaviors in response to these symptoms). However, medically unexplained symptoms remain a key feature in conversion disorder and pseudocyesis (other specified somatic symptom and related disorder) because it is possible to demonstrate definitively in such disorders that the symptoms are not consistent with medical pathophysiology.

It is important to note that some other mental disorders may initially manifest with primarily somatic symptoms (e.g., major depressive disorder, panic disorder). Such diagnoses may account for the somatic symptoms, or they may occur alongside one of the somatic symptom and related disorders in this chapter. There is also considerable medical comorbidity among somatizing individuals. Although somatic symptoms are frequently associated with psychological distress and psychopathology, some somatic symptom and related disorders can arise spontaneously, and their causes can remain obscure. Anxiety disorders and depressive disorders may accompany somatic symptom and related disorders. The somatic component adds severity and complexity to depressive and anxiety disorders and results in higher severity, functional impairment, and even refractoriness to traditional treatments. In rare instances, the degree of preoccupation may be so severe as to warrant consideration of a delusional disorder diagnosis.

A number of factors may contribute to somatic symptom and related disorders. These include genetic and biological vulnerability (e.g., increased sensitivity to pain), early traumatic experiences (e.g., violence, abuse, deprivation), and learning (e.g., attention obtained from illness, lack of reinforcement of nonsomatic expressions of distress), as well as cultural/social norms that devalue and stigmatize psychological suffering as compared with physical suffering. Differences in medical care across cultures affect the presentation, recognition, and management of these somatic presentations. Variations in symptom presentation are likely the result of the interaction of multiple factors within cultural contexts that affect how individuals identify and classify bodily sensations, perceive illness, and seek medical attention for them. Thus, somatic presentations can be viewed as expressions of personal suffering inserted in a cultural and social context.

All of these disorders are characterized by the prominent focus on somatic concerns and their initial presentation mainly in medical rather than mental health care settings. Somatic symptom disorder offers a more clinically useful method of characterizing individuals who may have been considered in the past for a diagnosis of somatization disorder. Furthermore, approximately 75% of individuals previously diagnosed with hypochondriasis are subsumed under the diagnosis of somatic symptom disorder. However, about 25% of individuals with hypochondriasis have high health anxiety in the absence of somatic symptoms, and many such individuals' symptoms would not qualify for an anxiety disorder diagnosis. The DSM-5 diagnosis of illness anxiety disorder is for this latter group of individuals. Illness anxiety disorder can be considered either in this diagnostic section or as an anxiety disorder. Because of the strong focus on somatic concerns, and because illness anxiety disorder is most often encountered in medical settings, for utility it is listed with the somatic symptom and related disorders. In conversion disorder, the essential feature is neurological symptoms that are found, after appropriate neurological assessment, to be incompatible with neurological pathophysiology. Psychological factors affecting other medical conditions is also included in this chapter. Its essential feature is the presence of one or more clinically significant psychological or behavioral factors that adversely affect a medical condition by increasing the risk for suffering, death, or disability. Like the other somatic symptom and related disorders, factitious disorder embodies persistent problems related to illness perception and identity. In the great majority of reported cases of factitious disorder, both imposed on self and imposed on another, individuals present with somatic symptoms and medical disease conviction. Consequently, DSM-5 factitious disorder is included among the somatic symptom and related disorders. Other specified somatic symptom and related disorder and unspecified somatic symptom and related disorder include conditions for which some, but not all, of the criteria for somatic symptom disorder or illness anxiety disorder are met, as well as pseudocyesis.

Somatic Symptom Disorder

Diagnostic Criteria 300.82 (F45.1)

A. One or more somatic symptoms that are distressing or result in significant disruption of daily life.

B. Excessive thoughts, feelings, or behaviors related to the somatic symptoms or associated health concerns as manifested by at least one of the following:

1. Disproportionate and persistent thoughts about the seriousness of one's symptoms.
2. Persistently high level of anxiety about health or symptoms.
3. Excessive time and energy devoted to these symptoms or health concerns.

C. Although any one somatic symptom may not be continuously present, the state of being symptomatic is persistent (typically more than 6 months).

Specify if:

With predominant pain (previously pain disorder): This specifier is for individuals whose somatic symptoms predominantly involve pain.

Specify if:

Persistent: A persistent course is characterized by severe symptoms, marked impairment, and long duration (more than 6 months).

Specify current severity:

Mild: Only one of the symptoms specified in Criterion B is fulfilled.

Moderate: Two or more of the symptoms specified in Criterion B are fulfilled.

Severe: Two or more of the symptoms specified in Criterion B are fulfilled, plus there are multiple somatic complaints (or one very severe somatic symptom).

Diagnostic Features

Individuals with somatic symptom disorder typically have multiple, current, somatic symptoms that are distressing or result in significant disruption of daily life (Criterion A), although sometimes only one severe symptom, most commonly pain, is present. Symptoms may be specific (e.g., localized pain) or relatively nonspecific (e.g., fatigue). The symptoms sometimes represent normal bodily sensations or discomfort that does not generally signify serious disease. Somatic symptoms without an evident medical explanation are not sufficient to make this diagnosis. The individual's suffering is authentic, whether or not it is medically explained.

The symptoms may or may not be associated with another medical condition. The diagnoses of somatic symptom disorder and a concurrent medical illness are not mutually exclusive, and these frequently occur together. For example, an individual may become seriously disabled by symptoms of somatic symptom disorder after an uncomplicated myocardial infarction even if the myocardial infarction itself did not result in any disability. If another medical condition or high risk for developing one is present (e.g., strong family history), the thoughts, feelings, and behaviors associated with this condition are excessive (Criterion B).

Individuals with somatic symptom disorder tend to have very high levels of worry about illness (Criterion B). They appraise their bodily symptoms as unduly threatening, harmful, or troublesome and often think the worst about their health. Even when there is evidence to the contrary, some patients still fear the medical seriousness of their symptoms. In severe somatic symptom disorder, health concerns may assume a central role in the individual's life, becoming a feature of his or her identity and dominating interpersonal relationships.

Individuals typically experience distress that is principally focused on somatic symptoms and their significance. When asked directly about their distress, some individuals describe it in relation to other aspects of their lives, while others deny any source of distress other than the somatic symptoms. Health-related quality of life is often impaired, both physically and mentally. In severe somatic symptom disorder, the impairment is marked, and when persistent, the disorder can lead to invalidism.

There is often a high level of medical care utilization, which rarely alleviates the individual's concerns. Consequently, the patient may seek care from multiple doctors for the same symptoms. These individuals often seem unresponsive to medical interventions, and new interventions may only exacerbate the presenting symptoms. Some individuals with the disorder seem unusually sensitive to medication side effects. Some feel that their medical assessment and treatment have been inadequate.

Associated Features Supporting Diagnosis

Cognitive features include attention focused on somatic symptoms, attribution of normal bodily sensations to physical illness (possibly with catastrophic interpretations), worry about illness, and fear that any physical activity may damage the body. The relevant associated behavioral features may include repeated bodily checking for abnormalities, repeated seeking of medical help and reassurance, and avoidance of physical activity. These behavioral features are most pronounced in severe, persistent somatic symptom disorder. These features are usually associated with frequent requests for medical help for different somatic symptoms. This may lead to medical consultations in which individuals are so focused on their concerns about somatic symptom(s) that they cannot be redirected to other matters. Any reassurance by the doctor that the symptoms are not indicative of serious physical illness tends to be short-lived and/or is experienced by the individuals as the doctor not taking their symptoms with due seriousness. As the focus on somatic symptoms is a primary feature of the disorder, individuals with somatic symptom disorder typically present to general medical health services rather than mental health services. The suggestion of referral to a mental health specialist may be met with surprise or even frank refusal by individuals with somatic symptom disorder.

Since somatic symptom disorder is associated with depressive disorders, there is an increased suicide risk. It is not known whether somatic symptom disorder is associated with suicide risk independent of its association with depressive disorders.

Prevalence

The prevalence of somatic symptom disorder is not known. However, the prevalence of somatic symptom disorder is expected to be higher than that of the more restrictive DSM-IV somatization disorder (<1%) but lower than that of undifferentiated somatoform disorder (approximately 19%). The prevalence of somatic symptom disorder in the general adult population may be around 5%–7%. Females tend to report more somatic symptoms than do males, and the prevalence of somatic symptom disorder is consequently likely to be higher in females.

Development and Course

In older individuals, somatic symptoms and concurrent medical illnesses are common, and a focus on Criterion B is crucial for making the diagnosis. Somatic symptom disorder may be underdiagnosed in older adults either because certain somatic symptoms (e.g., pain, fatigue) are considered part of normal aging or because illness worry is considered "understandable" in older adults who have more general medical illnesses and medications than do younger people. Concurrent depressive disorder is common in older people who present with numerous somatic symptoms.

In children, the most common symptoms are recurrent abdominal pain, headache, fatigue, and nausea. A single prominent symptom is more common in children than in adults. While young children may have somatic complaints, they rarely worry about "illness" per se prior to adolescence. The parents' response to the symptom is important, as this may determine the level of associated distress. It is the parent who may determine the interpretation of symptoms and the associated time off school and medical help seeking.

Risk and Prognostic Factors

Temperamental.   The personality trait of negative affectivity (neuroticism) has been identified as an independent correlate/risk factor of a high number of somatic symptoms. Comorbid anxiety or depression is common and may exacerbate symptoms and impairment.

Environmental.   Somatic symptom disorder is more frequent in individuals with few years of education and low socioeconomic status, and in those who have recently experienced stressful life events.

Course modifiers.   Persistent somatic symptoms are associated with demographic features (female sex, older age, fewer years of education, lower socioeconomic status, unemployment), a reported history of sexual abuse or other childhood adversity, concurrent chronic physical illness or psychiatric disorder (depression, anxiety, persistent depressive disorder [dysthymia], panic), social stress, and reinforcing social factors such as illness benefits. Cognitive factors that affect clinical course include sensitization to pain, heightened attention to bodily sensations, and attribution of bodily symptoms to a possible medical illness rather than recognizing them as a normal phenomenon or psychological stress.

Culture-Related Diagnostic Issues

Somatic symptoms are prominent in various "culture-bound syndromes." High numbers of somatic symptoms are found in population-based and primary care studies around the world, with a similar pattern of the most commonly reported somatic symptoms, impairment, and treatment seeking. The relationship between number of somatic symptoms and illness worry is similar in different cultures, and marked illness worry is associated with impairment and greater treatment seeking across cultures. The relationship between numerous somatic symptoms and depression appears to be very similar around the world and between different cultures within one country.

Despite these similarities, there are differences in somatic symptoms among cultures and ethnic groups. The description of somatic symptoms varies with linguistic and other local cultural factors. These somatic presentations have been described as "idioms of distress" because somatic symptoms may have special meanings and shape patient-clinician interactions in the particular cultural contexts. "Burnout," the sensation of heaviness or the complaints of "gas"; too much heat in the body; or burning in the head are examples of symptoms that are common in some cultures or ethnic groups but rare in others. Explanatory models also vary, and somatic symptoms may be attributed variously to particular family, work, or environmental stresses; general medical illness; the suppression of feelings of anger and resentment; or certain culture-specific phenomena, such as semen loss. There may also be differences in medical treatment seeking among cultural groups, in addition to differences due to variable access to medical care services. Seeking treatment for multiple somatic symptoms in general medical clinics is a worldwide phenomenon and occurs at similar rates among ethnic groups in the same country.

Functional Consequences of Somatic Symptom Disorder

The disorder is associated with marked impairment of health status. Many individuals with severe somatic symptom disorder are likely to have impaired health status scores more than 2 standard deviations below population norms.

Differential Diagnosis

If the somatic symptoms are consistent with another mental disorder (e.g., panic disorder), and the diagnostic criteria for that disorder are fulfilled, then that mental disorder should be considered as an alternative or additional diagnosis. If, as commonly occurs, the criteria for both somatic symptom disorder and another mental disorder diagnosis are fulfilled, then both should be coded, as both may require treatment.

Other medical conditions.   The presence of somatic symptoms of unclear etiology is not in itself sufficient to make the diagnosis of somatic symptom disorder. The symptoms of many individuals with disorders like irritable bowel syndrome or fibromyalgia would not satisfy the criterion necessary to diagnose somatic symptom disorder (Criterion B). Conversely, the presence of somatic symptoms of an established medical disorder (e.g., diabetes or heart disease) does not exclude the diagnosis of somatic symptom disorder if the criteria are otherwise met.

Panic disorder.   In panic disorder, somatic symptoms and anxiety about health tend to occur in acute episodes, whereas in somatic symptom disorder, anxiety and somatic symptoms are more persistent.

Generalized anxiety disorder.   Individuals with generalized anxiety disorder worry about multiple events, situations, or activities, only one of which may involve their health. The main focus is not usually somatic symptoms or fear of illness as it is in somatic symptom disorder.

Depressive disorders.   Depressive disorders are commonly accompanied by somatic symptoms. However, depressive disorders are differentiated from somatic symptom disorder by the core depressive symptoms of low (dysphoric) mood and anhedonia.

Illness anxiety disorder.   If the individual has extensive worries about health but no or minimal somatic symptoms, it may be more appropriate to consider illness anxiety disorder.

Conversion disorder (functional neurological symptom disorder).   In conversion disorder, the presenting symptom is loss of function (e.g., of a limb), whereas in somatic symptom disorder, the focus is on the distress that particular symptoms cause. The features listed under Criterion B of somatic symptom disorder may be helpful in differentiating the two disorders.

Delusional disorder.   In somatic symptom disorder, the individual's beliefs that somatic symptoms might reflect serious underlying physical illness are not held with delusional intensity. Nonetheless, the individual's beliefs concerning the somatic symptoms can be firmly held. In contrast, in delusional disorder, somatic subtype, the somatic symptom beliefs and behavior are stronger than those found in somatic symptom disorder.

Body dysmorphic disorder.   In body dysmorphic disorder, the individual is excessively concerned about, and preoccupied by, a perceived defect in his or her physical features. In contrast, in somatic symptom disorder, the concern about somatic symptoms reflects fear of underlying illness, not of a defect in appearance.

Obsessive-compulsive disorder.   In somatic symptom disorder, the recurrent ideas about somatic symptoms or illness are less intrusive, and individuals with this disorder do not exhibit the associated repetitive behaviors aimed at reducing anxiety that occur in obsessive-compulsive disorder.

Comorbidity

Somatic symptom disorder is associated with high rates of comorbidity with medical disorders as well as anxiety and depressive disorders. When a concurrent medical illness is present, the degree of impairment is more marked than would be expected from the physical illness alone. When an individual's symptoms meet diagnostic criteria for somatic symptom disorder, the disorder should be diagnosed; however, in view of the frequent comorbidity, especially with anxiety and depressive disorders, evidence for these concurrent diagnoses should be sought.

Illness Anxiety Disorder

Diagnostic Criteria	**300.7** (F45.21)

A. Preoccupation with having or acquiring a serious illness.

B. Somatic symptoms are not present or, if present, are only mild in intensity. If another medical condition is present or there is a high risk for developing a medical condition (e.g., strong family history is present), the preoccupation is clearly excessive or disproportionate.

C. There is a high level of anxiety about health, and the individual is easily alarmed about personal health status.

D. The individual performs excessive health-related behaviors (e.g., repeatedly checks his or her body for signs of illness) or exhibits maladaptive avoidance (e.g., avoids doctor appointments and hospitals).

E. Illness preoccupation has been present for at least 6 months, but the specific illness that is feared may change over that period of time.

F. The illness-related preoccupation is not better explained by another mental disorder, such as somatic symptom disorder, panic disorder, generalized anxiety disorder, body dysmorphic disorder, obsessive-compulsive disorder, or delusional disorder, somatic type.

Specify whether:

Care-seeking type: Medical care, including physician visits or undergoing tests and procedures, is frequently used.

Care-avoidant type: Medical care is rarely used.

Diagnostic Features

Most individuals with hypochondriasis are now classified as having somatic symptom disorder; however, in a minority of cases, the diagnosis of illness anxiety disorder applies instead. Illness anxiety disorder entails a preoccupation with having or acquiring a serious, undiagnosed medical illness (Criterion A). Somatic symptoms are not present or, if present, are only mild in intensity (Criterion B). A thorough evaluation fails to identify a serious medical condition that accounts for the individual's concerns. While the concern may be derived from a nonpathological physical sign or sensation, the individual's distress emanates not primarily from the physical complaint itself but rather from his or her anxiety about the meaning, significance, or cause of the complaint (i.e., the suspected medical diagnosis). If a physical sign or symptom is present, it is often a normal physiological sensation (e.g., orthostatic dizziness), a benign and self-limited dysfunction (e.g., transient tinnitus), or a bodily discomfort not generally considered indicative of disease (e.g., belching). If a diagnosable medical condition is present, the individual's anxiety and preoccupation are clearly excessive and disproportionate to the severity of the condition (Criterion B). Empirical evidence and existing literature pertain to previously defined DSM hypochondriasis, and it is unclear to what extent and how precisely they apply to the description of this new diagnosis.

The preoccupation with the idea that one is sick is accompanied by substantial anxiety about health and disease (Criterion C). Individuals with illness anxiety disorder are easily alarmed about illness, such as by hearing about someone else falling ill or reading a health-related news story. Their concerns about undiagnosed disease do not respond to appropriate medical reassurance, negative diagnostic tests, or benign course. The physician's attempts at reassurance and symptom palliation generally do not alleviate the individual's concerns and may heighten them. Illness concerns assume a prominent place in the individual's life, affecting daily activities, and may even result in invalidism. Illness becomes a central feature of the individual's identity and self-image, a frequent topic of social discourse, and a characteristic response to stressful life events. Individuals with the disorder often examine themselves repeatedly (e.g., examining one's throat in the mirror) (Criterion D). They research their suspected disease excessively (e.g., on the Internet) and repeatedly seek reassurance from family, friends, or physicians. This incessant worrying often becomes frustrating for others and may result in considerable strain within the family. In some cases, the anxiety leads to maladaptive avoidance of situations (e.g., visiting sick family members) or activities (e.g., exercise) that these individuals fear might jeopardize their health.

Associated Features Supporting Diagnosis

Because they believe they are medically ill, individuals with illness anxiety disorder are encountered far more frequently in medical than in mental health settings. The majority of individuals with illness anxiety disorder have extensive yet unsatisfactory medical care, though some may be too anxious to seek medical attention. They generally have elevated rates of medical utilization but do not utilize mental health services more than the general population. They often consult multiple physicians for the same problem and obtain repeatedly negative diagnostic test results. At times, medical attention leads to a paradoxical exacerbation of anxiety or to iatrogenic complications from diagnostic tests and procedures. Individuals with the disorder are generally dissatisfied with their medical care and find it unhelpful, often feeling they are not being taken seriously by physicians. At times, these concerns may be justified, since physicians sometimes are dismissive or respond with frustration or hostility. This response can occasionally result in a failure to diagnose a medical condition that is present.

Prevalence

Prevalence estimates of illness anxiety disorder are based on estimates of the DSM-III and DSM-IV diagnosis *hypochondriasis*. The 1- to 2-year prevalence of health anxiety and/or disease conviction in community surveys and population-based samples ranges from 1.3% to 10%. In ambulatory medical populations, the 6-month/1-year prevalence rates are between 3% and 8%. The prevalence of the disorder is similar in males and females.

Development and Course

The development and course of illness anxiety disorder are unclear. Illness anxiety disorder is generally thought to be a chronic and relapsing condition with an age at onset in early and middle adulthood. In population-based samples, health-related anxiety increases with age, but the ages of individuals with high health anxiety in medical settings do not appear to differ from those of other patients in those settings. In older individuals, health-related anxiety often focuses on memory loss; the disorder is thought to be rare in children.

Risk and Prognostic Factors

Environmental.   Illness anxiety disorder may sometimes be precipitated by a major life stress or a serious but ultimately benign threat to the individual's health. A history of childhood abuse or of a serious childhood illness may predispose to development of the disorder in adulthood.

Course modifiers.   Approximately one-third to one-half of individuals with illness anxiety disorder have a transient form, which is associated with less psychiatric comorbidity, more medical comorbidity, and less severe illness anxiety disorder.

Culture-Related Diagnostic Issues

The diagnosis should be made with caution in individuals whose ideas about disease are congruent with widely held, culturally sanctioned beliefs. Little is known about the phenomenology of the disorder across cultures, although the prevalence appears to be similar across different countries with diverse cultures.

Functional Consequences of Illness Anxiety Disorder

Illness anxiety disorder causes substantial role impairment and decrements in physical function and health-related quality of life. Health concerns often interfere with interpersonal relationships, disrupt family life, and damage occupational performance.

Differential Diagnosis

Other medical conditions.   The first differential diagnostic consideration is an underlying medical condition, including neurological or endocrine conditions, occult malignancies, and other diseases that affect multiple body systems. The presence of a medical condition does not rule out the possibility of coexisting illness anxiety disorder. If a medical condition is present, the health-related anxiety and disease concerns are clearly disproportionate to its seriousness. Transient preoccupations related to a medical condition do not constitute illness anxiety disorder.

Adjustment disorders.   Health-related anxiety is a normal response to serious illness and is not a mental disorder. Such nonpathological health anxiety is clearly related to the medical condition and is typically time-limited. If the health anxiety is severe enough, an adjustment disorder may be diagnosed. However, only when the health anxiety is of sufficient duration, severity, and distress can illness anxiety disorder be diagnosed. Thus, the diagnosis requires the continuous persistence of disproportionate health-related anxiety for at least 6 months.

Somatic symptom disorder.   Somatic symptom disorder is diagnosed when significant somatic symptoms are present. In contrast, individuals with illness anxiety disorder have minimal somatic symptoms and are primarily concerned with the idea they are ill.

Anxiety disorders.   In generalized anxiety disorder, individuals worry about multiple events, situations, or activities, only one of which may involve health. In panic disorder, the individual may be concerned that the panic attacks reflect the presence of a medical illness; however, although these individuals may have health anxiety, their anxiety is typically very acute and episodic. In illness anxiety disorder, the health anxiety and fears are more persistent and enduring. Individuals with illness anxiety disorder may experience panic attacks that are triggered by their illness concerns.

Obsessive-compulsive and related disorders.   Individuals with illness anxiety disorder may have intrusive thoughts about having a disease and also may have associated compulsive behaviors (e.g., seeking reassurance). However, in illness anxiety disorder, the preoccupations are usually focused on having a disease, whereas in obsessive-compulsive disorder (OCD), the thoughts are intrusive and are usually focused on fears of getting a disease in the future. Most individuals with OCD have obsessions or compulsions involving other concerns in addition to fears about contracting disease. In body dysmorphic disorder, concerns are limited to the individual's physical appearance, which is viewed as defective or flawed.

Major depressive disorder.   Some individuals with a major depressive episode ruminate about their health and worry excessively about illness. A separate diagnosis of illness anxiety disorder is not made if these concerns occur only during major depressive episodes. However, if excessive illness worry persists after remission of an episode of major depressive disorder, the diagnosis of illness anxiety disorder should be considered.

Psychotic disorders.   Individuals with illness anxiety disorder are not delusional and can acknowledge the possibility that the feared disease is not present. Their ideas do not attain the rigidity and intensity seen in the somatic delusions occurring in psychotic disorders (e.g., schizophrenia; delusional disorder, somatic type; major depressive disorder, with psychotic features). True somatic delusions are generally more bizarre (e.g., that an organ is rotting or dead) than the concerns seen in illness anxiety disorder. The concerns seen in illness anxiety disorder, though not founded in reality, are plausible.

Comorbidity

Because illness anxiety disorder is a new disorder, exact comorbidities are unknown. Hypochondriasis co-occurs with anxiety disorders (in particular, generalized anxiety disorder, panic disorder, and OCD) and depressive disorders. Approximately two-thirds of individuals with illness anxiety disorder are likely to have at least one other comorbid major mental disorder. Individuals with illness anxiety disorder may have an elevated risk for somatic symptom disorder and personality disorders.

Conversion Disorder (Functional Neurological Symptom Disorder)

Diagnostic Criteria

A. One or more symptoms of altered voluntary motor or sensory function.
B. Clinical findings provide evidence of incompatibility between the symptom and recognized neurological or medical conditions.
C. The symptom or deficit is not better explained by another medical or mental disorder.
D. The symptom or deficit causes clinically significant distress or impairment in social, occupational, or other important areas of functioning or warrants medical evaluation.

Coding note: The ICD-9-CM code for conversion disorder is **300.11,** which is assigned regardless of the symptom type. The ICD-10-CM code depends on the symptom type (see below).

Specify symptom type:

　(F44.4) With weakness or paralysis
　(F44.4) With abnormal movement (e.g., tremor, dystonic movement, myoclonus, gait disorder)
　(F44.4) With swallowing symptoms
　(F44.4) With speech symptom (e.g., dysphonia, slurred speech)
　(F44.5) With attacks or seizures
　(F44.6) With anesthesia or sensory loss
　(F44.6) With special sensory symptom (e.g., visual, olfactory, or hearing disturbance)
　(F44.7) With mixed symptoms

Specify if:
   Acute episode: Symptoms present for less than 6 months.
   Persistent: Symptoms occurring for 6 months or more.
Specify if:
   With psychological stressor *(specify stressor)*
   Without psychological stressor

Diagnostic Features

Many clinicians use the alternative names of "functional" (referring to abnormal central nervous system functioning) or "psychogenic" (referring to an assumed etiology) to describe the symptoms of conversion disorder (functional neurological symptom disorder). In conversion disorder, there may be one or more symptoms of various types. Motor symptoms include weakness or paralysis; abnormal movements, such as tremor or dystonic movements; gait abnormalities; and abnormal limb posturing. Sensory symptoms include altered, reduced, or absent skin sensation, vision, or hearing. Episodes of abnormal generalized limb shaking with apparent impaired or loss of consciousness may resemble epileptic seizures (also called *psychogenic* or *non-epileptic seizures*). There may be episodes of unresponsiveness resembling syncope or coma. Other symptoms include reduced or absent speech volume (dysphonia/aphonia), altered articulation (dysarthria), a sensation of a lump in the throat (globus), and diplopia.

Although the diagnosis requires that the symptom is not explained by neurological disease, it should not be made simply because results from investigations are normal or because the symptom is "bizarre." There must be clinical findings that show clear evidence of incompatibility with neurological disease. Internal inconsistency at examination is one way to demonstrate incompatibility (i.e., demonstrating that physical signs elicited through one examination method are no longer positive when tested a different way). Examples of such examination findings include

- Hoover's sign, in which weakness of hip extension returns to normal strength with contralateral hip flexion against resistance.
- Marked weakness of ankle plantar-flexion when tested on the bed in an individual who is able to walk on tiptoes;
- Positive findings on the tremor entrainment test. On this test, a unilateral tremor may be identified as functional if the tremor changes when the individual is distracted away from it. This may be observed if the individual is asked to copy the examiner in making a rhythmical movement with their unaffected hand and this causes the functional tremor to change such that it copies or "entrains" to the rhythm of the unaffected hand or the functional tremor is suppressed, or no longer makes a simple rhythmical movement.
- In attacks resembling epilepsy or syncope ("psychogenic" non-epileptic attacks), the occurrence of closed eyes with resistance to opening or a normal simultaneous electroencephalogram (although this alone does not exclude all forms of epilepsy or syncope).
- For visual symptoms, a tubular visual field (i.e., tunnel vision).

It is important to note that the diagnosis of conversion disorder should be based on the overall clinical picture and not on a single clinical finding.

Associated Features Supporting Diagnosis

A number of associated features can support the diagnosis of conversion disorder. There may be a history of multiple similar somatic symptoms. Onset may be associated with stress or trauma, either psychological or physical in nature. The potential etiological relevance of this stress or trauma may be suggested by a close temporal relationship. However, while assessment for stress and trauma is important, the diagnosis should not be withheld if none is found.

Conversion disorder is often associated with dissociative symptoms, such as depersonalization, derealization, and dissociative amnesia, particularly at symptom onset or during attacks.

The diagnosis of conversion disorder does not require the judgment that the symptoms are not intentionally produced (i.e., not feigned), as the definite absence of feigning may not be reliably discerned. The phenomenon of *la belle indifférence* (i.e., lack of concern about the nature or implications of the symptom) has been associated with conversion disorder but it is not specific for conversion disorder and should not be used to make the diagnosis. Similarly the concept of *secondary gain* (i.e., when individuals derive external benefits such as money or release from responsibilities) is also not specific to conversion disorder and particularly in the context of definite evidence for feigning, the diagnoses that should be considered instead would include factitious disorder or malingering (see the section "Differential Diagnosis" for this disorder).

Prevalence

Transient conversion symptoms are common, but the precise prevalence of the disorder is unknown. This is partly because the diagnosis usually requires assessment in secondary care, where it is found in approximately 5% of referrals to neurology clinics. The incidence of individual persistent conversion symptoms is estimated to be 2–5/100,000 per year.

Development and Course

Onset has been reported throughout the life course. The onset of non-epileptic attacks peaks in the third decade, and motor symptoms have their peak onset in the fourth decade. The symptoms can be transient or persistent. The prognosis may be better in younger children than in adolescents and adults.

Risk and Prognostic Factors

Temperamental.   Maladaptive personality traits are commonly associated with conversion disorder.

Environmental.   There may be a history of childhood abuse and neglect. Stressful life events are often, but not always, present.

Genetic and physiological.   The presence of neurological disease that causes similar symptoms is a risk factor (e.g., non-epileptic seizures are more common in patients who also have epilepsy).

Course modifiers.   Short duration of symptoms and acceptance of the diagnosis are positive prognostic factors. Maladaptive personality traits, the presence of comorbid physical disease, and the receipt of disability benefits may be negative prognostic factors.

Culture-Related Diagnostic Issues

Changes resembling conversion (and dissociative) symptoms are common in certain culturally sanctioned rituals. If the symptoms are fully explained within the particular cultural context and do not result in clinically significant distress or disability, then the diagnosis of conversion disorder is not made.

Gender-Related Diagnostic Issues

Conversion disorder is two to three times more common in females.

Functional Consequences of Conversion Disorder

Individuals with conversion symptoms may have substantial disability. The severity of disability can be similar to that experienced by individuals with comparable medical diseases.

Differential Diagnosis

If another mental disorder better explains the symptoms, that diagnosis should be made. However the diagnosis of conversion disorder may be made in the presence of another mental disorder.

Neurological disease. The main differential diagnosis is neurological disease that might better explain the symptoms. After a thorough neurological assessment, an unexpected neurological disease cause for the symptoms is rarely found at follow up. However, reassessment may be required if the symptoms appear to be progressive. Conversion disorder may coexist with neurological disease.

Somatic symptom disorder. Conversion disorder may be diagnosed in addition to somatic symptom disorder. Most of the somatic symptoms encountered in somatic symptom disorder cannot be demonstrated to be clearly incompatible with pathophysiology (e.g., pain, fatigue), whereas in conversion disorder, such incompatibility is required for the diagnosis. The excessive thoughts, feelings, and behaviors characterizing somatic symptom disorder are often absent in conversion disorder.

Factitious disorder and malingering. The diagnosis of conversion disorder does not require the judgment that the symptoms are *not* intentionally produced (i.e., not feigned), because assessment of conscious intention is unreliable. However definite evidence of feigning (e.g., clear evidence that loss of function is present during the examination but not at home) would suggest a diagnosis of factitious disorder if the individual's apparent aim is to assume the sick role or malingering if the aim is to obtain an incentive such as money.

Dissociative disorders. Dissociative symptoms are common in individuals with conversion disorder. If both conversion disorder and a dissociative disorder are present, both diagnoses should be made.

Body dysmorphic disorder. Individuals with body dysmorphic disorder are excessively concerned about a perceived defect in their physical features but do not complain of symptoms of sensory or motor functioning in the affected body part.

Depressive disorders. In depressive disorders, individuals may report general heaviness of their limbs, whereas the weakness of conversion disorder is more focal and prominent. Depressive disorders are also differentiated by the presence of core depressive symptoms.

Panic disorder. Episodic neurological symptoms (e.g., tremors and paresthesias) can occur in both conversion disorder and panic attacks. In panic attacks, the neurological symptoms are typically transient and acutely episodic with characteristic cardiorespiratory symptoms. Loss of awareness with amnesia for the attack and violent limb movements occur in non-epileptic attacks, but not in panic attacks.

Comorbidity

Anxiety disorders, especially panic disorder, and depressive disorders commonly co-occur with conversion disorder. Somatic symptom disorder may co-occur as well. Psychosis, substance use disorder, and alcohol misuse are uncommon. Personality disorders are more common in individuals with conversion disorder than in the general population. Neurological or other medical conditions commonly coexist with conversion disorder as well.

Psychological Factors Affecting Other Medical Conditions

Diagnostic Criteria   **316 (F54)**

A. A medical symptom or condition (other than a mental disorder) is present.

B. Psychological or behavioral factors adversely affect the medical condition in one of the following ways:

   1. The factors have influenced the course of the medical condition as shown by a close temporal association between the psychological factors and the development or exacerbation of, or delayed recovery from, the medical condition.

   2. The factors interfere with the treatment of the medical condition (e.g., poor adherence).

   3. The factors constitute additional well-established health risks for the individual.

   4. The factors influence the underlying pathophysiology, precipitating or exacerbating symptoms or necessitating medical attention.

C. The psychological and behavioral factors in Criterion B are not better explained by another mental disorder (e.g., panic disorder, major depressive disorder, posttraumatic stress disorder).

Specify current severity:

   Mild: Increases medical risk (e.g., inconsistent adherence with antihypertension treatment).

   Moderate: Aggravates underlying medical condition (e.g., anxiety aggravating asthma).

   Severe: Results in medical hospitalization or emergency room visit.

   Extreme: Results in severe, life-threatening risk (e.g., ignoring heart attack symptoms).

Diagnostic Features

The essential feature of psychological factors affecting other medical conditions is the presence of one or more clinically significant psychological or behavioral factors that adversely affect a medical condition by increasing the risk for suffering, death, or disability (Criterion B). These factors can adversely affect the medical condition by influencing its course or treatment, by constituting an additional well-established health risk factor, or by influencing the underlying pathophysiology to precipitate or exacerbate symptoms or to necessitate medical attention.

Psychological or behavioral factors include psychological distress, patterns of interpersonal interaction, coping styles, and maladaptive health behaviors, such as denial of symptoms or poor adherence to medical recommendations. Common clinical examples are anxiety-exacerbating asthma, denial of need for treatment for acute chest pain, and manipulation of insulin by an individual with diabetes wishing to lose weight. Many different psychological factors have been demonstrated to adversely influence medical conditions—for example, symptoms of depression or anxiety, stressful life events, relationship style, personality traits, and coping styles. The adverse effects can range from acute, with immediate medical consequences (e.g., Takotsubo cardiomyopathy) to chronic, occurring over a long period of time (e.g., chronic occupational stress increasing risk for hypertension). Affected medical conditions can be those with clear pathophysiology (e.g., diabetes, cancer, coronary disease), functional syndromes (e.g., migraine, irritable bowel syndrome, fibromyalgia), or idiopathic medical symptoms (e.g., pain, fatigue, dizziness).

This diagnosis should be reserved for situations in which the effect of the psychological factor on the medical condition is evident and the psychological factor has clinically significant effects on the course or outcome of the medical condition. Abnormal psychological or behavioral symptoms that develop in response to a medical condition are more properly coded as an adjustment disorder (a clinically significant psychological response to an identifiable stressor). There must be reasonable evidence to suggest an association between the psychological factors and the medical condition, although it may often not be possible to demonstrate direct causality or the mechanisms underlying the relationship.

Prevalence

The prevalence of psychological factors affecting other medical conditions is unclear. In U.S. private insurance billing data, it is a more common diagnosis than somatic symptom disorders.

Development and Course

Psychological factors affecting other medical conditions can occur across the lifespan. Particularly with young children, corroborative history from parents or school can assist the diagnostic evaluation. Some conditions are characteristic of particular life stages (e.g., in older individuals, the stress associated with acting as a caregiver for an ill spouse or partner).

Culture-Related Diagnostic Issues

Many differences between cultures may influence psychological factors and their effects on medical conditions, such as those in language and communication style, explanatory models of illness, patterns of seeking health care, service availability and organization, doctor-patient relationships and other healing practices, family and gender roles, and attitudes toward pain and death. Psychological factors affecting other medical conditions must be differentiated from culturally specific behaviors such as using faith or spiritual healers or other variations in illness management that are acceptable within a culture and represent an attempt to help the medical condition rather than interfere with it. These local practices may complement rather than obstruct evidence-based interventions. If they do not adversely affect outcomes, they should not be pathologized as psychological factors affecting other medical conditions.

Functional Consequences of Psychological Factors Affecting Other Medical Conditions

Psychological and behavioral factors have been demonstrated to affect the course of many medical diseases.

Differential Diagnosis

Mental disorder due to another medical condition. A temporal association between symptoms of a mental disorder and those of a medical condition is also characteristic of a mental disorder due to another medical condition, but the presumed causality is in the opposite direction. In a mental disorder due to another medical condition, the medical condition is judged to be causing the mental disorder through a direct physiological mechanism. In psychological factors affecting other medical conditions, the psychological or behavioral factors are judged to affect the course of the medical condition.

Adjustment disorders. Abnormal psychological or behavioral symptoms that develop in response to a medical condition are more properly coded as an adjustment disorder (a clinically significant psychological response to an identifiable stressor). For example, an individual with angina that is precipitated whenever he becomes enraged would be diagnosed as having psychological factors affecting other medical conditions, whereas an individual with angina who developed maladaptive anticipatory anxiety would be diagnosed as having an adjustment disorder with anxiety. In clinical practice, however, psychological factors and a medical condition are often mutually exacerbating (e.g., anxiety as both a precipitant and a consequence of angina), in which case the distinction is arbitrary. Other mental disorders frequently result in medical complications, most notably substance use disorders (e.g., alcohol use disorder, tobacco use disorder). If an individual has a coexisting major mental disorder that adversely affects or causes another medical condition, diagnoses of the mental disorder and the medical condition are usually sufficient. Psychological factors affecting other medical conditions is diagnosed when the psychological traits or behaviors do not meet criteria for a mental diagnosis.

Somatic symptom disorder.   Somatic symptom disorder is characterized by a combination of distressing somatic symptoms and excessive or maladaptive thoughts, feelings, and behavior in response to these symptoms or associated health concerns. The individual may or may not have a diagnosable medical condition. In contrast, in psychological factors affecting other medical conditions, the psychological factors adversely affect a medical condition; the individual's thoughts, feelings, and behavior are not necessarily excessive. The difference is one of emphasis, rather than a clear-cut distinction. In psychological factors affecting other medical conditions, the emphasis is on the exacerbation of the medical condition (e.g., an individual with angina that is precipitated whenever he becomes anxious). In somatic symptom disorder, the emphasis is on maladaptive thoughts, feelings, and behavior (e.g., an individual with angina who worries constantly that she will have a heart attack, takes her blood pressure multiple times per day, and restricts her activities).

Illness anxiety disorder.   Illness anxiety disorder is characterized by high illness anxiety that is distressing and/or disruptive to daily life with minimal somatic symptoms. The focus of clinical concern is the individual's worry about having a disease; in most cases, no serious disease is present. In psychological factors affecting other medical conditions, anxiety may be a relevant psychological factor affecting a medical condition, but the clinical concern is the adverse effects on the medical condition.

Comorbidity

By definition, the diagnosis of psychological factors affecting other medical conditions entails a relevant psychological or behavioral syndrome or trait and a comorbid medical condition.

Factitious Disorder

Diagnostic Criteria   **300.19 (F68.10)**

Factitious Disorder Imposed on Self

A. Falsification of physical or psychological signs or symptoms, or induction of injury or disease, associated with identified deception.
B. The individual presents himself or herself to others as ill, impaired, or injured.
C. The deceptive behavior is evident even in the absence of obvious external rewards.
D. The behavior is not better explained by another mental disorder, such as delusional disorder or another psychotic disorder.

Specify:
  Single episode
  Recurrent episodes (two or more events of falsification of illness and/or induction of injury)

Factitious Disorder Imposed on Another (Previously Factitious Disorder by Proxy)

A. Falsification of physical or psychological signs or symptoms, or induction of injury or disease, in another, associated with identified deception.

B. The individual presents another individual (victim) to others as ill, impaired, or injured.

C. The deceptive behavior is evident even in the absence of obvious external rewards.

D. The behavior is not better explained by another mental disorder, such as delusional disorder or another psychotic disorder.

Note: The perpetrator, not the victim, receives this diagnosis.

Specify:

Single episode

Recurrent episodes (two or more events of falsification of illness and/or induction of injury)

Recording Procedures

When an individual falsifies illness in another (e.g., children, adults, pets), the diagnosis is factitious disorder imposed on another. The perpetrator, not the victim, is given the diagnosis. The victim may be given an abuse diagnosis (e.g., 995.54 [T74.12X]; see the chapter "Other Conditions That May Be a Focus of Clinical Attention").

Diagnostic Features

The essential feature of factitious disorder is the falsification of medical or psychological signs and symptoms in oneself or others that are associated with the identified deception. Individuals with factitious disorder can also seek treatment for themselves or another following induction of injury or disease. The diagnosis requires demonstrating that the individual is taking surreptitious actions to misrepresent, simulate, or cause signs or symptoms of illness or injury in the absence of obvious external rewards. Methods of illness falsification can include exaggeration, fabrication, simulation, and induction. While a preexisting medical condition may be present, the deceptive behavior or induction of injury associated with deception causes others to view such individuals (or another) as more ill or impaired, and this can lead to excessive clinical intervention. Individuals with factitious disorder might, for example, report feelings of depression and suicidality following the death of a spouse despite the death not being true or the individual's not having a spouse; deceptively report episodes of neurological symptoms (e.g., seizures, dizziness, or blacking out); manipulate a laboratory test (e.g., by adding blood to urine) to falsely indicate an abnormality; falsify medical records to indicate an illness; ingest a substance (e.g., insulin or warfarin) to induce an abnormal laboratory result or illness; or physically injure themselves or induce illness in themselves or another (e.g., by injecting fecal material to produce an abscess or to induce sepsis).

Associated Features Supporting Diagnosis

Individuals with factitious disorder imposed on self or factitious disorder imposed on another are at risk for experiencing great psychological distress or functional impairment by causing harm to themselves and others. Family, friends, and health care professionals are also often adversely affected by their behavior. Factitious disorders have similarities to substance use disorders, eating disorders, impulse-control disorders, pedophilic disorder, and some other established disorders related to both the persistence of the behavior and the intentional efforts to conceal the disordered behavior through deception. Whereas some aspects of factitious disorders might represent criminal behavior (e.g., factitious disorder imposed on another, in which the parent's actions represent abuse and maltreatment of a child), such criminal behavior and mental illness are not mutually exclusive. The diagnosis of factitious disorder emphasizes the objective identification of falsification of signs and symptoms of illness, rather than an inference about intent or possible underlying motivation. Moreover, such behaviors, including the induction of injury or disease, are associated with deception.

Prevalence

The prevalence of factitious disorder is unknown, likely because of the role of deception in this population. Among patients in hospital settings, it is estimated that about 1% of individuals have presentations that meet the criteria for factitious disorder.

Development and Course

The course of factitious disorder is usually one of intermittent episodes. Single episodes and episodes that are characterized as persistent and unremitting are both less common. Onset is usually in early adulthood, often after hospitalization for a medical condition or a mental disorder. When imposed on another, the disorder may begin after hospitalization of the individual's child or other dependent. In individuals with recurrent episodes of falsification of signs and symptoms of illness and/or induction of injury, this pattern of successive deceptive contact with medical personnel, including hospitalizations, may become lifelong.

Differential Diagnosis

Caregivers who lie about abuse injuries in dependents solely to protect themselves from liability are not diagnosed with factitious disorder imposed on another because protection from liability is an external reward (Criterion C, the deceptive behavior is evident even in the absence of obvious external rewards). Such caregivers who, upon observation, analysis of medical records, and/or interviews with others, are found to lie more extensively than needed for immediate self-protection are diagnosed with factitious disorder imposed on another.

Somatic symptom disorder.   In somatic symptom disorder, there may be excessive attention and treatment seeking for perceived medical concerns, but there is no evidence that the individual is providing false information or behaving deceptively.

Malingering.   Malingering is differentiated from factitious disorder by the intentional reporting of symptoms for personal gain (e.g., money, time off work). In contrast, the diagnosis of factitious disorder requires the absence of obvious rewards.

Conversion disorder (functional neurological symptom disorder).   Conversion disorder is characterized by neurological symptoms that are inconsistent with neurological pathophysiology. Factitious disorder with neurological symptoms is distinguished from conversion disorder by evidence of deceptive falsification of symptoms.

Borderline personality disorder.   Deliberate physical self-harm in the absence of suicidal intent can also occur in association with other mental disorders such as borderline personality disorder. Factitious disorder requires that the induction of injury occur in association with deception.

Medical condition or mental disorder not associated with intentional symptom falsification.   Presentation of signs and symptoms of illness that do not conform to an identifiable medical condition or mental disorder increases the likelihood of the presence of a factitious disorder. However, the diagnosis of factitious disorder does not exclude the presence of true medical condition or mental disorder, as comorbid illness often occurs in the individual along with factitious disorder. For example, individuals who might manipulate blood sugar levels to produce symptoms may also have diabetes.

Other Specified Somatic Symptom and Related Disorder

300.89 (F45.8)

This category applies to presentations in which symptoms characteristic of a somatic symptom and related disorder that cause clinically significant distress or impairment in social, occupational, or other important areas of functioning predominate but do not meet the full criteria for any of the disorders in the somatic symptom and related disorders diagnostic class.

Examples of presentations that can be specified using the "other specified" designation include the following:

1. **Brief somatic symptom disorder:** Duration of symptoms is less than 6 months.
2. **Brief illness anxiety disorder:** Duration of symptoms is less than 6 months.
3. **Illness anxiety disorder without excessive health-related behaviors:** Criterion D for illness anxiety disorder is not met.
4. **Pseudocyesis:** A false belief of being pregnant that is associated with objective signs and reported symptoms of pregnancy.

Unspecified Somatic Symptom and Related Disorder

300.82 (F45.9)

This category applies to presentations in which symptoms characteristic of a somatic symptom and related disorder that cause clinically significant distress or impairment in social, occupational, or other important areas of functioning predominate but do not meet the full criteria for any of the disorders in the somatic symptom and related disorders diagnostic class. The unspecified somatic symptom and related disorder category should not be used unless there are decidedly unusual situations where there is insufficient information to make a more specific diagnosis.

Feeding and Eating Disorders

Feeding and eating disorders are characterized by a persistent disturbance of eating or eating-related behavior that results in the altered consumption or absorption of food and that significantly impairs physical health or psychosocial functioning. Diagnostic criteria are provided for pica, rumination disorder, avoidant/restrictive food intake disorder, anorexia nervosa, bulimia nervosa, and binge-eating disorder.

The diagnostic criteria for rumination disorder, avoidant/restrictive food intake disorder, anorexia nervosa, bulimia nervosa, and binge-eating disorder result in a classification scheme that is mutually exclusive, so that during a single episode, only one of these diagnoses can be assigned. The rationale for this approach is that, despite a number of common psychological and behavioral features, the disorders differ substantially in clinical course, outcome, and treatment needs. A diagnosis of pica, however, may be assigned in the presence of any other feeding and eating disorder.

Some individuals with disorders described in this chapter report eating-related symptoms resembling those typically endorsed by individuals with substance use disorders, such as craving and patterns of compulsive use. This resemblance may reflect the involvement of the same neural systems, including those implicated in regulatory self-control and reward, in both groups of disorders. However, the relative contributions of shared and distinct factors in the development and perpetuation of eating and substance use disorders remain insufficiently understood.

Finally, obesity is not included in DSM-5 as a mental disorder. Obesity (excess body fat) results from the long-term excess of energy intake relative to energy expenditure. A range of genetic, physiological, behavioral, and environmental factors that vary across individuals contributes to the development of obesity; thus, obesity is not considered a mental disorder. However, there are robust associations between obesity and a number of mental disorders (e.g., binge-eating disorder, depressive and bipolar disorders, schizophrenia). The side effects of some psychotropic medications contribute importantly to the development of obesity, and obesity may be a risk factor for the development of some mental disorders (e.g., depressive disorders).

Pica

Diagnostic Criteria

A. Persistent eating of nonnutritive, nonfood substances over a period of at least 1 month.
B. The eating of nonnutritive, nonfood substances is inappropriate to the developmental level of the individual.
C. The eating behavior is not part of a culturally supported or socially normative practice.
D. If the eating behavior occurs in the context of another mental disorder (e.g., intellectual disability [intellectual developmental disorder], autism spectrum disorder, schizophrenia) or medical condition (including pregnancy), it is sufficiently severe to warrant additional clinical attention.

Coding note: The ICD-9-CM code for pica is **307.52** and is used for children or adults. The ICD-10-CM codes for pica are **(F98.3)** in children and **(F50.89)** in adults.
Specify if:
   In remission: After full criteria for pica were previously met, the criteria have not been met for a sustained period of time.

Diagnostic Features

The essential feature of pica is the eating of one or more nonnutritive, nonfood substances on a persistent basis over a period of at least 1 month (Criterion A) that is severe enough to warrant clinical attention. Typical substances ingested tend to vary with age and availability and might include paper, soap, cloth, hair, string, wool, soil, chalk, talcum powder, paint, gum, metal, pebbles, charcoal or coal, ash, clay, starch, or ice. The term *nonfood* is included because the diagnosis of pica does not apply to ingestion of diet products that have minimal nutritional content. There is typically no aversion to food in general. The eating of nonnutritive, nonfood substances must be developmentally inappropriate (Criterion B) and not part of a culturally supported or socially normative practice (Criterion C). A minimum age of 2 years is suggested for a pica diagnosis to exclude developmentally normal mouthing of objects by infants that results in ingestion. The eating of nonnutritive, nonfood substances can be an associated feature of other mental disorders (e.g., intellectual disability [intellectual developmental disorder], autism spectrum disorder, schizophrenia). If the eating behavior occurs exclusively in the context of another mental disorder, a separate diagnosis of pica should be made only if the eating behavior is sufficiently severe to warrant additional clinical attention (Criterion D).

Associated Features Supporting Diagnosis

Although deficiencies in vitamins or minerals (e.g., zinc, iron) have been reported in some instances, often no specific biological abnormalities are found. In some cases, pica comes to clinical attention only following general medical complications (e.g., mechanical bowel problems; intestinal obstruction, such as that resulting from a bezoar; intestinal perforation; infections such as toxoplasmosis and toxocariasis as a result of ingesting feces or dirt; poisoning, such as by ingestion of lead-based paint).

Prevalence

The prevalence of pica is unclear. Among individuals with intellectual disability, the prevalence of pica appears to increase with the severity of the condition.

Development and Course

Onset of pica can occur in childhood, adolescence, or adulthood, although childhood onset is most commonly reported. Pica can occur in otherwise normally developing children, whereas in adults, it appears more likely to occur in the context of intellectual disability or other mental disorders. The eating of nonnutritive, nonfood substances may also manifest in pregnancy, when specific cravings (e.g., chalk or ice) might occur. The diagnosis of pica during pregnancy is only appropriate if such cravings lead to the ingestion of nonnutritive, nonfood substances to the extent that the eating of these substances poses potential medical risks. The course of the disorder can be protracted and can result in medical emergencies (e.g., intestinal obstruction, acute weight loss, poisoning). The disorder can potentially be fatal depending on substances ingested.

Risk and Prognostic Factors

Environmental.   Neglect, lack of supervision, and developmental delay can increase the risk for this condition.

Culture-Related Diagnostic Issues

In some populations, the eating of earth or other seemingly nonnutritive substances is believed to be of spiritual, medicinal, or other social value, or may be a culturally supported or socially normative practice. Such behavior does not warrant a diagnosis of pica (Criterion C).

Gender-Related Diagnostic Issues

Pica occurs in both males and females. It can occur in females during pregnancy; however, little is known about the course of pica in the postpartum period.

Diagnostic Markers

Abdominal flat plate radiography, ultrasound, and other scanning methods may reveal obstructions related to pica. Blood tests and other laboratory tests can be used to ascertain levels of poisoning or the nature of infection.

Functional Consequences of Pica

Pica can significantly impair physical functioning, but it is rarely the sole cause of impairment in social functioning. Pica often occurs with other disorders associated with impaired social functioning.

Differential Diagnosis

Eating of nonnutritive, nonfood substances may occur during the course of other mental disorders (e.g., autism spectrum disorder, schizophrenia) and in Kleine-Levin syndrome. In any such instance, an additional diagnosis of pica should be given only if the eating behavior is sufficiently persistent and severe to warrant additional clinical attention.

Anorexia nervosa.   Pica can usually be distinguished from the other feeding and eating disorders by the consumption of nonnutritive, nonfood substances. It is important to note, however, that some presentations of anorexia nervosa include ingestion of nonnutritive, nonfood substances, such as paper tissues, as a means of attempting to control appetite. In such cases, when the eating of nonnutritive, nonfood substances is primarily used as a means of weight control, anorexia nervosa should be the primary diagnosis.

Factitious disorder.   Some individuals with factitious disorder may intentionally ingest foreign objects as part of the pattern of falsification of physical symptoms. In such instances, there is an element of deception that is consistent with deliberate induction of injury or disease.

Nonsuicidal self-injury and nonsuicidal self-injury behaviors in personality disorders.
Some individuals may swallow potentially harmful items (e.g., pins, needles, knives) in the context of maladaptive behavior patterns associated with personality disorders or nonsuicidal self-injury.

Comorbidity

Disorders most commonly comorbid with pica are autism spectrum disorder and intellectual disability (intellectual developmental disorder), and, to a lesser degree, schizophrenia and obsessive-compulsive disorder. Pica can be associated with trichotillomania (hair-pulling disorder) and excoriation (skin-picking) disorder. In comorbid presentations, the hair or skin is typically ingested. Pica can also be associated with avoidant/restrictive food intake disorder, particularly in individuals with a strong sensory component to their presentation. When an individual is known to have pica, assessment should include consideration of the possibility of gastrointestinal complications, poisoning, infection, and nutritional deficiency.

Rumination Disorder

Diagnostic Criteria   **307.53 (F98.21)**

A. Repeated regurgitation of food over a period of at least 1 month. Regurgitated food may be re-chewed, re-swallowed, or spit out.

B. The repeated regurgitation is not attributable to an associated gastrointestinal or other medical condition (e.g., gastroesophageal reflux, pyloric stenosis).

C. The eating disturbance does not occur exclusively during the course of anorexia nervosa, bulimia nervosa, binge-eating disorder, or avoidant/restrictive food intake disorder.

D. If the symptoms occur in the context of another mental disorder (e.g., intellectual disability [intellectual developmental disorder] or another neurodevelopmental disorder), they are sufficiently severe to warrant additional clinical attention.

Specify if:

In remission: After full criteria for rumination disorder were previously met, the criteria have not been met for a sustained period of time.

Diagnostic Features

The essential feature of rumination disorder is the repeated regurgitation of food occurring after feeding or eating over a period of at least 1 month (Criterion A). Previously swallowed food that may be partially digested is brought up into the mouth without apparent nausea, involuntary retching, or disgust. The food may be re-chewed and then ejected from the mouth or re-swallowed. Regurgitation in rumination disorder should be frequent, occurring at least several times per week, typically daily. The behavior is not better explained by an associated gastrointestinal or other medical condition (e.g., gastroesophageal reflux, pyloric stenosis) (Criterion B) and does not occur exclusively during the course of anorexia nervosa, bulimia nervosa, binge-eating disorder, or avoidant/restrictive food intake disorder (Criterion C). If the symptoms occur in the context of another mental disorder (e.g., intellectual disability [intellectual developmental disorder], neurodevelopmental disorder), they must be sufficiently severe to warrant additional clinical attention (Criterion D) and should represent a primary aspect of the individual's presentation requiring intervention. The disorder may be diagnosed across the life span, particularly in individuals who also have intellectual disability. Many individuals with rumination disorder can be directly observed engaging in the behavior by the clinician. In other instances diagnosis can be made on the basis of self-report or corroborative information from parents or caregivers. Individuals may describe the behavior as habitual or outside of their control.

Associated Features Supporting Diagnosis

Infants with rumination disorder display a characteristic position of straining and arching the back with the head held back, making sucking movements with their tongue. They may give the impression of gaining satisfaction from the activity. They may be irritable and hungry between episodes of regurgitation. Weight loss and failure to make expected weight gains are common features in infants with rumination disorder. Malnutrition may occur despite the infant's apparent hunger and the ingestion of relatively large amounts of food, particularly in severe cases, when regurgitation immediately follows each feeding episode and regurgitated food is expelled. Malnutrition might also occur in older children and adults, particularly when the regurgitation is accompanied by restriction of intake. Adolescents and adults may attempt to disguise the regurgitation behavior by placing a hand over the mouth or coughing. Some will avoid eating with others because of the ac-knowledged social undesirability of the behavior. This may extend to an avoidance of eat-ing prior to social situations, such as work or school (e.g., avoiding breakfast because it may be followed by regurgitation).

Prevalence

Prevalence data for rumination disorder are inconclusive, but the disorder is commonly reported to be higher in certain groups, such as individuals with intellectual disability.

Development and Course

Onset of rumination disorder can occur in infancy, childhood, adolescence, or adulthood. The age at onset in infants is usually between ages 3 and 12 months. In infants, the disorder frequently remits spontaneously, but its course can be protracted and can result in medical emergencies (e.g., severe malnutrition). It can potentially be fatal, particularly in infancy. Rumination disorder can have an episodic course or occur continuously until treated. In infants, as well as in older individuals with intellectual disability (intellectual developmen-tal disorder) or other neurodevelopmental disorders, the regurgitation and rumination be-havior appears to have a self-soothing or self-stimulating function, similar to that of other repetitive motor behaviors such as head banging.

Risk and Prognostic Factors

Environmental.   Psychosocial problems such as lack of stimulation, neglect, stressful life situations, and problems in the parent-child relationship may be predisposing factors in infants and young children.

Functional Consequences of Rumination Disorder

Malnutrition secondary to repeated regurgitation may be associated with growth delay and have a negative effect on development and learning potential. Some older individuals with rumination disorder deliberately restrict their food intake because of the social un-desirability of regurgitation. They may therefore present with weight loss or low weight. In older children, adolescents, and adults, social functioning is more likely to be adversely affected.

Differential Diagnosis

Gastrointestinal conditions.   It is important to differentiate regurgitation in rumination disorder from other conditions characterized by gastroesophageal reflux or vomiting. Con-ditions such as gastroparesis, pyloric stenosis, hiatal hernia, and Sandifer syndrome in in-fants should be ruled out by appropriate physical examinations and laboratory tests.

Anorexia nervosa and bulimia nervosa.   Individuals with anorexia nervosa and bulimia nervosa may also engage in regurgitation with subsequent spitting out of food as a means of disposing of ingested calories because of concerns about weight gain.

Comorbidity

Regurgitation with associated rumination can occur in the context of a concurrent medical condition or another mental disorder (e.g., generalized anxiety disorder). When the regur-gitation occurs in this context, a diagnosis of rumination disorder is appropriate only when the severity of the disturbance exceeds that routinely associated with such conditions or disorders and warrants additional clinical attention.

Avoidant/Restrictive Food Intake Disorder

Diagnostic Criteria   **307.59** (F50.89)

A. An eating or feeding disturbance (e.g., apparent lack of interest in eating or food; avoidance based on the sensory characteristics of food; concern about aversive consequences of eating) as manifested by persistent failure to meet appropriate nutritional and/or energy needs associated with one (or more) of the following:

   1. Significant weight loss (or failure to achieve expected weight gain or faltering growth in children).
   2. Significant nutritional deficiency.
   3. Dependence on enteral feeding or oral nutritional supplements.
   4. Marked interference with psychosocial functioning.

B. The disturbance is not better explained by lack of available food or by an associated culturally sanctioned practice.

C. The eating disturbance does not occur exclusively during the course of anorexia nervosa or bulimia nervosa, and there is no evidence of a disturbance in the way in which one's body weight or shape is experienced.

D. The eating disturbance is not attributable to a concurrent medical condition or not better explained by another mental disorder. When the eating disturbance occurs in the context of another condition or disorder, the severity of the eating disturbance exceeds that routinely associated with the condition or disorder and warrants additional clinical attention.

Specify if:

   In remission: After full criteria for avoidant/restrictive food intake disorder were previously met, the criteria have not been met for a sustained period of time.

Diagnostic Features

Avoidant/restrictive food intake disorder replaces and extends the DSM-IV diagnosis of feeding disorder of infancy or early childhood. The main diagnostic feature of avoidant/restrictive food intake disorder is avoidance or restriction of food intake (Criterion A) manifested by clinically significant failure to meet requirements for nutrition or insufficient energy intake through oral intake of food. One or more of the following key features must be present: significant weight loss, significant nutritional deficiency (or related health impact), dependence on enteral feeding or oral nutritional supplements, or marked interference with psychosocial functioning. The determination of whether weight loss is significant (Criterion A1) is a clinical judgment; instead of losing weight, children and adolescents who have not completed growth may not maintain weight or height increases along their developmental trajectory.

Determination of significant nutritional deficiency (Criterion A2) is also based on clinical assessment (e.g., assessment of dietary intake, physical examination, and laboratory testing), and related impact on physical health can be of a similar severity to that seen in anorexia nervosa (e.g., hypothermia, bradycardia, anemia). In severe cases, particularly in infants, malnutrition can be life threatening. "Dependence" on enteral feeding or oral nutritional supplements (Criterion A3) means that supplementary feeding is required to sustain adequate intake. Examples of individuals requiring supplementary feeding include infants with failure to thrive who require nasogastric tube feeding, children with neurodevelopmental disorders who are dependent on nutritionally complete supplements, and individuals who rely on gastrostomy tube feeding or complete oral nutrition supplements in the absence of an underlying medical condition. Inability to participate in normal social activities, such as eating with others, or to sustain relationships as a result of the disturbance would indicate marked interference with psychosocial functioning (Criterion A4).

Avoidant/restrictive food intake disorder does not include avoidance or restriction of food intake related to lack of availability of food or to cultural practices (e.g., religious fasting or normal dieting) (Criterion B), nor does it include developmentally normal behaviors (e.g., picky eating in toddlers, reduced intake in older adults). The disturbance is not better explained by excessive concern about body weight or shape (Criterion C) or by concurrent medical factors or mental disorders (Criterion D).

In some individuals, food avoidance or restriction may be based on the sensory characteristics of qualities of food, such as extreme sensitivity to appearance, color, smell, texture, temperature, or taste. Such behavior has been described as "restrictive eating," "selective eating," "choosy eating," "perseverant eating," "chronic food refusal," and "food neophobia" and may manifest as refusal to eat particular brands of foods or to tolerate the smell of food being eaten by others. Individuals with heightened sensory sensitivities associated with autism may show similar behaviors.

Food avoidance or restriction may also represent a conditioned negative response associated with food intake following, or in anticipation of, an aversive experience, such as choking; a traumatic investigation, usually involving the gastrointestinal tract (e.g., esophagoscopy); or repeated vomiting. The terms *functional dysphagia* and *globus hystericus* have also been used for such conditions.

Associated Features Supporting Diagnosis

Several features may be associated with food avoidance or reduced food intake, including a lack of interest in eating or food, leading to weight loss or faltering growth. Very young infants may present as being too sleepy, distressed, or agitated to feed. Infants and young children may not engage with the primary caregiver during feeding or communicate hunger in favor of other activities. In older children and adolescents, food avoidance or restriction may be associated with more generalized emotional difficulties that do not meet diagnostic criteria for an anxiety, depressive, or bipolar disorder, sometimes called "food avoidance emotional disorder."

Development and Course

Food avoidance or restriction associated with insufficient intake or lack of interest in eating most commonly develops in infancy or early childhood and may persist in adulthood. Likewise, avoidance based on sensory characteristics of food tends to arise in the first decade of life but may persist into adulthood. Avoidance related to aversive consequences can arise at any age. The scant literature regarding long-term outcomes suggests that food avoidance or restriction based on sensory aspects is relatively stable and long-standing, but when persisting into adulthood, such avoidance/restriction can be associated with relatively normal functioning. There is currently insufficient evidence directly linking avoidant/restrictive food intake disorder and subsequent onset of an eating disorder.

Infants with avoidant/restrictive food intake disorder may be irritable and difficult to console during feeding, or may appear apathetic and withdrawn. In some instances, parent-child interaction may contribute to the infant's feeding problem (e.g., presenting food inappropriately, or interpreting the infant's behavior as an act of aggression or rejection). Inadequate nutritional intake may exacerbate the associated features (e.g., irritability, developmental lags) and further contribute to feeding difficulties. Associated factors include infant temperament or developmental impairments that reduce an infant's responsiveness to feeding. Coexisting parental psychopathology, or child abuse or neglect, is suggested if feeding and weight improve in response to changing caregivers. In infants, children, and prepubertal adolescents, avoidant/restrictive food intake disorder may be associated with growth delay, and the resulting malnutrition negatively affects development and learning potential. In older children, adolescents, and adults, social functioning tends to be adversely affected. Regardless of the age, family function may be affected, with heightened stress at mealtimes and in other feeding or eating contexts involving friends and relatives.

Avoidant/restrictive food intake disorder manifests more commonly in children than in adults, and there may be a long delay between onset and clinical presentation. Triggers for presentation vary considerably and include physical, social, and emotional difficulties.

Risk and Prognostic Factors

Temperamental. Anxiety disorders, autism spectrum disorder, obsessive-compulsive disorder, and attention-deficit/hyperactivity disorder may increase risk for avoidant or restrictive feeding or eating behavior characteristic of the disorder.

Environmental. Environmental risk factors for avoidant/restrictive food intake disorder include familial anxiety. Higher rates of feeding disturbances may occur in children of mothers with eating disorders.

Genetic and physiological. History of gastrointestinal conditions, gastroesophageal reflux disease, vomiting, and a range of other medical problems has been associated with feeding and eating behaviors characteristic of avoidant/restrictive food intake disorder.

Culture-Related Diagnostic Issues

Presentations similar to avoidant/restrictive food intake disorder occur in various populations, including in the United States, Canada, Australia, and Europe. Avoidant/restrictive food intake disorder should not be diagnosed when avoidance of food intake is solely related to specific religious or cultural practices.

Gender-Related Diagnostic Issues

Avoidant/restrictive food intake disorder is equally common in males and females in infancy and early childhood, but avoidant/restrictive food intake disorder comorbid with autism spectrum disorder has a male predominance. Food avoidance or restriction related to altered sensory sensitivities can occur in some physiological conditions, most notably pregnancy, but is not usually extreme and does not meet full criteria for the disorder.

Diagnostic Markers

Diagnostic markers include malnutrition, low weight, growth delay, and the need for artificial nutrition in the absence of any clear medical condition other than poor intake.

Functional Consequences of Avoidant/Restrictive Food Intake Disorder

Associated developmental and functional limitations include impairment of physical development and social difficulties that can have a significant negative impact on family function.

Differential Diagnosis

Appetite loss preceding restricted intake is a nonspecific symptom that can accompany a number of mental diagnoses. Avoidant/restrictive food intake disorder can be diagnosed concurrently with the disorders below if all criteria are met, and the eating disturbance requires specific clinical attention.

Other medical conditions (e.g., gastrointestinal disease, food allergies and intolerances, occult malignancies). Restriction of food intake may occur in other medical conditions, especially those with ongoing symptoms such as vomiting, loss of appetite, nausea, abdominal pain, or diarrhea. A diagnosis of avoidant/restrictive food intake disorder requires that the disturbance of intake is beyond that directly accounted for by physical symptoms consistent with a medical condition; the eating disturbance may also persist after being triggered by a medical condition and following resolution of the medical condition.

Underlying medical or comorbid mental conditions may complicate feeding and eating. Because older individuals, postsurgical patients, and individuals receiving chemotherapy often lose their appetite, an additional diagnosis of avoidant/restrictive food intake disorder requires that the eating disturbance is a primary focus for intervention.

Specific neurological/neuromuscular, structural, or congenital disorders and conditions associated with feeding difficulties.   Feeding difficulties are common in a number of congenital and neurological conditions often related to problems with oral/esophageal/pharyngeal structure and function, such as hypotonia of musculature, tongue protrusion, and unsafe swallowing. Avoidant/restrictive food intake disorder can be diagnosed in individuals with such presentations as long as all diagnostic criteria are met.

Reactive attachment disorder.   Some degree of withdrawal is characteristic of reactive attachment disorder and can lead to a disturbance in the caregiver-child relationship that can affect feeding and the child's intake. Avoidant/restrictive food intake disorder should be diagnosed concurrently only if all criteria are met for both disorders and the feeding disturbance is a primary focus for intervention.

Autism spectrum disorder.   Individuals with autism spectrum disorder often present with rigid eating behaviors and heightened sensory sensitivities. However, these features do not always result in the level of impairment that would be required for a diagnosis of avoidant/restrictive food intake disorder. Avoidant/restrictive food intake disorder should be diagnosed concurrently only if all criteria are met for both disorders and when the eating disturbance requires specific treatment.

Specific phobia, social anxiety disorder (social phobia), and other anxiety disorders. Specific phobia, other type, specifies "situations that may lead to choking or vomiting" and can represent the primary trigger for the fear, anxiety, or avoidance required for diagnosis. Distinguishing specific phobia from avoidant/restrictive food intake disorder can be difficult when a fear of choking or vomiting has resulted in food avoidance. Although avoidance or restriction of food intake secondary to a pronounced fear of choking or vomiting can be conceptualized as specific phobia, in situations when the eating problem becomes the primary focus of clinical attention, avoidant/restrictive food intake disorder becomes the appropriate diagnosis. In social anxiety disorder, the individual may present with a fear of being observed by others while eating, which can also occur in avoidant/restrictive food intake disorder.

Anorexia nervosa.   Restriction of energy intake relative to requirements leading to significantly low body weight is a core feature of anorexia nervosa. However, individuals with anorexia nervosa also display a fear of gaining weight or of becoming fat, or persistent behavior that interferes with weight gain, as well as specific disturbances in relation to perception and experience of their own body weight and shape. These features are not present in avoidant/restrictive food intake disorder, and the two disorders should not be diagnosed concurrently. Differential diagnosis between avoidant/restrictive food intake disorder and anorexia nervosa may be difficult, especially in late childhood and early adolescence, because these disorders may share a number of common symptoms (e.g., food avoidance, low weight). Differential diagnosis is also potentially difficult in individuals with anorexia nervosa who deny any fear of fatness but nonetheless engage in persistent behaviors that prevent weight gain and who do not recognize the medical seriousness of their low weight—a presentation sometimes termed "non-fat phobic anorexia nervosa." Full consideration of symptoms, course, and family history is advised, and diagnosis may be best made in the context of a clinical relationship over time. In some individuals, avoidant/restrictive food intake disorder might precede the onset of anorexia nervosa.

Obsessive-compulsive disorder.   Individuals with obsessive-compulsive disorder may present with avoidance or restriction of intake in relation to preoccupations with food or ritualized eating behavior. Avoidant/restrictive food intake disorder should be diagnosed concurrently only if all criteria are met for both disorders and when the aberrant eating is a major aspect of the clinical presentation requiring specific intervention.

Major depressive disorder.   In major depressive disorder, appetite might be affected to such an extent that individuals present with significantly restricted food intake, usually in relation to overall energy intake and often associated with weight loss. Usually appetite loss and related reduction of intake abate with resolution of mood problems. Avoidant/restrictive food intake disorder should only be used concurrently if full criteria are met for both disorders and when the eating disturbance requires specific treatment.

Schizophrenia spectrum disorders.   Individuals with schizophrenia, delusional disorder, or other psychotic disorders may exhibit odd eating behaviors, avoidance of specific foods because of delusional beliefs, or other manifestations of avoidant or restrictive intake. In some cases, delusional beliefs may contribute to a concern about negative consequences of ingesting certain foods. Avoidant/restrictive food intake disorder should be used concurrently only if all criteria are met for both disorders and when the eating disturbance requires specific treatment.

Factitious disorder or factitious disorder imposed on another.   Avoidant/restrictive food intake disorder should be differentiated from factitious disorder or factitious disorder imposed on another. In order to assume the sick role, some individuals with factitious disorder may intentionally describe diets that are much more restrictive than those they are actually able to consume, as well as complications of such behavior, such as a need for enteral feedings or nutritional supplements, an inability to tolerate a normal range of foods, and/or an inability to participate normally in age-appropriate situations involving food. The presentation may be impressively dramatic and engaging, and the symptoms reported inconsistently. In factitious disorder imposed on another, the caregiver describes symptoms consistent with avoidant/restrictive food intake disorder and may induce physical symptoms such as failure to gain weight. As with any diagnosis of factitious disorder imposed on another, the caregiver receives the diagnosis rather than the affected individual, and diagnosis should be made only on the basis of a careful, comprehensive assessment of the affected individual, the caregiver, and their interaction.

Comorbidity

The most commonly observed disorders comorbid with avoidant/restrictive food intake disorder are anxiety disorders, obsessive-compulsive disorder, and neurodevelopmental disorders (specifically autism spectrum disorder, attention-deficit/hyperactivity disorder, and intellectual disability [intellectual developmental disorder]).

Anorexia Nervosa

Diagnostic Criteria

A. Restriction of energy intake relative to requirements, leading to a significantly low body weight in the context of age, sex, developmental trajectory, and physical health. *Significantly low weight* is defined as a weight that is less than minimally normal or, for children and adolescents, less than that minimally expected.

B. Intense fear of gaining weight or of becoming fat, or persistent behavior that interferes with weight gain, even though at a significantly low weight.

C. Disturbance in the way in which one's body weight or shape is experienced, undue influence of body weight or shape on self-evaluation, or persistent lack of recognition of the seriousness of the current low body weight.

Coding note: The ICD-9-CM code for anorexia nervosa is **307.1,** which is assigned regardless of the subtype. The ICD-10-CM code depends on the subtype (see below).

Specify whether:

(F50.01) Restricting type: During the last 3 months, the individual has not engaged in recurrent episodes of binge eating or purging behavior (i.e., self-induced vomiting or the misuse of laxatives, diuretics, or enemas). This subtype describes presentations in which weight loss is accomplished primarily through dieting, fasting, and/or excessive exercise.

(F50.02) Binge-eating/purging type: During the last 3 months, the individual has engaged in recurrent episodes of binge eating or purging behavior (i.e., self-induced vomiting or the misuse of laxatives, diuretics, or enemas).

Specify if:

In partial remission: After full criteria for anorexia nervosa were previously met, Criterion A (low body weight) has not been met for a sustained period, but either Criterion B (intense fear of gaining weight or becoming fat or behavior that interferes with weight gain) or Criterion C (disturbances in self-perception of weight and shape) is still met.

In full remission: After full criteria for anorexia nervosa were previously met, none of the criteria have been met for a sustained period of time.

Specify current severity:

The minimum level of severity is based, for adults, on current body mass index (BMI) (see below) or, for children and adolescents, on BMI percentile. The ranges below are derived from World Health Organization categories for thinness in adults; for children and adolescents, corresponding BMI percentiles should be used. The level of severity may be increased to reflect clinical symptoms, the degree of functional disability, and the need for supervision.

Mild: BMI $\geq$ 17 kg/m^2
Moderate: BMI 16–16.99 kg/m^2
Severe: BMI 15–15.99 kg/m^2
Extreme: BMI < 15 kg/m^2

Subtypes

Most individuals with the binge-eating/purging type of anorexia nervosa who binge eat also purge through self-induced vomiting or the misuse of laxatives, diuretics, or enemas. Some individuals with this subtype of anorexia nervosa do not binge eat but do regularly purge after the consumption of small amounts of food.

Crossover between the subtypes over the course of the disorder is not uncommon; therefore, subtype description should be used to describe current symptoms rather than longitudinal course.

Diagnostic Features

There are three essential features of anorexia nervosa: persistent energy intake restriction; intense fear of gaining weight or of becoming fat, or persistent behavior that interferes with weight gain; and a disturbance in self-perceived weight or shape. The individual maintains a body weight that is below a minimally normal level for age, sex, developmental trajectory, and physical health (Criterion A). Individuals' body weights frequently meet this criterion following a significant weight loss, but among children and adolescents, there may alternatively be failure to make expected weight gain or to maintain a normal developmental trajectory (i.e., while growing in height) instead of weight loss.

Criterion A requires that the individual's weight be significantly low (i.e., less than minimally normal or, for children and adolescents, less than that minimally expected). Weight assessment can be challenging because normal weight range differs among individuals, and different thresholds have been published defining thinness or underweight status. Body mass index (BMI; calculated as weight in kilograms/height in meters^2) is a useful measure to assess body weight for height. For adults, a BMI of 18.5 kg/m^2 has been employed by the Centers for Disease Control and Prevention (CDC) and the World Health Organization (WHO) as the lower limit of normal body weight. Therefore, most adults with a BMI greater than or equal to 18.5 kg/m^2 would not be considered to have a significantly low body weight. On the other hand, a BMI of lower than 17.0 kg/m^2 has been considered by the WHO to indicate moderate or severe thinness; therefore, an individual with a BMI less than 17.0 kg/m^2 would likely be considered to have a significantly low weight. An adult with a BMI between 17.0 and 18.5 kg/m^2, or even above 18.5 kg/m^2, might be considered to have a significantly low weight if clinical history or other physiological information supports this judgment.

For children and adolescents, determining a BMI-for-age percentile is useful (see, e.g., the CDC BMI percentile calculator for children and teenagers). As for adults, it is not possible to provide definitive standards for judging whether a child's or an adolescent's weight is significantly low, and variations in developmental trajectories among youth limit the utility of simple numerical guidelines. The CDC has used a BMI-for-age below the 5th percentile as suggesting underweight; however, children and adolescents with a BMI above this benchmark may be judged to be significantly underweight in light of failure to maintain their expected growth trajectory. In summary, in determining whether Criterion A is met, the clinician should consider available numerical guidelines, as well as the individual's body build, weight history, and any physiological disturbances.

Individuals with this disorder typically display an intense fear of gaining weight or of becoming fat (Criterion B). This intense fear of becoming fat is usually not alleviated by weight loss. In fact, concern about weight gain may increase even as weight falls. Younger individuals with anorexia nervosa, as well as some adults, may not recognize or acknowledge a fear of weight gain. In the absence of another explanation for the significantly low weight, clinician inference drawn from collateral history, observational data, physical and laboratory findings, or longitudinal course either indicating a fear of weight gain or supporting persistent behaviors that prevent it may be used to establish Criterion B.

The experience and significance of body weight and shape are distorted in these individuals (Criterion C). Some individuals feel globally overweight. Others realize that they are thin but are still concerned that certain body parts, particularly the abdomen, buttocks, and thighs, are "too fat." They may employ a variety of techniques to evaluate their body size or weight, including frequent weighing, obsessive measuring of body parts, and persistent use of a mirror to check for perceived areas of "fat." The self-esteem of individuals with anorexia nervosa is highly dependent on their perceptions of body shape and weight. Weight loss is often viewed as an impressive achievement and a sign of extraordinary self-discipline, whereas weight gain is perceived as an unacceptable failure of self-control. Although some individuals with this disorder may acknowledge being thin, they often do not recognize the serious medical implications of their malnourished state.

Often, the individual is brought to professional attention by family members after marked weight loss (or failure to make expected weight gains) has occurred. If individuals seek help on their own, it is usually because of distress over the somatic and psychological sequelae of starvation. It is rare for an individual with anorexia nervosa to complain of weight loss per se. In fact, individuals with anorexia nervosa frequently either lack insight into or deny the problem. It is therefore often important to obtain information from family members or other sources to evaluate the history of weight loss and other features of the illness.

Associated Features Supporting Diagnosis

The semi-starvation of anorexia nervosa, and the purging behaviors sometimes associated with it, can result in significant and potentially life-threatening medical conditions. The nutritional compromise associated with this disorder affects most major organ systems and can produce a variety of disturbances. Physiological disturbances, including amenorrhea and vital sign abnormalities, are common. While most of the physiological disturbances associated with malnutrition are reversible with nutritional rehabilitation, some, including loss of bone mineral density, are often not completely reversible. Behaviors such as self-induced vomiting and misuse of laxatives, diuretics, and enemas may cause a number of disturbances that lead to abnormal laboratory findings; however, some individuals with anorexia nervosa exhibit no laboratory abnormalities.

When seriously underweight, many individuals with anorexia nervosa have depressive signs and symptoms such as depressed mood, social withdrawal, irritability, insomnia, and diminished interest in sex. Because these features are also observed in individuals without anorexia nervosa who are significantly undernourished, many of the depressive features may be secondary to the physiological sequelae of semi-starvation, although they may also be sufficiently severe to warrant an additional diagnosis of major depressive disorder.

Obsessive-compulsive features, both related and unrelated to food, are often prominent. Most individuals with anorexia nervosa are preoccupied with thoughts of food. Some collect recipes or hoard food. Observations of behaviors associated with other forms of starvation suggest that obsessions and compulsions related to food may be exacerbated by undernutrition. When individuals with anorexia nervosa exhibit obsessions and compulsions that are not related to food, body shape, or weight, an additional diagnosis of obsessive-compulsive disorder (OCD) may be warranted.

Other features sometimes associated with anorexia nervosa include concerns about eating in public, feelings of ineffectiveness, a strong desire to control one's environment, inflexible thinking, limited social spontaneity, and overly restrained emotional expression. Compared with individuals with anorexia nervosa, restricting type, those with binge-eating/purging type have higher rates of impulsivity and are more likely to abuse alcohol and other drugs.

A subgroup of individuals with anorexia nervosa show excessive levels of physical activity. Increases in physical activity often precede onset of the disorder, and over the course of the disorder increased activity accelerates weight loss. During treatment, excessive activity may be difficult to control, thereby jeopardizing weight recovery.

Individuals with anorexia nervosa may misuse medications, such as by manipulating dosage, in order to achieve weight loss or avoid weight gain. Individuals with diabetes mellitus may omit or reduce insulin doses in order to minimize carbohydrate metabolism.

Prevalence

The 12-month prevalence of anorexia nervosa among young females is approximately 0.4%. Less is known about prevalence among males, but anorexia nervosa is far less common in males than in females, with clinical populations generally reflecting approximately a 10:1 female-to-male ratio.

Development and Course

Anorexia nervosa commonly begins during adolescence or young adulthood. It rarely begins before puberty or after age 40, but cases of both early and late onset have been described. The onset of this disorder is often associated with a stressful life event, such as leaving home for college. The course and outcome of anorexia nervosa are highly variable. Younger individuals may manifest atypical features, including denying "fear of fat." Older individuals more likely have a longer duration of illness, and their clinical presentation may include more signs and symptoms of long-standing disorder. Clinicians should not exclude anorexia nervosa from the differential diagnosis solely on the basis of older age.

Many individuals have a period of changed eating behavior prior to full criteria for the disorder being met. Some individuals with anorexia nervosa recover fully after a single episode, with some exhibiting a fluctuating pattern of weight gain followed by relapse, and others experiencing a chronic course over many years. Hospitalization may be required to restore weight and to address medical complications. Most individuals with anorexia nervosa experience remission within 5 years of presentation. Among individuals admitted to hospitals, overall remission rates may be lower. The crude mortality rate (CMR) for anorexia nervosa is approximately 5% per decade. Death most commonly results from medical complications associated with the disorder itself or from suicide.

Risk and Prognostic Factors

Temperamental.   Individuals who develop anxiety disorders or display obsessional traits in childhood are at increased risk of developing anorexia nervosa.

Environmental.   Historical and cross-cultural variability in the prevalence of anorexia nervosa supports its association with cultures and settings in which thinness is valued. Occupations and avocations that encourage thinness, such as modeling and elite athletics, are also associated with increased risk.

Genetic and physiological.   There is an increased risk of anorexia nervosa and bulimia nervosa among first-degree biological relatives of individuals with the disorder. An increased risk of bipolar and depressive disorders has also been found among first-degree relatives of individuals with anorexia nervosa, particularly relatives of individuals with the binge-eating/purging type. Concordance rates for anorexia nervosa in monozygotic twins are significantly higher than those for dizygotic twins. A range of brain abnormalities has been described in anorexia nervosa using functional imaging technologies (functional magnetic resonance imaging, positron emission tomography). The degree to which these findings reflect changes associated with malnutrition versus primary abnormalities associated with the disorder is unclear.

Culture-Related Diagnostic Issues

Anorexia nervosa occurs across culturally and socially diverse populations, although available evidence suggests cross-cultural variation in its occurrence and presentation. Anorexia nervosa is probably most prevalent in post-industrialized, high-income countries such as in the United States, many European countries, Australia, New Zealand, and Japan, but its incidence in most low- and middle-income countries is uncertain. Whereas the prevalence of anorexia nervosa appears comparatively low among Latinos, African Americans, and Asians in the United States, clinicians should be aware that mental health service utilization among individuals with an eating disorder is significantly lower in these ethnic groups and that the low rates may reflect an ascertainment bias. The presentation of weight concerns among individuals with feeding and eating disorders varies substantially across cultural contexts. The absence of an expressed intense fear of weight gain, sometimes referred to as "fat phobia," appears to be relatively more common in populations in Asia, where the rationale for dietary restriction is commonly related to a more culturally sanctioned complaint such as gastrointestinal discomfort. Within the United States, presentations without a stated intense fear of weight gain may be comparatively more common among Latino groups.

Diagnostic Markers

The following laboratory abnormalities may be observed in anorexia nervosa; their presence may serve to increase diagnostic confidence.

Hematology.   Leukopenia is common, with the loss of all cell types but usually with apparent lymphocytosis. Mild anemia can occur, as well as thrombocytopenia and, rarely, bleeding problems.

Serum chemistry.   Dehydration may be reflected by an elevated blood urea nitrogen level. Hypercholesterolemia is common. Hepatic enzyme levels may be elevated. Hypomagnesemia, hypozincemia, hypophosphatemia, and hyperamylasemia are occasionally observed. Self-induced vomiting may lead to metabolic alkalosis (elevated serum bicarbonate), hypochloremia, and hypokalemia; laxative abuse may cause a mild metabolic acidosis.

Endocrine.   Serum thyroxine (T_4) levels are usually in the low-normal range; triiodothyronine (T_3) levels are decreased, while reverse T_3 levels are elevated. Females have low serum estrogen levels, whereas males have low levels of serum testosterone.

Electrocardiography.   Sinus bradycardia is common, and, rarely, arrhythmias are noted. Significant prolongation of the QTc interval is observed in some individuals.

Bone mass.   Low bone mineral density, with specific areas of osteopenia or osteoporosis, is often seen. The risk of fracture is significantly elevated.

Electroencephalography.   Diffuse abnormalities, reflecting a metabolic encephalopathy, may result from significant fluid and electrolyte disturbances.

Resting energy expenditure.   There is often a significant reduction in resting energy expenditure.

Physical signs and symptoms.   Many of the physical signs and symptoms of anorexia nervosa are attributable to starvation. Amenorrhea is commonly present and appears to be an indicator of physiological dysfunction. If present, amenorrhea is usually a consequence of the weight loss, but in a minority of individuals it may actually precede the weight loss. In prepubertal females, menarche may be delayed. In addition to amenorrhea, there may be complaints of constipation, abdominal pain, cold intolerance, lethargy, and excess energy.

   The most remarkable finding on physical examination is emaciation. Commonly, there is also significant hypotension, hypothermia, and bradycardia. Some individuals develop lanugo, a fine downy body hair. Some develop peripheral edema, especially during weight restoration or upon cessation of laxative and diuretic abuse. Rarely, petechiae or ecchymoses, usually on the extremities, may indicate a bleeding diathesis. Some individuals evidence a yellowing of the skin associated with hypercarotenemia. As may be seen in individuals with bulimia nervosa, individuals with anorexia nervosa who self-induce vomiting may have hypertrophy of the salivary glands, particularly the parotid glands, as well as dental enamel erosion. Some individuals may have scars or calluses on the dorsal surface of the hand from repeated contact with the teeth while inducing vomiting.

Suicide Risk

Suicide risk is elevated in anorexia nervosa, with rates reported as 12 per 100,000 per year. Comprehensive evaluation of individuals with anorexia nervosa should include assessment of suicide-related ideation and behaviors as well as other risk factors for suicide, including a history of suicide attempt(s).

Functional Consequences of Anorexia Nervosa

Individuals with anorexia nervosa may exhibit a range of functional limitations associated with the disorder. While some individuals remain active in social and professional functioning, others demonstrate significant social isolation and/or failure to fulfill academic or career potential.

Differential Diagnosis

Other possible causes of either significantly low body weight or significant weight loss should be considered in the differential diagnosis of anorexia nervosa, especially when the presenting features are atypical (e.g., onset after age 40 years).

Medical conditions (e.g., gastrointestinal disease, hyperthyroidism, occult malignancies, and acquired immunodeficiency syndrome [AIDS]). Serious weight loss may occur in medical conditions, but individuals with these disorders usually do not also manifest a disturbance in the way their body weight or shape is experienced or an intense fear of weight gain or persist in behaviors that interfere with appropriate weight gain. Acute weight loss associated with a medical condition can occasionally be followed by the onset or recurrence of anorexia nervosa, which can initially be masked by the comorbid medical condition. Rarely, anorexia nervosa develops after bariatric surgery for obesity.

Major depressive disorder. In major depressive disorder, severe weight loss may occur, but most individuals with major depressive disorder do not have either a desire for excessive weight loss or an intense fear of gaining weight.

Schizophrenia. Individuals with schizophrenia may exhibit odd eating behavior and occasionally experience significant weight loss, but they rarely show the fear of gaining weight and the body image disturbance required for a diagnosis of anorexia nervosa.

Substance use disorders. Individuals with substance use disorders may experience low weight due to poor nutritional intake but generally do not fear gaining weight and do not manifest body image disturbance. Individuals who abuse substances that reduce appetite (e.g., cocaine, stimulants) and who also endorse fear of weight gain should be carefully evaluated for the possibility of comorbid anorexia nervosa, given that the substance use may represent a persistent behavior that interferes with weight gain (Criterion B).

Social anxiety disorder (social phobia), obsessive-compulsive disorder, and body dysmorphic disorder. Some of the features of anorexia nervosa overlap with the criteria for social phobia, OCD, and body dysmorphic disorder. Specifically, individuals may feel humiliated or embarrassed to be seen eating in public, as in social phobia; may exhibit obsessions and compulsions related to food, as in OCD; or may be preoccupied with an imagined defect in bodily appearance, as in body dysmorphic disorder. If the individual with anorexia nervosa has social fears that are limited to eating behavior alone, the diagnosis of social phobia should not be made, but social fears unrelated to eating behavior (e.g., excessive fear of speaking in public) may warrant an additional diagnosis of social phobia. Similarly, an additional diagnosis of OCD should be considered only if the individual exhibits obsessions and compulsions unrelated to food (e.g., an excessive fear of contamination), and an additional diagnosis of body dysmorphic disorder should be considered only if the distortion is unrelated to body shape and size (e.g., preoccupation that one's nose is too big).

Bulimia nervosa. Individuals with bulimia nervosa exhibit recurrent episodes of binge eating, engage in inappropriate behavior to avoid weight gain (e.g., self-induced vomiting), and are overly concerned with body shape and weight. However, unlike individuals with anorexia nervosa, binge-eating/purging type, individuals with bulimia nervosa maintain body weight at or above a minimally normal level.

Avoidant/restrictive food intake disorder. Individuals with this disorder may exhibit significant weight loss or significant nutritional deficiency, but they do not have a fear of gaining weight or of becoming fat, nor do they have a disturbance in the way they experience their body shape and weight.

Comorbidity

Bipolar, depressive, and anxiety disorders commonly co-occur with anorexia nervosa. Many individuals with anorexia nervosa report the presence of either an anxiety disorder or symptoms prior to onset of their eating disorder. OCD is described in some individuals with anorexia nervosa, especially those with the restricting type. Alcohol use disorder and other substance use disorders may also be comorbid with anorexia nervosa, especially among those with the binge-eating/purging type.

Bulimia Nervosa

Diagnostic Criteria   307.51 (F50.2)

A. Recurrent episodes of binge eating. An episode of binge eating is characterized by both of the following:

  1. Eating, in a discrete period of time (e.g., within any 2-hour period), an amount of food that is definitely larger than what most individuals would eat in a similar period of time under similar circumstances.
  2. A sense of lack of control over eating during the episode (e.g., a feeling that one cannot stop eating or control what or how much one is eating).

B. Recurrent inappropriate compensatory behaviors in order to prevent weight gain, such as self-induced vomiting; misuse of laxatives, diuretics, or other medications; fasting; or excessive exercise.

C. The binge eating and inappropriate compensatory behaviors both occur, on average, at least once a week for 3 months.

D. Self-evaluation is unduly influenced by body shape and weight.

E. The disturbance does not occur exclusively during episodes of anorexia nervosa.

Specify if:

In partial remission: After full criteria for bulimia nervosa were previously met, some, but not all, of the criteria have been met for a sustained period of time.

In full remission: After full criteria for bulimia nervosa were previously met, none of the criteria have been met for a sustained period of time.

Specify current severity:

The minimum level of severity is based on the frequency of inappropriate compensatory behaviors (see below). The level of severity may be increased to reflect other symptoms and the degree of functional disability.

Mild: An average of 1–3 episodes of inappropriate compensatory behaviors per week.

Moderate: An average of 4–7 episodes of inappropriate compensatory behaviors per week.

Severe: An average of 8–13 episodes of inappropriate compensatory behaviors per week.

Extreme: An average of 14 or more episodes of inappropriate compensatory behaviors per week.

Diagnostic Features

There are three essential features of bulimia nervosa: recurrent episodes of binge eating (Criterion A), recurrent inappropriate compensatory behaviors to prevent weight gain (Criterion B), and self-evaluation that is unduly influenced by body shape and weight (Criterion D). To qualify for the diagnosis, the binge eating and inappropriate compensatory behaviors must occur, on average, at least once per week for 3 months (Criterion C).

An "episode of binge eating" is defined as eating, in a discrete period of time, an amount of food that is definitely larger than most individuals would eat in a similar period of time under similar circumstances (Criterion A1). The context in which the eating occurs may affect the clinician's estimation of whether the intake is excessive. For example, a quantity of food that might be regarded as excessive for a typical meal might be considered normal during a celebration or holiday meal. A "discrete period of time" refers to a limited period, usually less than 2 hours. A single episode of binge eating need not be restricted to one setting. For example, an individual may begin a binge in a restaurant and then continue to eat on returning home. Continual snacking on small amounts of food throughout the day would not be considered an eating binge.

An occurrence of excessive food consumption must be accompanied by a sense of lack of control (Criterion A2) to be considered an episode of binge eating. An indicator of loss of control is the inability to refrain from eating or to stop eating once started. Some individuals describe a dissociative quality during, or following, the binge-eating episodes. The impairment in control associated with binge eating may not be absolute; for example, an individual may continue binge eating while the telephone is ringing but will cease if a roommate or spouse unexpectedly enters the room. Some individuals report that their binge-eating episodes are no longer characterized by an acute feeling of loss of control but rather by a more generalized pattern of uncontrolled eating. If individuals report that they have abandoned efforts to control their eating, loss of control should be considered as present. Binge eating can also be planned in some instances.

The type of food consumed during binges varies both across individuals and for a given individual. Binge eating appears to be characterized more by an abnormality in the amount of food consumed than by a craving for a specific nutrient. However, during binges, individuals tend to eat foods they would otherwise avoid.

Individuals with bulimia nervosa are typically ashamed of their eating problems and attempt to conceal their symptoms. Binge eating usually occurs in secrecy or as inconspicuously as possible. The binge eating often continues until the individual is uncomfortably, or even painfully, full. The most common antecedent of binge eating is negative affect. Other triggers include interpersonal stressors; dietary restraint; negative feelings related to body weight, body shape, and food; and boredom. Binge eating may minimize or mitigate factors that precipitated the episode in the short-term, but negative self-evaluation and dysphoria often are the delayed consequences.

Another essential feature of bulimia nervosa is the recurrent use of inappropriate compensatory behaviors to prevent weight gain, collectively referred to as *purge behaviors* or *purging* (Criterion B). Many individuals with bulimia nervosa employ several methods to compensate for binge eating. Vomiting is the most common inappropriate compensatory behavior. The immediate effects of vomiting include relief from physical discomfort and reduction of fear of gaining weight. In some cases, vomiting becomes a goal in itself, and the individual will binge eat in order to vomit or will vomit after eating a small amount of food. Individuals with bulimia nervosa may use a variety of methods to induce vomiting, including the use of fingers or instruments to stimulate the gag reflex. Individuals generally become adept at inducing vomiting and are eventually able to vomit at will. Rarely, individuals consume syrup of ipecac to induce vomiting. Other purging behaviors include the misuse of laxatives and diuretics. A number of other compensatory methods may also be used in rare cases. Individuals with bulimia nervosa may misuse enemas following episodes of binge eating, but this is seldom the sole compensatory method employed. Individuals with this disorder may take thyroid hormone in an attempt to avoid weight gain. Individuals with diabetes mellitus and bulimia nervosa may omit or reduce insulin doses in order to reduce the metabolism of food consumed during eating binges. Individuals with bulimia nervosa may fast for a day or more or exercise excessively in an attempt to prevent weight gain. Exercise may be considered excessive when it significantly interferes with important activities, when it occurs at inappropriate times or in inappropriate settings, or when the individual continues to exercise despite injury or other medical complications.

Individuals with bulimia nervosa place an excessive emphasis on body shape or weight in their self-evaluation, and these factors are typically extremely important in determining self-esteem (Criterion D). Individuals with this disorder may closely resemble those with anorexia nervosa in their fear of gaining weight, in their desire to lose weight, and in the level of dissatisfaction with their bodies. However, a diagnosis of bulimia nervosa should not be given when the disturbance occurs only during episodes of anorexia nervosa (Criterion E).

Associated Features Supporting Diagnosis

Individuals with bulimia nervosa typically are within the normal weight or overweight range (body mass index [BMI] ≥ 18.5 and < 30 in adults). The disorder occurs but is uncommon among obese individuals. Between eating binges, individuals with bulimia nervosa typically restrict their total caloric consumption and preferentially select low-calorie ("diet") foods while avoiding foods that they perceive to be fattening or likely to trigger a binge.

Menstrual irregularity or amenorrhea often occurs among females with bulimia nervosa; it is uncertain whether such disturbances are related to weight fluctuations, to nutritional deficiencies, or to emotional distress. The fluid and electrolyte disturbances resulting from the purging behavior are sometimes sufficiently severe to constitute medically serious problems. Rare but potentially fatal complications include esophageal tears, gastric rupture, and cardiac arrhythmias. Serious cardiac and skeletal myopathies have been reported among individuals following repeated use of syrup of ipecac to induce vomiting. Individuals who chronically abuse laxatives may become dependent on their use to stimulate bowel movements. Gastrointestinal symptoms are commonly associated with bulimia nervosa, and rectal prolapse has also been reported among individuals with this disorder.

Prevalence

Twelve-month prevalence of bulimia nervosa among young females is 1%–1.5%. Point prevalence is highest among young adults since the disorder peaks in older adolescence and young adulthood. Less is known about the point prevalence of bulimia nervosa in males, but bulimia nervosa is far less common in males than it is in females, with an approximately 10:1 female-to-male ratio.

Development and Course

Bulimia nervosa commonly begins in adolescence or young adulthood. Onset before puberty or after age 40 is uncommon. The binge eating frequently begins during or after an episode of dieting to lose weight. Experiencing multiple stressful life events also can precipitate onset of bulimia nervosa.

Disturbed eating behavior persists for at least several years in a high percentage of clinic samples. The course may be chronic or intermittent, with periods of remission alternating with recurrences of binge eating. However, over longer-term follow-up, the symptoms of many individuals appear to diminish with or without treatment, although treatment clearly impacts outcome. Periods of remission longer than 1 year are associated with better long-term outcome.

Significantly elevated risk for mortality (all-cause and suicide) has been reported for individuals with bulimia nervosa. The CMR (crude mortality rate) for bulimia nervosa is nearly 2% per decade.

Diagnostic cross-over from initial bulimia nervosa to anorexia nervosa occurs in a minority of cases (10%–15%). Individuals who do experience cross-over to anorexia nervosa commonly will revert back to bulimia nervosa or have multiple occurrences of cross-overs between these disorders. A subset of individuals with bulimia nervosa continue to binge eat but no longer engage in inappropriate compensatory behaviors, and therefore their symptoms meet criteria for binge-eating disorder or other specified eating disorder. Diagnosis should be based on the current (i.e., past 3 months) clinical presentation.

Risk and Prognostic Factors

Temperamental.   Weight concerns, low self-esteem, depressive symptoms, social anxiety disorder, and overanxious disorder of childhood are associated with increased risk for the development of bulimia nervosa.

Environmental.   Internalization of a thin body ideal has been found to increase risk for developing weight concerns, which in turn increase risk for the development of bulimia nervosa. Individuals who experienced childhood sexual or physical abuse are at increased risk for developing bulimia nervosa.

Genetic and physiological.   Childhood obesity and early pubertal maturation increase risk for bulimia nervosa. Familial transmission of bulimia nervosa may be present, as well as genetic vulnerabilities for the disorder.

Course modifiers.   Severity of psychiatric comorbidity predicts worse long-term outcome of bulimia nervosa.

Culture-Related Diagnostic Issues

Bulimia nervosa has been reported to occur with roughly similar frequencies in most industrialized countries, including the United States, Canada, many European countries, Australia, Japan, New Zealand, and South Africa. In clinical studies of bulimia nervosa in the United States, individuals presenting with this disorder are primarily white. However, the disorder also occurs in other ethnic groups and with prevalence comparable to estimated prevalences observed in white samples.

Gender-Related Diagnostic Issues

Bulimia nervosa is far more common in females than in males. Males are especially underrepresented in treatment-seeking samples, for reasons that have not yet been systematically examined.

Diagnostic Markers

No specific diagnostic test for bulimia nervosa currently exists. However, several laboratory abnormalities may occur as a consequence of purging and may increase diagnostic certainty. These include fluid and electrolyte abnormalities, such as hypokalemia (which can provoke cardiac arrhythmias), hypochloremia, and hyponatremia. The loss of gastric acid through vomiting may produce a metabolic alkalosis (elevated serum bicarbonate), and the frequent induction of diarrhea or dehydration through laxative and diuretic abuse can cause metabolic acidosis. Some individuals with bulimia nervosa exhibit mildly elevated levels of serum amylase, probably reflecting an increase in the salivary isoenzyme.

Physical examination usually yields no physical findings. However, inspection of the mouth may reveal significant and permanent loss of dental enamel, especially from lingual surfaces of the front teeth due to recurrent vomiting. These teeth may become chipped and appear ragged and "moth-eaten." There may also be an increased frequency of dental caries. In some individuals, the salivary glands, particularly the parotid glands, may become notably enlarged. Individuals who induce vomiting by manually stimulating the gag reflex may develop calluses or scars on the dorsal surface of the hand from repeated contact with the teeth. Serious cardiac and skeletal myopathies have been reported among individuals following repeated use of syrup of ipecac to induce vomiting.

Suicide Risk

Suicide risk is elevated in bulimia nervosa. Comprehensive evaluation of individuals with this disorder should include assessment of suicide-related ideation and behaviors as well as other risk factors for suicide, including a history of suicide attempts.

Functional Consequences of Bulimia Nervosa

Individuals with bulimia nervosa may exhibit a range of functional limitations associated with the disorder. A minority of individuals report severe role impairment, with the social-life domain most likely to be adversely affected by bulimia nervosa.

Differential Diagnosis

Anorexia nervosa, binge-eating/purging type.   Individuals whose binge-eating behavior occurs only during episodes of anorexia nervosa are given the diagnosis anorexia nervosa, binge-eating/purging type, and should not be given the additional diagnosis of bulimia nervosa. For individuals with an initial diagnosis of anorexia nervosa who binge and purge but whose presentation no longer meets the full criteria for anorexia nervosa, binge-eating/purging type (e.g., when weight is normal), a diagnosis of bulimia nervosa should be given only when all criteria for bulimia nervosa have been met for at least 3 months.

Binge-eating disorder.   Some individuals binge eat but do not engage in regular inappropriate compensatory behaviors. In these cases, the diagnosis of binge-eating disorder should be considered.

Kleine-Levin syndrome.   In certain neurological or other medical conditions, such as Kleine-Levin syndrome, there is disturbed eating behavior, but the characteristic psychological features of bulimia nervosa, such as overconcern with body shape and weight, are not present.

Major depressive disorder, with atypical features.   Overeating is common in major depressive disorder, with atypical features, but individuals with this disorder do not engage in inappropriate compensatory behaviors and do not exhibit the excessive concern with body shape and weight characteristic of bulimia nervosa. If criteria for both disorders are met, both diagnoses should be given.

Borderline personality disorder.   Binge-eating behavior is included in the impulsive behavior criterion that is part of the definition of borderline personality disorder. If the criteria for both borderline personality disorder and bulimia nervosa are met, both diagnoses should be given.

Comorbidity

Comorbidity with mental disorders is common in individuals with bulimia nervosa, with most experiencing at least one other mental disorder and many experiencing multiple comorbidities. Comorbidity is not limited to any particular subset but rather occurs across a wide range of mental disorders. There is an increased frequency of depressive symptoms (e.g., low self-esteem) and bipolar and depressive disorders (particularly depressive disorders) in individuals with bulimia nervosa. In many individuals, the mood disturbance begins at the same time as or following the development of bulimia nervosa, and individuals often ascribe their mood disturbances to the bulimia nervosa. However, in some individuals, the mood disturbance clearly precedes the development of bulimia nervosa. There may also be an increased frequency of anxiety symptoms (e.g., fear of social situations) or anxiety disorders. These mood and anxiety disturbances frequently remit following effective treatment of the bulimia nervosa. The lifetime prevalence of substance use, particularly alcohol or stimulant use, is at least 30% among individuals with bulimia nervosa. Stimulant use often begins in an attempt to control appetite and weight. A substantial percentage of individuals with bulimia nervosa also have personality features that meet criteria for one or more personality disorders, most frequently borderline personality disorder.

Binge-Eating Disorder

Diagnostic Criteria   **307.51** (F50.81)

A. Recurrent episodes of binge eating. An episode of binge eating is characterized by both of the following:

   1. Eating, in a discrete period of time (e.g., within any 2-hour period), an amount of food that is definitely larger than what most people would eat in a similar period of time under similar circumstances.
   2. A sense of lack of control over eating during the episode (e.g., a feeling that one cannot stop eating or control what or how much one is eating).

B. The binge-eating episodes are associated with three (or more) of the following:

   1. Eating much more rapidly than normal.
   2. Eating until feeling uncomfortably full.
   3. Eating large amounts of food when not feeling physically hungry.
   4. Eating alone because of feeling embarrassed by how much one is eating.
   5. Feeling disgusted with oneself, depressed, or very guilty afterward.

C. Marked distress regarding binge eating is present.

D. The binge eating occurs, on average, at least once a week for 3 months.

E. The binge eating is not associated with the recurrent use of inappropriate compensatory behavior as in bulimia nervosa and does not occur exclusively during the course of bulimia nervosa or anorexia nervosa.

Specify if:

   In partial remission: After full criteria for binge-eating disorder were previously met, binge eating occurs at an average frequency of less than one episode per week for a sustained period of time.

   In full remission: After full criteria for binge-eating disorder were previously met, none of the criteria have been met for a sustained period of time.

Specify current severity:

The minimum level of severity is based on the frequency of episodes of binge eating (see below). The level of severity may be increased to reflect other symptoms and the degree of functional disability.

   Mild: 1–3 binge-eating episodes per week.
   Moderate: 4–7 binge-eating episodes per week.
   Severe: 8–13 binge-eating episodes per week.
   Extreme: 14 or more binge-eating episodes per week.

Diagnostic Features

The essential feature of binge-eating disorder is recurrent episodes of binge eating that must occur, on average, at least once per week for 3 months (Criterion D). An "episode of binge eating" is defined as eating, in a discrete period of time, an amount of food that is definitely larger than most people would eat in a similar period of time under similar circumstances (Criterion A1). The context in which the eating occurs may affect the clinician's estimation of whether the intake is excessive. For example, a quantity of food that might be regarded as excessive for a typical meal might be considered normal during a celebration or holiday meal. A "discrete period of time" refers to a limited period, usually less than 2 hours. A single episode of binge eating need not be restricted to one setting. For example, an individual may begin a binge in a restaurant and then continue to eat on returning home. Continual snacking on small amounts of food throughout the day would not be considered an eating binge.

An occurrence of excessive food consumption must be accompanied by a sense of lack of control (Criterion A2) to be considered an episode of binge eating. An indicator of loss of control is the inability to refrain from eating or to stop eating once started. Some individuals describe a dissociative quality during, or following, the binge-eating episodes. The impairment in control associated with binge eating may not be absolute; for example, an individual may continue binge eating while the telephone is ringing but will cease if a roommate or spouse unexpectedly enters the room. Some individuals report that their binge-eating episodes are no longer characterized by an acute feeling of loss of control but rather by a more generalized pattern of uncontrolled eating. If individuals report that they have abandoned efforts to control their eating, loss of control may still be considered as present. Binge eating can also be planned in some instances.

The type of food consumed during binges varies both across individuals and for a given individual. Binge eating appears to be characterized more by an abnormality in the amount of food consumed than by a craving for a specific nutrient.

Binge eating must be characterized by marked distress (Criterion C) and at least three of the following features: eating much more rapidly than normal; eating until feeling uncomfortably full; eating large amounts of food when not feeling physically hungry; eating alone because of feeling embarrassed by how much one is eating; and feeling disgusted with oneself, depressed, or very guilty afterward (Criterion B).

Individuals with binge-eating disorder are typically ashamed of their eating problems and attempt to conceal their symptoms. Binge eating usually occurs in secrecy or as inconspicuously as possible. The most common antecedent of binge eating is negative affect. Other triggers include interpersonal stressors; dietary restraint; negative feelings related to body weight, body shape, and food; and boredom. Binge eating may minimize or mitigate factors that precipitated the episode in the short-term, but negative self-evaluation and dysphoria often are the delayed consequences.

Associated Features Supporting Diagnosis

Binge-eating disorder occurs in normal-weight/overweight and obese individuals. It is reliably associated with overweight and obesity in treatment-seeking individuals. Nevertheless, binge-eating disorder is distinct from obesity. Most obese individuals do not engage in recurrent binge eating. In addition, compared with weight-matched obese individuals without binge-eating disorder, those with the disorder consume more calories in laboratory studies of eating behavior and have greater functional impairment, lower quality of life, more subjective distress, and greater psychiatric comorbidity.

Prevalence

Twelve-month prevalence of binge-eating disorder among U.S. adult (age 18 or older) females and males is 1.6% and 0.8%, respectively. The gender ratio is far less skewed in binge-eating disorder than in bulimia nervosa. Binge-eating disorder is as prevalent among females from racial or ethnic minority groups as has been reported for white females. The disorder is more prevalent among individuals seeking weight-loss treatment than in the general population.

Development and Course

Little is known about the development of binge-eating disorder. Both binge eating and loss-of-control eating without objectively excessive consumption occur in children and are associated with increased body fat, weight gain, and increases in psychological symptoms. Binge eating is common in adolescent and college-age samples. Loss-of-control eating or episodic binge eating may represent a prodromal phase of eating disorders for some individuals.

Dieting follows the development of binge eating in many individuals with binge-eating disorder. (This is in contrast to bulimia nervosa, in which dysfunctional dieting usually precedes the onset of binge eating.) Binge-eating disorder typically begins in adolescence or young adulthood but can begin in later adulthood. Individuals with binge-eating disorder who seek treatment usually are older than individuals with either bulimia nervosa or anorexia nervosa who seek treatment.

Remission rates in both natural course and treatment outcome studies are higher for binge-eating disorder than for bulimia nervosa or anorexia nervosa. Binge-eating disorder appears to be relatively persistent, and the course is comparable to that of bulimia nervosa in terms of severity and duration. Crossover from binge-eating disorder to other eating disorders is uncommon.

Risk and Prognostic Factors

Genetic and physiological.   Binge-eating disorder appears to run in families, which may reflect additive genetic influences.

Culture-Related Diagnostic Issues

Binge-eating disorder occurs with roughly similar frequencies in most industrialized countries, including the United States, Canada, many European countries, Australia, and New Zealand. In the United States, the prevalence of binge-eating disorder appears comparable among non-Latino whites, Latinos, Asians, and African Americans.

Functional Consequences of Binge-Eating Disorder

Binge-eating disorder is associated with a range of functional consequences, including social role adjustment problems, impaired health-related quality of life and life satisfaction, increased medical morbidity and mortality, and associated increased health care utilization compared with body mass index (BMI)–matched control subjects. It may also be associated with an increased risk for weight gain and the development of obesity.

Differential Diagnosis

Bulimia nervosa.   Binge-eating disorder has recurrent binge eating in common with bulimia nervosa but differs from the latter disorder in some fundamental respects. In terms of clinical presentation, the recurrent inappropriate compensatory behavior (e.g., purging, driven exercise) seen in bulimia nervosa is absent in binge-eating disorder. Unlike individuals with bulimia nervosa, individuals with binge-eating disorder typically do not show marked or sustained dietary restriction designed to influence body weight and shape between binge-eating episodes. They may, however, report frequent attempts at dieting. Binge-eating disorder also differs from bulimia nervosa in terms of response to treatment. Rates of improvement are consistently higher among individuals with binge-eating disorder than among those with bulimia nervosa.

Obesity.   Binge-eating disorder is associated with overweight and obesity but has several key features that are distinct from obesity. First, levels of overvaluation of body weight and shape are higher in obese individuals with the disorder than in those without the disorder. Second, rates of psychiatric comorbidity are significantly higher among obese individuals with the disorder compared with those without the disorder. Third, the long-term successful outcome of evidence-based psychological treatments for binge-eating disorder can be contrasted with the absence of effective long-term treatments for obesity.

Bipolar and depressive disorders.   Increases in appetite and weight gain are included in the criteria for major depressive episode and in the atypical features specifiers for depressive and bipolar disorders. Increased eating in the context of a major depressive episode may or may not be associated with loss of control. If the full criteria for both disorders are met, both diagnoses can be given. Binge eating and other symptoms of disordered eating are seen in association with bipolar disorder. If the full criteria for both disorders are met, both diagnoses should be given.

Borderline personality disorder.   Binge eating is included in the impulsive behavior criterion that is part of the definition of borderline personality disorder. If the full criteria for both disorders are met, both diagnoses should be given.

Comorbidity

Binge-eating disorder is associated with significant psychiatric comorbidity that is comparable to that of bulimia nervosa and anorexia nervosa. The most common comorbid disorders are bipolar disorders, depressive disorders, anxiety disorders, and, to a lesser degree, substance use disorders. The psychiatric comorbidity is linked to the severity of binge eating and not to the degree of obesity.

Other Specified Feeding or Eating Disorder

307.59 (F50.89)

This category applies to presentations in which symptoms characteristic of a feeding and eating disorder that cause clinically significant distress or impairment in social, occupational, or other important areas of functioning predominate but do not meet the full criteria for any of the disorders in the feeding and eating disorders diagnostic class. The other specified feeding or eating disorder category is used in situations in which the clinician chooses to communicate the specific reason that the presentation does not meet the criteria for any specific feeding and eating disorder. This is done by recording "other specified feeding or eating disorder" followed by the specific reason (e.g., "bulimia nervosa of low frequency").

Examples of presentations that can be specified using the "other specified" designation include the following:

1. **Atypical anorexia nervosa:** All of the criteria for anorexia nervosa are met, except that despite significant weight loss, the individual's weight is within or above the normal range.
2. **Bulimia nervosa (of low frequency and/or limited duration):** All of the criteria for bulimia nervosa are met, except that the binge eating and inappropriate compensatory behaviors occur, on average, less than once a week and/or for less than 3 months.
3. **Binge-eating disorder (of low frequency and/or limited duration):** All of the criteria for binge-eating disorder are met, except that the binge eating occurs, on average, less than once a week and/or for less than 3 months.
4. **Purging disorder:** Recurrent purging behavior to influence weight or shape (e.g., self-induced vomiting; misuse of laxatives, diuretics, or other medications) in the absence of binge eating.

5. **Night eating syndrome:** Recurrent episodes of night eating, as manifested by eating after awakening from sleep or by excessive food consumption after the evening meal. There is awareness and recall of the eating. The night eating is not better explained by external influences such as changes in the individual's sleep-wake cycle or by local social norms. The night eating causes significant distress and/or impairment in functioning. The disordered pattern of eating is not better explained by binge-eating disorder or another mental disorder, including substance use, and is not attributable to another medical disorder or to an effect of medication.

Unspecified Feeding or Eating Disorder

307.50 (F50.9)

This category applies to presentations in which symptoms characteristic of a feeding and eating disorder that cause clinically significant distress or impairment in social, occupational, or other important areas of functioning predominate but do not meet the full criteria for any of the disorders in the feeding and eating disorders diagnostic class. The unspecified feeding or eating disorder category is used in situations in which the clinician chooses *not* to specify the reason that the criteria are not met for a specific feeding and eating disorder, and includes presentations in which there is insufficient information to make a more specific diagnosis (e.g., in emergency room settings).

Elimination Disorders

Elimination disorders all involve the inappropriate elimination of urine or feces and are usually first diagnosed in childhood or adolescence. This group of disorders includes *enuresis*, the repeated voiding of urine into inappropriate places, and *encopresis*, the repeated passage of feces into inappropriate places. Subtypes are provided to differentiate nocturnal from diurnal (i.e., during waking hours) voiding for enuresis and the presence or absence of constipation and overflow incontinence for encopresis. Although there are minimum age requirements for diagnosis of both disorders, these are based on developmental age and not solely on chronological age. Both disorders may be voluntary or involuntary. Although these disorders typically occur separately, co-occurrence may also be observed.

Enuresis

Diagnostic Criteria   307.6 (F98.0)

A. Repeated voiding of urine into bed or clothes, whether involuntary or intentional.
B. The behavior is clinically significant as manifested by either a frequency of at least twice a week for at least 3 consecutive months or the presence of clinically significant distress or impairment in social, academic (occupational), or other important areas of functioning.
C. Chronological age is at least 5 years (or equivalent developmental level).
D. The behavior is not attributable to the physiological effects of a substance (e.g., a diuretic, an antipsychotic medication) or another medical condition (e.g., diabetes, spina bifida, a seizure disorder).

Specify whether:
Nocturnal only: Passage of urine only during nighttime sleep.
Diurnal only: Passage of urine during waking hours.
Nocturnal and diurnal: A combination of the two subtypes above.

Subtypes

The nocturnal-only subtype of enuresis, sometimes referred to as *monosymptomatic enuresis*, is the most common subtype and involves incontinence only during nighttime sleep, typically during the first one-third of the night. The diurnal-only subtype occurs in the absence of nocturnal enuresis and may be referred to simply as *urinary incontinence*. Individuals with this subtype can be divided into two groups. Individuals with "urge incontinence" have sudden urge symptoms and detrusor instability, whereas individuals with "voiding postponement" consciously defer micturition urges until incontinence results. The nocturnal-and-diurnal subtype is also known as *nonmonosymptomatic enuresis*.

Diagnostic Features

The essential feature of enuresis is repeated voiding of urine during the day or at night into bed or clothes (Criterion A). Most often the voiding is involuntary, but occasionally it may

355

be intentional. To qualify for a diagnosis of enuresis, the voiding of urine must occur at least twice a week for at least 3 consecutive months or must cause clinically significant distress or impairment in social, academic (occupational), or other important areas of functioning (Criterion B). The individual must have reached an age at which continence is expected (i.e., a chronological age of at least 5 years or, for children with developmental delays, a mental age of at least 5 years) (Criterion C). The urinary incontinence is not attributable to the physiological effects of a substance (e.g., a diuretic, an antipsychotic medication) or another medical condition (e.g., diabetes, spina bifida, a seizure disorder) (Criterion D).

Associated Features Supporting Diagnosis

During nocturnal enuresis, occasionally the voiding takes place during rapid eye movement (REM) sleep, and the child may recall a dream that involved the act of urinating. During daytime (diurnal) enuresis, the child defers voiding until incontinence occurs, sometimes because of a reluctance to use the toilet as a result of social anxiety or a preoccupation with school or play activity. The enuretic event most commonly occurs in the early afternoon on school days and may be associated with symptoms of disruptive behavior. The enuresis commonly persists after appropriate treatment of an associated infection.

Prevalence

The prevalence of enuresis is 5%–10% among 5-year-olds, 3%–5% among 10-year-olds, and around 1% among individuals 15 years or older.

Development and Course

Two types of course of enuresis have been described: a "primary" type, in which the individual has never established urinary continence, and a "secondary" type, in which the disturbance develops after a period of established urinary continence. There are no differences in prevalence of comorbid mental disorders between the two types. By definition, primary enuresis begins at age 5 years. The most common time for the onset of secondary enuresis is between ages 5 and 8 years, but it may occur at any time. After age 5 years, the rate of spontaneous remission is 5%–10% per year. Most children with the disorder become continent by adolescence, but in approximately 1% of cases the disorder continues into adulthood. Diurnal enuresis is uncommon after age 9 years. While occasional diurnal incontinence is not uncommon in middle childhood, it is substantially more common in those who also have persistent nocturnal enuresis. When enuresis persists into late childhood or adolescence, the frequency of incontinence may increase, whereas continence in early childhood is usually associated with a declining frequency of wet nights.

Risk and Prognostic Factors

Environmental.   A number of predisposing factors for enuresis have been suggested, including delayed or lax toilet training and psychosocial stress.

Genetic and physiological.   Enuresis has been associated with delays in the development of normal circadian rhythms of urine production, with resulting nocturnal polyuria or abnormalities of central vasopressin receptor sensitivity, and reduced functional bladder capacities with bladder hyperreactivity (unstable bladder syndrome). Nocturnal enuresis is a genetically heterogeneous disorder. Heritability has been shown in family, twin, and segregation analyses. Risk for childhood nocturnal enuresis is approximately 3.6 times higher in offspring of enuretic mothers and 10.1 times higher in the presence of paternal urinary incontinence. The risk magnitudes for nocturnal enuresis and diurnal incontinence are similar.

Culture-Related Diagnostic Issues

Enuresis has been reported in a variety of European, African, and Asian countries as well as in the United States. At a national level, prevalence rates are remarkably similar, and there is great similarity in the developmental trajectories found in different countries. There are very high rates of enuresis in orphanages and other residential institutions, likely related to the mode and environment in which toilet training occurs.

Gender-Related Diagnostic Issues

Nocturnal enuresis is more common in males. Diurnal incontinence is more common in females. The relative risk of having a child who develops enuresis is greater for previously enuretic fathers than for previously enuretic mothers.

Functional Consequences of Enuresis

The amount of impairment associated with enuresis is a function of the limitation on the child's social activities (e.g., ineligibility for sleep-away camp) or its effect on the child's self-esteem, the degree of social ostracism by peers, and the anger, punishment, and rejection on the part of caregivers.

Differential Diagnosis

Neurogenic bladder or another medical condition.   The diagnosis of enuresis is not made in the presence of a neurogenic bladder or another medical condition that causes polyuria or urgency (e.g., untreated diabetes mellitus or diabetes insipidus) or during an acute urinary tract infection. However, a diagnosis is compatible with such conditions if urinary incontinence was regularly present prior to the development of another medical condition or if it persists after the institution of appropriate treatment of the medical condition.

Medication side effects.   Enuresis may occur during treatment with antipsychotic medications, diuretics, or other medications that may induce incontinence. In this case, the diagnosis should not be made in isolation but may be noted as a medication side effect. However, a diagnosis of enuresis may be made if urinary incontinence was regularly present prior to treatment with the medication.

Comorbidity

Although most children with enuresis do not have a comorbid mental disorder, the prevalence of comorbid behavioral symptoms is higher in children with enuresis than in children without enuresis. Developmental delays, including speech, language, learning, and motor skills delays, are also present in a portion of children with enuresis. Encopresis, sleepwalking, and sleep terror disorder may be present. Urinary tract infections are more common in children with enuresis, especially the diurnal subtype, than in those who are continent.

Encopresis

Diagnostic Criteria	307.7 (F98.1)

A. Repeated passage of feces into inappropriate places (e.g., clothing, floor), whether involuntary or intentional.

B. At least one such event occurs each month for at least 3 months.

C. Chronological age is at least 4 years (or equivalent developmental level).

D. The behavior is not attributable to the physiological effects of a substance (e.g., laxatives) or another medical condition except through a mechanism involving constipation.

Specify whether:

With constipation and overflow incontinence: There is evidence of constipation on physical examination or by history.

Without constipation and overflow incontinence: There is no evidence of constipation on physical examination or by history.

Subtypes

Feces in the with constipation and overflow incontinence subtype are characteristically (but not invariably) poorly formed, and leakage can be infrequent to continuous, occurring mostly during the day and rarely during sleep. Only part of the feces is passed during toileting, and the incontinence resolves after treatment of the constipation.

In the without constipation and overflow incontinence subtype, feces are likely to be of normal form and consistency, and soiling is intermittent. Feces may be deposited in a prominent location. This is usually associated with the presence of oppositional defiant disorder or conduct disorder or may be the consequence of anal masturbation. Soiling without constipation appears to be less common than soiling with constipation.

Diagnostic Features

The essential feature of encopresis is repeated passage of feces into inappropriate places (e.g., clothing or floor) (Criterion A). Most often the passage is involuntary but occasionally may be intentional. The event must occur at least once a month for at least 3 months (Criterion B), and the chronological age of the child must be at least 4 years (or for children with developmental delays, the mental age must be at least 4 years) (Criterion C). The fecal incontinence must not be exclusively attributable to the physiological effects of a substance (e.g., laxatives) or another medical condition except through a mechanism involving constipation (Criterion D).

When the passage of feces is involuntary rather than intentional, it is often related to constipation, impaction, and retention with subsequent overflow. The constipation may develop for psychological reasons (e.g., anxiety about defecating in a particular place, a more general pattern of anxious or oppositional behavior), leading to avoidance of defecation. Physiological predispositions to constipation include ineffectual straining or paradoxical defecation dynamics, with contraction rather than relaxation of the external sphincter or pelvic floor during straining for defecation. Dehydration associated with a febrile illness, hypothyroidism, or a medication side effect can also induce constipation. Once constipation has developed, it may be complicated by an anal fissure, painful defecation, and further fecal retention. The consistency of the stool may vary. In some individuals the stool may be of normal or near-normal consistency. In other individuals—such as those with overflow incontinence secondary to fecal retention—it may be liquid.

Associated Features Supporting Diagnosis

The child with encopresis often feels ashamed and may wish to avoid situations (e.g., camp, school) that might lead to embarrassment. The amount of impairment is a function of the effect on the child's self-esteem, the degree of social ostracism by peers, and the anger, punishment, and rejection on the part of caregivers. Smearing feces may be deliberate or accidental, resulting from the child's attempt to clean or hide feces that were passed involuntarily. When the incontinence is clearly deliberate, features of oppositional defiant disorder or conduct disorder may also be present. Many children with encopresis and chronic constipation also have enuresis symptoms and may have associated urinary reflux in the bladder or ureters that may lead to chronic urinary infections, the symptoms of which may remit with treatment of the constipation.

Prevalence

It is estimated that approximately 1% of 5-year-olds have encopresis, and the disorder is more common in males than in females.

Development and Course

Encopresis is not diagnosed until a child has reached a chronological age of at least 4 years (or for children with developmental delays, a mental age of at least 4 years). Inadequate, inconsistent toilet training and psychosocial stress (e.g., entering school, the birth of a sibling) may be predisposing factors. Two types of course have been described: a "primary" type, in which the individual has never established fecal continence, and a "secondary" type, in which the disturbance develops after a period of established fecal continence. Encopresis can persist, with intermittent exacerbations, for years.

Risk and Prognostic Factors

Genetic and physiological.   Painful defecation can lead to constipation and a cycle of withholding behaviors that make encopresis more likely. Use of some medications (e.g., anticonvulsants, cough suppressants) may increase constipation and make encopresis more likely.

Diagnostic Markers

In addition to physical examination, gastrointestinal imaging (e.g., abdominal radiograph) may be informative to assess retained stool and gas in the colon. Additional tests, such as barium enema and anorectal manography, may be used to help exclude other medical conditions, such as Hirschsprung's disease.

Differential Diagnosis

A diagnosis of encopresis in the presence of another medical condition is appropriate only if the mechanism involves constipation that cannot be explained by other medical conditions. Fecal incontinence related to other medical conditions (e.g., chronic diarrhea, spina bifida, anal stenosis) would not warrant a DSM-5 diagnosis of encopresis.

Comorbidity

Urinary tract infections can be comorbid with encopresis and are more common in females.

Other Specified Elimination Disorder

This category applies to presentations in which symptoms characteristic of an elimination disorder that cause clinically significant distress or impairment in social, occupational, or other important areas of functioning predominate but do not meet the full criteria for any of the disorders in the elimination disorders diagnostic class. The other specified elimination disorder category is used in situations in which the clinician chooses to communicate the specific reason that the presentation does not meet the criteria for any specific elimination disorder. This is done by recording "other specified elimination disorder" followed by the specific reason (e.g., "low-frequency enuresis").

Coding note: Code **788.39 (N39.498)** for other specified elimination disorder with urinary symptoms; **787.60 (R15.9)** for other specified elimination disorder with fecal symptoms.

Unspecified Elimination Disorder

This category applies to presentations in which symptoms characteristic of an elimination disorder that cause clinically significant distress or impairment in social, occupational, or other important areas of functioning predominate but do not meet the full criteria for any of the disorders in the elimination disorders diagnostic class. The unspecified elimination disorder category is used in situations in which the clinician chooses *not* to specify the reason that the criteria are not met for a specific elimination disorder, and includes presentations in which there is insufficient information to make a more specific diagnosis (e.g., in emergency room settings).

Coding note: Code **788.30 (R32)** for unspecified elimination disorder with urinary symptoms; **787.60 (R15.9)** for unspecified elimination disorder with fecal symptoms.

Sleep-Wake Disorders

The DSM-5 classification of sleep-wake disorders is intended for use by general mental health and medical clinicians (those caring for adult, geriatric, and pediatric patients). Sleep-wake disorders encompass 10 disorders or disorder groups: insomnia disorder, hypersomnolence disorder, narcolepsy, breathing-related sleep disorders, circadian rhythm sleep-wake disorders, non–rapid eye movement (NREM) sleep arousal disorders, nightmare disorder, rapid eye movement (REM) sleep behavior disorder, restless legs syndrome, and substance/medication-induced sleep disorder. Individuals with these disorders typically present with sleep-wake complaints of dissatisfaction regarding the quality, timing, and amount of sleep. Resulting daytime distress and impairment are core features shared by all of these sleep-wake disorders.

The organization of this chapter is designed to facilitate differential diagnosis of sleep-wake complaints and to clarify when referral to a sleep specialist is appropriate for further assessment and treatment planning. The DSM-5 sleep disorders nosology uses a simple, clinically useful approach, while also reflecting scientific advances in epidemiology, genetics, pathophysiology, assessment, and interventions research since DSM-IV. In some cases (e.g., insomnia disorder), a "lumping" approach has been adopted, whereas in others (e.g., narcolepsy), a "splitting" approach has been taken, reflecting the availability of validators derived from epidemiological, neurobiological, and interventions research.

Sleep disorders are often accompanied by depression, anxiety, and cognitive changes that must be addressed in treatment planning and management. Furthermore, persistent sleep disturbances (both insomnia and excessive sleepiness) are established risk factors for the subsequent development of mental illnesses and substance use disorders. They may also represent a prodromal expression of an episode of mental illness, allowing the possibility of early intervention to preempt or to attenuate a full-blown episode.

The differential diagnosis of sleep-wake complaints necessitates a multidimensional approach, with consideration of possibly coexisting medical and neurological conditions. Coexisting clinical conditions are the rule, not the exception. Sleep disturbances furnish a clinically useful indicator of medical and neurological conditions that often coexist with depression and other common mental disorders. Prominent among these comorbidities are breathing-related sleep disorders, disorders of the heart and lungs (e.g., congestive heart failure, chronic obstructive pulmonary disease), neurodegenerative disorders (e.g., Alzheimer's disease), and disorders of the musculoskeletal system (e.g., osteoarthritis). These disorders not only may disturb sleep but also may themselves be worsened during sleep (e.g., prolonged apneas or electrocardiographic arrhythmias during REM sleep; confusional arousals in patients with dementing illness; seizures in persons with complex partial seizures). REM sleep behavior disorder is often an early indicator of neurodegenerative disorders (alpha synucleinopathies) like Parkinson's disease. For all of these reasons—related to differential diagnosis, clinical comorbidity, and facilitation of treatment planning—sleep disorders are included in DSM-5.

The approach taken to the classification of sleep-wake disorders in DSM-5 can be understood within the context of "lumping versus splitting." DSM-IV represented an effort to simplify sleep-wake disorders classification and thus aggregated diagnoses under broader, less differentiated labels. At the other pole, the *International Classification of Sleep Disorders,*

2nd Edition (ICSD-2) elaborated numerous diagnostic subtypes. DSM-IV was prepared for use by mental health and general medical clinicians who are not experts in sleep medicine. ICSD-2 reflected the science and opinions of the sleep specialist community and was prepared for use by specialists.

The weight of available evidence supports the superior performance characteristics (interrater reliability, as well as convergent, discriminant, and face validity) of simpler, less-differentiated approaches to diagnosis of sleep-wake disorders. The text accompanying each set of diagnostic criteria provides linkages to the corresponding disorders included in ICSD-2. The DSM-5 sleep-wake disorders classification also specifies corresponding non-psychiatric listings (e.g., neurology codes) from the *International Classification of Diseases* (ICD).

The field of sleep disorders medicine has progressed in this direction since the publication of DSM-IV. The use of biological validators is now embodied in the DSM-5 classification of sleep-wake disorders, particularly for disorders of excessive sleepiness, such as narcolepsy; for breathing-related sleep disorders, for which formal sleep studies (i.e., polysomnography) are indicated; and for restless legs syndrome, which can often coexist with periodic limb movements during sleep, detectable via polysomnography.

Insomnia Disorder

Diagnostic Criteria   307.42 (F51.01)

A. A predominant complaint of dissatisfaction with sleep quantity or quality, associated with one (or more) of the following symptoms:

1. Difficulty initiating sleep. (In children, this may manifest as difficulty initiating sleep without caregiver intervention.)
2. Difficulty maintaining sleep, characterized by frequent awakenings or problems returning to sleep after awakenings. (In children, this may manifest as difficulty returning to sleep without caregiver intervention.)
3. Early-morning awakening with inability to return to sleep.

B. The sleep disturbance causes clinically significant distress or impairment in social, occupational, educational, academic, behavioral, or other important areas of functioning.

C. The sleep difficulty occurs at least 3 nights per week.

D. The sleep difficulty is present for at least 3 months.

E. The sleep difficulty occurs despite adequate opportunity for sleep.

F. The insomnia is not better explained by and does not occur exclusively during the course of another sleep-wake disorder (e.g., narcolepsy, a breathing-related sleep disorder, a circadian rhythm sleep-wake disorder, a parasomnia).

G. The insomnia is not attributable to the physiological effects of a substance (e.g., a drug of abuse, a medication).

H. Coexisting mental disorders and medical conditions do not adequately explain the predominant complaint of insomnia.

Specify if:

With non–sleep disorder mental comorbidity, including substance use disorders
With other medical comorbidity
With other sleep disorder

Coding note: The code 307.42 (F51.01) applies to all three specifiers. Code also the relevant associated mental disorder, medical condition, or other sleep disorder immediately after the code for insomnia disorder in order to indicate the association.

Specify if:
> **Episodic:** Symptoms last at least 1 month but less than 3 months.
> **Persistent:** Symptoms last 3 months or longer.
> **Recurrent:** Two (or more) episodes within the space of 1 year.

Note: Acute and short-term insomnia (i.e., symptoms lasting less than 3 months but otherwise meeting all criteria with regard to frequency, intensity, distress, and/or impairment) should be coded as an other specified insomnia disorder.

Note. The diagnosis of insomnia disorder is given whether it occurs as an independent condition or is comorbid with another mental disorder (e.g., major depressive disorder), medical condition (e.g., pain), or another sleep disorder (e.g., a breathing-related sleep disorder). For instance, insomnia may develop its own course with some anxiety and depressive features but in the absence of criteria being met for any one mental disorder. Insomnia may also manifest as a clinical feature of a more predominant mental disorder. Persistent insomnia may even be a risk factor for depression and is a common residual symptom after treatment for this condition. With comorbid insomnia and a mental disorder, treatment may also need to target both conditions. Given these different courses, it is often impossible to establish the precise nature of the relationship between these clinical entities, and this relationship may change over time. Therefore, in the presence of insomnia and a comorbid disorder, it is not necessary to make a causal attribution between the two conditions. Rather, the diagnosis of insomnia disorder is made with concurrent specification of the clinically comorbid conditions. A concurrent insomnia diagnosis should only be considered when the insomnia is sufficiently severe to warrant independent clinical attention; otherwise, no separate diagnosis is necessary.

Diagnostic Features

The essential feature of insomnia disorder is dissatisfaction with sleep quantity or quality with complaints of difficulty initiating or maintaining sleep. The sleep complaints are accompanied by clinically significant distress or impairment in social, occupational, or other important areas of functioning. The sleep disturbance may occur during the course of another mental disorder or medical condition, or it may occur independently.

Different manifestations of insomnia can occur at different times of the sleep period. *Sleep-onset insomnia* (or *initial insomnia*) involves difficulty initiating sleep at bedtime. *Sleep maintenance insomnia* (or *middle insomnia*) involves frequent or prolonged awakenings throughout the night. *Late insomnia* involves early-morning awakening with an inability to return to sleep. Difficulty maintaining sleep is the most common single symptom of insomnia, followed by difficulty falling asleep, while a combination of these symptoms is the most common presentation overall. The specific type of sleep complaint often varies over time. Individuals who complain of difficulty falling asleep at one time may later complain of difficulty maintaining sleep, and vice versa. Symptoms of difficulty falling asleep and difficulty maintaining sleep can be quantified by the individual's retrospective self-report, sleep diaries, or other methods, such as actigraphy or polysomnography, but the diagnosis of insomnia disorder is based on the individual's subjective perception of sleep or a caretaker's report.

Nonrestorative sleep, a complaint of poor sleep quality that does not leave the individual rested upon awakening despite adequate duration, is a common sleep complaint usually occurring in association with difficulty initiating or maintaining sleep, or less frequently in isolation. This complaint can also be reported in association with other sleep disorders (e.g., breathing-related sleep disorder). When a complaint of nonrestorative sleep occurs in isolation (i.e., in the absence of difficulty initiating and/or maintaining sleep) but all diagnostic criteria with regard to frequency, duration, and daytime distress and impairments are otherwise met, a diagnosis of other specified insomnia disorder or unspecified insomnia disorder is made.

Aside from the frequency and duration criteria required to make the diagnosis, additional criteria are useful to quantify insomnia severity. These quantitative criteria, while arbitrary, are provided for illustrative purpose only. For instance, difficulty initiating sleep is defined by a subjective sleep latency greater than 20–30 minutes, and difficulty maintaining sleep is defined by a subjective time awake after sleep onset greater than 20–30 minutes. Although there is no standard definition of early-morning awakening, this symptom involves awakening at least 30 minutes before the scheduled time and before total sleep time reaches 6½ hours. It is essential to take into account not only the final awakening time but also the bedtime on the previous evening. Awakening at 4:00 A.M. does not have the same clinical significance in those who go to bed at 9:00 P.M. as in those who go to bed at 11:00 P.M. Such a symptom may also reflect an age-dependent decrease in the ability to sustain sleep or an age-dependent shift in the timing of the main sleep period.

Insomnia disorder involves daytime impairments as well as nighttime sleep difficulties. These include fatigue or, less commonly, daytime sleepiness; the latter is more common among older individuals and when insomnia is comorbid with another medical condition (e.g., chronic pain) or sleep disorder (e.g., sleep apnea). Impairment in cognitive performance may include difficulties with attention, concentration and memory, and even with performing simple manual skills. Associated mood disturbances are typically described as irritability or mood lability and less commonly as depressive or anxiety symptoms. Not all individuals with nighttime sleep disturbances are distressed or have functional impairment. For example, sleep continuity is often interrupted in healthy older adults who nevertheless identify themselves as good sleepers. A diagnosis of insomnia disorder should be reserved for those individuals with significant daytime distress or impairment related to their nighttime sleep difficulties.

Associated Features Supporting Diagnosis

Insomnia is often associated with physiological and cognitive arousal and conditioning factors that interfere with sleep. A preoccupation with sleep and distress due to the inability to sleep may lead to a vicious cycle: the more the individual strives to sleep, the more frustration builds and further impairs sleep. Thus, excessive attention and efforts to sleep, which override normal sleep-onset mechanisms, may contribute to the development of insomnia. Individuals with persistent insomnia may also acquire maladaptive sleep habits (e.g., spending excessive time in bed; following an erratic sleep schedule; napping) and cognitions (e.g., fear of sleeplessness; apprehensions of daytime impairments; clock monitoring) during the course of the disorder. Engaging in such activities in an environment in which the individual has frequently spent sleepless nights may further compound the conditioned arousal and perpetuate sleep difficulties. Conversely, the individual may fall asleep more easily when not trying to do so. Some individuals also report better sleep when away from their own bedrooms and their usual routines.

Insomnia may be accompanied by a variety of daytime complaints and symptoms, including fatigue, decreased energy, and mood disturbances. Symptoms of anxiety or depression that do not meet criteria for a specific mental disorder may be present, as well as an excessive focus on the perceived effects of sleep loss on daytime functioning.

Individuals with insomnia may have elevated scores on self-report psychological or personality inventories with profiles indicating mild depression and anxiety, a worrisome cognitive style, an emotion-focused and internalizing style of conflict resolution, and a somatic focus. Patterns of neurocognitive impairment among individuals with insomnia disorder are inconsistent, although there may be impairments in performing tasks of higher complexity and those requiring frequent changes in performance strategy. Individuals with insomnia often require more effort to maintain cognitive performance.

Prevalence

Population-based estimates indicate that about one-third of adults report insomnia symptoms, 10%–15% experience associated daytime impairments, and 6%–10% have symptoms that meet criteria for insomnia disorder. Insomnia disorder is the most prevalent of all sleep disorders. In primary care settings, approximately 10%–20% of individuals complain of significant insomnia symptoms. Insomnia is a more prevalent complaint among females than among males, with a gender ratio of about 1.44:1. Although insomnia can be a symptom or an independent disorder, it is most frequently observed as a comorbid condition with another medical condition or mental disorder. For instance, 40%–50% of individuals with insomnia also present with a comorbid mental disorder.

Development and Course

The onset of insomnia symptoms can occur at any time during life, but the first episode is more common in young adulthood. Less frequently, insomnia begins in childhood or adolescence. In women, new-onset insomnia may occur during menopause and persist even after other symptoms (e.g., hot flashes) have resolved. Insomnia may have a late-life onset, which is often associated with the onset of other health-related conditions.

Insomnia can be situational, persistent, or recurrent. Situational or acute insomnia usually lasts a few days or a few weeks and is often associated with life events or rapid changes in sleep schedules or environment. It usually resolves once the initial precipitating event subsides. For some individuals, perhaps those more vulnerable to sleep disturbances, insomnia may persist long after the initial triggering event, possibly because of conditioning factors and heightened arousal. The factors that precipitate insomnia may differ from those that perpetuate it. For example, an individual who is bedridden with a painful injury and has difficulty sleeping may then develop negative associations for sleep. Conditioned arousal may then persist and lead to persistent insomnia. A similar course may develop in the context of an acute psychological stress or a mental disorder. For instance, insomnia that occurs during an episode of major depressive disorder can become a focus of attention, with consequent negative conditioning, and persist even after resolution of the depressive episode. In some cases, insomnia may also have an insidious onset without any identifiable precipitating factor.

The course of insomnia may also be episodic, with recurrent episodes of sleep difficulties associated with the occurrence of stressful events. Chronicity rates range from 45% to 75% for follow-ups of 1–7 years. Even when the course of the insomnia has become chronic, there is night-to-night variability in sleep patterns, with an occasional restful night's sleep interspersed with several nights of poor sleep. The characteristics of insomnia may also change over time. Many individuals with insomnia have a history of "light" or easily disturbed sleep prior to onset of more persistent sleep problems.

Insomnia complaints are more prevalent among middle-age and older adults. The type of insomnia symptom changes as a function of age, with difficulties initiating sleep being more common among young adults and problems maintaining sleep occurring more frequently among middle-age and older individuals.

Difficulties initiating and maintaining sleep can also occur in children and adolescents, but there are more limited data on prevalence, risk factors, and comorbidity during these developmental phases of the lifespan. Sleep difficulties in childhood can result from conditioning factors (e.g., a child who does not learn to fall asleep or return to sleep without the presence of a parent) or from the absence of consistent sleep schedules and bedtime routines. Insomnia in adolescence is often triggered or exacerbated by irregular sleep schedules (e.g., phase delay). In both children and adolescents, psychological and medical factors can contribute to insomnia.

The increased prevalence of insomnia in older adults is partly explained by the higher incidence of physical health problems with aging. Changes in sleep patterns associated with the normal developmental process must be differentiated from those exceeding age-related changes. Although polysomnography is of limited value in the routine evaluation of insomnia, it may be more useful in the differential diagnosis among older adults because the etiologies of insomnia (e.g., sleep apnea) are more often identifiable in older individuals.

Risk and Prognostic Factors

While the risk and prognostic factors discussed in this section increase vulnerability to insomnia, sleep disturbances are more likely to occur when predisposed individuals are exposed to precipitating events, such as major life events (e.g., illness, separation) or less severe but more chronic daily stress. Most individuals resume normal sleep patterns after the initial triggering event has disappeared, but others—perhaps those more vulnerable to insomnia—continue experiencing persistent sleep difficulties. Perpetuating factors such as poor sleep habits, irregular sleep scheduling, and the fear of not sleeping feed into the insomnia problem and may contribute to a vicious cycle that may induce persistent insomnia.

Temperamental.   Anxiety or worry-prone personality or cognitive styles, increased arousal predisposition, and tendency to repress emotions can increase vulnerability to insomnia.

Environmental.   Noise, light, uncomfortably high or low temperature, and high altitude may also increase vulnerability to insomnia.

Genetic and physiological.   Female gender and advancing age are associated with increased vulnerability to insomnia. Disrupted sleep and insomnia display a familial disposition. The prevalence of insomnia is higher among monozygotic twins relative to dizygotic twins; it is also higher in first-degree family members compared with the general population. The extent to which this link is inherited through a genetic predisposition, learned by observations of parental models, or established as a by-product of another psychopathology remains undetermined.

Course modifiers.   Deleterious course modifiers include poor sleep hygiene practices (e.g., excessive caffeine use, irregular sleep schedules).

Gender-Related Diagnostic Issues

Insomnia is a more prevalent complaint among females than among males, with first onset often associated with the birth of a new child or with menopause. Despite higher prevalence among older females, polysomnographic studies suggest better preservation of sleep continuity and slow-wave sleep in older females than in older males.

Diagnostic Markers

Polysomnography usually shows impairments of sleep continuity (e.g., increased sleep latency and time awake after sleep onset and decreased sleep efficiency [percentage of time in bed asleep] and may show increased stage 1 sleep and decreased stages 3 and 4 sleep. The severity of these sleep impairments does not always match the individual's clinical presentation or subjective complaint of poor sleep, as individuals with insomnia often underestimate sleep duration and overestimate wakefulness relative to polysomnography. Quantitative electroencephalographic analyses may indicate that individuals with insomnia have greater high-frequency electroencephalography power relative to good sleepers both around the sleep onset period and during non–rapid eye movement sleep, a feature suggestive of increased cortical arousal. Individuals with insomnia disorder may have a lower sleep propensity and typically do not show increased daytime sleepiness on objective sleep laboratory measures compared with individuals without sleep disorders.

Other laboratory measures show evidence, although not consistently, of increased arousal and a generalized activation of the hypothalamic-pituitary-adrenal axis (e.g., increased cortisol levels, heart rate variability, reactivity to stress, metabolic rate). In general, findings are consistent with the hypothesis that increased physiological and cognitive arousal plays a significant role in insomnia disorder.

Individuals with insomnia disorder may appear either fatigued or haggard or, conversely, overaroused and "wired." However, there are no consistent or characteristic abnormalities on physical examination. There may be an increased incidence of stress-related psychophysiological symptoms (e.g., tension headache, muscle tension or pain, gastrointestinal symptoms).

Functional Consequences of Insomnia Disorder

Interpersonal, social, and occupational problems may develop as a result of insomnia or excessive concern with sleep, increased daytime irritability, and poor concentration. Decreased attention and concentration are common and may be related to higher rates of accidents observed in insomnia. Persistent insomnia is also associated with long-term consequences, including increased risks of major depressive disorder, hypertension, and myocardial infarction; increased absenteeism and reduced productivity at work; reduced quality of life; and increased economic burden.

Differential Diagnosis

Normal sleep variations. Normal sleep duration varies considerably across individuals. Some individuals who require little sleep ("short sleepers") may be concerned about their sleep duration. Short sleepers differ from individuals with insomnia disorder by the lack of difficulty falling or staying asleep and by the absence of characteristic daytime symptoms (e.g., fatigue, concentration problems, irritability). However, some short sleepers may desire or attempt to sleep for a longer period of time and, by prolonging time in bed, may create an insomnia-like sleep pattern. Clinical insomnia also should be distinguished from normal, age-related sleep changes. Insomnia must also be distinguished from sleep deprivation due to inadequate opportunity or circumstance for sleep resulting, for example, from an emergency or from professional or family obligations forcing the individual to stay awake.

Situational/acute insomnia. *Situational/acute insomnia* is a condition lasting a few days to a few weeks, often associated with life events or with changes in sleep schedules. These acute or short-term insomnia symptoms may also produce significant distress and interfere with social, personal, and occupational functioning. When such symptoms are frequent enough and meet all other criteria except for the 3-month duration, a diagnosis of other specified insomnia disorder or unspecified insomnia disorder is made.

Delayed sleep phase and shift work types of circadian rhythm sleep-wake disorder. Individuals with the delayed sleep phase type of circadian rhythm sleep-wake disorder report sleep-onset insomnia only when they try to sleep at socially normal times, but they do not report difficulty falling asleep or staying asleep when their bed and rising times are delayed and coincide with their endogenous circadian rhythm. Shift work type differs from insomnia disorder by the history of recent shift work.

Restless legs syndrome. Restless legs syndrome often produces difficulties initiating and maintaining sleep. However, an urge to move the legs and any accompanying unpleasant leg sensations are features that differentiate this disorder from insomnia disorder.

Breathing-related sleep disorders. Most individuals with a breathing-related sleep disorder have a history of loud snoring, breathing pauses during sleep, and excessive daytime sleepiness. Nonetheless, as many as 50% of individuals with sleep apnea may also report insomnia symptoms, a feature that is more common among females and older adults.

Narcolepsy. Narcolepsy may cause insomnia complaints but is distinguished from insomnia disorder by the predominance of symptoms of excessive daytime sleepiness, cataplexy, sleep paralysis, and sleep-related hallucinations.

Parasomnias. Parasomnias are characterized by a complaint of unusual behavior or events during sleep that may lead to intermittent awakenings and difficulty resuming sleep. However, it is these behavioral events, rather than the insomnia per se, that dominate the clinical picture.

Substance/medication-induced sleep disorder, insomnia type.   Substance/medication-induced sleep disorder, insomnia type, is distinguished from insomnia disorder by the fact that a substance (i.e., a drug of abuse, a medication, or exposure to a toxin) is judged to be etiologically related to the insomnia (see "Substance/Medication-Induced Sleep Disorder" later in this chapter). For example, insomnia occurring only in the context of heavy coffee consumption would be diagnosed as caffeine-induced sleep disorder, insomnia type, with onset during intoxication.

Comorbidity

Insomnia is a common comorbidity of many medical conditions, including diabetes, coronary heart disease, chronic obstructive pulmonary disease, arthritis, fibromyalgia, and other chronic pain conditions. The risk relationship appears to be bidirectional: insomnia increases the risk of medical conditions, and medical problems increase the risk of insomnia. The direction of the relationship is not always clear and may change over time; for this reason, comorbid insomnia is the preferred terminology in the presence of coexisting insomnia with another medical condition (or mental disorder).

Individuals with insomnia disorder frequently have a comorbid mental disorder, particularly bipolar, depressive, and anxiety disorders. Persistent insomnia represents a risk factor or an early symptom of subsequent bipolar, depressive, anxiety, and substance use disorders. Individuals with insomnia may misuse medications or alcohol to help with nighttime sleep, anxiolytics to combat tension or anxiety, and caffeine or other stimulants to combat excessive fatigue. In addition to worsening the insomnia, this type of substance use may in some cases progress to a substance use disorder.

Relationship to International Classification of Sleep Disorders

There are several distinct insomnia phenotypes relating to the perceived source of the insomnia that are recognized by the *International Classification of Sleep Disorders,* 2nd Edition (ICSD-2). These include *psychophysiological insomnia, idiopathic insomnia, sleep-state misperception,* and *inadequate sleep hygiene.* Despite their clinical appeal and heuristic value, there is limited evidence to support these distinct phenotypes.

Hypersomnolence Disorder

Diagnostic Criteria	307.44 (F51.11)

A. Self-reported excessive sleepiness (hypersomnolence) despite a main sleep period lasting at least 7 hours, with at least one of the following symptoms:
   1. Recurrent periods of sleep or lapses into sleep within the same day.
   2. A prolonged main sleep episode of more than 9 hours per day that is nonrestorative (i.e., unrefreshing).
   3. Difficulty being fully awake after abrupt awakening.
B. The hypersomnolence occurs at least three times per week, for at least 3 months.
C. The hypersomnolence is accompanied by significant distress or impairment in cognitive, social, occupational, or other important areas of functioning.
D. The hypersomnolence is not better explained by and does not occur exclusively during the course of another sleep disorder (e.g., narcolepsy, breathing-related sleep disorder, circadian rhythm sleep-wake disorder, or a parasomnia).
E. The hypersomnolence is not attributable to the physiological effects of a substance (e.g., a drug of abuse, a medication).

F. Coexisting mental and medical disorders do not adequately explain the predominant complaint of hypersomnolence.

Specify if:

With mental disorder, including substance use disorders
With medical condition
With another sleep disorder

Coding note: The code 307.44 (F51.11) applies to all three specifiers. Code also the relevant associated mental disorder, medical condition, or other sleep disorder immediately after the code for hypersomnolence disorder in order to indicate the association.

Specify if:

Acute: Duration of less than 1 month.
Subacute: Duration of 1–3 months.
Persistent: Duration of more than 3 months.

Specify current severity:

Specify severity based on degree of difficulty maintaining daytime alertness as manifested by the occurrence of multiple attacks of irresistible sleepiness within any given day occurring, for example, while sedentary, driving, visiting with friends, or working.

Mild: Difficulty maintaining daytime alertness 1–2 days/week.
Moderate: Difficulty maintaining daytime alertness 3–4 days/week.
Severe: Difficulty maintaining daytime alertness 5–7 days/week.

Diagnostic Features

Hypersomnolence is a broad diagnostic term and includes symptoms of excessive quantity of sleep (e.g., extended nocturnal sleep or involuntary daytime sleep), deteriorated quality of wakefulness (i.e., sleep propensity during wakefulness as shown by difficulty awakening or inability to remain awake when required), and sleep inertia (i.e., a period of impaired performance and reduced vigilance following awakening from the regular sleep episode or from a nap) (Criterion A). Individuals with this disorder fall asleep quickly and have a good sleep efficiency (>90%). They may have difficulty waking up in the morning, sometimes appearing confused, combative, or ataxic. This prolonged impairment of alertness at the sleep-wake transition is often referred to as *sleep inertia* (i.e., sleep drunkenness). It can also occur upon awakening from a daytime nap. During that period, the individual appears awake, but there is a decline in motor dexterity, behavior may be very inappropriate, and memory deficits, disorientation in time and space, and feelings of grogginess may occur. This period may last some minutes to hours.

The persistent need for sleep can lead to automatic behavior (usually of a very routine, low-complexity type) that the individual carries out with little or no subsequent recall. For example, individuals may find themselves having driven several miles from where they thought they were, unaware of the "automatic" driving they did in the preceding minutes. For some individuals with hypersomnolence disorder, the major sleep episode (for most individuals, nocturnal sleep) has a duration of 9 hours or more. However, the sleep is often nonrestorative and is followed by difficulty awakening in the morning. For other individuals with hypersomnolence disorder, the major sleep episode is of normal nocturnal sleep duration (6–9 hours). In these cases, the excessive sleepiness is characterized by several unintentional daytime naps. These daytime naps tend to be relatively long (often lasting 1 hour or more), are experienced as nonrestorative (i.e., unrefreshing), and do not lead to improved alertness. Individuals with hypersomnolence have daytime naps nearly everyday regardless of the nocturnal sleep duration. Subjective sleep quality may or may not be reported as good. Individuals typically feel sleepiness developing over a period of time, rather than experiencing a sudden sleep "attack." Unintentional sleep episodes typically occur in low-stimulation and low-activity situations (e.g., while attending lectures, reading, watching television, or driving long distances), but in more severe cases they can manifest in high-attention situations such as at work, in meetings, or at social gatherings.

Associated Features Supporting Diagnosis

Nonrestorative sleep, automatic behavior, difficulties awakening in the morning, and sleep inertia, although common in hypersomnolence disorder, may also be seen in a variety of conditions, including narcolepsy. Approximately 80% of individuals with hypersomnolence report that their sleep is nonrestorative, and as many have difficulties awakening in the morning. Sleep inertia, though less common (i.e., observed in 36%–50% of individuals with hypersomnolence disorder), is highly specific to hypersomnolence. Short naps (i.e., duration of less than 30 minutes) are often unrefreshing. Individuals with hypersomnolence often appear sleepy and may even fall asleep in the clinician's waiting area.

A subset of individuals with hypersomnolence disorder have a family history of hypersomnolence and also have symptoms of autonomic nervous system dysfunction, including recurrent vascular-type headaches, reactivity of the peripheral vascular system (Raynaud's phenomenon), and fainting.

Prevalence

Approximately 5%–10% of individuals who consult in sleep disorders clinics with complaints of daytime sleepiness are diagnosed as having hypersomnolence disorder. It is estimated that about 1% of the European and U.S. general population has episodes of sleep inertia. Hypersomnolence occurs with relatively equal frequency in males and females.

Development and Course

Hypersomnolence disorder has a persistent course, with a progressive evolution in the severity of symptoms. In most extreme cases, sleep episodes can last up to 20 hours. However, the average nighttime sleep duration is around 9½ hours. While many individuals with hypersomnolence are able to reduce their sleep time during working days, weekend and holiday sleep is greatly increased (by up to 3 hours). Awakenings are very difficult and accompanied by sleep inertia episodes in nearly 40% of cases. Hypersomnolence fully manifests in most cases in late adolescence or early adulthood, with a mean age at onset of 17–24 years. Individuals with hypersomnolence disorder are diagnosed, on average, 10–15 years after the appearance of the first symptoms. Pediatric cases are rare.

Hypersomnolence has a progressive onset, with symptoms beginning between ages 15 and 25 years, with a gradual progression over weeks to months. For most individuals, the course is then persistent and stable, unless treatment is initiated. The development of other sleep disorders (e.g., breathing-related sleep disorder) may worsen the degree of sleepiness. Although hyperactivity may be one of the presenting signs of daytime sleepiness in children, voluntary napping increases with age. This normal phenomenon is distinct from hypersomnolence.

Risk and Prognostic Factors

Environmental.   Hypersomnolence can be increased temporarily by psychological stress and alcohol use, but they have not been documented as environmental precipitating factors. Viral infections have been reported to have preceded or accompanied hypersomnolence in about 10% of cases. Viral infections, such as HIV pneumonia, infectious mononucleosis, and Guillain-Barré syndrome, can also evolve into hypersomnolence within months after the infection. Hypersomnolence can also appear within 6–18 months following a head trauma.

Genetic and physiological.   Hypersomnolence may be familial, with an autosomal-dominant mode of inheritance.

Diagnostic Markers

Nocturnal polysomnography demonstrates a normal to prolonged sleep duration, short sleep latency, and normal to increased sleep continuity. The distribution of rapid eye movement (REM) sleep is also normal. Sleep efficiency is mostly greater than 90%. Some individuals with hypersomnolence disorder have increased amounts of slow-wave sleep. The multiple sleep latency test documents sleep tendency, typically indicated by mean sleep latency values of less than 8 minutes. In hypersomnolence disorder, the mean sleep latency is typically less than 10 minutes and frequently 8 minutes or less. Sleep-onset REM periods (SOREMPs; i.e., the occurrence of REM sleep within 20 minutes of sleep onset) may be present but occur less than two times in four to five nap opportunities.

Functional Consequences of Hypersomnolence Disorder

The low level of alertness that occurs while an individual fights the need for sleep can lead to reduced efficiency, diminished concentration, and poor memory during daytime activities. Hypersomnolence can lead to significant distress and dysfunction in work and social relationships. Prolonged nocturnal sleep and difficulty awakening can result in difficulty in meeting morning obligations, such as arriving at work on time. Unintentional daytime sleep episodes can be embarrassing and even dangerous, if, for instance, the individual is driving or operating machinery when the episode occurs.

Differential Diagnosis

Normative variation in sleep.   "Normal" sleep duration varies considerably in the general population. "Long sleepers" (i.e., individuals who require a greater than average amount of sleep) do not have excessive sleepiness, sleep inertia, or automatic behavior when they obtain their required amount of nocturnal sleep. Sleep is reported to be refreshing. If social or occupational demands lead to shorter nocturnal sleep, daytime symptoms may appear. In hypersomnolence disorder, by contrast, symptoms of excessive sleepiness occur regardless of nocturnal sleep duration. An inadequate amount of nocturnal sleep, or *behaviorally induced insufficient sleep syndrome,* can produce symptoms of daytime sleepiness very similar to those of hypersomnolence. An average sleep duration of fewer than 7 hours per night strongly suggests inadequate nocturnal sleep, and an average of more than 9–10 hours of sleep per 24-hour period suggests hypersomnolence. Individuals with inadequate nocturnal sleep typically "catch up" with longer sleep durations on days when they are free from social or occupational demands or on vacations. Unlike hypersomnolence, insufficient nocturnal sleep is unlikely to persist unabated for decades. A diagnosis of hypersomnolence disorder should not be made if there is a question regarding the adequacy of nocturnal sleep duration. A diagnostic and therapeutic trial of sleep extension for 10–14 days can often clarify the diagnosis.

Poor sleep quality and fatigue.   Hypersomnolence disorder should be distinguished from excessive sleepiness related to insufficient sleep quantity or quality and fatigue (i.e., tiredness not necessarily relieved by increased sleep and unrelated to sleep quantity or quality). Excessive sleepiness and fatigue are difficult to differentiate and may overlap considerably.

Breathing-related sleep disorders.   Individuals with hypersomnolence and breathing-related sleep disorders may have similar patterns of excessive sleepiness. Breathing-related sleep disorders are suggested by a history of loud snoring, pauses in breathing during sleep, brain injury, or cardiovascular disease and by the presence of obesity, oropharyngeal anatomical abnormalities, hypertension, or heart failure on physical examination. Polysomnographic studies can confirm the presence of apneic events in breathing-related sleep disorder (and their absence in hypersomnolence disorder).

Circadian rhythm sleep-wake disorders.   Circadian rhythm sleep-wake disorders are often characterized by daytime sleepiness. A history of an abnormal sleep-wake schedule (with shifted or irregular hours) is present in individuals with a circadian rhythm sleep-wake disorder.

Parasomnias.   Parasomnias rarely produce the prolonged, undisturbed nocturnal sleep or daytime sleepiness characteristic of hypersomnolence disorder.

Other mental disorders.   Hypersomnolence disorder must be distinguished from mental disorders that include hypersomnolence as an essential or associated feature. In particular, complaints of daytime sleepiness may occur in a major depressive episode, with atypical features, and in the depressed phase of bipolar disorder. Assessment for other mental disorders is essential before a diagnosis of hypersomnolence disorder is considered. A diagnosis of hypersomnolence disorder can be made in the presence of another current or past mental disorder.

Comorbidity

Hypersomnolence can be associated with depressive disorders, bipolar disorders (during a depressive episode), and major depressive disorder, with seasonal pattern. Many individuals with hypersomnolence disorder have symptoms of depression that may meet criteria for a depressive disorder. This presentation may be related to the psychosocial consequences of persistent increased sleep need. Individuals with hypersomnolence disorder are also at risk for substance-related disorders, particularly related to self-medication with stimulants. This general lack of specificity may contribute to very heterogeneous profiles among individuals whose symptoms meet the same diagnostic criteria for hypersomnolence disorder. Neurodegenerative conditions, such as Alzheimer's disease, Parkinson's disease, and multiple system atrophy, may also be associated with hypersomnolence.

Relationship to International Classification of Sleep Disorders

The *International Classification of Sleep Disorders*, 2nd Edition (ICSD-2), differentiates nine subtypes of "hypersomnias of central origin," including recurrent hypersomnia (Kleine-Levin syndrome).

Narcolepsy

Diagnostic Criteria

A. Recurrent periods of an irrepressible need to sleep, lapsing into sleep, or napping occurring within the same day. These must have been occurring at least three times per week over the past 3 months.

B. The presence of at least one of the following:

1. Episodes of cataplexy, defined as either (a) or (b), occurring at least a few times per month:

   a. In individuals with long-standing disease, brief (seconds to minutes) episodes of sudden bilateral loss of muscle tone with maintained consciousness that are precipitated by laughter or joking.

    b. In children or in individuals within 6 months of onset, spontaneous grimaces or jaw-opening episodes with tongue thrusting or a global hypotonia, without any obvious emotional triggers.

2. Hypocretin deficiency, as measured using cerebrospinal fluid (CSF) hypocretin-1 immunoreactivity values (less than or equal to one-third of values obtained in healthy subjects tested using the same assay, or less than or equal to 110 pg/mL). Low CSF levels of hypocretin-1 must not be observed in the context of acute brain injury, inflammation, or infection.

3. Nocturnal sleep polysomnography showing rapid eye movement (REM) sleep latency less than or equal to 15 minutes, or a multiple sleep latency test showing a mean sleep latency less than or equal to 8 minutes and two or more sleep-onset REM periods.

Specify whether:

347.00 (G47.419) Narcolepsy without cataplexy but with hypocretin deficiency: Criterion B requirements of low CSF hypocretin-1 levels and positive polysomnography/multiple sleep latency test are met, but no cataplexy is present (Criterion B1 not met).

347.01 (G47.411) Narcolepsy with cataplexy but without hypocretin deficiency: In this rare subtype (less than 5% of narcolepsy cases), Criterion B requirements of cataplexy and positive polysomnography/multiple sleep latency test are met, but CSF hypocretin-1 levels are normal (Criterion B2 not met).

347.00 (G47.419) Autosomal dominant cerebellar ataxia, deafness, and narcolepsy: This subtype is caused by exon 21 DNA (cytosine-5)-methyltransferase-1 mutations and is characterized by late-onset (age 30–40 years) narcolepsy (with low or intermediate CSF hypocretin-1 levels), deafness, cerebellar ataxia, and eventually dementia.

347.00 (G47.419) Autosomal dominant narcolepsy, obesity, and type 2 diabetes: Narcolepsy, obesity, and type 2 diabetes and low CSF hypocretin-1 levels have been described in rare cases and are associated with a mutation in the myelin oligodendrocyte glycoprotein gene.

347.10 (G47.429) Narcolepsy secondary to another medical condition: This subtype is for narcolepsy that develops secondary to medical conditions that cause infectious (e.g., Whipple's disease, sarcoidosis), traumatic, or tumoral destruction of hypocretin neurons.

Coding note (for ICD-9-CM code 347.10 only): Code first the underlying medical condition (e.g., 040.2 Whipple's disease; 347.10 narcolepsy secondary to Whipple's disease).

Specify current severity:

Mild: Infrequent cataplexy (less than once per week), need for naps only once or twice per day, and less disturbed nocturnal sleep.

Moderate: Cataplexy once daily or every few days, disturbed nocturnal sleep, and need for multiple naps daily.

Severe: Drug-resistant cataplexy with multiple attacks daily, nearly constant sleepiness, and disturbed nocturnal sleep (i.e., movements, insomnia, and vivid dreaming).

Subtypes

In narcolepsy without cataplexy but with hypocretin deficiency, unclear "cataplexy-like" symptoms may be reported (e.g., the symptoms are not triggered by emotions and are unusually long lasting). In extremely rare cases, cerebrospinal fluid (CSF) levels of hypocretin-1 are low, and polysomnographic/multiple sleep latency test (MSLT) results are negative: repeating the test is advised before establishing the subtype diagnosis. In narcolepsy with cataplexy but without hypocretin deficiency, test results for human leukocyte antigen (HLA) DQB1*06:02 may be negative. Seizures, falls of other origin, and conversion disorder (functional neurological symptom disorder) should be excluded. In narcolepsy secondary to infectious (e.g., Whipple's disease, sarcoidosis), traumatic, or tumoral destruction of hypocretin neurons, test results for HLA DQB1*06:02 may be positive and may result from the insult triggering the autoimmune process. In other cases, the destruction of hypocretin neurons may be secondary to trauma or hypothalamic surgery. Head trauma or infections of the central nervous system can, however, produce transitory decreases in CSF hypocretin-1 levels without hypocretin cell loss, complicating the diagnosis.

Diagnostic Features

The essential features of sleepiness in narcolepsy are recurrent daytime naps or lapses into sleep. Sleepiness typically occurs daily but must occur at a minimum three times a week for at least 3 months (Criterion A). Narcolepsy generally produces cataplexy, which most commonly presents as brief episodes (seconds to minutes) of sudden, bilateral loss of muscle tone precipitated by emotions, typically laughing and joking. Muscles affected may include those of the neck, jaw, arms, legs, or whole body, resulting in head bobbing, jaw dropping, or complete falls. Individuals are awake and aware during cataplexy. To meet Criterion B1(a), cataplexy must be triggered by laughter or joking and must occur at least a few times per month when the condition is untreated or in the past.

Cataplexy should not be confused with "weakness" occurring in the context of athletic activities (physiological) or exclusively after unusual emotional triggers such as stress or anxiety (suggesting possible psychopathology). Episodes lasting hours or days, or those not triggered by emotions, are unlikely to be cataplexy, nor is rolling on the floor while laughing hysterically.

In children close to onset, genuine cataplexy can be atypical, affecting primarily the face, causing grimaces or jaw opening with tongue thrusting ("cataplectic faces"). Alternatively, cataplexy may present as low-grade continuous hypotonia, yielding a wobbling walk. In these cases, Criterion B1(b) can be met in children or in individuals within 6 months of a rapid onset.

Narcolepsy-cataplexy nearly always results from the loss of hypothalamic hypocretin (orexin)–producing cells, causing hypocretin deficiency (less than or equal to one-third of control values, or 110 pg/mL in most laboratories). Cell loss is likely autoimmune, and approximately 99% of affected individuals carry HLA-DQB1*06:02 (vs. 12%–38% of control subjects). Thus, checking for the presence of DQB1*06:02 prior to a lumbar puncture for evaluation of CSF hypocretin-1 immunoreactivity may be useful. Rarely, low CSF levels of hypocretin-1 occur without cataplexy, notably in youths who may develop cataplexy later. CSF hypocretin-1 measurement represents the gold standard, excepting associated severe conditions (neurological, inflammatory, infectious, trauma) that can interfere with the assay.

A nocturnal polysomnographic sleep study followed by an MSLT can also be used to confirm the diagnosis (Criterion B3). These tests must be performed after the individual has stopped all psychotropic medications, following 2 weeks of adequate sleep time (as documented with sleep diaries, actigraphy). Short rapid eye movement (REM) latency (sleep-onset REM period, REM latency less than or equal to 15 minutes) during polysomnography is sufficient to confirm the diagnosis and meets Criterion B3. Alternatively, the MSLT result must be positive, showing a mean sleep latency of less than or equal to 8 minutes and two or more sleep-onset REM periods in four to five naps.

Associated Features Supporting Diagnosis

When sleepiness is severe, automatic behaviors may occur, with the individual continuing his or her activities in a semi-automatic, hazelike fashion without memory or consciousness. Approximately 20%–60% of individuals experience vivid hypnagogic hallucinations before or upon falling asleep or hypnopompic hallucinations just after awakening. These hallucinations are distinct from the less vivid, nonhallucinatory dreamlike mentation at sleep onset that occurs in normal sleepers. Nightmares and vivid dreaming are also frequent in narcolepsy, as is REM sleep behavior disorder. Approximately 20%–60% of individuals experience sleep paralysis upon falling asleep or awakening, leaving them awake but unable to move or speak. However, many normal sleepers also report sleep paralysis, especially with stress or sleep deprivation. Nocturnal eating may occur. Obesity is common. Nocturnal sleep disruption with frequent long or short awakenings is common and can be disabling.

Individuals may appear sleepy or fall asleep in the waiting area or during clinical examination. During cataplexy, individuals may slump in a chair and have slurred speech or drooping eyelids. If the clinician has time to check reflexes during cataplexy (most attacks are less than 10 seconds), reflexes are abolished—an important finding distinguishing genuine cataplexy from conversion disorder.

Prevalence

Narcolepsy-cataplexy affects 0.02%–0.04% of the general population in most countries. Narcolepsy affects both genders, with possibly a slight male preponderance.

Development and Course

Onset is typically in children and adolescents/young adults but rarely in older adults. Two peaks of onset are suggested, at ages 15–25 years and ages 30–35 years. Onset can be abrupt or progressive (over years). Severity is highest when onset is abrupt in children, and then decreases with age or with treatment, so that symptoms such as cataplexy can occasionally disappear. Abrupt onset in young, prepubescent children can be associated with obesity and premature puberty, a phenotype more frequently observed since 2009. In adolescents, onset is more difficult to pinpoint. Onset in adults is often unclear, with some individuals reporting having had excessive sleepiness since birth. Once the disorder has manifested, the course is persistent and lifelong.

In 90% of cases, the first symptom to manifest is sleepiness or increased sleep, followed by cataplexy (within 1 year in 50% of cases, within 3 years in 85%). Sleepiness, hypnagogic hallucinations, vivid dreaming, and REM sleep behavior disorder (excessive movements during REM sleep) are early symptoms. Excessive sleep rapidly progresses to an inability to stay awake during the day, and to maintain good sleep at night, without a clear increase in total 24-hour sleep needs. In the first months, cataplexy may be atypical, especially in children. Sleep paralysis usually develops around puberty in children with prepubertal onset. Exacerbations of symptoms suggest lack of compliance with medications or development of a concurrent sleep disorder, notably sleep apnea.

Young children and adolescents with narcolepsy often develop aggression or behavioral problems secondary to sleepiness and/or nighttime sleep disruption. Workload and social pressure increase through high school and college, reducing available sleep time at night. Pregnancy does not seem to modify symptoms consistently. After retirement, individuals typically have more opportunity for napping, reducing the need for stimulants. Maintaining a regular schedule benefits individuals at all ages.

Risk and Prognostic Factors

Temperamental. Parasomnias, such as sleepwalking, bruxism, REM sleep behavior disorder, and enuresis, may be more common in individuals who develop narcolepsy. Individuals commonly report that they need more sleep than other family members.

Environmental. Group A streptococcal throat infection, influenza (notably pandemic H1N1 2009), or other winter infections are likely triggers of the autoimmune process, producing narcolepsy a few months later. Head trauma and abrupt changes in sleep-wake patterns (e.g., job changes, stress) may be additional triggers.

Genetic and physiological.   Monozygotic twins are 25%–32% concordant for narcolepsy. The prevalence of narcolepsy is 1%–2% in first-degree relatives (a 10- to 40-fold increase overall). Narcolepsy is strongly associated with DQB1*06:02 (99% vs. 12%–38% in control subjects of various ethnic groups; 25% in the general U.S. population). DQB1*03:01 increases, while DQB1*05:01, DQB1*06:01, and DQB1*06:03 reduce risk in the presence of DQB1*06:02, but the effect is small. Polymorphisms within the T-cell receptor alpha gene and other immune modulating genes also modulate risk slightly.

Culture-Related Diagnostic Issues

Narcolepsy has been described in all ethnic groups and in many cultures. Among African Americans, more cases present without cataplexy or with atypical cataplexy, complicating diagnosis, especially in the presence of obesity and obstructive sleep apnea.

Diagnostic Markers

Functional imaging suggests impaired hypothalamic responses to humorous stimuli. Nocturnal polysomnography followed by an MSLT is used to confirm the diagnosis of narcolepsy, especially when the disorder is first being diagnosed and before treatment has begun, and if hypocretin deficiency has not been documented biochemically. The polysomnography/MSLT should be performed after the individual is no longer taking any psychotropic drugs and after regular sleep-wake patterns, without shift work or sleep deprivation, have been documented.

A sleep-onset REM period during the polysomnography (REM sleep latency less than or equal to 15 minutes) is highly specific (approximately 1% positive in control subjects) but moderately sensitive (approximately 50%). A positive MSLT result displays an average sleep latency of less than or equal to 8 minutes, and sleep-onset REM periods in two or more naps on a four- or five-nap test. The MSLT result is positive in 90%–95% of individuals with narcolepsy versus 2%–4% of control subjects or individuals with other sleep disorders. Additional polysomnographic findings often include frequent arousals, decreased sleep efficiency, and increased stage 1 sleep. Periodic limb movements (found in about 40% of individuals with narcolepsy) and sleep apnea are often noted.

Hypocretin deficiency is demonstrated by measuring CSF hypocretin-1 immunoreactivity. The test is particularly useful in individuals with suspected conversion disorder and those without typical cataplexy, or in treatment-refractory cases. The diagnostic value of the test is not affected by medications, sleep deprivation, or circadian time, but the findings are uninterpretable when the individual is severely ill with a concurrent infection or head trauma or is comatose. CSF cytology, protein, and glucose are within normal range even when sampled within weeks of rapid onset. CSF hypocretin-1 in these incipient cases is typically already very diminished or undetectable.

Functional Consequences of Narcolepsy

Driving and working are impaired, and individuals with narcolepsy should avoid jobs that place themselves (e.g., working with machinery) or others (e.g., bus driver, pilot) in danger. Once the narcolepsy is controlled with therapy, patients can usually drive, although rarely long distances alone. Untreated individuals are also at risk for social isolation and accidental injury to themselves or others. Social relations may suffer as these individuals strive to avert cataplexy by exerting control over emotions.

Differential Diagnosis

Other hypersomnias.   Hypersomnolence and narcolepsy are similar with respect to the degree of daytime sleepiness, age at onset, and stable course over time but can be distinguished based on distinctive clinical and laboratory features. Individuals with hypersomnolence typically have longer and less disrupted nocturnal sleep, greater difficulty awakening, more persistent daytime sleepiness (as opposed to more discrete "sleep attacks" in narcolepsy), longer and less refreshing daytime sleep episodes, and little or no dreaming during daytime naps. By contrast, individuals with narcolepsy have cataplexy and recurrent intrusions of elements of REM sleep into the transition between sleep and wakefulness (e.g., sleep-related hallucinations and sleep paralysis). The MSLT typically demonstrates shorter sleep latencies (i.e., greater physiological sleepiness) as well as the presence of multiple sleep-onset REM periods in individuals with narcolepsy.

Sleep deprivation and insufficient nocturnal sleep. Sleep deprivation and insufficient nocturnal sleep are common in adolescents and shift workers. In adolescents, difficulties falling asleep at night are common, causing sleep deprivation. The MSLT result may be positive if conducted while the individual is sleep deprived or while his or her sleep is phase delayed.

Sleep apnea syndromes. Sleep apneas are especially likely in the presence of obesity. Because obstructive sleep apnea is more frequent than narcolepsy, cataplexy may be overlooked (or absent), and the individual is assumed to have obstructive sleep apnea unresponsive to usual therapies.

Major depressive disorder. Narcolepsy or hypersomnia may be associated or confused with depression. Cataplexy is not present in depression. The MSLT results are most often normal, and there is dissociation between subjective and objective sleepiness, as measured by the mean sleep latency during the MSLT.

Conversion disorder (functional neurological symptom disorder). Atypical features, such as long-lasting cataplexy or unusual triggers, may be present in conversion disorder (functional neurological symptom disorder). Individuals may report sleeping and dreaming, yet the MSLT does not show the characteristic sleep-onset REM period. Full-blown, long-lasting pseudocataplexy may occur during consultation, allowing the examining physician enough time to verify reflexes, which remain intact.

Attention-deficit/hyperactivity disorder or other behavioral problems. In children and adolescents, sleepiness can cause behavioral problems, including aggressiveness and inattention, leading to a misdiagnosis of attention-deficit/hyperactivity disorder.

Seizures. In young children, cataplexy can be misdiagnosed as seizures. Seizures are not commonly triggered by emotions, and when they are, the trigger is not usually laughing or joking. During a seizure, individuals are more likely to hurt themselves when falling. Seizures characterized by isolated atonia are rarely seen in isolation of other seizures, and they also have signatures on the electroencephalogram.

Chorea and movement disorders. In young children, cataplexy can be misdiagnosed as chorea or pediatric autoimmune neuropsychiatric disorders associated with streptococcal infections, especially in the context of a strep throat infection and high antistreptolysin O antibody levels. Some children may have an overlapping movement disorder close to onset of the cataplexy.

Schizophrenia. In the presence of florid and vivid hypnagogic hallucinations, individuals may think these experiences are real—a feature that suggests schizophrenia. Similarly, with stimulant treatment, persecutory delusions may develop. If cataplexy is present, the clinician should first assume that these symptoms are secondary to narcolepsy before considering a co-occurring diagnosis of schizophrenia.

Comorbidity

Narcolepsy can co-occur with bipolar, depressive, and anxiety disorders, and in rare cases with schizophrenia. Narcolepsy is also associated with increased body mass index or obesity, especially when the narcolepsy is untreated. Rapid weight gain is common in young children with a sudden disease onset. Comorbid sleep apnea should be considered if there is a sudden aggravation of preexisting narcolepsy.

Relationship to International Classification of Sleep Disorders

The *International Classification of Sleep Disorders*, 2nd Edition (ICSD-2), differentiates five subtypes of narcolepsy.

Breathing-Related Sleep Disorders

The breathing-related sleep disorders category encompasses three relatively distinct disorders: obstructive sleep apnea hypopnea, central sleep apnea, and sleep-related hypoventilation.

Obstructive Sleep Apnea Hypopnea

Diagnostic Criteria   **327.23 (G47.33)**

A. Either (1) or (2):

1. Evidence by polysomnography of at least five obstructive apneas or hypopneas per hour of sleep and either of the following sleep symptoms:

    a. Nocturnal breathing disturbances: snoring, snorting/gasping, or breathing pauses during sleep.
    b. Daytime sleepiness, fatigue, or unrefreshing sleep despite sufficient opportunities to sleep that is not better explained by another mental disorder (including a sleep disorder) and is not attributable to another medical condition.

2. Evidence by polysomnography of 15 or more obstructive apneas and/or hypopneas per hour of sleep regardless of accompanying symptoms.

Specify current severity:
   Mild: Apnea hypopnea index is less than 15.
   Moderate: Apnea hypopnea index is 15–30.
   Severe: Apnea hypopnea index is greater than 30.

Specifiers

Disease severity is measured by a count of the number of apneas plus hypopneas per hour of sleep (apnea hypopnea index) using polysomnography or other overnight monitoring. Overall severity is also informed by levels of nocturnal desaturation and sleep fragmentation (measured by brain cortical arousal frequency and sleep stages) and degree of associated symptoms and daytime impairment. However, the exact number and thresholds may vary according to the specific measurement techniques used, and these numbers may change over time. Regardless of the apnea hypopnea index (count) per se, the disorder is considered to be more severe when apneas and hypopneas are accompanied by significant oxygen hemoglobin desaturation (e.g., when more than 10% of the sleep time is spent at desaturation levels of less than 90%) or when sleep is severely fragmented as shown by an elevated arousal index (arousal index greater than 30) or reduced stages in deep sleep (e.g., percentage stage N3 [slow-wave sleep] less than 5%).

Diagnostic Features

Obstructive sleep apnea hypopnea is the most common breathing-related sleep disorder. It is characterized by repeated episodes of upper (pharyngeal) airway obstruction (apneas and hypopneas) during sleep. *Apnea* refers to the total absence of airflow, and *hypopnea* refers to a reduction in airflow. Each apnea or hypopnea represents a reduction in breathing of at least 10 seconds in duration in adults or two missed breaths in children and is typically associated with drops in oxygen saturation of 3% or greater and/or an electroencephalographic arousal. Both sleep-related (nocturnal) and wake-time symptoms are common. The cardinal symptoms of obstructive sleep apnea hypopnea are snoring and daytime sleepiness.

Obstructive sleep apnea hypopnea in adults is diagnosed on the basis of polysomnographic findings and symptoms. The diagnosis is based on symptoms of 1) nocturnal breathing disturbances (i.e., snoring, snorting/gasping, breathing pauses during sleep), or 2) daytime sleepiness, fatigue, or unrefreshing sleep despite sufficient opportunities to sleep that are not better explained by another mental disorder and not attributable to another medical condition, along with 3) evidence by polysomnography of five or more obstructive apneas or hypopneas per hour of sleep (Criterion A1). Diagnosis can be made in the absence of these symptoms if there is evidence by polysomnography of 15 or more obstructive apneas and/or hypopneas per hour of sleep (Criterion A2).

Specific attention to disturbed sleep occurring in association with snoring or breathing pauses and physical findings that increase risk of obstructive sleep apnea hypopnea (e.g., central obesity, crowded pharyngeal airway, elevated blood pressure) is needed to reduce the chance of misdiagnosing this treatable condition.

Associated Features Supporting Diagnosis

Because of the frequency of nocturnal awakenings that occur with obstructive sleep apnea hypopnea, individuals may report symptoms of insomnia. Other common, though nonspecific, symptoms of obstructive sleep apnea hypopnea are heartburn, nocturia, morning headaches, dry mouth, erectile dysfunction, and reduced libido. Rarely, individuals may complain of difficulty breathing while lying supine or sleeping. Hypertension may occur in more than 60% of individuals with obstructive sleep apnea hypopnea.

Prevalence

Obstructive sleep apnea hypopnea is a very common disorder, affecting at least 1%–2% of children, 2%–15% of middle-age adults, and more than 20% of older individuals. In the general community, prevalence rates of undiagnosed obstructive sleep apnea hypopnea may be very high in elderly individuals. Since the disorder is strongly associated with obesity, increases in obesity rates are likely to be accompanied by an increased prevalence of this disorder. Prevalence may be particularly high among males, older adults, and certain racial/ethnic groups. In adults, the male-to-female ratio of obstructive sleep apnea hypopnea ranges from 2:1 to 4:1. Gender differences decline in older age, possibly because of an increased prevalence in females after menopause. There is no gender difference among prepubertal children.

Development and Course

The age distribution of obstructive sleep apnea hypopnea likely follows a **J**-shaped distribution. There is a peak in children ages 3–8 years when the nasopharynx may be compromised by a relatively large mass of tonsillar tissue compared with the size of the upper airway. With growth of the airway and regression of lymphoid tissue during later childhood, there is reduction in prevalence. Then, as obesity prevalence increases in midlife and females enter menopause, obstructive sleep apnea hypopnea again increases. The course in older age is unclear; the disorder may level off after age 65 years, but in other individuals, prevalence may increase with aging. Because there is some age dependency of the occurrence of apneas and hypopneas, polysomnographic results must be interpreted in light of other clinical data. In particular, significant clinical symptoms of insomnia or hypersomnia should be investigated regardless of the individual's age.

Obstructive sleep apnea hypopnea usually has an insidious onset, gradual progression, and persistent course. Typically the loud snoring has been present for many years, often since childhood, but an increase in its severity may lead the individual to seek evaluation. Weight gain may precipitate an increase in symptoms. Although obstructive sleep apnea hypopnea can occur at any age, it most commonly manifests among individuals ages 40–60 years. Over 4–5 years, the average apnea hypopnea index increases in adults and older individuals by approximately two apneas/hypopneas per hour. The apnea hypopnea index is increased and incident obstructive sleep apnea hypopnea is greater among individuals who are older, who are male, or who have a higher baseline body mass index (BMI) or increase their BMI over time. Spontaneous resolution of obstructive sleep apnea hypopnea has been reported with weight loss, particularly after bariatric surgery. In children, seasonal variation in obstructive sleep apnea hypopnea has been observed, as has improvement with overall growth.

In young children, the signs and symptoms of obstructive sleep apnea hypopnea may be more subtle than in adults, making diagnosis more difficult to establish. Polysomnography is useful in confirming diagnosis. Evidence of fragmentation of sleep on the polysomnogram may not be as apparent as in studies of older individuals, possibly because of the high homeostatic drive in young individuals. Symptoms such as snoring are usually parent-reported and thus have reduced sensitivity. Agitated arousals and unusual sleep postures, such as sleeping on the hands and knees, may occur. Nocturnal enuresis also may occur and should raise the suspicion of obstructive sleep apnea hypopnea if it recurs in a child who was previously dry at night. Children may also manifest excessive daytime sleepiness, although this is not as common or pronounced as in adults. Daytime mouth breathing, difficulty in swallowing, and poor speech articulation are also common features in children. Children younger than 5 years more often present with nighttime symptoms, such as observed apneas or labored breathing, than with behavioral symptoms (i.e., the nighttime symptoms are more noticeable and more often bring the child to clinical attention). In children older than 5 years, daytime symptoms such as sleepiness and behavioral problems (e.g., impulsivity and hyperactivity), attention-deficit/hyperactivity disorder, learning difficulties, and morning headaches are more often the focus of concern. Children with obstructive sleep apnea hypopnea also may present with failure to thrive and developmental delays. In young children, obesity is a less common risk factor, while delayed growth and "failure to thrive" may be present.

Risk and Prognostic Factors

Genetic and physiological.   The major risk factors for obstructive sleep apnea hypopnea are obesity and male gender. Others include maxillary-mandibular retrognathia or micrognathia, positive family history of sleep apnea, genetic syndromes that reduce upper airway patency (e.g., Down syndrome, Treacher Collins syndrome), adenotonsillar hypertrophy (especially in young children), menopause (in females), and various endocrine syndromes (e.g., acromegaly). Compared with premenopausal females, males are at increased risk for obstructive sleep apnea hypopnea, possibly reflecting the influences of sex hormones on ventilatory control and body fat distribution, as well as because of gender differences in airway structure. Medications for mental disorders and medical conditions that tend to induce somnolence may worsen the course of apnea symptoms if these medications are not managed carefully.

Obstructive sleep apnea hypopnea has a strong genetic basis, as evidenced by the significant familial aggregation of the apnea hypopnea index. The prevalence of obstructive sleep apnea hypopnea is approximately twice as high among the first-degree relatives of probands with obstructive sleep apnea hypopnea as compared with members of control families. One-third of the variance in the apnea hypopnea index is explained by shared familial factors. Although genetic markers with diagnostic or prognostic value are not yet available for use, eliciting a family history of obstructive sleep apnea hypopnea should increase the clinical suspicion for the disorder.

Culture-Related Diagnostic Issues

There is a potential for sleepiness and fatigue to be reported differently across cultures. In some groups, snoring may be considered a sign of health and thus may not trigger concerns. Individuals of Asian ancestry may be at increased risk for obstructive sleep apnea hypopnea despite relatively low BMI, possibly reflecting the influence of craniofacial risk factors that narrow the nasopharynx.

Gender-Related Diagnostic Issues

Females may more commonly report fatigue rather than sleepiness and may underreport snoring.

Diagnostic Markers

Polysomnography provides quantitative data on frequency of sleep-related respiratory disturbances and associated changes in oxygen saturation and sleep continuity. Polysomnographic findings in children differ from those in adults in that children demonstrate labored breathing, partial obstructive hypoventilation with cyclical desaturations, hypercapnia and paradoxical movements. Apnea hypopnea index levels as low as 2 are used to define thresholds of abnormality in children.

Arterial blood gas measurements while the individual is awake are usually normal, but some individuals can have waking hypoxemia or hypercapnia. This pattern should alert the clinician to the possibility of coexisting lung disease or hypoventilation. Imaging procedures may reveal narrowing of the upper airway. Cardiac testing may show evidence of impaired ventricular function. Individuals with severe nocturnal oxygen desaturation may also have elevated hemoglobin or hematocrit values. Validated sleep measures (e.g., multiple sleep latency test [MSLT], maintenance of wakefulness test) may identify sleepiness.

Functional Consequences of Obstructive Sleep Apnea Hypopnea

More than 50% of individuals with moderate to severe obstructive sleep apnea hypopnea report symptoms of daytime sleepiness. A twofold increased risk of occupational accidents has been reported in association with symptoms of snoring and sleepiness. Motor vehicle crashes also have been reported to be as much as sevenfold higher among individuals with elevated apnea hypopnea index values. Clinicians should be cognizant of state government requirements for reporting this disorder, especially in relationship to commercial drivers. Reduced scores on measures of health-related quality of life are common in individuals with obstructive sleep apnea hypopnea, with the largest decrements observed in the physical and vitality subscales.

Differential Diagnosis

Primary snoring and other sleep disorders.   Individuals with obstructive sleep apnea hypopnea must be differentiated from individuals with primary snoring (i.e., otherwise asymptomatic individuals who snore and do not have abnormalities on overnight polysomnography). Individuals with obstructive sleep apnea hypopnea may additionally report nocturnal gasping and choking. The presence of sleepiness or other daytime symptoms not explained by other etiologies suggests the diagnosis of obstructive sleep apnea hypopnea, but this differentiation requires polysomnography. Definitive differential diagnosis between hypersomnia, central sleep apnea, sleep-related hypoventilation, and obstructive sleep apnea hypopnea also requires polysomnographic studies.

Obstructive sleep apnea hypopnea must be differentiated from other causes of sleepiness, such as narcolepsy, hypersomnia, and circadian rhythm sleep disorders. Obstructive sleep apnea hypopnea can be differentiated from narcolepsy by the absence of cataplexy, sleep-related hallucinations, and sleep paralysis and by the presence of loud snoring, gasping during sleep, or observed apneas in sleep. Daytime sleep episodes in narcolepsy are characteristically shorter, more refreshing, and more often associated with dreaming. Obstructive sleep apnea hypopnea shows characteristic apneas and hypopneas and oxygen desaturation during nocturnal polysomnographic studies. Narcolepsy results in multiple sleep-onset rapid eye movement (REM) periods during the MSLT. Narcolepsy, like obstructive sleep apnea hypopnea, may be associated with obesity, and some individuals have concurrent narcolepsy and obstructive sleep apnea hypopnea. A diagnosis of narcolepsy does not exclude the diagnosis of obstructive sleep apnea hypopnea, as the two conditions may co-occur.

Insomnia disorder.   For individuals complaining of difficulty initiating or maintaining sleep or early-morning awakenings, insomnia disorder can be differentiated from obstructive sleep apnea hypopnea by the absence of snoring and the absence of the history, signs, and symptoms characteristic of the latter disorder. However, insomnia and obstructive sleep apnea hypopnea may coexist, and if so, both disorders may need to be addressed concurrently to improve sleep.

Panic attacks.   Nocturnal panic attacks may include symptoms of gasping or choking during sleep that may be difficult to distinguish clinically from obstructive sleep apnea hypopnea. However, the lower frequency of episodes, intense autonomic arousal, and lack of excessive sleepiness differentiate nocturnal panic attacks from obstructive sleep apnea hypopnea. Polysomnography in individuals with nocturnal panic attacks does not reveal the typical pattern of apneas or oxygen desaturation characteristic of obstructive sleep apnea hypopnea. Individuals with obstructive sleep apnea hypopnea do not provide a history of daytime panic attacks.

Attention-deficit/hyperactivity disorder.   Attention-deficit/hyperactivity disorder in children may include symptoms of inattention, academic impairment, hyperactivity, and internalizing behaviors, all of which may also be symptoms of childhood obstructive sleep apnea hypopnea. The presence of other symptoms and signs of childhood obstructive sleep apnea hypopnea (e.g., labored breathing or snoring during sleep and adenotonsillar hypertrophy) would suggest the presence of obstructive sleep apnea hypopnea. Obstructive sleep apnea hypopnea and attention-deficit/hyperactivity disorder may commonly co-occur, and there may be causal links between them; therefore, risk factors such as enlarged tonsils, obesity, or a family history of sleep apnea may help alert the clinician to their co-occurrence.

Substance/medication-induced insomnia or hypersomnia.   Substance use and substance withdrawal (including medications) can produce insomnia or hypersomnia. A careful history is usually sufficient to identify the relevant substance/medication, and follow-up shows improvement of the sleep disturbance after discontinuation of the substance/medication. In other cases, the use of a substance/medication (e.g., alcohol, barbiturates, benzodiazepines, tobacco) has been shown to exacerbate obstructive sleep apnea hypopnea. An individual with symptoms and signs consistent with obstructive sleep apnea hypopnea should receive that diagnosis, even in the presence of concurrent substance use that is exacerbating the condition.

Comorbidity

Systemic hypertension, coronary artery disease, heart failure, stroke, diabetes, and increased mortality are consistently associated with obstructive sleep apnea hypopnea. Risk estimates vary from 30% to as much as 300% for moderate to severe obstructive sleep apnea hypopnea. Evidence of pulmonary hypertension and right heart failure (e.g., cor pulmonale, ankle edema, hepatic congestion) are rare in obstructive sleep apnea hypopnea and when present indicate either very severe disease or associated hypoventilation or cardiopulmonary comorbidities. Obstructive sleep apnea hypopnea also may occur with increased frequency in association with a number of medical or neurological conditions (e.g., cerebrovascular disease, Parkinson's disease). Physical findings reflect the co-occurrence of these conditions.

As many as one-third of individuals referred for evaluation of obstructive sleep apnea hypopnea report symptoms of depression, with as many of 10% having depression scores consistent with moderate to severe depression. Severity of obstructive sleep apnea hypopnea, as measured by the apnea hypopnea index, has been found to be correlated with severity of symptoms of depression. This association may be stronger in males than in females.

Relationship to International Classification of Sleep Disorders

The *International Classification of Sleep Disorders,* 2nd Edition (ICSD-2), differentiates 11 subtypes of "sleep-related breathing disorders," including primary central sleep apnea, obstructive sleep apnea, and sleep-related hypoventilation.

Central Sleep Apnea

Diagnostic Criteria

A. Evidence by polysomnography of five or more central apneas per hour of sleep.
B. The disorder is not better explained by another current sleep disorder.

Specify whether:

327.21 (G47.31) Idiopathic central sleep apnea: Characterized by repeated episodes of apneas and hypopneas during sleep caused by variability in respiratory effort but without evidence of airway obstruction.

786.04 (R06.3) Cheyne-Stokes breathing: A pattern of periodic crescendo-decrescendo variation in tidal volume that results in central apneas and hypopneas at a frequency of at least five events per hour, accompanied by frequent arousal.

780.57 (G47.37) Central sleep apnea comorbid with opioid use: The pathogenesis of this subtype is attributed to the effects of opioids on the respiratory rhythm generators in the medulla as well as the differential effects on hypoxic versus hypercapnic respiratory drive.

Coding note (for 780.57 [G47.37] code only): When an opioid use disorder is present, first code the opioid use disorder: 305.50 (F11.10) mild opioid use disorder or 304.00 (F11.20) moderate or severe opioid use disorder; then code 780.57 (G47.37) central sleep apnea comorbid with opioid use. When an opioid use disorder is not present (e.g., after a one-time heavy use of the substance), code only 780.57 (G47.37) central sleep apnea comorbid with opioid use.

Note: See the section "Diagnostic Features" in text.

Specify current severity:

Severity of central sleep apnea is graded according to the frequency of the breathing disturbances as well as the extent of associated oxygen desaturation and sleep fragmentation that occur as a consequence of repetitive respiratory disturbances.

Subtypes

Idiopathic central sleep apnea and Cheyne-Stokes breathing are characterized by increased gain of the ventilatory control system, also referred to as *high loop gain,* which leads to instability in ventilation and $PaCO_2$ levels. This instability is termed *periodic breathing* and can be recognized by hyperventilation alternating with hypoventilation. Individuals with these disorders typically have pCO_2 levels while awake that are slightly hypocapneic or normocapneic. Central sleep apnea may also manifest during initiation of treatment of obstructive sleep apnea hypopnea or may occur in association with obstructive sleep apnea hypopnea syndrome (termed *complex sleep apnea*). The occurrence of central sleep apnea in association with obstructive sleep apnea is also considered to be due to high loop gain. In contrast, the pathogenesis of central sleep apnea comorbid with opioid use has been attributed to the effects of opioids on the respiratory rhythm generators in the medulla as well as to its differential effects on hypoxic versus hypercapneic respiratory drive. These individuals may have elevated pCO_2 levels while awake. Individuals receiving chronic methadone maintenance therapy have been noted to have increased somnolence and depression, although the role of breathing disorders associated with opioid medication in causing these problems has not been studied.

Specifiers

An increase in the central apnea index (i.e., number of central apneas per hour of sleep) reflects an increase in severity of central sleep apnea. Sleep continuity and quality may be markedly impaired with reductions in restorative stages of non–rapid eye movement (REM) sleep (i.e., decreased slow-wave sleep [stage N3]). In individuals with severe Cheyne-Stokes breathing, the pattern can also be observed during resting wakefulness, a finding that is thought to be a poor prognostic marker for mortality.

Diagnostic Features

Central sleep apnea disorders are characterized by repeated episodes of apneas and hypopneas during sleep caused by variability in respiratory effort. These are disorders of ventilatory control in which respiratory events occur in a periodic or intermittent pattern. *Idiopathic central sleep apnea* is characterized by sleepiness, insomnia, and awakenings due to dyspnea in association with five or more central apneas per hour of sleep. Central sleep apnea occurring in individuals with heart failure, stroke, or renal failure typically have a breathing pattern called *Cheyne-Stokes breathing,* which is characterized by a pattern of periodic crescendo-decrescendo variation in tidal volume that results in central apneas and hypopneas occurring at a frequency of at least five events per hour that are accompanied by frequent arousals. Central and obstructive sleep apneas may coexist; the ratio of central to obstructive apneas/hypopneas may be used to identify which condition is predominant.

Alterations in neuromuscular control of breathing can occur in association with medications or substances used in individuals with mental health conditions, which can cause or exacerbate impairments of respiratory rhythm and ventilation. Individuals taking these medications have a sleep-related breathing disorder that could contribute to sleep disturbances and symptoms such as sleepiness, confusion, and depression. Specifically, *chronic use of long-acting opioid medications* is often associated with impairment of respiratory control leading to central sleep apnea.

Associated Features Supporting Diagnosis

Individuals with central sleep apnea hypopneas can manifest with sleepiness or insomnia. There can be complaints of sleep fragmentation, including awakening with dyspnea. Some individuals are asymptomatic. Obstructive sleep apnea hypopnea can coexist with Cheyne-Stokes breathing, and thus snoring and abruptly terminating apneas may be observed during sleep.

Prevalence

The prevalence of idiopathic central sleep apnea is unknown but thought to be rare. The prevalence of Cheyne-Stokes breathing is high in individuals with depressed cardiac ventricular ejection fraction. In individuals with an ejection fraction of less than 45%, the prevalence has been reported to be 20% or higher. The male-to-female ratio for prevalence is even more highly skewed toward males than for obstructive sleep apnea hypopnea. Prevalence increases with age, and most patients are older than 60 years. Cheyne-Stokes breathing occurs in approximately 20% of individuals with acute stroke. Central sleep apnea comorbid with opioid use occurs in approximately 30% of individuals taking chronic opioids for nonmalignant pain and similarly in individuals receiving methadone maintenance therapy.

Development and Course

The onset of Cheyne-Stokes breathing appears tied to the development of heart failure. The Cheyne-Stokes breathing pattern is associated with oscillations in heart rate, blood pressure and oxygen desaturation, and elevated sympathetic nervous system activity that can promote progression of heart failure. The clinical significance of Cheyne-Stokes breathing in the setting of stroke is not known, but Cheyne-Stokes breathing may be a transient finding that resolves with time after acute stroke. Central sleep apnea comorbid with opioid use has been documented with chronic use (i.e., several months).

Risk and Prognostic Factors

Genetic and physiological. Cheyne-Stokes breathing is frequently present in individuals with heart failure. The coexistence of atrial fibrillation further increases risk, as do older age and male gender. Cheyne-Stokes breathing is also seen in association with acute stroke and possibly renal failure. The underlying ventilatory instability in the setting of heart failure has been attributed to increased ventilatory chemosensitivity and hyperventilation due to pulmonary vascular congestion and circulatory delay. Central sleep apnea is seen in individuals taking long-acting opioids.

Diagnostic Markers

Physical findings seen in individuals with a Cheyne-Stokes breathing pattern relate to its risk factors. Findings consistent with heart failure, such as jugular venous distension, S_3 heart sound, lung crackles, and lower extremity edema, may be present. Polysomnography is used to characterize the breathing characteristics of each breathing-related sleep disorder subtype. Central sleep apneas are recorded when periods of breathing cessation for longer than 10 seconds occur. Cheyne-Stokes breathing is characterized by a pattern of periodic crescendo-decrescendo variation in tidal volume that results in central apneas and hypopneas occurring at a frequency of at least five events per hour that are accompanied by frequent arousals. The cycle length of Cheyne-Stokes breathing (or time from end of one central apnea to the end of the next apnea) is about 60 seconds.

Functional Consequences of Central Sleep Apnea

Idiopathic central sleep apnea has been reported to cause symptoms of disrupted sleep, including insomnia and sleepiness. Cheyne-Stokes breathing with comorbid heart failure has been associated with excessive sleepiness, fatigue, and insomnia, although many individuals may be asymptomatic. Coexistence of heart failure and Cheyne-Stokes breathing may be associated with increased cardiac arrhythmias and increased mortality or cardiac transplantation. Individuals with central sleep apnea comorbid with opioid use may present with symptoms of sleepiness or insomnia.

Differential Diagnosis

Idiopathic central sleep apnea must be distinguished from other breathing-related sleep disorders, other sleep disorders, and medical conditions and mental disorders that cause sleep fragmentation, sleepiness, and fatigue. This is achieved using polysomnography.

Other breathing-related sleep disorders and sleep disorders.   Central sleep apnea can be distinguished from obstructive sleep apnea hypopnea by the presence of at least five central apneas per hour of sleep. These conditions may co-occur, but central sleep apnea is considered to predominate when the ratio of central to obstructive respiratory events exceeds 50%.

Cheyne-Stokes breathing can be distinguished from other mental disorders, including other sleep disorders, and other medical conditions that cause sleep fragmentation, sleepiness, and fatigue based on the presence of a predisposing condition (e.g., heart failure or stroke) and signs and polysomnographic evidence of the characteristic breathing pattern. Polysomnographic respiratory findings can help distinguish Cheyne-Stokes breathing from insomnia due to other medical conditions. High-altitude periodic breathing has a pattern that resembles Cheyne-Stokes breathing but has a shorter cycle time, occurs only at high altitude, and is not associated with heart failure.

Central sleep apnea comorbid with opioid use can be differentiated from other types of breathing-related sleep disorders based on the use of long-acting opioid medications in conjunction with polysomnographic evidence of central apneas and periodic or ataxic breathing. It can be distinguished from insomnia due to drug or substance use based on polysomnographic evidence of central sleep apnea.

Comorbidity

Central sleep apnea disorders are frequently present in users of long-acting opioids, such as methadone. Individuals taking these medications have a sleep-related breathing disorder that could contribute to sleep disturbances and symptoms such as sleepiness, confusion, and depression. While the individual is asleep, breathing patterns such as central apneas, periodic apneas, and ataxic breathing may be observed. Obstructive sleep apnea hypopnea may coexist with central sleep apnea, and features consistent with this condition can also be present (see "Obstructive Sleep Apnea Hypopnea" earlier in this chapter). Cheyne-Stokes breathing is more commonly observed in association with conditions that include heart failure, stroke, and renal failure and is seen more frequently in individuals with atrial fibrillation. Individuals with Cheyne-Stokes breathing are more likely to be older, to be male, and to have lower weight than individuals with obstructive sleep apnea hypopnea.

Sleep-Related Hypoventilation

Diagnostic Criteria

A. Polysomnograpy demonstrates episodes of decreased respiration associated with elevated CO_2 levels. (**Note:** In the absence of objective measurement of CO_2, persistent low levels of hemoglobin oxygen saturation unassociated with apneic/hypopneic events may indicate hypoventilation.)

B. The disturbance is not better explained by another current sleep disorder.

Specify whether:

327.24 (G47.34) Idiopathic hypoventilation: This subtype is not attributable to any readily identified condition.

327.25 (G47.35) Congenital central alveolar hypoventilation: This subtype is a rare congenital disorder in which the individual typically presents in the perinatal period with shallow breathing, or cyanosis and apnea during sleep.

327.26 (G47.36) Comorbid sleep-related hypoventilation: This subtype occurs as a consequence of a medical condition, such as a pulmonary disorder (e.g., interstitial lung disease, chronic obstructive pulmonary disease) or a neuromuscular or chest wall disorder (e.g., muscular dystrophies, postpolio syndrome, cervical spinal cord injury, kyphoscoliosis), or medications (e.g., benzodiazepines, opiates). It also occurs with obesity (obesity hypoventilation disorder), where it reflects a combination of increased work of breathing due to reduced chest wall compliance and ventilation-perfusion mismatch and variably reduced ventilatory drive. Such individuals usually are characterized by body mass index of greater than 30 and hypercapnia during wakefulness (with a pCO_2 of greater than 45), without other evidence of hypoventilation.

Specify current severity:

Severity is graded according to the degree of hypoxemia and hypercarbia present during sleep and evidence of end organ impairment due to these abnormalities (e.g., right-sided heart failure). The presence of blood gas abnormalities during wakefulness is an indicator of greater severity.

Subtypes

Regarding obesity hypoventilation disorder, the prevalence of obesity hypoventilation in the general population is not known but is thought to be increasing in association with the increased prevalence of obesity and extreme obesity.

Diagnostic Features

Sleep-related hypoventilation can occur independently or, more frequently, comorbid with medical or neurological disorders, medication use, or substance use disorder. Although symptoms are not mandatory to make this diagnosis, individuals often report excessive daytime sleepiness, frequent arousals and awakenings during sleep, morning headaches, and insomnia complaints.

Associated Features Supporting Diagnosis

Individuals with sleep-related hypoventilation can present with sleep-related complaints of insomnia or sleepiness. Episodes of orthopnea can occur in individuals with diaphragm weakness. Headaches upon awakening may be present. During sleep, episodes of shallow breathing may be observed, and obstructive sleep apnea hypopnea or central sleep apnea may coexist. Consequences of ventilatory insufficiency, including pulmonary hypertension, cor pulmonale (right heart failure), polycythemia, and neurocognitive dysfunction, can be present. With progression of ventilatory insufficiency, blood gas abnormalities extend into wakefulness. Features of the medical condition causing sleep-related hypoventilation can also be present. Episodes of hypoventilation may be associated with frequent arousals or bradytachycardia. Individuals may complain of excessive sleepiness and insomnia or morning headaches or may present with findings of neurocognitive dysfunction or depression. Hypoventilation may not be present during wakefulness.

Prevalence

Idiopathic sleep-related hypoventilation in adults is very uncommon. The prevalence of congenital central alveolar hypoventilation is unknown, but the disorder is rare. Comorbid sleep-related hypoventilation (i.e., hypoventilation comorbid with other conditions, such as chronic obstructive pulmonary disease [COPD], neuromuscular disorders, or obesity) is more common.

Development and Course

Idiopathic sleep-related hypoventilation is thought to be a slowly progressive disorder of respiratory impairment. When this disorder occurs comorbidly with other disorders (e.g., COPD, neuromuscular disorders, obesity), disease severity reflects the severity of the underlying condition, and the disorder progresses as the condition worsens. Complications such as pulmonary hypertension, cor pulmonale, cardiac dysrhythmias, polycythemia, neurocognitive dysfunction, and worsening respiratory failure can develop with increasing severity of blood gas abnormalities.

Congenital central alveolar hypoventilation usually manifests at birth with shallow, erratic, or absent breathing. This disorder can also manifest during infancy, childhood, and adulthood because of variable penetrance of the *PHOX2B* mutation. Children with congenital central alveolar hypoventilation are more likely to have disorders of the autonomic nervous system, Hirschsprung's disease, neural crest tumors, and characteristic box-shaped face (i.e., the face is short relative to its width).

Risk and Prognostic Factors

Environmental.   Ventilatory drive can be reduced in individuals using central nervous system depressants, including benzodiazepines, opiates, and alcohol.

Genetic and physiological.   Idiopathic sleep-related hypoventilation is associated with reduced ventilatory drive due to a blunted chemoresponsiveness to CO_2 (reduced respiratory drive; i.e., "won't breathe"), reflecting underlying neurological deficits in centers governing the control of ventilation. More commonly, sleep-related hypoventilation is comorbid with another medical condition, such as a pulmonary disorder, a neuromuscular or chest wall disorder, or hypothyroidism, or with use of medications (e.g., benzodiazepines, opiates). In these conditions, the hypoventilation may be a consequence of increased work of breathing and/or impairment of respiratory muscle function (i.e., "can't breathe") or reduced respiratory drive (i.e., "won't breathe").

Neuromuscular disorders influence breathing through impairment of respiratory motor innervation or respiratory muscle function. They include conditions such as amyotrophic lateral sclerosis, spinal cord injury, diaphragmatic paralysis, myasthenia gravis, Lambert-Eaton syndrome, toxic or metabolic myopathies, postpolio syndrome, and Charcot-Marie-Tooth syndrome.

Congenital central alveolar hypoventilation is a genetic disorder attributable to mutations of *PHOX2B*, a gene that is crucial for the development of the embryonic autonomic nervous system and neural crest derivatives. Children with congenital central alveolar hypoventilation show blunted ventilatory responses to hypercapnia, especially in non–rapid eye movement sleep.

Gender-Related Diagnostic Issues

Gender distributions for sleep-related hypoventilation occurring in association with co-morbid conditions reflect the gender distributions of the comorbid conditions. For example, COPD is more frequently present in males and with increasing age.

Diagnostic Markers

Sleep-related hypoventilation is diagnosed using polysomnography showing sleep-related hypoxemia and hypercapnia that is not better explained by another breathing-related sleep disorder. The documentation of increased arterial pCO_2 levels to greater than 55 mmHg during sleep or a 10 mmHg or greater increase in pCO_2 levels (to a level that also exceeds 50 mmHg) during sleep in comparison to awake supine values, for 10 minutes or longer, is the gold standard for diagnosis. However, obtaining arterial blood gas determinations during sleep is impractical, and non-invasive measures of pCO_2 have not been adequately validated during sleep and are not widely used during polysomnography in adults. Prolonged and sustained decreases in oxygen saturation (oxygen saturation of less than 90% for more than 5 minutes with a nadir of at least 85%, or oxygen saturation of less than 90% for at least 30% of sleep time) in the absence of evidence of upper airway obstruction are often used as an indication of sleep-related hypoventilation; however, this finding is not specific, as there are other potential causes of hypoxemia, such as that due to lung disease.

Functional Consequences of Sleep-Related Hypoventilation

The consequences of sleep-related hypoventilation are related to the effects of chronic exposure to hypercapnia and hypoxemia. These blood gas derangements cause vasoconstriction of the pulmonary vasculature leading to pulmonary hypertension, which, if severe, can result in right-sided heart failure (cor pulmonale). Hypoxemia can lead to dysfunction of organs such as the brain, blood, and heart, leading to outcomes such as cognitive dysfunction, polycythemia, and cardiac arrhythmias. Hypercapnia can depress ventilatory drive, leading to progressive respiratory failure.

Differential Diagnosis

Other medical conditions affecting ventilation.   In adults, the idiopathic variety of sleep-related hypoventilation is very uncommon and is determined by excluding the presence of lung diseases, skeletal malformations, neuromuscular disorders, and other medical and neurological disorders or medications that affect ventilation. Sleep-related hypoventilation must be distinguished from other causes of sleep-related hypoxemia, such as that due to lung disease.

Other breathing-related sleep disorders.   Sleep-related hypoventilation can be distinguished from obstructive sleep apnea hypopnea and central sleep apnea based on clinical features and findings on polysomnography. Sleep-related hypoventilation typically shows more sustained periods of oxygen desaturation rather that the periodic episodes seen in obstructive sleep apnea hypopnea and central sleep apnea. Obstructive sleep apnea hypopnea and central sleep apnea also show a pattern of discrete episodes of repeated airflow decreases that can be absent in sleep-related hypoventilation.

Comorbidity

Sleep-related hypoventilation often occurs in association with a pulmonary disorder (e.g., interstitial lung disease, COPD), with a neuromuscular or chest wall disorder (e.g., muscular dystrophies, post-polio syndrome, cervical spinal cord injury, obesity, kyphoscoliosis), or, most relevant to the mental health provider, with medication use (e.g., benzodiazepines, opiates). Congenital central alveolar hypoventilation often occurs in association with autonomic dysfunction and may occur in association with Hirschsprung's disease. COPD, a disorder of lower airway obstruction usually associated with cigarette smoking, can result in sleep-related hypoventilation and hypoxemia. The presence of coexisting obstructive sleep apnea hypopnea is thought to exacerbate hypoxemia and hypercapnia during sleep and wakefulness. The relationship between congenital central alveolar hypoventilation and idiopathic sleep-related hypoventilation is unclear; in some individuals, idiopathic sleep-related hypoventilation may represent cases of late-onset congenital central alveolar hypoventilation.

Relationship to International Classification of Sleep Disorders

The *International Classification of Sleep Disorders,* 2nd Edition (ICSD-2), combines sleep-related hypoventilation and sleep-related hypoxemia under the category of sleep-related hypoventilation/hypoxemic syndromes. This approach to classification reflects the frequent co-occurrence of disorders that lead to hypoventilation and hypoxemia. In contrast, the classification used in DSM-5 reflects evidence that there are distinct sleep-related pathogenetic processes leading to hypoventilation.

Circadian Rhythm Sleep-Wake Disorders

Diagnostic Criteria

A. A persistent or recurrent pattern of sleep disruption that is primarily due to an alteration of the circadian system or to a misalignment between the endogenous circadian rhythm and the sleep–wake schedule required by an individual's physical environment or social or professional schedule.

B. The sleep disruption leads to excessive sleepiness or insomnia, or both.

C. The sleep disturbance causes clinically significant distress or impairment in social, occupational, and other important areas of functioning.

Coding note: For ICD-9-CM, code **307.45** for all subtypes. For ICD-10-CM, code is based on subtype.

Specify whether:

307.45 (G47.21) Delayed sleep phase type: A pattern of delayed sleep onset and awakening times, with an inability to fall asleep and awaken at a desired or conventionally acceptable earlier time.

Specify if:

Familial: A family history of delayed sleep phase is present.

Specify if:

Overlapping with non-24-hour sleep-wake type: Delayed sleep phase type may overlap with another circadian rhythm sleep-wake disorder, non-24-hour sleep-wake type.

307.45 (G47.22) Advanced sleep phase type: A pattern of advanced sleep onset and awakening times, with an inability to remain awake or asleep until the desired or conventionally acceptable later sleep or wake times.

Specify if:

Familial: A family history of advanced sleep phase is present.

307.45 (G47.23) Irregular sleep-wake type: A temporally disorganized sleep-wake pattern, such that the timing of sleep and wake periods is variable throughout the 24-hour period.

307.45 (G47.24) Non-24-hour sleep-wake type: A pattern of sleep-wake cycles that is not synchronized to the 24-hour environment, with a consistent daily drift (usually to later and later times) of sleep onset and wake times.

307.45 (G47.26) Shift work type: Insomnia during the major sleep period and/or excessive sleepiness (including inadvertent sleep) during the major awake period associated with a shift work schedule (i.e., requiring unconventional work hours).

307.45 (G47.20) Unspecified type

Specify if:

Episodic: Symptoms last at least 1 month but less than 3 months.

Persistent: Symptoms last 3 months or longer.

Recurrent: Two or more episodes occur within the space of 1 year.

Delayed Sleep Phase Type

Diagnostic Features

The delayed sleep phase type is based primarily on a history of a delay in the timing of the major sleep period (usually more than 2 hours) in relation to the desired sleep and wake-up time, resulting in symptoms of insomnia and excessive sleepiness. When allowed to set their own schedule, individuals with delayed sleep phase type exhibit normal sleep quality and duration for age. Symptoms of sleep-onset insomnia, difficulty waking in the morning, and excessive early day sleepiness are prominent.

Associated Features Supporting Diagnosis

Common associated features of delayed sleep phase type include a history of mental disorders or a concurrent mental disorder. Extreme and prolonged difficulty awakening with morning confusion is also common. Psychophysiological insomnia may develop as a result of maladaptive behaviors that impair sleep and increase arousal because of repeated attempts to fall asleep at an earlier time.

Prevalence

Prevalence of delayed sleep phase type in the general population is approximately 0.17% but appears to be greater than 7% in adolescents. Although the prevalence of familial delayed sleep phase type has not been established, a family history of delayed sleep phase is present in individuals with delayed sleep phase type.

Development and Course

Course is persistent, lasting longer than 3 months, with intermittent exacerbations throughout adulthood. Although age at onset is variable, symptoms begin typically in adolescence and early adulthood and persist for several months to years before diagnosis is established. Severity may decrease with age. Relapse of symptoms is common.

Clinical expression may vary across the lifespan depending on social, school, and work obligations. Exacerbation is usually triggered by a change in work or school schedule that requires an early rise time. Individuals who can alter their work schedules to accommodate the delayed circadian sleep and wake timing can experience remission of symptoms.

Increased prevalence in adolescence may be a consequence of both physiological and behavioral factors. Hormonal changes may be involved specifically, as delayed sleep phase is associated with the onset of puberty. Thus, delayed sleep phase type in adolescents should be differentiated from the common delay in the timing of circadian rhythms in this age group. In the familial form, the course is persistent and may not improve significantly with age.

Risk and Prognostic Factors

Genetic and physiological. Predisposing factors may include a longer than average circadian period, changes in light sensitivity, and impaired homeostatic sleep drive. Some individuals with delayed sleep phase type may be hypersensitive to evening light, which can serve as a delay signal to the circadian clock, or they may be hyposensitive to morning light such that its phase-advancing effects are reduced. Genetic factors may play a role in the pathogenesis of familial and sporadic forms of delayed sleep phase type, including mutations in circadian genes (e.g., *PER3, CKIe*).

Diagnostic Markers

Confirmation of the diagnosis includes a complete history and use of a sleep diary or actigraphy (i.e., a wrist-worn motion detector that monitors motor activity for prolonged periods and can be used as a proxy for sleep-wake patterns for at least 7 days). The period covered should include weekends, when social and occupational obligations are less strict, to ensure that the individual exhibits a consistently delayed sleep-wake pattern. Biomarkers such as salivary dim light melatonin onset should be obtained only when the diagnosis is unclear.

Functional Consequences of Delayed Sleep Phase Type

Excessive early day sleepiness is prominent. Extreme and prolonged difficulty awakening with morning confusion (i.e., sleep inertia) is also common. The severity of insomnia and excessive sleepiness symptoms varies substantially among individuals and largely depends on the occupational and social demands on the individual.

Differential Diagnosis

Normative variations in sleep. Delayed sleep phase type must be distinguished from "normal" sleep patterns in which an individual has a late schedule that does not cause personal, social, or occupational distress (most commonly seen in adolescents and young adults).

Other sleep disorders. Insomnia disorder and other circadian rhythm sleep-wake disorders should be included in the differential. Excessive sleepiness may also be caused by other sleep disturbances, such as breathing-related sleep disorders, insomnias, sleep-related movement disorders, and medical, neurological, and mental disorders. Overnight polysomnography may help in evaluating for other comorbid sleep disorders, such as sleep apnea. The circadian nature of delayed sleep phase type, however, should differentiate it from other disorders with similar complaints.

Comorbidity

Delayed sleep phase type is strongly associated with depression, personality disorder, and somatic symptom disorder or illness anxiety disorder. In addition, comorbid sleep disorders, such as insomnia disorder, restless legs syndrome, and sleep apnea, as well as depressive and bipolar disorders and anxiety disorders, can exacerbate symptoms of insomnia and excessive sleepiness. Delayed sleep phase type may overlap with another circadian rhythm sleep-wake disorder, non-24-hour sleep-wake type. Sighted individuals with non-24-hour sleep-wake type disorder commonly also have a history of delayed circadian sleep phase.

Advanced Sleep Phase Type

Specifiers

Advanced sleep phase type may be documented with the specified "familial." Although the prevalence of familial advanced sleep phase type has not been established, a family history of advanced sleep phase is present in individuals with advanced sleep phase type. In this type, specific mutations demonstrate an autosomal dominant mode of inheritance. In the familial form, onset of symptoms may occur earlier (during childhood and early adulthood), the course is persistent, and the severity of symptoms may increase with age.

Diagnostic Features

Advanced sleep phase type is characterized by sleep-wake times that are several hours earlier than desired or conventional times. Diagnosis is based primarily on a history of an advance in the timing of the major sleep period (usually more than 2 hours) in relation to the desired sleep and wake-up time, with symptoms of early morning insomnia and excessive daytime sleepiness. When allowed to set their schedule, individuals with advanced sleep phase type will exhibit normal sleep quality and duration for age.

Associated Features Supporting Diagnosis

Individuals with advanced sleep phase type are "morning types," having earlier sleep-wake times, with the timing of circadian biomarkers such as melatonin and core body temperature rhythms occurring 2–4 hours earlier than normal. When required to keep a conventional schedule requiring a delay of bedtime, these individuals will continue to have an early rise time, leading to persistent sleep deprivation and daytime sleepiness. Use of hypnotics or alcohol to combat sleep-maintenance insomnia and stimulants to reduce daytime sleepiness may lead to substance abuse in these individuals.

Prevalence

The estimated prevalence of advanced sleep phase type is approximately 1% in middle-age adults. Sleep-wake times and circadian phase advance in older individuals, probably accounting for increased prevalence in this population.

Development and Course

Onset is usually in late adulthood. In the familial form, onset can be earlier. The course is typically persistent, lasting more than 3 months, but the severity may increase depending on work and social schedules. The advanced sleep phase type is more common in older adults.

Clinical expression may vary across the lifespan depending on social, school, and work obligations. Individuals who can alter their work schedules to accommodate the advanced circadian sleep and wake timing can experience remission of symptoms. Increasing age tends to advance the sleep phase, however, it is unclear whether the common age-associated advanced sleep phase type is due solely to a change in circadian timing (as seen in the familial form) or also to age-related changes in the homeostatic regulation of sleep, resulting in earlier awakening. Severity, remission, and relapse of symptoms suggest lack of adherence to behavioral and environmental treatments designed to control sleep and wake structure and light exposure.

Risk and Prognostic Factors

Environmental. Decreased late afternoon/early evening exposure to light and/or exposure to early morning light due to early morning awakening can increase the risk of advanced sleep phase type by advancing circadian rhythms. By going to bed early, these individuals are not exposed to light in the phase delay region of the curve, resulting in perpetuation of advanced phase. In familial advanced sleep phase type, a shortening of the endogenous circadian period can result in an advanced sleep phase, although circadian period does not appear to systematically decrease with age.

Genetic and physiological. Advanced sleep phase type has demonstrated an autosomal dominant mode of inheritance, including a *PER2* gene mutation causing hypophosphorylation of the PER2 protein and a missense mutation in *CKI*.

Culture-Related Diagnostic Issues
African Americans may have a shorter circadian period and larger magnitude phase advances to light than do Caucasians, possibly increasing the risk for development of advanced sleep phase type in this population.

Diagnostic Markers
A sleep diary and actigraphy may be used as diagnostic markers, as described earlier for delayed sleep phase type.

Functional Consequences of Advanced Sleep Phase Type
Excessive sleepiness associated with advanced sleep phase can have a negative effect on cognitive performance, social interaction, and safety. Use of wake-promoting agents to combat sleepiness or sedatives for early morning awakening may increase potential for substance abuse.

Differential Diagnosis

Other sleep disorders. Behavioral factors such as irregular sleep schedules, voluntary early awakening, and exposure to light in the early morning should be considered, particularly in older adults. Careful attention should be paid to rule out other sleep-wake disorders, such as insomnia disorder, and other mental disorders and medical conditions that can cause early morning awakening.

Depressive and bipolar disorders. Because early morning awakening, fatigue, and sleepiness are prominent features of major depressive disorder, depressive and bipolar disorders must also be considered.

Comorbidity
Medical conditions and mental disorders with the symptom of early morning awakening, such as insomnia, can co-occur with the advance sleep phase type.

Irregular Sleep-Wake Type

Diagnostic Features
The diagnosis of irregular sleep-wake type is based primarily on a history of symptoms of insomnia at night (during the usual sleep period) and excessive sleepiness (napping) during the day. Irregular sleep-wake type is characterized by a lack of discernible sleep-wake

circadian rhythm. There is no major sleep period, and sleep is fragmented into at least three periods during the 24-hour day.

Associated Features Supporting Diagnosis

Individuals with irregular sleep-wake type typically present with insomnia or excessive sleepiness, depending on the time of day. Sleep and wake periods across 24 hours are fragmented, although the longest sleep period tends to occur between 2:00 A.M. and 6:00 A.M. and is usually less than 4 hours. A history of isolation or reclusion may occur in association with the disorder and contribute to the symptoms via a lack of external stimuli to help entrain a normal pattern. Individuals or their caregivers report frequent naps throughout the day. Irregular sleep-wake type is most commonly associated with neurodegenerative disorders, such as major neurocognitive disorder, and many neurodevelopmental disorders in children.

Prevalence

Prevalence of irregular sleep-wake type in the general population is unknown.

Development and Course

The course of irregular sleep-wake type is persistent. Age at onset is variable, but the disorder is more common in older adults.

Risk and Prognostic Factors

Temperamental. Neurodegenerative disorders, such as Alzheimer's disease, Parkinson's disease, and Huntington's disease, and neurodevelopmental disorders in children increase the risk for irregular sleep-wake type.

Environmental. Decreased exposure to environmental light and structured daytime activity can be associated with a low-amplitude circadian rhythm. Hospitalized individuals are especially prone to such weak external entraining stimuli, and even outside the hospital setting, individuals with major neurocognitive disorder (i.e., dementia) are exposed to significantly less bright light.

Diagnostic Markers

A detailed sleep history and a sleep diary (by a caregiver) or actigraphy help confirm the irregular sleep-wake pattern.

Functional Consequences of Irregular Sleep-Wake Type

Lack of a clearly discernible major sleep and wake period in irregular sleep-wake type results in insomnia or excessive sleepiness, depending on the time of day. Disruption of the caregiver's sleep also often occurs and is an important consideration.

Differential Diagnosis

Normative variations in sleep. Irregular sleep-wake type should be distinguished from a voluntary irregular sleep-wake schedule and poor sleep hygiene, which can result in insomnia and excessive sleepiness.

Other medical conditions and mental disorders. Other causes of insomnia and daytime sleepiness, including comorbid medical conditions and mental disorders or medication, should be considered.

Comorbidity

Irregular sleep-wake type is often comorbid with neurodegenerative and neurodevelopmental disorders, such as major neurocognitive disorder, intellectual disability (intellectual developmental disorder), and traumatic brain injury. It is also comorbid with other medical conditions and mental disorders in which there is social isolation and/or lack of light and structured activities.

Non-24-Hour Sleep-Wake Type

Diagnostic Features

The diagnosis of non-24-hour sleep-wake type is based primarily on a history of symptoms of insomnia or excessive sleepiness related to abnormal synchronization between the 24-hour light-dark cycle and the endogenous circadian rhythm. Individuals typically present with periods of insomnia, excessive sleepiness, or both, which alternate with short asymptomatic periods. Starting with the asymptomatic period, when the individual's sleep phase is aligned to the external environment, sleep latency will gradually increase and the individual will complain of sleep-onset insomnia. As the sleep phase continues to drift so that sleep time is now in the daytime, the individual will have trouble staying awake during the day and will complain of sleepiness. Because the circadian period is not aligned to the external 24-hour environment, symptoms will depend on when an individual tries to sleep in relation to the circadian rhythm of sleep propensity.

Associated Features Supporting Diagnosis

Non-24-hour sleep-wake type is most common among blind or visually impaired individuals who have decreased light perception. In sighted individuals, there is often a history of delayed sleep phase and of decreased exposure to light and structured social and physical activity. Sighted individuals with non-24-hour sleep-wake type also demonstrate increased sleep duration.

Prevalence

Prevalence of non-24-hour sleep-wake type in the general population is unclear, but the disorder appears rare in sighted individuals. The prevalence in blind individuals is estimated to be 50%.

Development and Course

Course of non-24-hour sleep-wake type is persistent, with intermittent remission and exacerbations due to changes in work and social schedules throughout the lifespan. Age at onset is variable, depending on the onset of visual impairment. In sighted individuals, because of the overlap with delayed sleep phase type, non-24-hour sleep-wake type may develop in adolescence or early adulthood. Remission and relapse of symptoms in blind and sighted individuals largely depend on adherence to treatments designed to control sleep and wake structure and light exposure.

Clinical expression may vary across the lifespan depending on social, school, and work obligations. In adolescents and adults, irregular sleep-wake schedules and exposure to light or lack of light at critical times of the day can exacerbate the effects of sleep loss and disrupt circadian entrainment. Consequently, symptoms of insomnia, daytime sleepiness, and school, professional, and interpersonal functioning may worsen.

Risk and Prognostic Factors

Environmental.   In sighted individuals, decreased exposure or sensitivity to light and social and physical activity cues may contribute to a free-running circadian rhythm. With the high frequency of mental disorders involving social isolation and cases of non-24-hour sleep-wake type developing after a change in sleep habits (e.g., night shift work, job loss), behavioral factors in combination with physiological tendency may precipitate and perpetuate this disorder in sighted individuals. Hospitalized individuals with neurological and psychiatric disorders can become insensitive to social cues, predisposing them to the development of non-24-hour sleep-wake type.

Genetic and physiological. Blindness is a risk factor for non-24-hour sleep-wake type. Non-24-hour sleep-wake type has been associated with traumatic brain injury.

Diagnostic Markers

Diagnosis is confirmed by history and sleep diary or actigraphy for an extended period. Sequential measurement of phase markers (e.g., melatonin) can help determine circadian phase in both sighted and blind individuals.

Functional Consequences of Non-24-Hour Sleep-Wake Type

Complaints of insomnia (sleep onset and sleep maintenance), excessive sleepiness, or both are prominent. The unpredictability of sleep and wake times (typically a daily delay drift) results in an inability to attend school or maintain a steady job and may increase potential for social isolation.

Differential Diagnosis

Circadian rhythm sleep-wake disorders. In sighted individuals, non-24-hour sleep-wake type should be differentiated from delayed sleep phase type, as individuals with delayed sleep phase type may display a similar progressive delay in sleep period for several days.

Depressive disorders. Depressive symptoms and depressive disorders may result in similar circadian dysregulation and symptoms.

Comorbidity

Blindness is often comorbid with non-24-hour sleep-wake type, as are depressive and bipolar disorders with social isolation.

Shift Work Type

Diagnostic Features

Diagnosis is primarily based on a history of the individual working outside of the normal 8:00 A.M. to 6:00 P.M. daytime window (particularly at night) on a regularly scheduled (i.e., non-overtime) basis. Symptoms of excessive sleepiness at work, and impaired sleep at home, on a persistent basis are prominent. Presence of both sets of symptoms are usually required for a diagnosis of shift work type. Typically, when the individual reverts to a day-work routine, symptoms resolve. Although the etiology is slightly different, individuals who travel across many time zones on a very frequent basis may experience effects similar to those experienced by individuals with shift work type who work rotating shifts.

Prevalence

The prevalence of shift work type is unclear, but the disorder is estimated to affect 5%–10% of the night worker population (16%–20% of the workforce). Prevalence rises with advancement into middle-age and beyond (Drake et al. 2004).

Development and Course

Shift work type can appear in individuals of any age but is more prevalent in individuals older than 50 years and typically worsens with the passage of time if the disruptive work hours persist. Although older adults may show similar rates of circadian phase adjustment to a change in routine as do younger adults, they appear to experience significantly more sleep disruption as a consequence of the circadian phase shift.

Risk and Prognostic Factors

Temperamental. Predisposing factors include a morning-type disposition, a need for long (i.e., more than 8 hours) sleep durations in order to feel well rested, and strong competing social and domestic needs (e.g., parents of young children). Individuals who are able to commit to a nocturnal lifestyle, with few competing day-oriented demands, appear at lower risk for shift work type.

Genetic and physiological. Because shift workers are more likely than day workers to be obese, obstructive sleep apnea may be present and may exacerbate the symptoms.

Diagnostic Markers

A history and sleep diary or actigraphy may be useful in diagnosis, as discussed earlier for delayed sleep phase type.

Functional Consequences of Shift Work Type

Individuals with shift work type not only may perform poorly at work but also appear to be at risk for accidents both at work and on the drive home. They may also be at risk for poor mental health (e.g., alcohol use disorder, substance use disorder, depression) and physical health (e.g., gastrointestinal disorders, cardiovascular disease, diabetes, cancer). Individuals with a history of bipolar disorder are particularly vulnerable to shift work type–related episodes of mania resulting from missed nights of sleep. Shift work type often results in interpersonal problems.

Differential Diagnosis

Normative variations in sleep with shift work. The diagnosis of shift work type, as opposed to the "normal" difficulties of shift work, must depend to some extent on the severity of symptoms and/or level of distress experienced by the individual. Presence of shift work type symptoms even when the individual is able to live on a day-oriented routine for several weeks at a time may suggest the presence of other sleep disorders, such as sleep apnea, insomnia, and narcolepsy, which should be ruled out.

Comorbidity

Shift work type has been associated with increased alcohol use disorder, other substance use disorders, and depression. A variety of physical health disorders (e.g., gastrointestinal disorders, cardiovascular disease, diabetes, cancer) have been found to be associated with prolonged exposure to shift work.

Relationship to International Classification of Sleep Disorders

The *International Classification of Sleep Disorders,* 2nd Edition (ICSD-2), differentiates nine circadian rhythm sleep disorders, including jet lag type.

Parasomnias

Parasomnias are disorders characterized by abnormal behavioral, experiential, or physiological events occurring in association with sleep, specific sleep stages, or sleep-wake transitions. The most common parasomnias—non–rapid eye movement (NREM) sleep arousal disorders and rapid eye movement (REM) sleep behavior disorder—represent admixtures of wakefulness and NREM sleep and wakefulness and REM sleep, respectively. These conditions serve as a reminder that sleep and wakefulness are not mutually exclusive and that sleep is not necessarily a global, whole-brain phenomenon.

Non–Rapid Eye Movement Sleep Arousal Disorders

Diagnostic Criteria

A. Recurrent episodes of incomplete awakening from sleep, usually occurring during the first third of the major sleep episode, accompanied by either one of the following:

  1. **Sleepwalking:** Repeated episodes of rising from bed during sleep and walking about. While sleepwalking, the individual has a blank, staring face; is relatively unresponsive to the efforts of others to communicate with him or her; and can be awakened only with great difficulty.

  2. **Sleep terrors:** Recurrent episodes of abrupt terror arousals from sleep, usually beginning with a panicky scream. There is intense fear and signs of autonomic arousal, such as mydriasis, tachycardia, rapid breathing, and sweating, during each episode. There is relative unresponsiveness to efforts of others to comfort the individual during the episodes.

B. No or little (e.g., only a single visual scene) dream imagery is recalled.

C. Amnesia for the episodes is present.

D. The episodes cause clinically significant distress or impairment in social, occupational, or other important areas of functioning.

E. The disturbance is not attributable to the physiological effects of a substance (e.g., a drug of abuse, a medication).

F. Coexisting mental and medical disorders do not explain the episodes of sleepwalking or sleep terrors.

Coding note: For ICD-9-CM, code **307.46** for all subtypes. For ICD-10-CM, code is based on subtype.

Specify whether:

  307.46 (F51.3) Sleepwalking type

  Specify if:

  With sleep-related eating

  With sleep-related sexual behavior (sexsomnia)

  307.46 (F51.4) Sleep terror type

Diagnostic Features

The essential feature of non–rapid eye movement (NREM) sleep arousal disorders is the repeated occurrence of incomplete arousals, usually beginning during the first third of the major sleep episode (Criterion A), that typically are brief, lasting 1–10 minutes, but may be protracted, lasting up to 1 hour. The maximum duration of an event is unknown. The eyes are typically open during these events. Many individuals exhibit both subtypes of arousals on different occasions, which underscores the unitary underlying pathophysiology. The subtypes reflect varying degrees of simultaneous occurrence of wakefulness and NREM sleep, resulting in complex behaviors arising from sleep with varying degrees of conscious awareness, motor activity, and autonomic activation.

The essential feature of *sleepwalking* is repeated episodes of complex motor behavior initiated during sleep, including rising from bed and walking about (Criterion A1). Sleep-walking episodes begin during any stage of NREM sleep, most commonly during slow-wave sleep and therefore most often occurring during the first third of the night. During episodes, the individual has reduced alertness and responsiveness, a blank stare, and relative unresponsiveness to communication with others or efforts by others to awaken the individual. If awakened during the episode (or on awakening the following morning), the individual has limited recall for the episode. After the episode, there may initially be a brief period of confusion or difficulty orienting, followed by full recovery of cognitive function and appropriate behavior.

The essential feature of *sleep terrors* is the repeated occurrence of precipitous awakenings from sleep, usually beginning with a panicky scream or cry (Criterion A2). Sleep terrors usually begin during the first third of the major sleep episode and last 1–10 minutes, but they may last considerably longer, particularly in children. The episodes are accompanied by impressive autonomic arousal and behavioral manifestations of intense fear. During an episode, the individual is difficult to awaken or comfort. If the individual awakens after the sleep terror, little or none of the dream, or only fragmentary, single images, are recalled. During a typical episode of sleep terrors, the individual abruptly sits up in bed screaming or crying, with a frightened expression and autonomic signs of intense anxiety (e.g., tachycardia, rapid breathing, sweating, dilation of the pupils). The individual may be inconsolable and is usually unresponsive to the efforts of others to awaken or comfort him or her. Sleep terrors are also called "night terrors" or "pavor nocturnus."

Associated Features Supporting Diagnosis

Sleepwalking episodes can include a wide variety of behaviors. Episodes may begin with confusion: the individual may simply sit up in bed, look about, or pick at the blanket or sheet. This behavior then becomes progressively complex. The individual may actually leave the bed and walk into closets, out of the room, and even out of buildings. Individuals may use the bathroom, eat, talk, or engage in more complex behaviors. Running and frantic attempts to escape some apparent threat can also occur. Most behaviors during sleep-walking episodes are routine and of low complexity. However, cases of unlocking doors and even operating machinery (driving an automobile) have been reported. Sleepwalking can also include inappropriate behavior (e.g., commonly, urinating in a closet or wastebasket). Most episodes last for several minutes to a half hour but may be more protracted. Inasmuch as sleep is a state of relative analgesia, painful injuries sustained during sleepwalking may not be appreciated until awakening after the fact.

There are two "specialized" forms of sleepwalking: sleep-related eating behavior and sleep-related sexual behavior (sexsomnia or sleep sex). Individuals with *sleep-related eating* experience unwanted recurrent episodes of eating with varying degrees of amnesia, ranging from no awareness to full awareness without the ability to not eat. During these episodes, inappropriate foods may be ingested. Individuals with sleep-related eating disorder may find evidence of their eating only the next morning. In *sexsomnia*, varying degrees of sexual activity (e.g., masturbation, fondling, groping, sexual intercourse) occur as complex behaviors arising from sleep without conscious awareness. This condition is more common in males and may result in serious interpersonal relationship problems or medicolegal consequences.

During a typical episode of sleep terrors, there is often a sense of overwhelming dread, with a compulsion to escape. Although fragmentary vivid dream images may occur, a story-like dream sequence (as in nightmares) is not reported. Most commonly, the individual does not awaken fully, but returns to sleep and has amnesia for the episode on awakening the next morning. Usually only one episode will occur on any one night. Occasionally several episodes may occur at intervals throughout the night. These events rarely arise during daytime naps.

Prevalence

Isolated or infrequent NREM sleep arousal disorders are very common in the general population. From 10% to 30% of children have had at least one episode of sleepwalking, and 2%–3% sleepwalk often. The prevalence of sleepwalking disorder, marked by repeated episodes and impairment or distress, is much lower, probably in the range of 1%–5%. The prevalence of sleepwalking episodes (not sleepwalking disorder) is 1.0%–7.0% among adults, with weekly to monthly episodes occurring in 0.5%–0.7%. The lifetime prevalence of sleepwalking in adults is 29.2%, with a past-year prevalence of sleepwalking of 3.6%.

The prevalence of sleep terrors in the general population is unknown. The prevalence of sleep terror episodes (as opposed to sleep terror disorder, in which there is recurrence and distress or impairment) is approximately 36.9% at 18 months of age, 19.7% at 30 months of age, and 2.2% in adults.

Development and Course

NREM sleep arousal disorders occur most commonly in childhood and diminish in frequency with increasing age. The onset of sleepwalking in adults with no prior history of sleepwalking as children should prompt a search for specific etiologies, such as obstructive sleep apnea, nocturnal seizures, or effect of medication.

Risk and Prognostic Factors

Environmental. Sedative use, sleep deprivation, sleep-wake schedule disruptions, fatigue, and physical or emotional stress increase the likelihood of episodes. Fever and sleep deprivation can produce an increased frequency of NREM sleep arousal disorders.

Genetic and physiological. A family history for sleepwalking or sleep terrors may occur in up to 80% of individuals who sleepwalk. The risk for sleepwalking is further increased (to as much as 60% of offspring) when both parents have a history of the disorder.

Individuals with sleep terrors frequently have a positive family history of either sleep terrors or sleepwalking, with as high as a 10-fold increase in the prevalence of the disorder among first-degree biological relatives. Sleep terrors are much more common in monozygotic twins as compared with dizygotic twins. The exact mode of inheritance is unknown.

Gender-Related Diagnostic Issues

Violent or sexual activity during sleepwalking episodes is more likely to occur in adults. Eating during sleepwalking episodes is more commonly seen in females. Sleepwalking occurs more often in females during childhood but more often in males during adulthood.

Older children and adults provide a more detailed recollection of fearful images associated with sleep terrors than do younger children, who are more likely to have complete amnesia or report only a vague sense of fear. Among children, sleep terrors are more common in males than in females. Among adults, the sex ratio is even.

Diagnostic Markers

NREM sleep arousal disorders arise from any stage of NREM sleep but most commonly from deep NREM sleep (slow-wave sleep). They are most likely to appear in the first third of the night and do not commonly occur during daytime naps. During the episode, the polysomnogram may be obscured with movement artifact. In the absence of such artifact, the electroencephalogram typically shows theta or alpha frequency activity during the episode, indicating partial or incomplete arousal.

Polysomnography in conjunction with audiovisual monitoring can be used to document episodes of sleepwalking. In the absence of actually capturing an event during a polysomnographic recording, there are no polysomnographic features that can serve as a marker for sleepwalking. Sleep deprivation may increase the likelihood of capturing an event. As a group, individuals who sleepwalk show instability of deep NREM sleep, but the overlap in findings with individuals who do not sleepwalk is great enough to preclude use of this indicator in establishing a diagnosis. Unlike arousals from REM sleep associated with nightmares, in which there is an increase in heart rate and respiration prior to the arousal, the NREM sleep arousals of sleep terrors begin precipitously from sleep, without anticipatory autonomic changes. The arousals are associated with impressive autonomic activity, with doubling or tripling of the heart rate. The pathophysiology is poorly understood, but there appears to be instability in the deeper stages of NREM sleep. Absent capturing an event during a formal sleep study, there are no reliable polysomnographic indicators of the tendency to experience sleep terrors.

Functional Consequences of Non-REM Sleep Arousal Disorders

For the diagnosis of a NREM sleep arousal disorder to be made, the individual or household members must experience clinically significant distress or impairment, although parasomnia symptoms may occur occasionally in nonclinical populations and would be subthreshold for the diagnosis. Embarrassment concerning the episodes can impair social relationships. Social isolation or occupational difficulties can result. The determination of a "disorder" depends on a number of factors, which may vary on an individual basis and will depend on the frequency of events, potential for violence or injurious behaviors, embarrassment, or disruption/distress of other household members. Severity determination is best made based on the nature or consequence of the behaviors rather than simply on frequency. Uncommonly, NREM sleep arousal disorders may result in serious injury to the individual or to someone trying to console the individual. Injuries to others are confined to those in close proximity; individuals are not "sought out." Typically, sleepwalking in both children and adults is not associated with significant mental disorders. For individuals with sleep-related eating behaviors, unknowingly preparing or eating food during the sleep period may create problems such as poor diabetes control, weight gain, injury (cuts and burns), or consequences of eating dangerous or toxic inedibles. NREM sleep arousal disorders may rarely result in violent or injurious behaviors with forensic implications.

Differential Diagnosis

Nightmare disorder.   In contrast to individuals with NREM sleep arousal disorders, individuals with nightmare disorder typically awaken easily and completely, report vivid storylike dreams accompanying the episodes, and tend to have episodes later in the night. NREM sleep arousal disorders occur during NREM sleep, whereas nightmares usually occur during REM sleep. Parents of children with NREM sleep arousal disorders may misinterpret reports of fragmentary imagery as nightmares.

Breathing-related sleep disorders.   Breathing disorders during sleep can also produce confusional arousals with subsequent amnesia. However, breathing-related sleep disorders are also characterized by characteristic symptoms of snoring, breathing pauses, and daytime sleepiness. In some individuals, a breathing-related sleep disorder may precipitate episodes of sleepwalking.

REM sleep behavior disorder.   REM sleep behavior disorder may be difficult to distinguish from NREM sleep arousal disorders. REM sleep behavior disorder is characterized by episodes of prominent, complex movements, often involving personal injury arising from sleep. In contrast to NREM sleep arousal disorders, REM sleep behavior disorder occurs during REM sleep. Individuals with REM sleep behavior disorder awaken easily and report more detailed and vivid dream content than do individuals with NREM sleep arousal disorders. They often report that they "act out dreams."

Parasomnia overlap syndrome.   Parasomnia overlap syndrome consists of clinical and polysomnographic features of both sleepwalking and REM sleep behavior disorder.

Sleep-related seizures.   Some types of seizures can produce episodes of very unusual behaviors that occur predominantly or exclusively during sleep. Nocturnal seizures may closely mimic NREM sleep arousal disorders but tend to be more stereotypic in nature, occur multiple times nightly, and be more likely to occur from daytime naps. The presence of sleep-related seizures does not preclude the presence of NREM sleep arousal disorders. Sleep-related seizures should be classified as a form of epilepsy.

Alcohol-induced blackouts.   Alcohol-induced blackouts may be associated with extremely complex behaviors in the absence of other suggestions of intoxication. They do not involve the loss of consciousness but rather reflect an isolated disruption of memory for events during a drinking episode. By history, these behaviors may be indistinguishable from those seen in NREM sleep arousal disorders.

Dissociative amnesia, with dissociative fugue.   Dissociative fugue may be extremely difficult to distinguish from sleepwalking. Unlike all other parasomnias, nocturnal dissociative fugue arises from a period of wakefulness during sleep, rather than precipitously from sleep without intervening wakefulness. A history of recurrent childhood physical or sexual abuse is usually present (but may be difficult to obtain).

Malingering or other voluntary behavior occurring during wakefulness.   As with dissociative fugue, malingering or other voluntary behavior occurring during wakefulness arises from wakefulness.

Panic disorder.   Panic attacks may also cause abrupt awakenings from deep NREM sleep accompanied by fearfulness, but these episodes produce rapid and complete awakening without the confusion, amnesia, or motor activity typical of NREM sleep arousal disorders.

Medication-induced complex behaviors.   Behaviors similar to those in NREM sleep arousal disorders can be induced by use of, or withdrawal from, substances or medications (e.g., benzodiazepines, nonbenzodiazepine sedative-hypnotics, opiates, cocaine, nicotine, antipsychotics, tricyclic antidepressants, chloral hydrate). Such behaviors may arise from the sleep period and may be extremely complex. The underlying pathophysiology appears to be a relatively isolated amnesia. In such cases, substance/medication-induced sleep disorder, parasomnia type, should be diagnosed (see "Substance/Medication-Induced Sleep Disorder" later in this chapter).

Night eating syndrome.   The sleep-related eating disorder form of sleepwalking is to be differentiated from night eating syndrome, in which there is a delay in the circadian rhythm of food ingestion and an association with insomnia and/or depression.

Comorbidity

In adults, there is an association between sleepwalking and major depressive episodes and obsessive-compulsive disorder. Children or adults with sleep terrors may have elevated scores for depression and anxiety on personality inventories.

Relationship to International Classification of Sleep Disorders

The *International Classification of Sleep Disorders,* 2nd Edition, includes "confusional arousal" as a NREM sleep arousal disorder.

Nightmare Disorder

Diagnostic Criteria   **307.47 (F51.5)**

A. Repeated occurrences of extended, extremely dysphoric, and well-remembered dreams that usually involve efforts to avoid threats to survival, security, or physical integrity and that generally occur during the second half of the major sleep episode.
B. On awakening from the dysphoric dreams, the individual rapidly becomes oriented and alert.
C. The sleep disturbance causes clinically significant distress or impairment in social, occupational, or other important areas of functioning.
D. The nightmare symptoms are not attributable to the physiological effects of a substance (e.g., a drug of abuse, a medication).
E. Coexisting mental and medical disorders do not adequately explain the predominant complaint of dysphoric dreams.

Specify if:
   During sleep onset

Specify if:
   With associated non–sleep disorder, including substance use disorders
   With associated other medical condition
   With associated other sleep disorder

   Coding note: The code 307.47 (F51.5) applies to all three specifiers. Code also the relevant associated mental disorder, medical condition, or other sleep disorder immediately after the code for nightmare disorder in order to indicate the association.

Specify if:
   Acute: Duration of period of nightmares is 1 month or less.
   Subacute: Duration of period of nightmares is greater than 1 month but less than 6 months.
   Persistent: Duration of period of nightmares is 6 months or greater.

Specify current severity:
   Severity can be rated by the frequency with which the nightmares occur:
   Mild: Less than one episode per week on average.
   Moderate: One or more episodes per week but less than nightly.
   Severe: Episodes nightly.

Diagnostic Features

Nightmares are typically lengthy, elaborate, storylike sequences of dream imagery that seem real and that incite anxiety, fear, or other dysphoric emotions. Nightmare content typically focuses on attempts to avoid or cope with imminent danger but may involve themes that evoke other negative emotions. Nightmares occurring after traumatic experiences may replicate the threatening situation ("replicative nightmares"), but most do not. On awakening, nightmares are well remembered and can be described in detail. They arise almost exclusively during rapid eye movement (REM) sleep and can thus occur through-out sleep but are more likely in the second half of the major sleep episode when dreaming is longer and more intense. Factors that increase early-night REM intensity, such as sleep fragmentation or deprivation, jet lag, and REM-sensitive medications, might facilitate nightmares earlier in the night, including at sleep onset.

Nightmares usually terminate with awakening and rapid return of full alertness. How-ever, the dysphoric emotions may persist into wakefulness and contribute to difficulty re-turning to sleep and lasting daytime distress. Some nightmares, known as "bad dreams," may not induce awakening and are recalled only later. If nightmares occur during sleep-onset REM periods (*hypnagogic*), the dysphoric emotion is frequently accompanied by a sense of being both awake and unable to move voluntarily (*isolated sleep paralysis*).

Associated Features Supporting Diagnosis

Mild autonomic arousal, including sweating, tachycardia, and tachypnea, may character-ize nightmares. Body movements and vocalizations are not characteristic because of REM sleep–related loss of skeletal muscle tone, but such behaviors may occur under situations of emotional stress or sleep fragmentation and in posttraumatic stress disorder (PTSD). When talking or emoting occurs, it is typically a brief event terminating the nightmare.

Individuals with frequent nightmares are at substantially greater risk for suicidal ide-ation and suicide attempts, even when gender and mental illness are taken into account.

Prevalence

Prevalence of nightmares increases through childhood into adolescence. From 1.3% to 3.9% of parents report that their preschool children have nightmares "often" or "always". Prevalence increases from ages 10 to 13 for both males and females but continues to in-crease to ages 20–29 for females (while decreasing for males), when it can be twice as high for females as for males. Prevalence decreases steadily with age for both sexes, but the gen-der difference remains. Among adults, prevalence of nightmares at least monthly is 6%, whereas prevalence for frequent nightmares is 1%–2%. Estimates often combine idio-pathic and posttraumatic nightmares indiscriminately.

Development and Course

Nightmares often begin between ages 3 and 6 years but reach a peak prevalence and se-verity in late adolescence or early adulthood. Nightmares most likely appear in children exposed to acute or chronic psychosocial stressors and thus may not resolve spontane-ously. In a minority, frequent nightmares persist into adulthood, becoming virtually a life-long disturbance. Although specific nightmare content may reflect the individual's age, the essential features of the disorder are the same across age groups.

Risk and Prognostic Factors

Temperamental.   Individuals who experience nightmares report more frequent past ad-verse events, but not necessarily trauma, and often display personality disturbances or psychiatric diagnosis.

Environmental.   Sleep deprivation or fragmentation, and irregular sleep-wake schedules that alter the timing, intensity, or quantity of REM sleep, can put individuals at risk for nightmares.

Genetic and physiological.   Twin studies have identified genetic effects on the disposi-tion to nightmares and their co-occurrence with other parasomnias (e.g., sleeptalking).

Course modifiers.   Adaptive parental bedside behaviors, such as soothing the child fol-lowing nightmares, may protect against developing chronic nightmares.

Culture-Related Diagnostic Issues

The significance attributed to nightmares may vary by culture, and sensitivity to such beliefs may facilitate disclosure.

Gender-Related Diagnostic Issues

Adult females report having nightmares more frequently than do adult males. Nightmare content differs by sex, with adult females tending to report themes of sexual harassment or of loved ones disappearing/dying, and adult males tending to report themes of physical aggression or war/terror.

Diagnostic Markers

Polysomnographic studies demonstrate abrupt awakenings from REM sleep, usually during the second half of the night, prior to report of a nightmare. Heart, respiratory, and eye movement rates may quicken or increase in variability before awakening. Nightmares following traumatic events may also arise during non-REM (NREM), particularly stage 2, sleep. The typical sleep of individuals with nightmares is mildly impaired (e.g., reduced efficiency, less slow-wave sleep, more awakenings), with more frequent periodic leg movements in sleep and relative sympathetic nervous system activation after REM sleep deprivation.

Functional Consequences of Nightmare Disorder

Nightmares cause more significant subjective distress than demonstrable social or occupational impairment. However, if awakenings are frequent or result in sleep avoidance, individuals may experience excessive daytime sleepiness, poor concentration, depression, anxiety, or irritability. Frequent childhood nightmares (e.g., several per week), may cause significant distress to parents and child.

Differential Diagnosis

Sleep terror disorder.   Both nightmare disorder and sleep terror disorder include awakenings or partial awakenings with fearfulness and autonomic activation, but the two disorders are differentiable. Nightmares typically occur later in the night, during REM sleep, and produce vivid, storylike, and clearly recalled dreams; mild autonomic arousal; and complete awakenings. Sleep terrors typically arise in the first third of the night during stage 3 or 4 NREM sleep and produce either no dream recall or images without an elaborate storylike quality. The terrors lead to partial awakenings that leave the individual confused, disoriented, and only partially responsive and with substantial autonomic arousal. There is usually amnesia for the event in the morning.

REM sleep behavior disorder.   The presence of complex motor activity during frightening dreams should prompt further evaluation for REM sleep behavior disorder, which occurs more typically among late middle-age males and, unlike nightmare disorder, is associated with often violent dream enactments and a history of nocturnal injuries. The dream disturbance of REM sleep behavior disorder is described by patients as nightmares but is controlled by appropriate medication.

Bereavement.   Dysphoric dreams may occur during bereavement but typically involve loss and sadness and are followed by self-reflection and insight, rather than distress, on awakening.

Narcolepsy.   Nightmares are a frequent complaint in narcolepsy, but the presence of excessive sleepiness and cataplexy differentiates this condition from nightmare disorder.

Nocturnal seizures.   Seizures may rarely manifest as nightmares and should be evaluated with polysomnography and continuous video electroencephalography. Nocturnal seizures usually involve stereotypical motor activity. Associated nightmares, if recalled, are often repetitive in nature or reflect epileptogenic features such as the content of diurnal auras (e.g., unmotivated dread), phosphenes, or ictal imagery. Disorders of arousal, especially confusional arousals, may also be present.

Breathing-related sleep disorders.   Breathing-related sleep disorders can lead to awakenings with autonomic arousal, but these are not usually accompanied by recall of nightmares.

Panic disorder.   Attacks arising during sleep can produce abrupt awakenings with autonomic arousal and fearfulness, but nightmares are typically not reported and symptoms are similar to panic attacks arising during wakefulness.

Sleep-related dissociative disorders.   Individuals may recall actual physical or emotional trauma as a "dream" during electroencephalography-documented awakenings.

Medication or substance use.   Numerous substances/medications can precipitate nightmares, including dopaminergics; beta-adrenergic antagonists and other antihypertensives; amphetamine, cocaine, and other stimulants; antidepressants; smoking cessation aids; and melatonin. Withdrawal of REM sleep–suppressant medications (e.g., antidepressants) and alcohol can produce REM sleep rebound accompanied by nightmares. If nightmares are sufficiently severe to warrant independent clinical attention, a diagnosis of substance/medication-induced sleep disorder should be considered.

Comorbidity

Nightmares may be comorbid with several medical conditions, including coronary heart disease, cancer, parkinsonism, and pain, and can accompany medical treatments, such as hemodialysis, or withdrawal from medications or substances of abuse. Nightmares frequently are comorbid with other mental disorders, including PTSD; insomnia disorder; schizophrenia; psychosis; mood, anxiety, adjustment, and personality disorders; and grief during bereavement. A concurrent nightmare disorder diagnosis should only be considered when independent clinical attention is warranted (i.e., Criteria A–C are met). Otherwise, no separate diagnosis is necessary. These conditions should be listed under the appropriate comorbid category specifier. However, nightmare disorder may be diagnosed as a separate disorder in individuals with PTSD if the nightmares are temporally unrelated to PTSD (i.e., preceding other PTSD symptoms or persisting after other PTSD symptoms have resolved).

Nightmares are normally characteristic of REM sleep behavior disorder, PTSD, and acute stress disorder, but nightmare disorder may be independently coded if nightmares preceded the condition and their frequency or severity necessitates independent clinical attention. The latter may be determined by asking whether nightmares were a problem before onset of the other disorder and whether they continued after other symptoms had remitted.

Relationship to International Classification of Sleep Disorders

The *International Classification of Sleep Disorders*, 2nd Edition (ICSD-2), presents similar diagnostic criteria for nightmare disorder.

Rapid Eye Movement Sleep Behavior Disorder

Diagnostic Criteria   **327.42 (G47.52)**

A. Repeated episodes of arousal during sleep associated with vocalization and/or complex motor behaviors.
B. These behaviors arise during rapid eye movement (REM) sleep and therefore usually occur more than 90 minutes after sleep onset, are more frequent during the later portions of the sleep period, and uncommonly occur during daytime naps.

C. Upon awakening from these episodes, the individual is completely awake, alert, and not confused or disoriented.

D. Either of the following:

1. REM sleep without atonia on polysomnographic recording.
2. A history suggestive of REM sleep behavior disorder and an established synuclein-opathy diagnosis (e.g., Parkinson's disease, multiple system atrophy).

E. The behaviors cause clinically significant distress or impairment in social, occupa-tional, or other important areas of functioning (which may include injury to self or the bed partner).

F. The disturbance is not attributable to the physiological effects of a substance (e.g., a drug of abuse, a medication) or another medical condition.

G. Coexisting mental and medical disorders do not explain the episodes.

Diagnostic Features

The essential feature of rapid eye movement (REM) sleep behavior disorder is repeated episodes of arousal, often associated with vocalizations and/or complex motor behaviors arising from REM sleep (Criterion A). These behaviors often reflect motor responses to the content of action-filled or violent dreams of being attacked or trying to escape from a threatening situation, which may be termed *dream enacting behaviors.* The vocalizations are often loud, emotion-filled, and profane. These behaviors may be very bothersome to the individual and the bed partner and may result in significant injury (e.g., falling, jumping, or flying out of bed; running, punching, thrusting, hitting, or kicking). Upon awakening, the individual is immediately awake, alert, and oriented (Criterion C) and is often able to recall dream mentation, which closely correlates with the observed behavior. The eyes typically remain closed during these events. The diagnosis of REM sleep behavior disor-der requires clinically significant distress or impairment (Criterion E); this determination will depend on a number of factors, including the frequency of events, the potential for vi-olence or injurious behaviors, embarrassment, and distress in other household members.

Associated Features Supporting Diagnosis

Severity determination is best made based on the nature or consequence of the behavior rather than simply on frequency. Although the behaviors are typically prominent and vi-olent, lesser behaviors may also occur.

Prevalence

The prevalence of REM sleep behavior disorder is approximately 0.38%–0.5% in the gen-eral population. Prevalence in patients with psychiatric disorders may be greater, possibly related to medications prescribed for the psychiatric disorder.

Development and Course

The onset of REM sleep behavior disorder may be gradual or rapid, and the course is usu-ally progressive. REM sleep behavior disorder associated with neurodegenerative disor-ders may improve as the underlying neurodegenerative disorder progresses. Because of the very high association with the later appearance of an underlying neurodegenerative disorder, most notably one of the synucleinopathies (Parkinson's disease, multiple system atrophy, or major or mild neurocognitive disorder with Lewy bodies), the neurological status of individuals with REM sleep behavior disorder should be closely monitored.

REM sleep behavior disorder overwhelmingly affects males older than 50 years, but in-creasingly this disorder is being identified in females and in younger individuals. Symptoms in young individuals, particularly young females, should raise the possibility of narcolepsy or medication-induced REM sleep behavior disorder.

Risk and Prognostic Factors

Genetic and physiological. Many widely prescribed medications, including tricyclic antidepressants, selective serotonin reuptake inhibitors, serotonin-norepinephrine reuptake inhibitors, and beta-blockers, may result in polysomnographic evidence of REM sleep without atonia and in frank REM sleep behavior disorder. It is not known whether the medications per se result in REM sleep behavior disorder or they unmask an underlying predisposition.

Diagnostic Markers

Associated laboratory findings from polysomnography indicate increased tonic and/or phasic electromyographic activity during REM sleep that is normally associated with muscle atonia. The increased muscle activity variably affects different muscle groups, mandating more extensive electromyographic monitoring than is employed in conventional sleep studies. For this reason, it is suggested that electromyographic monitoring include the submentalis, bilateral extensor digitorum, and bilateral anterior tibialis muscle groups. Continuous video monitoring is mandatory. Other polysomnographic findings may include very frequent periodic and aperiodic extremity electromyography activity during non-REM (NREM) sleep. This polysomnography observation, termed *REM sleep without atonia*, is present in virtually all cases of REM sleep behavior disorder but may also be an asymptomatic polysomnographic finding. Clinical dream-enacting behaviors coupled with the polysomnographic finding of REM without atonia is necessary for the diagnosis of REM sleep behavior disorder. REM sleep without atonia without a clinical history of dream-enacting behaviors is simply an asymptomatic polysomnographic observation. It is not known whether isolated REM sleep without atonia is a precursor to REM sleep behavior disorder.

Functional Consequences of Rapid Eye Movement Sleep Behavior Disorder

REM sleep behavior disorder may occur in isolated occasions in otherwise unaffected individuals. Embarrassment concerning the episodes can impair social relationships. Individuals may avoid situations in which others might become aware of the disturbance, visiting friends overnight, or sleeping with bed partners. Social isolation or occupational difficulties can result. Uncommonly, REM sleep behavior disorder may result in serious injury to the victim or to the bed partner.

Differential Diagnosis

Other parasomnias. Confusional arousals, sleepwalking, and sleep terrors can easily be confused with REM sleep behavior disorder. In general, these disorders occur in younger individuals. Unlike REM sleep behavior disorder, they arise from deep NREM sleep and therefore tend to occur in the early portion of the sleep period. Awakening from a confusional arousal is associated with confusion, disorientation, and incomplete recall of dream mentation accompanying the behavior. Polysomnographic monitoring in the disorders of arousal reveals normal REM atonia.

Nocturnal seizures. Nocturnal seizures may perfectly mimic REM sleep behavior disorder, but the behaviors are generally more stereotyped. Polysomnographic monitoring employing a full electroencephalographic seizure montage may differentiate the two. REM sleep without atonia is not present on polysomnographic monitoring.

Obstructive sleep apnea.   Obstructive sleep apnea may result in behaviors indistinguishable from REM sleep behavior disorder. Polysomnographic monitoring is necessary to differentiate between the two. In this case, the symptoms resolve following effective treatment of the obstructive sleep apnea, and REM sleep without atonia is not present on polysomnography monitoring.

Other specified dissociative disorder (sleep-related psychogenic dissociative disorder). Unlike virtually all other parasomnias, which arise precipitously from NREM or REM sleep, psychogenic dissociative behaviors arise from a period of well-defined wakefulness during the sleep period. Unlike REM sleep behavior disorder, this condition is more prevalent in young females.

Malingering.   Many cases of malingering in which the individual reports problematic sleep movements perfectly mimic the clinical features of REM sleep behavior disorder, and polysomnographic documentation is mandatory.

Comorbidity

REM sleep behavior disorder is present concurrently in approximately 30% of patients with narcolepsy. When it occurs in narcolepsy, the demographics reflect the younger age range of narcolepsy, with equal frequency in males and females. Based on findings from individuals presenting to sleep clinics, most individuals (>50%) with initially "idiopathic" REM sleep behavior disorder will eventually develop a neurodegenerative disease—most notably, one of the synucleinopathies (Parkinson's disease, multiple system atrophy, or major or mild neurocognitive disorder with Lewy bodies). REM sleep behavior disorder often predates any other sign of these disorders by many years (often more than a decade).

Relationship to International Classification of Sleep Disorders

REM sleep behavior disorder is virtually identical to REM sleep behavior disorder in the *International Classification of Sleep Disorders*, 2nd Edition (ICSD-2).

Restless Legs Syndrome

Diagnostic Criteria   **333.94 (G25.81)**

A. An urge to move the legs, usually accompanied by or in response to uncomfortable and unpleasant sensations in the legs, characterized by all of the following:

1. The urge to move the legs begins or worsens during periods of rest or inactivity.
2. The urge to move the legs is partially or totally relieved by movement.
3. The urge to move the legs is worse in the evening or at night than during the day, or occurs only in the evening or at night.

B. The symptoms in Criterion A occur at least three times per week and have persisted for at least 3 months.

C. The symptoms in Criterion A are accompanied by significant distress or impairment in social, occupational, educational, academic, behavioral, or other important areas of functioning.

D. The symptoms in Criterion A are not attributable to another mental disorder or medical condition (e.g., arthritis, leg edema, peripheral ischemia, leg cramps) and are not better explained by a behavioral condition (e.g., positional discomfort, habitual foot tapping).

E. The symptoms are not attributable to the physiological effects of a drug of abuse or medication (e.g., akathisia).

Diagnostic Features

Restless legs syndrome (RLS) is a sensorimotor, neurological sleep disorder characterized by a desire to move the legs or arms, usually associated with uncomfortable sensations typically described as creeping, crawling, tingling, burning, or itching (Criterion A). The diagnosis of RLS is based primarily on patient self-report and history. Symptoms are worse when the individual is at rest, and frequent movements of the legs occur in an effort to relieve the uncomfortable sensations. Symptoms are worse in the evening or night, and in some individuals they occur only in the evening or night. Evening worsening occurs independently of any differences in activity. It is important to differentiate RLS from other conditions such as positional discomfort and leg cramps (Criterion D).

The symptoms of RLS can delay sleep onset and awaken the individual from sleep and are associated with significant sleep fragmentation. The relief obtained from moving the legs may no longer be apparent in severe cases. RLS is associated with daytime sleepiness and is frequently accompanied by significant clinical distress or functional impairment.

Associated Features Supporting Diagnosis

Periodic leg movements in sleep (PLMS) can serve as corroborating evidence for RLS, with up to 90% of individuals diagnosed with RLS demonstrating PLMS when recordings are taken over multiple nights. Periodic leg movements during wakefulness are supportive of an RLS diagnosis. Reports of difficulty initiating and maintaining sleep and of excessive daytime sleepiness may also support the diagnosis of RLS. Additional supportive features include a family history of RLS among first-degree relatives and a reduction in symptoms, at least initially, with dopaminergic treatment.

Prevalence

Prevalence rates of RLS vary widely when broad criteria are utilized but range from 2% to 7.2% when more defined criteria are employed. When frequency of symptoms is at least three times per week with moderate or severe distress, the prevalence rate is 1.6%; when frequency of symptoms is a minimum of one time per week, the prevalence rate is 4.5%. Females are 1.5–2 times more likely than males to have RLS. RLS also increases with age. The prevalence of RLS may be lower in Asian populations.

Development and Course

The onset of RLS typically occurs in the second or third decade. Approximately 40% of individuals diagnosed with RLS during adulthood report having experienced symptoms before age 20 years, and 20% report having experienced symptoms before age 10 years. Prevalence rates of RLS increase steadily with age until about age 60 years, with symptoms remaining stable or decreasing slightly in older age groups. Compared with nonfamilial cases, familial RLS usually has a younger age at onset and a slower progressive course. The clinical course of RLS differs by age at onset. When onset occurs before age 45, there is often a slow progression of symptoms. In late-onset RLS, rapid progression is typical, and aggravating factors are common. Symptoms of RLS appear similar across the lifespan, remaining stable or decreasing slightly in older age groups.

Diagnosis of RLS in children can be difficult because of the self-report component. While Criterion A for adults assumes that the description of "urge to move" is by the patient, pediatric diagnosis requires a description in the child's own words rather than by a parent or caretaker. Typically children age 6 years or older are able to provide detailed, adequate descriptors of RLS. However, children rarely use or understand the word "urge," reporting instead that their legs "have to" or "got to" move. Also, potentially related to prolonged periods of sitting during class, two-thirds of children and adolescents report daytime leg sensations. Thus, for diagnostic Criterion A3, it is important to compare equal duration of sitting or lying down in the day to sitting or lying down in the evening or night. Nocturnal worsening tends to persist even in the context of pediatric RLS. As with RLS in adults, there is a significant negative impact on sleep, mood, cognition, and function. Impairment in children and adolescents is manifested more often in behavioral and educational domains.

Risk and Prognostic Factors

Genetic and physiological.   Predisposing factors include female gender, advancing age, genetic risk variants, and family history of RLS. Precipitating factors are often time-limited, such as iron deficiency, with most individuals resuming normal sleep patterns after the initial triggering event has disappeared. Genetic risk variants also play a role in RLS secondary to such disorders as uremia, suggesting that individuals with a genetic susceptibility develop RLS in the presence of further risk factors. RLS has a strong familial component.

There are defined pathophysiological pathways subserving RLS. Genome-wide association studies have found that RLS is significantly associated with common genetic variants in intronic or intergenic regions in *MEIS1*, *BTBD9*, and *MAP2K5* on chromosomes 2p, 6p, and 15q, respectively. The association of these three variants with RLS has been independently replicated. *BTBD9* confers a very large (80%) excessive risk when even a single allele is present. Because of the high frequency of this variant in individuals of European descent, the population attributable risk (PAR) approximates 50%. At-risk alleles associated with *MEIS1* and *BTBD9* are less common in individuals of African or Asian descent, perhaps suggesting lower risk for RLS in these populations.

Pathophysiological mechanisms in RLS also include disturbances in the central dopaminergic system and disturbances in iron metabolism. The endogenous opiate system may also be involved. Treatment effects of dopaminergic drugs (primarily D_2 and D_3 non-ergot agonists) provide further support that RLS is grounded in dysfunctional central dopaminergic pathways. While the effective treatment of RLS has also been shown to significantly reduce depressive symptoms, serotonergic antidepressants can induce or aggravate RLS in some individuals.

Gender-Related Diagnostic Issues

Although RLS is more prevalent in females than in males, there are no diagnostic differences according to gender. However, the prevalence of RLS during pregnancy is two to three times greater than in the general population. RLS associated with pregnancy peaks during the third trimester and improves or resolves in most cases soon after delivery. The gender difference in prevalence of RLS is explained at least in part by parity, with nulliparous females being at the same risk of RLS as age-matched males.

Diagnostic Markers

Polysomnography demonstrates significant abnormalities in RLS, commonly increased latency to sleep, and higher arousal index. Polysomnography with a preceding immobilization test may provide an indicator of the motor sign of RLS, periodic limb movements, under standard conditions of sleep and during quiet resting, both of which can provoke RLS symptoms.

Functional Consequences of Restless Legs Syndrome

Forms of RLS severe enough to significantly impair functioning or associated with mental disorders, including depression and anxiety, occur in approximately 2%–3% of the population.

Although the impact of milder symptoms is less well characterized, individuals with RLS complain of disruption in at least one activity of daily living, with up to 50% reporting a negative impact on mood, and 47.6% reporting a lack of energy. The most common consequences of RLS are sleep disturbance, including reduced sleep time, sleep fragmentation, and overall disturbance; depression, generalized anxiety disorder, panic disorder, and posttraumatic stress disorder; and quality-of-life impairments. RLS can result in daytime sleepiness or fatigue and is frequently accompanied by significant distress or impairment in affective, social, occupational, educational, academic, behavioral, or cognitive functioning.

Differential Diagnosis

The most important conditions in the differential diagnosis of RLS are leg cramps, positional discomfort, arthralgias/arthritis, myalgias, positional ischemia (numbness), leg edema, peripheral neuropathy, radiculopathy, and habitual foot tapping. "Knotting" of the muscle (cramps), relief with a single postural shift, limitation to joints, soreness to palpation (myalgias), and other abnormalities on physical examination are not characteristic of RLS. Unlike RLS, nocturnal leg cramps do not typically present with the desire to move the limbs nor are there frequent limb movements. Less common conditions to be differentiated from RLS include neuroleptic-induced akathisia, myelopathy, symptomatic venous insufficiency, peripheral artery disease, eczema, other orthopedic problems, and anxiety-induced restlessness. Worsening at night and periodic limb movements are more common in RLS than in medication-induced akathisia or peripheral neuropathy.

While is it important that RLS symptoms not be solely accounted for by another medical or behavioral condition, it should also be appreciated that any of these similar conditions can occur in an individual with RLS. This necessitates a separate focus on each possible condition in the diagnostic process and when assessing impact. For cases in which the diagnosis of RLS is not certain, evaluation for the supportive features of RLS, particularly PLMS or a family history of RLS, may be helpful. Clinical features, such as response to a dopaminergic agent and positive family history for RLS, can help with the differential diagnosis.

Comorbidity

Depressive disorders, anxiety disorders, and attentional disorders are commonly comorbid with RLS and are discussed in the section "Functional Consequences of Restless Legs Syndrome." The main medical disorder comorbid with RLS is cardiovascular disease. There may be an association with numerous other medical disorders, including hypertension, narcolepsy, migraine, Parkinson's disease, multiple sclerosis, peripheral neuropathy, obstructive sleep apnea, diabetes mellitus, fibromyalgia, osteoporosis, obesity, thyroid disease, and cancer. Iron deficiency, pregnancy, and chronic renal failure are also comorbid with RLS.

Relationship to International Classification of Sleep Disorders

The *International Classification of Sleep Disorders,* 2nd Edition (ICSD-2), presents similar diagnostic criteria for RLS but does not contain a criterion specifying frequency or duration of symptoms.

Substance/Medication-Induced Sleep Disorder

Diagnostic Criteria

A. A prominent and severe disturbance in sleep.
B. There is evidence from the history, physical examination, or laboratory findings of both (1) and (2):

   1. The symptoms in Criterion A developed during or soon after substance intoxication or after withdrawal from or exposure to a medication.
   2. The involved substance/medication is capable of producing the symptoms in Criterion A.

C. The disturbance is not better explained by a sleep disorder that is not substance/medication-induced. Such evidence of an independent sleep disorder could include the following:

   The symptoms precede the onset of the substance/medication use; the symptoms persist for a substantial period of time (e.g., about 1 month) after the cessation of acute withdrawal or severe intoxication; or there is other evidence suggesting the existence of an independent non-substance/medication-induced sleep disorder (e.g., a history of recurrent non-substance/medication-related episodes).

D. The disturbance does not occur exclusively during the course of a delirium.
E. The disturbance causes clinically significant distress or impairment in social, occupational, or other important areas of functioning.

Note: This diagnosis should be made instead of a diagnosis of substance intoxication or substance withdrawal only when the symptoms in Criterion A predominate in the clinical picture and when they are sufficiently severe to warrant clinical attention.

Coding note: The ICD-9-CM and ICD-10-CM codes for the [specific substance/medication]-induced sleep disorders are indicated in the table below. Note that the ICD-10-CM code depends on whether or not there is a comorbid substance use disorder present for the same class of substance. If a mild substance use disorder is comorbid with the substance-induced sleep disorder, the 4th position character is "1," and the clinician should record "mild [substance] use disorder" before the substance-induced sleep disorder (e.g., "mild cocaine use disorder with cocaine-induced sleep disorder"). If a moderate or severe substance use disorder is comorbid with the substance-induced sleep disorder, the 4th position character is "2," and the clinician should record "moderate [substance] use disorder" or "severe [substance] use disorder," depending on the severity of the comorbid substance use disorder. If there is no comorbid substance use disorder (e.g., after a one-time heavy use of the substance), then the 4th position character is "9," and the clinician should record only the substance-induced sleep disorder. A moderate or severe tobacco use disorder is required in order to code a tobacco-induced sleep disorder; it is not permissible to code a comorbid mild tobacco use disorder or no tobacco use disorder with a tobacco-induced sleep disorder.

Specify whether:
   Insomnia type: Characterized by difficulty falling asleep or maintaining sleep, frequent nocturnal awakenings, or nonrestorative sleep.
   Daytime sleepiness type: Characterized by predominant complaint of excessive sleepiness/fatigue during waking hours or, less commonly, a long sleep period.
   Parasomnia type: Characterized by abnormal behavioral events during sleep.
   Mixed type: Characterized by a substance/medication-induced sleep problem characterized by multiple types of sleep symptoms, but no symptom clearly predominates.

Specify if (see Table 1 in the chapter "Substance-Related and Addictive Disorders" for diagnoses associated with substance class):
   With onset during intoxication: This specifier should be used if criteria are met for intoxication with the substance/medication and symptoms developed during the intoxication period.
   With onset during discontinuation/withdrawal: This specifier should be used if criteria are met for discontinuation/withdrawal from the substance/medication and symptoms developed during, or shortly after, discontinuation of the substance/medication.

	ICD-9-CM	ICD-10-CM		
		With use disorder, mild	With use disorder, moderate or severe	Without use disorder
Alcohol	291.82	F10.182	F10.282	F10.982
Caffeine	292.85	F15.182	F15.282	F15.982
Cannabis	292.85	F12.188	F12.288	F12.988
Opioid	292.85	F11.182	F11.282	F11.982
Sedative, hypnotic, or anxiolytic	292.85	F13.182	F13.282	F13.982
Amphetamine (or other stimulant)	292.85	F15.182	F15.282	F15.982
Cocaine	292.85	F14.182	F14.282	F14.982
Tobacco	292.85	NA	F17.208	NA
Other (or unknown) substance	292.85	F19.182	F19.282	F19.982

Recording Procedures

ICD-9-CM. The name of the substance/medication-induced sleep disorder begins with the specific substance (e.g., cocaine, bupropion) that is presumed to be causing the sleep disturbance. The diagnostic code is selected from the table included in the criteria set, which is based on the drug class. For substances that do not fit into any of the classes (e.g., bupropion), the code for "other substance" should be used; and in cases in which a substance is judged to be an etiological factor but the specific class of substance is unknown, the category "unknown substance" should be used.

The name of the disorder is followed by the specification of onset (i.e., onset during intoxication, onset during discontinuation/withdrawal), followed by the subtype designation (i.e., insomnia type, daytime sleepiness type, parasomnia type, mixed type). Unlike the recording procedures for ICD-10-CM, which combine the substance-induced disorder and substance use disorder into a single code, for ICD-9-CM a separate diagnostic code is given for the substance use disorder. For example, in the case of insomnia occurring during withdrawal in a man with a severe lorazepam use disorder, the diagnosis is 292.85 lorazepam-induced sleep disorder, with onset during withdrawal, insomnia type. An additional diagnosis of 304.10 severe lorazepam use disorder is also given. When more than one substance is judged to play a significant role in the development of the sleep disturbance, each should be listed separately (e.g., 292.85 alcohol-induced sleep disorder, with onset during intoxication, insomnia type; 292.85 cocaine-induced sleep disorder, with onset during intoxication, insomnia type).

ICD-10-CM. The name of the substance/medication-induced sleep disorder begins with the specific substance (e.g., cocaine, bupropion) that is presumed to be causing the sleep disturbance. The diagnostic code is selected from the table included in the criteria set, which is based on the drug class and presence or absence of a comorbid substance use disorder. For substances that do not fit into any of the classes (e.g., bupropion), the code for "other substance" should be used; and in cases in which a substance is judged to be an etiological factor but the specific class of substance is unknown, the category "unknown substance" should be used.

When recording the name of the disorder, the comorbid substance use disorder (if any) is listed first, followed by the word "with," followed by the name of the substance-induced sleep disorder, followed by the specification of onset (i.e., onset during intoxication, onset during discontinuation/withdrawal), followed by the subtype designation (i.e., insomnia type, daytime sleepiness type, parasomnia type, mixed type). For example, in the case of insomnia occurring during withdrawal in a man with a severe lorazepam use disorder, the diagnosis is F13.282 severe lorazepam use disorder with lorazepam-induced sleep disorder, with onset during withdrawal, insomnia type. A separate diagnosis of the comorbid severe lorazepam use disorder is not given. If the substance-induced sleep disorder occurs without a comorbid substance use disorder (e.g., with medication use), no accompanying substance use disorder is noted (e.g., F19.982 bupropion-induced sleep disorder, with onset during medication use, insomnia type). When more than one substance is judged to play a significant role in the development of the sleep disturbance, each should be listed separately (e.g., F10.282 severe alcohol use disorder with alcohol-induced sleep disorder, with onset during intoxication, insomnia type; F14.282 severe cocaine use disorder with cocaine-induced sleep disorder, with onset during intoxication, insomnia type).

Diagnostic Features

The essential feature of substance/medication-induced sleep disorder is a prominent sleep disturbance that is sufficiently severe to warrant independent clinical attention (Criterion A) and that is judged to be primarily associated with the pharmacological effects of a substance (i.e., a drug of abuse, a medication, toxin exposure) (Criterion B). Depending on the substance involved, one of four types of sleep disturbances is reported. Insomnia type and daytime sleepiness type are most common, while parasomnia type is seen less often. The mixed type is noted when more than one type of sleep disturbance–related symptom is present and none predominates. The disturbance must not be better explained by another sleep disorder (Criterion C). A substance/medication-induced sleep disorder is distinguished from insomnia disorder or a disorder associated with excessive daytime sleepiness by considering onset and course. For drugs of abuse, there must be evidence of intoxication or withdrawal from the history, physical examination, or laboratory findings. Substance/medication-induced sleep disorder arises only in association with intoxication or discontinuation/withdrawal states, whereas other sleep disorders may precede the onset of substance use or occur during times of sustained abstinence. As discontinuation/withdrawal states for some substances can be protracted, onset of the sleep disturbance can occur 4 weeks after cessation of substance use, and the disturbance may have features atypical of other sleep disorders (e.g., atypical age at onset or course). The diagnosis is not made if the sleep disturbance occurs only during a delirium (Criterion D). The symptoms must cause clinically significant distress or impairment in social, occupational, or other important areas of functioning (Criterion E). This diagnosis should be made instead of a diagnosis of substance intoxication or substance withdrawal only when the symptoms in Criterion A predominate in the clinical picture and when the symptoms warrant independent clinical attention.

Associated Features Supporting Diagnosis

During periods of substance/medication use, intoxication, or withdrawal, individuals frequently complain of dysphoric mood, including depression and anxiety, irritability, cognitive impairment, inability to concentrate, and fatigue.

Prominent and severe sleep disturbances can occur in association with intoxication with the following classes of substances: alcohol; caffeine; cannabis; opioids; sedatives, hypnotics, or anxiolytics; stimulants (including cocaine); and other (or unknown) substances. Prominent and severe sleep disturbances can occur in association with withdrawal from the following classes of substances: alcohol; caffeine; cannabis; opioids; sedatives, hypnotics, or anxiolytics; stimulant (including cocaine); tobacco; and other (or unknown) substances. Some medications that invoke sleep disturbances include adrenergic agonists and antagonists, dopamine agonists and antagonists, cholinergic agonists and antagonists, serotonergic agonists and antagonists, antihistamines, and corticosteroids.

Alcohol.   Alcohol-induced sleep disorder typically occurs as insomnia type. During acute intoxication, alcohol produces an immediate sedative effect depending on dose, accompanied by increased stages 3 and 4 non–rapid eye movement (NREM) sleep and reduced rapid eye movement (REM) sleep. Following these initial effects, there may be increased wakefulness, restless sleep, and vivid and anxiety-laden dreams for the remaining sleep period. In parallel, stages 3 and 4 sleep are reduced, and wakefulness and REM sleep are increased. Alcohol can aggravate breathing-related sleep disorder. With habitual use, alcohol continues to show a short-lived sedative effect in the first half of the night, followed by sleep continuity disruption in the second half. During alcohol withdrawal, there is extremely disrupted sleep continuity, and an increased amount and intensity of REM sleep, associated frequently with vivid dreaming, which in extreme form, constitutes part of alcohol withdrawal delirium. After acute withdrawal, chronic alcohol users may continue to complain of light, fragmented sleep for weeks to years associated with a persistent deficit in slow-wave sleep.

Caffeine.   Caffeine-induced sleep disorder produces insomnia in a dose-dependent manner, with some individuals presenting with daytime sleepiness related to withdrawal.

Cannabis.   Acute administration of cannabis may shorten sleep latency, though arousing effects with increments in sleep latency also occur. Cannabis enhances slow-wave sleep and suppresses REM sleep after acute administration. In chronic users, tolerance to the sleep-inducing and slow-wave sleep–enhancing effects develops. Upon withdrawal, sleep difficulties and unpleasant dreams have been reported lasting for several weeks. Polysomnography studies demonstrate reduced slow-wave sleep and increased REM sleep during this phase.

Opioids.   Opioids may produce an increase in sleepiness and in subjective depth of sleep, and reduced REM sleep, during acute short-term use. With continued administration, tolerance to the sedative effects of opioids develops and there are complaints of insomnia. Consistent with their respiratory depressant effects, opioids exacerbate sleep apnea.

Sedative, hypnotic, or anxiolytic substances.   Sedatives, hypnotics, and anxiolytics (e.g., barbiturates, benzodiazepines receptor agonists, meprobamate, glutethimide, methyprylon) have similar effects as opioids on sleep. During acute intoxication, sedative-hypnotic drugs produce the expected increase in sleepiness and decrease in wakefulness. Chronic use (particularly of barbiturates and the older nonbarbiturate, nonbenzodiazepine drugs) may cause tolerance with subsequent return of insomnia. Daytime sleepiness may occur. Sedative-hypnotic drugs can increase the frequency and severity of obstructive sleep apnea events. Parasomnias are associated with use of benzodiazepine receptor agonists, especially when these medications are taken at higher doses and when they are combined with other sedative drugs. Abrupt discontinuation of chronic sedative, hypnotic, or anxiolytic use can lead to withdrawal but more commonly rebound insomnia, a condition of an exacerbation of insomnia upon drug discontinuation for 1–2 days reported to occur even with short-term use. Sedative, hypnotic, or anxiolytic drugs with short durations of action are most likely to produce complaints of rebound insomnia, whereas those with longer durations of action are more often associated with daytime sleepiness. Any sedative, hypnotic, or anxiolytic drug can potentially cause daytime sedation, withdrawal, or rebound insomnia.

Amphetamines and related substances and other stimulants.   Sleep disorders induced by amphetamine and related substances and other stimulants are characterized by insomnia during intoxication and excessive sleepiness during withdrawal. During acute intoxication, stimulants reduce the total amount of sleep, increase sleep latency and sleep continuity disturbances, and decrease REM sleep. Slow-wave sleep tends to be reduced. During withdrawal from chronic stimulant use, there is both prolonged nocturnal sleep duration and excessive daytime sleepiness. Multiple sleep latency tests may show increased daytime sleepiness during the withdrawal phase. Drugs like 3,4-methylenedioxymethamphetamine (MDMA; "ecstasy") and related substances lead to restless and disturbed sleep within 48 hours of intake; frequent use of these compounds is associated with persisting symptoms of anxiety, depression, and sleep disturbances, even during longer-term abstinence.

Tobacco.   Chronic tobacco consumption is associated primarily with symptoms of insomnia, decreased slow-wave sleep with a reduction of sleep efficiency, and increased daytime sleepiness. Withdrawal from tobacco can lead to impaired sleep. Individuals who smoke heavily may experience regular nocturnal awakenings caused by tobacco craving.

Other or unknown substances/medications.   Other substances/medications may produce sleep disturbances, particularly medications that affect the central or autonomic nervous systems (e.g., adrenergic agonists and antagonists, dopamine agonists and antagonists, cholinergic agonists and antagonists, serotonergic agonists and antagonists, antihistamines, corticosteroids).

Development and Course

Insomnia in children can be identified by either a parent or the child. Often the child has a clear sleep disturbance associated with initiation of a medication but may not report symptoms, although parents observe the sleep disturbances. The use of some illicit substances (e.g., cannabis, ecstasy) is prevalent in adolescence and early adulthood. Insomnia or any other sleep disturbance encountered in this age group should prompt careful consideration of whether the sleep disturbance is due to consumption of these substances. Help-seeking behavior for the sleep disturbance in these age groups is limited, and thus corroborative report may be elicited from a parent, caregiver, or teacher. Older individuals take more medications and are at increased risk for developing a substance/medication-induced sleep disorder. They may interpret sleep disturbance as part of normal aging and fail to report symptoms. Individuals with major neurocognitive disorder (e.g., dementia) are at risk for substance/medication-induced sleep disorders but may not report symptoms, making corroborative report from caregiver(s) particularly important.

Risk and Prognostic Factors

Risk and prognostic factors involved in substance abuse/dependence or medication use are normative for certain age groups. They are relevant for, and likely applicable to, the type of sleep disturbance encountered (see the chapter "Substance-Related and Addictive Disorders" for descriptions of respective substance use disorders).

Temperamental.   Substance use generally precipitates or accompanies insomnia in vulnerable individuals. Thus, presence of insomnia in response to stress or change in sleep environment or timing can represent a risk for developing substance/medication-induced sleep disorder. A similar risk may be present for individuals with other sleep disorders (e.g., individuals with hypersomnia who use stimulants).

Culture-Related Diagnostic Issues

The consumption of substances, including prescribed medications, may depend in part on cultural background and specific local drug regulations.

Gender-Related Diagnostic Issues

Gender-specific prevalences (i.e., females affected more than males at a ratio of about 2:1) exist for patterns of consumption of some substances (e.g., alcohol). The same amount and duration of consumption of a given substance may lead to highly different sleep-related outcomes in males and females based on, for example, gender-specific differences in hepatic functioning.

Diagnostic Markers

Each of the substance/medication-induced sleep disorders produces electroencephalographic sleep patterns that are associated with, but cannot be considered diagnostic of, other disorders. The electroencephalographic sleep profile for each substance is related to the stage of use, whether intake/intoxication, chronic use, or withdrawal following discontinuation of the substance. All-night polysomnography can help define the severity of insomnia complaints, while the multiple sleep latency test provides information about the severity of daytime sleepiness. Monitoring of nocturnal respiration and periodic limb movements with polysomnography may verify a substance's impact on nocturnal breathing and motor behavior. Sleep diaries for 2 weeks and actigraphy are considered helpful in confirming the presence of substance/medication-induced sleep disorder. Drug screening can be of use when the individual is not aware or unwilling to relate information about substance intake.

Functional Consequences of Substance/Medication-Induced Sleep Disorder

While there are many functional consequences associated with sleep disorders, the only unique consequence for substance/medication-induced sleep disorder is increased risk for relapse. The degree of sleep disturbance during alcohol withdrawal (e.g., REM sleep rebound predicts risk of relapse of drinking). Monitoring of sleep quality and daytime sleepiness during and after withdrawal may provide clinically meaningful information on whether an individual is at increased risk for relapse.

Differential Diagnosis

Substance intoxication or substance withdrawal. Sleep disturbances are commonly encountered in the context of substance intoxication or substance discontinuation/withdrawal. A diagnosis of substance/medication-induced sleep disorder should be made instead of a diagnosis of substance intoxication or substance withdrawal only when the sleep disturbance is predominant in the clinical picture and is sufficiently severe to warrant independent clinical attention.

Delirium. If the substance/medication-induced sleep disturbance occurs exclusively during the course of a delirium, it is not diagnosed separately.

Other sleep disorders. A substance/medication-induced sleep disorder is distinguished from another sleep disorder if a substance/medication is judged to be etiologically related to the symptoms. A substance/medication-induced sleep disorder attributed to a prescribed medication for a mental disorder or medical condition must have its onset while the individual is receiving the medication or during discontinuation, if there is a discontinuation/withdrawal syndrome associated with the medication. Once treatment is discontinued, the sleep disturbance will usually remit within days to several weeks. If symptoms persist beyond 4 weeks, other causes for the sleep disturbance–related symptoms should be considered. Not infrequently, individuals with another sleep disorder use medications or drugs of abuse to self-medicate their symptoms (e.g., alcohol for management of insomnia). If the substance/medication is judged to play a significant role in the exacerbation of the sleep disturbance, an additional diagnosis of a substance/medication-induced sleep disorder may be warranted.

Sleep disorder due to another medical condition. Substance/medication-induced sleep disorder and sleep disorder associated with another medical condition may produce similar symptoms of insomnia, daytime sleepiness, or a parasomnia. Many individuals with other medical conditions that cause sleep disturbance are treated with medications that may also cause sleep disturbances. The chronology of symptoms is the most important factor in distinguishing between these two sources of sleep symptoms. Difficulties with sleep that clearly preceded the use of any medication for treatment of a medical condition would suggest a diagnosis of sleep disorder associated with another medical condition. Conversely, sleep symptoms that appear only after the initiation of a particular medication/substance suggest a substance/medication-induced sleep disorder. If the disturbance is comorbid with another medical condition and is also exacerbated by substance use, both diagnoses (i.e., sleep disorder associated with another medical condition and substance/medication-induced sleep disorder) are given. When there is insufficient evidence to determine whether the sleep disturbance is attributable to a substance/medication or to another medical condition or is primary (i.e., not due to either a substance/medication or another medical condition), a diagnosis of other specified sleep-wake disorder or unspecified sleep-wake disorder is indicated.

Comorbidity

See the "Comorbidity" sections for other sleep disorders in this chapter, including insomnia, hypersomnolence, central sleep apnea, sleep-related hypoventilation, and circadian rhythm sleep-wake disorders, shift work type.

Relationship to International Classification of Sleep Disorders

The *International Classification of Sleep Disorders*, 2nd Edition (ICSD-2), lists sleep disorders "due to drug or substance" under their respective phenotypes (e.g., insomnia, hypersomnia).

Other Specified Insomnia Disorder

780.52 (G47.09)

This category applies to presentations in which symptoms characteristic of insomnia disorder that cause clinically significant distress or impairment in social, occupational, or other important areas of functioning predominate but do not meet the full criteria for insomnia disorder or any of the disorders in the sleep-wake disorders diagnostic class. The other specified insomnia disorder category is used in situations in which the clinician chooses to communicate the specific reason that the presentation does not meet the criteria for insomnia disorder or any specific sleep-wake disorder. This is done by recording "other specified insomnia disorder" followed by the specific reason (e.g., "brief insomnia disorder").

Examples of presentations that can be specified using the "other specified" designation include the following:

1. **Brief insomnia disorder:** Duration is less than 3 months.
2. **Restricted to nonrestorative sleep:** Predominant complaint is nonrestorative sleep unaccompanied by other sleep symptoms such as difficulty falling asleep or remaining asleep.

Unspecified Insomnia Disorder

780.52 (G47.00)

This category applies to presentations in which symptoms characteristic of insomnia disorder that cause clinically significant distress or impairment in social, occupational, or other important areas of functioning predominate but do not meet the full criteria for insomnia disorder or any of the disorders in the sleep-wake disorders diagnostic class. The unspecified insomnia disorder category is used in situations in which the clinician chooses *not* to specify the reason that the criteria are not met for insomnia disorder or a specific sleep-wake disorder, and includes presentations in which there is insufficient information to make a more specific diagnosis.

Other Specified Hypersomnolence Disorder

780.54 (G47.19)

This category applies to presentations in which symptoms characteristic of hypersomnolence disorder that cause clinically significant distress or impairment in social, occupational, or other important areas of functioning predominate but do not meet the full criteria for hypersomnolence disorder or any of the disorders in the sleep-wake disorders diagnostic class. The other specified hypersomnolence disorder category is used in situations in which the clinician chooses to communicate the specific reason that the presentation does not meet the criteria for hypersomnolence disorder or any specific sleep-wake disorder. This is done by recording "other specified hypersomnolence disorder" followed by the specific reason (e.g., "brief-duration hypersomnolence," as in Kleine-Levin syndrome).

Unspecified Hypersomnolence Disorder

780.54 (G47.10)

This category applies to presentations in which symptoms characteristic of hypersomnolence disorder that cause clinically significant distress or impairment in social, occupational, or other important areas of functioning predominate but do not meet the full criteria for hypersomnolence disorder or any of the disorders in the sleep-wake disorders diagnostic class. The unspecified hypersomnolence disorder category is used in situations in which the clinician chooses *not* to specify the reason that the criteria are not met for hypersomnolence disorder or a specific sleep-wake disorder, and includes presentations in which there is insufficient information to make a more specific diagnosis.

Other Specified Sleep-Wake Disorder

780.59 (G47.8)

This category applies to presentations in which symptoms characteristic of a sleep-wake disorder that cause clinically significant distress or impairment in social, occupational, or other important areas of functioning predominate but do not meet the full criteria for any of the disorders in the sleep-wake disorders diagnostic class and do not qualify for a diagnosis of other specified insomnia disorder or other specified hypersomnolence disorder. The other specified sleep-wake disorder category is used in situations in which the clinician chooses to communicate the specific reason that the presentation does not meet the criteria for any specific sleep-wake disorder. This is done by recording "other specified sleep-wake disorder" followed by the specific reason (e.g., "repeated arousals during rapid eye movement sleep without polysomnography or history of Parkinson's disease or other synucleinopathy").

Unspecified Sleep-Wake Disorder

780.59 (G47.9)

This category applies to presentations in which symptoms characteristic of a sleep-wake disorder that cause clinically significant distress or impairment in social, occupational, or other important areas of functioning predominate but do not meet the full criteria for any of the disorders in the sleep-wake disorders diagnostic class and do not qualify for a diagnosis of unspecified insomnia disorder or unspecified hypersomnolence disorder. The unspecified sleep-wake disorder category is used in situations in which the clinician chooses *not* to specify the reason that the criteria are not met for a specific sleep-wake disorder, and includes presentations in which there is insufficient information to make a more specific diagnosis.

Sexual Dysfunctions

Sexual dysfunctions include delayed ejaculation, erectile disorder, female orgasmic disorder, female sexual interest/arousal disorder, genito-pelvic pain/penetration disorder, male hypoactive sexual desire disorder, premature (early) ejaculation, substance/medication-induced sexual dysfunction, other specified sexual dysfunction, and unspecified sexual dysfunction. Sexual dysfunctions are a heterogeneous group of disorders that are typically characterized by a clinically significant disturbance in a person's ability to respond sexually or to experience sexual pleasure. An individual may have several sexual dysfunctions at the same time. In such cases, all of the dysfunctions should be diagnosed.

Clinical judgment should be used to determine if the sexual difficulties are the result of inadequate sexual stimulation; in these cases, there may still be a need for care, but a diagnosis of a sexual dysfunction would not be made. These cases may include, but are not limited to, conditions in which lack of knowledge about effective stimulation prevents the experience of arousal or orgasm.

Subtypes are used to designate the onset of the difficulty. In many individuals with sexual dysfunctions, the time of onset may indicate different etiologies and interventions. *Lifelong* refers to a sexual problem that has been present from first sexual experiences, and *acquired* applies to sexual disorders that develop after a period of relatively normal sexual function. *Generalized* refers to sexual difficulties that are not limited to certain types of stimulation, situations, or partners, and *situational* refers to sexual difficulties that only occur with certain types of stimulation, situations, or partners.

In addition to the lifelong/acquired and generalized/situational subtypes, a number of factors must be considered during the assessment of sexual dysfunction, given that they may be relevant to etiology and/or treatment, and that may contribute, to varying degrees, across individuals: 1) partner factors (e.g., partner's sexual problems; partner's health status); 2) relationship factors (e.g., poor communication; discrepancies in desire for sexual activity); 3) individual vulnerability factors (e.g., poor body image; history of sexual or emotional abuse), psychiatric comorbidity (e.g., depression, anxiety), or stressors (e.g., job loss, bereavement); 4) cultural or religious factors (e.g., inhibitions related to prohibitions against sexual activity or pleasure; attitudes toward sexuality); and 5) medical factors relevant to prognosis, course, or treatment.

Clinical judgment about the diagnosis of sexual dysfunction should take into consideration cultural factors that may influence expectations or engender prohibitions about the experience of sexual pleasure. Aging may be associated with a normative decrease in sexual response.

Sexual response has a requisite biological underpinning, yet is usually experienced in an intrapersonal, interpersonal, and cultural context. Thus, sexual function involves a complex interaction among biological, sociocultural, and psychological factors. In many clinical contexts, a precise understanding of the etiology of a sexual problem is unknown. Nonetheless, a sexual dysfunction diagnosis requires ruling out problems that are better explained by a nonsexual mental disorder, by the effects of a substance (e.g., drug or medication), by a medical condition (e.g., due to pelvic nerve damage), or by severe relationship distress, partner violence, or other stressors.

If the sexual dysfunction is mostly explainable by another nonsexual mental disorder (e.g., depressive or bipolar disorder, anxiety disorder, posttraumatic stress disorder, psychotic disorder), then only the other mental disorder diagnosis should be made. If the problem is thought to be better explained by the use/misuse or discontinuation of a drug or substance, it should be diagnosed accordingly as a substance/medication-induced sexual dysfunction. If the sexual dysfunction is attributable to another medical condition (e.g., peripheral neuropathy), the individual would not receive a psychiatric diagnosis. If severe relationship distress, partner violence, or significant stressors better explain the sexual difficulties, then a sexual dysfunction diagnosis is not made, but an appropriate V or Z code for the relationship problem or stressor may be listed. In many cases, a precise etiological relationship between another condition (e.g., a medical condition) and a sexual dysfunction cannot be established.

Delayed Ejaculation

Diagnostic Criteria   302.74 (F52.32)

A. Either of the following symptoms must be experienced on almost all or all occasions (approximately 75%–100%) of partnered sexual activity (in identified situational contexts or, if generalized, in all contexts), and without the individual desiring delay:

   1. Marked delay in ejaculation.
   2. Marked infrequency or absence of ejaculation.

B. The symptoms in Criterion A have persisted for a minimum duration of approximately 6 months.

C. The symptoms in Criterion A cause clinically significant distress in the individual.

D. The sexual dysfunction is not better explained by a nonsexual mental disorder or as a consequence of severe relationship distress or other significant stressors and is not attributable to the effects of a substance/medication or another medical condition.

Specify whether:

   Lifelong: The disturbance has been present since the individual became sexually active.
   Acquired: The disturbance began after a period of relatively normal sexual function.

Specify whether:

   Generalized: Not limited to certain types of stimulation, situations, or partners.
   Situational: Only occurs with certain types of stimulation, situations, or partners.

Specify current severity:

   Mild: Evidence of mild distress over the symptoms in Criterion A.
   Moderate: Evidence of moderate distress over the symptoms in Criterion A.
   Severe: Evidence of severe or extreme distress over the symptoms in Criterion A.

Diagnostic Features

The distinguishing feature of delayed ejaculation is a marked delay in or inability to achieve ejaculation (Criterion A). The man reports difficulty or inability to ejaculate despite the presence of adequate sexual stimulation and the desire to ejaculate. The presenting complaint usually involves partnered sexual activity. In most cases, the diagnosis will be made by self-report of the individual. The definition of "delay" does not have precise boundaries, as there is noconsensus as to what constitutes a reasonable time to reach orgasm or what is unacceptably long for most men and their sexual partners.

Associated Features Supporting Diagnosis

The man and his partner may report prolonged thrusting to achieve orgasm to the point of exhaustion or genital discomfort and then ceasing efforts. Some men may report avoiding sexual activity because of a repetitive pattern of difficulty ejaculating. Some sexual partners may report feeling less sexually attractive because their partner cannot ejaculate easily.

In addition to the subtypes "lifelong/acquired" and "generalized/situational," the following five factors must be considered during assessment and diagnosis of delayed ejaculation, given that they may be relevant to etiology and/or treatment: 1) partner factors (e.g., partner's sexual problems, partner's health status); 2) relationship factors (e.g., poor communication, discrepancies in desire for sexual activity); 3) individual vulnerability factors (e.g., poor body image; history of sexual or emotional abuse), psychiatric comorbidity (e.g., depression, anxiety), or stressors (e.g., job loss, bereavement); 4) cultural/religious factors (e.g., inhibitions related to prohibitions against sexual activity; attitudes toward sexuality); and 5) medical factors relevant to prognosis, course, or treatment. Each of these factors may contribute differently to the presenting symptoms of different men with this disorder.

Prevalence

Prevalence is unclear because of the lack of a precise definition of this syndrome. It is the least common male sexual complaint. Only 75% of men report always ejaculating during sexual activity, and less than 1% of men will complain of problems with reaching ejaculation that last more than 6 months.

Development and Course

Lifelong delayed ejaculation begins with early sexual experiences and continues throughout life. By definition, acquired delayed ejaculation begins after a period of normal sexual function. There is minimal evidence concerning the course of acquired delayed ejaculation. The prevalence of delayed ejaculation appears to remain relatively constant until around age 50 years, when the incidence begins to increase significantly. Men in their 80s report twice as much difficulty ejaculating as men younger than 59 years.

Risk and Prognostic Factors

Genetic and physiological.   Age-related loss of the fast-conducting peripheral sensory nerves and age-related decreased sex steroid secretion may be associated with the increase in delayed ejaculation in men older than 50 years.

Culture-Related Diagnostic Issues

Complaints of ejaculatory delay vary across countries and cultures. Such complaints are more common among men in Asian populations than in men living in Europe, Australia, or the United States. This variation may be attributable to cultural or genetic differences between cultures.

Functional Consequences of Delayed Ejaculation

Difficulty with ejaculation may contribute to difficulties in conception. Delayed ejaculation is often associated with considerable psychological distress in one or both partners.

Differential Diagnosis

Another medical condition.   The major differential diagnosis is between delayed ejaculation fully explained by another medical illness or injury and delayed ejaculation with a psychogenic, idiopathic, or combined psychological and medical etiology. A situational aspect to the complaint is suggestive of a psychological basis for the problem (e.g., men who can ejaculate during sexual activity with one sex but not the other; men who can ejaculate with one partner but not another of the same sex; men with paraphilic arousal patterns; men who require highly ritualized activity to ejaculate during partnered sexual activity). Another medical illness or injury may produce delays in ejaculation independent of psychological issues. For example, inability to ejaculate can be caused by interruption of the nerve supply to the genitals, such as can occur after traumatic surgical injury to the lumbar sympathetic ganglia, abdominoperitoneal surgery, or lumbar sympathectomy. Ejaculation is thought to be under autonomic nervous system control involving the hypogastric (sympathetic) and pudendal (parasympathetic) nerves. A number of neurodegenerative diseases, such as multiple sclerosis and diabetic and alcoholic neuropathy, can cause inability to ejaculate. Delayed ejaculation should also be differentiated from retrograde ejaculation (i.e., ejaculation into the bladder), which may follow transurethral prostatic resection.

Substance/medication use.   A number of pharmacological agents, such as antidepressants, antipsychotics, alpha sympathetic drugs, and opioid drugs, can cause ejaculatory problems.

Dysfunction with orgasm.   It is important in the history to ascertain whether the complaint concerns delayed ejaculation or the sensation of orgasm, or both. Ejaculation occurs in the genitals, whereas the experience of orgasm is believed to be primarily subjective. Ejaculation and orgasm usually occur together but not always. For example, a man with a normal ejaculatory pattern may complain of decreased pleasure (i.e., anhedonic ejaculation). Such a complaint would not be coded as delayed ejaculation but could be coded as other specified sexual dysfunction or unspecified sexual dysfunction.

Comorbidity

There is some evidence to suggest that delayed ejaculation may be more common in severe forms of major depressive disorder.

Erectile Disorder

Diagnostic Criteria   **302.72 (F52.21)**

A. At least one of the three following symptoms must be experienced on almost all or all (approximately 75%–100%) occasions of sexual activity (in identified situational contexts or, if generalized, in all contexts):
   1. Marked difficulty in obtaining an erection during sexual activity.
   2. Marked difficulty in maintaining an erection until the completion of sexual activity.
   3. Marked decrease in erectile rigidity.
B. The symptoms in Criterion A have persisted for a minimum duration of approximately 6 months.
C. The symptoms in Criterion A cause clinically significant distress in the individual.
D. The sexual dysfunction is not better explained by a nonsexual mental disorder or as a consequence of severe relationship distress or other significant stressors and is not attributable to the effects of a substance/medication or another medical condition.

Specify whether:
   Lifelong: The disturbance has been present since the individual became sexually active.
   Acquired: The disturbance began after a period of relatively normal sexual function.
Specify whether:
   Generalized: Not limited to certain types of stimulation, situations, or partners.
   Situational: Only occurs with certain types of stimulation, situations, or partners.

Specify current severity:
  Mild: Evidence of mild distress over the symptoms in Criterion A.
  Moderate: Evidence of moderate distress over the symptoms in Criterion A.
  Severe: Evidence of severe or extreme distress over the symptoms in Criterion A.

Diagnostic Features

The essential feature of erectile disorder is the repeated failure to obtain or maintain erections during partnered sexual activities (Criterion A). A careful sexual history is necessary to ascertain that the problem has been present for a significant duration of time (i.e., at least approximately 6 months) and occurs on the majority of sexual occasions (i.e., at least 75% of the time). Symptoms may occur only in specific situations involving certain types of stimulation or partners, or they may occur in a generalized manner in all types of situations, stimulation, or partners.

Associated Features Supporting Diagnosis

Many men with erectile disorder may have low self-esteem, low self-confidence, and a decreased sense of masculinity, and may experience depressed affect. Fear and/or avoidance of future sexual encounters may occur. Decreased sexual satisfaction and reduced sexual desire in the individual's partner are common.

In addition to the subtypes "lifelong/acquired" and "generalized/situational," the following five factors must be considered during assessment and diagnosis of erectile disorder given that they may be relevant to etiology and/or treatment: 1) partner factors (e.g., partner's sexual problems, partner's health status); 2) relationship factors (e.g., poor communication, discrepancies in desire for sexual activity); 3) individual vulnerability factors (e.g., poor body image, history of sexual or emotional abuse), psychiatric comorbidity (e.g., depression, anxiety), or stressors (e.g., job loss, bereavement); 4) cultural/religious factors (e.g., inhibitions related to prohibitions against sexual activity; attitudes toward sexuality); and 5) medical factors relevant to prognosis, course, or treatment. Each of these factors may contribute differently to the presenting symptoms of different men with this disorder.

Prevalence

The prevalence of lifelong versus acquired erectile disorder is unknown. There is a strong age-related increase in both prevalence and incidence of problems with erection, particularly after age 50 years. Approximately 13%–21% of men ages 40–80 years complain of occasional problems with erections. Approximately 2% of men younger than age 40–50 years complain of frequent problems with erections, whereas 40%–50% of men older than 60–70 years may have significant problems with erections. About 20% of men fear erectile problems on their first sexual experience, whereas approximately 8% experienced erectile problems that hindered penetration during their first sexual experience.

Development and Course

Erectile failure on first sexual attempt has been found to be related to having sex with a previously unknown partner, concomitant use of drugs or alcohol, not wanting to have sex, and peer pressure. There is minimal evidence regarding the persistence of such problems after the first attempt. It is assumed that most of these problems spontaneously remit without professional intervention, but some men may continue to have episodic problems. In contrast, acquired erectile disorder is often associated with biological factors such as diabetes and cardiovascular disease. Acquired erectile disorder is likely to be persistent in most men.

The natural history of lifelong erectile disorder is unknown. Clinical observation supports the association of lifelong erectile disorder with psychological factors that are self-limiting or responsive to psychological interventions, whereas, as noted above, acquired erectile disorder is more likely to be related to biological factors and to be persistent. The incidence of erectile disorder increases with age. A minority of men diagnosed as having moderate erectile failure may experience spontaneous remission of symptoms without medical intervention. Distress associated with erectile disorder is lower in older men as compared with younger men.

Risk and Prognostic Factors

Temperamental.   Neurotic personality traits may be associated with erectile problems in college students, and submissive personality traits may be associated with erectile problems in men age 40 years and older. *Alexithymia* (i.e., deficits in cognitive processing of emotions) is common in men diagnosed with "psychogenic" erectile dysfunction. Erectile problems are common in men diagnosed with depression and posttraumatic stress disorder.

Course modifiers.   Risk factors for acquired erectile disorder include age, smoking tobacco, lack of physical exercise, diabetes, and decreased desire.

Culture-Related Diagnostic Issues

Complaints of erectile disorder have been found to vary across countries. It is unclear to what extent these differences represent differences in cultural expectations as opposed to genuine differences in the frequency of erectile failure.

Diagnostic Markers

Nocturnal penile tumescence testing and measured erectile turgidity during sleep can be employed to help differentiate organic from psychogenic erectile problems on the assumption that adequate erections during rapid eye movement sleep indicate a psychological etiology to the problem. A number of other diagnostic procedures may be employed depending on the clinician's assessment of their relevance given the individual's age, comorbid medical problems, and clinical presentation. Doppler ultrasonography and intravascular injection of vasoactive drugs, as well as invasive diagnostic procedures such as dynamic infusion cavernosography, can be used to assess vascular integrity. Pudendal nerve conduction studies, including somatosensory evoked potentials, can be employed when a peripheral neuropathy is suspected. In men also complaining of decreased sexual desire, serum bioavailable or free testosterone is frequently assessed to determine if the difficulty is secondary to endocrinological factors. Thyroid function may also be assessed. Determination of fasting serum glucose is useful to screen for the presence of diabetes mellitus. The assessment of serum lipids is important, as erectile disorder in men 40 years and older is predictive of the future risk of coronary artery disease.

Functional Consequences of Erectile Disorder

Erectile disorder can interfere with fertility and produce both individual and interpersonal distress. Fear and/or avoidance of sexual encounters may interfere with the ability to develop intimate relationships.

Differential Diagnosis

Nonsexual mental disorders.   Major depressive disorder and erectile disorder are closely associated, and erectile disorder accompanying severe depressive disorder may occur.

Normal erectile function.   The differential should include consideration of normal erectile function in men with excessive expectations.

Substance/medication use.   Another major differential diagnosis is whether the erectile problem is secondary to substance/medication use. An onset that coincides with the beginning of substance/medication use and that dissipates with discontinuation of the substance/medication or dose reduction is suggestive of a substance/medication-induced sexual dysfunction.

Another medical condition.   The most difficult aspect of the differential diagnosis of erectile disorder is ruling out erectile problems that are fully explained by medical factors. Such cases would not receive a diagnosis of a mental disorder. The distinction between erectile disorder as a mental disorder and erectile dysfunction as the result of another medical condition is usually unclear, and many cases will have complex, interactive biological and psychiatric etiologies. If the individual is older than 40–50 years and/or has concomitant medical problems, the differential diagnosis should include medical etiologies, especially vascular disease. The presence of an organic disease known to cause erectile problems does not confirm a causal relationship. For example, a man with diabetes mellitus can develop erectile disorder in response to psychological stress. In general, erectile dysfunction due to organic factors is generalized and gradual in onset. An exception would be erectile problems after traumatic injury to the nervous innervation of the genital organs (e.g., spinal cord injury). Erectile problems that are situational and inconsistent and that have an acute onset after a stressful life event are most often due to psychological events. An age of less than 40 years is also suggestive of a psychological etiology to the difficulty.

Other sexual dysfunctions.   Erectile disorder may coexist with premature (early) ejaculation and male hypoactive sexual desire disorder.

Comorbidity

Erectile disorder can be comorbid with other sexual diagnoses, such as premature (early) ejaculation and male hypoactive sexual desire disorder, as well as with anxiety and depressive disorders. Erectile disorder is common in men with lower urinary tract symptoms related to prostatic hypertrophy. Erectile disorder may be comorbid with dyslipidemia, cardiovascular disease, hypogonadism, multiple sclerosis, diabetes mellitus, and other diseases that interfere with the vascular, neurological, or endocrine function necessary for normal erectile function.

Relationship to International Classification of Diseases

Erectile response is coded as failure of genital response in ICD-10 (F2.2).

Female Orgasmic Disorder

Diagnostic Criteria	**302.73 (F52.31)**

A. Presence of either of the following symptoms and experienced on almost all or all (approximately 75%–100%) occasions of sexual activity (in identified situational contexts or, if generalized, in all contexts):

1. Marked delay in, marked infrequency of, or absence of orgasm.
2. Markedly reduced intensity of orgasmic sensations.

B. The symptoms in Criterion A have persisted for a minimum duration of approximately 6 months.

C. The symptoms in Criterion A cause clinically significant distress in the individual.

D. The sexual dysfunction is not better explained by a nonsexual mental disorder or as a consequence of severe relationship distress (e.g., partner violence) or other significant stressors and is not attributable to the effects of a substance/medication or another medical condition.

Specify whether:

Lifelong: The disturbance has been present since the individual became sexually active.

Acquired: The disturbance began after a period of relatively normal sexual function.

Specify whether:

Generalized: Not limited to certain types of stimulation, situations, or partners.

Situational: Only occurs with certain types of stimulation, situations, or partners.

Specify if:

Never experienced an orgasm under any situation.

Specify current severity:

Mild: Evidence of mild distress over the symptoms in Criterion A.

Moderate: Evidence of moderate distress over the symptoms in Criterion A.

Severe: Evidence of severe or extreme distress over the symptoms in Criterion A.

Diagnostic Features

Female orgasmic disorder is characterized by difficulty experiencing orgasm and/or markedly reduced intensity of orgasmic sensations (Criterion A). Women show wide variability in the type or intensity of stimulation that elicits orgasm. Similarly, subjective descriptions of orgasm are extremely varied, suggesting that it is experienced in very different ways, both across women and on different occasions by the same woman. For a diagnosis of female orgasmic disorder, symptoms must be experienced on almost all or all (approximately 75%–100%) occasions of sexual activity (in identified situational contexts or, if generalized, in all contexts) and have a minimum duration of approximately 6 months. The use of the minimum severity and duration criteria is intended to distinguish transient orgasm difficulties from more persistent orgasmic dysfunction. The inclusion of "approximately" in Criterion B allows for clinician judgment in cases in which symptom duration does not meet the recommended 6-month threshold.

For a woman to have a diagnosis of female orgasmic disorder, clinically significant distress must accompany the symptoms (Criterion C). In many cases of orgasm problems, the causes are multifactorial or cannot be determined. If female orgasmic disorder is deemed to be better explained by another mental disorder, the effects of a substance/medication, or a medical condition, then a diagnosis of female orgasmic disorder would not be made. Finally, if interpersonal or significant contextual factors, such as severe relationship distress, intimate partner violence, or other significant stressors, are present, then a diagnosis of female orgasmic disorder would not be made.

Many women require clitoral stimulation to reach orgasm, and a relatively small proportion of women report that they always experience orgasm during penile-vaginal intercourse. Thus, a woman's experiencing orgasm through clitoral stimulation but not during intercourse does not meet criteria for a clinical diagnosis of female orgasmic disorder. It is also important to consider whether orgasmic difficulties are the result of inadequate sexual stimulation; in these cases, there may still be a need for care, but a diagnosis of female orgasmic disorder would not be made.

Associated Features Supporting Diagnosis

Associations between specific patterns of personality traits or psychopathology and orgasmic dysfunction have generally not been supported. Compared with women without the disorder, some women with female orgasmic disorder may have greater difficulty communicating about sexual issues. Overall sexual satisfaction, however, is not strongly correlated with orgasmic experience. Many women report high levels of sexual satisfaction despite rarely or never experiencing orgasm. Orgasmic difficulties in women often co-occur with problems related to sexual interest and arousal.

In addition to the subtypes "lifelong/acquired" and "generalized/situational," the following five factors must be considered during assessment and diagnosis of female orgasmic disorder given that they may be relevant to etiology and/or treatment: 1) partner factors (e.g., partner's sexual problems, partner's health status); 2) relationship factors (e.g., poor communication, discrepancies in desire for sexual activity); 3) individual vulnerability factors (e.g., poor body image, history of sexual or emotional abuse), psychiatric comorbidity (e.g., depression, anxiety), or stressors (e.g., job loss, bereavement); (4) cultural/religious factors (e.g., inhibitions related to prohibitions against sexual activity; attitudes toward sexuality); and 5) medical factors relevant to prognosis, course, or treatment. Each of these factors may contribute differently to the presenting symptoms of different women with this disorder.

Prevalence

Reported prevalence rates for female orgasmic problems in women vary widely, from 10% to 42%, depending on multiple factors (e.g., age, culture, duration, and severity of symptoms); however, these estimates do not take into account the presence of distress. Only a proportion of women experiencing orgasm difficulties also report associated distress. Variation in how symptoms are assessed (e.g., the duration of symptoms and the recall period) also influence prevalence rates. Approximately 10% of women do not experience orgasm throughout their lifetime.

Development and Course

By definition, lifelong female orgasmic disorder indicates that the orgasmic difficulties have always been present, whereas the acquired subtype would be assigned if the woman's orgasmic difficulties developed after a period of normal orgasmic functioning.

A woman's first experience of orgasm can occur any time from the prepubertal period to well into adulthood. Women show a more variable pattern in age at first orgasm than do men, and women's reports of having experienced orgasm increase with age. Many women learn to experience orgasm as they experience a wide variety of stimulation and acquire more knowledge about their bodies. Women's rates of orgasm consistency (defined as "usually or always" experiencing orgasm) are higher during masturbation than during sexual activity with a partner.

Risk and Prognostic Factors

Temperamental.   A wide range of psychological factors, such as anxiety and concerns about pregnancy, can potentially interfere with a woman's ability to experience orgasm.

Environmental.   There is a strong association between relationship problems, physical health, and mental health and orgasm difficulties in women. Sociocultural factors (e.g., gender role expectations and religious norms) are also important influences on the experience of orgasmic difficulties.

Genetic and physiological.   Many physiological factors may influence a woman's experience of orgasm, including medical conditions and medications. Conditions such as multiple sclerosis, pelvic nerve damage from radical hysterectomy, and spinal cord injury can all influence orgasmic functioning in women. Selective serotonin reuptake inhibitors are known to delay or inhibit orgasm in women. Women with vulvovaginal atrophy (characterized by symptoms such as vaginal dryness, itching, and pain) are significantly more likely to report orgasm difficulties than are women without this condition. Menopausal status is not consistently associated with the likelihood of orgasm difficulties. There may be a significant genetic contribution to variation in female orgasmic function. However, psychological, sociocultural, and physiological factors likely interact in complex ways to influence women's experience of orgasm and of orgasm difficulties.

Culture-Related Diagnostic Issues

The degree to which lack of orgasm in women is regarded as a problem that requires treatment may vary depending on cultural context. In addition, women differ in how important orgasm is to their sexual satisfaction. There may be marked sociocultural and generational differences in women's orgasmic ability. For example, the prevalence of inability to reach orgasm has ranged from 17.7% (in Northern Europe) to 42.2% (in Southeast Asia).

Diagnostic Markers

Although measurable physiological changes occur during female orgasm, including changes in hormones, pelvic floor musculature, and brain activation, there is significant variability in these indicators of orgasm across women. In clinical situations, the diagnosis of female orgasmic disorder is based on a woman's self-report.

Functional Consequences of Female Orgasmic Disorder

The functional consequences of female orgasmic disorder are unclear. Although there is a strong association between relationship problems and orgasmic difficulties in women, it is unclear whether relationship factors are risk factors for orgasmic difficulties or are consequences of those difficulties.

Differential Diagnosis

Nonsexual mental disorders.   Nonsexual mental disorders, such as major depressive disorder, which is characterized by markedly diminished interest or pleasure in all, or almost all, activities, may explain female orgasmic disorder. If the orgasmic difficulties are better explained by another mental disorder, then a diagnosis of female orgasmic disorder would not be made.

Substance/medication-induced sexual dysfunction.   Substance/medication use may explain the orgasmic difficulties.

Another medical condition.   If the disorder is due to another medical condition (e.g., multiple sclerosis, spinal cord injury), then a diagnosis of female orgasmic disorder would not be made.

Interpersonal factors.   If interpersonal or significant contextual factors, such as severe relationship distress, intimate partner violence, or other significant stressors, are associated with the orgasmic difficulties, then a diagnosis of female orgasmic disorder would not be made.

Other sexual dysfunctions.   Female orgasmic disorder may occur in association with other sexual dysfunctions (e.g., female sexual interest/arousal disorder). The presence of another sexual dysfunction does not rule out a diagnosis of female orgasmic disorder. Occasional orgasmic difficulties that are short-term or infrequent and are not accompanied by clinically significant distress or impairment are not diagnosed as female orgasmic disorder. A diagnosis is also not appropriate if the problems are the result of inadequate sexual stimulation.

Comorbidity

Women with female orgasmic disorder may have co-occurring sexual interest/arousal difficulties. Women with diagnoses of other nonsexual mental disorders, such as major depressive disorder, may experience lower sexual interest/arousal, and this may indirectly increase the likelihood of orgasmic difficulties.

Female Sexual Interest/Arousal Disorder

Diagnostic Criteria   **302.72** (F52.22)

A. Lack of, or significantly reduced, sexual interest/arousal, as manifested by at least three of the following:

1. Absent/reduced interest in sexual activity.
2. Absent/reduced sexual/erotic thoughts or fantasies.
3. No/reduced initiation of sexual activity, and typically unreceptive to a partner's attempts to initiate.
4. Absent/reduced sexual excitement/pleasure during sexual activity in almost all or all (approximately 75%–100%) sexual encounters (in identified situational contexts or, if generalized, in all contexts).
5. Absent/reduced sexual interest/arousal in response to any internal or external sexual/erotic cues (e.g., written, verbal, visual).
6. Absent/reduced genital or nongenital sensations during sexual activity in almost all or all (approximately 75%–100%) sexual encounters (in identified situational contexts or, if generalized, in all contexts).

B. The symptoms in Criterion A have persisted for a minimum duration of approximately 6 months.

C. The symptoms in Criterion A cause clinically significant distress in the individual.

D. The sexual dysfunction is not better explained by a nonsexual mental disorder or as a consequence of severe relationship distress (e.g., partner violence) or other significant stressors and is not attributable to the effects of a substance/medication or another medical condition.

Specify whether:

   Lifelong: The disturbance has been present since the individual became sexually active.

   Acquired: The disturbance began after a period of relatively normal sexual function.

Specify whether:

   Generalized: Not limited to certain types of stimulation, situations, or partners.

   Situational: Only occurs with certain types of stimulation, situations, or partners.

Specify current severity:

   Mild: Evidence of mild distress over the symptoms in Criterion A.

   Moderate: Evidence of moderate distress over the symptoms in Criterion A.

   Severe: Evidence of severe or extreme distress over the symptoms in Criterion A.

Diagnostic Features

In assessing female sexual interest/arousal disorder, interpersonal context must be taken into account. A "desire discrepancy," in which a woman has lower desire for sexual activity than her partner, is not sufficient to diagnose female sexual interest/arousal disorder. In order for the criteria for the disorder to be met, there must be absence or reduced frequency or intensity of at least three of six indicators (Criterion A) for a minimum duration of approximately 6 months (Criterion B). There may be different symptom profiles across women, as well as variability in how sexual interest and arousal are expressed. For example, in one woman, sexual interest/arousal disorder may be expressed as a lack of interest in sexual activity, an absence of erotic or sexual thoughts, and reluctance to initiate sexual activity and respond to a partner's sexual invitations. In another woman, an inability to become sexually excited, to respond to sexual stimuli with sexual desire, and a corresponding lack of signs of physical sexual arousal may be the primary features. Because sexual desire and arousal frequently coexist and are elicited in response to adequate sexual cues, the criteria for female sexual interest/arousal disorder take into account that difficulties in desire and arousal often simultaneously characterize the complaints of women with this disorder. Short-term changes in sexual interest or arousal are common and may be adaptive responses to events in a woman's life and do not represent a sexual dysfunction. Diagnosis of female sexual interest/arousal disorder requires a minimum duration of symptoms of approximately 6 months as a reflection that the symptoms must be a persistent problem. The estimation of persistence may be determined by clinical judgment when a duration of 6 months cannot be ascertained precisely.

There may be absent or reduced frequency or intensity of interest in sexual activity (Criterion A1), which was previously termed *hypoactive sexual desire disorder*. The frequency or intensity of sexual and erotic thoughts or fantasies may be absent or reduced (Criterion A2). The expression of fantasies varies widely across women and may include memories of past sexual experiences. The normative decline in sexual thoughts with age should be taken into account when this criterion is being assessed. Absence or reduced frequency of initiating sexual activity and of receptivity to a partner's sexual invitations (Criterion A3) is a behaviorally focused criterion. A couple's beliefs and preferences for sexual initiation patterns are highly relevant to the assessment of this criterion. There may be absent or reduced sexual excitement or pleasure during sexual activity in almost all or all (approximately 75%–100%) sexual encounters (Criterion A4). Lack of pleasure is a common presenting clinical complaint in women with low desire. Among women who report low sexual desire, there are fewer sexual or erotic cues that elicit sexual interest or arousal (i.e., there is a lack of "responsive desire"). Assessment of the adequacy of sexual stimuli will assist in determining if there is a difficulty with responsive sexual desire (Criterion A5). Frequency or intensity of genital or nongenital sensations during sexual activity may be reduced or absent (Criterion A6). This may include reduced vaginal lubrication/vasocongestion, but because physiological measures of genital sexual response do not differentiate women who report sexual arousal concerns from those who do not, the self-report of reduced or absent genital or nongenital sensations is sufficient.

For a diagnosis of female sexual interest/arousal disorder to be made, clinically significant distress must accompany the symptoms in Criterion A. Distress may be experienced as a result of the lack of sexual interest/arousal or as a result of significant interference in a woman's life and well-being. If a lifelong lack of sexual desire is better explained by one's self-identification as "asexual," then a diagnosis of female sexual interest/arousal disorder would not be made.

Associated Features Supporting Diagnosis

Female sexual interest/arousal disorder is frequently associated with problems in experiencing orgasm, pain experienced during sexual activity, infrequent sexual activity, and couple-level discrepancies in desire. Relationship difficulties and mood disorders are also frequently associated features of female sexual interest/arousal disorder. Unrealistic expectations and norms regarding the "appropriate" level of sexual interest or arousal, along with poor sexual techniques and lack of information about sexuality, may also be evident in women diagnosed with female sexual interest/arousal disorder. The latter, as well as normative beliefs about gender roles, are important factors to consider.

In addition to the subtypes "lifelong/acquired" and "generalized/situational," the following five factors must be considered during assessment and diagnosis of female sexual interest/arousal disorder given that they may be relevant to etiology and/or treatment: 1) partner factors (e.g., partner's sexual problems, partner's health status); 2) relationship factors (e.g., poor communication, discrepancies in desire for sexual activity); 3) individual vulnerability factors (e.g., poor body image, history of sexual or emotional abuse), psychiatric comorbidity (e.g., depression, anxiety), or stressors (e.g., job loss, bereavement); 4) cultural/religious factors (e.g., inhibitions related to prohibitions against sexual activity; attitudes toward sexuality); and

5) medical factors relevant to prognosis, course, or treatment. Note that each of these factors may contribute differently to the presenting symptoms of different women with this disorder.

Prevalence

The prevalence of female sexual interest/arousal disorder, as defined in this manual, is unknown. The prevalence of low sexual desire and of problems with sexual arousal (with and without associated distress), as defined by DSM-IV or ICD-10, may vary markedly in relation to age, cultural setting, duration of symptoms, and presence of distress. Regarding duration of symptoms, there are striking differences in prevalence estimates between short-term and persistent problems related to lack of sexual interest. When distress about sexual functioning is required, prevalence estimates are markedly lower. Some older women report less distress about low sexual desire than younger women, although sexual desire may decrease with age.

Development and Course

By definition, lifelong female sexual interest/arousal disorder suggests that the lack of sexual interest or arousal has been present for the woman's entire sexual life. For Criteria A3, A4, and A6, which assess functioning during sexual activity, a subtype of lifelong would mean presence of symptoms since the individual's first sexual experiences. The acquired subtype would be assigned if the difficulties with sexual interest or arousal developed after a period of nonproblematic sexual functioning. Adaptive and normative changes in sexual functioning may result from partner-related, interpersonal, or personal events and may be transient in nature. However, persistence of symptoms for approximately 6 months or more would constitute a sexual dysfunction.

There are normative changes in sexual interest and arousal across the life span. Furthermore, women in relationships of longer duration are more likely to report engaging in sex despite no obvious feelings of sexual desire at the outset of a sexual encounter compared with women in shorter-duration relationships. Vaginal dryness in older women is related to age and menopausal status.

Risk and Prognostic Factors

Temperamental.   Temperamental factors include negative cognitions and attitudes about sexuality and past history of mental disorders. Differences in propensity for sexual excitation and sexual inhibition may also predict the likelihood of developing sexual problems.

Environmental.   Environmental factors include relationship difficulties, partner sexual functioning, and developmental history, such as early relationships with caregivers and childhood stressors.

Genetic and physiological.   Some medical conditions (e.g., diabetes mellitus, thyroid dysfunction) can be risk factors for female sexual interest/arousal disorder. There appears to be a strong influence of genetic factors on vulnerability to sexual problems in women. Psychophysiological research using vaginal photoplethysmography has not found differences between women with and without perceived lack of genital arousal.

Culture-Related Diagnostic Issues

There is marked variability in prevalence rates of low desire across cultures. Lower rates of sexual desire may be more common among East Asian women compared with Euro-Canadian women. Although the lower levels of sexual desire and arousal found in men and women from East Asian countries compared with Euro-American groups may reflect less interest in sex in those cultures, the possibility remains that such group differences are an artifact of the measures used to quantify desire. A judgment about whether low sexual desire reported by a woman from a certain ethnocultural group meets criteria for female sexual interest/arousal disorder must take into account the fact that different cultures may pathologize some behaviors and not others.

Gender-Related Diagnostic Issues

By definition, the diagnosis of female sexual interest/arousal disorder is only given to women. Distressing difficulties with sexual desire in men would be considered under male hypoactive sexual desire disorder.

Functional Consequences of Female Sexual Interest/Arousal Disorder

Difficulties in sexual interest/arousal are often associated with decreased relationship satisfaction.

Differential Diagnosis

Nonsexual mental disorders.   Nonsexual mental disorders, such as major depressive disorder, in which there is "markedly diminished interest or pleasure in all, or almost all, activities most of the day, nearly every day," may explain the lack of sexual interest/arousal. If the lack of interest or arousal is completely attributable to another mental disorder, then a diagnosis of female sexual interest/arousal disorder would not be made.

Substance/medication use.   Substance or medication use may explain the lack of interest/arousal.

Another medical condition.   If the sexual symptoms are considered to be almost exclusively associated with the effects of another medical condition (e.g., diabetes mellitus, endothelial disease, thyroid dysfunction, central nervous system disease), then a diagnosis of female sexual interest/arousal disorder would not be made.

Interpersonal factors.   If interpersonal or significant contextual factors, such as severe relationship distress, intimate partner violence, or other significant stressors, explain the sexual interest/arousal symptoms, then a diagnosis of female sexual interest/arousal disorder would not be made.

Other sexual dysfunctions.   The presence of another sexual dysfunction does not rule out a diagnosis of female sexual interest/arousal disorder. It is common for women to experience more than one sexual dysfunction. For example, the presence of chronic genital pain may lead to a lack of desire for the (painful) sexual activity. Lack of interest and arousal during sexual activity may impair orgasmic ability. For some women, all aspects of the sexual response may be unsatisfying and distressing.

Inadequate or absent sexual stimuli.   When differential diagnoses are being considered, it is important to assess the adequacy of sexual stimuli within the woman's sexual experience. In cases where inadequate or absent sexual stimuli are contributing to the clinical picture, there may be evidence for clinical care, but a sexual dysfunction diagnosis would not be made. Similarly, transient and adaptive alterations in sexual functioning that are secondary to a significant life or personal event must be considered in the differential diagnosis.

Comorbidity

Comorbidity between sexual interest/arousal problems and other sexual difficulties is extremely common. Sexual distress and dissatisfaction with sex life are also highly correlated in women with low sexual desire. Distressing low desire is associated with depression, thyroid problems, anxiety, urinary incontinence, and other medical factors. Arthritis and inflammatory or irritable bowel disease are also associated with sexual arousal problems. Low desire appears to be comorbid with depression, sexual and physical abuse in adulthood, global mental functioning, and use of alcohol.

Genito-Pelvic Pain/Penetration Disorder

Diagnostic Criteria   302.76 (F52.6)

A. Persistent or recurrent difficulties with one (or more) of the following:
    1. Vaginal penetration during intercourse.
    2. Marked vulvovaginal or pelvic pain during vaginal intercourse or penetration attempts.
    3. Marked fear or anxiety about vulvovaginal or pelvic pain in anticipation of, during, or as a result of vaginal penetration.
    4. Marked tensing or tightening of the pelvic floor muscles during attempted vaginal penetration.

B. The symptoms in Criterion A have persisted for a minimum duration of approximately 6 months.

C. The symptoms in Criterion A cause clinically significant distress in the individual.

D. The sexual dysfunction is not better explained by a nonsexual mental disorder or as a consequence of a severe relationship distress (e.g., partner violence) or other significant stressors and is not attributable to the effects of a substance/medication or another medical condition.

Specify whether:
Lifelong: The disturbance has been present since the individual became sexually active.
Acquired: The disturbance began after a period of relatively normal sexual function.

Specify current severity:
Mild: Evidence of mild distress over the symptoms in Criterion A.
Moderate: Evidence of moderate distress over the symptoms in Criterion A.
Severe: Evidence of severe or extreme distress over the symptoms in Criterion A.

Diagnostic Features

Genito-pelvic pain/penetration disorder refers to four commonly comorbid symptom dimensions: 1) difficulty having intercourse, 2) genito-pelvic pain, 3) fear of pain or vaginal penetration, and 4) tension of the pelvic floor muscles (Criterion A). Because major difficulty in any one of these symptom dimensions is often sufficient to cause clinically significant distress, a diagnosis can be made on the basis of marked difficulty in only one symptom dimension. However, all four symptom dimensions should be assessed even if a diagnosis can be made on the basis of only one symptom dimension.

Marked difficulty having vaginal intercourse/penetration (Criterion A1) can vary from a total inability to experience vaginal penetration in any situation (e.g., intercourse, gynecological examinations, tampon insertion) to the ability to easily experience penetration in one situation and but not in another. Although the most common clinical situation is when a woman is unable to experience intercourse or penetration with a partner, difficulties in undergoing required gynecological examinations may also be present. *Marked vulvovaginal or pelvic pain during vaginal intercourse or penetration attempts* (Criterion A2) refers to pain occurring in different locations in the genito-pelvic area. Location of pain as well as intensity should be assessed. Typically, pain can be characterized as superficial (vulvovaginal or occurring during penetration) or deep (pelvic; i.e., not felt until deeper penetration). The intensity of the pain is often not linearly related to distress or interference with sexual intercourse or other sexual activities. Some genito-pelvic pain only occurs when provoked (i.e., by intercourse or mechanical stimulation); other genito-pelvic pain may be spontaneous as well as provoked. Genito-pelvic pain can also be usefully characterized qualitatively (e.g., "burning," "cutting," "shooting," "throbbing"). The pain may persist for a period after intercourse is completed and may also occur during urination. Typically, the pain experienced during sexual intercourse can be reproduced during a gynecological examination.

Marked fear or anxiety about vulvovaginal or pelvic pain either in anticipation of, or during, or as a result of vaginal penetration (Criterion A3) is commonly reported by women who have regularly experienced pain during sexual intercourse. This "normal" reaction may lead to avoidance of sexual/intimate situations. In other cases, this marked fear does not appear to be closely related to the experience of pain but nonetheless leads to avoidance of intercourse and vaginal penetration situations. Some have described this as similar to a phobic reaction except that the phobic object may be vaginal penetration or the fear of pain.

Marked tensing or tightening of the pelvic floor muscles during attempted vaginal penetration (Criterion A4) can vary from reflexive-like spasm of the pelvic floor in response to attempted vaginal entry to "normal/voluntary" muscle guarding in response to the anticipated or the repeated experience of pain or to fear or anxiety. In the case of "normal/guarding" reactions, penetration may be possible under circumstances of relaxation. The characterization and assessment of pelvic floor dysfunction is often best undertaken by a specialist gynecologist or by a pelvic floor physical therapist.

Associated Features Supporting Diagnosis

Genito-pelvic pain/penetration disorder is frequently associated with other sexual dysfunctions, particularly reduced sexual desire and interest (female sexual interest/arousal disorder). Sometimes desire and interest are preserved in sexual situations that are not painful or do not require penetration. Even when individuals with genito-pelvic pain/penetration disorder report sexual interest/motivation, there is often behavioral avoidance of sexual situations and opportunities. Avoidance of gynecological examinations despite medical recommendations is also frequent. The pattern of avoidance is similar to that seen in phobic disorders. It is common for women who have not succeeded in having sexual intercourse to come for treatment only when they wish to conceive. Many women with genito-pelvic pain/penetration disorder will experience associated relationship/marital problems; they also often report that the symptoms significantly diminish their feelings of femininity.

In addition to the subtype "lifelong/acquired," five factors should be considered during assessment and diagnosis of genito-pelvic pain/penetration disorder because they may be relevant to etiology and/or treatment: 1) partner factors (e.g., partner's sexual problems, partner's health status); 2) relationship factors (e.g., poor communication, discrepancies in desire for sexual activity); 3) individual vulnerability factors (e.g., poor body image, history of sexual or emotional abuse), psychiatric comorbidity (e.g., depression, anxiety), or stressors (e.g., job loss, bereavement); 4) cultural/religious factors (e.g., inhibitions related to prohibitions against sexual activity; attitudes toward sexuality); and 5) medical factors relevant to prognosis, course, or treatment. Each of these factors may contribute differently to the presenting symptoms of different women with this disorder.

There are no valid physiological measures of any of the component symptom dimensions of genito-pelvic pain/penetration disorder. Validated psychometric inventories may be used to formally assess the pain and anxiety components related to genito-pelvic pain/penetration disorder.

Prevalence

The prevalence of genito-pelvic pain/penetration disorder is unknown. However, approximately 15% of women in North America report recurrent pain during intercourse. Difficulties having intercourse appear to be a frequent referral to sexual dysfunction clinics and to specialist clinicians.

Development and Course

The development and course of genito-pelvic pain/penetration disorder is unclear. Because women generally do not seek treatment until they experience problems in sexual functioning, it can, in general, be difficult to characterize genito-pelvic pain/penetration disorder as life-long (primary) or acquired (secondary). Although women typically come to clinical attention after the initiation of sexual activity, there are often earlier clinical signs. For example, difficulty with or the avoidance of use of tampons is an important predictor of later problems. Difficulties with vaginal penetration (inability or fear or pain) may not be obvious until sexual intercourse is attempted. Even once intercourse is attempted, the frequency of attempts may not be significant or regular. In cases where it is difficult to establish whether symptomatology is lifelong or acquired, it is useful to determine the presence of any consistent period of successful pain-, fear-, and tension-free intercourse. If the experience of such a period can be established, then genito-pelvic pain/penetration disorder can be characterized as acquired. Once symptomatology is well established for a period of approximately 6 months, the probability of spontaneous and significant symptomatic remission appears to diminish.

Complaints related to genito-pelvic pain peak during early adulthood and in the peri- and postmenopausal period. Women with complaints about difficulty having intercourse appear to be primarily premenopausal. There may also be an increase in genito-pelvic pain–related symptoms in the postpartum period.

Risk and Prognostic Factors

Environmental.   Sexual and/or physical abuse have often been cited as predictors of the DSM-IV-defined sexual pain disorders dyspareunia and vaginismus. This is a matter of controversy in the current literature.

Genetic and physiological.   Women experiencing superficial pain during sexual intercourse often report the onset of the pain after a history of vaginal infections. Even after the infections have resolved and there are no known residual physical findings, the pain persists. Pain during tampon insertion or the inability to insert tampons before any sexual contact has been attempted is an important risk factor for genito-pelvic pain/penetration disorder.

Culture-Related Diagnostic Issues

In the past, inadequate sexual education and religious orthodoxy have often been considered to be culturally related predisposing factors to the DSM-IV diagnosis of vaginismus. This perception appears to be confirmed by recent reports from Turkey, a primarily Muslim country, indicating a strikingly high prevalence for the disorder. However, most available research, although limited in scope, does not support this notion.

Gender-Related Diagnostic Issues

By definition, the diagnosis of genito-pelvic pain/penetration disorder is only given to women. There is relatively new research concerning urological chronic pelvic pain syndrome in men, suggesting that men may experience some similar problems. The research and clinical experience are not sufficiently developed yet to justify the application of this diagnosis to men. Other specified sexual dysfunction or unspecified sexual dysfunction may be diagnosed in men appearing to fit this pattern.

Functional Consequences of Genito-Pelvic Pain/Penetration Disorder

Functional difficulties in genito-pelvic pain/penetration disorder are often associated with interference in relationship satisfaction and sometimes with the ability to conceive via penile/vaginal intercourse.

Differential Diagnosis

Another medical condition.   In many instances, women with genito-pelvic pain/penetration disorder will also be diagnosed with another medical condition (e.g., lichen sclerosus, endometriosis, pelvic inflammatory disease, vulvovaginal atrophy). In some cases, treating the medical condition may alleviate the genito-pelvic pain/penetration disorder. Much of the time, this is not the case. There are no reliable tools or diagnostic methods to allow clinicians to know whether the medical condition or genito-pelvic pain/penetration disorder is primary. Often, the associated medical conditions are difficult to diagnose and treat. For example, the increased incidence of postmenopausal pain during intercourse may sometimes be attributable to vaginal dryness or vulvovaginal atrophy associated with declining estrogen levels. The relationship, however, between vulvovaginal atrophy/dryness, estrogen, and pain is not well understood.

Somatic symptom and related disorders.   Some women with genito-pelvic pain/penetration disorder may also be diagnosable with somatic symptom disorder. Since both genito-pelvic pain/penetration disorder and the somatic symptom and related disorders are new diagnoses, it is not yet clear whether they can be reliably differentiated. Some women diagnosed with genito-pelvic pain/penetration disorder will also be diagnosed with a specific phobia.

Inadequate sexual stimuli.   It is important that the clinician, in considering differential diagnoses, assess the adequacy of sexual stimuli within the woman's sexual experience. Sexual situations in which there is inadequate foreplay or arousal may lead to difficulties in penetration, pain, or avoidance. Erectile dysfunction or premature ejaculation in the male partner may result in difficulties with penetration. These conditions should be carefully assessed. In some situations, a diagnosis of genito-pelvic pain/penetration disorder may not be appropriate.

Comorbidity

Comorbidity between genito-pelvic pain/penetration disorder and other sexual difficulties appears to be common. Comorbidity with relationship distress is also common. This is not surprising, since in Western cultures the inability to have (pain-free) intercourse with a desired partner and the avoidance of sexual opportunities may be either a contributing factor to or the result of other sexual or relationship problems. Because pelvic floor symptoms are implicated in the diagnosis of genito-pelvic pain/penetration disorder, there is likely to be a higher prevalence of other disorders related to the pelvic floor or reproductive organs (e.g., interstitial cystitis, constipation, vaginal infection, endometriosis, irritable bowel syndrome).

Male Hypoactive Sexual Desire Disorder

Diagnostic Criteria   **302.71 (F52.0)**

A. Persistently or recurrently deficient (or absent) sexual/erotic thoughts or fantasies and desire for sexual activity. The judgment of deficiency is made by the clinician, taking into account factors that affect sexual functioning, such as age and general and sociocultural contexts of the individual's life.

B. The symptoms in Criterion A have persisted for a minimum duration of approximately 6 months.

C. The symptoms in Criterion A cause clinically significant distress in the individual.

D. The sexual dysfunction is not better explained by a nonsexual mental disorder or as a consequence of severe relationship distress or other significant stressors and is not attributable to the effects of a substance/medication or another medical condition.

Specify whether:
>   **Lifelong:** The disturbance has been present since the individual became sexually active.
>   **Acquired:** The disturbance began after a period of relatively normal sexual function.

Specify whether:
>   **Generalized:** Not limited to certain types of stimulation, situations, or partners.
>   **Situational:** Only occurs with certain types of stimulation, situations, or partners.

Specify current severity:
>   **Mild:** Evidence of mild distress over the symptoms in Criterion A.
>   **Moderate:** Evidence of moderate distress over the symptoms in Criterion A.
>   **Severe:** Evidence of severe or extreme distress over the symptoms in Criterion A.

Diagnostic Features

When an assessment for male hypoactive sexual desire disorder is being made, interpersonal context must be taken into account. A "desire discrepancy," in which a man has lower desire for sexual activity than his partner, is not sufficient to diagnose male hypoactive sexual desire disorder. Both low/absent desire for sex and deficient/absent sexual thoughts or fantasies are required for a diagnosis of the disorder. There may be variation across men in how sexual desire is expressed.

The lack of desire for sex and deficient/absent erotic thoughts or fantasies must be persistent or recurrent and must occur for a minimum duration of approximately 6 months. The inclusion of this duration criterion is meant to safeguard against making a diagnosis in cases in which a man's low sexual desire may represent an adaptive response to adverse life conditions (e.g., concern about a partner's pregnancy when the man is considering terminating the relationship). The introduction of "approximately" in Criterion B allows for clinician judgment in cases in which symptom duration does not meet the recommended 6-month threshold.

Associated Features Supporting Diagnosis

Male hypoactive sexual desire disorder is sometimes associated with erectile and/or ejaculatory concerns. For example, persistent difficulties obtaining an erection may lead a man to lose interest in sexual activity. Men with hypoactive sexual desire disorder often report that they no longer initiate sexual activity and that they are minimally receptive to a partner's attempt to initiate. Sexual activities (e.g., masturbation or partnered sexual activity) may sometimes occur even in the presence of low sexual desire. Relationship-specific preferences regarding patterns of sexual initiation must be taken into account when making a diagnosis of male hypoactive sexual desire disorder. Although men are more likely to initiate sexual activity, and thus low desire may be characterized by a pattern of non-initiation, many men may prefer to have their partner initiate sexual activity. In such situations, the man's lack of receptivity to a partner's initiation should be considered when evaluating low desire.

In addition to the subtypes "lifelong/acquired" and "generalized/situational," the following five factors must be considered during assessment and diagnosis of male hypoactive sexual desire disorder given that they may be relevant to etiology and/or treatment: 1) partner factors (e.g., partner's sexual problems, partner's health status); 2) relationship factors (e.g., poor communication, discrepancies in desire for sexual activity); 3) individual vulnerability factors (e.g., poor body image, history of sexual or emotional abuse), psychiatric comorbidity (e.g., depression, anxiety), or stressors (e.g., job loss, bereavement); 4) cultural/religious factors (e.g., inhibitions related to prohibitions against sexual activity; attitudes toward sexuality); and 5) medical factors relevant to prognosis, course, or treatment. Each of these factors may contribute differently to the presenting symptoms of different men with this disorder.

Prevalence

The prevalence of male hypoactive sexual desire disorder varies depending on country of origin and method of assessment. Approximately 6% of younger men (ages 18–24 years) and 41% of older men (ages 66–74 years) have problems with sexual desire. However, a persistent lack of interest in sex, lasting 6 months or more, affects only a small proportion of men ages 16–44 (1.8%).

Development and Course

By definition, lifelong male hypoactive sexual desire disorder indicates that low or no sexual desire has always been present, whereas the acquired subtype would be assigned if the man's low desire developed after a period of normal sexual desire. There is a requirement that low desire persist for approximately 6 months or more; thus, short-term changes in sexual desire should not be diagnosed as male hypoactive sexual desire disorder.

There is a normative age-related decline in sexual desire. Like women, men identify a variety of triggers for their sexual desire, and they describe a wide range of reasons that they choose to engage in sexual activity. Although erotic visual cues may be more potent elicitors of desire in younger men, the potency of sexual cues may decrease with age and must be considered when evaluating men for hypoactive sexual desire disorder.

Risk and Prognostic Factors

Temperamental.   Mood and anxiety symptoms appear to be strong predictors of low desire in men. Up to half of men with a past history of psychiatric symptoms may have moderate or severe loss of desire, compared with only 15% of those without such a history. A man's feelings about himself, his perception of his partner's sexual desire toward him, feelings of being emotionally connected, and contextual variables may all negatively (as well as positively) affect sexual desire.

Environmental.   Alcohol use may increase the occurrence of low desire. Among gay men, self-directed homophobia, interpersonal problems, attitudes, lack of adequate sex education, and trauma resulting from early life experiences must be taken into account in explaining the low desire. Social and cultural contextual factors should also be considered.

Genetic and physiological.   Endocrine disorders such as hyperprolactinemia significantly affect sexual desire in men. Age is a significant risk factor for low desire in men. It is unclear whether or not men with low desire also have abnormally low levels of testosterone; however, among hypogonadal men, low desire is common. There also may be a critical threshold below which testosterone will affect sexual desire in men and above which there is little effect of testosterone on men's desire.

Culture-Related Diagnostic Issues

There is marked variability in prevalence rates of low desire across cultures, ranging from 12.5% in Northern European men to 28% in Southeast Asian men ages 40–80 years. Just as there are higher rates of low desire among East Asian subgroups of women, men of East Asian ancestry also have higher rates of low desire. Guilt about sex may mediate this association between East Asian ethnicity and sexual desire in men.

Gender-Related Diagnostic Issues

In contrast to the classification of sexual disorders in women, desire and arousal disorders have been retained as separate constructs in men. Despite some similarities in the experience of desire across men and women, and the fact that desire fluctuates over time and is dependent on contextual factors, men do report a significantly higher intensity and frequency of sexual desire compared with women.

Differential Diagnosis

Nonsexual mental disorders. Nonsexual mental disorders, such as major depressive disorder, which is characterized by "markedly diminished interest or pleasure in all, or almost all, activities," may explain the lack of sexual desire. If the lack of desire is better explained by another mental disorder, then a diagnosis of male hypoactive sexual desire disorder would not be made.

Substance/medication use. Substance/medication use may explain the lack of sexual desire.

Another medical condition. If the low/absent desire and deficient/absent erotic thoughts or fantasies are better explained by the effects of another medical condition (e.g., hypogonadism, diabetes mellitus, thyroid dysfunction, central nervous system disease), then a diagnosis of male hypoactive sexual desire disorder would not be made.

Interpersonal factors. If interpersonal or significant contextual factors, such as severe relationship distress or other significant stressors, are associated with the loss of desire in the man, then a diagnosis of male hypoactive sexual desire disorder would not be made.

Other sexual dysfunctions. The presence of another sexual dysfunction does not rule out a diagnosis of male hypoactive sexual desire disorder; there is some evidence that up to one-half of men with low sexual desire also have erectile difficulties, and slightly fewer may also have early ejaculation difficulties. If the man's low desire is explained by self-identification as an asexual, then a diagnosis of male hypoactive sexual desire disorder is not made.

Comorbidity

Depression and other mental disorders, as well as endocrinological factors, are often comorbid with male hypoactive sexual desire disorder.

Premature (Early) Ejaculation

Diagnostic Criteria | 302.75 (F52.4)

A. A persistent or recurrent pattern of ejaculation occurring during partnered sexual activity within approximately 1 minute following vaginal penetration and before the individual wishes it.

Note: Although the diagnosis of premature (early) ejaculation may be applied to individuals engaged in nonvaginal sexual activities, specific duration criteria have not been established for these activities.

B. The symptom in Criterion A must have been present for at least 6 months and must be experienced on almost all or all (approximately 75%–100%) occasions of sexual activity (in identified situational contexts or, if generalized, in all contexts).

C. The symptom in Criterion A causes clinically significant distress in the individual.

D. The sexual dysfunction is not better explained by a nonsexual mental disorder or as a consequence of severe relationship distress or other significant stressors and is not attributable to the effects of a substance/medication or another medical condition.

Specify whether:

Lifelong: The disturbance has been present since the individual became sexually active.

Acquired: The disturbance began after a period of relatively normal sexual function.

Specify whether:
>   **Generalized:** Not limited to certain types of stimulation, situations, or partners.
>   **Situational:** Only occurs with certain types of stimulation, situations, or partners.

Specify current severity:
>   **Mild:** Ejaculation occurring within approximately 30 seconds to 1 minute of vaginal penetration.
>   **Moderate:** Ejaculation occurring within approximately 15–30 seconds of vaginal penetration.
>   **Severe:** Ejaculation occurring prior to sexual activity, at the start of sexual activity, or within approximately 15 seconds of vaginal penetration.

Diagnostic Features

Premature (early) ejaculation is manifested by ejaculation that occurs prior to or shortly after vaginal penetration, operationalized by an individual's estimate of ejaculatory latency (i.e., elapsed time before ejaculation) after vaginal penetration. Estimated and measured intravaginal ejaculatory latencies are highly correlated as long as the ejaculatory latency is of short duration; therefore, self-reported estimates of ejaculatory latency are sufficient for diagnostic purposes. A 60-second intravaginal ejaculatory latency time is an appropriate cutoff for the diagnosis of lifelong premature (early) ejaculation in heterosexual men. There are insufficient data to determine if this duration criterion can be applied to acquired premature (early) ejaculation. The durational definition may apply to males of varying sexual orientations, since ejaculatory latencies appear to be similar across men of different sexual orientations and across different sexual activities.

Associated Features Supporting Diagnosis

Many males with premature (early) ejaculation complain of a sense of lack of control over ejaculation and report apprehension about their anticipated inability to delay ejaculation on future sexual encounters.

The following factors may be relevant in the evaluation of any sexual dysfunction: 1) partner factors (e.g., partner's sexual problems, partner's health status); 2) relationship factors (e.g., poor communication, discrepancies in desire for sexual activity); 3) individual vulnerability factors (e.g., poor body image, history of sexual or emotional abuse), psychiatric comorbidity (e.g., depression, anxiety), and stressors (e.g., job loss, bereavement); 4) cultural/religious factors (e.g., inhibitions related to prohibitions against sexual activity; attitudes toward sexuality); and 5) medical factors relevant to prognosis, course, or treatment.

Prevalence

Estimates of the prevalence of premature (early) ejaculation vary widely depending on the definition utilized. Internationally, more than 20%–30% of men ages 18–70 years report concern about how rapidly they ejaculate. With the new definition of premature (early) ejaculation (i.e., ejaculation occurring within approximately 1 minute of vaginal penetration), only 1%–3% of men would be diagnosed with the disorder. Prevalence of premature (early) ejaculation may increase with age.

Development and Course

By definition, lifelong premature (early) ejaculation starts during a male's initial sexual experiences and persists thereafter. Some men may experience premature (early) ejaculation during their initial sexual encounters but gain ejaculatory control over time. It is the persistence of ejaculatory problems for longer than 6 months that determines the diagnosis of premature (early) ejaculation. In contrast, some men develop the disorder after a period of having a normal ejaculatory latency, known as *acquired premature (early) ejaculation*. There is far less known about acquired premature (early) ejaculation than about lifelong premature (early) ejaculation. The acquired form likely has a later onset, usually appearing during or after the fourth decade of life. Lifelong is relatively stable throughout life. Little is known about the course of acquired premature (early) ejaculation. Reversal of medical conditions such as hyperthyroidism and prostatitis appears to restore ejaculatory latencies to baseline values. Lifelong premature (early) ejaculation begins with early sexual experiences and persists throughout an individual's life. In approximately 20% of men with premature (early) ejaculation, ejaculatory latencies decrease further with age. Age and relationship length have been found to be negatively associated with prevalence of premature (early) ejaculation.

Risk and Prognostic Factors

Temperamental.   Premature (early) ejaculation may be more common in men with anxiety disorders, especially social anxiety disorder (social phobia).

Genetic and physiological.   There is a moderate genetic contribution to lifelong premature (early) ejaculation. Premature (early) ejaculation may be associated with dopamine transporter gene polymorphism or serotonin transporter gene polymorphism. Thyroid disease, prostatitis, and drug withdrawal are associated with acquired premature (early) ejaculation. Positron emission tomography measures of regional cerebral blood flow during ejaculation have shown primary activation in the mesocephalic transition zone, including the ventral tegmental area.

Culture-Related Diagnostic Issues

Perception of what constitutes a normal ejaculatory latency is different in many cultures. Measured ejaculatory latencies may differ in some countries. Such differences may be explained by cultural or religious factors as well as genetic differences between populations.

Gender-Related Diagnostic Issues

Premature (early) ejaculation is a sexual disorder in males. Males and their sexual partners may differ in their perception of what constitutes an acceptable ejaculatory latency. There may be increasing concerns in females about early ejaculation in their sexual partners, which may be a reflection of changing societal attitudes concerning female sexual activity.

Diagnostic Markers

Ejaculatory latency is usually monitored in research settings by the sexual partner utilizing a timing device (e.g., stopwatch), though this is not ideal in real-life sexual situations. For vaginal intercourse, the time between intravaginal penetration and ejaculation is measured.

Functional Consequences of
Premature (Early) Ejaculation

A pattern of premature (early) ejaculation may be associated with decreased self-esteem, a sense of lack of control, and adverse consequences for partner relationships. It may also cause personal distress in the sexual partner and decreased sexual satisfaction in the sexual partner. Ejaculation prior to penetration may be associated with difficulties in conception.

Differential Diagnosis

Substance/medication-induced sexual dysfunction.   When problems with premature ejaculation are due exclusively to substance use, intoxication, or withdrawal, substance/medication-induced sexual dysfunction should be diagnosed.

Ejaculatory concerns that do not meet diagnostic criteria.   It is necessary to identify males with normal ejaculatory latencies who desire longer ejaculatory latencies and males who have episodic premature (early) ejaculation (e.g., during the first sexual encounter with a new partner when a short ejaculatory latency may be common or normative). Neither of these situations would lead to a diagnosis of premature (early) ejaculation, even though these situations may be distressing to some males.

Comorbidity

Premature (early) ejaculation may be associated with erectile problems. In many cases, it may be difficult to determine which difficulty preceded the other. Lifelong premature (early) ejaculation may be associated with certain anxiety disorders. Acquired premature (early) ejaculation may be associated with prostatitis, thyroid disease, or drug withdrawal (e.g., during opioid withdrawal).

Substance/Medication-Induced Sexual Dysfunction

Diagnostic Criteria

A. A clinically significant disturbance in sexual function is predominant in the clinical picture.
B. There is evidence from the history, physical examination, or laboratory findings of both (1) and (2):
    1. The symptoms in Criterion A developed during or soon after substance intoxication or withdrawal or after exposure to a medication.
    2. The involved substance/medication is capable of producing the symptoms in Criterion A.
C. The disturbance is not better explained by a sexual dysfunction that is not substance/medication-induced. Such evidence of an independent sexual dysfunction could include the following:

    The symptoms precede the onset of the substance/medication use; the symptoms persist for a substantial period of time (e.g., about 1 month) after the cessation of acute withdrawal or severe intoxication; or there is other evidence suggesting the existence of an independent non-substance/medication-induced sexual dysfunction (e.g., a history of recurrent non-substance/medication-related episodes).

D. The disturbance does not occur exclusively during the course of a delirium.
E. The disturbance causes clinically significant distress in the individual.

Note: This diagnosis should be made instead of a diagnosis of substance intoxication or substance withdrawal only when the symptoms in Criterion A predominate in the clinical picture and are sufficiently severe to warrant clinical attention.

Coding note: The ICD-9-CM and ICD-10-CM codes for the [specific substance/medication]-induced sexual dysfunctions are indicated in the table below. Note that the ICD-10-CM code depends on whether or not there is a comorbid substance use disorder present for the same class of substance. If a mild substance use disorder is comorbid with the substance-induced sexual dysfunction, the 4th position character is "1," and the clinician should record "mild [substance] use disorder" before the substance-induced sexual dysfunction (e.g., "mild cocaine use disorder with cocaine-induced sexual dysfunction"). If a moderate or severe substance use disorder is comorbid with the substance-induced sexual dysfunction, the 4th position character is "2," and the clinician should record "moderate [substance] use disorder" or "severe [substance] use disorder," depending on the severity of the comorbid substance use disorder. If there is no comorbid substance use disorder (e.g., after a one-time heavy use of the substance), then the 4th position character is "9," and the clinician should record only the substance-induced sexual dysfunction.

		ICD-10-CM		
	ICD-9-CM	With use disorder, mild	With use disorder, moderate or severe	Without use disorder
Alcohol	291.89	F10.181	F10.281	F10.981
Opioid	292.89	F11.181	F11.281	F11.981
Sedative, hypnotic, or anxiolytic	292.89	F13.181	F13.281	F13.981
Amphetamine (or other stimulant)	292.89	F15.181	F15.281	F15.981
Cocaine	292.89	F14.181	F14.281	F14.981
Other (or unknown) substance	292.89	F19.181	F19.281	F19.981

Specify if (see Table 1 in the chapter "Substance-Related and Addictive Disorders" for diagnoses associated with substance class):

With onset during intoxication: If the criteria are met for intoxication with the substance and the symptoms develop during intoxication.

With onset during withdrawal: If criteria are met for withdrawal from the substance and the symptoms develop during, or shortly after, withdrawal.

With onset after medication use: Symptoms may appear either at initiation of medication or after a modification or change in use.

Specify current severity:

Mild: Occurs on 25%–50% of occasions of sexual activity.

Moderate: Occurs on 50%–75% of occasions of sexual activity.

Severe: Occurs on 75% or more of occasions of sexual activity.

Recording Procedures

ICD-9-CM. The name of the substance/medication-induced sexual dysfunction begins with the specific substance (e.g., alcohol, fluoxetine) that is presumed to be causing the sexual dysfunction. The diagnostic code is selected from the table included in the criteria set, which is based on the drug class. For substances that do not fit into any of the classes (e.g., fluoxetine), the code for "other substance" should be used; and in cases in which a substance is judged to be an etiological factor but the specific class of substance is unknown, the category "unknown substance" should be used.

The name of the disorder is followed by the specification of onset (i.e., onset during intoxication, onset during withdrawal, with onset after medication use), followed by the severity specifier (e.g., mild, moderate, severe). Unlike the recording procedures for ICD-10-CM, which combine the substance-induced disorder and substance use disorder into a single code, for ICD-9-CM a separate diagnostic code is given for the substance use disorder. For example, in the case of erectile dysfunction occurring during intoxication in a man with a severe alcohol use disorder, the diagnosis is 291.89 alcohol-induced sexual dysfunction, with onset during intoxication, moderate. An additional diagnosis of 303.90 severe alcohol use disorder is also given. When more than one substance is judged to play a significant role in the development of the sexual dysfunction, each should be listed separately (e.g., 292.89 cocaine-induced sexual dysfunction with onset during intoxication, moderate; 292.89 fluoxetine-induced sexual dysfunction, with onset after medication use).

ICD-10-CM. The name of the substance/medication-induced sexual dysfunction begins with the specific substance (e.g., alcohol, fluoxetine) that is presumed to be causing the sexual dysfunction. The diagnostic code is selected from the table included in the criteria set, which is based on the drug class and presence or absence of a comorbid substance use disorder. For substances that do not fit into any of the classes (e.g., fluoxetine), the code for "other substance" should be used; and in cases in which a substance is judged to be an etiological factor but the specific class of substance is unknown, the category "unknown substance" should be used.

When recording the name of the disorder, the comorbid substance use disorder (if any) is listed first, followed by the word "with," followed by the name of the substance-induced sexual dysfunction, followed by the specification of onset (i.e., onset during intoxication, onset during withdrawal, with onset after medication use), followed by the severity specifier (e.g., mild, moderate, severe). For example, in the case of erectile dysfunction occurring during intoxication in a man with a severe alcohol use disorder, the diagnosis is F10.281 moderate alcohol use disorder with alcohol-induced sexual dysfunction, with onset during intoxication, moderate. A separate diagnosis of the comorbid severe alcohol use disorder is not given. If the substance-induced sexual dysfunction occurs without a comorbid substance use disorder (e.g., after a one-time heavy use of the substance), no accompanying substance use disorder is noted (e.g., F15.981 amphetamine-induced sexual dysfunction, with onset during intoxication). When more than one substance is judged to play a significant role in the development of the sexual dysfunction, each should be listed separately (e.g., F14.181 mild cocaine use disorder with cocaine-induced sexual dysfunction, with onset during intoxication, moderate; F19.981 fluoxetine-induced sexual dysfunction, with onset after medication use, moderate).

Diagnostic Features

The major feature is a disturbance in sexual function that has a temporal relationship with substance/medication initiation, dose increase, or substance/medication discontinuation.

Associated Features Supporting Diagnosis

Sexual dysfunctions can occur in association with intoxication with the following classes of substances: alcohol; opioids; sedatives, hypnotics, or anxiolytics; stimulants (including cocaine); and other (or unknown) substances. Sexual dysfunctions can occur in association with withdrawal from the following classes of substances: alcohol; opioids; sedatives, hypnotics, or anxiolytics; and other (or unknown) substances. Medications that can induce sexual dysfunctions include antidepressants, antipsychotics, and hormonal contraceptives.

The most commonly reported side effect of antidepressant drugs is difficulty with orgasm or ejaculation. Problems with desire and erection are less frequent. Approximately 30% of sexual complaints are clinically significant. Certain agents, such as bupropion and mirtazapine, appear not to be associated with sexual side effects.

The sexual problems associated with antipsychotic drugs, including problems with sexual desire, erection, lubrication, ejaculation, or orgasm, have occurred with typical as well as atypical agents. However, problems are less common with prolactin-sparing antipsychotics than with agents that cause significant prolactin elevation.

Although the effects of mood stabilizers on sexual function are unclear, it is possible that lithium and anticonvulsants, with the possible exception of lamotrigine, have adverse effects on sexual desire. Problems with orgasm may occur with gabapentin. Similarly, there may be a higher prevalence of erectile and orgasmic problems associated with benzodiazepines. There have not been such reports with buspirone.

Many nonpsychiatric medications, such as cardiovascular, cytotoxic, gastrointestinal, and hormonal agents, are associated with disturbances in sexual function. Illicit substance use is associated with decreased sexual desire, erectile dysfunction, and difficulty reaching orgasm. Sexual dysfunctions are also seen in individuals receiving methadone but are seldom reported by patients receiving buprenorphine. Chronic alcohol abuse and chronic nicotine abuse are associated with erectile problems.

Prevalence

The prevalence and the incidence of substance/medication-induced sexual dysfunction are unclear, likely because of underreporting of treatment-emergent sexual side effects. Data on substance/medication-induced sexual dysfunction typically concern the effects of antidepressant drugs. The prevalence of antidepressant-induced sexual dysfunction varies in part depending on the specific agent. Approximately 25%–80% of individuals taking monoamine oxidase inhibitors, tricyclic antidepressants, serotonergic antidepressants, and combined serotonergic-adrenergic antidepressants report sexual side effects. There are differences in the incidence of sexual side effects between some serotonergic and combined adrenergic-serotonergic antidepressants, although it is unclear if these differences are clinically significant.

Approximately 50% of individuals taking antipsychotic medications will experience adverse sexual side effects, including problems with sexual desire, erection, lubrication, ejaculation, or orgasm. The incidence of these side effects among different antipsychotic agents is unclear.

Exact prevalence and incidence of sexual dysfunctions among users of nonpsychiatric medications such as cardiovascular, cytotoxic, gastrointestinal, and hormonal agents are unknown. Elevated rates of sexual dysfunction have been reported with methadone or high-dose opioid drugs for pain. There are increased rates of decreased sexual desire, erectile dysfunction, and difficulty reaching orgasm associated with illicit substance use. The prevalence of sexual problems appears related to chronic drug abuse and appears higher in individuals who abuse heroin (approximately 60%–70%) than in individuals who abuse amphetamines or 3,4-methylenedioxymethamphetamine (i.e., MDMA, ecstasy). Elevated rates of sexual dysfunction are also seen in individuals receiving methadone but are seldom reported by patients receiving buprenorphine. Chronic alcohol abuse and chronic nicotine abuse are related to higher rates of erectile problems.

Development and Course

The onset of antidepressant-induced sexual dysfunction may be as early as 8 days after the agent is first taken. Approximately 30% of individuals with mild to moderate orgasm delay will experience spontaneous remission of the dysfunction within 6 months. In some cases, serotonin reuptake inhibitor–induced sexual dysfunction may persist after the agent is discontinued. The time to onset of sexual dysfunction after initiation of antipsychotic drugs or drugs of abuse is unknown. It is probable that the adverse effects of nicotine and alcohol may not appear until after years of use. Premature (early) ejaculation can sometimes occur after cessation of opioid use. There is some evidence that disturbances in sexual function related to substance/medication use increase with age.

Culture-Related Diagnostic Issues

There may be an interaction among cultural factors, the influence of medications on sexual functioning, and the response of the individual to those changes.

Gender-Related Diagnostic Issues

Some gender differences in sexual side effects may exist.

Functional Consequences of Substance/Medication-Induced Sexual Dysfunction

Medication-induced sexual dysfunction may result in medication noncompliance.

Differential Diagnosis

Non-substance/medication-induced sexual dysfunctions. Many mental conditions, such as depressive, bipolar, anxiety, and psychotic disorders, are associated with disturbances of sexual function. Thus, differentiating a substance/medication-induced sexual dysfunction from a manifestation of the underlying mental disorder can be quite difficult. The diagnosis is usually established if a close relationship between substance/medication initiation or discontinuation is observed. A clear diagnosis can be established if the problem occurs after substance/medication initiation, dissipates with substance/medication discontinuation, and recurs with introduction of the same agent. Most substance/medication-induced side effects occur shortly after initiation or discontinuation. Sexual side effects that only occur after chronic use of a substance/medication may be extremely difficult to diagnose with certainty.

Other Specified Sexual Dysfunction

302.79 (F52.8)

This category applies to presentations in which symptoms characteristic of a sexual dysfunction that cause clinically significant distress in the individual predominate but do not meet the full criteria for any of the disorders in the sexual dysfunctions diagnostic class. The other specified sexual dysfunction category is used in situations in which the clinician chooses to communicate the specific reason that the presentation does not meet the criteria for any specific sexual dysfunction. This is done by recording "other specified sexual dysfunction" followed by the specific reason (e.g., "sexual aversion").

Unspecified Sexual Dysfunction

302.70 (F52.9)

This category applies to presentations in which symptoms characteristic of a sexual dysfunction that cause clinically significant distress in the individual predominate but do not meet the full criteria for any of the disorders in the sexual dysfunctions diagnostic class. The unspecified sexual dysfunction category is used in situations in which the clinician chooses *not* to specify the reason that the criteria are not met for a specific sexual dysfunction, and includes presentations for which there is insufficient information to make a more specific diagnosis.

Gender Dysphoria

In this chapter, there is one overarching diagnosis of gender dysphoria, with separate developmentally appropriate criteria sets for children and for adolescents and adults. The area of sex and gender is highly controversial and has led to a proliferation of terms whose meanings vary over time and within and between disciplines. An additional source of confusion is that in English "sex" connotes both male/female and sexuality. This chapter employs constructs and terms as they are widely used by clinicians from various disciplines with specialization in this area. In this chapter, *sex* and *sexual* refer to the biological indicators of male and female (understood in the context of reproductive capacity), such as in sex chromosomes, gonads, sex hormones, and nonambiguous internal and external genitalia. Disorders of sex development denote conditions of inborn somatic deviations of the reproductive tract from the norm and/or discrepancies among the biological indicators of male and female. *Cross-sex* hormone treatment denotes the use of feminizing hormones in an individual assigned male at birth based on traditional biological indicators or the use of masculinizing hormones in an individual assigned female at birth.

The need to introduce the term *gender* arose with the realization that for individuals with conflicting or ambiguous biological indicators of sex (i.e., "intersex"), the lived role in society and/or the identification as male or female could not be uniformly associated with or predicted from the biological indicators and, later, that some individuals develop an identity as female or male at variance with their uniform set of classical biological indicators. Thus, *gender* is used to denote the public (and usually legally recognized) lived role as boy or girl, man or woman, but, in contrast to certain social constructionist theories, biological factors are seen as contributing, in interaction with social and psychological factors, to gender development. *Gender assignment* refers to the initial assignment as male or female. This occurs usually at birth and, thereby, yields the "natal gender." *Gender-atypical* refers to somatic features or behaviors that are not typical (in a statistical sense) of individuals with the same assigned gender in a given society and historical era; for behavior, *gender-nonconforming* is an alternative descriptive term. *Gender reassignment* denotes an official (and usually legal) change of gender. *Gender identity* is a category of social identity and refers to an individual's identification as male, female, or, occasionally, some category other than male or female. *Gender dysphoria* as a general descriptive term refers to an individual's affective/cognitive discontent with the assigned gender but is more specifically defined when used as a diagnostic category. *Transgender* refers to the broad spectrum of individuals who transiently or persistently identify with a gender different from their natal gender. *Transsexual* denotes an individual who seeks, or has undergone, a social transition from male to female or female to male, which in many, but not all, cases also involves a somatic transition by cross-sex hormone treatment and genital surgery (*sex reassignment surgery*).

Gender dysphoria refers to the distress that may accompany the incongruence between one's experienced or expressed gender and one's assigned gender. Although not all individuals will experience distress as a result of such incongruence, many are distressed if the desired physical interventions by means of hormones and/or surgery are not available. The current term is more descriptive than the previous DSM-IV term *gender identity disorder* and focuses on dysphoria as the clinical problem, not identity per se.

Gender Dysphoria

Diagnostic Criteria

Gender Dysphoria in Children   302.6 (F64.2)

A. A marked incongruence between one's experienced/expressed gender and assigned gender, of at least 6 months' duration, as manifested by at least six of the following (one of which must be Criterion A1):

1. A strong desire to be of the other gender or an insistence that one is the other gender (or some alternative gender different from one's assigned gender).
2. In boys (assigned gender), a strong preference for cross-dressing or simulating female attire; or in girls (assigned gender), a strong preference for wearing only typical masculine clothing and a strong resistance to the wearing of typical feminine clothing.
3. A strong preference for cross-gender roles in make-believe play or fantasy play.
4. A strong preference for the toys, games, or activities stereotypically used or engaged in by the other gender.
5. A strong preference for playmates of the other gender.
6. In boys (assigned gender), a strong rejection of typically masculine toys, games, and activities and a strong avoidance of rough-and-tumble play; or in girls (assigned gender), a strong rejection of typically feminine toys, games, and activities.
7. A strong dislike of one's sexual anatomy.
8. A strong desire for the primary and/or secondary sex characteristics that match one's experienced gender.

B. The condition is associated with clinically significant distress or impairment in social, school, or other important areas of functioning.

Specify if:

With a disorder of sex development (e.g., a congenital adrenogenital disorder such as 255.2 [E25.0] congenital adrenal hyperplasia or 259.50 [E34.50] androgen insensitivity syndrome).

Coding note: Code the disorder of sex development as well as gender dysphoria.

Gender Dysphoria in Adolescents and Adults   302.85 (F64.0)

A. A marked incongruence between one's experienced/expressed gender and assigned gender, of at least 6 months' duration, as manifested by at least two of the following:

1. A marked incongruence between one's experienced/expressed gender and primary and/or secondary sex characteristics (or in young adolescents, the anticipated secondary sex characteristics).
2. A strong desire to be rid of one's primary and/or secondary sex characteristics because of a marked incongruence with one's experienced/expressed gender (or in young adolescents, a desire to prevent the development of the anticipated secondary sex characteristics).
3. A strong desire for the primary and/or secondary sex characteristics of the other gender.
4. A strong desire to be of the other gender (or some alternative gender different from one's assigned gender).
5. A strong desire to be treated as the other gender (or some alternative gender different from one's assigned gender).
6. A strong conviction that one has the typical feelings and reactions of the other gender (or some alternative gender different from one's assigned gender).

B. The condition is associated with clinically significant distress or impairment in social, occupational, or other important areas of functioning.

Specify if:

With a disorder of sex development (e.g., a congenital adrenogenital disorder such as 255.2 [E25.0] congenital adrenal hyperplasia or 259.50 [E34.50] androgen insensitivity syndrome).

Coding note: Code the disorder of sex development as well as gender dysphoria.

Specify if:

Posttransition: The individual has transitioned to full-time living in the desired gender (with or without legalization of gender change) and has undergone (or is preparing to have) at least one cross-sex medical procedure or treatment regimen—namely, regular cross-sex hormone treatment or gender reassignment surgery confirming the desired gender (e.g., penectomy, vaginoplasty in a natal male; mastectomy or phalloplasty in a natal female).

Specifiers

The posttransition specifier may be used in the context of continuing treatment procedures that serve to support the new gender assignment.

Diagnostic Features

Individuals with gender dysphoria have a marked incongruence between the gender they have been assigned to (usually at birth, referred to as *natal gender*) and their experienced/expressed gender. This discrepancy is the core component of the diagnosis. There must also be evidence of distress about this incongruence. Experienced gender may include alternative gender identities beyond binary stereotypes. Consequently, the distress is not limited to a desire to simply be of the other gender, but may include a desire to be of an alternative gender, provided that it differs from the individual's assigned gender.

Gender dysphoria manifests itself differently in different age groups. Prepubertal natal girls with gender dysphoria may express the wish to be a boy, assert they are a boy, or assert they will grow up to be a man. They prefer boys' clothing and hairstyles, are often perceived by strangers as boys, and may ask to be called by a boy's name. Usually, they display intense negative reactions to parental attempts to have them wear dresses or other feminine attire. Some may refuse to attend school or social events where such clothes are required. These girls may demonstrate marked cross-gender identification in role-playing, dreams, and fantasies. Contact sports, rough-and-tumble play, traditional boyhood games, and boys as playmates are most often preferred. They show little interest in stereotypically feminine toys (e.g., dolls) or activities (e.g., feminine dress-up or role-play). Occasionally, they refuse to urinate in a sitting position. Some natal girls may express a desire to have a penis or claim to have a penis or that they will grow one when older. They may also state that they do not want to develop breasts or menstruate.

Prepubertal natal boys with gender dysphoria may express the wish to be a girl or assert they are a girl or that they will grow up to be a woman. They have a preference for dressing in girls' or women's clothes or may improvise clothing from available materials (e.g., using towels, aprons, and scarves for long hair or skirts). These children may role-play female figures (e.g., playing "mother") and often are intensely interested in female fantasy figures. Traditional feminine activities, stereotypical games, and pastimes (e.g., "playing house"; drawing feminine pictures; watching television or videos of favorite female characters) are most often preferred. Stereotypical female-type dolls (e.g., Barbie) are often favorite toys, and girls are their preferred playmates. They avoid rough-and-tumble play and competitive sports and have little interest in stereotypically masculine toys (e.g., cars, trucks). Some may pretend not to have a penis and insist on sitting to urinate. More rarely, they may state that they find their penis or testes disgusting, that they wish them removed, or that they have, or wish to have, a vagina.

In young adolescents with gender dysphoria, clinical features may resemble those of children or adults with the condition, depending on developmental level. As secondary sex characteristics of young adolescents are not yet fully developed, these individuals may not state dislike of them, but they are concerned about imminent physical changes.

In adults with gender dysphoria, the discrepancy between experienced gender and physical sex characteristics is often, but not always, accompanied by a desire to be rid of primary and/or secondary sex characteristics and/or a strong desire to acquire some primary and/or secondary sex characteristics of the other gender. To varying degrees, adults with gender dysphoria may adopt the behavior, clothing, and mannerisms of the experienced gender. They feel uncomfortable being regarded by others, or functioning in society, as members of their assigned gender. Some adults may have a strong desire to be of a different gender and treated as such, and they may have an inner certainty to feel and respond as the experienced gender without seeking medical treatment to alter body characteristics. They may find other ways to resolve the incongruence between experienced/ expressed and assigned gender by partially living in the desired role or by adopting a gender role neither conventionally male nor conventionally female.

Associated Features Supporting Diagnosis

When visible signs of puberty develop, natal boys may shave their legs at the first signs of hair growth. They sometimes bind their genitals to make erections less visible. Girls may bind their breasts, walk with a stoop, or use loose sweaters to make breasts less visible. Increasingly, adolescents request, or may obtain without medical prescription and supervision, hormonal suppressors ("blockers") of gonadal steroids (e.g., gonadotropin-releasing hormone [GnRH] analog, spironolactone). Clinically referred adolescents often want hormone treatment and many also wish for gender reassignment surgery. Adolescents living in an accepting environment may openly express the desire to be and be treated as the experienced gender and dress partly or completely as the experienced gender, have a hairstyle typical of the experienced gender, preferentially seek friendships with peers of the other gender, and/or adopt a new first name consistent with the experienced gender. Older adolescents, when sexually active, usually do not show or allow partners to touch their sexual organs. For adults with an aversion toward their genitals, sexual activity is constrained by the preference that their genitals not be seen or touched by their partners. Some adults may seek hormone treatment (sometimes without medical prescription and supervision) and gender reassignment surgery. Others are satisfied with either hormone treatment or surgery alone.

Adolescents and adults with gender dysphoria before gender reassignment are at increased risk for suicidal ideation, suicide attempts, and suicides. After gender reassignment, adjustment may vary, and suicide risk may persist.

Prevalence

For natal adult males, prevalence ranges from 0.005% to 0.014%, and for natal females, from 0.002% to 0.003%. Since not all adults seeking hormone treatment and surgical reassignment attend specialty clinics, these rates are likely modest underestimates. Sex differences in rate of referrals to specialty clinics vary by age group. In children, sex ratios of natal boys to girls range from 2:1 to 4.5:1. In adolescents, the sex ratio is close to parity; in adults, the sex ratio favors natal males, with ratios ranging from 1:1 to 6.1:1. In two countries, the sex ratio appears to favor natal females (Japan: 2.2:1; Poland: 3.4:1).

Development and Course

Because expression of gender dysphoria varies with age, there are separate criteria sets for children versus adolescents and adults. Criteria for children are defined in a more concrete, behavioral manner than those for adolescents and adults. Many of the core criteria draw on well-documented behavioral gender differences between typically developing boys and girls. Young children are less likely than older children, adolescents, and adults to express extreme and persistent anatomic dysphoria. In adolescents and adults, incongruence between experienced gender and somatic sex is a central feature of the diagnosis. Factors related to distress and impairment also vary with age. A very young child may show signs of distress (e.g., intense crying) only when parents tell the child that he or she is "really" not a member of the other gender but only "desires" to be. Distress may not be manifest in social environments supportive of the child's desire to live in the role of the other gender and may emerge only if the desire is interfered with. In adolescents and adults, distress may manifest because of strong incongruence between experienced gender and somatic sex. Such distress may, however, be mitigated by supportive environments and knowledge that biomedical treatments exist to reduce incongruence. Impairment (e.g., school refusal, development of depression, anxiety, and substance abuse) may be a consequence of gender dysphoria.

Gender dysphoria without a disorder of sex development.   For clinic-referred children, onset of cross-gender behaviors is usually between ages 2 and 4 years. This corresponds to the developmental time period in which most typically developing children begin expressing gendered behaviors and interests. For some preschool-age children, both pervasive cross-gender behaviors and the expressed desire to be the other gender may be present, or, more rarely, labeling oneself as a member of the other gender may occur. In some cases, the expressed desire to be the other gender appears later, usually at entry into elementary school. A small minority of children express discomfort with their sexual anatomy or will state the desire to have a sexual anatomy corresponding to the experienced gender ("anatomic dysphoria"). Expressions of anatomic dysphoria become more common as children with gender dysphoria approach and anticipate puberty.

Rates of persistence of gender dysphoria from childhood into adolescence or adulthood vary. In natal males, persistence has ranged from 2.2% to 30%. In natal females, persistence has ranged from 12% to 50%. Persistence of gender dysphoria is modestly correlated with dimensional measures of severity ascertained at the time of a childhood baseline assessment. In one sample of natal males, lower socioeconomic background was also modestly correlated with persistence. It is unclear if particular therapeutic approaches to gender dysphoria in children are related to rates of long-term persistence. Extant follow-up samples consisted of children receiving no formal therapeutic intervention or receiving therapeutic interventions of various types, ranging from active efforts to reduce gender dysphoria to a more neutral, "watchful waiting" approach. It is unclear if children "encouraged" or supported to live socially in the desired gender will show higher rates of persistence, since such children have not yet been followed longitudinally in a systematic manner. For both natal male and female children showing persistence, almost all are sexually attracted to individuals of their natal sex. For natal male children whose gender dysphoria does not persist, the majority are *androphilic* (sexually attracted to males) and often self-identify as gay or homosexual (ranging from 63% to 100%). In natal female children whose gender dysphoria does not persist, the percentage who are *gynephilic* (sexually attracted to females) and self-identify as lesbian is lower (ranging from 32% to 50%).

In both adolescent and adult natal males, there are two broad trajectories for development of gender dysphoria: early onset and late onset. *Early-onset gender dysphoria* starts in childhood and continues into adolescence and adulthood; or, there is an intermittent period in which the gender dysphoria desists and these individuals self-identify as gay or homosexual, followed by recurrence of gender dysphoria. *Late-onset gender dysphoria* occurs around puberty or much later in life. Some of these individuals report having had a desire to be of the other gender in childhood that was not expressed verbally to others. Others do not recall any signs of childhood gender dysphoria. For adolescent males with late-onset gender dysphoria, parents often report surprise because they did not see signs of gender dysphoria during childhood. Expressions of anatomic dysphoria are more common and salient in adolescents and adults once secondary sex characteristics have developed.

Adolescent and adult natal males with early-onset gender dysphoria are almost always sexually attracted to men (androphilic). Adolescents and adults with late-onset gender dysphoria frequently engage in transvestic behavior with sexual excitement. The majority of these individuals are gynephilic or sexually attracted to other posttransition natal males with late-onset gender dysphoria. A substantial percentage of adult males with late-onset gender dysphoria cohabit with or are married to natal females. After gender transition, many self-identify as lesbian. Among adult natal males with gender dysphoria, the early-onset group seeks out clinical care for hormone treatment and reassignment surgery at an earlier age than does the late-onset group. The late-onset group may have more fluctuations in the degree of gender dysphoria and be more ambivalent about and less likely satisfied after gender reassignment surgery.

In both adolescent and adult natal females, the most common course is the early-onset form of gender dysphoria. The late-onset form is much less common in natal females compared with natal males. As in natal males with gender dysphoria, there may have been a period in which the gender dysphoria desisted and these individuals self-identified as lesbian; however, with recurrence of gender dysphoria, clinical consultation is sought, often with the desire for hormone treatment and reassignment surgery. Parents of natal adolescent females with the late-onset form also report surprise, as no signs of childhood gender dysphoria were evident. Expressions of anatomic dysphoria are much more common and salient in adolescents and adults than in children.

Adolescent and adult natal females with early-onset gender dysphoria are almost always gynephilic. Adolescents and adults with the late-onset form of gender dysphoria are usually androphilic and after gender transition self-identify as gay men. Natal females with the late-onset form do not have co-occurring transvestic behavior with sexual excitement.

Gender dysphoria in association with a disorder of sex development.   Most individuals with a disorder of sex development who develop gender dysphoria have already come to medical attention at an early age. For many, starting at birth, issues of gender assignment were raised by physicians and parents. Moreover, as infertility is quite common for this group, physicians are more willing to perform cross-sex hormone treatments and genital surgery before adulthood.

Disorders of sex development in general are frequently associated with gender-atypical behavior starting in early childhood. However, in the majority of cases, this does not lead to gender dysphoria. As individuals with a disorder of sex development become aware of their medical history and condition, many experience uncertainty about their gender, as opposed to developing a firm conviction that they are another gender. However, most do not progress to gender transition. Gender dysphoria and gender transition may vary considerably as a function of a disorder of sex development, its severity, and assigned gender.

Risk and Prognostic Factors

Temperamental.   For individuals with gender dysphoria without a disorder of sex development, atypical gender behavior among individuals with early-onset gender dysphoria develops in early preschool age, and it is possible that a high degree of atypicality makes the development of gender dysphoria and its persistence into adolescence and adulthood more likely.

Environmental.   Among individuals with gender dysphoria without a disorder of sex development, males with gender dysphoria (in both childhood and adolescence) more commonly have older brothers than do males without the condition. Additional predisposing factors under consideration, especially in individuals with late-onset gender dysphoria (adolescence, adulthood), include habitual fetishistic transvestism developing into autogynephilia (i.e., sexual arousal associated with the thought or image of oneself as a woman) and other forms of more general social, psychological, or developmental problems.

Genetic and physiological. For individuals with gender dysphoria without a disorder of sex development, some genetic contribution is suggested by evidence for (weak) familiality of transsexualism among nontwin siblings, increased concordance for transsexualism in monozygotic compared with dizygotic same-sex twins, and some degree of heritability of gender dysphoria. As to endocrine findings, no endogenous systemic abnormalities in sex-hormone levels have been found in 46,XY individuals, whereas there appear to be increased androgen levels (in the range found in hirsute women but far below normal male levels) in 46,XX individuals. Overall, current evidence is insufficient to label gender dysphoria without a disorder of sex development as a form of intersexuality limited to the central nervous system.

In gender dysphoria associated with a disorder of sex development, the likelihood of later gender dysphoria is increased if prenatal production and utilization (via receptor sensitivity) of androgens are grossly atypical relative to what is usually seen in individuals with the same assigned gender. Examples include 46,XY individuals with a history of normal male prenatal hormone milieu but inborn nonhormonal genital defects (as in cloacal bladder exstrophy or penile agenesis) and who have been assigned to the female gender. The likelihood of gender dysphoria is further enhanced by additional, prolonged, highly gender-atypical postnatal androgen exposure with somatic virilization as may occur in female-raised and noncastrated 46,XY individuals with 5-alpha reductase-2 deficiency or 17-beta-hydroxysteroid dehydrogenase-3 deficiency or in female-raised 46,XX individuals with classical congenital adrenal hyperplasia with prolonged periods of non-adherence to glucocorticoid replacement therapy. However, the prenatal androgen milieu is more closely related to gendered behavior than to gender identity. Many individuals with disorders of sex development and markedly gender-atypical behavior do not develop gender dysphoria. Thus, gender-atypical behavior by itself should not be interpreted as an indicator of current or future gender dysphoria. There appears to be a higher rate of gender dysphoria and patient-initiated gender change from assigned female to male than from assigned male to female in 46,XY individuals with a disorder of sex development.

Culture-Related Diagnostic Issues

Individuals with gender dysphoria have been reported across many countries and cultures. The equivalent of gender dysphoria has also been reported in individuals living in cultures with institutionalized gender categories other than male or female. It is unclear whether with these individuals the diagnostic criteria for gender dysphoria would be met.

Diagnostic Markers

Individuals with a somatic disorder of sex development show some correlation of final gender identity outcome with the degree of prenatal androgen production and utilization. However, the correlation is not robust enough for the biological factor, where ascertainable, to replace a detailed and comprehensive diagnostic interview evaluation for gender dysphoria.

Functional Consequences of Gender Dysphoria

Preoccupation with cross-gender wishes may develop at all ages after the first 2–3 years of childhood and often interfere with daily activities. In older children, failure to develop age-typical same-sex peer relationships and skills may lead to isolation from peer groups and to distress. Some children may refuse to attend school because of teasing and harassment or pressure to dress in attire associated with their assigned sex. Also in adolescents and adults, preoccupation with cross-gender wishes often interferes with daily activities. Relationship difficulties, including sexual relationship problems, are common, and functioning at school or at work may be impaired. Gender dysphoria, along with atypical gender expression, is associated with high levels of stigmatization, discrimination, and victimization, leading to negative self-concept, increased rates of mental disorder comorbidity, school dropout, and economic marginalization, including unemployment, with attendant social and mental health risks, especially in individuals from resource-poor family backgrounds. In addition, these individuals' access to health services and mental health services may be impeded by structural barriers, such as institutional discomfort or inexperience in working with this patient population.

Differential Diagnosis

Nonconformity to gender roles.   Gender dysphoria should be distinguished from simple nonconformity to stereotypical gender role behavior by the strong desire to be of another gender than the assigned one and by the extent and pervasiveness of gender-variant activities and interests. The diagnosis is not meant to merely describe nonconformity to stereotypical gender role behavior (e.g., "tomboyism" in girls, "girly-boy" behavior in boys, occasional cross-dressing in adult men). Given the increased openness of atypical gender expressions by individuals across the entire range of the transgender spectrum, it is important that the clinical diagnosis be limited to those individuals whose distress and impairment meet the specified criteria.

Transvestic disorder.   Transvestic disorder occurs in heterosexual (or bisexual) adolescent and adult males (rarely in females) for whom cross-dressing behavior generates sexual excitement and causes distress and/or impairment without drawing their primary gender into question. It is occasionally accompanied by gender dysphoria. An individual with transvestic disorder who also has clinically significant gender dysphoria can be given both diagnoses. In many cases of late-onset gender dysphoria in gynephilic natal males, transvestic behavior with sexual excitement is a precursor.

Body dysmorphic disorder.   An individual with body dysmorphic disorder focuses on the alteration or removal of a specific body part because it is perceived as abnormally formed, not because it represents a repudiated assigned gender. When an individual's presentation meets criteria for both gender dysphoria and body dysmorphic disorder, both diagnoses can be given. Individuals wishing to have a healthy limb amputated (termed by some *body integrity identity disorder*) because it makes them feel more "complete" usually do not wish to change gender, but rather desire to live as an amputee or a disabled person.

Schizophrenia and other psychotic disorders.   In schizophrenia, there may rarely be delusions of belonging to some other gender. In the absence of psychotic symptoms, insistence by an individual with gender dysphoria that he or she is of some other gender is not considered a delusion. Schizophrenia (or other psychotic disorders) and gender dysphoria may co-occur.

Other clinical presentations.   Some individuals with an emasculinization desire who develop an alternative, nonmale/nonfemale gender identity do have a presentation that meets criteria for gender dysphoria. However, some males seek castration and/or penectomy for aesthetic reasons or to remove psychological effects of androgens without changing male identity; in these cases, the criteria for gender dysphoria are not met.

Comorbidity

Clinically referred children with gender dysphoria show elevated levels of emotional and behavioral problems—most commonly, anxiety, disruptive and impulse-control, and depressive disorders. In prepubertal children, increasing age is associated with having more behavioral or emotional problems; this is related to the increasing non-acceptance of gender-variant behavior by others. In older children, gender-variant behavior often leads to peer ostracism, which may lead to more behavioral problems. The prevalence of mental health problems differs among cultures; these differences may also be related to differences in attitudes toward gender variance in children. However, also in some non-Western cultures, anxiety has been found to be relatively common in individuals with gender dysphoria, even in cultures with accepting attitudes toward gender-variant behavior. Autism spectrum disorder is more prevalent in clinically referred children with gender dysphoria than in the general population. Clinically referred adolescents with gender dysphoria appear to have comorbid mental disorders, with anxiety and depressive disorders being the most common. As in children, autism spectrum disorder is more prevalent in clinically referred adolescents with gender dysphoria than in the general population. Clinically referred adults with gender dysphoria may have coexisting mental health problems, most commonly anxiety and depressive disorders.

Other Specified Gender Dysphoria

302.6 (F64.8)

This category applies to presentations in which symptoms characteristic of gender dysphoria that cause clinically significant distress or impairment in social, occupational, or other important areas of functioning predominate but do not meet the full criteria for gender dysphoria. The other specified gender dysphoria category is used in situations in which the clinician chooses to communicate the specific reason that the presentation does not meet the criteria for gender dysphoria. This is done by recording "other specified gender dysphoria" followed by the specific reason (e.g., "brief gender dysphoria").

An example of a presentation that can be specified using the "other specified" designation is the following:

The current disturbance meets symptom criteria for gender dysphoria, but the duration is less than 6 months.

Unspecified Gender Dysphoria

302.6 (F64.9)

This category applies to presentations in which symptoms characteristic of gender dysphoria that cause clinically significant distress or impairment in social, occupational, or other important areas of functioning predominate but do not meet the full criteria for gender dysphoria. The unspecified gender dysphoria category is used in situations in which the clinician chooses *not* to specify the reason that the criteria are not met for gender dysphoria, and includes presentations in which there is insufficient information to make a more specific diagnosis.

Disruptive, Impulse-Control, and Conduct Disorders

Disruptive, impulse-control, and conduct disorders include conditions involving problems in the self-control of emotions and behaviors. While other disorders in DSM-5 may also involve problems in emotional and/or behavioral regulation, the disorders in this chapter are unique in that these problems are manifested in behaviors that violate the rights of others (e.g., aggression, destruction of property) and/or that bring the individual into significant conflict with societal norms or authority figures. The underlying causes of the problems in the self-control of emotions and behaviors can vary greatly across the disorders in this chapter and among individuals within a given diagnostic category.

The chapter includes oppositional defiant disorder, intermittent explosive disorder, conduct disorder, antisocial personality disorder (which is described in the chapter "Personality Disorders"), pyromania, kleptomania, and other specified and unspecified disruptive, impulse-control, and conduct disorders. Although all the disorders in the chapter involve problems in both emotional and behavioral regulation, the source of variation among the disorders is the relative emphasis on problems in the two types of self-control. For example, the criteria for conduct disorder focus largely on poorly controlled behaviors that violate the rights of others or that violate major societal norms. Many of the behavioral symptoms (e.g., aggression) can be a result of poorly controlled emotions such as anger. At the other extreme, the criteria for intermittent explosive disorder focus largely on such poorly controlled emotion, outbursts of anger that are disproportionate to the interpersonal or other provocation or to other psychosocial stressors. Intermediate in impact to these two disorders is oppositional defiant disorder, in which the criteria are more evenly distributed between emotions (anger and irritation) and behaviors (argumentativeness and defiance). Pyromania and kleptomania are less commonly used diagnoses characterized by poor impulse control related to specific behaviors (fire setting or stealing) that relieve internal tension. Other specified disruptive, impulse-control, and conduct disorder is a category for conditions in which there are symptoms of conduct disorder, oppositional defiant disorder, or other disruptive, impulse-control, and conduct disorders, but the number of symptoms does not meet the diagnostic threshold for any of the disorders in this chapter, even though there is evidence of clinically significant impairment associated with the symptoms.

The disruptive, impulse-control, and conduct disorders all tend to be more common in males than in females, although the relative degree of male predominance may differ both across disorders and within a disorder at different ages. The disorders in this chapter tend to have first onset in childhood or adolescence. In fact, it is very rare for either conduct disorder or oppositional defiant disorder to first emerge in adulthood. There is a developmental relationship between oppositional defiant disorder and conduct disorder, in that most cases of conduct disorder previously would have met criteria for oppositional defiant disorder, at least in those cases in which conduct disorder emerges prior to adolescence. However, most children with oppositional defiant disorder do not eventually develop conduct disorder. Furthermore, children with oppositional defiant disorder are at risk for eventually developing other problems besides conduct disorder, including anxiety and depressive disorders.

Many of the symptoms that define the disruptive, impulse-control, and conduct disorders are behaviors that can occur to some degree in typically developing individuals. Thus, it is critical that the frequency, persistence, pervasiveness across situations, and im-

461

pairment associated with the behaviors indicative of the diagnosis be considered relative to what is normative for a person's age, gender, and culture when determining if they are symptomatic of a disorder.

The disruptive, impulse-control, and conduct disorders have been linked to a common externalizing spectrum associated with the personality dimensions labeled as *disinhibition* and (inversely) *constraint* and, to a lesser extent, negative emotionality. These shared personality dimensions could account for the high level of comorbidity among these disorders and their frequent comorbidity with substance use disorders and antisocial personality disorder. However, the specific nature of the shared diathesis that constitutes the externalizing spectrum remains unknown.

Oppositional Defiant Disorder

Diagnostic Criteria   313.81 (F91.3)

A. A pattern of angry/irritable mood, argumentative/defiant behavior, or vindictiveness lasting at least 6 months as evidenced by at least four symptoms from any of the following categories, and exhibited during interaction with at least one individual who is not a sibling.

Angry/Irritable Mood

1. Often loses temper.
2. Is often touchy or easily annoyed.
3. Is often angry and resentful.

Argumentative/Defiant Behavior

4. Often argues with authority figures or, for children and adolescents, with adults.
5. Often actively defies or refuses to comply with requests from authority figures or with rules.
6. Often deliberately annoys others.
7. Often blames others for his or her mistakes or misbehavior.

Vindictiveness

8. Has been spiteful or vindictive at least twice within the past 6 months.

Note: The persistence and frequency of these behaviors should be used to distinguish a behavior that is within normal limits from a behavior that is symptomatic. For children younger than 5 years, the behavior should occur on most days for a period of at least 6 months unless otherwise noted (Criterion A8). For individuals 5 years or older, the behavior should occur at least once per week for at least 6 months, unless otherwise noted (Criterion A8). While these frequency criteria provide guidance on a minimal level of frequency to define symptoms, other factors should also be considered, such as whether the frequency and intensity of the behaviors are outside a range that is normative for the individual's developmental level, gender, and culture.

B. The disturbance in behavior is associated with distress in the individual or others in his or her immediate social context (e.g., family, peer group, work colleagues), or it impacts negatively on social, educational, occupational, or other important areas of functioning.

C. The behaviors do not occur exclusively during the course of a psychotic, substance use, depressive, or bipolar disorder. Also, the criteria are not met for disruptive mood dysregulation disorder.

Specify current severity:

  Mild: Symptoms are confined to only one setting (e.g., at home, at school, at work, with peers).

Moderate: Some symptoms are present in at least two settings.
Severe: Some symptoms are present in three or more settings.

Specifiers

It is not uncommon for individuals with oppositional defiant disorder to show symptoms only at home and only with family members. However, the pervasiveness of the symptoms is an indicator of the severity of the disorder.

Diagnostic Features

The essential feature of oppositional defiant disorder is a frequent and persistent pattern of angry/irritable mood, argumentative/defiant behavior, or vindictiveness (Criterion A). It is not unusual for individuals with oppositional defiant disorder to show the behavioral features of the disorder without problems of negative mood. However, individuals with the disorder who show the angry/irritable mood symptoms typically show the behavioral features as well.

The symptoms of oppositional defiant disorder may be confined to only one setting, and this is most frequently the home. Individuals who show enough symptoms to meet the diagnostic threshold, even if it is only at home, may be significantly impaired in their social functioning. However, in more severe cases, the symptoms of the disorder are present in multiple settings. Given that the pervasiveness of symptoms is an indicator of the severity of the disorder, it is critical that the individual's behavior be assessed across multiple settings and relationships. Because these behaviors are common among siblings, they must be observed during interactions with persons other than siblings. Also, because symptoms of the disorder are typically more evident in interactions with adults or peers whom the individual knows well, they may not be apparent during a clinical examination.

The symptoms of oppositional defiant disorder can occur to some degree in individuals without this disorder. There are several key considerations for determining if the behaviors are symptomatic of oppositional defiant disorder. First, the diagnostic threshold of four or more symptoms within the preceding 6 months must be met. Second, the persistence and frequency of the symptoms should exceed what is normative for an individual's age, gender, and culture. For example, it is not unusual for preschool children to show temper tantrums on a weekly basis. Temper outbursts for a preschool child would be considered a symptom of oppositional defiant disorder only if they occurred on most days for the preceding 6 months, if they occurred with at least three other symptoms of the disorder, and if the temper outbursts contributed to the significant impairment associated with the disorder (e.g., led to destruction of property during outbursts, resulted in the child being asked to leave a preschool).

The symptoms of the disorder often are part of a pattern of problematic interactions with others. Furthermore, individuals with this disorder typically do not regard themselves as angry, oppositional, or defiant. Instead, they often justify their behavior as a response to unreasonable demands or circumstances. Thus, it can be difficult to disentangle the relative contribution of the individual with the disorder to the problematic interactions he or she experiences. For example, children with oppositional defiant disorder may have experienced a history of hostile parenting, and it is often impossible to determine if the child's behavior caused the parents to act in a more hostile manner toward the child, if the parents' hostility led to the child's problematic behavior, or if there was some combination of both. Whether or not the clinician can separate the relative contributions of potential causal factors should not influence whether or not the diagnosis is made. In the event that the child may be living in particularly poor conditions where neglect or mistreatment may occur (e.g., in institutional settings), clinical attention to reducing the contribution of the environment may be helpful.

Associated Features Supporting Diagnosis

In children and adolescents, oppositional defiant disorder is more prevalent in families in which child care is disrupted by a succession of different caregivers or in families in which harsh, inconsistent, or neglectful child-rearing practices are common. Two of the most common co-occurring conditions with oppositional defiant disorder are attention-deficit/ hyperactivity disorder (ADHD) and conduct disorder (see the section "Comorbidity" for this disorder). Oppositional defiant disorder has been associated with increased risk for suicide attempts, even after comorbid disorders are controlled for.

Prevalence

The prevalence of oppositional defiant disorder ranges from 1% to 11%, with an average prevalence estimate of around 3.3%. The rate of oppositional defiant disorder may vary depending on the age and gender of the child. The disorder appears to be somewhat more prevalent in males than in females (1.4:1) prior to adolescence. This male predominance is not consistently found in samples of adolescents or adults.

Development and Course

The first symptoms of oppositional defiant disorder usually appear during the preschool years and rarely later than early adolescence. Oppositional defiant disorder often precedes the development of conduct disorder, especially for those with the childhood-onset type of conduct disorder. However, many children and adolescents with oppositional defiant disorder do not subsequently develop conduct disorder. Oppositional defiant disorder also conveys risk for the development of anxiety disorders and major depressive disorder, even in the absence of conduct disorder. The defiant, argumentative, and vindictive symptoms carry most of the risk for conduct disorder, whereas the angry-irritable mood symptoms carry most of the risk for emotional disorders.

Manifestations of the disorder across development appear consistent. Children and adolescents with oppositional defiant disorder are at increased risk for a number of problems in adjustment as adults, including antisocial behavior, impulse-control problems, substance abuse, anxiety, and depression.

Many of the behaviors associated with oppositional defiant disorder increase in frequency during the preschool period and in adolescence. Thus, it is especially critical during these development periods that the frequency and intensity of these behaviors be evaluated against normative levels before it is decided that they are symptoms of oppositional defiant disorder.

Risk and Prognostic Features

Temperamental.   Temperamental factors related to problems in emotional regulation (e.g., high levels of emotional reactivity, poor frustration tolerance) have been predictive of the disorder.

Environmental.   Harsh, inconsistent, or neglectful child-rearing practices are common in families of children and adolescents with oppositional defiant disorder, and these parenting practices play an important role in many causal theories of the disorder.

Genetic and physiological.   A number of neurobiological markers (e.g., lower heart rate and skin conductance reactivity; reduced basal cortisol reactivity; abnormalities in the prefrontal cortex and amygdala) have been associated with oppositional defiant disorder. However, the vast majority of studies have not separated children with oppositional defiant disorder from those with conduct disorder. Thus, it is unclear whether there are markers specific to oppositional defiant disorder.

Culture-Related Diagnostic Issues

The prevalence of the disorder in children and adolescents is relatively consistent across countries that differ in race and ethnicity.

Functional Consequences of Oppositional Defiant Disorder

When oppositional defiant disorder is persistent throughout development, individuals with the disorder experience frequent conflicts with parents, teachers, supervisors, peers, and romantic partners. Such problems often result in significant impairments in the individual's emotional, social, academic, and occupational adjustment.

Differential Diagnosis

Conduct disorder.   Conduct disorder and oppositional defiant disorder are both related to conduct problems that bring the individual in conflict with adults and other authority figures (e.g., teachers, work supervisors). The behaviors of oppositional defiant disorder are typically of a less severe nature than those of conduct disorder and do not include aggression toward people or animals, destruction of property, or a pattern of theft or deceit. Furthermore, oppositional defiant disorder includes problems of emotional dysregulation (i.e., angry and irritable mood) that are not included in the definition of conduct disorder.

Attention-deficit/hyperactivity disorder.   ADHD is often comorbid with oppositional defiant disorder. To make the additional diagnosis of oppositional defiant disorder, it is important to determine that the individual's failure to conform to requests of others is not solely in situations that demand sustained effort and attention or demand that the individual sit still.

Depressive and bipolar disorders.   Depressive and bipolar disorders often involve negative affect and irritability. As a result, a diagnosis of oppositional defiant disorder should not be made if the symptoms occur exclusively during the course of a mood disorder.

Disruptive mood dysregulation disorder.   Oppositional defiant disorder shares with disruptive mood dysregulation disorder the symptoms of chronic negative mood and temper outbursts. However, the severity, frequency, and chronicity of temper outbursts are more severe in individuals with disruptive mood dysregulation disorder than in those with oppositional defiant disorder. Thus, only a minority of children and adolescents whose symptoms meet criteria for oppositional defiant disorder would also be diagnosed with disruptive mood dysregulation disorder. When the mood disturbance is severe enough to meet criteria for disruptive mood dysregulation disorder, a diagnosis of oppositional defiant disorder is not given, even if all criteria for oppositional defiant disorder are met.

Intermittent explosive disorder.   Intermittent explosive disorder also involves high rates of anger. However, individuals with this disorder show serious aggression toward others that is not part of the definition of oppositional defiant disorder.

Intellectual disability (intellectual developmental disorder).   In individuals with intellectual disability, a diagnosis of oppositional defiant disorder is given only if the oppositional behavior is markedly greater than is commonly observed among individuals of comparable mental age and with comparable severity of intellectual disability.

Language disorder.   Oppositional defiant disorder must also be distinguished from a failure to follow directions that is the result of impaired language comprehension (e.g., hearing loss).

Social anxiety disorder (social phobia).   Oppositional defiant disorder must also be distinguished from defiance due to fear of negative evaluation associated with social anxiety disorder.

Comorbidity

Rates of oppositional defiant disorder are much higher in samples of children, adolescents, and adults with ADHD, and this may be the result of shared temperamental risk factors. Also, oppositional defiant disorder often precedes conduct disorder, although this appears to be most common in children with the childhood-onset subtype. Individuals with oppositional defiant disorder are also at increased risk for anxiety disorders and major depressive disorder, and this seems largely attributable to the presence of the angry-irritable mood symptoms. Adolescents and adults with oppositional defiant disorder also show a higher rate of substance use disorders, although it is unclear if this association is independent of the comorbidity with conduct disorder.

Intermittent Explosive Disorder

Diagnostic Criteria   **312.34 (F63.81)**

A. Recurrent behavioral outbursts representing a failure to control aggressive impulses as manifested by either of the following:

   1. Verbal aggression (e.g., temper tantrums, tirades, verbal arguments or fights) or physical aggression toward property, animals, or other individuals, occurring twice weekly, on average, for a period of 3 months. The physical aggression does not result in damage or destruction of property and does not result in physical injury to animals or other individuals.

   2. Three behavioral outbursts involving damage or destruction of property and/or physical assault involving physical injury against animals or other individuals occurring within a 12-month period.

B. The magnitude of aggressiveness expressed during the recurrent outbursts is grossly out of proportion to the provocation or to any precipitating psychosocial stressors.

C. The recurrent aggressive outbursts are not premeditated (i.e., they are impulsive and/or anger-based) and are not committed to achieve some tangible objective (e.g., money, power, intimidation).

D. The recurrent aggressive outbursts cause either marked distress in the individual or impairment in occupational or interpersonal functioning, or are associated with financial or legal consequences.

E. Chronological age is at least 6 years (or equivalent developmental level).

F. The recurrent aggressive outbursts are not better explained by another mental disorder (e.g., major depressive disorder, bipolar disorder, disruptive mood dysregulation disorder, a psychotic disorder, antisocial personality disorder, borderline personality disorder) and are not attributable to another medical condition (e.g., head trauma, Alzheimer's disease) or to the physiological effects of a substance (e.g., a drug of abuse, a medication). For children ages 6–18 years, aggressive behavior that occurs as part of an adjustment disorder should not be considered for this diagnosis.

Note: This diagnosis can be made in addition to the diagnosis of attention-deficit/hyperactivity disorder, conduct disorder, oppositional defiant disorder, or autism spectrum disorder when recurrent impulsive aggressive outbursts are in excess of those usually seen in these disorders and warrant independent clinical attention.

Diagnostic Features

The impulsive (or anger-based) aggressive outbursts in intermittent explosive disorder have a rapid onset and, typically, little or no prodromal period. Outbursts typically last for less than 30 minutes and commonly occur in response to a minor provocation by a close intimate or associate. Individuals with intermittent explosive disorder often have less severe episodes of verbal and/or nondamaging, nondestructive, or noninjurious physical assault (Criterion A1) in between more severe destructive/assaultive episodes (Criterion A2). Criterion A1 defines frequent (i.e., twice weekly, on average, for a period of 3 months) aggressive outbursts characterized by temper tantrums, tirades, verbal arguments or fights, or assault without damage to objects or without injury to animals or other individuals. Criterion A2 defines infrequent (i.e., three in a 1-year period) impulsive aggressive outbursts characterized by damaging or destroying an object, regardless of its tangible value, or by assaulting/striking or otherwise causing physical injury to an animal or to another individual. Regardless of the nature of the impulsive aggressive outburst, the core feature of intermittent explosive disorder is failure to control impulsive aggressive behavior in response to subjectively experienced provocation (i.e., psychosocial stressor) that would not typically result in an aggressive outburst (Criterion B). The aggressive outbursts are generally impulsive and/or anger-based, rather than premeditated or instrumental (Criterion C) and are associated with significant distress or impairment in psychosocial function (Criterion D). A diagnosis of intermittent explosive disorder should not be given to individuals younger than 6 years, or the equivalent developmental level (Criterion E), or to individuals whose aggressive outbursts are better explained by another mental disorder (Criterion F). A diagnosis of intermittent explosive disorder should not be given to individuals with disruptive mood dysregulation disorder or to individuals whose impulsive aggressive outbursts are attributable to another medical condition or to the physiological effects of a substance (Criterion F). In addition, children ages 6–18 years should not receive this diagnosis when impulsive aggressive outbursts occur in the context of an adjustment disorder (Criterion F).

Associated Features Supporting Diagnosis

Mood disorders (unipolar), anxiety disorders, and substance use disorders are associated with intermittent explosive disorder, although onset of these disorders is typically later than that of intermittent explosive disorder.

Prevalence

One-year prevalence data for intermittent explosive disorder in the United States is about 2.7% (narrow definition). Intermittent explosive disorder is more prevalent among younger individuals (e.g., younger than 35–40 years), compared with older individuals (older than 50 years), and in individuals with a high school education or less.

Development and Course

The onset of recurrent, problematic, impulsive aggressive behavior is most common in late childhood or adolescence and rarely begins for the first time after age 40 years. The core features of intermittent explosive disorder, typically, are persistent and continue for many years.

The course of the disorder may be episodic, with recurrent periods of impulsive aggressive outbursts. Intermittent explosive disorder appears to follow a chronic and persistent course over many years. It also appears to be quite common regardless of the presence or absence of attention-deficit/hyperactivity disorder (ADHD) or disruptive, impulse-control, and conduct disorders (e.g., conduct disorder, oppositional defiant disorder).

Risk and Prognostic Factors

Environmental.   Individuals with a history of physical and emotional trauma during the first two decades of life are at increased risk for intermittent explosive disorder.

Genetic and physiological.   First-degree relatives of individuals with intermittent explosive disorder are at increased risk for intermittent explosive disorder, and twin studies have demonstrated a substantial genetic influence for impulsive aggression.

Research provides neurobiological support for the presence of serotonergic abnormalities, globally and in the brain, specifically in areas of the limbic system (anterior cingulate) and orbitofrontal cortex in individuals with intermittent explosive disorder. Amygdala responses to anger stimuli, during functional magnetic resonance imaging scanning, are greater in individuals with intermittent explosive disorder compared with healthy individuals.

Culture-Related Diagnostic Issues

The lower prevalence of intermittent explosive disorder in some regions (Asia, Middle East) or countries (Romania, Nigeria), compared with the United States, suggests that information about recurrent, problematic, impulsive aggressive behaviors either is not elicited on questioning or is less likely to be present, because of cultural factors.

Gender-Related Diagnostic Issues

In some studies the prevalence of intermittent explosive disorder is greater in males than in females (odds ratio = 1.4–2.3); other studies have found no gender difference.

Functional Consequences of Intermittent Explosive Disorder

Social (e.g., loss of friends, relatives, marital instability), occupational (e.g., demotion, loss of employment), financial (e.g., due to value of objects destroyed), and legal (e.g., civil suits as a result of aggressive behavior against person or property; criminal charges for assault) problems often develop as a result of intermittent explosive disorder.

Differential Diagnosis

A diagnosis of intermittent explosive disorder should not be made when Criteria A1 and/or A2 are only met during an episode of another mental disorder (e.g., major depressive disorder, bipolar disorder, psychotic disorder), or when impulsive aggressive outbursts are attributable to another medical condition or to the physiological effects of a substance or medication. This diagnosis also should not be made, particularly in children and adolescents ages 6–18 years, when the impulsive aggressive outbursts occur in the context of an adjustment disorder. Other examples in which recurrent, problematic, impulsive aggressive outbursts may, or may not, be diagnosed as intermittent explosive disorder include the following.

Disruptive mood dysregulation disorder.   In contrast to intermittent explosive disorder, disruptive mood dysregulation disorder is characterized by a persistently negative mood state (i.e., irritability, anger) most of the day, nearly every day, between impulsive aggressive outbursts. A diagnosis of disruptive mood dysregulation disorder can only be given when the onset of recurrent, problematic, impulsive aggressive outbursts is before age 10 years. Finally, a diagnosis of disruptive mood dysregulation disorder should not be made for the first time after age 18 years. Otherwise, these diagnoses are mutually exclusive.

Antisocial personality disorder or borderline personality disorder.   Individuals with antisocial personality disorder or borderline personality disorder often display recurrent, problematic impulsive aggressive outbursts. However, the level of impulsive aggression in individuals with antisocial personality disorder or borderline personality disorder is lower than that in individuals with intermittent explosive disorder.

Delirium, major neurocognitive disorder, and personality change due to another medical condition, aggressive type. A diagnosis of intermittent explosive disorder should not be made when aggressive outbursts are judged to result from the physiological effects of another diagnosable medical condition (e.g., brain injury associated with a change in personality characterized by aggressive outbursts; complex partial epilepsy). Nonspecific abnormalities on neurological examination (e.g., "soft signs") and nonspecific electroencephalographic changes are compatible with a diagnosis of intermittent explosive disorder unless there is a diagnosable medical condition that better explains the impulsive aggressive outbursts.

Substance intoxication or substance withdrawal. A diagnosis of intermittent explosive disorder should not be made when impulsive aggressive outbursts are nearly always associated with intoxication with or withdrawal from substances (e.g., alcohol, phencyclidine, cocaine and other stimulants, barbiturates, inhalants). However, when a sufficient number of impulsive aggressive outbursts also occur in the absence of substance intoxication or withdrawal, and these warrant independent clinical attention, a diagnosis of intermittent explosive disorder may be given.

Attention-deficit/hyperactivity disorder, conduct disorder, oppositional defiant disorder, or autism spectrum disorder. Individuals with any of these childhood-onset disorders may exhibit impulsive aggressive outbursts. Individuals with ADHD are typically impulsive and, as a result, may also exhibit impulsive aggressive outbursts. While individuals with conduct disorder can exhibit impulsive aggressive outbursts, the form of aggression characterized by the diagnostic criteria is proactive and predatory. Aggression in oppositional defiant disorder is typically characterized by temper tantrums and verbal arguments with authority figures, whereas impulsive aggressive outbursts in intermittent explosive disorder are in response to a broader array of provocation and include physical assault. The level of impulsive aggression in individuals with a history of one or more of these disorders has been reported as lower than that in comparable individuals whose symptoms also meet intermittent explosive disorder Criteria A through E. Accordingly, if Criteria A through E are also met, and the impulsive aggressive outbursts warrant independent clinical attention, a diagnosis of intermittent explosive disorder may be given.

Comorbidity

Depressive disorders, anxiety disorders, and substance use disorders are most commonly comorbid with intermittent explosive disorder. In addition, individuals with antisocial personality disorder or borderline personality disorder, and individuals with a history of disorders with disruptive behaviors (e.g., ADHD, conduct disorder, oppositional defiant disorder), are at greater risk for comorbid intermittent explosive disorder.

Conduct Disorder

Diagnostic Criteria

A. A repetitive and persistent pattern of behavior in which the basic rights of others or major age-appropriate societal norms or rules are violated, as manifested by the presence of at least three of the following 15 criteria in the past 12 months from any of the categories below, with at least one criterion present in the past 6 months:

Aggression to People and Animals

1. Often bullies, threatens, or intimidates others.
2. Often initiates physical fights.
3. Has used a weapon that can cause serious physical harm to others (e.g., a bat, brick, broken bottle, knife, gun).

4. Has been physically cruel to people.
5. Has been physically cruel to animals.
6. Has stolen while confronting a victim (e.g., mugging, purse snatching, extortion, armed robbery).
7. Has forced someone into sexual activity.

Destruction of Property

8. Has deliberately engaged in fire setting with the intention of causing serious damage.
9. Has deliberately destroyed others' property (other than by fire setting).

Deceitfulness or Theft

10. Has broken into someone else's house, building, or car.
11. Often lies to obtain goods or favors or to avoid obligations (i.e., "cons" others).
12. Has stolen items of nontrivial value without confronting a victim (e.g., shoplifting, but without breaking and entering; forgery).

Serious Violations of Rules

13. Often stays out at night despite parental prohibitions, beginning before age 13 years.
14. Has run away from home overnight at least twice while living in the parental or parental surrogate home, or once without returning for a lengthy period.
15. Is often truant from school, beginning before age 13 years.

B. The disturbance in behavior causes clinically significant impairment in social, academic, or occupational functioning.

C. If the individual is age 18 years or older, criteria are not met for antisocial personality disorder.

Specify whether:

312.81 (F91.1) Childhood-onset type: Individuals show at least one symptom characteristic of conduct disorder prior to age 10 years.

312.82 (F91.2) Adolescent-onset type: Individuals show no symptom characteristic of conduct disorder prior to age 10 years.

312.89 (F91.9) Unspecified onset: Criteria for a diagnosis of conduct disorder are met, but there is not enough information available to determine whether the onset of the first symptom was before or after age 10 years.

Specify if:

With limited prosocial emotions: To qualify for this specifier, an individual must have displayed at least two of the following characteristics persistently over at least 12 months and in multiple relationships and settings. These characteristics reflect the individual's typical pattern of interpersonal and emotional functioning over this period and not just occasional occurrences in some situations. Thus, to assess the criteria for the specifier, multiple information sources are necessary. In addition to the individual's self-report, it is necessary to consider reports by others who have known the individual for extended periods of time (e.g., parents, teachers, co-workers, extended family members, peers).

Lack of remorse or guilt: Does not feel bad or guilty when he or she does something wrong (exclude remorse when expressed only when caught and/or facing punishment). The individual shows a general lack of concern about the negative consequences of his or her actions. For example, the individual is not remorseful after hurting someone or does not care about the consequences of breaking rules.

Callous—lack of empathy: Disregards and is unconcerned about the feelings of others. The individual is described as cold and uncaring. The person appears more concerned about the effects of his or her actions on himself or herself, rather than their effects on others, even when they result in substantial harm to others.

Unconcerned about performance: Does not show concern about poor/problematic performance at school, at work, or in other important activities. The individual does not put forth the effort necessary to perform well, even when expectations are clear, and typically blames others for his or her poor performance.

Shallow or deficient affect: Does not express feelings or show emotions to others, except in ways that seem shallow, insincere, or superficial (e.g., actions contradict the emotion displayed; can turn emotions "on" or "off" quickly) or when emotional expressions are used for gain (e.g., emotions displayed to manipulate or intimidate others).

Specify current severity:

Mild: Few if any conduct problems in excess of those required to make the diagnosis are present, and conduct problems cause relatively minor harm to others (e.g., lying, truancy, staying out after dark without permission, other rule breaking).

Moderate: The number of conduct problems and the effect on others are intermediate between those specified in "mild" and those in "severe" (e.g., stealing without confronting a victim, vandalism).

Severe: Many conduct problems in excess of those required to make the diagnosis are present, or conduct problems cause considerable harm to others (e.g., forced sex, physical cruelty, use of a weapon, stealing while confronting a victim, breaking and entering).

Subtypes

Three subtypes of conduct disorder are provided based on the age at onset of the disorder. Onset is most accurately estimated with information from both the youth and the caregiver; estimates are often 2 years later than actual onset. Both subtypes can occur in a mild, moderate, or severe form. An unspecified-onset subtype is designated when there is insufficient information to determine age at onset.

In childhood-onset conduct disorder, individuals are usually male, frequently display physical aggression toward others, have disturbed peer relationships, may have had oppositional defiant disorder during early childhood, and usually have symptoms that meet full criteria for conduct disorder prior to puberty. Many children with this subtype also have concurrent attention-deficit/hyperactivity disorder (ADHD) or other neurodevelopmental difficulties. Individuals with childhood-onset type are more likely to have persistent conduct disorder into adulthood than are those with adolescent-onset type. As compared with individuals with childhood-onset type, individuals with adolescent-onset conduct disorder are less likely to display aggressive behaviors and tend to have more normative peer relationships (although they often display conduct problems in the company of others). These individuals are less likely to have conduct disorder that persists into adulthood. The ratio of males to females with conduct disorder is more balanced for the adolescent-onset type than for the childhood-onset type.

Specifiers

A minority of individuals with conduct disorder exhibit characteristics that qualify for the "with limited prosocial emotions" specifier. The indicators of this specifier are those that have often been labeled as callous and unemotional traits in research. Other personality features, such as thrill seeking, fearlessness, and insensitivity to punishment, may also distinguish those with characteristics described in the specifier. Individuals with characteristics described in this specifier may be more likely than other individuals with conduct disorder to engage in aggression that is planned for instrumental gain. Individuals with conduct disorder of any subtype or any level of severity can have characteristics that qualify for the specifier "with limited prosocial emotions," although individuals with the specifier are more likely to have childhood-onset type and a severity specifier rating of severe.

Although the validity of self-report to assess the presence of the specifier has been supported in some research contexts, individuals with conduct disorder with this specifier may not readily admit to the traits in a clinical interview. Thus, to assess the criteria for the specifier, multiple information sources are necessary. Also, because the indicators of the specifier are characteristics that reflect the individual's typical pattern of interpersonal and emotional functioning, it is important to consider reports by others who have known the individual for extended periods of time and across relationships and settings (e.g., parents, teachers, co-workers, extended family members, peers).

Diagnostic Features

The essential feature of conduct disorder is a repetitive and persistent pattern of behavior in which the basic rights of others or major age-appropriate societal norms or rules are violated (Criterion A). These behaviors fall into four main groupings: aggressive conduct that causes or threatens physical harm to other people or animals (Criteria A1–A7); non-aggressive conduct that causes property loss or damage (Criteria A8–A9); deceitfulness or theft (Criteria A10–A12); and serious violations of rules (Criteria A13–A15). Three or more characteristic behaviors must have been present during the past 12 months, with at least one behavior present in the past 6 months. The disturbance in behavior causes clinically significant impairment in social, academic, or occupational functioning (Criterion B). The behavior pattern is usually present in a variety of settings, such as home, at school, or in the community. Because individuals with conduct disorder are likely to minimize their conduct problems, the clinician often must rely on additional informants. However, informants' knowledge of the individual's conduct problems may be limited if they have inadequately supervised the individual or the individual has concealed symptom behaviors.

Individuals with conduct disorder often initiate aggressive behavior and react aggressively to others. They may display bullying, threatening, or intimidating behavior (including bullying via messaging on Web-based social media) (Criterion A1); initiate frequent physical fights (Criterion A2); use a weapon that can cause serious physical harm (e.g., a bat, brick, broken bottle, knife, gun) (Criterion A3); be physically cruel to people (Criterion A4) or animals (Criterion A5); steal while confronting a victim (e.g., mugging, purse snatching, extortion, armed robbery) (Criterion A6); or force someone into sexual activity (Criterion A7). Physical violence may take the form of rape, assault, or, in rare cases, homicide. Deliberate destruction of others' property may include deliberate fire setting with the intention of causing serious damage (Criterion A8) or deliberate destroying of other people's property in other ways (e.g., smashing car windows, vandalizing school property) (Criterion A9). Acts of deceitfulness or theft may include breaking into someone else's house, building, or car (Criterion A10); frequently lying or breaking promises to obtain goods or favors or to avoid debts or obligations (e.g., "conning" other individuals) (Criterion A11); or stealing items of nontrivial value without confronting the victim (e.g., shoplifting, forgery, fraud) (Criterion A12).

Individuals with conduct disorder may also frequently commit serious violations of rules (e.g., school, parental, workplace). Children with conduct disorder often have a pattern, beginning before age 13 years, of staying out late at night despite parental prohibitions (Criterion A13). Children may also show a pattern of running away from home overnight (Criterion A14). To be considered a symptom of conduct disorder, the running away must have occurred at least twice (or only once if the individual did not return for a lengthy period). Runaway episodes that occur as a direct consequence of physical or sexual abuse do not typically qualify for this criterion. Children with conduct disorder may often be truant from school, beginning prior to age 13 years (Criterion A15).

Associated Features Supporting Diagnosis

Especially in ambiguous situations, aggressive individuals with conduct disorder frequently misperceive the intentions of others as more hostile and threatening than is the case and respond with aggression that they then feel is reasonable and justified. Personality features of trait negative emotionality and poor self-control, including poor frustration tolerance, irritability, temper outbursts, suspiciousness, insensitivity to punishment, thrill seeking, and recklessness, frequently co-occur with conduct disorder. Substance misuse is often an associated feature, particularly in adolescent females. Suicidal ideation, suicide attempts, and completed suicide occur at a higher-than-expected rate in individuals with conduct disorder.

Prevalence

One-year population prevalence estimates range from 2% to more than 10%, with a median of 4%. The prevalence of conduct disorder appears to be fairly consistent across various countries that differ in race and ethnicity. Prevalence rates rise from childhood to adolescence and are higher among males than among females. Few children with impairing conduct disorder receive treatment.

Development and Course

The onset of conduct disorder may occur as early as the preschool years, but the first significant symptoms usually emerge during the period from middle childhood through middle adolescence. Oppositional defiant disorder is a common precursor to the childhood-onset type of conduct disorder. Conduct disorder may be diagnosed in adults, however, symptoms of conduct disorder usually emerge in childhood or adolescence, and onset is rare after age 16 years. The course of conduct disorder after onset is variable. In a majority of individuals, the disorder remits by adulthood. Many individuals with conduct disorder—particularly those with adolescent-onset type and those with few and milder symptoms—achieve adequate social and occupational adjustment as adults. However, the early-onset type predicts a worse prognosis and an increased risk of criminal behavior, conduct disorder, and substance-related disorders in adulthood. Individuals with conduct disorder are at risk for later mood disorders, anxiety disorders, posttraumatic stress disorder, impulse-control disorders, psychotic disorders, somatic symptom disorders, and substance-related disorders as adults.

Symptoms of the disorder vary with age as the individual develops increased physical strength, cognitive abilities, and sexual maturity. Symptom behaviors that emerge first tend to be less serious (e.g., lying, shoplifting), whereas conduct problems that emerge last tend to be more severe (e.g., rape, theft while confronting a victim). However, there are wide differences among individuals, with some engaging in the more damaging behaviors at an early age (which is predictive of a worse prognosis). When individuals with conduct disorder reach adulthood, symptoms of aggression, property destruction, deceitfulness, and rule violation, including violence against co-workers, partners, and children, may be exhibited in the workplace and the home, such that antisocial personality disorder may be considered.

Risk and Prognostic Factors

Temperamental. Temperamental risk factors include a difficult undercontrolled infant temperament and lower-than-average intelligence, particularly with regard to verbal IQ.

Environmental. Family-level risk factors include parental rejection and neglect, inconsistent child-rearing practices, harsh discipline, physical or sexual abuse, lack of supervision, early institutional living, frequent changes of caregivers, large family size, parental criminality, and certain kinds of familial psychopathology (e.g., substance-related disorders). Community-level risk factors include peer rejection, association with a delinquent peer group, and neighborhood exposure to violence. Both types of risk factors tend to be more common and severe among individuals with the childhood-onset subtype of conduct disorder.

Genetic and physiological.   Conduct disorder is influenced by both genetic and environmental factors. The risk is increased in children with a biological or adoptive parent or a sibling with conduct disorder. The disorder also appears to be more common in children of biological parents with severe alcohol use disorder, depressive and bipolar disorders, or schizophrenia or biological parents who have a history of ADHD or conduct disorder. Family history particularly characterizes individuals with the childhood-onset subtype of conduct disorder. Slower resting heart rate has been reliably noted in individuals with conduct disorder compared with those without the disorder, and this marker is not characteristic of any other mental disorder. Reduced autonomic fear conditioning, particularly low skin conductance, is also well documented. However, these psychophysiological findings are not diagnostic of the disorder. Structural and functional differences in brain areas associated with affect regulation and affect processing, particularly frontotemporal-limbic connections involving the brain's ventral prefrontal cortex and amygdala, have been consistently noted in individuals with conduct disorder compared with those without the disorder. However, neuroimaging findings are not diagnostic of the disorder.

Course modifiers.   Persistence is more likely for individuals with behaviors that meet criteria for the childhood-onset subtype and qualify for the specifier "with limited prosocial emotions". The risk that conduct disorder will persist is also increased by co-occurring ADHD and by substance abuse.

Culture-Related Diagnostic Issues

Conduct disorder diagnosis may at times be potentially misapplied to individuals in settings where patterns of disruptive behavior are viewed as near-normative (e.g., in very threatening, high-crime areas or war zones). Therefore, the context in which the undesirable behaviors have occurred should be considered.

Gender-Related Diagnostic Issues

Males with a diagnosis of conduct disorder frequently exhibit fighting, stealing, vandalism, and school discipline problems. Females with a diagnosis of conduct disorder are more likely to exhibit lying, truancy, running away, substance use, and prostitution. Whereas males tend to exhibit both physical aggression and relational aggression (behavior that harms social relationships of others), females tend to exhibit relatively more relational aggression.

Functional Consequences of Conduct Disorder

Conduct disorder behaviors may lead to school suspension or expulsion, problems in work adjustment, legal difficulties, sexually transmitted diseases, unplanned pregnancy, and physical injury from accidents or fights. These problems may preclude attendance in ordinary schools or living in a parental or foster home. Conduct disorder is often associated with an early onset of sexual behavior, alcohol use, tobacco smoking, use of illegal substances, and reckless and risk-taking acts. Accident rates appear to be higher among individuals with conduct disorder compared with those without the disorder. These functional consequences of conduct disorder may predict health difficulties when individuals reach midlife. It is not uncommon for individuals with conduct disorder to come into contact with the criminal justice system for engaging in illegal behavior. Conduct disorder is a common reason for treatment referral and is frequently diagnosed in mental health facilities for children, especially in forensic practice. It is associated with impairment that is more severe and chronic than that experienced by other clinic-referred children.

Differential Diagnosis

Oppositional defiant disorder.   Conduct disorder and oppositional defiant disorder are both related to symptoms that bring the individual in conflict with adults and other authority figures (e.g., parents, teachers, work supervisors). The behaviors of oppositional defiant disorder are typically of a less severe nature than those of individuals with conduct disorder and do not include aggression toward individuals or animals, destruction of property, or a pattern of theft or deceit. Furthermore, oppositional defiant disorder includes problems of emotional dysregulation (i.e., angry and irritable mood) that are not included in the definition of conduct disorder. When criteria are met for both oppositional defiant disorder and conduct disorder, both diagnoses can be given.

Attention-deficit/hyperactivity disorder. Although children with ADHD often exhibit hyperactive and impulsive behavior that may be disruptive, this behavior does not by itself violate societal norms or the rights of others and therefore does not usually meet criteria for conduct disorder. When criteria are met for both ADHD and conduct disorder, both diagnoses should be given.

Depressive and bipolar disorders. Irritability, aggression, and conduct problems can occur in children or adolescents with a major depressive disorder, a bipolar disorder, or disruptive mood dysregulation disorder. The behavioral problems associated with these mood disorders can usually be distinguished from the pattern of conduct problems seen in conduct disorder based on their course. Specifically, persons with conduct disorder will display substantial levels of aggressive or non-aggressive conduct problems during periods in which there is no mood disturbance, either historically (i.e., a history of conduct problems predating the onset of the mood disturbance) or concurrently (i.e., display of some conduct problems that are premeditated and do not occur during periods of intense emotional arousal). In those cases in which criteria for conduct disorder and a mood disorder are met, both diagnoses can be given.

Intermittent explosive disorder. Both conduct disorder and intermittent explosive disorder involve high rates of aggression. However, the aggression in individuals with intermittent explosive disorder is limited to impulsive aggression and is not premeditated, and it is not committed in order to achieve some tangible objective (e.g., money, power, intimidation). Also, the definition of intermittent explosive disorder does not include the non-aggressive symptoms of conduct disorder. If criteria for both disorders are met, the diagnosis of intermittent explosive disorder should be given only when the recurrent impulsive aggressive outbursts warrant independent clinical attention.

Adjustment disorders. The diagnosis of an adjustment disorder (with disturbance of conduct or with mixed disturbance of emotions and conduct) should be considered if clinically significant conduct problems that do not meet the criteria for another specific disorder develop in clear association with the onset of a psychosocial stressor and do not resolve within 6 months of the termination of the stressor (or its consequences). Conduct disorder is diagnosed only when the conduct problems represent a repetitive and persistent pattern that is associated with impairment in social, academic, or occupational functioning.

Comorbidity

ADHD and oppositional defiant disorder are both common in individuals with conduct disorder, and this comorbid presentation predicts worse outcomes. Individuals who show the personality features associated with antisocial personality disorder often violate the basic rights of others or violate major age-appropriate societal norms, and as a result their pattern of behavior often meets criteria for conduct disorder. Conduct disorder may also co-occur with one or more of the following mental disorders: specific learning disorder, anxiety disorders, depressive or bipolar disorders, and substance-related disorders. Academic achievement, particularly in reading and other verbal skills, is often below the level expected on the basis of age and intelligence and may justify the additional diagnosis of specific learning disorder or a communication disorder.

Antisocial Personality Disorder

Criteria and text for antisocial personality disorder can be found in the chapter "Personality Disorders." Because this disorder is closely connected to the spectrum of "externalizing" conduct disorders in this chapter, as well as to the disorders in the adjoining chapter "Substance-Related and Addictive Disorders," it is dual coded here as well as in the chapter "Personality Disorders."

Pyromania

Diagnostic Criteria   **312.33 (F63.1)**

A. Deliberate and purposeful fire setting on more than one occasion.
B. Tension or affective arousal before the act.
C. Fascination with, interest in, curiosity about, or attraction to fire and its situational contexts (e.g., paraphernalia, uses, consequences).
D. Pleasure, gratification, or relief when setting fires or when witnessing or participating in their aftermath.
E. The fire setting is not done for monetary gain, as an expression of sociopolitical ideology, to conceal criminal activity, to express anger or vengeance, to improve one's living circumstances, in response to a delusion or hallucination, or as a result of impaired judgment (e.g., in major neurocognitive disorder, intellectual disability [intellectual developmental disorder], substance intoxication).
F. The fire setting is not better explained by conduct disorder, a manic episode, or antisocial personality disorder.

Diagnostic Features

The essential feature of pyromania is the presence of multiple episodes of deliberate and purposeful fire setting (Criterion A). Individuals with this disorder experience tension or affective arousal before setting a fire (Criterion B). There is a fascination with, interest in, curiosity about, or attraction to fire and its situational contexts (e.g., paraphernalia, uses, consequences) (Criterion C). Individuals with this disorder are often regular "watchers" at fires in their neighborhoods, may set off false alarms, and derive pleasure from institutions, equipment, and personnel associated with fire. They may spend time at the local fire department, set fires to be affiliated with the fire department, or even become firefighters. Individuals with this disorder experience pleasure, gratification, or relief when setting the fire, witnessing its effects, or participating in its aftermath (Criterion D). The fire setting is not done for monetary gain, as an expression of sociopolitical ideology, to conceal criminal activity, to express anger or vengeance, to improve one's living circumstances, or in response to a delusion or a hallucination (Criterion E). The fire setting does not result from impaired judgment (e.g., in major neurocognitive disorder or intellectual disability [intellectual developmental disorder]). The diagnosis is not made if the fire setting is better explained by conduct disorder, a manic episode, or antisocial personality disorder (Criterion F).

Associated Features Supporting Diagnosis

Individuals with pyromania may make considerable advance preparation for starting a fire. They may be indifferent to the consequences to life or property caused by the fire, or they may derive satisfaction from the resulting property destruction. The behaviors may lead to property damage, legal consequences, or injury or loss of life to the fire setter or to others. Individuals who impulsively set fires (who may or may not have pyromania) often have a current or past history of alcohol use disorder.

Prevalence

The population prevalence of pyromania is not known. The lifetime prevalence of fire setting, which is just one component of pyromania and not sufficient for a diagnosis by itself, was reported as 1.13% in a population sample, but the most common comorbidities were antisocial personality disorder, substance use disorder, bipolar disorder, and pathological gambling (gambling disorder). In contrast, pyromania as a primary diagnosis appears to be very rare. Among a sample of persons reaching the criminal system with repeated fire setting, only 3.3% had symptoms that met full criteria for pyromania.

Development and Course

There are insufficient data to establish a typical age at onset of pyromania. The relationship between fire setting in childhood and pyromania in adulthood has not been documented. In individuals with pyromania, fire-setting incidents are episodic and may wax and wane in frequency. Longitudinal course is unknown. Although fire setting is a major problem in children and adolescents (over 40% of those arrested for arson offenses in the United States are younger than 18 years), pyromania in childhood appears to be rare. Juvenile fire setting is usually associated with conduct disorder, attention-deficit/hyperactivity disorder, or an adjustment disorder.

Gender-Related Diagnostic Issues

Pyromania occurs much more often in males, especially those with poorer social skills and learning difficulties.

Differential Diagnosis

Other causes of intentional fire setting.   It is important to rule out other causes of fire setting before giving the diagnosis of pyromania. Intentional fire setting may occur for profit, sabotage, or revenge; to conceal a crime; to make a political statement (e.g., an act of terrorism or protest); or to attract attention or recognition (e.g., setting a fire in order to discover it and save the day). Fire setting may also occur as part of developmental experimentation in childhood (e.g., playing with matches, lighters, or fire).

Other mental disorders.   A separate diagnosis of pyromania is not given when fire setting occurs as part of conduct disorder, a manic episode, or antisocial personality disorder, or if it occurs in response to a delusion or a hallucination (e.g., in schizophrenia) or is attributable to the physiological effects of another medical condition (e.g., epilepsy). The diagnosis of pyromania should also not be given when fire setting results from impaired judgment associated with major neurocognitive disorder, intellectual disability, or substance intoxication.

Comorbidity

There appears to be a high co-occurrence of substance use disorders, gambling disorder, depressive and bipolar disorders, and other disruptive, impulse-control, and conduct disorders with pyromania.

Kleptomania

Diagnostic Criteria   **312.32** (F63.2)

A. Recurrent failure to resist impulses to steal objects that are not needed for personal use or for their monetary value.
B. Increasing sense of tension immediately before committing the theft.
C. Pleasure, gratification, or relief at the time of committing the theft.
D. The stealing is not committed to express anger or vengeance and is not in response to a delusion or a hallucination.
E. The stealing is not better explained by conduct disorder, a manic episode, or antisocial personality disorder.

Diagnostic Features

The essential feature of kleptomania is the recurrent failure to resist impulses to steal items even though the items are not needed for personal use or for their monetary value (Criterion A). The individual experiences a rising subjective sense of tension before the theft (Criterion B) and feels pleasure, gratification, or relief when committing the theft (Criterion C). The stealing is not committed to express anger or vengeance, is not done in response to a delusion or hallucination (Criterion D), and is not better explained by conduct disorder, a manic episode, or antisocial personality disorder (Criterion E). The objects are stolen despite the fact that they are typically of little value to the individual, who could have afforded to pay for them and often gives them away or discards them. Occasionally the individual may hoard the stolen objects or surreptitiously return them. Although individuals with this disorder will generally avoid stealing when immediate arrest is probable (e.g., in full view of a police officer), they usually do not preplan the thefts or fully take into account the chances of apprehension. The stealing is done without assistance from, or collaboration with, others.

Associated Features Supporting Diagnosis

Individuals with kleptomania typically attempt to resist the impulse to steal, and they are aware that the act is wrong and senseless. The individual frequently fears being apprehended and often feels depressed or guilty about the thefts. Neurotransmitter pathways associated with behavioral addictions, including those associated with the serotonin, dopamine, and opioid systems, appear to play a role in kleptomania as well.

Prevalence

Kleptomania occurs in about 4%–24% of individuals arrested for shoplifting. Its prevalence in the general population is very rare, at approximately 0.3%–0.6%. Females outnumber males at a ratio of 3:1.

Development and Course

Age at onset of kleptomania is variable, but the disorder often begins in adolescence. However, the disorder may begin in childhood, adolescence, or adulthood, and in rare cases in late adulthood. There is little systematic information on the course of kleptomania, but three typical courses have been described: sporadic with brief episodes and long periods of remission; episodic with protracted periods of stealing and periods of remission; and chronic with some degree of fluctuation. The disorder may continue for years, despite multiple convictions for shoplifting.

Risk and Prognostic Factors

Genetic and physiological.   There are no controlled family history studies of kleptomania. However, first-degree relatives of individuals with kleptomania may have higher rates of obsessive-compulsive disorder than the general population. There also appears to be a higher rate of substance use disorders, including alcohol use disorder, in relatives of individuals with kleptomania than in the general population.

Functional Consequences of Kleptomania

The disorder may cause legal, family, career, and personal difficulties.

Differential Diagnosis

Ordinary theft.   Kleptomania should be distinguished from ordinary acts of theft or shoplifting. Ordinary theft (whether planned or impulsive) is deliberate and is motivated by the usefulness of the object or its monetary worth. Some individuals, especially adolescents, may also steal on a dare, as an act of rebellion, or as a rite of passage. The diagnosis is not made unless other characteristic features of kleptomania are also present. Kleptomania is exceedingly rare, whereas shoplifting is relatively common.

Malingering.   In malingering, individuals may simulate the symptoms of kleptomania to avoid criminal prosecution.

Antisocial personality disorder and conduct disorder.   Antisocial personality disorder and conduct disorder are distinguished from kleptomania by a general pattern of antisocial behavior.

Manic episodes, psychotic episodes, and major neurocognitive disorder.   Kleptomania should be distinguished from intentional or inadvertent stealing that may occur during a manic episode, in response to delusions or hallucinations (as in, e.g., schizophrenia), or as a result of a major neurocognitive disorder.

Comorbidity

Kleptomania may be associated with compulsive buying as well as with depressive and bipolar disorders (especially major depressive disorder), anxiety disorders, eating disorders (particularly bulimia nervosa), personality disorders, substance use disorders (especially alcohol use disorder), and other disruptive, impulse-control, and conduct disorders.

Other Specified Disruptive, Impulse-Control, and Conduct Disorder

312.89 (F91.8)

This category applies to presentations in which symptoms characteristic of a disruptive, impulse-control, and conduct disorder that cause clinically significant distress or impairment in social, occupational, or other important areas of functioning predominate but do not meet the full criteria for any of the disorders in the disruptive, impulse-control, and conduct disorders diagnostic class. The other specified disruptive, impulse-control, and conduct disorder category is used in situations in which the clinician chooses to communicate the specific reason that the presentation does not meet the criteria for any specific disruptive, impulse-control, and conduct disorder. This is done by recording "other specified disruptive, impulse-control, and conduct disorder" followed by the specific reason (e.g., "recurrent behavioral outbursts of insufficient frequency").

Unspecified Disruptive, Impulse-Control, and Conduct Disorder

312.9 (F91.9)

This category applies to presentations in which symptoms characteristic of a disruptive, impulse-control, and conduct disorder that cause clinically significant distress or impairment in social, occupational, or other important areas of functioning predominate but do not meet the full criteria for any of the disorders in the disruptive, impulse-control, and conduct disorders diagnostic class. The unspecified disruptive, impulse-control, and conduct disorder category is used in situations in which the clinician chooses *not* to specify the reason that the criteria are not met for a specific disruptive, impulse-control, and conduct disorder, and includes presentations in which there is insufficient information to make a more specific diagnosis (e.g., in emergency room settings).

Substance-Related and Addictive Disorders

The substance-related disorders encompass 10 separate classes of drugs: alcohol; caffeine; cannabis; hallucinogens (with separate categories for phencyclidine [or similarly acting arylcyclohexylamines] and other hallucinogens); inhalants; opioids; sedatives, hypnotics, and anxiolytics; stimulants (amphetamine-type substances, cocaine, and other stimulants); tobacco; and other (or unknown) substances. These 10 classes are not fully distinct. All drugs that are taken in excess have in common direct activation of the brain reward system, which is involved in the reinforcement of behaviors and the production of memories. They produce such an intense activation of the reward system that normal activities may be neglected. Instead of achieving reward system activation through adaptive behaviors, drugs of abuse directly activate the reward pathways. The pharmacological mechanisms by which each class of drugs produces reward are different, but the drugs typically activate the system and produce feelings of pleasure, often referred to as a "high." Furthermore, individuals with lower levels of self-control, which may reflect impairments of brain inhibitory mechanisms, may be particularly predisposed to develop substance use disorders, suggesting that the roots of substance use disorders for some persons can be seen in behaviors long before the onset of actual substance use itself.

In addition to the substance-related disorders, this chapter also includes gambling disorder, reflecting evidence that gambling behaviors activate reward systems similar to those activated by drugs of abuse and produce some behavioral symptoms that appear comparable to those produced by the substance use disorders. Other excessive behavioral patterns, such as Internet gaming, have also been described, but the research on these and other behavioral syndromes is less clear. Thus, groups of repetitive behaviors, which some term *behavioral addictions,* with such subcategories as "sex addiction," "exercise addiction," or "shopping addiction," are not included because at this time there is insufficient peer-reviewed evidence to establish the diagnostic criteria and course descriptions needed to identify these behaviors as mental disorders.

The substance-related disorders are divided into two groups: substance use disorders and substance-induced disorders. The following conditions may be classified as substance-induced: intoxication, withdrawal, and other substance/medication-induced mental disorders (psychotic disorders, bipolar and related disorders, depressive disorders, anxiety disorders, obsessive-compulsive and related disorders, sleep disorders, sexual dysfunctions, delirium, and neurocognitive disorders).

The current section begins with a general discussion of criteria sets for a substance use disorder, substance intoxication and withdrawal, and other substance/medication-induced mental disorders, at least some of which are applicable across classes of substances. Reflecting some unique aspects of the 10 substance classes relevant to this chapter, the remainder of the chapter is organized by the class of substance and describes their unique aspects. To facilitate differential diagnosis, the text and criteria for the remaining substance/medication-induced mental disorders are included with disorders with which they share phenomenology (e.g., substance/medication-induced depressive disorder is in the chapter "Depressive Disorders"). The broad diagnostic categories associated with each specific group of substances are shown in Table 1.

TABLE 1 Diagnoses associated with substance class

	Psychotic disorders	Bipolar disorders	Depressive disorders	Anxiety disorders	Obsessive-compulsive and related disorders	Sleep disorders	Sexual dysfunctions	Delirium	Neuro-cognitive disorders	Substance use disorders	Substance intoxication	Substance withdrawal
Alcohol	I/W	I/W	I/W	I/W		I/W	I/W	I/W	I/W/P	X	X	X
Caffeine				I		I/W					X	X
Cannabis	I			I		I/W		I		X	X	X
Hallucinogens												
Phencyclidine	I	I	I	I				I		X	X	
Other hallucinogens	I*	I	I	I				I		X	X	
Inhalants	I		I	I				I	I/P	X	X	
Opioids			I/W	W		I/W	I/W	I/W		X	X	X
Sedatives, hypnotics, or anxiolytics	I/W	I/W	I/W	W		I/W	I/W	I/W	I/W/P	X	X	X
Stimulants**	I	I/W	I/W	I/W	I/W	I/W	I	I		X	X	X
Tobacco						W				X		X
Other (or unknown)	I/W	I/W	I/W	I/W	I/W	I/W	I/W	I/W	I/W/P	X	X	X

Note. X = The category is recognized in DSM-5.
I = The specifier "with onset during intoxication" may be noted for the category.
W = The specifier "with onset during withdrawal" may be noted for the category.
I/W = Either "with onset during intoxication" or "with onset during withdrawal" may be noted for the category.
P = The disorder is persisting.
* Also hallucinogen persisting perception disorder (flashbacks).
**Includes amphetamine-type substances, cocaine, and other or unspecified stimulants.

Substance-Related Disorders

Substance Use Disorders

Features

The essential feature of a substance use disorder is a cluster of cognitive, behavioral, and physiological symptoms indicating that the individual continues using the substance despite significant substance-related problems. As seen in Table 1, the diagnosis of a substance use disorder can be applied to all 10 classes included in this chapter except caffeine. For certain classes some symptoms are less salient, and in a few instances not all symptoms apply (e.g., withdrawal symptoms are not specified for phencyclidine use disorder, other hallucinogen use disorder, or inhalant use disorder).

An important characteristic of substance use disorders is an underlying change in brain circuits that may persist beyond detoxification, particularly in individuals with severe disorders. The behavioral effects of these brain changes may be exhibited in the repeated relapses and intense drug craving when the individuals are exposed to drug-related stimuli. These persistent drug effects may benefit from long-term approaches to treatment.

Overall, the diagnosis of a substance use disorder is based on a pathological pattern of behaviors related to use of the substance. To assist with organization, Criterion A criteria can be considered to fit within overall groupings of *impaired control, social impairment, risky use,* and *pharmacological criteria.* Impaired control over substance use is the first criteria grouping (Criteria 1–4). The individual may take the substance in larger amounts or over a longer period than was originally intended (Criterion 1). The individual may express a persistent desire to cut down or regulate substance use and may report multiple unsuccessful efforts to decrease or discontinue use (Criterion 2). The individual may spend a great deal of time obtaining the substance, using the substance, or recovering from its effects (Criterion 3). In some instances of more severe substance use disorders, virtually all of the individual's daily activities revolve around the substance. Craving (Criterion 4) is manifested by an intense desire or urge for the drug that may occur at any time but is more likely when in an environment where the drug previously was obtained or used. Craving has also been shown to involve classical conditioning and is associated with activation of specific reward structures in the brain. Craving is queried by asking if there has ever been a time when they had such strong urges to take the drug that they could not think of anything else. Current craving is often used as a treatment outcome measure because it may be a signal of impending relapse.

Social impairment is the second grouping of criteria (Criteria 5–7). Recurrent substance use may result in a failure to fulfill major role obligations at work, school, or home (Criterion 5). The individual may continue substance use despite having persistent or recurrent social or interpersonal problems caused or exacerbated by the effects of the substance (Criterion 6). Important social, occupational, or recreational activities may be given up or reduced because of substance use (Criterion 7). The individual may withdraw from family activities and hobbies in order to use the substance.

Risky use of the substance is the third grouping of criteria (Criteria 8–9). This may take the form of recurrent substance use in situations in which it is physically hazardous (Criterion 8). The individual may continue substance use despite knowledge of having a persistent or recurrent physical or psychological problem that is likely to have been caused or exacerbated by the substance (Criterion 9). The key issue in evaluating this criterion is not the existence of the problem, but rather the individual's failure to abstain from using the substance despite the difficulty it is causing.

Pharmacological criteria are the final grouping (Criteria 10 and 11). Tolerance (Criterion 10) is signaled by requiring a markedly increased dose of the substance to achieve the desired effect or a markedly reduced effect when the usual dose is consumed. The degree to which tolerance develops varies greatly across different individuals as well as across substances and may involve a variety of central nervous system effects. For example, tolerance to respiratory depression and tolerance to sedating and motor coordination may develop at different rates, depending on the substance. Tolerance may be difficult to determine by history alone, and laboratory tests may be helpful (e.g., high blood levels of the substance coupled with little evidence of intoxication suggest that tolerance is likely). Tolerance must also be distinguished from individual variability in the initial sensitivity to the effects of particular substances. For example, some first-time alcohol drinkers show very little evidence of intoxication with three or four drinks, whereas others of similar weight and drinking histories have slurred speech and incoordination.

Withdrawal (Criterion 11) is a syndrome that occurs when blood or tissue concentrations of a substance decline in an individual who had maintained prolonged heavy use of the substance. After developing withdrawal symptoms, the individual is likely to consume the substance to relieve the symptoms. Withdrawal symptoms vary greatly across the classes of substances, and separate criteria sets for withdrawal are provided for the drug classes. Marked and generally easily measured physiological signs of withdrawal are common with alcohol, opioids, and sedatives, hypnotics, and anxiolytics. Withdrawal signs and symptoms with stimulants (amphetamines and cocaine), as well as tobacco and cannabis, are often present but may be less apparent. Significant withdrawal has *not* been documented in humans after repeated use of phencyclidine, other hallucinogens, and inhalants; therefore, this criterion is not included for these substances. Neither tolerance nor withdrawal is necessary for a diagnosis of a substance use disorder. However, for most classes of substances, a past history of withdrawal is associated with a more severe clinical course (i.e., an earlier onset of a substance use disorder, higher levels of substance intake, and a greater number of substance-related problems).

Symptoms of tolerance and withdrawal occurring during appropriate medical treatment with prescribed medications (e.g., opioid analgesics, sedatives, stimulants) are specifically *not* counted when diagnosing a substance use disorder. The appearance of normal, expected pharmacological tolerance and withdrawal during the course of medical treatment has been known to lead to an erroneous diagnosis of "addiction" even when these were the only symptoms present. Individuals whose *only* symptoms are those that occur as a result of medical treatment (i.e., tolerance and withdrawal as part of medical care when the medications are taken as prescribed) should not receive a diagnosis solely on the basis of these symptoms. However, prescription medications can be used inappropriately, and a substance use disorder can be correctly diagnosed when there are other symptoms of compulsive, drug-seeking behavior.

Severity and Specifiers

Substance use disorders occur in a broad range of severity, from mild to severe, with severity based on the number of symptom criteria endorsed. As a general estimate of severity, a *mild* substance use disorder is suggested by the presence of two to three symptoms, *moderate* by four to five symptoms, and *severe* by six or more symptoms. Changing severity across time is also reflected by reductions or increases in the frequency and/or dose of substance use, as assessed by the individual's own report, report of knowledgeable others, clinician's observations, and biological testing. The following course specifiers and descriptive features specifiers are also available for substance use disorders: "in early remission," "in sustained remission," "on maintenance therapy," and "in a controlled environment." Definitions of each are provided within respective criteria sets.

Recording Procedures for Substance Use Disorders

The clinician should use the code that applies to the class of substances but record the name of the *specific substance*. For example, the clinician should record 304.10 (F13.20) moderate alprazolam use disorder (rather than moderate sedative, hypnotic, or anxiolytic use disorder) or 305.70 (F15.10) mild methamphetamine use disorder (rather than mild stimulant use disorder). For substances that do not fit into any of the classes (e.g., anabolic steroids), the appropriate code for "other substance use disorder" should be used and the specific substance indicated (e.g., 305.90 [F19.10] mild anabolic steroid use disorder). If the substance taken by the individual is unknown, the code for the class "other (or unknown)" should be used (e.g., 304.90 [F19.20] severe unknown substance use disorder). If criteria are met for more than one substance use disorder, all should be diagnosed (e.g., 304.00 [F11.20] severe heroin use disorder; 304.20 [F14.20] moderate cocaine use disorder).

The appropriate ICD-10-CM code for a substance use disorder depends on whether there is a comorbid substance-induced disorder (including intoxication and withdrawal). In the above example, the diagnostic code for moderate alprazolam use disorder, F13.20, reflects the absence of a comorbid alprazolam-induced mental disorder. Because ICD-10-CM codes for substance-induced disorders indicate both the presence (or absence) and severity of the substance use disorder, ICD-10-CM codes for substance use disorders can be used only in the absence of a substance-induced disorder. See the individual substance-specific sections for additional coding information.

Note that the word *addiction* is not applied as a diagnostic term in this classification, although it is in common usage in many countries to describe severe problems related to compulsive and habitual use of substances. The more neutral term *substance use disorder* is used to describe the wide range of the disorder, from a mild form to a severe state of chronically relapsing, compulsive drug taking. Some clinicians will choose to use the word *addiction* to describe more extreme presentations, but the word is omitted from the official DSM-5 substance use disorder diagnostic terminology because of its uncertain definition and its potentially negative connotation.

Substance-Induced Disorders

The overall category of substance-induced disorders includes intoxication, withdrawal, and other substance/medication-induced mental disorders (e.g., substance-induced psychotic disorder, substance-induced depressive disorder).

Substance Intoxication and Withdrawal

Criteria for substance intoxication are included within the substance-specific sections of this chapter. The essential feature is the development of a reversible substance-specific syndrome due to the recent ingestion of a substance (Criterion A). The clinically significant problematic behavioral or psychological changes associated with intoxication (e.g., belligerence, mood lability, impaired judgment) are attributable to the physiological effects of the substance on the central nervous system and develop during or shortly after use of the substance (Criterion B). The symptoms are not attributable to another medical condition and are not better explained by another mental disorder (Criterion D). Substance intoxication is common among those with a substance use disorder but also occurs frequently in individuals without a substance use disorder. This category does *not* apply to tobacco.

The most common changes in intoxication involve disturbances of perception, wakefulness, attention, thinking, judgment, psychomotor behavior, and interpersonal behavior. Short-term, or "acute," intoxications may have different signs and symptoms than sustained, or "chronic," intoxications. For example, moderate cocaine doses may initially produce gregariousness, but social withdrawal may develop if such doses are frequently repeated over days or weeks.

When used in the physiological sense, the term *intoxication* is broader than substance intoxication as defined here. Many substances may produce physiological or psychological changes that are not necessarily problematic. For example, an individual with tachycardia from substance use has a physiological effect, but if this is the only symptom in the absence of problematic behavior, the diagnosis of intoxication would not apply. Intoxication may sometimes persist beyond the time when the substance is detectable in the body. This may be due to enduring central nervous system effects, the recovery of which takes longer than the time for elimination of the substance. These longer-term effects of intoxication must be distinguished from withdrawal (i.e., symptoms initiated by a decline in blood or tissue concentrations of a substance).

Criteria for substance withdrawal are included within the substance-specific sections of this chapter. The essential feature is the development of a substance-specific problematic behavioral change, with physiological and cognitive concomitants, that is due to the cessation of, or reduction in, heavy and prolonged substance use (Criterion A). The substance-specific syndrome causes clinically significant distress or impairment in social, occupational, or other important areas of functioning (Criterion C). The symptoms are not due to another medical condition and are not better explained by another mental disorder (Criterion D). Withdrawal is usually, but not always, associated with a substance use disorder. Most individuals with withdrawal have an urge to re-administer the substance to reduce the symptoms.

Route of Administration and Speed of Substance Effects

Routes of administration that produce more rapid and efficient absorption into the bloodstream (e.g., intravenous, smoking, intranasal "snorting") tend to result in a more intense intoxication and an increased likelihood of an escalating pattern of substance use leading to withdrawal. Similarly, rapidly acting substances are more likely than slower-acting substances to produce immediate intoxication.

Duration of Effects

Within the same drug category, relatively short-acting substances tend to have a higher potential for the development of withdrawal than do those with a longer duration of action. However, longer-acting substances tend to have longer withdrawal duration. The half-life of the substance parallels aspects of withdrawal: the longer the duration of action, the longer the time between cessation and the onset of withdrawal symptoms and the longer the withdrawal duration. In general, the longer the acute withdrawal period, the less intense the syndrome tends to be.

Use of Multiple Substances

Substance intoxication and withdrawal often involve several substances used simultaneously or sequentially. In these cases, each diagnosis should be recorded separately.

Associated Laboratory Findings

Laboratory analyses of blood and urine samples can help determine recent use and the specific substances involved. However, a positive laboratory test result does not by itself indicate that the individual has a pattern of substance use that meets criteria for a substance-induced or substance use disorder, and a negative test result does not by itself rule out a diagnosis.

Laboratory tests can be useful in identifying withdrawal. If the individual presents with withdrawal from an unknown substance, laboratory tests may help identify the substance and may also be helpful in differentiating withdrawal from other mental disorders.

In addition, normal functioning in the presence of high blood levels of a substance suggests considerable tolerance.

Development and Course

Individuals ages 18–24 years have relatively high prevalence rates for the use of virtually every substance. Intoxication is usually the initial substance-related disorder and often begins in the teens. Withdrawal can occur at any age as long as the relevant drug has been taken in sufficient doses over an extended period of time.

Recording Procedures for Intoxication and Withdrawal

The clinician should use the code that applies to the class of substances but record the name of the *specific substance.* For example, the clinician should record 292.0 (F13.239) secobarbital withdrawal (rather than sedative, hypnotic, or anxiolytic withdrawal) or 292.89 (F15.129) methamphetamine intoxication (rather than stimulant intoxication). Note that the appropriate ICD-10-CM diagnostic code for intoxication depends on whether there is a comorbid substance use disorder. In this case, the F15.129 code for methamphetamine indicates the presence of a comorbid mild methamphetamine use disorder. If there had been no comorbid methamphetamine use disorder, the diagnostic code would have been F15.929. ICD-10-CM coding rules require that all withdrawal codes imply a comorbid moderate to severe substance use disorder for that substance. In the above case, the code for secobarbital withdrawal (F13.239) indicates the comorbid presence of a moderate to severe secobarbital use disorder. See the coding note for the substance-specific intoxication and withdrawal syndromes for the actual coding options.

For substances that do not fit into any of the classes (e.g., anabolic steroids), the appropriate code for "other substance intoxication" should be used and the specific substance indicated (e.g., 292.89 [F19.929] anabolic steroid intoxication). If the substance taken by the individual is unknown, the code for the class "other (or unknown)" should be used (e.g., 292.89 [F19.929] unknown substance intoxication). If there are symptoms or problems associated with a particular substance but criteria are not met for any of the substance-specific disorders, the unspecified category can be used (e.g., 292.9 [F12.99] unspecified cannabis-related disorder).

As noted above, the substance-related codes in ICD-10-CM combine the substance use disorder aspect of the clinical picture and the substance-induced aspect into a single combined code. Thus, if both heroin withdrawal and moderate heroin use disorder are present, the single code F11.23 is given to cover both presentations. In ICD-9-CM, separate diagnostic codes (292.0 and 304.00) are given to indicate withdrawal and a moderate heroin use disorder, respectively. See the individual substance-specific sections for additional coding information.

Substance/Medication-Induced Mental Disorders

The substance/medication-induced mental disorders are potentially severe, usually temporary, but sometimes persisting central nervous system (CNS) syndromes that develop in the context of the effects of substances of abuse, medications, or several toxins. They are distinguished from the substance use disorders, in which a cluster of cognitive, behavioral, and physiological symptoms contribute to the continued use of a substance despite significant substance-related problems. The substance/medication-induced mental disorders may be induced by the 10 classes of substances that produce substance use disorders, or by a great variety of other medications used in medical treatment. Each substance-induced mental disorder is described in the relevant chapter (e.g., "Depressive Disorders," "Neurocognitive Disorders"), and therefore, only a brief description is offered here. All substance/medication-induced disorders share common characteristics. It is important to recognize these common features to aid in the detection of these disorders. These features are described as follows:

A. The disorder represents a clinically significant symptomatic presentation of a relevant mental disorder.
B. There is evidence from the history, physical examination, or laboratory findings of both of the following:
   1. The disorder developed during or within 1 month of a substance intoxication or withdrawal or taking a medication; and
   2. The involved substance/medication is capable of producing the mental disorder.
C. The disorder is not better explained by an independent mental disorder (i.e., one that is not substance- or medication-induced). Such evidence of an independent mental disorder could include the following:
   1. The disorder preceded the onset of severe intoxication or withdrawal or exposure to the medication; or
   2. The full mental disorder persisted for a substantial period of time (e.g., at least 1 month) after the cessation of acute withdrawal or severe intoxication or taking the medication. This criterion does not apply to substance-induced neurocognitive disorders or hallucinogen persisting perception disorder, which persist beyond the cessation of acute intoxication or withdrawal.
D. The disorder does not occur exclusively during the course of a delirium.
E. The disorder causes clinically significant distress or impairment in social, occupational, or other important areas of functioning.

Features

Some generalizations can be made regarding the categories of substances capable of producing clinically relevant substance-induced mental disorders. In general, the more sedating drugs (sedative, hypnotics, or anxiolytics, and alcohol) can produce prominent and clinically significant depressive disorders during intoxication, while anxiety conditions are likely to be observed during withdrawal syndromes from these substances. Also, during intoxication, the more stimulating substances (e.g., amphetamines and cocaine) are likely to be associated with substance-induced psychotic disorders and substance-induced anxiety disorders, with substance-induced major depressive episodes observed during withdrawal. Both the more sedating and more stimulating drugs are likely to produce significant but temporary sleep and sexual disturbances. An overview of the relationship between specific categories of substances and specific psychiatric syndromes is presented in Table 1.

The medication-induced conditions include what are often idiosyncratic CNS reactions or relatively extreme examples of side effects for a wide range of medications taken for a variety of medical concerns. These include neurocognitive complications of anesthetics, antihistamines, antihypertensives, and a variety of other medications and toxins (e.g., organophosphates, insecticides, carbon monoxide), as described in the chapter on neurocognitive disorders. Psychotic syndromes may be temporarily experienced in the context of anticholinergic, cardiovascular, and steroid drugs, as well as during use of stimulant-like and depressant-like prescription or over-the-counter drugs. Temporary but severe mood disturbances can be observed with a wide range of medications, including steroids, antihypertensives, disulfiram, and any prescription or over-the-counter depressant or stimulant-like substances. A similar range of medications can be associated with temporary anxiety syndromes, sexual dysfunctions, and conditions of disturbed sleep.

In general, to be considered a substance/medication-induced mental disorder, there must be evidence that the disorder being observed is not likely to be better explained by an independent mental condition. The latter are most likely to be seen if the mental disorder was present before the severe intoxication or withdrawal or medication administration, or, with the exception of several substance-induced persisting disorders listed in Table 1, continued more than 1 month after cessation of acute withdrawal, severe intoxication, or use of the medications. When symptoms are only observed during a delirium (e.g., alcohol withdrawal delirium), the mental disorder should be diagnosed as a delirium, and the psychiatric syndrome occurring during the delirium should not also be diagnosed separately, as many symptoms (including disturbances in mood, anxiety, and reality testing) are commonly seen during agitated, confused states. The features associated with each relevant major mental disorder are similar whether observed with independent or substance/medication-induced mental disorders. However, individuals with substance/medication-induced mental disorders are likely to also demonstrate the associated features seen with the specific category of substance or medication, as listed in other subsections of this chapter.

Development and Course

Substance-induced mental disorders develop in the context of intoxication or withdrawal from substances of abuse, and medication-induced mental disorders are seen with prescribed or over-the-counter medications that are taken at the suggested doses. Both conditions are usually temporary and likely to disappear within 1 month or so of cessation of acute withdrawal, severe intoxication, or use of the medication. Exceptions to these generalizations occur for certain long-duration substance-induced disorders: substance-associated neurocognitive disorders that relate to conditions such as alcohol-induced neurocognitive disorder, inhalant-induced neurocognitive disorder, and sedative-, hypnotic-, or anxiolytic-induced neurocognitive disorder; and hallucinogen persisting perception disorder ("flashbacks"; see the section "Hallucinogen-Related Disorders" later in this chapter). However, most other substance/medication-induced mental disorders, regardless of the severity of the symptoms, are likely to improve relatively quickly with abstinence and unlikely to remain clinically relevant for more than 1 month after complete cessation of use.

As is true of many consequences of heavy substance use, some individuals are more and others less prone toward specific substance-induced disorders. Similar types of predispositions may make some individuals more likely to develop psychiatric side effects of some types of medications, but not others. However, it is unclear whether individuals with family histories or personal prior histories with independent psychiatric syndromes are more likely to develop the induced syndrome once the consideration is made as to whether the quantity and frequency of the substance was sufficient to lead to the development of a substance-induced syndrome.

There are indications that the intake of substances of abuse or some medications with psychiatric side effects in the context of a preexisting mental disorder is likely to result in an intensification of the preexisting independent syndrome. The risk for substance/medication-induced mental disorders is likely to increase with both the quantity and the frequency of consumption of the relevant substance.

The symptom profiles for the substance/medication-induced mental disorders resemble independent mental disorders. While the symptoms of substance/medication-induced mental disorders can be identical to those of independent mental disorders (e.g., delusions, hallucinations, psychoses, major depressive episodes, anxiety syndromes), and although they can have the same severe consequences (e.g., suicide), most induced mental disorders are likely to improve in a matter of days to weeks of abstinence.

The substance/medication-induced mental disorders are an important part of the differential diagnoses for the independent psychiatric conditions. The importance of recognizing an induced mental disorder is similar to the relevance of identifying the possible role of some medical conditions and medication reactions before diagnosing an independent mental disorder. Symptoms of substance- and medication-induced mental disorders may be identical cross-sectionally to those of independent mental disorders but have different treatments and prognoses from the independent condition.

Functional Consequences of Substance/Medication-Induced Mental Disorders

The same consequences related to the relevant independent mental disorder (e.g., suicide attempts) are likely to apply to the substance/medication-induced mental disorders, but these are likely to disappear within 1 month after abstinence. Similarly, the same functional consequences associated with the relevant substance use disorder are likely to be seen for the substance-induced mental disorders.

Recording Procedures for Substance/Medication-Induced Mental Disorders

Coding notes and separate recording procedures for ICD-9-CM and ICD-10-CM codes for other specific substance/medication-induced mental disorders are provided in other chapters of the manual with disorders with which they share phenomenology (see the substance/medication-induced mental disorders in these chapters: "Schizophrenia Spectrum and Other Psychotic Disorders," "Bipolar and Related Disorders," "Depressive Disorders," "Anxiety Disorders," "Obsessive-Compulsive and Related Disorders," "Sleep-Wake Disorders," "Sexual Dysfunctions," and "Neurocognitive Disorders"). Generally, for ICD-9-CM, if a mental disorder is induced by a substance use disorder, a separate diagnostic code is given for the specific substance use disorder, in addition to the code for the substance/medication-induced mental disorder. For ICD-10-CM, a single code combines the substance-induced mental disorder with the substance use disorder. A separate diagnosis of the comorbid substance use disorder is not given, although the name and severity of the specific substance use disorder (when present) are used when recording the substance/medication-induced mental disorder. ICD-10-CM codes are also provided for situations in which the substance/medication-induced mental disorder is not induced by a substance use disorder (e.g., when a disorder is induced by one-time use of a substance or medication). Additional information needed to record the diagnostic name of the substance/medication-induced mental disorder is provided in the section "Recording Procedures" for each substance/medication-induced mental disorder in its respective chapter.

Alcohol-Related Disorders

Alcohol Use Disorder
Alcohol Intoxication
Alcohol Withdrawal
Other Alcohol-Induced Disorders
Unspecified Alcohol-Related Disorder

Alcohol Use Disorder

Diagnostic Criteria

A. A problematic pattern of alcohol use leading to clinically significant impairment or distress, as manifested by at least two of the following, occurring within a 12-month period:

1. Alcohol is often taken in larger amounts or over a longer period than was intended.
2. There is a persistent desire or unsuccessful efforts to cut down or control alcohol use.

3. A great deal of time is spent in activities necessary to obtain alcohol, use alcohol, or recover from its effects.
4. Craving, or a strong desire or urge to use alcohol.
5. Recurrent alcohol use resulting in a failure to fulfill major role obligations at work, school, or home.
6. Continued alcohol use despite having persistent or recurrent social or interpersonal problems caused or exacerbated by the effects of alcohol.
7. Important social, occupational, or recreational activities are given up or reduced because of alcohol use.
8. Recurrent alcohol use in situations in which it is physically hazardous.
9. Alcohol use is continued despite knowledge of having a persistent or recurrent physical or psychological problem that is likely to have been caused or exacerbated by alcohol.
10. Tolerance, as defined by either of the following:
    a. A need for markedly increased amounts of alcohol to achieve intoxication or desired effect.
    b. A markedly diminished effect with continued use of the same amount of alcohol.
11. Withdrawal, as manifested by either of the following:
    a. The characteristic withdrawal syndrome for alcohol (refer to Criteria A and B of the criteria set for alcohol withdrawal, pp. 499–500).
    b. Alcohol (or a closely related substance, such as a benzodiazepine) is taken to relieve or avoid withdrawal symptoms.

Specify if:

In early remission: After full criteria for alcohol use disorder were previously met, none of the criteria for alcohol use disorder have been met for at least 3 months but for less than 12 months (with the exception that Criterion A4, "Craving, or a strong desire or urge to use alcohol," may be met).

In sustained remission: After full criteria for alcohol use disorder were previously met, none of the criteria for alcohol use disorder have been met at any time during a period of 12 months or longer (with the exception that Criterion A4, "Craving, or a strong desire or urge to use alcohol," may be met).

Specify if:

In a controlled environment: This additional specifier is used if the individual is in an environment where access to alcohol is restricted.

Code based on current severity: Note for ICD-10-CM codes: If an alcohol intoxication, alcohol withdrawal, or another alcohol-induced mental disorder is also present, do not use the codes below for alcohol use disorder. Instead, the comorbid alcohol use disorder is indicated in the 4th character of the alcohol-induced disorder code (see the coding note for alcohol intoxication, alcohol withdrawal, or a specific alcohol-induced mental disorder). For example, if there is comorbid alcohol intoxication and alcohol use disorder, only the alcohol intoxication code is given, with the 4th character indicating whether the comorbid alcohol use disorder is mild, moderate, or severe: F10.129 for mild alcohol use disorder with alcohol intoxication or F10.229 for a moderate or severe alcohol use disorder with alcohol intoxication.

Specify current severity:

305.00 (F10.10) Mild: Presence of 2–3 symptoms.

303.90 (F10.20) Moderate: Presence of 4–5 symptoms.

303.90 (F10.20) Severe: Presence of 6 or more symptoms.

Specifiers

"In a controlled environment" applies as a further specifier of remission if the individual is both in remission and in a controlled environment (i.e., in early remission in a controlled environment or in sustained remission in a controlled environment). Examples of these environments are closely supervised and substance-free jails, therapeutic communities, and locked hospital units.

Severity of the disorder is based on the number of diagnostic criteria endorsed. For a given individual, changes in severity of alcohol use disorder across time are also reflected by reductions in the frequency (e.g., days of use per month) and/or dose (e.g., number of standard drinks consumed per day) of alcohol used, as assessed by the individual's self-report, report of knowledgeable others, clinician observations, and, when practical, biological testing (e.g., elevations in blood tests as described in the section "Diagnostic Markers" for this disorder).

Diagnostic Features

Alcohol use disorder is defined by a cluster of behavioral and physical symptoms, which can include withdrawal, tolerance, and craving. Alcohol withdrawal is characterized by withdrawal symptoms that develop approximately 4–12 hours after the reduction of intake following prolonged, heavy alcohol ingestion. Because withdrawal from alcohol can be unpleasant and intense, individuals may continue to consume alcohol despite adverse consequences, often to avoid or to relieve withdrawal symptoms. Some withdrawal symptoms (e.g., sleep problems) can persist at lower intensities for months and can contribute to relapse. Once a pattern of repetitive and intense use develops, individuals with alcohol use disorder may devote substantial periods of time to obtaining and consuming alcoholic beverages.

Craving for alcohol is indicated by a strong desire to drink that makes it difficult to think of anything else and that often results in the onset of drinking. School and job performance may also suffer either from the aftereffects of drinking or from actual intoxication at school or on the job; child care or household responsibilities may be neglected; and alcohol-related absences may occur from school or work. The individual may use alcohol in physically hazardous circumstances (e.g., driving an automobile, swimming, operating machinery while intoxicated). Finally, individuals with an alcohol use disorder may continue to consume alcohol despite the knowledge that continued consumption poses significant physical (e.g., blackouts, liver disease), psychological (e.g., depression), social, or interpersonal problems (e.g., violent arguments with spouse while intoxicated, child abuse).

Associated Features Supporting Diagnosis

Alcohol use disorder is often associated with problems similar to those associated with other substances (e.g., cannabis; cocaine; heroin; amphetamines; sedatives, hypnotics, or anxiolytics). Alcohol may be used to alleviate the unwanted effects of these other substances or to substitute for them when they are not available. Symptoms of conduct problems, depression, anxiety, and insomnia frequently accompany heavy drinking and sometimes precede it.

Repeated intake of high doses of alcohol can affect nearly every organ system, especially the gastrointestinal tract, cardiovascular system, and the central and peripheral nervous systems. Gastrointestinal effects include gastritis, stomach or duodenal ulcers, and, in about 15% of individuals who use alcohol heavily, liver cirrhosis and/or pancreatitis. There is also an increased rate of cancer of the esophagus, stomach, and other parts of the gastrointestinal tract. One of the most commonly associated conditions is low-grade hypertension. Cardiomyopathy and other myopathies are less common but occur at an increased rate among those who drink very heavily. These factors, along with marked increases in levels of triglycerides and low-density lipoprotein cholesterol, contribute to an elevated risk of heart disease. Peripheral neuropathy may be evidenced by muscular weakness, paresthesias, and decreased peripheral sensation. More persistent central nervous system effects include cognitive deficits, severe memory impairment, and degenerative changes in the cerebellum. These effects are related to the direct effects of alcohol or of trauma and to vitamin deficiencies (particularly of the B vitamins, including thiamine). One devastating central nervous system effect is the relatively rare alcohol-induced persisting amnestic disorder, or Wernicke-Korsakoff syndrome, in which the ability to encode new memory is severely impaired. This condition would now be described within the chapter "Neurocognitive Disorders" and would be termed a *substance/medication-induced neurocognitive disorder.*

Alcohol use disorder is an important contributor to suicide risk during severe intoxication and in the context of a temporary alcohol-induced depressive and bipolar disorder. There is an increased rate of suicidal behavior as well as of completed suicide among individuals with the disorder.

Prevalence

Alcohol use disorder is a common disorder. In the United States, the 12-month prevalence of alcohol use disorder is estimated to be 4.6% among 12- to 17-year-olds and 8.5% among adults age 18 years and older in the United States. Rates of the disorder are greater among adult men (12.4%) than among adult women (4.9%). Twelve-month prevalence of alcohol use disorder among adults decreases in middle age, being greatest among individuals 18- to 29-years-old (16.2%) and lowest among individuals age 65 years and older (1.5%).

Twelve-month prevalence varies markedly across race/ethnic subgroups of the U.S. population. For 12- to 17-year-olds, rates are greatest among Hispanics (6.0%) and Native Americans and Alaska Natives (5.7%) relative to whites (5.0%), African Americans (1.8%), and Asian Americans and Pacific Islanders (1.6%). In contrast, among adults, the 12-month prevalence of alcohol use disorder is clearly greater among Native Americans and Alaska Natives (12.1%) than among whites (8.9%), Hispanics (7.9%), African Americans (6.9%), and Asian Americans and Pacific Islanders (4.5%).

Development and Course

The first episode of alcohol intoxication is likely to occur during the mid-teens. Alcohol-related problems that do not meet full criteria for a use disorder or isolated problems may occur prior to age 20 years, but the age at onset of an alcohol use disorder with two or more of the criteria clustered together peaks in the late teens or early to mid 20s. The large majority of individuals who develop alcohol-related disorders do so by their late 30s. The first evidence of withdrawal is not likely to appear until after many other aspects of an alcohol use disorder have developed. An earlier onset of alcohol use disorder is observed in adolescents with preexisting conduct problems and those with an earlier onset of intoxication.

Alcohol use disorder has a variable course that is characterized by periods of remission and relapse. A decision to stop drinking, often in response to a crisis, is likely to be followed by a period of weeks or more of abstinence, which is often followed by limited periods of controlled or nonproblematic drinking. However, once alcohol intake resumes, it is highly likely that consumption will rapidly escalate and that severe problems will once again develop.

Alcohol use disorder is often erroneously perceived as an intractable condition, perhaps based on the fact that individuals who present for treatment typically have a history of many years of severe alcohol-related problems. However, these most severe cases represent only a small proportion of individuals with this disorder, and the typical individual with the disorder has a much more promising prognosis.

Among adolescents, conduct disorder and repeated antisocial behavior often co-occur with alcohol- and with other substance-related disorders. While most individuals with alcohol use disorder develop the condition before age 40 years, perhaps 10% have later onset. Age-related physical changes in older individuals result in increased brain susceptibility to the depressant effects of alcohol; decreased rates of liver metabolism of a variety of substances, including alcohol; and decreased percentages of body water. These changes can cause older people to develop more severe intoxication and subsequent problems at lower levels of consumption. Alcohol-related problems in older people are also especially likely to be associated with other medical complications.

Risk and Prognostic Factors

Environmental.   Environmental risk and prognostic factors may include cultural attitudes toward drinking and intoxication, the availability of alcohol (including price), acquired personal experiences with alcohol, and stress levels. Additional potential mediators of how alcohol problems develop in predisposed individuals include heavier peer substance use, exaggerated positive expectations of the effects of alcohol, and suboptimal ways of coping with stress.

Genetic and physiological.   Alcohol use disorder runs in families, with 40%–60% of the variance of risk explained by genetic influences. The rate of this condition is three to four times higher in close relatives of individuals with alcohol use disorder, with values highest for individuals with a greater number of affected relatives, closer genetic relationships to the affected person, and higher severity of the alcohol-related problems in those relatives. A significantly higher rate of alcohol use disorders exists in the monozygotic twin than in the dizygotic twin of an individual with the condition. A three- to fourfold increase in risk has been observed in children of individuals with alcohol use disorder, even when these children were given up for adoption at birth and raised by adoptive parents who did not have the disorder.

Recent advances in our understanding of genes that operate through intermediate characteristics (or phenotypes) to affect the risk of alcohol use disorder can help to identify individuals who might be at particularly low or high risk for alcohol use disorder. Among the low-risk phenotypes are the acute alcohol-related skin flush (seen most prominently in Asians). High vulnerability is associated with preexisting schizophrenia or bipolar disorder, as well as impulsivity (producing enhanced rates of all substance use disorders and gambling disorder), and a high risk specifically for alcohol use disorder is associated with a low level of response (low sensitivity) to alcohol. A number of gene variations may account for low response to alcohol or modulate the dopamine reward systems; it is important to note, however, that any one gene variation is likely to explain only 1%–2% of the risk for these disorders.

Course modifiers.   In general, high levels of impulsivity are associated with an earlier onset and more severe alcohol use disorder.

Culture-Related Diagnostic Issues

In most cultures, alcohol is the most frequently used intoxicating substance and contributes to considerable morbidity and mortality. An estimated 3.8% of all global deaths and 4.6% of global disability-adjusted life-years are attributable to alcohol. In the United States, 80% of adults (age 18 years and older) have consumed alcohol at some time in their lives, and 65% are current drinkers (last 12 months). An estimated 3.6% of the world population (15–64 years old) has a current (12-month) alcohol use disorder, with a lower prevalence (1.1%) found in the African region, a higher rate (5.2%) found in the American region (North, South, and Central America and the Caribbean), and the highest rate (10.9%) found in the Eastern Europe region.

Polymorphisms of genes for the alcohol-metabolizing enzymes alcohol dehydrogenase and aldehyde dehydrogenase are most often seen in Asians and affect the response to alcohol. When consuming alcohol, individuals with these gene variations can experience a flushed face and palpitations, reactions that can be so severe as to limit or preclude future alcohol consumption and diminish the risk for alcohol use disorder. These gene variations are seen in as many as 40% of Japanese, Chinese, Korean, and related groups worldwide and are related to lower risks for the disorder.

Despite small variations regarding individual criterion items, the diagnostic criteria perform equally well across most race/ethnicity groups.

Gender-Related Diagnostic Issues

Males have higher rates of drinking and related disorders than females. However, because females generally weigh less than males, have more fat and less water in their bodies, and metabolize less alcohol in their esophagus and stomach, they are likely to develop higher blood alcohol levels per drink than males. Females who drink heavily may also be more vulnerable than males to some of the physical consequences associated with alcohol, including liver disease.

Diagnostic Markers

Individuals whose heavier drinking places them at elevated risk for alcohol use disorder can be identified both through standardized questionnaires and by elevations in blood test results likely to be seen with regular heavier drinking. These measures do not establish a diagnosis of an alcohol-related disorder but can be useful in highlighting individuals for whom more information should be gathered. The most direct test available to measure alcohol consumption cross-sectionally is *blood alcohol concentration*, which can also be used to judge tolerance to alcohol. For example, an individual with a concentration of 150 mg of ethanol per deciliter (dL) of blood who does not show signs of intoxication can be presumed to have acquired at least some degree of tolerance to alcohol. At 200 mg/dL, most nontolerant individuals demonstrate severe intoxication.

Regarding laboratory tests, one sensitive laboratory indicator of heavy drinking is a modest elevation or high-normal levels (>35 units) of gamma-glutamyltransferase (GGT). This may be the only laboratory finding. At least 70% of individuals with a high GGT level are persistent heavy drinkers (i.e., consuming eight or more drinks daily on a regular basis). A second test with comparable or even higher levels of sensitivity and specificity is carbohydrate-deficient transferrin (CDT), with levels of 20 units or higher useful in identifying individuals who regularly consume eight or more drinks daily. Since both GGT and CDT levels return toward normal within days to weeks of stopping drinking, both state markers may be useful in monitoring abstinence, especially when the clinician observes increases, rather than decreases, in these values over time—a finding indicating that the person is likely to have returned to heavy drinking. The combination of tests for CDT and GGT may have even higher levels of sensitivity and specificity than either test used alone. Additional useful tests include the mean corpuscular volume (MCV), which may be elevated to high-normal values in individuals who drink heavily—a change that is due to the direct toxic effects of alcohol on erythropoiesis. Although the MCV can be used to help identify those who drink heavily, it is a poor method of monitoring abstinence because of the long half-life of red blood cells. Liver function tests (e.g., alanine aminotransferase [ALT] and alkaline phosphatase) can reveal liver injury that is a consequence of heavy drinking. Other potential markers of heavy drinking that are more nonspecific for alcohol but can help the clinician think of the possible effects of alcohol include elevations in blood levels or lipids (e.g., triglycerides and high-density lipoprotein cholesterol) and high-normal levels of uric acid.

Additional diagnostic markers relate to signs and symptoms that reflect the consequences often associated with persistent heavy drinking. For example, dyspepsia, nausea, and bloating can accompany gastritis, and hepatomegaly, esophageal varices, and hemorrhoids may reflect alcohol-induced changes in the liver. Other physical signs of heavy drinking include tremor, unsteady gait, insomnia, and erectile dysfunction. Males with chronic alcohol use disorder may exhibit decreased testicular size and feminizing effects associated with reduced testosterone levels. Repeated heavy drinking in females is associated with menstrual irregularities and, during pregnancy, spontaneous abortion and fetal alcohol syndrome. Individuals with preexisting histories of epilepsy or severe head trauma are more likely to develop alcohol-related seizures. Alcohol withdrawal may be associated with nausea, vomiting, gastritis, hematemesis, dry mouth, puffy blotchy complexion, and mild peripheral edema.

Functional Consequences of Alcohol Use Disorder

The diagnostic features of alcohol use disorder highlight major areas of life functioning likely to be impaired. These include driving and operating machinery, school and work, interpersonal relationships and communication, and health. Alcohol-related disorders contribute to absenteeism from work, job-related accidents, and low employee productivity. Rates are elevated in homeless individuals, perhaps reflecting a downward spiral in social and occupational functioning, although most individuals with alcohol use disorder continue to live with their families and function within their jobs.

Alcohol use disorder is associated with a significant increase in the risk of accidents, violence, and suicide. It is estimated that one in five intensive care unit admissions in some urban hospitals is related to alcohol and that 40% of individuals in the United States experience an alcohol-related adverse event at some time in their lives, with alcohol accounting for up to 55% of fatal driving events. Severe alcohol use disorder, especially in individuals with antisocial personality disorder, is associated with the commission of criminal acts, including homicide. Severe problematic alcohol use also contributes to disinhibition and feelings of sadness and irritability, which contribute to suicide attempts and completed suicides.

Unanticipated alcohol withdrawal in hospitalized individuals for whom a diagnosis of alcohol use disorder has been overlooked can add to the risks and costs of hospitalization and to time spent in the hospital.

Differential Diagnosis

Nonpathological use of alcohol.   The key element of alcohol use disorder is the use of heavy doses of alcohol with resulting repeated and significant distress or impaired functioning. While most drinkers sometimes consume enough alcohol to feel intoxicated, only a minority (less than 20%) ever develop alcohol use disorder. Therefore, drinking, even daily, in low doses and occasional intoxication do not by themselves make this diagnosis.

Sedative, hypnotic, or anxiolytic use disorder.   The signs and symptoms of alcohol use disorder are similar to those seen in sedative, hypnotic, or anxiolytic use disorder. The two must be distinguished, however, because the course may be different, especially in relation to medical problems.

Conduct disorder in childhood and adult antisocial personality disorder.   Alcohol use disorder, along with other substance use disorders, is seen in the majority of individuals with antisocial personality and preexisting conduct disorder. Because these diagnoses are associated with an early onset of alcohol use disorder as well as a worse prognosis, it is important to establish both conditions.

Comorbidity

Bipolar disorders, schizophrenia, and antisocial personality disorder are associated with a markedly increased rate of alcohol use disorder, and several anxiety and depressive disorders may relate to alcohol use disorder as well. At least a part of the reported association between depression and moderate to severe alcohol use disorder may be attributable to temporary, alcohol-induced comorbid depressive symptoms resulting from the acute effects of intoxication or withdrawal. Severe, repeated alcohol intoxication may also suppress immune mechanisms and predispose individuals to infections and increase the risk for cancers.

Alcohol Intoxication

Diagnostic Criteria

A. Recent ingestion of alcohol.
B. Clinically significant problematic behavioral or psychological changes (e.g., inappropriate sexual or aggressive behavior, mood lability, impaired judgment) that developed during, or shortly after, alcohol ingestion.
C. One (or more) of the following signs or symptoms developing during, or shortly after, alcohol use:
   1. Slurred speech.
   2. Incoordination.
   3. Unsteady gait.
   4. Nystagmus.
   5. Impairment in attention or memory.
   6. Stupor or coma.
D. The signs or symptoms are not attributable to another medical condition and are not better explained by another mental disorder, including intoxication with another substance.

Coding note: The ICD-9-CM code is **303.00.** The ICD-10-CM code depends on whether there is a comorbid alcohol use disorder. If a mild alcohol use disorder is comorbid, the ICD-10-CM code is **F10.129,** and if a moderate or severe alcohol use disorder is comorbid, the ICD-10-CM code is **F10.229.** If there is no comorbid alcohol use disorder, then the ICD-10-CM code is **F10.929.**

Diagnostic Features

The essential feature of alcohol intoxication is the presence of clinically significant problematic behavioral or psychological changes (e.g., inappropriate sexual or aggressive behavior, mood lability, impaired judgment, impaired social or occupational functioning) that develop during, or shortly after, alcohol ingestion (Criterion B). These changes are accompanied by evidence of impaired functioning and judgment and, if intoxication is intense, can result in a life-threatening coma. The symptoms must not be attributable to another medical condition (e.g., diabetic ketoacidosis), are not a reflection of conditions such as delirium, and are not related to intoxication with other depressant drugs (e.g., benzodiazepines) (Criterion D). The levels of incoordination can interfere with driving abilities and performance of usual activities to the point of causing accidents. Evidence of alcohol use can be obtained by smelling alcohol on the individual's breath, eliciting a history from the individual or another observer, and, when needed, having the individual provide breath, blood, or urine samples for toxicology analyses.

Associated Features Supporting Diagnosis

Alcohol intoxication is sometimes associated with amnesia for the events that occurred during the course of the intoxication ("blackouts"). This phenomenon may be related to the presence of a high blood alcohol level and, perhaps, to the rapidity with which this level is reached. During even mild alcohol intoxication, different symptoms are likely to be observed at different time points. Evidence of mild intoxication with alcohol can be seen in most individuals after approximately two drinks (each standard drink is approximately 10–12 grams of ethanol and raises the blood alcohol concentration approximately 20 mg/dL). Early in the drinking period, when blood alcohol levels are rising, symptoms often include talkativeness, a sensation of well-being, and a bright, expansive mood. Later, especially when blood alcohol levels are falling, the individual is likely to become progressively more depressed, withdrawn, and cognitively impaired. At very high blood alcohol levels (e.g., 200–300 mg/dL), an individual who has not developed tolerance for alcohol is likely to fall asleep and enter a first stage of anesthesia. Higher blood alcohol levels (e.g., in excess of 300–400 mg/dL) can cause inhibition of respiration and pulse and even death in nontolerant individuals. The duration of intoxication depends on how much alcohol was consumed over what period of time. In general, the body is able to metabolize approximately one drink per hour, so that the blood alcohol level generally decreases at a rate of 15–20 mg/dL per hour. Signs and symptoms of intoxication are likely to be more intense when the blood alcohol level is rising than when it is falling.

Alcohol intoxication is an important contributor to suicidal behavior. There appears to be an increased rate of suicidal behavior, as well as of completed suicide, among persons intoxicated by alcohol.

Prevalence

The large majority of alcohol consumers are likely to have been intoxicated to some degree at some point in their lives. For example, in 2010, 44% of 12th-grade students admitted to having been "drunk in the past year," with more than 70% of college students reporting the same.

Development and Course

Intoxication usually occurs as an episode usually developing over minutes to hours and typically lasting several hours. In the United States, the average age at first intoxication is approximately 15 years, with the highest prevalence at approximately 18–25 years. Frequency and intensity usually decrease with further advancing age. The earlier the onset of regular intoxication, the greater the likelihood the individual will go on to develop alcohol use disorder.

Risk and Prognostic Factors

Temperamental.   Episodes of alcohol intoxication increase with personality characteristics of sensation seeking and impulsivity.

Environmental.   Episodes of alcohol intoxication increase with a heavy drinking environment.

Culture-Related Diagnostic Issues

The major issues parallel the cultural differences regarding the use of alcohol overall. Thus, college fraternities and sororities may encourage alcohol intoxication. This condition is also frequent on certain dates of cultural significance (e.g., New Year's Eve) and, for some subgroups, during specific events (e.g., wakes following funerals). Other subgroups encourage drinking at religious celebrations (e.g., Jewish and Catholic holidays), while still others strongly discourage all drinking or intoxication (e.g., some religious groups, such as Mormons, fundamentalist Christians, and Muslims).

Gender-Related Diagnostic Issues

Historically, in many Western societies, acceptance of drinking and drunkenness is more tolerated for males, but such gender differences may be much less prominent in recent years, especially during adolescence and young adulthood.

Diagnostic Markers

Intoxication is usually established by observing an individual's behavior and smelling alcohol on the breath. The degree of intoxication increases with an individual's blood or breath alcohol level and with the ingestion of other substances, especially those with sedating effects.

Functional Consequences of Alcohol Intoxication

Alcohol intoxication contributes to the more than 30,000 alcohol-related drinking deaths in the United States each year. In addition, intoxication with this drug contributes to huge costs associated with drunk driving, lost time from school or work, as well as interpersonal arguments and physical fights.

Differential Diagnosis

Other medical conditions. Several medical (e.g., diabetic acidosis) and neurological conditions (e.g., cerebellar ataxia, multiple sclerosis) can temporarily resemble alcohol intoxication.

Sedative, hypnotic, or anxiolytic intoxication. Intoxication with sedative, hypnotic, or anxiolytic drugs or with other sedating substances (e.g., antihistamines, anticholinergic drugs) can be mistaken for alcohol intoxication. The differential requires observing alcohol on the breath, measuring blood or breath alcohol levels, ordering a medical workup, and gathering a good history. The signs and symptoms of sedative-hypnotic intoxication are very similar to those observed with alcohol and include similar problematic behavioral or psychological changes. These changes are accompanied by evidence of impaired functioning and judgment—which, if intense, can result in a life-threatening coma—and levels of incoordination that can interfere with driving abilities and with performing usual activities. However, there is no smell as there is with alcohol, but there is likely to be evidence of misuse of the depressant drug in the blood or urine toxicology analyses.

Comorbidity

Alcohol intoxication may occur comorbidly with other substance intoxication, especially in individuals with conduct disorder or antisocial personality disorder.

Alcohol Withdrawal

Diagnostic Criteria

A. Cessation of (or reduction in) alcohol use that has been heavy and prolonged.

B. Two (or more) of the following, developing within several hours to a few days after the cessation of (or reduction in) alcohol use described in Criterion A:

1. Autonomic hyperactivity (e.g., sweating or pulse rate greater than 100 bpm).
2. Increased hand tremor.
3. Insomnia.
4. Nausea or vomiting.
5. Transient visual, tactile, or auditory hallucinations or illusions.
6. Psychomotor agitation.
7. Anxiety.
8. Generalized tonic-clonic seizures.

C. The signs or symptoms in Criterion B cause clinically significant distress or impairment in social, occupational, or other important areas of functioning.

D. The signs or symptoms are not attributable to another medical condition and are not better explained by another mental disorder, including intoxication or withdrawal from another substance.

Specify if:

With perceptual disturbances: This specifier applies in the rare instance when hallucinations (usually visual or tactile) occur with intact reality testing, or auditory, visual, or tactile illusions occur in the absence of a delirium.

Coding note: The ICD-9-CM code is **291.81.** The ICD-10-CM code for alcohol withdrawal without perceptual disturbances is **F10.239,** and the ICD-10-CM code for alcohol withdrawal with perceptual disturbances is **F10.232.** Note that the ICD-10-CM code indicates the comorbid presence of a moderate or severe alcohol use disorder, reflecting the fact that alcohol withdrawal can only occur in the presence of a moderate or severe alcohol use disorder. It is not permissible to code a comorbid mild alcohol use disorder with alcohol withdrawal.

Specifiers

When hallucinations occur in the absence of delirium (i.e., in a clear sensorium), a diagnosis of substance/medication-induced psychotic disorder should be considered.

Diagnostic Features

The essential feature of alcohol withdrawal is the presence of a characteristic withdrawal syndrome that develops within several hours to a few days after the cessation of (or reduction in) heavy and prolonged alcohol use (Criteria A and B). The withdrawal syndrome includes two or more of the symptoms reflecting autonomic hyperactivity and anxiety listed in Criterion B, along with gastrointestinal symptoms.

Withdrawal symptoms cause clinically significant distress or impairment in social, occupational, or other important areas of functioning (Criterion C). The symptoms must not be attributable to another medical condition and are not better explained by another mental disorder (e.g., generalized anxiety disorder), including intoxication or withdrawal from another substance (e.g., sedative, hypnotic, or anxiolytic withdrawal) (Criterion D).

Symptoms can be relieved by administering alcohol or benzodiazepines (e.g., diazepam). The withdrawal symptoms typically begin when blood concentrations of alcohol decline sharply (i.e., within 4–12 hours) after alcohol use has been stopped or reduced. Reflecting the relatively fast metabolism of alcohol, symptoms of alcohol withdrawal usually peak in intensity during the second day of abstinence and are likely to improve markedly by the fourth or fifth day. Following acute withdrawal, however, symptoms of anxiety, insomnia, and autonomic dysfunction may persist for up to 3–6 months at lower levels of intensity.

Fewer than 10% of individuals who develop alcohol withdrawal will ever develop dramatic symptoms (e.g., severe autonomic hyperactivity, tremors, alcohol withdrawal delirium). Tonic-clonic seizures occur in fewer than 3% of individuals.

Associated Features Supporting Diagnosis

Although confusion and changes in consciousness are not core criteria for alcohol withdrawal, alcohol withdrawal delirium (see "Delirium" in the chapter "Neurocognitive Disorders") may occur in the context of withdrawal. As is true for any agitated, confused state, regardless of the cause, in addition to a disturbance of consciousness and cognition, withdrawal delirium can include visual, tactile, or (rarely) auditory hallucinations (delirium tremens). When alcohol withdrawal delirium develops, it is likely that a clinically relevant medical condition may be present (e.g., liver failure, pneumonia, gastrointestinal bleeding, sequelae of head trauma, hypoglycemia, an electrolyte imbalance, postoperative status).

Prevalence

It is estimated that approximately 50% of middle-class, highly functional individuals with alcohol use disorder have ever experienced a full alcohol withdrawal syndrome. Among individuals with alcohol use disorder who are hospitalized or homeless, the rate of alcohol withdrawal may be greater than 80%. Less than 10% of individuals in withdrawal ever demonstrate alcohol withdrawal delirium or withdrawal seizures.

Development and Course

Acute alcohol withdrawal occurs as an episode usually lasting 4–5 days and only after extended periods of heavy drinking. Withdrawal is relatively rare in individuals younger than 30 years, and the risk and severity increase with increasing age.

Risk and Prognostic Factors

Environmental. The probability of developing alcohol withdrawal increases with the quantity and frequency of alcohol consumption. Most individuals with this condition are drinking daily, consuming large amounts (approximately more than eight drinks per day) for multiple days. However, there are large inter-individual differences, with enhanced risks for individuals with concurrent medical conditions, those with family histories of alcohol withdrawal (i.e., a genetic component), those with prior withdrawals, and individuals who consume sedative, hypnotic, or anxiolytic drugs.

Diagnostic Markers

Autonomic hyperactivity in the context of moderately high but falling blood alcohol levels and a history of prolonged heavy drinking indicate a likelihood of alcohol withdrawal.

Functional Consequences of Alcohol Withdrawal

Symptoms of withdrawal may serve to perpetuate drinking behaviors and contribute to relapse, resulting in persistently impaired social and occupational functioning. Symptoms requiring medically supervised detoxification result in hospital utilization and loss of work productivity. Overall, the presence of withdrawal is associated with greater functional impairment and poor prognosis.

Differential Diagnosis

Other medical conditions. The symptoms of alcohol withdrawal can also be mimicked by some medical conditions (e.g., hypoglycemia and diabetic ketoacidosis). Essential tremor, a disorder that frequently runs in families, may erroneously suggest the tremulousness associated with alcohol withdrawal.

Sedative, hypnotic, or anxiolytic withdrawal. Sedative, hypnotic, or anxiolytic withdrawal produces a syndrome very similar to that of alcohol withdrawal.

Comorbidity

Withdrawal is more likely to occur with heavier alcohol intake, and that might be most often observed in individuals with conduct disorder and antisocial personality disorder. Withdrawal states are also more severe in older individuals, individuals who are also dependent on other depressant drugs (sedative-hypnotics), and individuals who have had more alcohol withdrawal experiences in the past.

Other Alcohol-Induced Disorders

The following alcohol-induced disorders are described in other chapters of the manual with disorders with which they share phenomenology (see the substance/medication-induced mental disorders in these chapters): alcohol-induced psychotic disorder ("Schizophrenia Spectrum and Other Psychotic Disorders"); alcohol-induced bipolar disorder ("Bipolar and Related Disorders"); alcohol-induced depressive disorder ("Depressive Disorders"); alcohol-induced anxiety disorder ("Anxiety Disorders"); alcohol-induced sleep disorder ("Sleep-Wake Disorders"); alcohol-induced sexual dysfunction ("Sexual Dysfunctions"); and alcohol-induced major or mild neurocognitive disorder ("Neurocognitive Disorders"). For alcohol intoxication delirium and alcohol withdrawal delirium, see the criteria and discussion of delirium in the chapter "Neurocognitive Disorders." These alcohol-induced disorders are diagnosed instead of alcohol intoxication or alcohol withdrawal only when the symptoms are sufficiently severe to warrant independent clinical attention.

Features

The symptom profiles for an alcohol-induced condition resemble independent mental disorders as described elsewhere in DSM-5. However, the alcohol-induced disorder is temporary and observed after severe intoxication with and/or withdrawal from alcohol. While the symptoms can be identical to those of independent mental disorders (e.g., psychoses, major depressive disorder), and while they can have the same severe consequences (e.g., suicide attempts), alcohol-induced conditions are likely to improve without formal treatment in a matter of days to weeks after cessation of severe intoxication and/or withdrawal.

Each alcohol-induced mental disorder is listed in the relevant diagnostic section and therefore only a brief description is offered here. Alcohol-induced disorders must have developed in the context of severe intoxication and/or withdrawal from the substance capable of producing the mental disorder. In addition, there must be evidence that the disorder being observed is not likely to be better explained by another non-alcohol-induced mental disorder. The latter is likely to occur if the mental disorder was present before the severe intoxication or withdrawal, or continued more than 1 month after the cessation of severe intoxication and/or withdrawal. When symptoms are observed only during a delirium, they should be considered part of the delirium and not diagnosed separately, as many symptoms (including disturbances in mood, anxiety, and reality testing) are commonly seen during agitated, confused states. The alcohol-induced disorder must be clinically relevant, causing significant levels of distress or significant functional impairment. Finally, there are indications that the intake of substances of abuse in the context of a preexisting mental disorder are likely to result in an intensification of the preexisting independent syndrome.

The features associated with each relevant major mental disorder (e.g., psychotic episodes, major depressive disorder) are similar whether observed with an independent or an alcohol-induced condition. However, individuals with alcohol-induced disorders are likely to also demonstrate the associated features seen with an alcohol use disorder, as listed in the subsections of this chapter.

Rates of alcohol-induced disorders vary somewhat by diagnostic category. For example, the lifetime risk for major depressive episodes in individuals with alcohol use disorder is approximately 40%, but only about one-third to one-half of these represent independent major depressive syndromes observed outside the context of intoxication. Similar rates of alcohol-induced sleep and anxiety conditions are likely, but alcohol-induced psychotic episodes are fairly rare.

Development and Course

Once present, the symptoms of an alcohol-induced condition are likely to remain clinically relevant as long as the individual continues to experience severe intoxication and/or withdrawal. While the symptoms are identical to those of independent mental disorders (e.g., psychoses, major depressive disorder), and while they can have the same severe consequences (e.g., suicide attempts), all alcohol-induced syndromes other than alcohol-induced neurocognitive disorder, amnestic confabulatory type (alcohol-induced persisting amnestic disorder), regardless of the severity of the symptoms, are likely to improve relatively quickly and unlikely to remain clinically relevant for more than 1 month after cessation of severe intoxication and/or withdrawal.

The alcohol-induced disorders are an important part of the differential diagnoses for the independent mental conditions. Independent schizophrenia, major depressive disorder, bipolar disorder, and anxiety disorders, such as panic disorder, are likely to be associated with much longer-lasting periods of symptoms and often require longer-term medications to optimize the probability of improvement or recovery. The alcohol-induced conditions, on the other hand, are likely to be much shorter in duration and disappear within several days to 1 month after cessation of severe intoxication and/or withdrawal, even without psychotropic medications.

The importance of recognizing an alcohol-induced disorder is similar to the relevance of identifying the possible role of some endocrine conditions and medication reactions before diagnosing an independent mental disorder. In light of the high prevalence of alcohol use disorders worldwide, it is important that these alcohol-induced diagnoses be considered before independent mental disorders are diagnosed.

Unspecified Alcohol-Related Disorder

291.9 (F10.99)

This category applies to presentations in which symptoms characteristic of an alcohol-related disorder that cause clinically significant distress or impairment in social, occupational, or other important areas of functioning predominate but do not meet the full criteria for any specific alcohol-related disorder or any of the disorders in the substance-related and addictive disorders diagnostic class.

Caffeine-Related Disorders

Caffeine Intoxication
Caffeine Withdrawal
Other Caffeine-Induced Disorders
Unspecified Caffeine-Related Disorder

Caffeine Intoxication

Diagnostic Criteria   305.90 (F15.929)

A. Recent consumption of caffeine (typically a high dose well in excess of 250 mg).
B. Five (or more) of the following signs or symptoms developing during, or shortly after, caffeine use:

   1. Restlessness.
   2. Nervousness.

   3. Excitement.
   4. Insomnia.
   5. Flushed face.
   6. Diuresis.
   7. Gastrointestinal disturbance.
   8. Muscle twitching.
   9. Rambling flow of thought and speech.
   10. Tachycardia or cardiac arrhythmia.
   11. Periods of inexhaustibility.
   12. Psychomotor agitation.
C. The signs or symptoms in Criterion B cause clinically significant distress or impairment in social, occupational, or other important areas of functioning.
D. The signs or symptoms are not attributable to another medical condition and are not better explained by another mental disorder, including intoxication with another substance.

Diagnostic Features

Caffeine can be consumed from a number of different sources, including coffee, tea, caffeinated soda, "energy" drinks, over-the-counter analgesics and cold remedies, energy aids (e.g., drinks), weight-loss aids, and chocolate. Caffeine is also increasingly being used as an additive to vitamins and to food products. More than 85% of children and adults consume caffeine regularly. Some caffeine users display symptoms consistent with problematic use, including tolerance and withdrawal (see "Caffeine Withdrawal" later in this chapter); the data are not available at this time to determine the clinical significance of a caffeine use disorder and its prevalence. In contrast, there is evidence that caffeine withdrawal and caffeine intoxication are clinically significant and sufficiently prevalent.

The essential feature of caffeine intoxication is recent consumption of caffeine and five or more signs or symptoms that develop during or shortly after caffeine use (Criteria A and B). Symptoms include restlessness, nervousness, excitement, insomnia, flushed face, diuresis, and gastrointestinal complaints, which can occur with low doses (e.g., 200 mg) in vulnerable individuals such as children, the elderly, or individuals who have not been exposed to caffeine previously. Symptoms that generally appear at levels of more than 1 g/ day include muscle twitching, rambling flow of thought and speech, tachycardia or cardiac arrhythmia, periods of inexhaustibility, and psychomotor agitation. Caffeine intoxication may not occur despite high caffeine intake because of the development of tolerance. The signs or symptoms must cause clinically significant distress or impairment in social, occupational, or other important areas of functioning (Criterion C). The signs or symptoms must not be attributable to another medical condition and are not better explained by another mental disorder (e.g., an anxiety disorder) or intoxication with another substance (Criterion D).

Associated Features Supporting Diagnosis

Mild sensory disturbances (e.g., ringing in the ears and flashes of light) may occur with high doses of caffeine. Although large doses of caffeine can increase heart rate, smaller doses can slow heart rate. Whether excess caffeine intake can cause headaches is unclear. On physical examination, agitation, restlessness, sweating, tachycardia, flushed face, and increased bowel motility may be seen. Caffeine blood levels may provide important information for diagnosis, particularly when the individual is a poor historian, although these levels are not diagnostic by themselves in view of the individual variation in response to caffeine.

Prevalence

The prevalence of caffeine intoxication in the general population is unclear. In the United States, approximately 7% of individuals in the population may experience five or more symptoms along with functional impairment consistent with a diagnosis of caffeine intoxication.

Development and Course

Consistent with a half-life of caffeine of approximately 4–6 hours, caffeine intoxication symptoms usually remit within the first day or so and do not have any known long-lasting consequences. However, individuals who consume very high doses of caffeine (i.e., 5–10 g) may require immediate medical attention, as such doses can be lethal.

With advancing age, individuals are likely to demonstrate increasingly intense reactions to caffeine, with greater complaints of interference with sleep or feelings of hyperarousal. Caffeine intoxication among young individuals after consumption of highly caffeinated products, including energy drinks, has been observed. Children and adolescents may be at increased risk for caffeine intoxication because of low body weight, lack of tolerance, and lack of knowledge about the pharmacological effects of caffeine.

Risk and Prognostic Factors

Environmental. Caffeine intoxication is often seen among individuals who use caffeine less frequently or in those who have recently increased their caffeine intake by a substantial amount. Furthermore, oral contraceptives significantly decrease the elimination of caffeine and consequently may increase the risk of intoxication.

Genetic and physiological. Genetic factors may affect risk of caffeine intoxication.

Functional Consequences of Caffeine Intoxication

Impairment from caffeine intoxication may have serious consequences, including dysfunction at work or school, social indiscretions, or failure to fulfill role obligations. Moreover, extremely high doses of caffeine can be fatal. In some cases, caffeine intoxication may precipitate a caffeine-induced disorder.

Differential Diagnosis

Other mental disorders. Caffeine intoxication may be characterized by symptoms (e.g., panic attacks) that resemble primary mental disorders. To meet criteria for caffeine intoxication, the symptoms must not be associated with another medical condition or another mental disorder, such as an anxiety disorder, that could better explain them. Manic episodes; panic disorder; generalized anxiety disorder; amphetamine intoxication; sedative, hypnotic, or anxiolytic withdrawal or tobacco withdrawal; sleep disorders; and medication-induced side effects (e.g., akathisia) can cause a clinical picture that is similar to that of caffeine intoxication.

Other caffeine-induced disorders. The temporal relationship of the symptoms to increased caffeine use or to abstinence from caffeine helps to establish the diagnosis. Caffeine intoxication is differentiated from caffeine-induced anxiety disorder, with onset during intoxication (see "Substance/Medication-Induced Anxiety Disorder" in the chapter "Anxiety Disorders"), and caffeine-induced sleep disorder, with onset during intoxication (see "Substance/Medication-Induced Sleep Disorder" in the chapter "Sleep-Wake Disorders"), by the fact that the symptoms in these latter disorders are in excess of those usually associated with caffeine intoxication and are severe enough to warrant independent clinical attention.

Comorbidity

Typical dietary doses of caffeine have not been consistently associated with medical problems. However, heavy use (e.g., >400 mg) can cause or exacerbate anxiety and somatic symptoms and gastrointestinal distress. With acute, extremely high doses of caffeine, grand mal seizures and respiratory failure may result in death. Excessive caffeine use is associated with depressive disorders, bipolar disorders, eating disorders, psychotic disorders, sleep disorders, and substance-related disorders, whereas individuals with anxiety disorders are more likely to avoid caffeine.

Caffeine Withdrawal

Diagnostic Criteria   **292.0** (F15.93)

A. Prolonged daily use of caffeine.
B. Abrupt cessation of or reduction in caffeine use, followed within 24 hours by three (or more) of the following signs or symptoms:
   1. Headache.
   2. Marked fatigue or drowsiness.
   3. Dysphoric mood, depressed mood, or irritability.
   4. Difficulty concentrating.
   5. Flu-like symptoms (nausea, vomiting, or muscle pain/stiffness).
C. The signs or symptoms in Criterion B cause clinically significant distress or impairment in social, occupational, or other important areas of functioning.
D. The signs or symptoms are not associated with the physiological effects of another medical condition (e.g., migraine, viral illness) and are not better explained by another mental disorder, including intoxication or withdrawal from another substance.

Diagnostic Features

The essential feature of caffeine withdrawal is the presence of a characteristic withdrawal syndrome that develops after the abrupt cessation of (or substantial reduction in) prolonged daily caffeine ingestion (Criterion B). The caffeine withdrawal syndrome is indicated by three or more of the following (Criterion B): headache; marked fatigue or drowsiness; dysphoric mood, depressed mood, or irritability; difficulty concentrating; and flu-like symptoms (nausea, vomiting, or muscle pain/stiffness). The withdrawal syndrome causes clinical significant distress or impairment in social, occupational, or other important areas of functioning (Criterion C). The symptoms must not be associated with the physiological effects of another medical condition and are not better explained by another mental disorder (Criterion D).

Headache is the hallmark feature of caffeine withdrawal and may be diffuse, gradual in development, throbbing, severe, and sensitive to movement. However, other symptoms of caffeine withdrawal can occur in the absence of headache. Caffeine is the most widely used behaviorally active drug in the world and is present in many different types of beverages (e.g., coffee, tea, maté, soft drinks, energy drinks), foods, energy aids, medications, and dietary supplements. Because caffeine ingestion is often integrated into social customs and daily rituals (e.g., coffee break, tea time), some caffeine consumers may be unaware of their physical dependence on caffeine. Thus, caffeine withdrawal symptoms could be unexpected and misattributed to other causes (e.g., the flu, migraine). Furthermore, caffeine withdrawal symptoms may occur when individuals are required to abstain from foods and beverages prior to medical procedures or when a usual caffeine dose is missed because of a change in routine (e.g., during travel, weekends).

The probability and severity of caffeine withdrawal generally increase as a function of usual daily caffeine dose. However, there is large variability among individuals and within individuals across different episodes in the incidence, severity, and time course of withdrawal symptoms. Caffeine withdrawal symptoms may occur after abrupt cessation of relatively low chronic daily doses of caffeine (i.e., 100 mg).

Associated Features Supporting Diagnosis

Caffeine abstinence has been shown to be associated with impaired behavioral and cognitive performance (e.g., sustained attention). Electroencephalographic studies have shown that caffeine withdrawal symptoms are significantly associated with increases in theta power and decreases in beta-2 power. Decreased motivation to work and decreased sociability have also been reported during caffeine withdrawal. Increased analgesic use during caffeine withdrawal has been documented.

Prevalence

More than 85% of adults and children in the United States regularly consume caffeine, with adult caffeine consumers ingesting about 280 mg/day on average. The incidence and prevalence of the caffeine withdrawal syndrome in the general population are unclear. In the United States, headache may occur in approximately 50% of cases of caffeine abstinence. In attempts to permanently stop caffeine use, more than 70% of individuals may experience at least one caffeine withdrawal symptom (47% may experience headache), and 24% may experience headache plus one or more other symptoms as well as functional impairment due to withdrawal. Among individuals who abstain from caffeine for at least 24 hours but are not trying to permanently stop caffeine use, 11% may experience headache plus one or more other symptoms as well as functional impairment. Caffeine consumers can decrease the incidence of caffeine withdrawal by using caffeine daily or only infrequently (e.g., no more than 2 consecutive days). Gradual reduction in caffeine over a period of days or weeks may decrease the incidence and severity of caffeine withdrawal.

Development and Course

Symptoms usually begin 12–24 hours after the last caffeine dose and peak after 1–2 days of abstinence. Caffeine withdrawal symptoms last for 2–9 days, with the possibility of withdrawal headaches occurring for up to 21 days. Symptoms usually remit rapidly (within 30–60 minutes) after re-ingestion of caffeine.

Caffeine is unique in that it is a behaviorally active drug that is consumed by individuals of nearly all ages. Rates of caffeine consumption and overall level of caffeine consumption increase with age until the early to mid-30s and then level off. Although caffeine withdrawal among children and adolescents has been documented, relatively little is known about risk factors for caffeine withdrawal among this age group. The use of highly caffeinated energy drinks is increasing with in young individuals, which could increase the risk for caffeine withdrawal.

Risk and Prognostic Factors

Temperamental.   Heavy caffeine use has been observed among individuals with mental disorders, including eating disorders; smokers; prisoners; and drug and alcohol abusers. Thus, these individuals could be at higher risk for caffeine withdrawal upon acute caffeine abstinence.

Environmental.   The unavailability of caffeine is an environmental risk factor for incipient withdrawal symptoms. While caffeine is legal and usually widely available, there are conditions in which caffeine use may be restricted, such as during medical procedures, pregnancy, hospitalizations, religious observances, wartime, travel, and research participation. These external environmental circumstances may precipitate a withdrawal syndrome in vulnerable individuals.

Genetic and physiological factors.   Genetic factors appear to increase vulnerability to caffeine withdrawal, but no specific genes have been identified.

Course modifiers.   Caffeine withdrawal symptoms usually remit within 30–60 minutes of reexposure to caffeine. Doses of caffeine significantly less than one's usual daily dose may be sufficient to prevent or attenuate caffeine withdrawal symptoms (e.g., consumption of 25 mg by an individual who typically consumes 300 mg).

Culture-Related Diagnostic Issues

Habitual caffeine consumers who fast for religious reasons may be at increased risk for caffeine withdrawal.

Functional Consequences of Caffeine Withdrawal Disorder

Caffeine withdrawal symptoms can vary from mild to extreme, at times causing functional impairment in normal daily activities. Rates of functional impairment range from 10% to 55% (median 13%), with rates as high as 73% found among individuals who also show other problematic features of caffeine use. Examples of functional impairment include being unable to work, exercise, or care for children; staying in bed all day; missing religious services; ending a vacation early; and cancelling a social gathering. Caffeine withdrawal headaches may be described by individuals as "the worst headaches" ever experienced. Decrements in cognitive and motor performance have also been observed.

Differential Diagnosis

Other medical disorders and medical side effects.   Several disorders should be considered in the differential diagnosis of caffeine withdrawal. Caffeine withdrawal can mimic migraine and other headache disorders, viral illnesses, sinus conditions, tension, other drug withdrawal states (e.g., from amphetamines, cocaine), and medication side effects. The final determination of caffeine withdrawal should rest on a determination of the pattern and amount consumed, the time interval between caffeine abstinence and onset of symptoms, and the particular clinical features presented by the individual. A challenge dose of caffeine followed by symptom remission may be used to confirm the diagnosis.

Comorbidity

Caffeine withdrawal may be associated with major depressive disorder, generalized anxiety disorder, panic disorder, antisocial personality disorder in adults, moderate to severe alcohol use disorder, and cannabis and cocaine use.

Other Caffeine-Induced Disorders

The following caffeine-induced disorders are described in other chapters of the manual with disorders with which they share phenomenology (see the substance/medication-induced mental disorders in these chapters): caffeine-induced anxiety disorder ("Anxiety Disorders") and caffeine-induced sleep disorder ("Sleep-Wake Disorders"). These caffeine-induced disorders are diagnosed instead of caffeine intoxication or caffeine withdrawal only when the symptoms are sufficiently severe to warrant independent clinical attention.

Unspecified Caffeine-Related Disorder

292.9 (F15.99)

This category applies to presentations in which symptoms characteristic of a caffeine-related disorder that cause clinically significant distress or impairment in social, occupational, or other important areas of functioning predominate but do not meet the full criteria for any specific caffeine-related disorder or any of the disorders in the substance-related and addictive disorders diagnostic class.

Cannabis-Related Disorders

Cannabis Use Disorder
Cannabis Intoxication
Cannabis Withdrawal
Other Cannabis-Induced Disorders
Unspecified Cannabis-Related Disorder

Cannabis Use Disorder

Diagnostic Criteria

A. A problematic pattern of cannabis use leading to clinically significant impairment or distress, as manifested by at least two of the following, occurring within a 12-month period:

1. Cannabis is often taken in larger amounts or over a longer period than was intended.
2. There is a persistent desire or unsuccessful efforts to cut down or control cannabis use.
3. A great deal of time is spent in activities necessary to obtain cannabis, use cannabis, or recover from its effects.
4. Craving, or a strong desire or urge to use cannabis.
5. Recurrent cannabis use resulting in a failure to fulfill major role obligations at work, school, or home.
6. Continued cannabis use despite having persistent or recurrent social or interpersonal problems caused or exacerbated by the effects of cannabis.
7. Important social, occupational, or recreational activities are given up or reduced because of cannabis use.
8. Recurrent cannabis use in situations in which it is physically hazardous.
9. Cannabis use is continued despite knowledge of having a persistent or recurrent physical or psychological problem that is likely to have been caused or exacerbated by cannabis.
10. Tolerance, as defined by either of the following:
    a. A need for markedly increased amounts of cannabis to achieve intoxication or desired effect.
    b. Markedly diminished effect with continued use of the same amount of cannabis.
11. Withdrawal, as manifested by either of the following:
    a. The characteristic withdrawal syndrome for cannabis (refer to Criteria A and B of the criteria set for cannabis withdrawal, pp. 517–518).

b. Cannabis (or a closely related substance) is taken to relieve or avoid withdrawal symptoms.

Specify if:

In early remission: After full criteria for cannabis use disorder were previously met, none of the criteria for cannabis use disorder have been met for at least 3 months but for less than 12 months (with the exception that Criterion A4, "Craving, or a strong desire or urge to use cannabis," may be met).

In sustained remission: After full criteria for cannabis use disorder were previously met, none of the criteria for cannabis use disorder have been met at any time during a period of 12 months or longer (with the exception that Criterion A4, "Craving, or a strong desire or urge to use cannabis," may be present).

Specify if:

In a controlled environment: This additional specifier is used if the individual is in an environment where access to cannabis is restricted.

Code based on current severity: Note for ICD-10-CM codes: If a cannabis intoxication, cannabis withdrawal, or another cannabis-induced mental disorder is also present, do not use the codes below for cannabis use disorder. Instead, the comorbid cannabis use disorder is indicated in the 4th character of the cannabis-induced disorder code (see the coding note for cannabis intoxication, cannabis withdrawal, or a specific cannabis-induced mental disorder). For example, if there is comorbid cannabis-induced anxiety disorder and cannabis use disorder, only the cannabis-induced anxiety disorder code is given, with the 4th character indicating whether the comorbid cannabis use disorder is mild, moderate, or severe: F12.180 for mild cannabis use disorder with cannabis-induced anxiety disorder or F12.280 for a moderate or severe cannabis use disorder with cannabis-induced anxiety disorder.

Specify current severity:

305.20 (F12.10) Mild: Presence of 2–3 symptoms.
304.30 (F12.20) Moderate: Presence of 4–5 symptoms.
304.30 (F12.20) Severe: Presence of 6 or more symptoms.

Specifiers

"In a controlled environment" applies as a further specifier of remission if the individual is both in remission and in a controlled environment (i.e., in early remission in a controlled environment or in sustained remission in a controlled environment). Examples of these environments are closely supervised and substance-free jails, therapeutic communities, and locked hospital units.

Changing severity across time in an individual may also be reflected by changes in the frequency (e.g., days of use per month or times used per day) and/or dose (e.g., amount used per episode) of cannabis, as assessed by individual self-report, report of knowledgeable others, clinician's observations, and biological testing.

Diagnostic Features

Cannabis use disorder and the other cannabis-related disorders include problems that are associated with substances derived from the cannabis plant and chemically similar synthetic compounds. Over time, this plant material has accumulated many names (e.g., weed, pot, herb, grass, reefer, mary jane, dagga, dope, bhang, skunk, boom, gangster, kif, and ganja). A concentrated extraction of the cannabis plant that is also commonly used is hashish. *Cannabis* is the generic and perhaps the most appropriate scientific term for the psychoactive substance(s) derived from the plant, and as such it is used in this manual to refer to all forms of cannabis-like substances, including synthetic cannabinoid compounds.

Synthetic oral formulations (pill/capsules) of delta-9-tetrahydrocannabinol (delta-9-THC) are available by prescription for a number of approved medical indications (e.g., for nausea and vomiting caused by chemotherapy; for anorexia and weight loss in individuals with AIDS). Other synthetic cannabinoid compounds have been manufactured and distributed for nonmedical use in the form of plant material that has been sprayed with a cannabinoid formulation (e.g., K2, Spice, JWH-018, JWH-073).

The cannabinoids have diverse effects in the brain, prominent among which are actions on CB1 and CB2 cannabinoid receptors that are found throughout the central nervous system. Endogenous ligands for these receptors behave essentially like neurotransmitters. The potency of cannabis (delta-9-THC concentration) that is generally available varies greatly, ranging from 1% to approximately 15% in typical cannabis plant material and 10%–20% in hashish. During the past two decades, a steady increase in the potency of seized cannabis has been observed.

Cannabis is most commonly smoked via a variety of methods: pipes, water pipes (bongs or hookahs), cigarettes (joints or reefers), or, most recently, in the paper from hollowed out cigars (blunts). Cannabis is also sometimes ingested orally, typically by mixing it into food. More recently, devices have been developed in which cannabis is "vaporized." Vaporization involves heating the plant material to release psychoactive cannabinoids for inhalation. As with other psychoactive substances, smoking (and vaporization) typically produces more rapid onset and more intense experiences of the desired effects.

Individuals who regularly use cannabis can develop all the general diagnostic features of a substance use disorder. Cannabis use disorder is commonly observed as the only substance use disorder experienced by the individual; however, it also frequently occurs concurrently with other types of substance use disorders (i.e., alcohol, cocaine, opioid). In cases for which multiple types of substances are used, many times the individual may minimize the symptoms related to cannabis, as the symptoms may be less severe or cause less harm than those directly related to the use of the other substances. Pharmacological and behavioral tolerance to most of the effects of cannabis has been reported in individuals who use cannabis persistently. Generally, tolerance is lost when cannabis use is discontinued for a significant period of time (i.e., for at least several months).

New to DSM-5 is the recognition that abrupt cessation of daily or near-daily cannabis use often results in the onset of a cannabis withdrawal syndrome. Common symptoms of withdrawal include irritability, anger or aggression, anxiety, depressed mood, restlessness, sleep difficulty, and decreased appetite or weight loss. Although typically not as severe as alcohol or opioid withdrawal, the cannabis withdrawal syndrome can cause significant distress and contribute to difficulty quitting or relapse among those trying to abstain.

Individuals with cannabis use disorder may use cannabis throughout the day over a period of months or years, and thus may spend many hours a day under the influence. Others may use less frequently, but their use causes recurrent problems related to family, school, work, or other important activities (e.g., repeated absences at work; neglect of family obligations). Periodic cannabis use and intoxication can negatively affect behavioral and cognitive functioning and thus interfere with optimal performance at work or school, or place the individual at increased physical risk when performing activities that could be physically hazardous (e.g., driving a car; playing certain sports; performing manual work activities, including operating machinery). Arguments with spouses or parents over the use of cannabis in the home, or its use in the presence of children, can adversely impact family functioning and are common features of those with cannabis use disorder. Last, individuals with cannabis use disorder may continue using despite knowledge of physical problems (e.g., chronic cough related to smoking) or psychological problems (e.g., excessive sedation or exacerbation of other mental health problems) associated with its use.

Whether or not cannabis is being used for legitimate medical reasons may also affect diagnosis. When a substance is taken as indicated for a medical condition, symptoms of tolerance and withdrawal will naturally occur and should not be used as the primary criteria for determining a diagnosis of a substance use disorder. Although medical uses of cannabis remain controversial and equivocal, use for medical circumstances should be considered when a diagnosis is being made.

Associated Features Supporting Diagnosis

Individuals who regularly use cannabis often report that it is being used to cope with mood, sleep, pain, or other physiological or psychological problems, and those diagnosed with cannabis use disorder frequently do have concurrent other mental disorders. Careful assessment typically reveals reports of cannabis use contributing to exacerbation of these same symptoms, as well as other reasons for frequent use (e.g., to experience euphoria, to forget about problems, in response to anger, as an enjoyable social activity). Related to this issue, some individuals who use cannabis multiple times per day for the aforementioned reasons do not perceive themselves as (and thus do not report) spending an excessive amount of time under the influence or recovering from the effects of cannabis, despite being intoxicated on cannabis or coming down from it effects for the majority of most days. An important marker of a substance use disorder diagnosis, particularly in milder cases, is continued use despite a clear risk of negative consequences to other valued activities or relationships (e.g., school, work, sport activity, partner or parent relationship).

Because some cannabis users are motivated to minimize their amount or frequency of use, it is important to be aware of common signs and symptoms of cannabis use and intoxication so as to better assess the extent of use. As with other substances, experienced users of cannabis develop behavioral and pharmacological tolerance such that it can be difficult to detect when they are under the influence. Signs of acute and chronic use include red eyes (conjunctival injection), cannabis odor on clothing, yellowing of finger tips (from smoking joints), chronic cough, burning of incense (to hide the odor), and exaggerated craving and impulse for specific foods, sometimes at unusual times of the day or night.

Prevalence

Cannabinoids, especially cannabis, are the most widely used illicit psychoactive substances in the United States. The 12-month prevalence of cannabis use disorder (DSM-IV abuse and dependence rates combined) is approximately 3.4% among 12- to 17-year-olds and 1.5% among adults age 18 years and older. Rates of cannabis use disorder are greater among adult males (2.2%) than among adult females (0.8%) and among 12- to 17-year-old males (3.8%) than among 12- to 17-year-old females (3.0%). Twelve-month prevalence rates of cannabis use disorder among adults decrease with age, with rates highest among 18- to 29-year-olds (4.4%) and lowest among individuals age 65 years and older (0.01%). The high prevalence of cannabis use disorder likely reflects the much more widespread use of cannabis relative to other illicit drugs rather than greater addictive potential.

Ethnic and racial differences in prevalence are moderate. Twelve-month prevalences of cannabis use disorder vary markedly across racial-ethnic subgroups in the United States. For 12- to 17-year-olds, rates are highest among Native American and Alaska Natives (7.1%) compared with Hispanics (4.1%), whites (3.4%), African Americans (2.7%), and Asian Americans and Pacific Islanders (0.9%). Among adults, the prevalence of cannabis use disorder is also highest among Native Americans and Alaska Natives (3.4%) relative to rates among African Americans (1.8%), whites (1.4%), Hispanics (1.2%), and Asian and Pacific Islanders (1.2%). During the past decade the prevalence of cannabis use disorder has increased among adults and adolescents. Gender differences in cannabis use disorder generally are concordant with those in other substance use disorders. Cannabis use disorder is more commonly observed in males, although the magnitude of this difference is less among adolescents.

Development and Course

The onset of cannabis use disorder can occur at any time during or following adolescence, but onset is most commonly during adolescence or young adulthood. Although much less frequent, onset of cannabis use disorder in the preteen years or in the late 20s or older can occur. Recent acceptance by some of the use and availability of "medical marijuana" may increase the rate of onset of cannabis use disorder among older adults.

Generally, cannabis use disorder develops over an extended period of time, although the progression appears to be more rapid in adolescents, particularly those with pervasive conduct problems. Most people who develop a cannabis use disorder typically establish a pattern of cannabis use that gradually increases in both frequency and amount. Cannabis, along with tobacco and alcohol, is traditionally the first substance that adolescents try. Many perceive cannabis use as less harmful than alcohol or tobacco use, and this perception likely contributes to increased use. Moreover, cannabis intoxication does not typically result in as severe behavioral and cognitive dysfunction as does significant alcohol intoxication, which may increase the probability of more frequent use in more diverse situations than with alcohol. These factors likely contribute to the potential rapid transition from cannabis use to a cannabis use disorder among some adolescents and the common pattern of using throughout the day that is commonly observed among those with more severe cannabis use disorder.

Cannabis use disorder among preteens, adolescents, and young adults is typically expressed as excessive use with peers that is a component of a pattern of other delinquent behaviors usually associated with conduct problems. Milder cases primarily reflect continued use despite clear problems related to disapproval of use by other peers, school administration, or family, which also places the youth at risk for physical or behavioral consequences. In more severe cases, there is a progression to using alone or using throughout the day such that use interferes with daily functioning and takes the place of previously established, prosocial activities.

With adolescent users, changes in mood stability, energy level, and eating patterns are commonly observed. These signs and symptoms are likely due to the direct effects of cannabis use (intoxication) and the subsequent effects following acute intoxication (coming down), as well as attempts to conceal use from others. School-related problems are commonly associated with cannabis use disorder in adolescents, particularly a dramatic drop in grades, truancy, and reduced interest in general school activities and outcomes.

Cannabis use disorder among adults typically involves well-established patterns of daily cannabis use that continue despite clear psychosocial or medical problems. Many adults have experienced repeated desire to stop or have failed at repeated cessation attempts. Milder adult cases may resemble the more common adolescent cases in that cannabis use is not as frequent or heavy but continues despite potential significant consequences of sustained use. The rate of use among middle-age and older adults appears to be increasing, likely because of a cohort effect resulting from high prevalence of use in the late 1960s and the 1970s.

Early onset of cannabis use (e.g., prior to age 15 years) is a robust predictor of the development of cannabis use disorder and other types of substance use disorders and mental disorders during young adulthood. Such early onset is likely related to concurrent other externalizing problems, most notably conduct disorder symptoms. However, early onset is also a predictor of internalizing problems and as such probably reflects a general risk factor for the development of mental health disorders.

Risk and Prognostic Factors

Temperamental. A history of conduct disorder in childhood or adolescence and antisocial personality disorder are risk factors for the development of many substance-related disorders, including cannabis-related disorders. Other risk factors include externalizing or internalizing disorders during childhood or adolescence. Youths with high behavioral disinhibition scores show early-onset substance use disorders, including cannabis use disorder, multiple substance involvement, and early conduct problems.

Environmental.   Risk factors include academic failure, tobacco smoking, unstable or abusive family situation, use of cannabis among immediate family members, a family history of a substance use disorder, and low socioeconomic status. As with all substances of abuse, the ease of availability of the substance is a risk factor; cannabis is relatively easy to obtain in most cultures, which increases the risk of developing a cannabis use disorder.

Genetic and physiological.   Genetic influences contribute to the development of cannabis use disorders. Heritable factors contribute between 30% and 80% of the total variance in risk of cannabis use disorders. It should be noted that common genetic and shared environmental influences between cannabis and other types of substance use disorders suggest a common genetic basis for adolescent substance use and conduct problems.

Culture-Related Diagnostic Issues

Cannabis is probably the world's most commonly used illicit substance. Occurrence of cannabis use disorder across countries is unknown, but the prevalence rates are likely similar among developed countries. It is frequently among the first drugs of experimentation (often in the teens) of all cultural groups in the United States.

Acceptance of cannabis for medical purposes varies widely across and within cultures. Cultural factors (acceptability and legal status) that might impact diagnosis relate to differential consequences across cultures for detection of use (i.e., arrest, school suspensions, or employment suspension). The general change in substance use disorder diagnostic criteria from DSM-IV to DSM-5 (i.e., removal of the recurrent substance-related legal problems criterion) mitigates this concern to some degree.

Diagnostic Markers

Biological tests for cannabinoid metabolites are useful for determining if an individual has recently used cannabis. Such testing is helpful in making a diagnosis, particularly in milder cases if an individual denies using while others (family, work, school) purport concern about a substance use problem. Because cannabinoids are fat soluble, they persist in bodily fluids for extended periods of time and are excreted slowly. Expertise in urine testing methods is needed to reliably interpret results.

Functional Consequences of Cannabis Use Disorder

Functional consequences of cannabis use disorder are part of the diagnostic criteria. Many areas of psychosocial, cognitive, and health functioning may be compromised in relation to cannabis use disorder. Cognitive function, particularly higher executive function, appears to be compromised in cannabis users, and this relationship appears to be dose dependent (both acutely and chronically). This may contribute to increased difficulty at school or work. Cannabis use has been related to a reduction in prosocial goal-directed activity, which some have labeled an *amotivational syndrome,* that manifests itself in poor school performance and employment problems. These problems may be related to pervasive intoxication or recovery from the effects of intoxication. Similarly, cannabis-associated problems with social relationships are commonly reported in those with cannabis use disorder. Accidents due to engagement in potentially dangerous behaviors while under the influence (e.g., driving, sport, recreational or employment activities) are also of concern. Cannabis smoke contains high levels of carcinogenic compounds that place chronic users at risk for respiratory illnesses similar to those experienced by tobacco smokers. Chronic cannabis use may contribute to the onset or exacerbation of many other mental disorders. In particular, concern has been raised about cannabis use as a causal factor in schizophrenia and other psychotic disorders. Cannabis use can contribute to the onset of an acute psychotic episode, can exacerbate some symptoms, and can adversely affect treatment of a major psychotic illness.

Differential Diagnosis

Nonproblematic use of cannabis.   The distinction between nonproblematic use of cannabis and cannabis use disorder can be difficult to make because social, behavioral, or psychological problems may be difficult to attribute to the substance, especially in the context of use of other substances. Also, denial of heavy cannabis use and the attribution that cannabis is related to or causing substantial problems are common among individuals who are referred to treatment by others (i.e., school, family, employer, criminal justice system).

Other mental disorders.   Cannabis-induced disorder may be characterized by symptoms (e.g., anxiety) that resemble primary mental disorders (e.g., generalized anxiety disorder vs. cannabis-induced anxiety disorder, with generalized anxiety, with onset during intoxication). Chronic intake of cannabis can produce a lack of motivation that resembles persistent depressive disorder (dysthymia). Acute adverse reactions to cannabis should be differentiated from the symptoms of panic disorder, major depressive disorder, delusional disorder, bipolar disorder, or schizophrenia, paranoid type. Physical examination will usually show an increased pulse and conjunctival injection. Urine toxicological testing can be helpful in making a diagnosis.

Comorbidity

Cannabis has been commonly thought of as a "gateway" drug because individuals who frequently use cannabis have a much greater lifetime probability than nonusers of using what are commonly considered more dangerous substances, like opioids or cocaine. Cannabis use and cannabis use disorder are highly comorbid with other substance use disorders. Co-occurring mental conditions are common in cannabis use disorder. Cannabis use has been associated with poorer life satisfaction; increased mental health treatment and hospitalization; and higher rates of depression, anxiety disorders, suicide attempts, and conduct disorder. Individuals with past-year or lifetime cannabis use disorder have high rates of alcohol use disorder (greater than 50%) and tobacco use disorder (53%). Rates of other substance use disorders are also likely to be high among individuals with cannabis use disorder. Among those seeking treatment for a cannabis use disorder, 74% report problematic use of a secondary or tertiary substance: alcohol (40%), cocaine (12%), methamphetamine (6%), and heroin or other opiates (2%). Among those younger than 18 years, 61% reported problematic use of a secondary substance: alcohol (48%), cocaine (4%), methamphetamine (2%), and heroin or other opiates (2%). Cannabis use disorder is also often observed as a secondary problem among those with a primary diagnosis of other substance use disorders, with approximately 25%–80% of those in treatment for another substance use disorder reporting use of cannabis.

Individuals with past-year or lifetime diagnoses of cannabis use disorder also have high rates of concurrent mental disorders other than substance use disorders. Major depressive disorder (11%), any anxiety disorder (24%), and bipolar I disorder (13%) are quite common among individuals with a past-year diagnosis of a cannabis use disorder, as are antisocial (30%), obsessive-compulsive, (19%), and paranoid (18%) personality disorders. Approximately 33% of adolescents with cannabis use disorder have internalizing disorders (e.g., anxiety, depression, posttraumatic stress disorder), and 60% have externalizing disorders (e.g., conduct disorder, attention-deficit/hyperactivity disorder).

Although cannabis use can impact multiple aspects of normal human functioning, including the cardiovascular, immune, neuromuscular, ocular, reproductive, and respiratory systems, as well as appetite and cognition/perception, there are few clear medical conditions that commonly co-occur with cannabis use disorder. The most significant health effects of cannabis involve the respiratory system, and chronic cannabis smokers exhibit high rates of respiratory symptoms of bronchitis, sputum production, shortness of breath, and wheezing.

Cannabis Intoxication

Diagnostic Criteria

A. Recent use of cannabis.

B. Clinically significant problematic behavioral or psychological changes (e.g., impaired motor coordination, euphoria, anxiety, sensation of slowed time, impaired judgment, social withdrawal) that developed during, or shortly after, cannabis use.

C. Two (or more) of the following signs or symptoms developing within 2 hours of cannabis use:

   1. Conjunctival injection.
   2. Increased appetite.
   3. Dry mouth.
   4. Tachycardia.

D. The signs or symptoms are not attributable to another medical condition and are not better explained by another mental disorder, including intoxication with another substance.

Specify if:

With perceptual disturbances: Hallucinations with intact reality testing or auditory, visual, or tactile illusions occur in the absence of a delirium.

Coding note: The ICD-9-CM code is **292.89.** The ICD-10-CM code depends on whether or not there is a comorbid cannabis use disorder and whether or not there are perceptual disturbances.

For cannabis intoxication, without perceptual disturbances: If a mild cannabis use disorder is comorbid, the ICD-10-CM code is **F12.129,** and if a moderate or severe cannabis use disorder is comorbid, the ICD-10-CM code is **F12.229.** If there is no comorbid cannabis use disorder, then the ICD-10-CM code is **F12.929.**

For cannabis intoxication, with perceptual disturbances: If a mild cannabis use disorder is comorbid, the ICD-10-CM code is **F12.122,** and if a moderate or severe cannabis use disorder is comorbid, the ICD-10-CM code is **F12.222.** If there is no comorbid cannabis use disorder, then the ICD-10-CM code is **F12.922.**

Specifiers

When hallucinations occur in the absence of intact reality testing, a diagnosis of substance/medication-induced psychotic disorder should be considered.

Diagnostic Features

The essential feature of cannabis intoxication is the presence of clinically significant problematic behavioral or psychological changes that develop during, or shortly after, cannabis use (Criterion B). Intoxication typically begins with a "high" feeling followed by symptoms that include euphoria with inappropriate laughter and grandiosity, sedation, lethargy, impairment in short-term memory, difficulty carrying out complex mental processes, impaired judgment, distorted sensory perceptions, impaired motor performance, and the sensation that time is passing slowly. Occasionally, anxiety (which can be severe), dysphoria, or social withdrawal occurs. These psychoactive effects are accompanied by two or more of the following signs, developing within 2 hours of cannabis use: conjuncti-val injection, increased appetite, dry mouth, and tachycardia (Criterion C).

Intoxication develops within minutes if the cannabis is smoked but may take a few hours to develop if the cannabis is ingested orally. The effects usually last 3–4 hours, with the duration being somewhat longer when the substance is ingested orally. The magnitude of the behavioral and physiological changes depends on the dose, the method of adminis-tration, and the characteristics of the individual using the substance, such as rate of absorp-tion, tolerance, and sensitivity to the effects of the substance. Because most cannabinoids, including delta-9-tetrahydrocannabinol (delta-9-THC), are fat soluble, the effects of canna-bis or hashish may occasionally persist or reoccur for 12–24 hours because of the slow re-lease of psychoactive substances from fatty tissue or to enterohepatic circulation.

Prevalence

The prevalence of actual episodes of cannabis intoxication in the general population is un-known. However, it is probable that most cannabis users would at some time meet criteria for cannabis intoxication. Given this, the prevalence of cannabis users and the prevalence of individuals experiencing cannabis intoxication are likely similar.

Functional Consequences of Cannabis Intoxication

Impairment from cannabis intoxication may have serious consequences, including dys-function at work or school, social indiscretions, failure to fulfill role obligations, traffic ac-cidents, and having unprotected sex. In rare cases, cannabis intoxication may precipitate a psychosis that may vary in duration.

Differential Diagnosis

Note that if the clinical presentation includes hallucinations in the absence of intact reality testing, a diagnosis of substance/medication-induced psychotic disorder should be con-sidered.

Other substance intoxication.   Cannabis intoxication may resemble intoxication with other types of substances. However, in contrast to cannabis intoxication, alcohol intoxica-tion and sedative, hypnotic, or anxiolytic intoxication frequently decrease appetite, in-crease aggressive behavior, and produce nystagmus or ataxia. Hallucinogens in low doses may cause a clinical picture that resembles cannabis intoxication. Phencyclidine, like can-nabis, can be smoked and also causes perceptual changes, but phencyclidine intoxication is much more likely to cause ataxia and aggressive behavior.

Other cannabis-induced disorders.   Cannabis intoxication is distinguished from the other cannabis-induced disorders (e.g., cannabis-induced anxiety disorder, with onset during intoxication) because the symptoms in these latter disorders predominate the clinical pre-sentation and are severe enough to warrant independent clinical attention.

Cannabis Withdrawal

Diagnostic Criteria	292.0 (F12.288)

A. Cessation of cannabis use that has been heavy and prolonged (i.e., usually daily or almost daily use over a period of at least a few months).

B. Three (or more) of the following signs and symptoms develop within approximately 1 week after Criterion A:

1. Irritability, anger, or aggression.
2. Nervousness or anxiety.
3. Sleep difficulty (e.g., insomnia, disturbing dreams).
4. Decreased appetite or weight loss.
5. Restlessness.
6. Depressed mood.
7. At least one of the following physical symptoms causing significant discomfort: abdominal pain, shakiness/tremors, sweating, fever, chills, or headache.

C. The signs or symptoms in Criterion B cause clinically significant distress or impairment in social, occupational, or other important areas of functioning.

D. The signs or symptoms are not attributable to another medical condition and are not better explained by another mental disorder, including intoxication or withdrawal from another substance.

Coding note: The ICD-9-CM code is 292.0. The ICD-10-CM code for cannabis withdrawal is F12.288. Note that the ICD-10-CM code indicates the comorbid presence of a moderate or severe cannabis use disorder, reflecting the fact that cannabis withdrawal can only occur in the presence of a moderate or severe cannabis use disorder. It is not permissible to code a comorbid mild cannabis use disorder with cannabis withdrawal.

Diagnostic Features

The essential feature of cannabis withdrawal is the presence of a characteristic withdrawal syndrome that develops after the cessation of or substantial reduction in heavy and prolonged cannabis use. In addition to the symptoms in Criterion B, the following may also be observed postabstinence: fatigue, yawning, difficulty concentrating, and rebound periods of increased appetite and hypersomnia that follow initial periods of loss of appetite and insomnia. For the diagnosis, withdrawal symptoms must cause clinically significant distress or impairment in social, occupational, or other important areas of functioning (Criterion C). Many cannabis users report smoking cannabis or taking other substances to help relieve withdrawal symptoms, and many report that withdrawal symptoms make quitting difficult or have contributed to relapse. The symptoms typically are not of sufficient severity to require medical attention, but medication or behavioral strategies may help alleviate symptoms and improve prognosis in those trying to quit using cannabis.

Cannabis withdrawal is commonly observed in individuals seeking treatment for cannabis use as well as in heavy cannabis users who are not seeking treatment. Among individuals who have used cannabis regularly during some period of their lifetime, up to one-third report having experienced cannabis withdrawal. Among adults and adolescents enrolled in treatment or heavy cannabis users, 50%–95% report cannabis withdrawal. These findings indicate that cannabis withdrawal occurs among a substantial subset of regular cannabis users who try to quit.

Development and Course

The amount, duration, and frequency of cannabis smoking that is required to produce an associated withdrawal disorder during a quit attempt are unknown. Most symptoms have their onset within the first 24–72 hours of cessation, peak within the first week, and last approximately 1–2 weeks. Sleep difficulties may last more than 30 days. Cannabis withdrawal has been documented among adolescents and adults. Withdrawal tends to be more common and severe among adults, most likely related to the more persistent and greater frequency and quantity of use among adults.

Risk and Prognostic Factors

Environmental.   Most likely, the prevalence and severity of cannabis withdrawal are greater among heavier cannabis users, and particularly among those seeking treatment for cannabis use disorders. Withdrawal severity also appears to be positively related to the severity of comorbid symptoms of mental disorders.

Functional Consequences of Cannabis Withdrawal

Cannabis users report using cannabis to relieve withdrawal symptoms, suggesting that withdrawal might contribute to ongoing expression of cannabis use disorder. Worse outcomes may be associated with greater withdrawal. A substantial proportion of adults and adolescents in treatment for moderate to severe cannabis use disorder acknowledge moderate to severe withdrawal symptoms, and many complain that these symptoms make cessation more difficult. Cannabis users report having relapsed to cannabis use or initiating use of other drugs (e.g., tranquilizers) to provide relief from cannabis withdrawal symptoms. Last, individuals living with cannabis users observe significant withdrawal effects, suggesting that such symptoms are disruptive to daily living.

Differential Diagnosis

Because many of the symptoms of cannabis withdrawal are also symptoms of other substance withdrawal syndromes or of depressive or bipolar disorders, careful evaluation should focus on ensuring that the symptoms are not better explained by cessation from another substance (e.g., tobacco or alcohol withdrawal), another mental disorder (generalized anxiety disorder, major depressive disorder), or another medical condition.

Other Cannabis-Induced Disorders

The following cannabis-induced disorders are described in other chapters of the manual with disorders with which they share phenomenology (see the substance/medication-induced mental disorders in these chapters): cannabis-induced psychotic disorder ("Schizophrenia Spectrum and Other Psychotic Disorders"); cannabis-induced anxiety disorder ("Anxiety Disorders"); and cannabis-induced sleep disorder ("Sleep-Wake Disorders"). For cannabis intoxication delirium, see the criteria and discussion of delirium in the chapter "Neurocognitive Disorders." These cannabis-induced disorders are diagnosed instead of cannabis intoxication or cannabis withdrawal when the symptoms are sufficiently severe to warrant independent clinical attention.

Unspecified Cannabis-Related Disorder

292.9 (F12.99)

This category applies to presentations in which symptoms characteristic of a cannabis-related disorder that cause clinically significant distress or impairment in social, occupational, or other important areas of functioning predominate but do not meet the full criteria for any specific cannabis-related disorder or any of the disorders in the substance-related and addictive disorders diagnostic class.

Hallucinogen-Related Disorders

Phencyclidine Use Disorder
Other Hallucinogen Use Disorder
Phencyclidine Intoxication
Other Hallucinogen Intoxication
Hallucinogen Persisting Perception Disorder
Other Phencyclidine-Induced Disorders
Other Hallucinogen-Induced Disorders
Unspecified Phencyclidine-Related Disorder
Unspecified Hallucinogen-Related Disorder

Phencyclidine Use Disorder

Diagnostic Criteria

A. A pattern of phencyclidine (or a pharmacologically similar substance) use leading to clinically significant impairment or distress, as manifested by at least two of the following, occurring within a 12-month period:

1. Phencyclidine is often taken in larger amounts or over a longer period than was intended.
2. There is a persistent desire or unsuccessful efforts to cut down or control phencyclidine use.
3. A great deal of time is spent in activities necessary to obtain phencyclidine, use the phencyclidine, or recover from its effects.
4. Craving, or a strong desire or urge to use phencyclidine.
5. Recurrent phencyclidine use resulting in a failure to fulfill major role obligations at work, school, or home (e.g., repeated absences from work or poor work performance related to phencyclidine use; phencyclidine-related absences, suspensions, or expulsions from school; neglect of children or household).
6. Continued phencyclidine use despite having persistent or recurrent social or interpersonal problems caused or exacerbated by the effects of the phencyclidine (e.g., arguments with a spouse about consequences of intoxication; physical fights).
7. Important social, occupational, or recreational activities are given up or reduced because of phencyclidine use.
8. Recurrent phencyclidine use in situations in which it is physically hazardous (e.g., driving an automobile or operating a machine when impaired by a phencyclidine).
9. Phencyclidine use is continued despite knowledge of having a persistent or recurrent physical or psychological problem that is likely to have been caused or exacerbated by the phencyclidine.
10. Tolerance, as defined by either of the following:

    a. A need for markedly increased amounts of the phencyclidine to achieve intoxication or desired effect.
    b. A markedly diminished effect with continued use of the same amount of the phencyclidine.

Note: Withdrawal symptoms and signs are not established for phencyclidines, and so this criterion does not apply. (Withdrawal from phencyclidines has been reported in animals but not documented in human users.)

Specify if:

In early remission: After full criteria for phencyclidine use disorder were previously met, none of the criteria for phencyclidine use disorder have been met for at least 3 months but for less than 12 months (with the exception that Criterion A4, "Craving, or a strong desire or urge to use the phencyclidine," may be met).

In sustained remission: After full criteria for phencyclidine use disorder were previously met, none of the criteria for phencyclidine use disorder have been met at any time during a period of 12 months or longer (with the exception that Criterion A4, "Craving, or a strong desire or urge to use the phencyclidine," may be met).

Specify if:

In a controlled environment: This additional specifier is used if the individual is in an environment where access to phencyclidines is restricted.

Coding based on current severity: Note for ICD-10-CM codes: If a phencyclidine intoxication or another phencyclidine-induced mental disorder is also present, do not use the codes below for phencyclidine use disorder. Instead, the comorbid phencyclidine use disorder is indicated in the 4th character of the phencyclidine-induced disorder code (see the coding note for phencyclidine intoxication or a specific phencyclidine-induced mental disorder). For example, if there is comorbid phencyclidine-induced psychotic disorder, only the phencyclidine-induced psychotic disorder code is given, with the 4th character indicating whether the comorbid phencyclidine use disorder is mild, moderate, or severe: F16.159 for mild phencyclidine use disorder with phencyclidine-induced psychotic disorder or F16.259 for a moderate or severe phencyclidine use disorder with phencyclidine-induced psychotic disorder.

Specify current severity:

305.90 (F16.10) Mild: Presence of 2–3 symptoms.

304.60 (F16.20) Moderate: Presence of 4–5 symptoms.

304.60 (F16.20) Severe: Presence of 6 or more symptoms.

Specifiers

"In a controlled environment" applies as a further specifier of remission if the individual is both in remission and in a controlled environment (i.e., in early remission in a controlled environment or in sustained remission in a controlled environment). Examples of these environments are closely supervised and substance-free jails, therapeutic communities, and locked hospital units.

Diagnostic Features

The phencyclidines (or phencyclidine-like substances) include phencyclidine (e.g., PCP, "angel dust") and less potent but similarly acting compounds such as ketamine, cyclohexamine, and dizocilpine. These substances were first developed as dissociative anesthetics in the 1950s and became street drugs in the 1960s. They produce feelings of separation from mind and body (hence "dissociative") in low doses, and at high doses, stupor and coma can result. These substances are most commonly smoked or taken orally, but they may also be snorted or injected. Although the primary psychoactive effects of PCP last for a few hours, the total elimination rate of this drug from the body typically extends 8 days or longer. The hallucinogenic effects in vulnerable individuals may last for weeks and may precipitate a persistent psychotic episode resembling schizophrenia. Ketamine has been observed to have utility in the treatment of major depressive disorder. Withdrawal symptoms have not been clearly established in humans, and therefore the withdrawal criterion is not included in the diagnosis of phencyclidine use disorder.

Associated Features Supporting Diagnosis

Phencyclidine may be detected in urine for up to 8 days or even longer at very high doses. In addition to laboratory tests to detect its presence, characteristic symptoms resulting from intoxication with phencyclidine or related substances may aid in its diagnosis. Phencyclidine is likely to produce dissociative symptoms, analgesia, nystagmus, and hypertension, with risk of hypotension and shock. Violent behavior can also occur with phencyclidine use, as intoxicated persons may believe that they are being attacked. Residual symptoms following use may resemble schizophrenia.

Prevalence

The prevalence of phencyclidine use disorder is unknown. Approximately 2.5% of the population reports having ever used phencyclidine. The proportion of users increases with age, from 0.3% of 12- to 17-year-olds, to 1.3% of 18- to 25-year-olds, to 2.9% of those age 26 years and older reporting ever using phencyclidine. There appears to have been an increase among 12th graders in both ever used (to 2.3% from 1.8%) and past-year use (to 1.3% from 1.0%) of phencyclidine. Past-year use of ketamine appears relatively stable among 12th graders (1.6%–1.7% over the past 3 years).

Risk and Prognostic Factors

There is little information about risk factors for phencyclidine use disorder. Among individuals admitted to substance abuse treatment, those for whom phencyclidine was the primary substance were younger than those admitted for other substance use, had lower educational levels, and were more likely to be located in the West and Northeast regions of the United States, compared with other admissions.

Culture-Related Diagnostic Issues

Ketamine use in youths ages 16–23 years has been reported to be more common among whites (0.5%) than among other ethnic groups (range 0%–0.3%). Among individuals admitted to substance abuse treatment, those for whom phencyclidine was the primary substance were predominantly black (49%) or Hispanic (29%).

Gender-Related Diagnostic Issues

Males make up about three-quarters of those with phencyclidine-related emergency room visits.

Diagnostic Markers

Laboratory testing may be useful, as phencyclidine is present in the urine in intoxicated individuals up to 8 days after ingestion. The individual's history, along with certain physical signs, such as nystagmus, analgesia and prominent hypertension, may aid in distinguishing the phencyclidine clinical picture from that of other hallucinogens.

Functional Consequences of Phencyclidine Use Disorder

In individuals with phencyclidine use disorder, there may be physical evidence of injuries from accidents, fights, and falls. Chronic use of phencyclidine may lead to deficits in memory, speech, and cognition that may last for months. Cardiovascular and neurological toxicities (e.g., seizures, dystonias, dyskinesias, catalepsy, hypothermia or hyperthermia) may result from intoxication with phencyclidine. Other consequences include intracranial hemorrhage, rhabdomyolysis, respiratory problems, and (occasionally) cardiac arrest.

Differential Diagnosis

Other substance use disorders. Distinguishing the effects of phencyclidine from those of other substances is important, since it may be a common additive to other substances (e.g., cannabis, cocaine).

Schizophrenia and other mental disorders. Some of the effects of phencyclidine and related substance use may resemble symptoms of other psychiatric disorders, such as psychosis (schizophrenia), low mood (major depressive disorder), violent aggressive behaviors (conduct disorder, antisocial personality disorder). Discerning whether these behaviors occurred before the intake of the drug is important in the differentiation of acute drug effects from preexisting mental disorder. Phencyclidine-induced psychotic disorder should be considered when there is impaired reality testing in individuals experiencing disturbances in perception resulting from ingestion of phencyclidine.

Other Hallucinogen Use Disorder

Diagnostic Criteria

A. A problematic pattern of hallucinogen (other than phencyclidine) use leading to clinically significant impairment or distress, as manifested by at least two of the following, occurring within a 12-month period:

1. The hallucinogen is often taken in larger amounts or over a longer period than was intended.
2. There is a persistent desire or unsuccessful efforts to cut down or control hallucinogen use.
3. A great deal of time is spent in activities necessary to obtain the hallucinogen, use the hallucinogen, or recover from its effects.
4. Craving, or a strong desire or urge to use the hallucinogen.
5. Recurrent hallucinogen use resulting in a failure to fulfill major role obligations at work, school, or home (e.g., repeated absences from work or poor work performance related to hallucinogen use; hallucinogen-related absences, suspensions, or expulsions from school; neglect of children or household).
6. Continued hallucinogen use despite having persistent or recurrent social or interpersonal problems caused or exacerbated by the effects of the hallucinogen (e.g., arguments with a spouse about consequences of intoxication; physical fights).
7. Important social, occupational, or recreational activities are given up or reduced because of hallucinogen use.
8. Recurrent hallucinogen use in situations in which it is physically hazardous (e.g., driving an automobile or operating a machine when impaired by the hallucinogen).
9. Hallucinogen use is continued despite knowledge of having a persistent or recurrent physical or psychological problem that is likely to have been caused or exacerbated by the hallucinogen.
10. Tolerance, as defined by either of the following:
    a. A need for markedly increased amounts of the hallucinogen to achieve intoxication or desired effect.
    b. A markedly diminished effect with continued use of the same amount of the hallucinogen.

Note: Withdrawal symptoms and signs are not established for hallucinogens, and so this criterion does not apply.

Specify **the particular hallucinogen.**

Specify if:

In early remission: After full criteria for other hallucinogen use disorder were previously met, none of the criteria for other hallucinogen use disorder have been met for at least 3 months but for less than 12 months (with the exception that Criterion A4, "Craving, or a strong desire or urge to use the hallucinogen," may be met).

In sustained remission: After full criteria for other hallucinogen use disorder were previously met, none of the criteria for other hallucinogen use disorder have been met at any time during a period of 12 months or longer (with the exception that Criterion A4, "Craving, or a strong desire or urge to use the hallucinogen," may be met).

Specify if:

In a controlled environment: This additional specifier is used if the individual is in an environment where access to hallucinogens is restricted.

Coding based on current severity: Note for ICD-10-CM codes: If a hallucinogen intoxication or another hallucinogen-induced mental disorder is also present, do not use the codes below for hallucinogen use disorder. Instead, the comorbid hallucinogen use disorder is indicated in the 4th character of the hallucinogen-induced disorder code (see the coding note for hallucinogen intoxication or specific hallucinogen-induced mental disorder). For example, if there is comorbid hallucinogen-induced psychotic disorder and hallucinogen use disorder, only the hallucinogen-induced psychotic disorder code is given, with the 4th character indicating whether the comorbid hallucinogen use disorder is mild, moderate, or severe: F16.159 for mild hallucinogen use disorder with hallucinogen-induced psychotic disorder or F16.259 for a moderate or severe hallucinogen use disorder with hallucinogen-induced psychotic disorder.

Specify current severity:

305.30 (F16.10) Mild: Presence of 2–3 symptoms.

304.50 (F16.20) Moderate: Presence of 4–5 symptoms.

304.50 (F16.20) Severe: Presence of 6 or more symptoms.

Specifiers

"In a controlled environment" applies as a further specifier of remission if the individual is both in remission and in a controlled environment (i.e., in early remission in a controlled environment or in sustained remission in a controlled environment). Examples of these environments are closely supervised and substance-free jails, therapeutic communities, and locked hospital units.

Diagnostic Features

Hallucinogens comprise a diverse group of substances that, despite having different chemical structures and possibly involving different molecular mechanisms, produce similar alterations of perception, mood, and cognition in users. Hallucinogens included are phenylalkylamines (e.g., mescaline, DOM [2,5-dimethoxy-4-methylamphetamine], and MDMA [3,4-methylenedioxymethamphetamine; also called "ecstasy"]); the indoleamines, including psilocybin (i.e., psilocin) and dimethyltryptamine (DMT); and the ergolines, such as LSD (lysergic acid diethylamide) and morning glory seeds. In addition, miscellaneous other ethnobotanical compounds are classified as "hallucinogens," of which *Salvia divinorum* and jimsonweed are two examples. Excluded from the hallucinogen group are cannabis and its active compound, delta-9-tetrahydrocannabinol (THC) (see the section "Cannabis-Related Disorders"). These substances can have hallucinogenic effects but are diagnosed separately because of significant differences in their psychological and behavioral effects.

Hallucinogens are usually taken orally, although some forms are smoked (e.g., DMT, salvia) or (rarely) taken intranasally or by injection (e.g., ecstasy). Duration of effects varies across types of hallucinogens. Some of these substances (i.e., LSD, MDMA) have a long half-life and extended duration such that users may spend hours to days using and/or recovering from the effects of these drugs. However, other hallucinogenic drugs (e.g., DMT, salvia) are short acting. Tolerance to hallucinogens develops with repeated use and has been reported to have both autonomic and psychological effects. Cross-tolerance exists between LSD and other hallucinogens (e.g., psilocybin, mescaline) but does not extend to other drug categories such as amphetamines and cannabis.

MDMA/ecstasy as a hallucinogen may have distinctive effects attributable to both its hallucinogenic and its stimulant properties. Among heavy ecstasy users, continued use despite physical or psychological problems, tolerance, hazardous use, and spending a great deal of time obtaining the substance are the most commonly reported criteria—over 50% in adults and over 30% in a younger sample, while legal problems related to substance use and persistent desire/inability to quit are rarely reported. As found for other substances, diagnostic criteria for other hallucinogen use disorder are arrayed along a single continuum of severity.

One of the generic criteria for substance use disorders, a clinically significant withdrawal syndrome, has not been consistently documented in humans, and therefore the diagnosis of hallucinogen withdrawal syndrome is not included in DSM-5. However, there is evidence of withdrawal from MDMA, with endorsement of two or more withdrawal symptoms observed in 59%–98% in selected samples of ecstasy users. Both psychological and physical problems have been commonly reported as withdrawal problems.

Associated Features Supporting Diagnosis

The characteristic symptom features of some of the hallucinogens can aid in diagnosis if urine or blood toxicology results are not available. For example, individuals who use LSD tend to experience visual hallucinations that can be frightening. Individuals intoxicated with hallucinogens may exhibit a temporary increase in suicidality.

Prevalence

Of all substance use disorders, other hallucinogen use disorder is one of the rarest. The 12-month prevalence is estimated to be 0.5% among 12- to 17-year-olds and 0.1% among adults age 18 and older in the United States. Rates are higher in adult males (0.2%) compared with females (0.1%), but the opposite is observed in adolescent samples ages 12–17, in which the 12-month rate is slightly higher in females (0.6%) than in males (0.4%). Rates are highest in individuals younger than 30 years, with the peak occurring in individuals ages 18–29 years (0.6%) and decreasing to virtually 0.0% among individuals age 45 and older.

There are marked ethnic differences in 12-month prevalence of other hallucinogen use disorder. Among youths ages 12–17 years, 12-month prevalence is higher among Native Americans and Alaska Natives (1.2%) than among Hispanics (0.6%), whites (0.6%), African Americans (0.2%), and Asian Americans and Pacific Islanders (0.2%). Among adults, 12-month prevalence of other hallucinogen use disorder is similar for Native Americans and Alaska Natives, whites, and Hispanics (all 0.2%) but somewhat lower for Asian Americans and Pacific Islanders (0.07%) and African Americans (0.03%). Past-year prevalence is higher in clinical samples (e.g., 19% in adolescents in treatment). Among individuals currently using hallucinogens in the general population, 7.8% (adult) to 17% (adolescent) had a problematic pattern of use that met criteria for past-year other hallucinogen use disorder. Among select groups of individuals who use hallucinogens (e.g., recent heavy ecstasy use), 73.5% of adults and 77% of adolescents have a problematic pattern of use that may meet other hallucinogen use disorder criteria.

Development and Course

Unlike most substances where an early age at onset is associated with elevations in risk for the corresponding use disorder, it is unclear whether there is an association of an early age at onset with elevations in risk for other hallucinogen use disorder. However, patterns of drug consumption have been found to differ by age at onset, with early-onset ecstasy users more likely to be polydrug users than their later-onset counterparts. There may be a disproportionate influence of use of specific hallucinogens on risk of developing other hallucinogen use disorder, with use of ecstasy/MDMA increasing the risk of the disorder relative to use of other hallucinogens.

Little is known regarding the course of other hallucinogen use disorder, but it is generally thought to have low incidence, low persistence, and high rates of recovery. Adolescents are especially at risk for using these drugs, and it is estimated that 2.7% of youths ages 12–17 years have used one or more of these drugs in the past 12 months, with 44% having used ecstasy/MDMA. Other hallucinogen use disorder is a disorder observed primarily in individuals younger than 30 years, with rates vanishingly rare among older adults.

Risk and Prognostic Factors

Temperamental. In adolescents but not consistently in adults, MDMA use is associated with an elevated rate of other hallucinogen use disorder. Other substance use disorders, particularly alcohol, tobacco, and cannabis, and major depressive disorder are associated with elevated rates of other hallucinogen use disorder. Antisocial personality disorder may be elevated among individuals who use more than two other drugs in addition to hallucinogens, compared with their counterparts with less extensive use history. The influence of adult antisocial behaviors—but not conduct disorder or antisocial personality disorder—on other hallucinogen use disorder may be stronger in females than in males. Use of specific hallucinogens (e.g., salvia) is prominent among individuals ages 18–25 years with other risk-taking behaviors and illegal activities. Cannabis use has also been implicated as a precursor to initiation of use of hallucinogens (e.g., ecstasy), along with early use of alcohol and tobacco. Higher drug use by peers and high sensation seeking have also been associated with elevated rates of ecstasy use. MDMA/ecstasy use appears to signify a more severe group of hallucinogen users.

Genetic and physiological. Among male twins, total variance due to additive genetics has been estimated to range from 26% to 79%, with inconsistent evidence for shared environmental influences.

Culture-Related Diagnostic Issues

Historically, hallucinogens have been used as part of established religious practices, such as the use of peyote in the Native American Church and in Mexico. Ritual use by indigenous populations of psilocybin obtained from certain types of mushrooms has occurred in South America, Mexico, and some areas in the United States, or of ayahuasca in the Santo Daime and União de Vegetal sects. Regular use of peyote as part of religious rituals is not linked to neuropsychological or psychological deficits. For adults, no race or ethnicity differences for the full criteria or for any individual criterion are apparent at this time.

Gender-Related Diagnostic Issues

In adolescents, females may be less likely than males to endorse "hazardous use," and female gender may be associated with increased odds of other hallucinogen use disorder.

Diagnostic Markers

Laboratory testing can be useful in distinguishing among the different hallucinogens. However, because some agents (e.g., LSD) are so potent that as little as 75 micrograms can produce severe reactions, typical toxicological examination will not always reveal which substance has been used.

Functional Consequences of Other Hallucinogen Use Disorder

There is evidence for long-term neurotoxic effects of MDMA/ecstasy use, including impairments in memory, psychological function, and neuroendocrine function; serotonin system dysfunction; and sleep disturbance; as well as adverse effects on brain microvasculature, white matter maturation, and damage to axons. Use of MDMA/ecstasy may diminish functional connectivity among brain regions.

Differential Diagnosis

Other substance use disorders.   The effects of hallucinogens must be distinguished from those of other substances (e.g., amphetamines), especially because contamination of the hallucinogens with other drugs is relatively common.

Schizophrenia.   Schizophrenia also must be ruled out, as some affected individuals (e.g., individuals with schizophrenia who exhibit paranoia) may falsely attribute their symptoms to use of hallucinogens.

Other mental disorders or medical conditions.   Other potential disorders or conditions to consider include panic disorder, depressive and bipolar disorders, alcohol or sedative withdrawal, hypoglycemia and other metabolic conditions, seizure disorder, stroke, ophthalmological disorder, and central nervous system tumors. Careful history of drug taking, collateral reports from family and friends (if possible), age, clinical history, physical examination, and toxicology reports should be useful in arriving at the final diagnostic decision.

Comorbidity

Adolescents who use MDMA/ecstasy and other hallucinogens, as well as adults who have recently used ecstasy, have a higher prevalence of other substance use disorders compared with nonhallucinogen substance users. Individuals who use hallucinogens exhibit elevations of nonsubstance mental disorders (especially anxiety, depressive, and bipolar disorders), particularly with use of ecstasy and salvia. Rates of antisocial personality disorder (but not conduct disorder) are significantly elevated among individuals with other hallucinogen use disorder, as are rates of adult antisocial behavior. However, it is unclear whether the mental illnesses may be precursors to rather than consequences of other hallucinogen use disorder (see the section "Risk and Prognostic Factors" for this disorder). Both adults and adolescents who use ecstasy are more likely than other drug users to be polydrug users and to have other drug use disorders.

Phencyclidine Intoxication

Diagnostic Criteria

A. Recent use of phencyclidine (or a pharmacologically similar substance).
B. Clinically significant problematic behavioral changes (e.g., belligerence, assaultiveness, impulsiveness, unpredictability, psychomotor agitation, impaired judgment) that developed during, or shortly after, phencyclidine use.
C. Within 1 hour, two (or more) of the following signs or symptoms:

   Note: When the drug is smoked, "snorted," or used intravenously, the onset may be particularly rapid.

   1. Vertical or horizontal nystagmus.
   2. Hypertension or tachycardia.

3. Numbness or diminished responsiveness to pain.
4. Ataxia.
5. Dysarthria.
6. Muscle rigidity.
7. Seizures or coma.
8. Hyperacusis.

D. The signs or symptoms are not attributable to another medical condition and are not better explained by another mental disorder, including intoxication with another substance.

Coding note: The ICD-9-CM code is **292.89.** The ICD-10-CM code depends on whether there is a comorbid phencyclidine use disorder. If a mild phencyclidine use disorder is comorbid, the ICD-10-CM code is **F16.129,** and if a moderate or severe phencyclidine use disorder is comorbid, the ICD-10-CM code is **F16.229.** If there is no comorbid phencyclidine use disorder, then the ICD-10-CM code is **F16.929.**

Note: In addition to the section "Functional Consequences of Phencyclidine Intoxication," see the corresponding section in phencyclidine use disorder.

Diagnostic Features

Phencyclidine intoxication reflects the clinically significant behavioral changes that occur shortly after ingestion of this substance (or a pharmacologically similar substance). The most common clinical presentations of phencyclidine intoxication include disorientation, confusion without hallucinations, hallucinations or delusions, a catatonic-like syndrome, and coma of varying severity. The intoxication typically lasts for several hours but, depending on the type of clinical presentation and whether other drugs besides phencyclidine were consumed, may last for several days or longer.

Prevalence

Use of phencyclidine or related substances may be taken as an estimate of the prevalence of intoxication. Approximately 2.5% of the population reports having ever used phencyclidine. Among high school students, 2.3% of 12th graders report ever using phencyclidine, with 57% having used in the past 12 months. This represents an increase from prior to 2011. Past-year use of ketamine, which is assessed separately from other substances, has remained stable over time, with about 1.7% of 12th graders reporting use.

Diagnostic Markers

Laboratory testing may be useful, as phencyclidine is detectable in urine for up to 8 days following use, although the levels are only weakly associated with an individual's clinical presentation and may therefore not be useful for case management. Creatine phosphokinase and aspartate aminotransferase levels may be elevated.

Functional Consequences of Phencyclidine Intoxication

Phencyclidine intoxication produces extensive cardiovascular and neurological (e.g., seizures, dystonias, dyskinesias, catalepsy, hypothermia or hyperthermia) toxicity.

Differential Diagnosis

In particular, in the absence of intact reality testing (i.e., without insight into any perceptual abnormalities), an additional diagnosis of phencyclidine-induced psychotic disorder should be considered.

Other substance intoxication. Phencyclidine intoxication should be differentiated from intoxication due to other substances, including other hallucinogens; amphetamine, cocaine, or other stimulants; and anticholinergics, as well as withdrawal from benzodiazepines. Nystagmus and bizarre and violent behavior may distinguish intoxication due to phencyclidine from that due to other substances. Toxicological tests may be useful in making this distinction, since phencyclidine is detectable in urine for up to 8 days after use. However, there is a weak correlation between quantitative toxicology levels of phencyclidine and clinical presentation that diminishes the utility of the laboratory findings for patient management.

Other conditions. Other conditions to be considered include schizophrenia, depression, withdrawal from other drugs (e.g., sedatives, alcohol), certain metabolic disorders like hypoglycemia and hyponatremia, central nervous system tumors, seizure disorders, sepsis, neuroleptic malignant syndrome, and vascular insults.

Other Hallucinogen Intoxication

Diagnostic Criteria

A. Recent use of a hallucinogen (other than phencyclidine).
B. Clinically significant problematic behavioral or psychological changes (e.g., marked anxiety or depression, ideas of reference, fear of "losing one's mind," paranoid ideation, impaired judgment) that developed during, or shortly after, hallucinogen use.
C. Perceptual changes occurring in a state of full wakefulness and alertness (e.g., subjective intensification of perceptions, depersonalization, derealization, illusions, hallucinations, synesthesias) that developed during, or shortly after, hallucinogen use.
D. Two (or more) of the following signs developing during, or shortly after, hallucinogen use:
    1. Pupillary dilation.
    2. Tachycardia.
    3. Sweating.
    4. Palpitations.
    5. Blurring of vision.
    6. Tremors.
    7. Incoordination.
E. The signs or symptoms are not attributable to another medical condition and are not better explained by another mental disorder, including intoxication with another substance.

Coding note: The ICD-9-CM code is **292.89.** The ICD-10-CM code depends on whether there is a comorbid hallucinogen use disorder. If a mild hallucinogen use disorder is comorbid, the ICD-10-CM code is **F16.129,** and if a moderate or severe hallucinogen use disorder is comorbid, the ICD-10-CM code is **F16.229.** If there is no comorbid hallucinogen use disorder, then the ICD-10-CM code is **F16.929.**

Note: For information on Associated Features Supporting Diagnosis and Culture-Related Diagnostic Issues, see the corresponding sections in other hallucinogen use disorder.

Diagnostic Features
Other hallucinogen intoxication reflects the clinically significant behavioral or psychological changes that occur shortly after ingestion of a hallucinogen. Depending on the specific hallucinogen, the intoxication may last only minutes (e.g., for salvia) or several hours or longer (e.g., for LSD [lysergic acid diethylamide] or MDMA [3,4-methylenedioxymethamphetamine]).

Prevalence

The prevalence of other hallucinogen intoxication may be estimated by use of those substances. In the United States, 1.8% of individuals age 12 years or older report using hallucinogens in the past year. Use is more prevalent among younger individuals, with 3.1% of 12- to 17-year-olds and 7.1% of 18- to 25-year-olds using hallucinogens in the past year, compared with only 0.7% of individuals age 26 years or older. Twelve-month prevalence for hallucinogen use is more common in males (2.4%) than in females (1.2%), and even more so among 18- to 25-year-olds (9.2% for males vs. 5.0% for females). In contrast, among individuals ages 12–17 years, there are no gender differences (3.1% for both genders). These figures may be used as proxy estimates for gender-related differences in the prevalence of other hallucinogen intoxication.

Suicide Risk

Other hallucinogen intoxication may lead to increased suicidality, although suicide is rare among users of hallucinogens.

Functional Consequences of Other Hallucinogen Intoxication

Other hallucinogen intoxication can have serious consequences. The perceptual disturbances and impaired judgment associated with other hallucinogen intoxication can result in injuries or fatalities from automobile crashes, physical fights, or unintentional self-injury (e.g., attempts to "fly" from high places). Environmental factors and the personality and expectations of the individual using the hallucinogen may contribute to the nature of and severity of hallucinogen intoxication. Continued use of hallucinogens, particularly MDMA, has also been linked with neurotoxic effects.

Differential Diagnosis

Other substance intoxication.   Other hallucinogen intoxication should be differentiated from intoxication with amphetamines, cocaine, or other stimulants; anticholinergics; inhalants; and phencyclidine. Toxicological tests are useful in making this distinction, and determining the route of administration may also be useful.

Other conditions.   Other disorders and conditions to be considered include schizophrenia, depression, withdrawal from other drugs (e.g., sedatives, alcohol), certain metabolic disorders (e.g., hypoglycemia), seizure disorders, tumors of the central nervous system, and vascular insults.

Hallucinogen persisting perception disorder.   Other hallucinogen intoxication is distinguished from hallucinogen persisting perception disorder because the symptoms in the latter continue episodically or continuously for weeks (or longer) after the most recent intoxication.

Other hallucinogen-induced disorders.   Other hallucinogen intoxication is distinguished from the other hallucinogen-induced disorders (e.g., hallucinogen-induced anxiety disorder, with onset during intoxication) because the symptoms in these latter disorders predominate the clinical presentation and are severe enough to warrant independent clinical attention.

Hallucinogen Persisting Perception Disorder

Diagnostic Criteria	292.89 (F16.983)

A. Following cessation of use of a hallucinogen, the reexperiencing of one or more of the perceptual symptoms that were experienced while intoxicated with the hallucinogen (e.g., geometric hallucinations, false perceptions of movement in the peripheral visual fields, flashes of color, intensified colors, trails of images of moving objects, positive afterimages, halos around objects, macropsia and micropsia).

B. The symptoms in Criterion A cause clinically significant distress or impairment in social, occupational, or other important areas of functioning.

C. The symptoms are not attributable to another medical condition (e.g., anatomical lesions and infections of the brain, visual epilepsies) and are not better explained by another mental disorder (e.g., delirium, major neurocognitive disorder, schizophrenia) or hypnopompic hallucinations.

Diagnostic Features

The hallmark of hallucinogen persisting perception disorder is the reexperiencing, when the individual is sober, of the perceptual disturbances that were experienced while the individual was intoxicated with the hallucinogen (Criterion A). The symptoms may include any perceptual perturbations, but visual disturbances tend to be predominant. Typical of the abnormal visual perceptions are geometric hallucinations, false perceptions of movement in the peripheral visual fields, flashes of color, intensified colors, trails of images of moving objects (i.e., images left suspended in the path of a moving object as seen in stroboscopic photography), perceptions of entire objects, positive afterimages (i.e., a same-colored or complementary-colored "shadow" of an object remaining after removal of the object), halos around objects, or misperception of images as too large (macropsia) or too small (micropsia). Duration of the visual disturbances may be episodic or nearly continuous and must cause clinically significant distress or impairment in social, occupational, or other important areas of functioning (Criterion B). The disturbances may last for weeks, months, or years. Other explanations for the disturbances (e.g., brain lesions, preexisting psychosis, seizure disorders, migraine aura without headaches) must be ruled out (Criterion C).

Hallucinogen persisting perception disorder occurs primarily after LSD (lysergic acid diethylamide) use, but not exclusively. There does not appear to be a strong correlation between hallucinogen persisting perception disorder and number of occasions of hallucinogen use, with some instances of hallucinogen persisting perception disorder occurring in individuals with minimal exposure to hallucinogens. Some instances of hallucinogen persisting perception disorder may be triggered by use of other substances (e.g., cannabis or alcohol) or in adaptation to dark environments.

Associated Features Supporting Diagnosis

Reality testing remains intact in individuals with hallucinogen persisting perception disorder (i.e., the individual is aware that the disturbance is linked to the effect of the drug). If this is not the case, another disorder might better explain the abnormal perceptions.

Prevalence

Prevalence estimates of hallucinogen persisting perception disorder are unknown. Initial prevalence estimates of the disorder among individuals who use hallucinogens is approximately 4.2%.

Development and Course

Little is known about the development of hallucinogen persisting perception disorder. Its course, as suggested by its name, is persistent, lasting for weeks, months, or even years in certain individuals.

Risk and Prognostic Factors

There is little evidence regarding risk factors for hallucinogen persisting perception disorder, although genetic factors have been suggested as a possible explanation underlying the susceptibility to LSD effects in this condition.

Functional Consequences of Hallucinogen Persisting Perception Disorder

Although hallucinogen persisting perception disorder remains a chronic condition in some cases, many individuals with the disorder are able to suppress the disturbances and continue to function normally.

Differential Diagnosis

Conditions to be ruled out include schizophrenia, other drug effects, neurodegenerative disorders, stroke, brain tumors, infections, and head trauma. Neuroimaging results in hallucinogen persisting perception disorder cases are typically negative. As noted earlier, reality testing remains intact (i.e., the individual is aware that the disturbance is linked to the effect of the drug); if this is not the case, another disorder (e.g., psychotic disorder, another medical condition) might better explain the abnormal perceptions.

Comorbidity

Common comorbid mental disorders accompanying hallucinogen persisting perception disorder are panic disorder, alcohol use disorder, and major depressive disorder.

Other Phencyclidine-Induced Disorders

Other phencyclidine-induced disorders are described in other chapters of the manual with disorders with which they share phenomenology (see the substance/medication-induced mental disorders in these chapters): phencyclidine-induced psychotic disorder ("Schizophrenia Spectrum and Other Psychotic Disorders"); phencyclidine-induced bipolar disorder ("Bipolar and Related Disorders"); phencyclidine-induced depressive disorder ("Depressive Disorders"); and phencyclidine-induced anxiety disorder ("Anxiety Disorders"). For phencyclidine-induced intoxication delirium, see the criteria and discussion of delirium in the chapter "Neurocognitive Disorders." These phencyclidine-induced disorders are diagnosed instead of phencyclidine intoxication only when the symptoms are sufficiently severe to warrant independent clinical attention.

Other Hallucinogen-Induced Disorders

The following other hallucinogen-induced disorders are described in other chapters of the manual with disorders with which they share phenomenology (see the substance/medication-induced mental disorders in these chapters): other hallucinogen–induced psychotic disorder ("Schizophrenia Spectrum and Other Psychotic Disorders"); other hallucinogen–induced bipolar disorder ("Bipolar and Related Disorders"); other hallucinogen–induced depressive disorder ("Depressive Disorders"); and other hallucinogen–induced anxiety disorder ("Anxiety Disorders"). For other hallucinogen intoxication delirium, see the criteria and discussion of delirium in the chapter "Neurocognitive Disorders." These hallucinogen-induced disorders are diagnosed instead of other hallucinogen intoxication only when the symptoms are sufficiently severe to warrant independent clinical attention.

Unspecified Phencyclidine-Related Disorder

292.9 (F16.99)

This category applies to presentations in which symptoms characteristic of a phencyclidine-related disorder that cause clinically significant distress or impairment in social, occupational, or other important areas of functioning predominate but do not meet the full criteria for any specific phencyclidine-related disorder or any of the disorders in the substance-related and addictive disorders diagnostic class.

Unspecified Hallucinogen-Related Disorder

292.9 (F16.99)

This category applies to presentations in which symptoms characteristic of a hallucinogen-related disorder that cause clinically significant distress or impairment in social, occupational, or other important areas of functioning predominate but do not meet the full criteria for any specific hallucinogen-related disorder or any of the disorders in the substance-related and addictive disorders diagnostic class.

Inhalant-Related Disorders

Inhalant Use Disorder
Inhalant Intoxication
Other Inhalant-Induced Disorders
Unspecified Inhalant-Related Disorder

Inhalant Use Disorder

Diagnostic Criteria

A. A problematic pattern of use of a hydrocarbon-based inhalant substance leading to clinically significant impairment or distress, as manifested by at least two of the following, occurring within a 12-month period:

1. The inhalant substance is often taken in larger amounts or over a longer period than was intended.
2. There is a persistent desire or unsuccessful efforts to cut down or control use of the inhalant substance.

3. A great deal of time is spent in activities necessary to obtain the inhalant substance, use it, or recover from its effects.
4. Craving, or a strong desire or urge to use the inhalant substance.
5. Recurrent use of the inhalant substance resulting in a failure to fulfill major role obligations at work, school, or home.
6. Continued use of the inhalant substance despite having persistent or recurrent social or interpersonal problems caused or exacerbated by the effects of its use.
7. Important social, occupational, or recreational activities are given up or reduced because of use of the inhalant substance.
8. Recurrent use of the inhalant substance in situations in which it is physically hazardous.
9. Use of the inhalant substance is continued despite knowledge of having a persistent or recurrent physical or psychological problem that is likely to have been caused or exacerbated by the substance.
10. Tolerance, as defined by either of the following:
    a. A need for markedly increased amounts of the inhalant substance to achieve intoxication or desired effect.
    b. A markedly diminished effect with continued use of the same amount of the inhalant substance.

Specify **the particular inhalant:** When possible, the particular substance involved should be named (e.g., "solvent use disorder").

Specify if:

In early remission: After full criteria for inhalant use disorder were previously met, none of the criteria for inhalant use disorder have been met for at least 3 months but for less than 12 months (with the exception that Criterion A4, "Craving, or a strong desire or urge to use the inhalant substance," may be met).

In sustained remission: After full criteria for inhalant use disorder were previously met, none of the criteria for inhalant use disorder have been met at any time during a period of 12 months or longer (with the exception that Criterion A4, "Craving, or a strong desire or urge to use the inhalant substance," may be met).

Specify if:

In a controlled environment: This additional specifier is used if the individual is in an environment where access to inhalant substances is restricted.

Coding based on current severity: Note for ICD-10-CM codes: If an inhalant intoxication or another inhalant-induced mental disorder is also present, do not use the codes below for inhalant use disorder. Instead, the comorbid inhalant use disorder is indicated in the 4th character of the inhalant-induced disorder code (see the coding note for inhalant intoxication or a specific inhalant-induced mental disorder). For example, if there is comorbid inhalant-induced depressive disorder and inhalant use disorder, only the inhalant-induced depressive disorder code is given, with the 4th character indicating whether the comorbid inhalant use disorder is mild, moderate, or severe: F18.14 for mild inhalant use disorder with inhalant-induced depressive disorder or F18.24 for a moderate or severe inhalant use disorder with inhalant-induced depressive disorder.

Specify current severity:

305.90 (F18.10) Mild: Presence of 2–3 symptoms.

304.60 (F18.20) Moderate: Presence of 4–5 symptoms.

304.60 (F18.20) Severe: Presence of 6 or more symptoms.

Specifiers

This manual recognizes volatile hydrocarbon use meeting the above diagnostic criteria as inhalant use disorder. Volatile hydrocarbons are toxic gases from glues, fuels, paints, and other volatile compounds. When possible, the particular substance involved should be named (e.g., "toluene use disorder"). However, most compounds that are inhaled are a mixture of several substances that can produce psychoactive effects, and it is often difficult to ascertain the exact substance responsible for the disorder. Unless there is clear evidence that a single, unmixed substance has been used, the general term inhalant should be used in recording the diagnosis. Disorders arising from inhalation of nitrous oxide or of amyl-, butyl-, or isobutylnitrite are considered as other (or unknown) substance use disorder.

"In a controlled environment" applies as a further specifier of remission if the individual is both in remission and in a controlled environment (i.e., in early remission in a controlled environment or in sustained remission in a controlled environment). Examples of these environments are closely supervised and substance-free jails, therapeutic communities, and locked hospital units.

The severity of individuals' inhalant use disorder is assessed by the number of diagnostic criteria endorsed. Changing severity of individuals' inhalant use disorder across time is reflected by reductions in the frequency (e.g., days used per month) and/or dose (e.g., tubes of glue per day) used, as assessed by the individual's self-report, report of others, clinician's observations, and biological testing (when practical).

Diagnostic Features

Features of inhalant use disorder include repeated use of an inhalant substance despite the individual's knowing that the substance is causing serious problems for the individual (Criterion A9). Those problems are reflected in the diagnostic criteria.

Missing work or school or inability to perform typical responsibilities at work or school (Criterion A5), and continued use of the inhalant substance even though it causes arguments with family or friends, fights, and other social or interpersonal problems (Criterion A6), may be seen in inhalant use disorder. Limiting family contact, work or school obligations, or recreational activities (e.g., sports, games, hobbies) may also occur (Criterion A7). Use of inhalants when driving or operating dangerous equipment (Criterion A8) is also seen.

Tolerance (Criterion A10) and mild withdrawal are each reported by about 10% of individuals who use inhalants, and a few individuals use inhalants to avoid withdrawal. However, because the withdrawal symptoms are mild, this manual neither recognizes a diagnosis of inhalant withdrawal nor counts withdrawal complaints as a diagnostic criterion for inhalant use disorder.

Associated Features Supporting Diagnosis

A diagnosis of inhalant use disorder is supported by recurring episodes of intoxication with negative results in standard drug screens (which do not detect inhalants); possession, or lingering odors, of inhalant substances; peri-oral or peri-nasal "glue-sniffer's rash"; association with other individuals known to use inhalants; membership in groups with prevalent inhalant use (e.g., some native or aboriginal communities, homeless children in street gangs); easy access to certain inhalant substances; paraphernalia possession; presence of the disorder's characteristic medical complications (e.g., brain white matter pathology, rhabdomyolysis); and the presence of multiple substance use disorders. Inhalant use and inhalant use disorder are associated with past suicide attempts, especially among adults reporting previous episodes of low mood or anhedonia.

Prevalence

About 0.4% of Americans ages 12–17 years have a pattern of use that meets criteria for inhalant use disorder in the past 12 months. Among those youths, the prevalence is highest in Native Americans and lowest in African Americans. Prevalence falls to about 0.1% among Americans ages 18–29 years, and only 0.02% when all Americans 18 years or older are considered, with almost no females and a preponderance of European Americans. Of course, in isolated subgroups, prevalence may differ considerably from these overall rates.

Development and Course

About 10% of 13-year-old American children report having used inhalants at least once; that percentage remains stable through age 17 years. Among those 12- to 17-year-olds who use inhalants, the more-used substances include glue, shoe polish, or toluene; gasoline or lighter fluid; or spray paints.

Only 0.4% of 12- to 17-year-olds progress to inhalant use disorder; those youths tend to exhibit multiple other problems. The declining prevalence of inhalant use disorder after adolescence indicates that this disorder usually remits in early adulthood.

Volatile hydrocarbon use disorder is rare in prepubertal children, most common in adolescents and young adults, and uncommon in older persons. Calls to poison-control centers for "intentional abuse" of inhalants peak with calls involving individuals at age 14 years. Of adolescents who use inhalants, perhaps one-fifth develop inhalant use disorder; a few die from inhalant-related accidents, or "sudden sniffing death". But the disorder apparently remits in many individuals after adolescence. Prevalence declines dramatically among individuals in their 20s. Those with inhalant use disorder extending into adulthood often have severe problems: substance use disorders, antisocial personality disorder, and suicidal ideation with attempts.

Risk and Prognostic Factors

Temperamental. Predictors of progression from nonuse of inhalants, to use, to inhalant use disorder include comorbid non-inhalant substance use disorders and either conduct disorder or antisocial personality disorder. Other predictors are earlier onset of inhalant use and prior use of mental health services.

Environmental. Inhalant gases are widely and legally available, increasing the risk of misuse. Childhood maltreatment or trauma also is associated with youthful progression from inhalant non-use to inhalant use disorder.

Genetic and physiological. *Behavioral disinhibition* is a highly heritable general propensity to not constrain behavior in socially acceptable ways, to break social norms and rules, and to take dangerous risks, pursuing rewards excessively despite dangers of adverse consequences. Youths with strong behavioral disinhibition show risk factors for inhalant use disorder: early-onset substance use disorder, multiple substance involvement, and early conduct problems. Because behavioral disinhibition is under strong genetic influence, youths in families with substance and antisocial problems are at elevated risk for inhalant use disorder.

Culture-Related Diagnostic Issues

Certain native or aboriginal communities have experienced a high prevalence of inhalant problems. Also, in some countries, groups of homeless children in street gangs have extensive inhalant use problems.

Gender-Related Diagnostic Issues

Although the prevalence of inhalant use disorder is almost identical in adolescent males and females, the disorder is very rare among adult females.

Diagnostic Markers

Urine, breath, or saliva tests may be valuable for assessing concurrent use of non-inhalant substances by individuals with inhalant use disorder. However, technical problems and the considerable expense of analyses make frequent biological testing for inhalants themselves impractical.

Functional Consequences of Inhalant Use Disorder

Because of inherent toxicity, use of butane or propane is not infrequently fatal. Moreover, any inhaled volatile hydrocarbons may produce "sudden sniffing death" from cardiac arrhythmia. Fatalities may occur even on the first inhalant exposure and are not thought to be dose-related. Volatile hydrocarbon use impairs neurobehavioral function and causes various neurological, gastrointestinal, cardiovascular, and pulmonary problems.

Long-term inhalant users are at increased risk for tuberculosis, HIV/AIDS, sexually transmitted diseases, depression, anxiety, bronchitis, asthma, and sinusitis. Deaths may occur from respiratory depression, arrhythmias, asphyxiation, aspiration of vomitus, or accident and injury.

Differential Diagnosis

Inhalant exposure (unintentional) from industrial or other accidents.   This designation is used when findings suggest repeated or continuous inhalant exposure but the involved individual and other informants deny any history of purposeful inhalant use.

Inhalant use (intentional), without meeting criteria for inhalant use disorder.   Inhalant use is common among adolescents, but for most of those individuals, the inhalant use does not meet the diagnostic standard of two or more Criterion A items for inhalant use disorder in the past year.

Inhalant intoxication, without meeting criteria for inhalant use disorder.   Inhalant intoxication occurs frequently during inhalant use disorder but also may occur among individuals whose use does not meet criteria for inhalant use disorder, which requires at least two of the 10 diagnostic criteria in the past year.

Inhalant-induced disorders (i.e., inhalant-induced psychotic disorder, depressive disorder, anxiety disorder, neurocognitive disorder, other inhalant-induced disorders) without meeting criteria for inhalant use disorder.   Criteria are met for a psychotic, depressive, anxiety, or major neurocognitive disorder, and there is evidence from history, physical examination, or laboratory findings that the deficits are etiologically related to the effects of inhalant substances. Yet, criteria for inhalant use disorder may not be met (i.e., fewer than 2 of the 10 criteria were present).

Other substance use disorders, especially those involving sedating substances (e.g., alcohol, benzodiazepines, barbiturates).   Inhalant use disorder commonly co-occurs with other substance use disorders, and the symptoms of the disorders may be similar and overlapping. To disentangle symptom patterns, it is helpful to inquire about which symptoms persisted during periods when some of the substances were not being used.

Other toxic, metabolic, traumatic, neoplastic, or infectious disorders impairing central or peripheral nervous system function.   Individuals with inhalant use disorder may present with symptoms of pernicious anemia, subacute combined degeneration of the spinal cord, psychosis, major or minor cognitive disorder, brain atrophy, leukoencephalopathy, and many other nervous system disorders. Of course, these disorders also may occur in the absence of inhalant use disorder. A history of little or no inhalant use helps to exclude inhalant use disorder as the source of these problems.

Disorders of other organ systems.   Individuals with inhalant use disorder may present with symptoms of hepatic or renal damage, rhabdomyolysis, methemoglobinemia, or symptoms of other gastrointestinal, cardiovascular, or pulmonary diseases. A history of little or no inhalant use helps to exclude inhalant use disorder as the source of such medical problems.

Comorbidity

Individuals with inhalant use disorder receiving clinical care often have numerous other substance use disorders. Inhalant use disorder commonly co-occurs with adolescent conduct disorder and adult antisocial personality disorder. Adult inhalant use and inhalant use disorder also are strongly associated with suicidal ideation and suicide attempts.

Inhalant Intoxication

Diagnostic Criteria

A. Recent intended or unintended short-term, high-dose exposure to inhalant substances, including volatile hydrocarbons such as toluene or gasoline.

B. Clinically significant problematic behavioral or psychological changes (e.g., belligerence, assaultiveness, apathy, impaired judgment) that developed during, or shortly after, exposure to inhalants.

C. Two (or more) of the following signs or symptoms developing during, or shortly after, inhalant use or exposure:

1. Dizziness.
2. Nystagmus.
3. Incoordination.
4. Slurred speech.
5. Unsteady gait.
6. Lethargy.
7. Depressed reflexes.
8. Psychomotor retardation.
9. Tremor.
10. Generalized muscle weakness.
11. Blurred vision or diplopia.
12. Stupor or coma.
13. Euphoria.

D. The signs or symptoms are not attributable to another medical condition and are not better explained by another mental disorder, including intoxication with another substance.

Coding note: The ICD-9-CM code is **292.89.** The ICD-10-CM code depends on whether there is a comorbid inhalant use disorder. If a mild inhalant use disorder is comorbid, the ICD-10-CM code is **F18.129,** and if a moderate or severe inhalant use disorder is comorbid, the ICD-10-CM code is **F18.229.** If there is no comorbid inhalant use disorder, then the ICD-10-CM code is **F18.929.**

Note: For information on Development and Course, Risk and Prognostic Factors, Culture-Related Diagnostic Issues, and Diagnostic Markers, see the corresponding sections in inhalant use disorder.

Diagnostic Features

Inhalant intoxication is an inhalant-related, clinically significant mental disorder that develops during, or immediately after, intended or unintended inhalation of a volatile hydrocarbon substance. Volatile hydrocarbons are toxic gases from glues, fuels, paints, and other volatile compounds. When it is possible to do so, the particular substance involved should be named (e.g., toluene intoxication). Among those who do, the intoxication clears within a few minutes to a few hours after the exposure ends. Thus, inhalant intoxication usually occurs in brief episodes that may recur.

Associated Features Supporting Diagnosis

Inhalant intoxication may be indicated by evidence of possession, or lingering odors, of inhalant substances (e.g., glue, paint thinner, gasoline, butane lighters); apparent intoxication occurring in the age range with the highest prevalence of inhalant use (12–17 years); and apparent intoxication with negative results from the standard drug screens that usually fail to identify inhalants.

Prevalence

The prevalence of actual episodes of inhalant intoxication in the general population is unknown, but it is probable that most inhalant users would at some time exhibit use that would meet criteria for inhalant intoxication disorder. Therefore, the prevalence of inhalant use and the prevalence of inhalant intoxication disorder are likely similar. In 2009 and 2010, inhalant use in the past year was reported by 0.8% of all Americans older than 12 years; the prevalence was highest in younger age groups (3.6% for individuals 12 to 17 years old, and 1.7% for individuals 18 to 25 years old).

Gender-Related Diagnostic Issues

Gender differences in the prevalence of inhalant intoxication in the general population are unknown. However, if it is assumed that most inhalant users eventually experience inhalant intoxication, gender differences in the prevalence of inhalant *users* likely approximate those in the proportions of males and females experiencing inhalant intoxication. Regarding gender differences in the prevalence of inhalant users in the United States, 1% of males older than 12 years and 0.7% of females older than 12 years have used inhalants in the previous year, but in the younger age groups more females than males have used inhalants (e.g., among 12- to 17-year-olds, 3.6% of males and 4.2% of females).

Functional Consequences of Inhalant Intoxication

Use of inhaled substances in a closed container, such as a plastic bag over the head, may lead to unconsciousness, anoxia, and death. Separately, "sudden sniffing death," likely from cardiac arrhythmia or arrest, may occur with various volatile inhalants. The enhanced toxicity of certain volatile inhalants, such as butane or propane, also causes fatalities. Although inhalant intoxication itself is of short duration, it may produce persisting medical and neurological problems, especially if the intoxications are frequent.

Differential Diagnosis

Inhalant exposure, without meeting the criteria for inhalant intoxication disorder. The individual intentionally or unintentionally inhaled substances, but the dose was insufficient for the diagnostic criteria for inhalant use disorder to be met.

Intoxication and other substance/medication-induced disorders from other substances, especially from sedating substances (e.g., alcohol, benzodiazepines, barbiturates). These disorders may have similar signs and symptoms, but the intoxication is attributable to other intoxicants that may be identified via a toxicology screen. Differentiating the source of the intoxication may involve discerning evidence of inhalant exposure as described for inhalant use disorder. A diagnosis of inhalant intoxication may be suggested by possession, or lingering odors, of inhalant substances (e.g., glue, paint thinner, gasoline, butane lighters,); paraphernalia possession (e.g., rags or bags for concentrating glue fumes); perioral or perinasal "glue-sniffer's rash"; reports from family or friends that the intoxicated individual possesses or uses inhalants; apparent intoxication despite negative results on standard drug screens (which usually fail to identify inhalants); apparent intoxication occurring in that age range with the highest prevalence of inhalant use (12–17 years); association with others known to use inhalants; membership in certain small communities with prevalent inhalant use (e.g., some native or aboriginal communities, homeless street children and adolescents); or unusual access to certain inhalant substances.

Other inhalant-related disorders.   Episodes of inhalant intoxication do occur during, but are not identical with, other inhalant-related disorders. Those inhalant-related disorders are recognized by their respective diagnostic criteria: inhalant use disorder, inhalant-induced neurocognitive disorder, inhalant-induced psychotic disorder, inhalant-induced depressive disorder, inhalant-induced anxiety disorder, and other inhalant-induced disorders.

Other toxic, metabolic, traumatic, neoplastic, or infectious disorders that impair brain function and cognition.   Numerous neurological and other medical conditions may produce the clinically significant behavioral or psychological changes (e.g., belligerence, assaultiveness, apathy, impaired judgment) that also characterize inhalant intoxication.

Other Inhalant-Induced Disorders

The following inhalant-induced disorders are described in other chapters of the manual with disorders with which they share phenomenology (see the substance/medication-induced mental disorders in these chapters): inhalant-induced psychotic disorder ("Schizophrenia Spectrum and Other Psychotic Disorders"); inhalant-induced depressive disorder ("Depressive Disorders"); inhalant-induced anxiety disorder ("Anxiety Disorders"); and inhalant-induced major or mild neurocognitive disorder ("Neurocognitive Disorders"). For inhalant intoxication delirium, see the criteria and discussion of delirium in the chapter "Neurocognitive Disorders." These inhalant-induced disorders are diagnosed instead of inhalant intoxication only when symptoms are sufficiently severe to warrant independent clinical attention.

Unspecified Inhalant-Related Disorder

292.9 (F18.99)

This category applies to presentations in which symptoms characteristic of an inhalant-related disorder that cause clinically significant distress or impairment in social, occupational, or other important areas of functioning predominate but do not meet the full criteria for any specific inhalant-related disorder or any of the disorders in the substance-related and addictive disorders diagnostic class.

Opioid-Related Disorders

Opioid Use Disorder
Opioid Intoxication
Opioid Withdrawal
Other Opioid-Induced Disorders
Unspecified Opioid-Related Disorder

Opioid Use Disorder

Diagnostic Criteria

A. A problematic pattern of opioid use leading to clinically significant impairment or distress, as manifested by at least two of the following, occurring within a 12-month period:

1. Opioids are often taken in larger amounts or over a longer period than was intended.
2. There is a persistent desire or unsuccessful efforts to cut down or control opioid use.
3. A great deal of time is spent in activities necessary to obtain the opioid, use the opioid, or recover from its effects.
4. Craving, or a strong desire or urge to use opioids.
5. Recurrent opioid use resulting in a failure to fulfill major role obligations at work, school, or home.
6. Continued opioid use despite having persistent or recurrent social or interpersonal problems caused or exacerbated by the effects of opioids.
7. Important social, occupational, or recreational activities are given up or reduced because of opioid use.
8. Recurrent opioid use in situations in which it is physically hazardous.
9. Continued opioid use despite knowledge of having a persistent or recurrent physical or psychological problem that is likely to have been caused or exacerbated by the substance.
10. Tolerance, as defined by either of the following:
    a. A need for markedly increased amounts of opioids to achieve intoxication or desired effect.
    b. A markedly diminished effect with continued use of the same amount of an opioid.

    Note: This criterion is not considered to be met for those taking opioids solely under appropriate medical supervision.
11. Withdrawal, as manifested by either of the following:
    a. The characteristic opioid withdrawal syndrome (refer to Criteria A and B of the criteria set for opioid withdrawal, pp. 547–548).
    b. Opioids (or a closely related substance) are taken to relieve or avoid withdrawal symptoms.

    Note: This criterion is not considered to be met for those individuals taking opioids solely under appropriate medical supervision.

Specify if:
   In early remission: After full criteria for opioid use disorder were previously met, none of the criteria for opioid use disorder have been met for at least 3 months but for less than 12 months (with the exception that Criterion A4, "Craving, or a strong desire or urge to use opioids," may be met).
   In sustained remission: After full criteria for opioid use disorder were previously met, none of the criteria for opioid use disorder have been met at any time during a period of 12 months or longer (with the exception that Criterion A4, "Craving, or a strong desire or urge to use opioids," may be met).

Specify if:
   On maintenance therapy: This additional specifier is used if the individual is taking a prescribed agonist medication such as methadone or buprenorphine and none of the criteria for opioid use disorder have been met for that class of medication (except tolerance to, or withdrawal from, the agonist). This category also applies to those individ-

uals being maintained on a partial agonist, an agonist/antagonist, or a full antagonist such as oral naltrexone or depot naltrexone.

In a controlled environment: This additional specifier is used if the individual is in an environment where access to opioids is restricted.

Coding based on current severity: Note for ICD-10-CM codes: If an opioid intoxication, opioid withdrawal, or another opioid-induced mental disorder is also present, do not use the codes below for opioid use disorder. Instead, the comorbid opioid use disorder is indicated in the 4th character of the opioid-induced disorder code (see the coding note for opioid intoxication, opioid withdrawal, or a specific opioid-induced mental disorder). For example, if there is comorbid opioid-induced depressive disorder and opioid use disorder, only the opioid-induced depressive disorder code is given, with the 4th character indicating whether the comorbid opioid use disorder is mild, moderate, or severe: F11.14 for mild opioid use disorder with opioid-induced depressive disorder or F11.24 for a moderate or severe opioid use disorder with opioid-induced depressive disorder.

Specify current severity:

305.50 (F11.10) Mild: Presence of 2–3 symptoms.

304.00 (F11.20) Moderate: Presence of 4–5 symptoms.

304.00 (F11.20) Severe: Presence of 6 or more symptoms.

Specifiers

The "on maintenance therapy" specifier applies as a further specifier of remission if the individual is both in remission and receiving maintenance therapy. "In a controlled environment" applies as a further specifier of remission if the individual is both in remission and in a controlled environment (i.e., in early remission in a controlled environment or in sustained remission in a controlled environment). Examples of these environments are closely supervised and substance-free jails, therapeutic communities, and locked hospital units.

Changing severity across time in an individual is also reflected by reductions in the frequency (e.g., days of use per month) and/or dose (e.g., injections or number of pills) of an opioid, as assessed by the individual's self-report, report of knowledgeable others, clinician's observations, and biological testing.

Diagnostic Features

Opioid use disorder includes signs and symptoms that reflect compulsive, prolonged self-administration of opioid substances that are used for no legitimate medical purpose or, if another medical condition is present that requires opioid treatment, that are used in doses greatly in excess of the amount needed for that medical condition. (For example, an individual prescribed analgesic opioids for pain relief at adequate dosing will use significantly more than prescribed and not only because of persistent pain.) Individuals with opioid use disorder tend to develop such regular patterns of compulsive drug use that daily activities are planned around obtaining and administering opioids. Opioids are usually purchased on the illegal market but may also be obtained from physicians by falsifying or exaggerating general medical problems or by receiving simultaneous prescriptions from several physicians. Health care professionals with opioid use disorder will often obtain opioids by writing prescriptions for themselves or by diverting opioids that have been prescribed for patients or from pharmacy supplies. Most individuals with opioid use disorder have significant levels of tolerance and will experience withdrawal on abrupt discontinuation of opioid substances. Individuals with opioid use disorder often develop conditioned responses to drug-related stimuli (e.g., craving on seeing any heroin powder–like substance)—a phenomenon that occurs with most drugs that cause intense psychological changes. These responses probably contribute to relapse, are difficult to extinguish, and typically persist long after detoxification is completed.

Associated Features Supporting Diagnosis

Opioid use disorder can be associated with a history of drug-related crimes (e.g., possession or distribution of drugs, forgery, burglary, robbery, larceny, receiving stolen goods). Among health care professionals and individuals who have ready access to controlled substances, there is often a different pattern of illegal activities involving problems with state licensing boards, professional staffs of hospitals, or other administrative agencies. Marital difficulties (including divorce), unemployment, and irregular employment are often associated with opioid use disorder at all socioeconomic levels.

Prevalence

The 12-month prevalence of opioid use disorder is approximately 0.37% among adults age 18 years and older in the community population. This may be an underestimate because of the large number of incarcerated individuals with opioid use disorders. Rates are higher in males than in females (0.49% vs. 0.26%), with the male-to-female ratio typically being 1.5:1 for opioids other than heroin (i.e., available by prescription) and 3:1 for heroin. Female adolescents may have a higher likelihood of developing opioid use disorders. The prevalence decreases with age, with the prevalence highest (0.82%) among adults age 29 years or younger, and decreasing to 0.09% among adults age 65 years and older. Among adults, the prevalence of opioid use disorder is lower among African Americans at 0.18% and over-represented among Native Americans at 1.25%. It is close to average among whites (0.38%), Asian or Pacific Islanders (0.35%), and Hispanics (0.39%).

Among individuals in the United States ages 12–17 years, the overall 12-month prevalence of opioid use disorder in the community population is approximately 1.0%, but the prevalence of heroin use disorder is less than 0.1%. By contrast, analgesic use disorder is prevalent in about 1.0% of those ages 12–17 years, speaking to the importance of opioid analgesics as a group of substances with significant health consequences.

The 12-month prevalence of problem opioid use in European countries in the community population ages 15–64 years is between 0.1% and 0.8%. The average prevalence of problem opioid use in the European Union and Norway is between 0.36% and 0.44%.

Development and Course

Opioid use disorder can begin at any age, but problems associated with opioid use are most commonly first observed in the late teens or early 20s. Once opioid use disorder develops, it usually continues over a period of many years, even though brief periods of abstinence are frequent. In treated populations, relapse following abstinence is common. Even though relapses do occur, and while some long-term mortality rates may be as high as 2% per year, about 20%–30% of individuals with opioid use disorder achieve long-term abstinence. An exception concerns that of military service personnel who became dependent on opioids in Vietnam; over 90% of this population who had been dependent on opioids during deployment in Vietnam achieved abstinence after they returned, but they experienced increased rates of alcohol or amphetamine use disorder as well as increased suicidality.

Increasing age is associated with a decrease in prevalence as a result of early mortality and the remission of symptoms after age 40 years (i.e., "maturing out"). However, many individuals continue have presentations that meet opioid use disorder criteria for decades.

Risk and Prognostic Factors

Genetic and physiological.   The risk for opioid use disorder can be related to individual, family, peer, and social environmental factors, but within these domains, genetic factors play a particularly important role both directly and indirectly. For instance, impulsivity and novelty seeking are individual temperaments that relate to the propensity to develop a substance use disorder but may themselves be genetically determined. Peer factors may relate to genetic predisposition in terms of how an individual selects his or her environment.

Culture-Related Diagnostic Issues

Despite small variations regarding individual criterion items, opioid use disorder diagnostic criteria perform equally well across most race/ethnicity groups. Individuals from ethnic minority populations living in economically deprived areas have been overrepresented among individuals with opioid use disorder. However, over time, opioid use disorder is seen more often among white middle-class individuals, especially females, suggesting that differences in use reflect the availability of opioid drugs and that other social factors may impact prevalence. Medical personnel who have ready access to opioids may be at increased risk for opioid use disorder.

Diagnostic Markers

Routine urine toxicology test results are often positive for opioid drugs in individuals with opioid use disorder. Urine test results remain positive for most opioids (e.g., heroin, morphine, codeine, oxycodone, propoxyphene) for 12–36 hours after administration. Fentanyl is not detected by standard urine tests but can be identified by more specialized procedures for several days. Methadone, buprenorphine (or buprenorphine/naloxone combination), and LAAM (L-alpha-acetylmethadol) have to be specifically tested for and will not cause a positive result on routine tests for opiates. They can be detected for several days up to more than 1 week. Laboratory evidence of the presence of other substances (e.g., cocaine, marijuana, alcohol, amphetamines, benzodiazepines) is common. Screening test results for hepatitis A, B, and C virus are positive in as many as 80%–90% of injection opioid users, either for hepatitis antigen (signifying active infection) or for hepatitis antibody (signifying past infection). HIV is prevalent in injection opioid users as well. Mildly elevated liver function test results are common, either as a result of resolving hepatitis or from toxic injury to the liver due to contaminants that have been mixed with the injected opioid. Subtle changes in cortisol secretion patterns and body temperature regulation have been observed for up to 6 months following opioid detoxification.

Suicide Risk

Similar to the risk generally observed for all substance use disorders, opioid use disorder is associated with a heightened risk for suicide attempts and completed suicides. Particularly notable are both accidental and deliberate opioid overdoses. Some suicide risk factors overlap with risk factors for an opioid use disorder. In addition, repeated opioid intoxication or withdrawal may be associated with severe depressions that, although temporary, can be intense enough to lead to suicide attempts and completed suicides. Available data suggest that nonfatal accidental opioid overdose (which is common) and attempted suicide are distinct clinically significant problems that should not be mistaken for each other.

Functional Consequences of Opioid Use Disorder

Opioid use is associated with a lack of mucous membrane secretions, causing dry mouth and nose. Slowing of gastrointestinal activity and a decrease in gut motility can produce severe constipation. Visual acuity may be impaired as a result of pupillary constriction with acute administration. In individuals who inject opioids, sclerosed veins ("tracks") and puncture marks on the lower portions of the upper extremities are common. Veins sometimes become so severely sclerosed that peripheral edema develops, and individuals switch to injecting in veins in the legs, neck, or groin. When these veins become unusable, individuals often inject directly into their subcutaneous tissue ("skin-popping"), resulting in cellulitis, abscesses, and circular-appearing scars from healed skin lesions. Tetanus and *Clostridium botulinum* infections are relatively rare but extremely serious consequences of injecting opioids, especially with contaminated needles. Infections may also occur in other organs and include bacterial endocarditis, hepatitis, and HIV infection. Hepatitis C infections, for example, may occur in up to 90% of persons who inject opioids. In addition, the prevalence of HIV infection can be high among individuals who inject drugs, a large proportion of whom are individuals with opioid use disorder. HIV infection rates have been reported to be as high as 60% among heroin users with opioid use disorder in some areas of the United States or the Russian Federation. However, the incidence may also be 10% or less in other areas, especially those where access to clean injection material and paraphernalia is facilitated.

Tuberculosis is a particularly serious problem among individuals who use drugs intravenously, especially those who are dependent on heroin; infection is usually asymptomatic and evident only by the presence of a positive tuberculin skin test. However, many cases of active tuberculosis have been found, especially among those who are infected with HIV. These individuals often have a newly acquired infection but also are likely to experience reactivation of a prior infection because of impaired immune function.

Individuals who sniff heroin or other opioids into the nose ("snorting") often develop irritation of the nasal mucosa, sometimes accompanied by perforation of the nasal septum. Difficulties in sexual functioning are common. Males often experience erectile dysfunction during intoxication or chronic use. Females commonly have disturbances of reproductive function and irregular menses.

In relation to infections such as cellulitis, hepatitis, HIV infection, tuberculosis, and endocarditis, opioid use disorder is associated with a mortality rate as high as 1.5%–2% per year. Death most often results from overdose, accidents, injuries, AIDS, or other general medical complications. Accidents and injuries due to violence that is associated with buying or selling drugs are common. In some areas, violence accounts for more opioid-related deaths than overdose or HIV infection. Physiological dependence on opioids may occur in about half of the infants born to females with opioid use disorder; this can produce a severe withdrawal syndrome requiring medical treatment. Although low birth weight is also seen in children of mothers with opioid use disorder, it is usually not marked and is generally not associated with serious adverse consequences.

Differential Diagnosis

Opioid-induced mental disorders.   Opioid-induced disorders occur frequently in individuals with opioid use disorder. Opioid-induced disorders may be characterized by symptoms (e.g., depressed mood) that resemble primary mental disorders (e.g., persistent depressive disorder [dysthymia] vs. opioid-induced depressive disorder, with depressive features, with onset during intoxication). Opioids are less likely to produce symptoms of mental disturbance than are most other drugs of abuse. Opioid intoxication and opioid withdrawal are distinguished from the other opioid-induced disorders (e.g., opioid-induced depressive disorder, with onset during intoxication) because the symptoms in these latter disorders predominate the clinical presentation and are severe enough to warrant independent clinical attention.

Other substance intoxication.   Alcohol intoxication and sedative, hypnotic, or anxiolytic intoxication can cause a clinical picture that resembles that for opioid intoxication. A diagnosis of alcohol or sedative, hypnotic, or anxiolytic intoxication can usually be made based on the absence of pupillary constriction or the lack of a response to naloxone challenge. In some cases, intoxication may be due both to opioids and to alcohol or other sedatives. In these cases, the naloxone challenge will not reverse all of the sedative effects.

Other withdrawal disorders.   The anxiety and restlessness associated with opioid withdrawal resemble symptoms seen in sedative-hypnotic withdrawal. However, opioid withdrawal is also accompanied by rhinorrhea, lacrimation, and pupillary dilation, which are not seen in sedative-type withdrawal. Dilated pupils are also seen in hallucinogen intoxication and stimulant intoxication. However, other signs or symptoms of opioid withdrawal, such as nausea, vomiting, diarrhea, abdominal cramps, rhinorrhea, or lacrimation, are not present.

Comorbidity

The most common medical conditions associated with opioid use disorder are viral (e.g., HIV, hepatitis C virus) and bacterial infections, particularly among users of opioids by injection. These infections are less common in opioid use disorder with prescription opioids. Opioid use disorder is often associated with other substance use disorders, especially those involving tobacco, alcohol, cannabis, stimulants, and benzodiazepines, which are often taken to reduce symptoms of opioid withdrawal or craving for opioids, or to enhance the effects of administered opioids. Individuals with opioid use disorder are at risk for the development of mild to moderate depression that meets symptomatic and duration criteria for persistent depressive disorder (dysthymia) or, in some cases, for major depressive disorder. These symptoms may represent an opioid-induced depressive disorder or an exacerbation of a preexisting primary depressive disorder. Periods of depression are especially common during chronic intoxication or in association with physical or psychosocial stressors that are related to the opioid use disorder. Insomnia is common, especially during withdrawal. Antisocial personality disorder is much more common in individuals with opioid use disorder than in the general population. Posttraumatic stress disorder is also seen with increased frequency. A history of conduct disorder in childhood or adolescence has been identified as a significant risk factor for substance-related disorders, especially opioid use disorder.

Opioid Intoxication

Diagnostic Criteria

A. Recent use of an opioid.

B. Clinically significant problematic behavioral or psychological changes (e.g., initial euphoria followed by apathy, dysphoria, psychomotor agitation or retardation, impaired judgment) that developed during, or shortly after, opioid use.

C. Pupillary constriction (or pupillary dilation due to anoxia from severe overdose) and one (or more) of the following signs or symptoms developing during, or shortly after, opioid use:

1. Drowsiness or coma.
2. Slurred speech.
3. Impairment in attention or memory.

D. The signs or symptoms are not attributable to another medical condition and are not better explained by another mental disorder, including intoxication with another substance.

Specify if:

With perceptual disturbances: This specifier may be noted in the rare instance in which hallucinations with intact reality testing or auditory, visual, or tactile illusions occur in the absence of a delirium.

Coding note: The ICD-9-CM code is **292.89.** The ICD-10-CM code depends on whether or not there is a comorbid opioid use disorder and whether or not there are perceptual disturbances.

For opioid intoxication without perceptual disturbances: If a mild opioid use disorder is comorbid, the ICD-10-CM code is **F11.129,** and if a moderate or severe opioid use disorder is comorbid, the ICD-10-CM code is **F11.229.** If there is no comorbid opioid use disorder, then the ICD-10-CM code is **F11.929.**

For opioid intoxication with perceptual disturbances: If a mild opioid use disorder is comorbid, the ICD-10-CM code is **F11.122,** and if a moderate or severe opioid use disorder is comorbid, the ICD-10-CM code is **F11.222.** If there is no comorbid opioid use disorder, then the ICD-10-CM code is **F11.922.**

Diagnostic Features

The essential feature of opioid intoxication is the presence of clinically significant problematic behavioral or psychological changes (e.g., initial euphoria followed by apathy, dysphoria, psychomotor agitation or retardation, impaired judgment) that develop during, or shortly after, opioid use (Criteria A and B). Intoxication is accompanied by pupillary constriction (unless there has been a severe overdose with consequent anoxia and pupillary dilation) and one or more of the following signs: drowsiness (described as being "on the nod"), slurred speech, and impairment in attention or memory (Criterion C); drowsiness may progress to coma. Individuals with opioid intoxication may demonstrate inattention to the environment, even to the point of ignoring potentially harmful events. The signs or symptoms must not be attributable to another medical condition and are not better explained by another mental disorder (Criterion D).

Differential Diagnosis

Other substance intoxication.   Alcohol intoxication and sedative-hypnotic intoxication can cause a clinical picture that resembles opioid intoxication. A diagnosis of alcohol or sedative-hypnotic intoxication can usually be made based on the absence of pupillary constriction or the lack of a response to a naloxone challenge. In some cases, intoxication may be due both to opioids and to alcohol or other sedatives. In these cases, the naloxone challenge will not reverse all of the sedative effects.

Other opioid-related disorders.   Opioid intoxication is distinguished from the other opioid-induced disorders (e.g., opioid-induced depressive disorder, with onset during intoxication) because the symptoms in the latter disorders predominate in the clinical presentation and meet full criteria for the relevant disorder.

Opioid Withdrawal

Diagnostic Criteria   **292.0 (F11.23)**

A. Presence of either of the following:
   1. Cessation of (or reduction in) opioid use that has been heavy and prolonged (i.e., several weeks or longer).
   2. Administration of an opioid antagonist after a period of opioid use.

B. Three (or more) of the following developing within minutes to several days after Criterion A:
   1. Dysphoric mood.
   2. Nausea or vomiting.
   3. Muscle aches.
   4. Lacrimation or rhinorrhea.
   5. Pupillary dilation, piloerection, or sweating.

   6. Diarrhea.
   7. Yawning.
   8. Fever.
   9. Insomnia.

C. The signs or symptoms in Criterion B cause clinically significant distress or impairment in social, occupational, or other important areas of functioning.

D. The signs or symptoms are not attributable to another medical condition and are not better explained by another mental disorder, including intoxication or withdrawal from another substance.

Coding note: The ICD-9-CM code is 292.0. The ICD-10-CM code for opioid withdrawal is F11.23. Note that the ICD-10-CM code indicates the comorbid presence of a moderate or severe opioid use disorder, reflecting the fact that opioid withdrawal can only occur in the presence of a moderate or severe opioid use disorder. It is not permissible to code a comorbid mild opioid use disorder with opioid withdrawal.

Diagnostic Features

The essential feature of opioid withdrawal is the presence of a characteristic withdrawal syndrome that develops after the cessation of (or reduction in) opioid use that has been heavy and prolonged (Criterion A1). The withdrawal syndrome can also be precipitated by administration of an opioid antagonist (e.g., naloxone or naltrexone) after a period of opioid use (Criterion A2). This may also occur after administration of an opioid partial agonist such as buprenorphine to a person currently using a full opioid agonist.

Opioid withdrawal is characterized by a pattern of signs and symptoms that are opposite to the acute agonist effects. The first of these are subjective and consist of complaints of anxiety, restlessness, and an "achy feeling" that is often located in the back and legs, along with irritability and increased sensitivity to pain. Three or more of the following must be present to make a diagnosis of opioid withdrawal: dysphoric mood; nausea or vomiting; muscle aches; lacrimation or rhinorrhea; pupillary dilation, piloerection, or increased sweating; diarrhea; yawning; fever; and insomnia (Criterion B). Piloerection and fever are associated with more severe withdrawal and are not often seen in routine clinical practice because individuals with opioid use disorder usually obtain substances before withdrawal becomes that far advanced. These symptoms of opioid withdrawal must cause clinically significant distress or impairment in social, occupational, or other important areas of functioning (Criterion C). The symptoms must not be attributable to another medical condition and are not better explained by another mental disorder (Criterion D). Meeting diagnostic criteria for opioid withdrawal alone is not sufficient for a diagnosis of opioid use disorder, but concurrent symptoms of craving and drug-seeking behavior are suggestive of comorbid opioid use disorder. ICD-10-CM codes only allow a diagnosis of opioid withdrawal in the presence of comorbid moderate to severe opioid use disorder.

The speed and severity of withdrawal associated with opioids depend on the half-life of the opioid used. Most individuals who are physiologically dependent on short-acting drugs such as heroin begin to have withdrawal symptoms within 6–12 hours after the last dose. Symptoms may take 2–4 days to emerge in the case of longer-acting drugs such as methadone, LAAM (L-alpha-acetylmethadol), or buprenorphine. Acute withdrawal symptoms for a short-acting opioid such as heroin usually peak within 1–3 days and gradually subside over a period of 5–7 days. Less acute withdrawal symptoms can last for weeks to months. These more chronic symptoms include anxiety, dysphoria, anhedonia, and insomnia.

Associated Features Supporting Diagnosis

Males with opioid withdrawal may experience piloerection, sweating, and spontaneous ejaculations while awake. Opioid withdrawal is distinct from opioid use disorder and does not necessarily occur in the presence of the drug-seeking behavior associated with opioid use disorder. Opioid withdrawal may occur in any individual after cessation of repeated use of an opioid, whether in the setting of medical management of pain, during opioid agonist therapy for opioid use disorder, in the context of private recreational use, or following attempts to self-treat symptoms of mental disorders with opioids.

Prevalence

Among individuals from various clinical settings, opioid withdrawal occurred in 60% of individuals who had used heroin at least once in the prior 12 months.

Development and Course

Opioid withdrawal is typical in the course of an opioid use disorder. It can be part of an escalating pattern in which an opioid is used to reduce withdrawal symptoms, in turn leading to more withdrawal at a later time. For persons with an established opioid use disorder, withdrawal and attempts to relieve withdrawal are typical.

Differential Diagnosis

Other withdrawal disorders.   The anxiety and restlessness associated with opioid withdrawal resemble symptoms seen in sedative-hypnotic withdrawal. However, opioid withdrawal is also accompanied by rhinorrhea, lacrimation, and pupillary dilation, which are not seen in sedative-type withdrawal.

Other substance intoxication.   Dilated pupils are also seen in hallucinogen intoxication and stimulant intoxication. However, other signs or symptoms of opioid withdrawal, such as nausea, vomiting, diarrhea, abdominal cramps, rhinorrhea, and lacrimation, are not present.

Other opioid-induced disorders.   Opioid withdrawal is distinguished from the other opioid-induced disorders (e.g., opioid-induced depressive disorder, with onset during withdrawal) because the symptoms in these latter disorders are in excess of those usually associated with opioid withdrawal and meet full criteria for the relevant disorder.

Other Opioid-Induced Disorders

The following opioid-induced disorders are described in other chapters of the manual with disorders with which they share phenomenology (see the substance/medication-induced mental disorders in these chapters): opioid-induced depressive disorder ("Depressive Disorders"); opioid-induced anxiety disorder ("Anxiety Disorders"); opioid-induced sleep disorder ("Sleep-Wake Disorders"); and opioid-induced sexual dysfunction ("Sexual Dysfunctions"). For opioid intoxication delirium and opioid withdrawal delirium, see the criteria and discussion of delirium in the chapter "Neurocognitive Disorders." These opioid-induced disorders are diagnosed instead of opioid intoxication or opioid withdrawal only when the symptoms are sufficiently severe to warrant independent clinical attention.

Unspecified Opioid-Related Disorder

292.9 (F11.99)

This category applies to presentations in which symptoms characteristic of an opioid-related disorder that cause clinically significant distress or impairment in social, occupational, or other important areas of functioning predominate but do not meet the full criteria for any specific opioid-related disorder or any of the disorders in the substance-related and addictive disorders diagnostic class.

Sedative-, Hypnotic-, or Anxiolytic-Related Disorders

Sedative, Hypnotic, or Anxiolytic Use Disorder

Sedative, Hypnotic, or Anxiolytic Intoxication

Sedative, Hypnotic, or Anxiolytic Withdrawal

Other Sedative-, Hypnotic-, or Anxiolytic-Induced Disorders

Unspecified Sedative-, Hypnotic-, or Anxiolytic-Related Disorder

Sedative, Hypnotic, or Anxiolytic Use Disorder

Diagnostic Criteria

A. A problematic pattern of sedative, hypnotic, or anxiolytic use leading to clinically significant impairment or distress, as manifested by at least two of the following, occurring within a 12-month period:

1. Sedatives, hypnotics, or anxiolytics are often taken in larger amounts or over a longer period than was intended.
2. There is a persistent desire or unsuccessful efforts to cut down or control sedative, hypnotic, or anxiolytic use.
3. A great deal of time is spent in activities necessary to obtain the sedative, hypnotic, or anxiolytic; use the sedative, hypnotic, or anxiolytic; or recover from its effects.
4. Craving, or a strong desire or urge to use the sedative, hypnotic, or anxiolytic.
5. Recurrent sedative, hypnotic, or anxiolytic use resulting in a failure to fulfill major role obligations at work, school, or home (e.g., repeated absences from work or poor work performance related to sedative, hypnotic, or anxiolytic use; sedative-, hypnotic-, or anxiolytic-related absences, suspensions, or expulsions from school; neglect of children or household).
6. Continued sedative, hypnotic, or anxiolytic use despite having persistent or recurrent social or interpersonal problems caused or exacerbated by the effects of sedatives, hypnotics, or anxiolytics (e.g., arguments with a spouse about consequences of intoxication; physical fights).
7. Important social, occupational, or recreational activities are given up or reduced because of sedative, hypnotic, or anxiolytic use.

8. Recurrent sedative, hypnotic, or anxiolytic use in situations in which it is physically hazardous (e.g., driving an automobile or operating a machine when impaired by sedative, hypnotic, or anxiolytic use).

9. Sedative, hypnotic, or anxiolytic use is continued despite knowledge of having a persistent or recurrent physical or psychological problem that is likely to have been caused or exacerbated by the sedative, hypnotic, or anxiolytic.

10. Tolerance, as defined by either of the following:

    a. A need for markedly increased amounts of the sedative, hypnotic, or anxiolytic to achieve intoxication or desired effect.

    b. A markedly diminished effect with continued use of the same amount of the sedative, hypnotic, or anxiolytic.

    Note: This criterion is not considered to be met for individuals taking sedatives, hypnotics, or anxiolytics under medical supervision.

11. Withdrawal, as manifested by either of the following:

    a. The characteristic withdrawal syndrome for sedatives, hypnotics, or anxiolytics (refer to Criteria A and B of the criteria set for sedative, hypnotic, or anxiolytic withdrawal, pp. 557–558).

    b. Sedatives, hypnotics, or anxiolytics (or a closely related substance, such as alcohol) are taken to relieve or avoid withdrawal symptoms.

    Note: This criterion is not considered to be met for individuals taking sedatives, hypnotics, or anxiolytics under medical supervision.

Specify if:

In early remission: After full criteria for sedative, hypnotic, or anxiolytic use disorder were previously met, none of the criteria for sedative, hypnotic, or anxiolytic use disorder have been met for at least 3 months but for less than 12 months (with the exception that Criterion A4, "Craving, or a strong desire or urge to use the sedative, hypnotic, or anxiolytic," may be met).

In sustained remission: After full criteria for sedative, hypnotic, or anxiolytic use disorder were previously met, none of the criteria for sedative, hypnotic, or anxiolytic use disorder have been met at any time during a period of 12 months or longer (with the exception that Criterion A4, "Craving, or a strong desire or urge to use the sedative, hypnotic, or anxiolytic," may be met).

Specify if:

In a controlled environment: This additional specifier is used if the individual is in an environment where access to sedatives, hypnotics, or anxiolytics is restricted.

Coding based on current severity: Note for ICD-10-CM codes: If a sedative, hypnotic, or anxiolytic intoxication; sedative, hypnotic, or anxiolytic withdrawal; or another sedative-, hypnotic-, or anxiolytic-induced mental disorder is also present, do not use the codes below for sedative, hypnotic, or anxiolytic use disorder. Instead the comorbid sedative, hypnotic, or anxiolytic use disorder is indicated in the 4th character of the sedative-, hypnotic-, or anxiolytic-induced disorder (see the coding note for sedative, hypnotic, or anxiolytic intoxication; sedative, hypnotic, or anxiolytic withdrawal; or specific sedative-, hypnotic-, or anxiolytic-induced mental disorder). For example, if there is comorbid sedative-, hypnotic-, or anxiolytic-induced depressive disorder and sedative, hypnotic, or anxiolytic use disorder, only the sedative-, hypnotic-, or anxiolytic-induced depressive disorder code is given with the 4th character indicating whether the comorbid sedative, hypnotic, or anxiolytic use disorder is mild, moderate, or severe: F13.14 for mild sedative, hypnotic, or anxiolytic use disorder with sedative-, hypnotic-, or anxiolytic-induced depressive disorder or F13.24 for a moderate or severe sedative, hypnotic, or anxiolytic use disorder with sedative-, hypnotic-, or anxiolytic-induced depressive disorder.

Specify current severity:
   305.40 (F13.10) Mild: Presence of 2–3 symptoms.
   304.10 (F13.20) Moderate: Presence of 4–5 symptoms.
   304.10 (F13.20) Severe: Presence of 6 or more symptoms.

Specifiers

"In a controlled environment" applies as a further specifier of remission if the individual is both in remission and in a controlled environment (i.e., in early remission in a controlled environment or in sustained remission in a controlled environment). Examples of these environments are closely supervised and substance-free jails, therapeutic communities, and locked hospital units.

Diagnostic Features

Sedative, hypnotic, or anxiolytic substances include benzodiazepines, benzodiazepine-like drugs (e.g., zolpidem, zaleplon), carbamates (e.g., glutethimide, meprobamate), barbiturates (e.g., secobarbital), and barbiturate-like hypnotics (e.g., glutethimide, methaqualone). This class of substances includes all prescription sleeping medications and almost all prescription antianxiety medications. Nonbenzodiazepine antianxiety agents (e.g., buspirone, gepirone) are not included in this class because they do not appear to be associated with significant misuse.

Like alcohol, these agents are brain depressants and can produce similar substance/medication-induced and substance use disorders. Sedative, hypnotic, or anxiolytic substances are available both by prescription and illegally. Some individuals who obtain these substances by prescription will develop a sedative, hypnotic, or anxiolytic use disorder, while others who misuse these substances or use them for intoxication will not develop a use disorder. In particular, sedatives, hypnotics, or anxiolytics with rapid onset and/or short to intermediate lengths of action may be taken for intoxication purposes, although longer acting substances in this class may be taken for intoxication as well.

Craving (Criterion A4), either while using or during a period of abstinence, is a typical feature of sedative, hypnotic, or anxiolytic use disorder. Misuse of substances from this class may occur on its own or in conjunction with use of other substances. For example, individuals may use intoxicating doses of sedatives or benzodiazepines to "come down" from cocaine or amphetamines or use high doses of benzodiazepines in combination with methadone to "boost" its effects.

Repeated absences or poor work performance, school absences, suspensions or expulsions, and neglect of children or household (Criterion A5) may be related to sedative, hypnotic, or anxiolytic use disorder, as may the continued use of the substances despite arguments with a spouse about consequences of intoxication or despite physical fights (Criterion A6). Limiting contact with family or friends, avoiding work or school, or stopping participation in hobbies, sports, or games (Criterion A7) and recurrent sedative, hypnotic, or anxiolytic use when driving an automobile or operating a machine when impaired by sedative, hypnotic, or anxiolytic use (Criterion A8) are also seen in sedative, hypnotic, or anxiolytic use disorder.

Very significant levels of tolerance and withdrawal can develop to the sedative, hypnotic, or anxiolytic. There may be evidence of tolerance and withdrawal in the absence of a diagnosis of a sedative, hypnotic, or anxiolytic use disorder in an individual who has abruptly discontinued use of benzodiazepines that were taken for long periods of time at prescribed and therapeutic doses. In these cases, an additional diagnosis of sedative, hypnotic, or anxiolytic use disorder is made only if other criteria are met. That is, sedative, hypnotic, or anxiolytic medications may be prescribed for appropriate medical purposes, and depending on the dose regimen, these drugs may then produce tolerance and withdrawal. If these drugs are prescribed or recommended for appropriate medical purposes, and if they are used as prescribed, the resulting tolerance or withdrawal does not meet the criteria for diagnosing a substance use disorder. However, it is necessary to determine whether the drugs were appropriately prescribed and used (e.g., falsifying medical symptoms to obtain the medication; using more medication than prescribed; obtaining the medication from several doctors without informing them of the others' involvement).

Given the unidimensional nature of the symptoms of sedative, hypnotic, or anxiolytic use disorder, severity is based on the number of criteria endorsed.

Associated Features Supporting Diagnosis

Sedative, hypnotic, or anxiolytic use disorder is often associated with other substance use disorders (e.g., alcohol, cannabis, opioid, stimulant use disorders). Sedatives are often used to alleviate the unwanted effects of these other substances. With repeated use of the substance, tolerance develops to the sedative effects, and a progressively higher dose is used. However, tolerance to brain stem depressant effects develops much more slowly, and as the individual takes more substance to achieve euphoria or other desired effects, there may be a sudden onset of respiratory depression and hypotension, which may result in death. Intense or repeated sedative, hypnotic, or anxiolytic intoxication may be associated with severe depression that, although temporary, can lead to suicide attempt and completed suicide.

Prevalence

The 12-month prevalences of DSM-IV sedative, hypnotic, or anxiolytic use disorder are estimated to be 0.3% among 12- to 17-year-olds and 0.2% among adults age 18 years and older. Rates of DSM-IV sedative, hypnotic, or anxiolytic use disorder are slightly greater among adult males (0.3%) than among adult females, but for 12- to 17-year-olds, the rate for females (0.4%) exceeds that for males (0.2%). The 12-month prevalence of DSM-IV sedative, hypnotic, or anxiolytic use disorder decreases as a function of age and is greatest among 18- to 29-year-olds (0.5%) and lowest among individuals 65 years and older (0.04%).

Twelve-month prevalence of sedative, hypnotic, or anxiolytic use disorder varies across racial/ethnic subgroups of the U.S. population. For 12- to 17-year-olds, rates are greatest among whites (0.3%) relative to African Americans (0.2%), Hispanics (0.2%), Native Americans (0.1%), and Asian Americans and Pacific Islanders (0.1%). Among adults, 12-month prevalence is greatest among Native Americans and Alaska Natives (0.8%), with rates of approximately 0.2% among African Americans, whites, and Hispanics and 0.1% among Asian Americans and Pacific Islanders.

Development and Course

The usual course of sedative, hypnotic, or anxiolytic use disorder involves individuals in their teens or 20s who escalate their occasional use of sedative, hypnotic, or anxiolytic agents to the point at which they develop problems that meet criteria for a diagnosis. This pattern may be especially likely among individuals who have other substance use disorders (e.g., alcohol, opioids, stimulants). An initial pattern of intermittent use socially (e.g., at parties) can lead to daily use and high levels of tolerance. Once this occurs, an increasing level of interpersonal difficulties, as well as increasingly severe episodes of cognitive dysfunction and physiological withdrawal, can be expected.

The second and less frequently observed clinical course begins with an individual who originally obtained the medication by prescription from a physician, usually for the treatment of anxiety, insomnia, or somatic complaints. As either tolerance or a need for higher doses of the medication develops, there is a gradual increase in the dose and frequency of self-administration. The individual is likely to continue to justify use on the basis of his or her original symptoms of anxiety or insomnia, but substance-seeking behavior becomes more prominent, and the individual may seek out multiple physicians to obtain sufficient supplies of the medication. Tolerance can reach high levels, and withdrawal (including seizures and withdrawal delirium) may occur.

As with many substance use disorders, sedative, hypnotic, or anxiolytic use disorder generally has an onset during adolescence or early adult life. There is an increased risk for misuse and problems from many psychoactive substances as individuals age. In particular, cognitive impairment increases as a side effect with age, and the metabolism of sedatives, hypnotics, or anxiolytics decreases with age among older individuals. Both acute and chronic toxic effects of these substances, especially effects on cognition, memory, and motor coordination, are likely to increase with age as a consequence of pharmacodynamic and pharmacokinetic age-related changes. Individuals with major neurocognitive disorder (dementia) are more likely to develop intoxication and impaired physiological functioning at lower doses.

Deliberate intoxication to achieve a "high" is most likely to be observed in teenagers and individuals in their 20s. Problems associated with sedatives, hypnotics, or anxiolytics are also seen in individuals in their 40s and older who escalate the dose of prescribed medications. In older individuals, intoxication can resemble a progressive dementia.

Risk and Prognostic Factors

Temperamental.   Impulsivity and novelty seeking are individual temperaments that relate to the propensity to develop a substance use disorder but may themselves be genetically determined.

Environmental.   Since sedatives, hypnotics, or anxiolytics are all pharmaceuticals, a key risk factor relates to availability of the substances. In the United States, the historical patterns of sedative, hypnotic, or anxiolytic misuse relate to the broad prescribing patterns. For instance, a marked decrease in prescription of barbiturates was associated with an increase in benzodiazepine prescribing. Peer factors may relate to genetic predisposition in terms of how individuals select their environment. Other individuals at heightened risk might include those with alcohol use disorder who may receive repeated prescriptions in response to their complaints of alcohol-related anxiety or insomnia.

Genetic and physiological.   As for other substance use disorders, the risk for sedative, hypnotic, or anxiolytic use disorder can be related to individual, family, peer, social, and environmental factors. Within these domains, genetic factors play a particularly important role both directly and indirectly. Overall, across development, genetic factors seem to play a larger role in the onset of sedative, hypnotic, or anxiolytic use disorder as individuals age through puberty into adult life.

Course modifiers.   Early onset of use is associated with greater likelihood for developing a sedative, hypnotic, or anxiolytic use disorder.

Culture-Related Diagnostic Issues

There are marked variations in prescription patterns (and availability) of this class of substances in different countries, which may lead to variations in prevalence of sedative, hypnotic, or anxiolytic use disorders.

Gender-Related Diagnostic Issues

Females may be at higher risk than males for prescription drug misuse of sedative, hypnotic, or anxiolytic substances.

Diagnostic Markers

Almost all sedative, hypnotic, or anxiolytic substances can be identified through laboratory evaluations of urine or blood (the latter of which can quantify the amounts of these agents in the body). Urine tests are likely to remain positive for up to approximately 1 week after the use of long-acting substances, such as diazepam or flurazepam.

Functional Consequences of Sedative, Hypnotic, or Anxiolytic Use Disorder

The social and interpersonal consequences of sedative, hypnotic, or anxiolytic use disorder mimic those of alcohol in terms of the potential for disinhibited behavior. Accidents, interpersonal difficulties (such as arguments or fights), and interference with work or school performance are all common outcomes. Physical examination is likely to reveal evidence of a mild decrease in most aspects of autonomic nervous system functioning, including a slower pulse, a slightly decreased respiratory rate, and a slight drop in blood pressure (most likely to occur with postural changes). At high doses, sedative, hypnotic, or anxiolytic substances can be lethal, particularly when mixed with alcohol, although the lethal dosage varies considerably among the specific substances. Overdoses may be associated with a deterioration in vital signs that signals an impending medical emergency (e.g., respiratory arrest from barbiturates). There may be consequences of trauma (e.g., internal bleeding or a subdural hematoma) from accidents that occur while intoxicated. Intravenous use of these substances can result in medical complications related to the use of contaminated needles (e.g., hepatitis and HIV).

Acute intoxication can result in accidental injuries and automobile accidents. For elderly individuals, even short-term use of these sedating medications at prescribed doses can be associated with an increased risk for cognitive problems and falls. The disinhibiting effects of these agents, like alcohol, may potentially contribute to overly aggressive behavior, with subsequent interpersonal and legal problems. Accidental or deliberate overdoses, similar to those observed for alcohol use disorder or repeated alcohol intoxication, can occur. In contrast to their wide margin of safety when used alone, benzodiazepines taken in combination with alcohol can be particularly dangerous, and accidental overdoses are reported commonly. Accidental overdoses have also been reported in individuals who deliberately misuse barbiturates and other nonbenzodiazepine sedatives (e.g., methaqualone), but since these agents are much less available than the benzodiazepines, the frequency of overdosing is low in most settings.

Differential Diagnosis

Other mental disorders or medical conditions.   Individuals with sedative-, hypnotic-, or anxiolytic-induced disorders may present with symptoms (e.g., anxiety) that resemble primary mental disorders (e.g., generalized anxiety disorder vs. sedative-, hypnotic-, or anxiolytic-induced anxiety disorder, with onset during withdrawal). The slurred speech, incoordination, and other associated features characteristic of sedative, hypnotic, or anxiolytic intoxication could be the result of another medical condition (e.g., multiple sclerosis) or of a prior head trauma (e.g., a subdural hematoma).

Alcohol use disorder.   Sedative, hypnotic, or anxiolytic use disorder must be differentiated from alcohol use disorder.

Clinically appropriate use of sedative, hypnotic, or anxiolytic medications.   Individuals may continue to take benzodiazepine medication according to a physician's direction for a legitimate medical indication over extended periods of time. Even if physiological signs of tolerance or withdrawal are manifested, many of these individuals do not develop symptoms that meet the criteria for sedative, hypnotic, or anxiolytic use disorder because they are not preoccupied with obtaining the substance and its use does not interfere with their performance of usual social or occupational roles.

Comorbidity

Nonmedical use of sedative, hypnotic, or anxiolytic agents is associated with alcohol use disorder, tobacco use disorder, and, generally, illicit drug use. There may also be an overlap between sedative, hypnotic, or anxiolytic use disorder and antisocial personality disorder; depressive, bipolar, and anxiety disorders; and other substance use disorders, such as alcohol use disorder and illicit drug use disorders. Antisocial behavior and antisocial personality disorder are especially associated with sedative, hypnotic, or anxiolytic use disorder when the substances are obtained illegally.

Sedative, Hypnotic, or Anxiolytic Intoxication

Diagnostic Criteria

A. Recent use of a sedative, hypnotic, or anxiolytic.

B. Clinically significant maladaptive behavioral or psychological changes (e.g., inappropriate sexual or aggressive behavior, mood lability, impaired judgment) that developed during, or shortly after, sedative, hypnotic, or anxiolytic use.

C. One (or more) of the following signs or symptoms developing during, or shortly after, sedative, hypnotic, or anxiolytic use:

   1. Slurred speech.
   2. Incoordination.
   3. Unsteady gait.
   4. Nystagmus.
   5. Impairment in cognition (e.g., attention, memory).
   6. Stupor or coma.

D. The signs or symptoms are not attributable to another medical condition and are not better explained by another mental disorder, including intoxication with another substance.

Coding note: The ICD-9-CM code is **292.89.** The ICD-10-CM code depends on whether there is a comorbid sedative, hypnotic, or anxiolytic use disorder. If a mild sedative, hypnotic, or anxiolytic use disorder is comorbid, the ICD-10-CM code is **F13.129,** and if a moderate or severe sedative, hypnotic, or anxiolytic use disorder is comorbid, the ICD-10-CM code is **F13.229.** If there is no comorbid sedative, hypnotic, or anxiolytic use disorder, then the ICD-10-CM code is **F13.929.**

Note: For information on Development and Course; Risk and Prognostic Factors; Culture-Related Diagnostic Issues; Diagnostic Markers; Functional Consequences of Sedative, Hypnotic, or Anxiolytic Intoxication; and Comorbidity, see the corresponding sections in sedative, hypnotic, or anxiolytic use disorder.

Diagnostic Features

The essential feature of sedative, hypnotic, or anxiolytic intoxication is the presence of clinically significant maladaptive behavioral or psychological changes (e.g., inappropriate sexual or aggressive behavior, mood lability, impaired judgment, impaired social or occupational functioning) that develop during, or shortly after, use of a sedative, hypnotic, or anxiolytic (Criteria A and B). As with other brain depressants, such as alcohol, these behaviors may be accompanied by slurred speech, incoordination (at levels that can interfere with driving abilities and with performing usual activities to the point of causing falls or automobile accidents), an unsteady gait, nystagmus, impairment in cognition (e.g., attentional or memory problems), and stupor or coma (Criterion C). Memory impairment is a prominent feature of sedative, hypnotic, or anxiolytic intoxication and is most often characterized by an anterograde amnesia that resembles "alcoholic blackouts," which can be disturbing to the individual. The symptoms must not be attributable to another medical condition and are not better explained by another mental disorder (Criterion D). Intoxication may occur in individuals who are receiving these substances by prescription, are borrowing the medication from friends or relatives, or are deliberately taking the substance to achieve intoxication.

Associated Features Supporting Diagnosis

Associated features include taking more medication than prescribed, taking multiple different medications, or mixing sedative, hypnotic, or anxiolytic agents with alcohol, which can markedly increase the effects of these agents.

Prevalence

The prevalence of sedative, hypnotic, or anxiolytic intoxication in the general population is unclear. However, it is probable that most nonmedical users of sedatives, hypnotics, or anxiolytics would at some time have signs or symptoms that meet criteria for sedative, hypnotic, or anxiolytic intoxication; if so, then the prevalence of nonmedical sedative, hypnotic, or anxiolytic use in the general population may be similar to the prevalence of sedative, hypnotic, or anxiolytic intoxication. For example, tranquilizers are used nonmedically by 2.2% of Americans older than 12 years.

Differential Diagnosis

Alcohol use disorders.   Since the clinical presentations may be identical, distinguishing sedative, hypnotic, or anxiolytic intoxication from alcohol use disorders requires evidence for recent ingestion of sedative, hypnotic, or anxiolytic medications by self-report, informant report, or toxicological testing. Many individuals who misuse sedatives, hypnotics, or anxiolytics may also misuse alcohol and other substances, and so multiple intoxication diagnoses are possible.

Alcohol intoxication.   Alcohol intoxication may be distinguished from sedative, hypnotic, or anxiolytic intoxication by the smell of alcohol on the breath. Otherwise, the features of the two disorders may be similar.

Other sedative-, hypnotic-, or anxiolytic-induced disorders.   Sedative, hypnotic, or anxiolytic intoxication is distinguished from the other sedative-, hypnotic-, or anxiolytic-induced disorders (e.g., sedative-, hypnotic-, or anxiolytic-induced anxiety disorder, with onset during withdrawal) because the symptoms in the latter disorders predominate in the clinical presentation and are severe enough to warrant clinical attention.

Neurocognitive disorders.   In situations of cognitive impairment, traumatic brain injury, and delirium from other causes, sedatives, hypnotics, or anxiolytics may be intoxicating at quite low dosages. The differential diagnosis in these complex settings is based on the predominant syndrome. An additional diagnosis of sedative, hypnotic, or anxiolytic intoxication may be appropriate even if the substance has been ingested at a low dosage in the setting of these other (or similar) co-occurring conditions.

Sedative, Hypnotic, or Anxiolytic Withdrawal

Diagnostic Criteria

A. Cessation of (or reduction in) sedative, hypnotic, or anxiolytic use that has been prolonged.

B. Two (or more) of the following, developing within several hours to a few days after the cessation of (or reduction in) sedative, hypnotic, or anxiolytic use described in Criterion A:

1. Autonomic hyperactivity (e.g., sweating or pulse rate greater than 100 bpm).
2. Hand tremor.

3. Insomnia.
4. Nausea or vomiting.
5. Transient visual, tactile, or auditory hallucinations or illusions.
6. Psychomotor agitation.
7. Anxiety.
8. Grand mal seizures.

C. The signs or symptoms in Criterion B cause clinically significant distress or impairment in social, occupational, or other important areas of functioning.

D. The signs or symptoms are not attributable to another medical condition and are not better explained by another mental disorder, including intoxication or withdrawal from another substance.

Specify if:

With perceptual disturbances: This specifier may be noted when hallucinations with intact reality testing or auditory, visual, or tactile illusions occur in the absence of a delirium.

Coding note: The ICD-9-CM code is **292.0.** The ICD-10-CM code for sedative, hypnotic, or anxiolytic withdrawal depends on whether or not there is a comorbid moderate or severe sedative, hypnotic, or anxiolytic use disorder and whether or not there are perceptual disturbances. For sedative, hypnotic, or anxiolytic withdrawal without perceptual disturbances, the ICD-10-CM code is **F13.239.** For sedative, hypnotic, or anxiolytic withdrawal with perceptual disturbances, the ICD-10-CM code is **F13.232.** Note that the ICD-10-CM codes indicate the comorbid presence of a moderate or severe sedative, hypnotic, or anxiolytic use disorder, reflecting the fact that sedative, hypnotic, or anxiolytic withdrawal can only occur in the presence of a moderate or severe sedative, hypnotic, or anxiolytic use disorder. It is not permissible to code a comorbid mild sedative, hypnotic, or anxiolytic use disorder with sedative, hypnotic, or anxiolytic withdrawal.

Note: For information on Development and Course; Risk and Prognostic Factors; Culture-Related Diagnostic Issues; Functional Consequences of Sedative, Hypnotic, or Anxiolytic Withdrawal; and Comorbidity, see the corresponding sections in sedative, hypnotic, or anxiolytic use disorder.

Diagnostic Features

The essential feature of sedative, hypnotic, or anxiolytic withdrawal is the presence of a characteristic syndrome that develops after a marked decrease in or cessation of intake after several weeks or more of regular use (Criteria A and B). This withdrawal syndrome is characterized by two or more symptoms (similar to alcohol withdrawal) that include autonomic hyperactivity (e.g., increases in heart rate, respiratory rate, blood pressure, or body temperature, along with sweating); a tremor of the hands; insomnia; nausea, sometimes accompanied by vomiting; anxiety; and psychomotor agitation. A grand mal seizure may occur in perhaps as many as 20%–30% of individuals undergoing untreated withdrawal from these substances. In severe withdrawal, visual, tactile, or auditory hallucinations or illusions can occur but are usually in the context of a delirium. If the individual's reality testing is intact (i.e., he or she knows the substance is causing the hallucinations) and the illusions occur in a clear sensorium, the specifier "with perceptual disturbances" can be noted. When hallucinations occur in the absence of intact reality testing, a diagnosis of substance/medication-induced psychotic disorder should be considered. The symptoms cause clinically significant distress or impairment in social, occupational, or other important areas of functioning (Criterion C). The symptoms must not be attributable to another medical condition and are not better explained by another mental disorder (e.g., alcohol withdrawal or generalized anxiety disorder) (Criterion D). Relief of withdrawal symptoms with administration of any sedative-hypnotic agent would support a diagnosis of sedative, hypnotic, or anxiolytic withdrawal.

Associated Features Supporting Diagnosis

The timing and severity of the withdrawal syndrome will differ depending on the specific substance and its pharmacokinetics and pharmacodynamics. For example, withdrawal from shorter-acting substances that are rapidly absorbed and that have no active metabolites (e.g., triazolam) can begin within hours after the substance is stopped; withdrawal from substances with long-acting metabolites (e.g., diazepam) may not begin for 1–2 days or longer. The withdrawal syndrome produced by substances in this class may be characterized by the development of a delirium that can be life-threatening. There may be evidence of tolerance and withdrawal in the absence of a diagnosis of a substance use disorder in an individual who has abruptly discontinued benzodiazepines that were taken for long periods of time at prescribed and therapeutic doses. However, ICD-10-CM codes only allow a diagnosis of sedative, hypnotic, or anxiolytic withdrawal in the presence of comorbid moderate to severe sedative, hypnotic, or anxiolytic use disorder.

The time course of the withdrawal syndrome is generally predicted by the half-life of the substance. Medications whose actions typically last about 10 hours or less (e.g., lorazepam, oxazepam, temazepam) produce withdrawal symptoms within 6–8 hours of decreasing blood levels that peak in intensity on the second day and improve markedly by the fourth or fifth day. For substances with longer half-lives (e.g., diazepam), symptoms may not develop for more than 1 week, peak in intensity during the second week, and decrease markedly during the third or fourth week. There may be additional longer-term symptoms at a much lower level of intensity that persist for several months.

The longer the substance has been taken and the higher the dosages used, the more likely it is that there will be severe withdrawal. However, withdrawal has been reported with as little as 15 mg of diazepam (or its equivalent in other benzodiazepines) when taken daily for several months. Doses of approximately 40 mg of diazepam (or its equivalent) daily are more likely to produce clinically relevant withdrawal symptoms, and even higher doses (e.g., 100 mg of diazepam) are more likely to be followed by withdrawal seizures or delirium. Sedative, hypnotic, or anxiolytic withdrawal delirium is characterized by disturbances in consciousness and cognition, with visual, tactile, or auditory hallucinations. When present, sedative, hypnotic, or anxiolytic withdrawal delirium should be diagnosed instead of withdrawal.

Prevalence

The prevalence of sedative, hypnotic, or anxiolytic withdrawal is unclear.

Diagnostic Markers

Seizures and autonomic instability in the setting of a history of prolonged exposure to sedative, hypnotic, or anxiolytic medications suggest a high likelihood of sedative, hypnotic, or anxiolytic withdrawal.

Differential Diagnosis

Other medical disorders.   The symptoms of sedative, hypnotic, or anxiolytic withdrawal may be mimicked by other medical conditions (e.g., hypoglycemia, diabetic ketoacidosis). If seizures are a feature of the sedative, hypnotic, or anxiolytic withdrawal, the differential diagnosis includes the various causes of seizures (e.g., infections, head injury, poisonings).

Essential tremor.   Essential tremor, a disorder that frequently runs in families, may erroneously suggest the tremulousness associated with sedative, hypnotic, or anxiolytic withdrawal.

Alcohol withdrawal.   Alcohol withdrawal produces a syndrome very similar to that of sedative, hypnotic, or anxiolytic withdrawal.

Other sedative-, hypnotic-, or anxiolytic-induced disorders.   Sedative, hypnotic, or anxiolytic withdrawal is distinguished from the other sedative-, hypnotic-, or anxiolytic-induced disorders (e.g., sedative-, hypnotic-, or anxiolytic-induced anxiety disorder, with onset during withdrawal) because the symptoms in the latter disorders predominate in the clinical presentation and are severe enough to warrant clinical attention.

Anxiety disorders.   Recurrence or worsening of an underlying anxiety disorder produces a syndrome similar to sedative, hypnotic, or anxiolytic withdrawal. Withdrawal would be suspected with an abrupt reduction in the dosage of a sedative, hypnotic, or anxiolytic medication. When a taper is under way, distinguishing the withdrawal syndrome from the underlying anxiety disorder can be difficult. As with alcohol, lingering withdrawal symptoms (e.g., anxiety, moodiness, and trouble sleeping) can be mistaken for non-substance/medication-induced anxiety or depressive disorders (e.g., generalized anxiety disorder).

Other Sedative-, Hypnotic-, or Anxiolytic-Induced Disorders

The following sedative-, hypnotic-, or anxiolytic-induced disorders are described in other chapters of the manual with disorders with which they share phenomenology (see the substance/medication-induced mental disorders in these chapters): sedative-, hypnotic-, or anxiolytic-induced psychotic disorder ("Schizophrenia Spectrum and Other Psychotic Disorders"); sedative-, hypnotic-, or anxiolytic-induced bipolar disorder ("Bipolar and Related Disorders"); sedative-, hypnotic-, or anxiolytic-induced depressive disorder ("Depressive Disorders"); sedative-, hypnotic-, or anxiolytic-induced anxiety disorder ("Anxiety Disorders"); sedative-, hypnotic-, or anxiolytic-induced sleep disorder ("Sleep-Wake Disorders"); sedative-, hypnotic-, or anxiolytic-induced sexual dysfunction ("Sexual Dysfunctions"); and sedative-, hypnotic-, or anxiolytic-induced major or mild neurocognitive disorder ("Neurocognitive Disorders"). For sedative, hypnotic, or anxiolytic intoxication delirium and sedative, hypnotic, or anxiolytic withdrawal delirium, see the criteria and discussion of delirium in the chapter "Neurocognitive Disorders." These sedative-, hypnotic-, or anxiolytic-induced disorders are diagnosed instead of sedative, hypnotic, or anxiolytic intoxication or sedative, hypnotic, or anxiolytic withdrawal only when the symptoms are sufficiently severe to warrant independent clinical attention.

Unspecified Sedative-, Hypnotic-, or Anxiolytic-Related Disorder

292.9 (F13.99)

This category applies to presentations in which symptoms characteristic of a sedative-, hypnotic-, or anxiolytic-related disorder that cause clinically significant distress or impairment in social, occupational, or other important areas of functioning predominate but do not meet the full criteria for any specific sedative-, hypnotic-, or anxiolytic-related disorder or any of the disorders in the substance-related and addictive disorders diagnostic class.

Stimulant-Related Disorders

Stimulant Use Disorder
Stimulant Intoxication
Stimulant Withdrawal
Other Stimulant-Induced Disorders
Unspecified Stimulant-Related Disorder

Stimulant Use Disorder

Diagnostic Criteria

A. A pattern of amphetamine-type substance, cocaine, or other stimulant use leading to clinically significant impairment or distress, as manifested by at least two of the following, occurring within a 12-month period:

1. The stimulant is often taken in larger amounts or over a longer period than was intended.
2. There is a persistent desire or unsuccessful efforts to cut down or control stimulant use.
3. A great deal of time is spent in activities necessary to obtain the stimulant, use the stimulant, or recover from its effects.
4. Craving, or a strong desire or urge to use the stimulant.
5. Recurrent stimulant use resulting in a failure to fulfill major role obligations at work, school, or home.
6. Continued stimulant use despite having persistent or recurrent social or interpersonal problems caused or exacerbated by the effects of the stimulant.
7. Important social, occupational, or recreational activities are given up or reduced because of stimulant use.
8. Recurrent stimulant use in situations in which it is physically hazardous.
9. Stimulant use is continued despite knowledge of having a persistent or recurrent physical or psychological problem that is likely to have been caused or exacerbated by the stimulant.
10. Tolerance, as defined by either of the following:
    a. A need for markedly increased amounts of the stimulant to achieve intoxication or desired effect.
    b. A markedly diminished effect with continued use of the same amount of the stimulant.

    Note: This criterion is not considered to be met for those taking stimulant medications solely under appropriate medical supervision, such as medications for attention-deficit/hyperactivity disorder or narcolepsy.
11. Withdrawal, as manifested by either of the following:
    a. The characteristic withdrawal syndrome for the stimulant (refer to Criteria A and B of the criteria set for stimulant withdrawal, p. 569).
    b. The stimulant (or a closely related substance) is taken to relieve or avoid withdrawal symptoms.

Note: This criterion is not considered to be met for those taking stimulant medications solely under appropriate medical supervision, such as medications for attention-deficit/hyperactivity disorder or narcolepsy.

Specify if:

In early remission: After full criteria for stimulant use disorder were previously met, none of the criteria for stimulant use disorder have been met for at least 3 months but for less than 12 months (with the exception that Criterion A4, "Craving, or a strong desire or urge to use the stimulant," may be met).

In sustained remission: After full criteria for stimulant use disorder were previously met, none of the criteria for stimulant use disorder have been met at any time during a period of 12 months or longer (with the exception that Criterion A4, "Craving, or a strong desire or urge to use the stimulant," may be met).

Specify if:

In a controlled environment: This additional specifier is used if the individual is in an environment where access to stimulants is restricted.

Coding based on current severity: Note for ICD-10-CM codes: If an amphetamine intoxication, amphetamine withdrawal, or another amphetamine-induced mental disorder is also present, do not use the codes below for amphetamine use disorder. Instead, the comorbid amphetamine use disorder is indicated in the 4th character of the amphetamine-induced disorder code (see the coding note for amphetamine intoxication, amphetamine withdrawal, or a specific amphetamine-induced mental disorder). For example, if there is comorbid amphetamine-type or other stimulant-induced depressive disorder and amphetamine-type or other stimulant use disorder, only the amphetamine-type or other stimulant-induced depressive disorder code is given, with the 4th character indicating whether the comorbid amphetamine-type or other stimulant use disorder is mild, moderate, or severe: F15.14 for mild amphetamine-type or other stimulant use disorder with amphetamine-type or other stimulant-induced depressive disorder or F15.24 for a moderate or severe amphetamine-type or other stimulant use disorder with amphetamine-type or other stimulant-induced depressive disorder. Similarly, if there is comorbid cocaine-induced depressive disorder and cocaine use disorder, only the cocaine-induced depressive disorder code is given, with the 4th character indicating whether the comorbid cocaine use disorder is mild, moderate, or severe: F14.14 for mild cocaine use disorder with cocaine-induced depressive disorder or F14.24 for a moderate or severe cocaine use disorder with cocaine-induced depressive disorder.

Specify current severity:

Mild: Presence of 2–3 symptoms.

    305.70 (F15.10) Amphetamine-type substance
    305.60 (F14.10) Cocaine
    305.70 (F15.10) Other or unspecified stimulant

Moderate: Presence of 4–5 symptoms.

    304.40 (F15.20) Amphetamine-type substance
    304.20 (F14.20) Cocaine
    304.40 (F15.20) Other or unspecified stimulant

Severe: Presence of 6 or more symptoms.

    304.40 (F15.20) Amphetamine-type substance
    304.20 (F14.20) Cocaine
    304.40 (F15.20) Other or unspecified stimulant

Specifiers

"In a controlled environment" applies as a further specifier of remission if the individual is both in remission and in a controlled environment (i.e., in early remission in a controlled environment or in sustained remission in a controlled environment). Examples of these environments are closely supervised and substance-free jails, therapeutic communities, and locked hospital units.

Diagnostic Features

The amphetamine and amphetamine-type stimulants include substances with a substituted-phenylethylamine structure, such as amphetamine, dextroamphetamine, and methamphetamine. Also included are those substances that are structurally different but have similar effects, such as methylphenidate. These substances are usually taken orally or intravenously, although methamphetamine is also taken by the nasal route. In addition to the synthetic amphetamine-type compounds, there are naturally occurring, plant-derived stimulants such as *khât*. Amphetamines and other stimulants may be obtained by prescription for the treatment of obesity, attention-deficit/hyperactivity disorder, and narcolepsy. Consequently, prescribed stimulants may be diverted into the illegal market. The effects of amphetamines and amphetamine-like drugs are similar to those of cocaine, such that the criteria for stimulant use disorder are presented here as a single disorder with the ability to specify the particular stimulant used by the individual. Cocaine may be consumed in several preparations (e.g., coca leaves, coca paste, cocaine hydrochloride, and cocaine alkaloids such as freebase and crack) that differ in potency because of varying levels of purity and speed of onset. However, in all forms of the substance, cocaine is the active ingredient. Cocaine hydrochloride powder is usually "snorted" through the nostrils or dissolved in water and injected intravenously.

Individuals exposed to amphetamine-type stimulants or cocaine can develop stimulant use disorder as rapidly as 1 week, although the onset is not always this rapid. Regardless of the route of administration, tolerance occurs with repeated use. Withdrawal symptoms, particularly hypersomnia, increased appetite, and dysphoria, can occur and can enhance craving. Most individuals with stimulant use disorder have experienced tolerance or withdrawal.

Use patterns and course are similar for disorders involving amphetamine-type stimulants and cocaine, as both substances are potent central nervous system stimulants with similar psychoactive and sympathomimetic effects. Amphetamine-type stimulants are longer acting than cocaine and thus are used fewer times per day. Usage may be chronic or episodic, with binges punctuated by brief non-use periods. Aggressive or violent behavior is common when high doses are smoked, ingested, or administered intravenously. Intense temporary anxiety resembling panic disorder or generalized anxiety disorder, as well as paranoid ideation and psychotic episodes that resemble schizophrenia, is seen with high-dose use.

Withdrawal states are associated with temporary but intense depressive symptoms that can resemble a major depressive episode; the depressive symptoms usually resolve within 1 week. Tolerance to amphetamine-type stimulants develops and leads to escalation of the dose. Conversely, some users of amphetamine-type stimulants develop sensitization, characterized by enhanced effects.

Associated Features Supporting Diagnosis

When injected or smoked, stimulants typically produce an instant feeling of well-being, confidence, and euphoria. Dramatic behavioral changes can rapidly develop with stimulant use disorder. Chaotic behavior, social isolation, aggressive behavior, and sexual dysfunction can result from long-term stimulant use disorder.

Individuals with acute intoxication may present with rambling speech, headache, transient ideas of reference, and tinnitus. There may be paranoid ideation, auditory hallucinations in a clear sensorium, and tactile hallucinations, which the individual usually recognizes as drug effects. Threats or acting out of aggressive behavior may occur. Depression, suicidal ideation, irritability, anhedonia, emotional lability, or disturbances in attention and concentration commonly occur during withdrawal. Mental disturbances associated with cocaine use usually resolve hours to days after cessation of use but can persist for 1 month. Physiological changes during stimulant withdrawal are opposite to those of the intoxication phase, sometimes including bradycardia. Temporary depressive symptoms may meet symptomatic and duration criteria for major depressive episode. Histories consistent with repeated panic attacks, social anxiety disorder (social phobia)–like behavior, and generalized anxiety–like syndromes are common, as are eating disorders. One extreme instance of stimulant toxicity is stimulant-induced psychotic disorder, a disorder that resembles schizophrenia, with delusions and hallucinations.

Individuals with stimulant use disorder often develop conditioned responses to drug-related stimuli (e.g., craving on seeing any white powderlike substance). These responses contribute to relapse, are difficult to extinguish, and persist after detoxification.

Depressive symptoms with suicidal ideation or behavior can occur and are generally the most serious problems seen during stimulant withdrawal.

Prevalence

Stimulant use disorder: amphetamine-type stimulants.   Estimated 12-month prevalence of amphetamine-type stimulant use disorder in the United States is 0.2% among 12- to 17-year-olds and 0.2% among individuals 18 years and older. Rates are similar among adult males and females (0.2%), but among 12- to 17-year-olds, the rate for females (0.3%) is greater than that for males (0.1%). Intravenous stimulant use has a male-to-female ratio of 3:1 or 4:1, but rates are more balanced among non-injecting users, with males representing 54% of primary treatment admissions. Twelve-month prevalence is greater among 18- to 29-year-olds (0.4%) compared with 45- to 64-year-olds (0.1%). For 12- to 17-year-olds, rates are highest among whites and African Americans (0.3%) compared with Hispanics (0.1%) and Asian Americans and Pacific Islanders (0.01%), with amphetamine-type stimulant use disorder virtually absent among Native Americans. Among adults, rates are highest among Native Americans and Alaska Natives (0.6%) compared with whites (0.2%) and Hispanics (0.2%), with amphetamine-type stimulant use disorder virtually absent among African Americans and Asian Americans and Pacific Islanders. Past-year nonprescribed use of prescription stimulants occurred among 5%–9% of children through high school, with 5%–35% of college-age persons reporting past-year use.

Stimulant use disorder: cocaine.   Estimated 12-month prevalence of cocaine use disorder in the United States is 0.2% among 12- to 17-year-olds and 0.3% among individuals 18 years and older. Rates are higher among males (0.4%) than among females (0.1%). Rates are highest among 18- to 29-year-olds (0.6%) and lowest among 45- to 64-year-olds (0.1%). Among adults, rates are greater among Native Americans (0.8%) compared with African Americans (0.4%), Hispanics (0.3%), whites (0.2%), and Asian Americans and Pacific Islanders (0.1%). In contrast, for 12- to 17-year-olds, rates are similar among Hispanics (0.2%), whites (0.2%), and Asian Americans and Pacific Islanders (0.2%); and lower among African Americans (0.02%); with cocaine use disorder virtually absent among Native Americans and Alaska Natives.

Development and Course

Stimulant use disorders occur throughout all levels of society and are more common among individuals ages 12–25 years compared with individuals 26 years and older. First regular use among individuals in treatment occurs, on average, at approximately age 23 years. For primary methamphetamine–primary treatment admissions, the average age is 31 years.

Some individuals begin stimulant use to control weight or to improve performance in school, work, or athletics. This includes obtaining medications such as methylphenidate or amphetamine salts prescribed to others for the treatment of attention-deficit/hyperactivity disorder. Stimulant use disorder can develop rapidly with intravenous or smoked administration; among primary admissions for amphetamine-type stimulant use, 66% reported smoking, 18% reported injecting, and 10% reported snorting.

Patterns of stimulant administration include episodic or daily (or almost daily) use. Episodic use tends to be separated by 2 or more days of non-use (e.g., intense use over a weekend or on one or more weekdays). "Binges" involve continuous high-dose use over hours or days and are often associated with physical dependence. Binges usually terminate only when stimulant supplies are depleted or exhaustion ensues. Chronic daily use may involve high or low doses, often with an increase in dose over time.

Stimulant smoking and intravenous use are associated with rapid progression to severe-level stimulant use disorder, often occurring over weeks to months. Intranasal use of cocaine and oral use of amphetamine-type stimulants result in more gradual progression occurring over months to years. With continuing use, there is a diminution of pleasurable effects due to tolerance and an increase in dysphoric effects.

Risk and Prognostic Factors

Temperamental.   Comorbid bipolar disorder, schizophrenia, antisocial personality disorder, and other substance use disorders are risk factors for developing stimulant use disorder and for relapse to cocaine use in treatment samples. Also, impulsivity and similar personality traits may affect treatment outcomes. Childhood conduct disorder and adult antisocial personality disorder are associated with the later development of stimulant-related disorders.

Environmental.   Predictors of cocaine use among teenagers include prenatal cocaine exposure, postnatal cocaine use by parents, and exposure to community violence during childhood. For youths, especially females, risk factors include living in an unstable home environment, having a psychiatric condition, and associating with dealers and users.

Culture-Related Diagnostic Issues

Stimulant use–attendant disorders affect all racial/ethnic, socioeconomic, age, and gender groups. Diagnostic issues may be related to societal consequences (e.g., arrest, school suspensions, employment suspension). Despite small variations, cocaine and other stimulant use disorder diagnostic criteria perform equally across gender and race/ethnicity groups.

Chronic use of cocaine impairs cardiac left ventricular function in African Americans. Approximately 66% of individuals admitted for primary methamphetamine/amphetamine-related disorders are non-Hispanic white, followed by 21% of Hispanic origin, 3% Asian and Pacific Islander, and 3% non-Hispanic black.

Diagnostic Markers

Benzoylecgonine, a metabolite of cocaine, typically remains in the urine for 1–3 days after a single dose and may be present for 7–12 days in individuals using repeated high doses. Mildly elevated liver function tests can be present in cocaine injectors or users with concomitant alcohol use. There are no neurobiological markers of diagnostic utility. Discontinuation of chronic cocaine use may be associated with electroencephalographic changes, suggesting persistent abnormalities; alterations in secretion patterns of prolactin; and downregulation of dopamine receptors.

Short-half-life amphetamine-type stimulants (MDMA [3,4-methylenedioxy-*N*-methylamphetamine], methamphetamine) can be detected for 1–3 days, and possibly up to 4 days depending on dosage and metabolism. Hair samples can be used to detect presence of amphetamine-type stimulants for up to 90 days. Other laboratory findings, as well as physical findings and other medical conditions (e.g., weight loss, malnutrition; poor hygiene), are similar for both cocaine and amphetamine-type stimulant use disorder.

Functional Consequences of Stimulant Use Disorder

Various medical conditions may occur depending on the route of administration. Intranasal users often develop sinusitis, irritation, bleeding of the nasal mucosa, and a perforated nasal septum. Individuals who smoke the drugs are at increased risk for respiratory problems (e.g., coughing, bronchitis, and pneumonitis). Injectors have puncture marks and "tracks," most commonly on their forearms. Risk of HIV infection increases with frequent intravenous injections and unsafe sexual activity. Other sexually transmitted diseases, hepatitis, and tuberculosis and other lung infections are also seen. Weight loss and malnutrition are common.

Chest pain may be a common symptom during stimulant intoxication. Myocardial infarction, palpitations and arrhythmias, sudden death from respiratory or cardiac arrest, and stroke have been associated with stimulant use among young and otherwise healthy individuals. Seizures can occur with stimulant use. Pneumothorax can result from performing Valsalva-like maneuvers done to better absorb inhaled smoke. Traumatic injuries due to violent behavior are common among individuals trafficking drugs. Cocaine use is associated with irregularities in placental blood flow, abruptio placentae, premature labor and delivery, and an increased prevalence of infants with very low birth weights.

Individuals with stimulant use disorder may become involved in theft, prostitution, or drug dealing in order to acquire drugs or money for drugs.

Neurocognitive impairment is common among methamphetamine users. Oral health problems include "meth mouth" with gum disease, tooth decay, and mouth sores related to the toxic effects of smoking the drug and to bruxism while intoxicated. Adverse pulmonary effects appear to be less common for amphetamine-type stimulants because they are smoked fewer times per day. Emergency department visits are common for stimulant-related mental disorder symptoms, injury, skin infections, and dental pathology.

Differential Diagnosis

Primary mental disorders.   Stimulant-induced disorders may resemble primary mental disorders (e.g., major depressive disorder) (for discussion of this differential diagnosis, see "Stimulant Withdrawal"). The mental disturbances resulting from the effects of stimulants should be distinguished from the symptoms of schizophrenia; depressive and bipolar disorders; generalized anxiety disorder; and panic disorder.

Phencyclidine intoxication.   Intoxication with phencyclidine ("PCP" or "angel dust") or synthetic "designer drugs" such as mephedrone (known by different names, including "bath salts") may cause a similar clinical picture and can only be distinguished from stimulant intoxication by the presence of cocaine or amphetamine-type substance metabolites in a urine or plasma sample.

Stimulant intoxication and withdrawal.   Stimulant intoxication and withdrawal are distinguished from the other stimulant-induced disorders (e.g., anxiety disorder, with onset during intoxication) because the symptoms in the latter disorders predominate the clinical presentation and are severe enough to warrant independent clinical attention.

Comorbidity

Stimulant-related disorders often co-occur with other substance use disorders, especially those involving substances with sedative properties, which are often taken to reduce insomnia, nervousness, and other unpleasant side effects. Cocaine users often use alcohol, while amphetamine-type stimulant users often use cannabis. Stimulant use disorder may be associated with posttraumatic stress disorder, antisocial personality disorder, attention-deficit/hyperactivity disorder, and gambling disorder. Cardiopulmonary problems are often present in individuals seeking treatment for cocaine-related problems, with chest pain being the most common. Medical problems occur in response to adulterants used as "cutting" agents. Cocaine users who ingest cocaine cut with levamisole, an antimicrobial and veterinary medication, may experience agranulocytosis and febrile neutropenia.

Stimulant Intoxication

Diagnostic Criteria

A. Recent use of an amphetamine-type substance, cocaine, or other stimulant.

B. Clinically significant problematic behavioral or psychological changes (e.g., euphoria or affective blunting; changes in sociability; hypervigilance; interpersonal sensitivity; anxiety, tension, or anger; stereotyped behaviors; impaired judgment) that developed during, or shortly after, use of a stimulant.

C. Two (or more) of the following signs or symptoms, developing during, or shortly after, stimulant use:

1. Tachycardia or bradycardia.
2. Pupillary dilation.
3. Elevated or lowered blood pressure.
4. Perspiration or chills.
5. Nausea or vomiting.
6. Evidence of weight loss.
7. Psychomotor agitation or retardation.
8. Muscular weakness, respiratory depression, chest pain, or cardiac arrhythmias.
9. Confusion, seizures, dyskinesias, dystonias, or coma.

D. The signs or symptoms are not attributable to another medical condition and are not better explained by another mental disorder, including intoxication with another substance.

Specify **the specific intoxicant** (i.e., amphetamine-type substance, cocaine, or other stimulant).

Specify if:

With perceptual disturbances: This specifier may be noted when hallucinations with intact reality testing or auditory, visual, or tactile illusions occur in the absence of a delirium.

Coding note: The ICD-9-CM code is **292.89.** The ICD-10-CM code depends on whether the stimulant is an amphetamine, cocaine, or other stimulant; whether there is a comorbid amphetamine, cocaine, or other stimulant use disorder; and whether or not there are perceptual disturbances.

For amphetamine, cocaine, or other stimulant intoxication, without perceptual disturbances: If a mild amphetamine or other stimulant use disorder is comorbid, the ICD-10-CM code is **F15.129,** and if a moderate or severe amphetamine or other stimulant use disorder is comorbid, the ICD-10-CM code is **F15.229.** If there is no comorbid amphetamine or other stimulant use disorder, then the ICD-10-CM code is **F15.929.** Similarly, if a mild cocaine use disorder is comorbid, the ICD-10-CM code is **F14.129,** and if a moderate or severe cocaine use disorder is comorbid, the ICD-10-CM code is **F14.229.** If there is no comorbid cocaine use disorder, then the ICD-10-CM code is **F14.929.**

For amphetamine, cocaine, or other stimulant intoxication, with perceptual disturbances: If a mild amphetamine or other stimulant use disorder is comorbid, the ICD-10-CM code is **F15.122,** and if a moderate or severe amphetamine or other stimulant use disorder is comorbid, the ICD-10-CM code is **F15.222.** If there is no comorbid amphetamine or other stimulant use disorder, then the ICD-10-CM code is **F15.922.** Similarly, if a mild cocaine use disorder is comorbid, the ICD-10-CM code is **F14.122,** and if a moderate or severe cocaine use disorder is comorbid, the ICD-10-CM code is **F14.222.** If there is no comorbid cocaine use disorder, then the ICD-10-CM code is **F14.922.**

Diagnostic Features

The essential feature of stimulant intoxication, related to amphetamine-type stimulants and cocaine, is the presence of clinically significant behavioral or psychological changes that develop during, or shortly after, use of stimulants (Criteria A and B). Auditory hallucinations may be prominent, as may paranoid ideation, and these symptoms must be distinguished from an independent psychotic disorder such as schizophrenia. Stimulant intoxication usually begins with a "high" feeling and includes one or more of the following: euphoria with enhanced vigor, gregariousness, hyperactivity, restlessness, hypervigilance, interpersonal sensitivity, talkativeness, anxiety, tension, alertness, grandiosity, stereotyped and repetitive behavior, anger, impaired judgment, and, in the case of chronic intoxication, affective blunting with fatigue or sadness and social withdrawal. These behavioral and psychological changes are accompanied by two or more of the following signs and symptoms that develop during or shortly after stimulant use: tachycardia or bradycardia; pupillary dilation; elevated or lowered blood pressure; perspiration or chills; nausea or vomiting; evidence of weight loss; psychomotor agitation or retardation; muscular weakness, respiratory depression, chest pain, or cardiac arrhythmias; and confusion, seizures, dyskinesias, dystonias, or coma (Criterion C). Intoxication, either acute or chronic, is often associated with impaired social or occupational functioning. Severe intoxication can lead to convulsions, cardiac arrhythmias, hyperpyrexia, and death. For the diagnosis of stimulant intoxication to be made, the symptoms must not be attributable to another medical condition and not better explained by another mental disorder (Criterion D). While stimulant intoxication occurs in individuals with stimulant use disorders, intoxication is not a criterion for stimulant use disorder, which is confirmed by the presence of two of the 11 diagnostic criteria for use disorder.

Associated Features Supporting Diagnosis

The magnitude and direction of the behavioral and physiological changes depend on many variables, including the dose used and the characteristics of the individual using the substance or the context (e.g., tolerance, rate of absorption, chronicity of use, context in which it is taken). Stimulant effects such as euphoria, increased pulse and blood pressure, and psychomotor activity are most commonly seen. Depressant effects such as sadness, bradycardia, decreased blood pressure, and decreased psychomotor activity are less common and generally emerge only with chronic high-dose use.

Differential Diagnosis

Stimulant-induced disorders. Stimulant intoxication is distinguished from the other stimulant-induced disorders (e.g., stimulant-induced depressive disorder, bipolar disorder, psychotic disorder, anxiety disorder) because the severity of the intoxication symptoms exceeds that associated with the stimulant-induced disorders, and the symptoms warrant independent clinical attention. Stimulant intoxication delirium would be distinguished by a disturbance in level of awareness and change in cognition.

Other mental disorders. Salient mental disturbances associated with stimulant intoxication should be distinguished from the symptoms of schizophrenia, paranoid type; bipolar and depressive disorders; generalized anxiety disorder; and panic disorder as described in DSM-5.

Stimulant Withdrawal

Diagnostic Criteria

A. Cessation of (or reduction in) prolonged amphetamine-type substance, cocaine, or other stimulant use.

B. Dysphoric mood and two (or more) of the following physiological changes, developing within a few hours to several days after Criterion A:

   1. Fatigue.
   2. Vivid, unpleasant dreams.
   3. Insomnia or hypersomnia.
   4. Increased appetite.
   5. Psychomotor retardation or agitation.

C. The signs or symptoms in Criterion B cause clinically significant distress or impairment in social, occupational, or other important areas of functioning.

D. The signs or symptoms are not attributable to another medical condition and are not better explained by another mental disorder, including intoxication or withdrawal from another substance.

Specify **the specific substance that causes the withdrawal syndrome** (i.e., amphetamine-type substance, cocaine, or other stimulant).

Coding note: The ICD-9-CM code is **292.0.** The ICD-10-CM code depends on whether the stimulant is an amphetamine, cocaine, or other stimulant. The ICD-10-CM code for amphetamine or an other stimulant withdrawal is **F15.23,** and the ICD-10-CM for cocaine withdrawal is **F14.23.** Note that the ICD-10-CM code indicates the comorbid presence of a moderate or severe amphetamine, cocaine, or other stimulant use disorder, reflecting the fact that amphetamine, cocaine, or other stimulant withdrawal can only occur in the presence of a moderate or severe amphetamine, cocaine, or other stimulant use disorder. It is not permissible to code a comorbid mild amphetamine, cocaine, or other stimulant use disorder with amphetamine, cocaine, or other stimulant withdrawal.

Diagnostic Features

The essential feature of stimulant withdrawal is the presence of a characteristic withdrawal syndrome that develops within a few hours to several days after the cessation of (or marked reduction in) stimulant use (generally high dose) that has been prolonged (Criterion A). The withdrawal syndrome is characterized by the development of dysphoric mood accompanied by two or more of the following physiological changes: fatigue, vivid and unpleasant dreams, insomnia or hypersomnia, increased appetite, and psychomotor retardation or agitation (Criterion B). Bradycardia is often present and is a reliable measure of stimulant withdrawal.

Anhedonia and drug craving can often be present but are not part of the diagnostic criteria. These symptoms cause clinically significant distress or impairment in social, occupational, or other important areas of functioning (Criterion C). The symptoms must not be attributable to another medical condition and are not better explained by another mental disorder (Criterion D).

Associated Features Supporting Diagnosis

Acute withdrawal symptoms ("a crash") are often seen after periods of repetitive high-dose use ("runs" or "binges"). These periods are characterized by intense and unpleasant feelings of lassitude and depression and increased appetite, generally requiring several days of rest and recuperation. Depressive symptoms with suicidal ideation or behavior can occur and are generally the most serious problems seen during "crashing" or other forms of stimulant withdrawal. The majority of individuals with stimulant use disorder experience a withdrawal syndrome at some point, and virtually all individuals with the disorder report tolerance.

Differential Diagnosis

Stimulant use disorder and other stimulant-induced disorders.   Stimulant withdrawal is distinguished from stimulant use disorder and from the other stimulant-induced disorders (e.g., stimulant-induced intoxication delirium, depressive disorder, bipolar disorder, psychotic disorder, anxiety disorder, sexual dysfunction, sleep disorder) because the symptoms of withdrawal predominate the clinical presentation and are severe enough to warrant independent clinical attention.

Other Stimulant-Induced Disorders

The following stimulant-induced disorders (which include amphetamine-, cocaine-, and other stimulant–induced disorders) are described in other chapters of the manual with disorders with which they share phenomenology (see the substance/medication-induced mental disorders in these chapters): stimulant-induced psychotic disorder ("Schizophrenia Spectrum and Other Psychotic Disorders"); stimulant-induced bipolar disorder ("Bipolar and Related Disorders"); stimulant-induced depressive disorder ("Depressive Disorders"); stimulant-induced anxiety disorder ("Anxiety Disorders"); stimulant-induced obsessive-compulsive disorder ("Obsessive-Compulsive and Related Disorders"); stimulant-induced sleep disorder ("Sleep-Wake Disorders"); and stimulant-induced sexual dysfunction ("Sexual Dysfunctions"). For stimulant intoxication delirium, see the criteria and discussion of delirium in the chapter "Neurocognitive Disorders." These stimulant-induced disorders are diagnosed instead of stimulant intoxication or stimulant withdrawal only when the symptoms are sufficiently severe to warrant independent clinical attention.

Unspecified Stimulant-Related Disorder

This category applies to presentations in which symptoms characteristic of a stimulant-related disorder that cause clinically significant distress or impairment in social, occupational, or other important areas of functioning predominate but do not meet the full criteria for any specific stimulant-related disorder or any of the disorders in the substance-related and addictive disorders diagnostic class.

Coding note: The ICD-9-CM code is **292.9.** The ICD-10-CM code depends on whether the stimulant is an amphetamine, cocaine, or another stimulant. The ICD-10-CM code for an unspecified amphetamine- or other stimulant-related disorder is **F15.99.** The ICD-10-CM code for an unspecified cocaine-related disorder is **F14.99.**

Tobacco-Related Disorders

Tobacco Use Disorder
Tobacco Withdrawal
Other Tobacco-Induced Disorders
Unspecified Tobacco-Related Disorder

Tobacco Use Disorder

Diagnostic Criteria

A. A problematic pattern of tobacco use leading to clinically significant impairment or distress, as manifested by at least two of the following, occurring within a 12-month period:

1. Tobacco is often taken in larger amounts or over a longer period than was intended.
2. There is a persistent desire or unsuccessful efforts to cut down or control tobacco use.
3. A great deal of time is spent in activities necessary to obtain or use tobacco.
4. Craving, or a strong desire or urge to use tobacco.
5. Recurrent tobacco use resulting in a failure to fulfill major role obligations at work, school, or home (e.g., interference with work).
6. Continued tobacco use despite having persistent or recurrent social or interpersonal problems caused or exacerbated by the effects of tobacco (e.g., arguments with others about tobacco use).
7. Important social, occupational, or recreational activities are given up or reduced because of tobacco use.
8. Recurrent tobacco use in situations in which it is physically hazardous (e.g., smoking in bed).
9. Tobacco use is continued despite knowledge of having a persistent or recurrent physical or psychological problem that is likely to have been caused or exacerbated by tobacco.
10. Tolerance, as defined by either of the following:
    a. A need for markedly increased amounts of tobacco to achieve the desired effect.
    b. A markedly diminished effect with continued use of the same amount of tobacco.
11. Withdrawal, as manifested by either of the following:
    a. The characteristic withdrawal syndrome for tobacco (refer to Criteria A and B of the criteria set for tobacco withdrawal).
    b. Tobacco (or a closely related substance, such as nicotine) is taken to relieve or avoid withdrawal symptoms.

Specify if:
In early remission: After full criteria for tobacco use disorder were previously met, none of the criteria for tobacco use disorder have been met for at least 3 months but for less than 12 months (with the exception that Criterion A4, "Craving, or a strong desire or urge to use tobacco," may be met).
In sustained remission: After full criteria for tobacco use disorder were previously met, none of the criteria for tobacco use disorder have been met at any time during a period of 12 months or longer (with the exception that Criterion A4, "Craving, or a strong desire or urge to use tobacco," may be met).

Specify if:

> **On maintenance therapy:** The individual is taking a long-term maintenance medication, such as nicotine replacement medication, and no criteria for tobacco use disorder have been met for that class of medication (except tolerance to, or withdrawal from, the nicotine replacement medication).
>
> **In a controlled environment:** This additional specifier is used if the individual is in an environment where access to tobacco is restricted.

Coding based on current severity: Note for ICD-10-CM codes: If a tobacco withdrawal or tobacco-induced sleep disorder is also present, do not use the codes below for tobacco use disorder. Instead, the comorbid tobacco use disorder is indicated in the 4th character of the tobacco-induced disorder code (see the coding note for tobacco withdrawal or tobacco-induced sleep disorder). For example, if there is comorbid tobacco-induced sleep disorder and tobacco use disorder, only the tobacco-induced sleep disorder code is given, with the 4th character indicating whether the comorbid tobacco use disorder is moderate or severe: F17.208 for moderate or severe tobacco use disorder with tobacco-induced sleep disorder. It is not permissible to code a comorbid mild tobacco use disorder with a tobacco-induced sleep disorder.

Specify current severity:

> **305.1 (Z72.0) Mild:** Presence of 2–3 symptoms.
> **305.1 (F17.200) Moderate:** Presence of 4–5 symptoms.
> **305.1 (F17.200) Severe:** Presence of 6 or more symptoms.

Specifiers

"On maintenance therapy" applies as a further specifier to individuals being maintained on other tobacco cessation medication (e.g., bupropion, varenicline) and as a further specifier of remission if the individual is both in remission and on maintenance therapy. "In a controlled environment" applies as a further specifier of remission if the individual is both in remission and in a controlled environment (i.e., in early remission in a controlled environment or in sustained remission in a controlled environment). Examples of these environments are closely supervised and substance-free jails, therapeutic communities, and locked hospital units.

Diagnostic Features

Tobacco use disorder is common among individuals who use cigarettes and smokeless tobacco daily and is uncommon among individuals who do not use tobacco daily or who use nicotine medications. Tolerance to tobacco is exemplified by the disappearance of nausea and dizziness after repeated intake and with a more intense effect of tobacco the first time it is used during the day. Cessation of tobacco use can produce a well-defined withdrawal syndrome. Many individuals with tobacco use disorder use tobacco to relieve or to avoid withdrawal symptoms (e.g., after being in a situation where use is restricted). Many individuals who use tobacco have tobacco-related physical symptoms or diseases and continue to smoke. The large majority report craving when they do not smoke for several hours. Spending excessive time using tobacco can be exemplified by chain-smoking (i.e., smoking one cigarette after another with no time between cigarettes). Because tobacco sources are readily and legally available, and because nicotine intoxication is very rare, spending a great deal of time attempting to procure tobacco or recovering from its effects is uncommon. Giving up important social, occupational, or recreational activities can occur when an individual forgoes an activity because it occurs in tobacco use–restricted areas. Use of tobacco rarely results in failure to fulfill major role obligations (e.g., interference with work, interference with home obligations), but persistent social or interpersonal problems (e.g., having arguments with others about tobacco use, avoiding social situations because of others' disapproval of tobacco use) or use that is physically hazardous (e.g., smoking in bed, smoking around flammable chemicals) occur at an intermediate prevalence. Although these criteria are less often endorsed by tobacco users, if endorsed, they can indicate a more severe disorder.

Associated Features Supporting Diagnosis

Smoking within 30 minutes of waking, smoking daily, smoking more cigarettes per day, and waking at night to smoke are associated with tobacco use disorder. Environmental cues can evoke craving and withdrawal. Serious medical conditions, such as lung and other cancers, cardiac and pulmonary disease, perinatal problems, cough, shortness of breath, and accelerated skin aging, often occur.

Prevalence

Cigarettes are the most commonly used tobacco product, representing over 90% of tobacco/nicotine use. In the United States, 57% of adults have never been smokers, 22% are former smokers, and 21% are current smokers. Approximately 20% of current U.S. smokers are nondaily smokers. The prevalence of smokeless tobacco use is less than 5%, and the prevalence of tobacco use in pipes and cigars is less than 1%.

DSM-IV nicotine dependence criteria can be used to estimate the prevalence of tobacco use disorder, but since they are a subset of tobacco use disorder criteria, the prevalence of tobacco use disorder will be somewhat greater. The 12-month prevalence of DSM-IV nicotine dependence in the United States is 13% among adults age 18 years and older. Rates are similar among adult males (14%) and females (12%) and decline in age from 17% among 18- to 29-year-olds to 4% among individuals age 65 years and older. The prevalence of current nicotine dependence is greater among Native American and Alaska Natives (23%) than among whites (14%) but is less among African Americans (10%), Asian Americans and Pacific Islanders (6%), and Hispanics (6%). The prevalence among current daily smokers is approximately 50%.

In many developing nations, the prevalence of smoking is much greater in males than in females, but this is not the case in developed nations. However, there often is a lag in the demographic transition such that smoking increases in females at a later time.

Development and Course

The majority of U.S. adolescents experiment with tobacco use, and by age 18 years, about 20% smoke at least monthly. Most of these individuals become daily tobacco users. Initiation of smoking after age 21 years is rare. In general, some of the tobacco use disorder criteria symptoms occur soon after beginning tobacco use, and many individuals' pattern of use meets current tobacco use disorder criteria by late adolescence. More than 80% of individuals who use tobacco attempt to quit at some time, but 60% relapse within 1 week and less than 5% remain abstinent for life. However, most individuals who use tobacco make multiple attempts such that one-half of tobacco users eventually abstain. Individuals who use tobacco who do quit usually do not do so until after age 30 years. Although nondaily smoking in the United States was previously rare, it has become more prevalent in the last decade, especially among younger individuals who use tobacco.

Risk and Prognostic Factors

Temperamental.   Individuals with externalizing personality traits are more likely to initiate tobacco use. Children with attention-deficit/hyperactivity disorder or conduct disorder, and adults with depressive, bipolar, anxiety, personality, psychotic, or other substance use disorders, are at higher risk of starting and continuing tobacco use and of tobacco use disorder.

Environmental.   Individuals with low incomes and low educational levels are more likely to initiate tobacco use and are less likely to stop.

Genetic and physiological.   Genetic factors contribute to the onset of tobacco use, the continuation of tobacco use, and the development of tobacco use disorder, with a degree of heritability equivalent to that observed with other substance use disorders (i.e., about 50%). Some of this risk is specific to tobacco, and some is common with the vulnerability to developing any substance use disorder.

Culture-Related Diagnostic Issues

Cultures and subcultures vary widely in their acceptance of the use of tobacco. The prevalence of tobacco use declined in the United States from the 1960s through the 1990s, but this decrease has been less evident in African American and Hispanic populations. Also, smoking in developing countries is more prevalent than in developed nations. The degree to which these cultural differences are due to income, education, and tobacco control activities in a country is unclear. Non-Hispanic white smokers appear to be more likely to develop tobacco use disorder than are smokers. Some ethnic differences may be biologically based. African American males tend to have higher nicotine blood levels for a given number of cigarettes, and this might contribute to greater difficulty in quitting. Also, the speed of nicotine metabolism is significantly different for whites compared with African Americans and can vary by genotypes associated with ethnicities.

Diagnostic Markers

Carbon monoxide in the breath, and nicotine and its metabolite cotinine in blood, saliva, or urine, can be used to measure the extent of current tobacco or nicotine use; however, these are only weakly related to tobacco use disorder.

Functional Consequences of Tobacco Use Disorder

Medical consequences of tobacco use often begin when tobacco users are in their 40s and usually become progressively more debilitating over time. One-half of smokers who do not stop using tobacco will die early from a tobacco-related illness, and smoking-related morbidity occurs in more than one-half of tobacco users. Most medical conditions result from exposure to carbon monoxide, tars, and other non-nicotine components of tobacco. The major predictor of reversibility is duration of smoking. Secondhand smoke increases the risk of heart disease and cancer by 30%. Long-term use of nicotine medications does not appear to cause medical harm.

Comorbidity

The most common medical diseases from smoking are cardiovascular illnesses, chronic obstructive pulmonary disease, and cancers. Smoking also increases perinatal problems, such as low birth weight and miscarriage. The most common psychiatric comorbidities are alcohol/substance, depressive, bipolar, anxiety, personality, and attention-deficit/hyperactivity disorders. In individuals with current tobacco use disorder, the prevalence of current alcohol, drug, anxiety, depressive, bipolar, and personality disorders ranges from 22% to 32%. Nicotine-dependent smokers are 2.7–8.1 times more likely to have these disorders than nondependent smokers, never-smokers, or ex-smokers.

Tobacco Withdrawal

Diagnostic Criteria   **292.0 (F17.203)**

A. Daily use of tobacco for at least several weeks.

B. Abrupt cessation of tobacco use, or reduction in the amount of tobacco used, followed within 24 hours by four (or more) of the following signs or symptoms:

1. Irritability, frustration, or anger.
2. Anxiety.
3. Difficulty concentrating.
4. Increased appetite.
5. Restlessness.
6. Depressed mood.
7. Insomnia.

C. The signs or symptoms in Criterion B cause clinically significant distress or impairment in social, occupational, or other important areas of functioning.

D. The signs or symptoms are not attributed to another medical condition and are not better explained by another mental disorder, including intoxication or withdrawal from another substance.

Coding note: The ICD-9-CM code is 292.0. The ICD-10-CM code for tobacco withdrawal is F17.203. Note that the ICD-10-CM code indicates the comorbid presence of a moderate or severe tobacco use disorder, reflecting the fact that tobacco withdrawal can only occur in the presence of a moderate or severe tobacco use disorder. It is not permissible to code a comorbid mild tobacco use disorder with tobacco withdrawal.

Diagnostic Features

Withdrawal symptoms impair the ability to stop tobacco use. The symptoms after abstinence from tobacco are in large part due to nicotine deprivation. Symptoms are much more intense among individuals who smoke cigarettes or use smokeless tobacco than among those who use nicotine medications. This difference in symptom intensity is likely due to the more rapid onset and higher levels of nicotine with cigarette smoking. Tobacco withdrawal is common among daily tobacco users who stop or reduce but can also occur among nondaily users. Typically, heart rate decreases by 5–12 beats per minute in the first few days after stopping smoking, and weight increases an average of 4–7 lb (2–3 kg) over the first year after stopping smoking. Tobacco withdrawal can produce clinically significant mood changes and functional impairment.

Associated Features Supporting Diagnosis

Craving for sweet or sugary foods and impaired performance on tasks requiring vigilance are associated with tobacco withdrawal. Abstinence can increase constipation, coughing, dizziness, dreaming/nightmares, nausea, and sore throat. Smoking increases the metabolism of many medications used to treat mental disorders; thus, cessation of smoking can increase the blood levels of these medications, and this can produce clinically significant outcomes. This effect appears to be due not to nicotine but rather to other compounds in tobacco.

Prevalence

Approximately 50% of tobacco users who quit for 2 or more days will have symptoms that meet criteria for tobacco withdrawal. The most commonly endorsed signs and symptoms are anxiety, irritability, and difficulty concentrating. The least commonly endorsed symptoms are depression and insomnia.

Development and Course

Tobacco withdrawal usually begins within 24 hours of stopping or cutting down on tobacco use, peaks at 2–3 days after abstinence, and lasts 2–3 weeks. Tobacco withdrawal symptoms can occur among adolescent tobacco users, even prior to daily tobacco use. Prolonged symptoms beyond 1 month are uncommon.

Risk and Prognostic Factors

Temperamental.   Smokers with depressive disorders, bipolar disorders, anxiety disorders, attention-deficit/hyperactivity disorder, and other substance use disorders have more severe withdrawal.

Genetic and physiological.   Genotype can influence the probability of withdrawal upon abstinence.

Diagnostic Markers

Carbon monoxide in the breath, and nicotine and its metabolite cotinine in blood, saliva, or urine, can be used to measure the extent of tobacco or nicotine use but are only weakly related to tobacco withdrawal.

Functional Consequences of Tobacco Withdrawal

Abstinence from cigarettes can cause clinically significant distress. Withdrawal impairs the ability to stop or control tobacco use. Whether tobacco withdrawal can prompt a new mental disorder or recurrence of a mental disorder is debatable, but if this occurs, it would be in a small minority of tobacco users.

Differential Diagnosis

The symptoms of tobacco withdrawal overlap with those of other substance withdrawal syndromes (e.g., alcohol withdrawal; sedative, hypnotic, or anxiolytic withdrawal; stimulant withdrawal; caffeine withdrawal; opioid withdrawal); caffeine intoxication; anxiety, depressive, bipolar, and sleep disorders; and medication-induced akathisia. Admission to smoke-free inpatient units or voluntary smoking cessation can induce withdrawal symptoms that mimic, intensify, or disguise other disorders or adverse effects of medications used to treat mental disorders (e.g., irritability thought to be due to alcohol withdrawal could be due to tobacco withdrawal). Reduction in symptoms with the use of nicotine medications confirms the diagnosis.

Other Tobacco-Induced Disorders

Tobacco-induced sleep disorder is discussed in the chapter "Sleep-Wake Disorders" (see "Substance/Medication-Induced Sleep Disorder").

Unspecified Tobacco-Related Disorder

292.9 (F17.209)

This category applies to presentations in which symptoms characteristic of a tobacco-related disorder that cause clinically significant distress or impairment in social, occupational, or other important areas of functioning predominate but do not meet the full criteria for any specific tobacco-related disorder or any of the disorders in the substance-related and addictive disorders diagnostic class.

Other (or Unknown) Substance–Related Disorders

Other (or Unknown) Substance Use Disorder
Other (or Unknown) Substance Intoxication
Other (or Unknown) Substance Withdrawal
Other (or Unknown) Substance–Induced Disorders
Unspecified Other (or Unknown) Substance–Related Disorder

Other (or Unknown) Substance Use Disorder

Diagnostic Criteria

A. A problematic pattern of use of an intoxicating substance not able to be classified within the alcohol; caffeine; cannabis; hallucinogen (phencyclidine and others); inhalant; opioid; sedative, hypnotic, or anxiolytic; stimulant; or tobacco categories and leading to clinically significant impairment or distress, as manifested by at least two of the following, occurring within a 12-month period:

  1. The substance is often taken in larger amounts or over a longer period than was intended.
  2. There is a persistent desire or unsuccessful efforts to cut down or control use of the substance.
  3. A great deal of time is spent in activities necessary to obtain the substance, use the substance, or recover from its effects.
  4. Craving, or a strong desire or urge to use the substance.
  5. Recurrent use of the substance resulting in a failure to fulfill major role obligations at work, school, or home.
  6. Continued use of the substance despite having persistent or recurrent social or interpersonal problems caused or exacerbated by the effects of its use.
  7. Important social, occupational, or recreational activities are given up or reduced because of use of the substance.
  8. Recurrent use of the substance in situations in which it is physically hazardous.
  9. Use of the substance is continued despite knowledge of having a persistent or recurrent physical or psychological problem that is likely to have been caused or exacerbated by the substance.

10. Tolerance, as defined by either of the following:

    a. A need for markedly increased amounts of the substance to achieve intoxication or desired effect.

    b. A markedly diminished effect with continued use of the same amount of the substance.

11. Withdrawal, as manifested by either of the following:

    a. The characteristic withdrawal syndrome for other (or unknown) substance (refer to Criteria A and B of the criteria sets for other [or unknown] substance withdrawal, p. 583).

    b. The substance (or a closely related substance) is taken to relieve or avoid withdrawal symptoms.

Specify if:

In early remission: After full criteria for other (or unknown) substance use disorder were previously met, none of the criteria for other (or unknown) substance use disorder have been met for at least 3 months but for less than 12 months (with the exception that Criterion A4, "Craving, or a strong desire or urge to use the substance," may be met).

In sustained remission: After full criteria for other (or unknown) substance use disorder were previously met, none of the criteria for other (or unknown) substance use disorder have been met at any time during a period of 12 months or longer (with the exception that Criterion A4, "Craving, or a strong desire or urge to use the substance," may be met).

Specify if:

In a controlled environment: This additional specifier is used if the individual is in an environment where access to the substance is restricted.

Coding based on current severity: Note for ICD-10-CM codes: If an other (or unknown) substance intoxication, other (or unknown) substance withdrawal, or another other (or unknown) substance–induced mental disorder is present, do not use the codes below for other (or unknown) substance use disorder. Instead, the comorbid other (or unknown) substance use disorder is indicated in the 4th character of the other (or unknown) substance–induced disorder code (see the coding note for other (or unknown) substance intoxication, other (or unknown) substance withdrawal, or specific other (or unknown) substance–induced mental disorder). For example, if there is comorbid other (or unknown) substance–induced depressive disorder and other (or unknown) substance use disorder, only the other (or unknown) substance–induced depressive disorder code is given, with the 4th character indicating whether the comorbid other (or unknown) substance use disorder is mild, moderate, or severe: F19.14 for other (or unknown) substance use disorder with other (or unknown) substance–induced depressive disorder or F19.24 for a moderate or severe other (or unknown) substance use disorder with other (or unknown) substance–induced depressive disorder.

Specify current severity:

305.90 (F19.10) Mild: Presence of 2–3 symptoms.

304.90 (F19.20) Moderate: Presence of 4–5 symptoms.

304.90 (F19.20) Severe: Presence of 6 or more symptoms.

Specifiers

"In a controlled environment" applies as a further specifier of remission if the individual is both in remission and in a controlled environment (i.e., in early remission in a controlled environment or in sustained remission in a controlled environment). Examples of these environments are closely supervised and substance-free jails, therapeutic communities, and locked hospital units.

Diagnostic Features

The diagnostic class other (or unknown) substance use and related disorders comprises substance-related disorders unrelated to alcohol; caffeine; cannabis; hallucinogens (phencyclidine and others); inhalants; opioids; sedative, hypnotics, or anxiolytics; stimulants (including amphetamine and cocaine); or tobacco. Such substances include anabolic steroids; nonsteroidal anti-inflammatory drugs; cortisol; antiparkinsonian medications; antihistamines; nitrous oxide; amyl-, butyl-, or isobutyl-nitrites; betel nut, which is chewed in many cultures to produce mild euphoria and a floating sensation; kava (from a South Pacific pepper plant), which produces sedation, incoordination, weight loss, mild hepatitis, and lung abnormalities; or cathinones (including *khât* plant agents and synthetic chemical derivatives) that produce stimulant effects. Unknown substance-related disorders are associated with unidentified substances, such as intoxications in which the individual cannot identify the ingested drug, or substance use disorders involving either new, black market drugs not yet identified or familiar drugs illegally sold under false names.

Other (or unknown) substance use disorder is a mental disorder in which repeated use of an other or unknown substance typically continues, despite the individual's knowing that the substance is causing serious problems for the individual. Those problems are reflected in the diagnostic criteria. When the substance is known, it should be reflected in the name of the disorder upon coding (e.g., nitrous oxide use disorder).

Associated Features Supporting Diagnosis

A diagnosis of other (or unknown) substance use disorder is supported by the individual's statement that the substance involved is not among the nine classes listed in this chapter; by recurring episodes of intoxication with negative results in standard drug screens (which may not detect new or rarely used substances); or by the presence of symptoms characteristic of an unidentified substance that has newly appeared in the individual's community.

Because of increased access to nitrous oxide ("laughing gas"), membership in certain populations is associated with diagnosis of nitrous oxide use disorder. The role of this gas as an anesthetic agent leads to misuse by some medical and dental professionals. Its use as a propellant for commercial products (e.g., whipped cream dispensers) contributes to misuse by food service workers. With recent widespread availability of the substance in "whippet" cartridges for use in home whipped cream dispensers, nitrous oxide misuse by adolescents and young adults is significant, especially among those who also inhale volatile hydrocarbons. Some continuously using individuals, inhaling from as many as 240 whippets per day, may present with serious medical complications and mental conditions, including myeloneuropathy, spinal cord subacute combined degeneration, peripheral neuropathy, and psychosis. These conditions are also associated with a diagnosis of nitrous oxide use disorder.

Use of amyl-, butyl-, and isobutyl nitrite gases has been observed among homosexual men and some adolescents, especially those with conduct disorder. Membership in these populations may be associated with a diagnosis of amyl-, butyl-, or isobutyl-nitrite use disorder. However, it has not been determined that these substances produce a substance use disorder. Despite tolerance, these gases may not alter behavior through central effects, and they may be used only for their peripheral effects.

Substance use disorders generally are associated with elevated risks of suicide, but there is no evidence of unique risk factors for suicide with other (or unknown) substance use disorder.

Prevalence

Based on extremely limited data, the prevalence of other (or unknown) substance use disorder is likely lower than that of use disorders involving the nine substance classes in this chapter.

Development and Course

No single pattern of development or course characterizes the pharmacologically varied other (or unknown) substance use disorders. Often unknown substance use disorders will be reclassified when the unknown substance eventually is identified.

Risk and Prognostic Factors

Risk and prognostic factors for other (or unknown) substance use disorders are thought to be similar to those for most substance use disorders and include the presence of any other substance use disorders, conduct disorder, or antisocial personality disorder in the individual or the individual's family; early onset of substance problems; easy availability of the substance in the individual's environment; childhood maltreatment or trauma; and evidence of limited early self-control and behavioral disinhibition.

Culture-Related Diagnostic Issues

Certain cultures may be associated with other (or unknown) substance use disorders involving specific indigenous substances within the cultural region, such as betel nut.

Diagnostic Markers

Urine, breath, or saliva tests may correctly identify a commonly used substance falsely sold as a novel product. However, routine clinical tests usually cannot identify truly unusual or new substances, which may require testing in specialized laboratories.

Differential Diagnosis

Use of other or unknown substances without meeting criteria for other (or unknown) substance use disorder.   Use of unknown substances is not rare among adolescents, but most use does not meet the diagnostic standard of two or more criteria for other (or unknown) substance use disorder in the past year.

Substance use disorders.   Other (or unknown) substance use disorder may co-occur with various substance use disorders, and the symptoms of the disorders may be similar and overlapping. To disentangle symptom patterns, it is helpful to inquire about which symptoms persisted during periods when some of the substances were not being used.

Other (or unknown) substance/medication-induced disorder.   This diagnosis should be differentiated from instances when the individual's symptoms meet full criteria for one of the following disorders, and that disorder is caused by an other or unknown substance: delirium, major or mild neurocognitive disorder, psychotic disorder, depressive disorder, anxiety disorder, sexual dysfunction, or sleep disorder.

Other medical conditions.   Individuals with substance use disorders, including other (or unknown) substance use disorder, may present with symptoms of many medical disorders. These disorders also may occur in the absence of other (or unknown) substance use disorder. A history of little or no use of other or unknown substances helps to exclude other (or unknown) substance use disorder as the source of these problems.

Comorbidity

Substance use disorders, including other (or unknown) substance use disorder, are commonly comorbid with one another, with adolescent conduct disorder and adult antisocial personality disorder, and with suicidal ideation and suicide attempts.

Other (or Unknown) Substance Intoxication

Diagnostic Criteria

A. The development of a reversible substance-specific syndrome attributable to recent ingestion of (or exposure to) a substance that is not listed elsewhere or is unknown.

B. Clinically significant problematic behavioral or psychological changes that are attributable to the effect of the substance on the central nervous system (e.g., impaired motor coordination, psychomotor agitation or retardation, euphoria, anxiety, belligerence, mood lability, cognitive impairment, impaired judgment, social withdrawal) and develop during, or shortly after, use of the substance.

C. The signs or symptoms are not attributable to another medical condition and are not better explained by another mental disorder, including intoxication with another substance.

Coding note: The ICD-9-CM code is **292.89.** The ICD-10-CM code depends on whether there is a comorbid other (or unknown) substance use disorder involving the same substance. If a mild other (or unknown) substance use disorder is comorbid, the ICD-10-CM code is **F19.129,** and if a moderate or severe other (or unknown) substance use disorder is comorbid, the ICD-10-CM code is **F19.229.** If there is no comorbid other (or unknown) substance use disorder involving the same substance, then the ICD-10-CM code is **F19.929.**

Note: For information on Risk and Prognostic Factors, Culture-Related Diagnostic Issues, and Diagnostic Markers, see the corresponding sections in other (or unknown) substance use disorder.

Diagnostic Features

Other (or unknown) substance intoxication is a clinically significant mental disorder that develops during, or immediately after, use of either a) a substance not elsewhere addressed in this chapter (i.e., alcohol; caffeine; cannabis; phencyclidine and other hallucinogens; inhalants; opioids; sedatives, hypnotics, or anxiolytics; stimulants; or tobacco) or b) an unknown substance. If the substance is known, it should be reflected in the name of the disorder upon coding.

Application of the diagnostic criteria for other (or unknown) substance intoxication is very challenging. Criterion A requires development of a reversible "substance-specific syndrome," but if the substance is unknown, that syndrome usually will be unknown. To resolve this conflict, clinicians may ask the individual or obtain collateral history as to whether the individual has experienced a similar episode after using substances with the same "street" name or from the same source. Similarly, hospital emergency departments sometimes recognize over a few days numerous presentations of a severe, unfamiliar intoxication syndrome from a newly available, previously unknown substance. Because of the great variety of intoxicating substances, Criterion B can provide only broad examples of signs and symptoms from some intoxications, with no threshold for the number of symptoms required for a diagnosis; clinical judgment guides those decisions. Criterion C requires ruling out other medical conditions, mental disorders, or intoxications.

Prevalence

The prevalence of other (or unknown) substance intoxication is unknown.

Development and Course

Intoxications usually appear and then peak minutes to hours after use of the substance, but the onset and course vary with the substance and the route of administration. Generally, substances used by pulmonary inhalation and intravenous injection have the most rapid onset of action, while those ingested by mouth and requiring metabolism to an active product are much slower. (For example, after ingestion of certain mushrooms, the first signs of an eventually fatal intoxication may not appear for a few days.) Intoxication effects usually resolve within hours to a very few days. However, the body may completely eliminate an anesthetic gas such as nitrous oxide just minutes after use ends. At the other extreme, some "hit-and-run" intoxicating substances poison systems, leaving permanent impairments. For example, MPTP (1-methyl-4-phenyl-1,2,3,6-tetrahydropyridine), a contaminating by-product in the synthesis of a certain opioid, kills dopaminergic cells and induces permanent parkinsonism in users who sought opioid intoxication.

Functional Consequences of Other (or Unknown) Substance Intoxication

Impairment from intoxication with any substance may have serious consequences, including dysfunction at work, social indiscretions, problems in interpersonal relationships, failure to fulfill role obligations, traffic accidents, fighting, high-risk behaviors (i.e., having unprotected sex), and substance or medication overdose. The pattern of consequences will vary with the particular substance.

Differential Diagnosis

Use of other or unknown substance, without meeting criteria for other (or unknown) substance intoxication.   The individual used an other or unknown substance(s), but the dose was insufficient to produce symptoms that meet the diagnostic criteria required for the diagnosis.

Substance intoxication or other substance/medication-induced disorders.   Familiar substances may be sold in the black market as novel products, and individuals may experience intoxication from those substances. History, toxicology screens, or chemical testing of the substance itself may help to identify it.

Different types of other (or unknown) substance–related disorders.   Episodes of other (or unknown) substance intoxication may occur during, but are distinct from, other (or unknown) substance use disorder, unspecified other (or unknown) substance–related disorder, and other (or unknown) substance–induced disorders.

Other toxic, metabolic, traumatic, neoplastic, vascular, or infectious disorders that impair brain function and cognition.   Numerous neurological and other medical conditions may produce rapid onset of signs and symptoms mimicking those of intoxications, including the examples in Criterion B. Paradoxically, drug withdrawals also must be ruled out, because, for example, lethargy may indicate withdrawal from one drug or intoxication with another drug.

Comorbidity

As with all substance-related disorders, adolescent conduct disorder, adult antisocial personality disorder, and other substance use disorders tend to co-occur with other (or unknown) substance intoxication.

Other (or Unknown) Substance Withdrawal

Diagnostic Criteria   **292.0 (F19.239)**

A. Cessation of (or reduction in) use of a substance that has been heavy and prolonged.

B. The development of a substance-specific syndrome shortly after the cessation of (or reduction in) substance use.

C. The substance-specific syndrome causes clinically significant distress or impairment in social, occupational, or other important areas of functioning.

D. The symptoms are not attributable to another medical condition and are not better explained by another mental disorder, including withdrawal from another substance.

E. The substance involved cannot be classified under any of the other substance categories (alcohol; caffeine; cannabis; opioids; sedatives, hypnotics, or anxiolytics; stimulants; or tobacco) or is unknown.

Coding note: The ICD-9-CM code is 292.0. The ICD-10-CM code for other (or unknown) substance withdrawal is F19.239. Note that the ICD-10-CM code indicates the comorbid presence of a moderate or severe other (or unknown) substance use disorder. It is not permissible to code a comorbid mild other (or unknown) substance use disorder with other (or unknown) substance withdrawal.

Note: For information on Risk and Prognostic Factors and Diagnostic Markers, see the corresponding sections in other (or unknown) substance use disorder.

Diagnostic Features

Other (or unknown) substance withdrawal is a clinically significant mental disorder that develops during, or within a few hours to days after, reducing or terminating dosing with a substance (Criteria A and B). Although recent dose reduction or termination usually is clear in the history, other diagnostic procedures are very challenging if the drug is unknown. Criterion B requires development of a "substance-specific syndrome" (i.e., the individual's signs and symptoms must correspond with the known withdrawal syndrome for the recently stopped drug)—a requirement that rarely can be met with an unknown substance. Consequently, clinical judgment must guide such decisions when information is this limited. Criterion D requires ruling out other medical conditions, mental disorders, or withdrawals from familiar substances. When the substance is known, it should be reflected in the name of the disorder upon coding (e.g., betel nut withdrawal).

Prevalence

The prevalence of other (or unknown) substance withdrawal is unknown.

Development and Course

Withdrawal signs commonly appear some hours after use of the substance is terminated, but the onset and course vary greatly, depending on the dose typically used by the person and the rate of elimination of the specific substance from the body. At peak severity, withdrawal symptoms from some substances involve only moderate levels of discomfort, whereas withdrawal from other substances may be fatal. Withdrawal-associated dysphoria often motivates relapse to substance use. Withdrawal symptoms slowly abate over days, weeks, or months, depending on the particular drug and doses to which the individual became tolerant.

Culture-Related Diagnostic Issues

Culture-related issues in diagnosis will vary with the particular substance.

Functional Consequences of Other (or Unknown) Substance Withdrawal

Withdrawal from any substance may have serious consequences, including physical signs and symptoms (e.g., malaise, vital sign changes, abdominal distress, headache), intense drug craving, anxiety, depression, agitation, psychotic symptoms, or cognitive impairments. These consequences may lead to problems such as dysfunction at work, problems in interpersonal relationships, failure to fulfill role obligations, traffic accidents, fighting, high-risk behavior (e.g., having unprotected sex), suicide attempts, and substance or medication overdose. The pattern of consequences will vary with the particular substance.

Differential Diagnosis

Dose reduction after extended dosing, but not meeting the criteria for other (or unknown) substance withdrawal. The individual used other (or unknown) substances, but the dose that was used was insufficient to produce symptoms that meet the criteria required for the diagnosis.

Substance withdrawal or other substance/medication-induced disorders. Familiar substances may be sold in the black market as novel products, and individuals may experience withdrawal when discontinuing those substances. History, toxicology screens, or chemical testing of the substance itself may help to identify it.

Different types of other (or unknown) substance–related disorders. Episodes of other (or unknown) substance withdrawal may occur during, but are distinct from, other (or unknown) substance use disorder, unspecified other (or unknown) substance–related disorder, and unspecified other (or unknown) substance–induced disorders.

Other toxic, metabolic, traumatic, neoplastic, vascular, or infectious disorders that impair brain function and cognition. Numerous neurological and other medical conditions may produce rapid onset of signs and symptoms mimicking those of withdrawals. Paradoxically, drug intoxications also must be ruled out, because, for example, lethargy may indicate withdrawal from one drug or intoxication with another drug.

Comorbidity

As with all substance-related disorders, adolescent conduct disorder, adult antisocial personality disorder, and other substance use disorders likely co-occur with other (or unknown) substance withdrawal.

Other (or Unknown) Substance–Induced Disorders

Because the category of other or unknown substances is inherently ill-defined, the extent and range of induced disorders are uncertain. Nevertheless, other (or unknown) substance–induced disorders are possible and are described in other chapters of the manual with disorders with which they share phenomenology (see the substance/medication-induced mental disorders in these chapters): other (or unknown) substance–induced psychotic disorder ("Schizophrenia Spectrum and Other Psychotic Disorders"); other (or unknown substance–induced bipolar disorder ("Bipolar and Related Disorders"); other (or unknown) substance–induced depressive disorder ("Depressive Disorders"); other (or unknown) substance–induced anxiety disorders ("Anxiety Disorders"); other (or unknown) substance–induced obsessive-compulsive disorder ("Obsessive-Compulsive and Related Disorders"); other (or unknown) substance–induced sleep disorder ("Sleep-Wake

Disorders"); other (or unknown) substance–induced sexual dysfunction ("Sexual Dysfunctions"); and other (or unknown) substance/medication–induced major or mild neurocognitive disorder ("Neurocognitive Disorders"). For other (or unknown) substance–induced intoxication delirium and other (or unknown) substance–induced withdrawal delirium, see the criteria and discussion of delirium in the chapter "Neurocognitive Disorders." These other (or unknown) substance–induced disorders are diagnosed instead of other (or unknown) substance intoxication or other (or unknown) substance withdrawal only when the symptoms are sufficiently severe to warrant independent clinical attention.

Unspecified Other (or Unknown) Substance–Related Disorder

292.9 (F19.99)

This category applies to presentations in which symptoms characteristic of an other (or unknown) substance–related disorder that cause clinically significant distress or impairment in social, occupational, or other important areas of functioning predominate but do not meet the full criteria for any specific other (or unknown) substance–related disorder or any of the disorders in the substance-related disorders diagnostic class.

Non-Substance-Related Disorders

Gambling Disorder

Diagnostic Criteria   312.31 (F63.0)

A. Persistent and recurrent problematic gambling behavior leading to clinically significant impairment or distress, as indicated by the individual exhibiting four (or more) of the following in a 12-month period:

1. Needs to gamble with increasing amounts of money in order to achieve the desired excitement.
2. Is restless or irritable when attempting to cut down or stop gambling.
3. Has made repeated unsuccessful efforts to control, cut back, or stop gambling.
4. Is often preoccupied with gambling (e.g., having persistent thoughts of reliving past gambling experiences, handicapping or planning the next venture, thinking of ways to get money with which to gamble).
5. Often gambles when feeling distressed (e.g., helpless, guilty, anxious, depressed).
6. After losing money gambling, often returns another day to get even ("chasing" one's losses).
7. Lies to conceal the extent of involvement with gambling.
8. Has jeopardized or lost a significant relationship, job, or educational or career opportunity because of gambling.
9. Relies on others to provide money to relieve desperate financial situations caused by gambling.

B. The gambling behavior is not better explained by a manic episode.

Specify if:

Episodic: Meeting diagnostic criteria at more than one time point, with symptoms subsiding between periods of gambling disorder for at least several months.

Persistent: Experiencing continuous symptoms, to meet diagnostic criteria for multiple years.

Specify if:

In early remission: After full criteria for gambling disorder were previously met, none of the criteria for gambling disorder have been met for at least 3 months but for less than 12 months.

In sustained remission: After full criteria for gambling disorder were previously met, none of the criteria for gambling disorder have been met during a period of 12 months or longer.

Specify current severity:

Mild: 4–5 criteria met.

Moderate: 6–7 criteria met.

Severe: 8–9 criteria met.

Note: Although some behavioral conditions that do not involve ingestion of substances have similarities to substance-related disorders, only one disorder—gambling disorder—has sufficient data to be included in this section.

Specifiers

Severity is based on the number of criteria endorsed. Individuals with mild gambling disorder may exhibit only 4–5 of the criteria, with the most frequently endorsed criteria usually related to preoccupation with gambling and "chasing" losses. Individuals with moderately severe gambling disorder exhibit more of the criteria (i.e., 6–7). Individuals with the most severe form will exhibit all or most of the nine criteria (i.e., 8–9). Jeopardizing relationships or career opportunities due to gambling and relying on others to provide money for gambling losses are typically the least often endorsed criteria and most often occur among those with more severe gambling disorder. Furthermore, individuals presenting for treatment of gambling disorder typically have moderate to severe forms of the disorder.

Diagnostic Features

Gambling involves risking something of value in the hopes of obtaining something of greater value. In many cultures, individuals gamble on games and events, and most do so without experiencing problems. However, some individuals develop substantial impairment related to their gambling behaviors. The essential feature of gambling disorder is persistent and recurrent maladaptive gambling behavior that disrupts personal, family, and/or vocational pursuits (Criterion A). Gambling disorder is defined as a cluster of four or more of the symptoms listed in Criterion A occurring at any time in the same 12-month period.

A pattern of "chasing one's losses" may develop, with an urgent need to keep gambling (often with the placing of larger bets or the taking of greater risks) to undo a loss or series of losses. The individual may abandon his or her gambling strategy and try to win back losses all at once. Although many gamblers may "chase" for short periods of time, it is the frequent, and often long-term, "chase" that is characteristic of gambling disorder (Criterion A6). Individuals may lie to family members, therapists, or others to conceal the extent of involvement with gambling; these instances of deceit may also include, but are not limited to, covering up illegal behaviors such as forgery, fraud, theft, or embezzlement to obtain money with which to gamble (Criterion A7). Individuals may also engage in "bailout" behavior, turning to family or others for help with a desperate financial situation that was caused by gambling (Criterion A9).

Associated Features Supporting Diagnosis

Distortions in thinking (e.g., denial, superstitions, a sense of power and control over the outcome of chance events, overconfidence) may be present in individuals with gambling disorder. Many individuals with gambling disorder believe that money is both the cause of and the solution to their problems. Some individuals with gambling disorder are impulsive, competitive, energetic, restless, and easily bored; they may be overly concerned with the approval of others and may be generous to the point of extravagance when winning. Other individuals with gambling disorder are depressed and lonely, and they may gamble when feeling helpless, guilty, or depressed. Up to half of individuals in treatment for gambling disorder have suicidal ideation, and about 17% have attempted suicide.

Prevalence

The past-year prevalence rate of gambling disorder is about 0.2%–0.3% in the general population. In the general population, the lifetime prevalence rate is about 0.4%–1.0%. For females, the lifetime prevalence rate of gambling disorder is about 0.2%, and for males it is about 0.6%. The lifetime prevalence of pathological gambling among African Americans is about 0.9%, among whites about 0.4%, and among Hispanics about 0.3%.

Development and Course

The onset of gambling disorder can occur during adolescence or young adulthood, but in other individuals it manifests during middle or even older adulthood. Generally, gambling disorder develops over the course of years, although the progression appears to be more rapid in females than in males. Most individuals who develop a gambling disorder evidence a pattern of gambling that gradually increases in both frequency and amount of wagering. Certainly, milder forms can develop into more severe cases. Most individuals with gambling disorder report that one or two types of gambling are most problematic for them, although some individuals participate in many forms of gambling. Individuals are likely to engage in certain types of gambling (e.g., buying scratch tickets daily) more frequently than others (e.g., playing slot machines or blackjack at the casino weekly). Frequency of gambling can be related more to the type of gambling than to the severity of the overall gambling disorder. For example, purchasing a single scratch ticket each day may not be problematic, while less frequent casino, sports, or card gambling may be part of a gambling disorder. Similarly, amounts of money spent wagering are not in themselves indicative of gambling disorder. Some individuals can wager thousands of dollars per month and not have a problem with gambling, while others may wager much smaller amounts but experience substantial gambling-related difficulties.

Gambling patterns may be regular or episodic, and gambling disorder can be persistent or in remission. Gambling can increase during periods of stress or depression and during periods of substance use or abstinence. There may be periods of heavy gambling and severe problems, times of total abstinence, and periods of nonproblematic gambling. Gambling disorder is sometimes associated with spontaneous, long-term remissions. Nevertheless, some individuals underestimate their vulnerability to develop gambling disorder or to return to gambling disorder following remission. When in a period of remission, they may incorrectly assume that they will have no problem regulating gambling and that they may gamble on some forms nonproblematically, only to experience a return to gambling disorder.

Early expression of gambling disorder is more common among males than among females. Individuals who begin gambling in youth often do so with family members or friends. Development of early-life gambling disorder appears to be associated with impulsivity and substance abuse. Many high school and college students who develop gambling disorder grow out of the disorder over time, although it remains a lifelong problem for some. Mid- and later-life onset of gambling disorder is more common among females than among males.

There are age and gender variations in the type of gambling activities and the prevalence rates of gambling disorder. Gambling disorder is more common among younger and middle-age persons than among older adults. Among adolescents and young adults, the disorder is more prevalent in males than in females. Younger individuals prefer different forms of gambling (e.g., sports betting), while older adults are more likely to develop problems with slot machine and bingo gambling. Although the proportions of individuals who seek treatment for gambling disorder are low across all age groups, younger individuals are especially unlikely to present for treatment.

Males are more likely to begin gambling earlier in life and to have a younger age at onset of gambling disorder than females, who are more likely to begin gambling later in life and to develop gambling disorder in a shorter time frame. Females with gambling disorder are more likely than males with gambling disorder to have depressive, bipolar, and anxiety disorders. Females also have a later age at onset of the disorder and seek treatment sooner, although rates of treatment seeking are low (<10%) among individuals with gambling disorder regardless of gender.

Risk and Prognostic Factors

Temperamental.   Gambling that begins in childhood or early adolescence is associated with increased rates of gambling disorder. Gambling disorder also appears to aggregate with antisocial personality disorder, depressive and bipolar disorders, and other substance use disorders, particularly with alcohol disorders.

Genetic and physiological.   Gambling disorder can aggregate in families, and this effect appears to relate to both environmental and genetic factors. Gambling problems are more frequent in monozygotic than in dizygotic twins. Gambling disorder is also more prevalent among first-degree relatives of individuals with moderate to severe alcohol use disorder than among the general population.

Course modifiers.   Many individuals, including adolescents and young adults, are likely to resolve their problems with gambling disorder over time, although a strong predictor of future gambling problems is prior gambling problems.

Culture-Related Diagnostic Issues

Individuals from specific cultures and races/ethnicities are more likely to participate in some types of gambling activities than others (e.g., pai gow, cockfights, blackjack, horse racing). Prevalence rates of gambling disorder are higher among African Americans than among European Americans, with rates for Hispanic Americans similar to those of European Americans. Indigenous populations have high prevalence rates of gambling disorder.

Gender-Related Diagnostic Issues

Males develop gambling disorder at higher rates than females, although this gender gap may be narrowing. Males tend to wager on different forms of gambling than females, with cards, sports, and horse race gambling more prevalent among males, and slot machine and bingo gambling more common among females.

Functional Consequences of Gambling Disorder

Areas of psychosocial, health, and mental health functioning may be adversely affected by gambling disorder. Specifically, individuals with gambling disorder may, because of their involvement with gambling, jeopardize or lose important relationships with family members or friends. Such problems may occur from repeatedly lying to others to cover up the extent of gambling or from requesting money that is used for gambling or to pay off gambling debts. Employment or educational activities may likewise be adversely impacted by gambling disorder; absenteeism or poor work or school performance can occur with gambling disorder, as individuals may gamble during work or school hours or be preoccupied with gambling or its adverse consequence when they should be working or studying. Individuals with gambling disorder have poor general health and utilize medical services at high rates.

Differential Diagnosis

Nondisordered gambling. Gambling disorder must be distinguished from professional and social gambling. In professional gambling, risks are limited and discipline is central. Social gambling typically occurs with friends or colleagues and lasts for a limited period of time, with acceptable losses. Some individuals can experience problems associated with gambling (e.g., short-term chasing behavior and loss of control) that do not meet the full criteria for gambling disorder.

Manic episode. Loss of judgment and excessive gambling may occur during a manic episode. An additional diagnosis of gambling disorder should be given only if the gambling behavior is not better explained by manic episodes (e.g., a history of maladaptive gambling behavior at times other than during a manic episode). Alternatively, an individual with gambling disorder may, during a period of gambling, exhibit behavior that resembles a manic episode, but once the individual is away from the gambling, these manic-like features dissipate.

Personality disorders. Problems with gambling may occur in individuals with antisocial personality disorder and other personality disorders. If the criteria are met for both disorders, both can be diagnosed.

Other medical conditions. Some patients taking dopaminergic medications (e.g., for Parkinson's disease) may experience urges to gamble. If such symptoms dissipate when dopaminergic medications are reduced in dosage or ceased, then a diagnosis of gambling disorder would not be indicated.

Comorbidity

Gambling disorder is associated with poor general health. In addition, some specific medical diagnoses, such as tachycardia and angina, are more common among individuals with gambling disorder than in the general population, even when other substance use disorders, including tobacco use disorder, are controlled for. Individuals with gambling disorder have high rates of comorbidity with other mental disorders, such as substance use disorders, depressive disorders, anxiety disorders, and personality disorders. In some individuals, other mental disorders may precede gambling disorder and be either absent or present during the manifestation of gambling disorder. Gambling disorder may also occur prior to the onset of other mental disorders, especially anxiety disorders and substance use disorders.

Neurocognitive Disorders

The neurocognitive disorders (NCDs) (referred to in DSM-IV as "Dementia, Delirium, Amnestic, and Other Cognitive Disorders") begin with delirium, followed by the syndromes of major NCD, mild NCD, and their etiological subtypes. The major or mild NCD subtypes are NCD due to Alzheimer's disease; vascular NCD; NCD with Lewy bodies; NCD due to Parkinson's disease; frontotemporal NCD; NCD due to traumatic brain injury; NCD due to HIV infection; substance/medication-induced NCD; NCD due to Huntington's disease; NCD due to prion disease; NCD due to another medical condition; NCD due to multiple etiologies; and unspecified NCD. The NCD category encompasses the group of disorders in which the primary clinical deficit is in cognitive function, and that are acquired rather than developmental. Although cognitive deficits are present in many if not all mental disorders (e.g., schizophrenia, bipolar disorders), only disorders whose core features are cognitive are included in the NCD category. The NCDs are those in which impaired cognition has not been present since birth or very early life, and thus represents a decline from a previously attained level of functioning.

The NCDs are unique among DSM-5 categories in that these are syndromes for which the underlying pathology, and frequently the etiology as well, can potentially be determined. The various underlying disease entities have all been the subject of extensive research, clinical experience, and expert consensus on diagnostic criteria. The DSM-5 criteria for these disorders have been developed in close consultation with the expert groups for each of the disease entities and align as closely as possible with the current consensus criteria for each of them. The potential utility of biomarkers is also discussed in relation to diagnosis. Dementia is subsumed under the newly named entity *major neurocognitive disorder*, although the term *dementia* is not precluded from use in the etiological subtypes in which that term is standard. Furthermore, DSM-5 recognizes a less severe level of cognitive impairment, *mild neurocognitive disorder*, which can also be a focus of care, and which in DSM-IV was subsumed under "Cognitive Disorder Not Otherwise Specified." Diagnostic criteria are provided for both these syndromic entities, followed by diagnostic criteria for the different etiological subtypes. Several of the NCDs frequently coexist with one another, and their relationships may be multiply characterized under different chapter subheadings, including "Differential Diagnosis" (e.g., NCD due to Alzheimer's disease vs. vascular NCD), "Risk and Prognostic Factors" (e.g., vascular pathology increasing the clinical expression of Alzheimer's disease), and/or "Comorbidity" (e.g., mixed Alzheimer's disease–vascular pathology).

The term *dementia* is retained in DSM-5 for continuity and may be used in settings where physicians and patients are accustomed to this term. Although dementia is the customary term for disorders like the degenerative dementias that usually affect older adults, the term *neurocognitive disorder* is widely used and often preferred for conditions affecting younger individuals, such as impairment secondary to traumatic brain injury or HIV infection. Furthermore, the major NCD definition is somewhat broader than the term *dementia*, in that individuals with substantial decline in a single domain can receive this diagnosis, most notably the DSM-IV category of "Amnestic Disorder," which would now be diagnosed as major NCD due to another medical condition and for which the term *dementia* would not be used.

Neurocognitive Domains

The criteria for the various NCDs are all based on defined cognitive domains. Table 1 provides for each of the key domains a working definition, examples of symptoms or observations regarding impairments in everyday activities, and examples of assessments. The domains thus defined, along with guidelines for clinical thresholds, form the basis on which the NCDs, their levels, and their subtypes may be diagnosed.

TABLE 1 Neurocognitive domains

Cognitive domain	Examples of symptoms or observations	Examples of assessments
Complex attention (sustained attention, divided attention, selective attention, processing speed)	*Major:* Has increased difficulty in environments with multiple stimuli (TV, radio, conversation); is easily distracted by competing events in the environment. Is unable to attend unless input is restricted and simplified. Has difficulty holding new information in mind, such as recalling phone numbers or addresses just given, or reporting what was just said. Is unable to perform mental calculations. All thinking takes longer than usual, and components to be processed must be simplified to one or a few. *Mild:* Normal tasks take longer than previously. Begins to find errors in routine tasks; finds work needs more double-checking than previously. Thinking is easier when not competing with other things (radio, TV, other conversations, cell phone, driving).	*Sustained attention:* Maintenance of attention over time (e.g., pressing a button every time a tone is heard, and over a period of time). *Selective attention:* Maintenance of attention despite competing stimuli and/or distractors: hearing numbers and letters read and asked to count only letters. *Divided attention:* Attending to two tasks within the same time period: rapidly tapping while learning a story being read. Processing speed can be quantified on any task by timing it (e.g., time to put together a design of blocks; time to match symbols with numbers; speed in responding, such as counting speed or serial 3 speed).
Executive function (planning, decision making, working memory, responding to feedback/error correction, overriding habits/inhibition, mental flexibility)	*Major:* Abandons complex projects. Needs to focus on one task at a time. Needs to rely on others to plan instrumental activities of daily living or make decisions. *Mild:* Increased effort required to complete multistage projects. Has increased difficulty multitasking or difficulty resuming a task interrupted by a visitor or phone call. May complain of increased fatigue from the extra effort required to organize, plan, and make decisions. May report that large social gatherings are more taxing or less enjoyable because of increased effort required to follow shifting conversations.	*Planning:* Ability to find the exit to a maze; interpret a sequential picture or object arrangement. *Decision making:* Performance of tasks that assess process of deciding in the face of competing alternatives (e.g., simulated gambling). *Working memory:* Ability to hold information for a brief period and to manipulate it (e.g., adding up a list of numbers or repeating a series of numbers or words backward). *Feedback/error utilization:* Ability to benefit from feedback to infer the rules for solving a problem. *Overriding habits/inhibition:* Ability to choose a more complex and effortful solution to be correct (e.g., looking away from the direction indicated by an arrow; naming the color of a word's font rather than naming the word). *Mental/cognitive flexibility:* Ability to shift between two concepts, tasks, or response rules (e.g., from number to letter, from verbal to key-press response, from adding numbers to ordering numbers, from ordering objects by size to ordering by color).

TABLE 1 Neurocognitive domains *(continued)*

Cognitive domain	Examples of symptoms or observations	Examples of assessments
Learning and memory (immediate memory, recent memory [including free recall, cued recall, and recognition memory], very-long-term memory [semantic; autobiographical], implicit learning)	*Major:* Repeats self in conversation, often within the same conversation. Cannot keep track of short list of items when shopping or of plans for the day. Requires frequent reminders to orient to task at hand. *Mild:* Has difficulty recalling recent events, and relies increasingly on list making or calendar. Needs occasional reminders or re-reading to keep track of characters in a movie or novel. Occasionally may repeat self over a few weeks to the same person. Loses track of whether bills have already been paid. **Note:** Except in severe forms of major neurocognitive disorder, semantic, autobiographical, and implicit memory are relatively preserved, compared with recent memory.	*Immediate memory span:* Ability to repeat a list of words or digits. **Note:** Immediate memory sometimes subsumed under "working memory" (see "Executive Function"). *Recent memory:* Assesses the process of encoding new information (e.g., word lists, a short story, or diagrams). The aspects of recent memory that can be tested include 1) free recall (the person is asked to recall as many words, diagrams, or elements of a story as possible); 2) cued recall (examiner aids recall by providing semantic cues such as "List all the food items on the list" or "Name all of the children from the story"); and 3) recognition memory (examiner asks about specific items—e.g., "Was 'apple' on the list?" or "Did you see this diagram or figure?"). Other aspects of memory that can be assessed include semantic memory (memory for facts), autobiographical memory (memory for personal events or people), and implicit (procedural) learning (unconscious learning of skills).
Language (expressive language [including naming, word finding, fluency, and grammar, and syntax] and receptive language)	*Major:* Has significant difficulties with expressive or receptive language. Often uses general-use phrases such as "that thing" and "you know what I mean," and prefers general pronouns rather than names. With severe impairment, may not even recall names of closer friends and family. Idiosyncratic word usage, grammatical errors, and spontaneity of output and economy of utterances occur. Stereotypy of speech occurs; echolalia and automatic speech typically precede mutism. *Mild:* Has noticeable word-finding difficulty. May substitute general for specific terms. May avoid use of specific names of acquaintances. Grammatical errors involve subtle omission or incorrect use of articles, prepositions, auxiliary verbs, etc.	*Expressive language:* Confrontational naming (identification of objects or pictures); fluency (e.g., name as many items as possible in a semantic [e.g., animals] or phonemic [e.g., words starting with "f"] category in 1 minute). *Grammar and syntax* (e.g., omission or incorrect use of articles, prepositions, auxiliary verbs): Errors observed during naming and fluency tests are compared with norms to assess frequency of errors and compare with normal slips of the tongue. *Receptive language:* Comprehension (word definition and object-pointing tasks involving animate and inanimate stimuli): performance of actions/activities according to verbal command.

TABLE 1 Neurocognitive domains (continued)

Cognitive domain	Examples of symptoms or observations	Examples of assessments
Perceptual-motor (includes abilities subsumed under the terms *visual perception, visuoconstructional, perceptual-motor, praxis,* and *gnosis*)	*Major:* Has significant difficulties with previously familiar activities (using tools, driving motor vehicle), navigating in familiar environments; is often more confused at dusk, when shadows and lowering levels of light change perceptions. *Mild:* May need to rely more on maps or others for directions. Uses notes and follows others to get to a new place. May find self lost or turned around when not concentrating on task. Is less precise in parking. Needs to expend greater effort for spatial tasks such as carpentry, assembly, sewing, or knitting.	*Visual perception:* Line bisection tasks can be used to detect basic visual defect or attentional neglect. Motor-free perceptual tasks (including facial recognition) require the identification and/or matching of figures—best when tasks cannot be verbally mediated (e.g., figures are not objects); some require the decision of whether a figure can be "real" or not based on dimensionality. *Visuoconstructional:* Assembly of items requiring hand-eye coordination, such as drawing, copying, and block assembly. *Perceptual-motor:* Integrating perception with purposeful movement (e.g., inserting blocks into a form board without visual cues; rapidly inserting pegs into a slotted board). *Praxis:* Integrity of learned movements, such as ability to imitate gestures (wave goodbye) or pantomime use of objects to command ("Show me how you would use a hammer"). *Gnosis:* Perceptual integrity of awareness and recognition, such as recognition of faces and colors.
Social cognition (recognition of emotions, theory of mind)	*Major:* Behavior clearly out of acceptable social range; shows insensitivity to social standards of modesty in dress or of political, religious, or sexual topics of conversation. Focuses excessively on a topic despite group's disinterest or direct feedback. Behavioral intention without regard to family or friends. Makes decisions without regard to safety (e.g., inappropriate clothing for weather or social setting). Typically, has little insight into these changes. *Mild:* Has subtle changes in behavior or attitude, often described as a change in personality, such as less ability to recognize social cues or read facial expressions, decreased empathy, increased extraversion or introversion, decreased inhibition, or subtle or episodic apathy or restlessness.	*Recognition of emotions:* Identification of emotion in images of faces representing a variety of both positive and negative emotions. *Theory of mind:* Ability to consider another person's mental state (thoughts, desires, intentions) or experience—story cards with questions to elicit information about the mental state of the individuals portrayed, such as "Where will the girl look for the lost bag?" or "Why is the boy sad?"

Delirium

Diagnostic Criteria

A. A disturbance in attention (i.e., reduced ability to direct, focus, sustain, and shift attention) and awareness (reduced orientation to the environment).

B. The disturbance develops over a short period of time (usually hours to a few days), represents a change from baseline attention and awareness, and tends to fluctuate in severity during the course of a day.

C. An additional disturbance in cognition (e.g., memory deficit, disorientation, language, visuospatial ability, or perception).

D. The disturbances in Criteria A and C are not better explained by another preexisting, established, or evolving neurocognitive disorder and do not occur in the context of a severely reduced level of arousal, such as coma.

E. There is evidence from the history, physical examination, or laboratory findings that the disturbance is a direct physiological consequence of another medical condition, substance intoxication or withdrawal (i.e., due to a drug of abuse or to a medication), or exposure to a toxin, or is due to multiple etiologies.

Specify whether:

Substance intoxication delirium: This diagnosis should be made instead of substance intoxication when the symptoms in Criteria A and C predominate in the clinical picture and when they are sufficiently severe to warrant clinical attention.

Coding note: The ICD-9-CM and ICD-10-CM codes for the [specific substance] intoxication delirium are indicated in the table below. Note that the ICD-10-CM code depends on whether or not there is a comorbid substance use disorder present for the same class of substance. If a mild substance use disorder is comorbid with the substance intoxication delirium, the 4th position character is "1," and the clinician should record "mild [substance] use disorder" before the substance intoxication delirium (e.g., "mild cocaine use disorder with cocaine intoxication delirium"). If a moderate or severe substance use disorder is comorbid with the substance intoxication delirium, the 4th position character is "2," and the clinician should record "moderate [substance] use disorder" or "severe [substance] use disorder," depending on the severity of the comorbid substance use disorder. If there is no comorbid substance use disorder (e.g., after a one-time heavy use of the substance), then the 4th position character is "9," and the clinician should record only the substance intoxication delirium.

| | | ICD-10-CM | | |
	ICD-9-CM	With use disorder, mild	With use disorder, moderate or severe	Without use disorder
Alcohol	291.0	F10.121	F10.221	F10.921
Cannabis	292.81	F12.121	F12.221	F12.921
Phencyclidine	292.81	F16.121	F16.221	F16.921
Other hallucinogen	292.81	F16.121	F16.221	F16.921
Inhalant	292.81	F18.121	F18.221	F18.921
Opioid	292.81	F11.121	F11.221	F11.921

	ICD-9-CM	ICD-10-CM		
		With use disorder, mild	With use disorder, moderate or severe	Without use disorder
Sedative, hypnotic, or anxiolytic	292.81	F13.121	F13.221	F13.921
Amphetamine (or other stimulant)	292.81	F15.121	F15.221	F15.921
Cocaine	292.81	F14.121	F14.221	F14.921
Other (or unknown) substance	292.81	F19.121	F19.221	F19.921

Substance withdrawal delirium: This diagnosis should be made instead of substance withdrawal when the symptoms in Criteria A and C predominate in the clinical picture and when they are sufficiently severe to warrant clinical attention.

Code [specific substance] withdrawal delirium: **291.0 (F10.231)** alcohol; **292.0 (F11.23)** opioid; **292.0 (F13.231)** sedative, hypnotic, or anxiolytic; **292.0 (F19.231)** other (or unknown) substance/medication.

Medication-induced delirium: This diagnosis applies when the symptoms in Criteria A and C arise as a side effect of a medication taken as prescribed.

Coding note: The ICD-9-CM code for [specific medication]-induced delirium is **292.81.** The ICD-10-CM code depends on the type of medication. If the medication is an opioid taken as prescribed, the code is **F11.921.** If the medication is a sedative, hypnotic, or anxiolytic taken as prescribed, the code is **F13.921.** If the medication is an amphetamine-type or other stimulant taken as prescribed, the code is **F15.921.** For medications that do not fit into any of the classes (e.g., dexamethasone) and in cases in which a substance is judged to be an etiological factor but the specific class of substance is unknown, the code is **F19.921.**

293.0 (F05) Delirium due to another medical condition: There is evidence from the history, physical examination, or laboratory findings that the disturbance is attributable to the physiological consequences of another medical condition.

Coding note: Include the name of the other medical condition in the name of the delirium (e.g., 293.0 [F05] delirium due to hepatic encephalopathy). The other medical condition should also be coded and listed separately immediately before the delirium due to another medical condition (e.g., 572.2 [K72.90] hepatic encephalopathy; 293.0 [F05] delirium due to hepatic encephalopathy).

293.0 (F05) Delirium due to multiple etiologies: There is evidence from the history, physical examination, or laboratory findings that the delirium has more than one etiology (e.g., more than one etiological medical condition; another medical condition plus substance intoxication or medication side effect).

Coding note: Use multiple separate codes reflecting specific delirium etiologies (e.g., 572.2 [K72.90] hepatic encephalopathy, 293.0 [F05] delirium due to hepatic failure; 291.0 [F10.231] alcohol withdrawal delirium). Note that the etiological medical condition both appears as a separate code that precedes the delirium code and is substituted into the delirium due to another medical condition rubric.

Specify if:
    Acute: Lasting a few hours or days.
    Persistent: Lasting weeks or months.

Specify if:

Hyperactive: The individual has a hyperactive level of psychomotor activity that may be accompanied by mood lability, agitation, and/or refusal to cooperate with medical care.

Hypoactive: The individual has a hypoactive level of psychomotor activity that may be accompanied by sluggishness and lethargy that approaches stupor.

Mixed level of activity: The individual has a normal level of psychomotor activity even though attention and awareness are disturbed. Also includes individuals whose activity level rapidly fluctuates.

Recording Procedures

Substance intoxication delirium

ICD-9-CM. The name of the substance/medication intoxication delirium begins with the specific substance (e.g., cocaine, dexamethasone) that is presumed to be causing the delirium. The diagnostic code is selected from the table included in the criteria set, which is based on the drug class. For substances that do not fit into any of the classes (e.g., dexamethasone), the code for "other substance" should be used; and in cases in which a substance is judged to be an etiological factor but the specific class of substance is unknown, the category "unknown substance" should be used.

The name of the disorder is followed by the course (i.e., acute, persistent), followed by the specifier indicating level of psychomotor activity (i.e., hyperactive, hypoactive, mixed level of activity). Unlike the recording procedures for ICD-10-CM, which combine the substance/medication intoxication delirium and substance use disorder into a single code, for ICD-9-CM a separate diagnostic code is given for the substance use disorder. For example, in the case of acute hyperactive intoxication delirium occurring in a man with a severe cocaine use disorder, the diagnosis is 292.81 cocaine intoxication delirium, acute, hyperactive. An additional diagnosis of 304.20 severe cocaine use disorder is also given. If the intoxication delirium occurs without a comorbid substance use disorder (e.g., after a one-time heavy use of the substance), no accompanying substance use disorder is noted (e.g., 292.81 phencyclidine intoxication delirium, acute, hypoactive).

ICD-10-CM. The name of the substance/medication intoxication delirium begins with the specific substance (e.g., cocaine, dexamethasone) that is presumed to be causing the delirium. The diagnostic code is selected from the table included in the criteria set, which is based on the drug class and presence or absence of a comorbid substance use disorder. For substances that do not fit into any of the classes (e.g., dexamethasone), the code for "other substance" should be used; and in cases in which a substance is judged to be an etiological factor but the specific class of substance is unknown, the category "unknown substance" should be used.

When recording the name of the disorder, the comorbid substance use disorder (if any) is listed first, followed by the word "with," followed by the name of the substance intoxication delirium, followed by the course (i.e., acute, persistent), followed by the specifier indicating level of psychomotor activity (i.e., hyperactive, hypoactive, mixed level of activity). For example, in the case of acute hyperactive intoxication delirium occurring in a man with a severe cocaine use disorder, the diagnosis is F14.221 severe cocaine use disorder with cocaine intoxication delirium, acute, hyperactive. A separate diagnosis of the comorbid severe cocaine use disorder is not given. If the intoxication delirium occurs without a comorbid substance use disorder (e.g., after a one-time heavy use of the substance), no accompanying substance use disorder is noted (e.g., F16.921 phencyclidine intoxication delirium, acute, hypoactive).

Substance withdrawal delirium

ICD-9-CM. The name of the substance/medication withdrawal delirium begins with the specific substance (e.g., alcohol) that is presumed to be causing the withdrawal delirium. The diagnostic code is selected from substance-specific codes included in the coding note included in the criteria set. The name of the disorder is followed by the course (i.e., acute, persistent), followed by the specifier indicating level of psychomotor activity (i.e., hyperactive, hypoactive, mixed level of activity). Unlike the recording procedures for ICD-10-CM, which combine the substance/medication withdrawal delirium and substance use disorder into a single code, for ICD-9-CM a separate diagnostic code is given for the substance use disorder. For example, in the case of acute hyperactive withdrawal delirium occurring in a man with a severe alcohol use disorder, the diagnosis is 291.0 alcohol withdrawal delirium, acute, hyperactive. An additional diagnosis of 303.90 severe alcohol use disorder is also given.

ICD-10-CM.   The name of the substance/medication withdrawal delirium begins with the specific substance (e.g., alcohol) that is presumed to be causing the withdrawal delirium. The diagnostic code is selected from substance-specific codes included in the coding note included in the criteria set. When recording the name of the disorder, the comorbid moderate or severe substance use disorder (if any) is listed first, followed by the word "with," followed by the substance withdrawal delirium, followed by the course (i.e., acute, persistent), followed by the specifier indicating level of psychomotor activity (i.e., hyperactive, hypoactive, mixed level of activity). For example, in the case of acute hyperactive withdrawal delirium occurring in a man with a severe alcohol use disorder, the diagnosis is F10.231 severe alcohol use disorder with alcohol withdrawal delirium, acute, hyperactive. A separate diagnosis of the comorbid severe alcohol use disorder is not given.

Medication-induced delirium.   The name of the medication-induced delirium begins with the specific substance (e.g., dexamethasone) that is presumed to be causing the delirium. The name of the disorder is followed by the course (i.e., acute, persistent), followed by the specifier indicating level of psychomotor activity (i.e., hyperactive, hypoactive, mixed level of activity). For example, in the case of acute hyperactive medication-induced delirium occurring in a man using dexamethasone as prescribed, the diagnosis is 292.81 (F19.921) dexamethasone-induced delirium, acute, hyperactive.

Specifiers

Regarding course, in hospital settings, delirium usually lasts about 1 week, but some symptoms often persist even after individuals are discharged from the hospital.

Individuals with delirium may rapidly switch between hyperactive and hypoactive states. The hyperactive state may be more common or more frequently recognized and often is associated with medication side effects and drug withdrawal. The hypoactive state may be more frequent in older adults.

Diagnostic Features

The essential feature of delirium is a disturbance of attention or awareness that is accompanied by a change in baseline cognition that cannot be better explained by a preexisting or evolving neurocognitive disorder (NCD). The disturbance in attention (Criterion A) is manifested by reduced ability to direct, focus, sustain, and shift attention. Questions must be repeated because the individual's attention wanders, or the individual may perseverate with an answer to a previous question rather than appropriately shift attention. The individual is easily distracted by irrelevant stimuli. The disturbance in awareness is manifested by a reduced orientation to the environment or at times even to oneself.

The disturbance develops over a short period of time, usually hours to a few days, and tends to fluctuate during the course of the day, often with worsening in the evening and night when external orienting stimuli decrease (Criterion B). There is evidence from the history, physical examination, or laboratory findings that the disturbance is a physiological consequence of an underlying medical condition, substance intoxication or withdrawal, use of a medication, or a toxin exposure, or a combination of these factors (Criterion E). The etiology should be coded according to the etiologically appropriate subtype (i.e., substance or medication intoxication, substance withdrawal, another medical condition, or multiple etiologies). Delirium often occurs in the context of an underlying NCD. The impaired brain function of individuals with mild and major NCD renders them more vulnerable to delirium.

There is an accompanying change in at least one other area that may include memory and learning (particularly recent memory), disorientation (particularly to time and place), alteration in language, or perceptual distortion or a perceptual-motor disturbance (Criterion C). The perceptual disturbances accompanying delirium include misinterpretations, illusions, or hallucinations; these disturbances are typically visual, but may occur in other modalities as well, and range from simple and uniform to highly complex. Normal attention/arousal, delirium, and coma lie on a continuum, with coma defined as the lack of any response to verbal stimuli. The ability to evaluate cognition to diagnose delirium depends on there being a level of arousal sufficient for response to verbal stimulation; hence, delirium should not be diagnosed in the context of coma (Criterion D). Many noncomatose patients have a reduced level of arousal. Those patients who show only minimal responses to verbal stimulation are incapable of engaging with attempts at standardized testing or even interview. This inability to engage should be classified as severe inattention. Low-arousal states (of acute onset) should be recognized as indicating severe inattention and cognitive change, and hence delirium. They are clinically indistinguishable from delirium diagnosed on the basis of inattention or cognitive change elicited through cognitive testing and interview.

Associated Features Supporting Diagnosis

Delirium is often associated with a disturbance in the sleep-wake cycle. This disturbance can include daytime sleepiness, nighttime agitation, difficulty falling asleep, excessive sleepiness throughout the day, or wakefulness throughout the night. In some cases, complete reversal of the night-day sleep-wake cycle can occur. Sleep-wake cycle disturbances are very common in delirium and have been proposed as a core criterion for the diagnosis.

The individual with delirium may exhibit emotional disturbances, such as anxiety, fear, depression, irritability, anger, euphoria, and apathy. There may be rapid and unpredictable shifts from one emotional state to another. The disturbed emotional state may also be evident in calling out, screaming, cursing, muttering, moaning, or making other sounds. These behaviors are especially prevalent at night and under conditions in which stimulation and environmental cues are lacking.

Prevalence

The prevalence of delirium is highest among hospitalized older individuals and varies depending on the individuals' characteristics, setting of care, and sensitivity of the detection method. The prevalence of delirium in the community overall is low (1%–2%) but increases with age, rising to 14% among individuals older than 85 years. The prevalence is 10%–30% in older individuals presenting to emergency departments, where the delirium often indicates a medical illness.

The prevalence of delirium when individuals are admitted to the hospital ranges from 14% to 24%, and estimates of the incidence of delirium arising during hospitalization range from 6% to 56% in general hospital populations. Delirium occurs in 15%–53% of older individuals postoperatively and in 70%–87% of those in intensive care. Delirium occurs in up to 60% of individuals in nursing homes or post–acute care settings and in up to 83% of all individuals at the end of life.

Development and Course

While the majority of individuals with delirium have a full recovery with or without treatment, early recognition and intervention usually shortens the duration of the delirium. Delirium may progress to stupor, coma, seizures, or death, particularly if the underlying cause remains untreated. Mortality among hospitalized individuals with delirium is high, and as many as 40% of individuals with delirium, particularly those with malignancies and other significant underlying medical illness, die within a year after diagnosis.

Risk and Prognostic Factors

Environmental.   Delirium may be increased in the context of functional impairment, immobility, a history of falls, low levels of activity, and use of drugs and medications with psychoactive properties (particularly alcohol and anticholinergics).

Genetic and physiological.   Both major and mild NCDs can increase the risk for delirium and complicate the course. Older individuals are especially susceptible to delirium compared with younger adults. Susceptibility to delirium in infancy and through childhood may be greater than in early and middle adulthood. In childhood, delirium may be related to febrile illnesses and certain medications (e.g., anticholinergics).

Diagnostic Markers

In addition to laboratory findings characteristic of underlying medical conditions (or intoxication or withdrawal states), there is often generalized slowing on electroencephalography, and fast activity is occasionally found (e.g., in some cases of alcohol withdrawal delirium). However, electroencephalography is insufficiently sensitive and specific for diagnostic use.

Functional Consequences of Delirium

Delirium itself is associated with increased functional decline and risk of institutional placement. Hospitalized individuals 65 years or older with delirium have three times the risk of nursing home placement and about three times the functional decline as hospitalized patients without delirium at both discharge and 3 months postdischarge.

Differential Diagnosis

Psychotic disorders and bipolar and depressive disorders with psychotic features. Delirium that is characterized by vivid hallucinations, delusions, language disturbances, and agitation must be distinguished from brief psychotic disorder, schizophrenia, schizophreniform disorder, and other psychotic disorders, as well as from bipolar and depressive disorders with psychotic features.

Acute stress disorder.   Delirium associated with fear, anxiety, and dissociative symptoms, such as depersonalization, must be distinguished from acute stress disorder, which is precipitated by exposure to a severely traumatic event.

Malingering and factitious disorder.   Delirium can be distinguished from these disorders on the basis of the often atypical presentation in malingering and factitious disorder and the absence of another medical condition or substance that is etiologically related to the apparent cognitive disturbance.

Other neurocognitive disorders.   The most common differential diagnostic issue when evaluating confusion in older adults is disentangling symptoms of delirium and dementia. The clinician must determine whether the individual has delirium; a delirium superimposed on a preexisting NCD, such as that due to Alzheimer's disease; or an NCD without delirium. The traditional distinction between delirium and dementia according to acuteness of onset and temporal course is particularly difficult in those elderly individuals who had a prior NCD that may not have been recognized, or who develop persistent cognitive impairment following an episode of delirium.

Other Specified Delirium

780.09 (R41.0)

This category applies to presentations in which symptoms characteristic of delirium that cause clinically significant distress or impairment in social, occupational, or other important areas of functioning predominate but do not meet the full criteria for delirium or any of the disorders in the neurocognitive disorders diagnostic class. The other specified delirium category is used in situations in which the clinician chooses to communicate the specific reason that the presentation does not meet the criteria for delirium or any specific neurocognitive disorder. This is done by recording "other specified delirium" followed by the specific reason (e.g., "attenuated delirium syndrome").

An example of a presentation that can be specified using the "other specified" designation is the following:

Attenuated delirium syndrome: This syndrome applies in cases of delirium in which the severity of cognitive impairment falls short of that required for the diagnosis, or in which some, but not all, diagnostic criteria for delirium are met.

Unspecified Delirium

780.09 (R41.0)

This category applies to presentations in which symptoms characteristic of delirium that cause clinically significant distress or impairment in social, occupational, or other important areas of functioning predominate but do not meet the full criteria for delirium or any of the disorders in the neurocognitive disorders diagnostic class. The unspecified delirium category is used in situations in which the clinician chooses *not* to specify the reason that the criteria are not met for delirium, and includes presentations for which there is insufficient information to make a more specific diagnosis (e.g., in emergency room settings).

Major and Mild Neurocognitive Disorders

Major Neurocognitive Disorder

Diagnostic Criteria

A. Evidence of significant cognitive decline from a previous level of performance in one or more cognitive domains (complex attention, executive function, learning and memory, language, perceptual-motor, or social cognition) based on:

1. Concern of the individual, a knowledgeable informant, or the clinician that there has been a significant decline in cognitive function; and

2. A substantial impairment in cognitive performance, preferably documented by standardized neuropsychological testing or, in its absence, another quantified clinical assessment.

B. The cognitive deficits interfere with independence in everyday activities (i.e., at a minimum, requiring assistance with complex instrumental activities of daily living such as paying bills or managing medications).

C. The cognitive deficits do not occur exclusively in the context of a delirium.

D. The cognitive deficits are not better explained by another mental disorder (e.g., major depressive disorder, schizophrenia).

Specify whether due to:
   Alzheimer's disease (pp. 611–614)
   Frontotemporal lobar degeneration (pp. 614–618)
   Lewy body disease (pp. 618–621)
   Vascular disease (pp. 621–624)
   Traumatic brain injury (pp. 624–627)
   Substance/medication use (pp. 627–632)
   HIV infection (pp. 632–634)
   Prion disease (pp. 634–636)
   Parkinson's disease (pp. 636–638)
   Huntington's disease (pp. 638–641)
   Another medical condition (pp. 641–642)
   Multiple etiologies (pp. 642–643)
   Unspecified (p. 643)

Coding note: Code based on medical or substance etiology. In some cases, there is need for an additional code for the etiological medical condition, which must immediately precede the diagnostic code for major neurocognitive disorder, as follows:

Etiological subtype	Associated etiological medical code for major neurocognitive disorder[a]	Major neurocognitive disorder code[b]	Mild neurocognitive disorder code[c]
Alzheimer's disease	Probable: 331.0 (G30.9) Possible: no additional medical code	Probable: 294.1x (F02.8x) Possible: 331.9 (G31.9)[c]	331.83 (G31.84) (Do not use additional code for Alzheimer's disease.)
Frontotemporal lobar degeneration	Probable: 331.19 (G31.09) Possible: no additional medical code	Probable: 294.1x (F02.8x) Possible: 331.9 (G31.9)[c]	331.83 (G31.84) (Do not use additional code for frontotemporal disease.)
Lewy body disease	Probable: 331.82 (G31.83) Possible: no additional medical code	Probable: 294.1x (F02.8x) Possible: 331.9 (G31.9)[c]	331.83 (G31.84) (Do not use additional code for Lewy body disease.)
Vascular disease	No additional medical code	Probable: 290.40 (F01.5x) Possible: 331.9 (G31.9)[c]	331.83 (G31.84) (Do not use additional code for the vascular disease.)
Traumatic brain injury	907.0 (S06.2X9S)	294.1x (F02.8x)	331.83 (G31.84) (Do not use additional code for the traumatic brain injury.)
Substance/ medication-induced	No additional medical code	Code based on the type of substance causing the major neurocognitive disorder[c, d]	Code based on the type of substance causing the mild neurocognitive disorder[d]

Etiological subtype	Associated etiological medical code for major neurocognitive disorder[a]	Major neurocognitive disorder code[b]	Mild neurocognitive disorder code[c]
HIV infection	042 (B20)	294.1x (F02.8x)	331.83 (G31.84) (Do not use additional code for HIV infection.)
Prion disease	046.79 (A81.9)	294.1x (F02.8x)	331.83 (G31.84) (Do not use additional code for prion disease.)
Parkinson's disease	Probable: 332.0 (G20) Possible: No additional medical code	Probable: 294.1x (F02.8x) Possible: 331.9 (G31.9)[c]	331.83 (G31.84) (Do not use additional code for Parkinson's disease.)
Huntington's disease	333.4 (G10)	294.1x (F02.8x)	331.83 (G31.84) (Do not use additional code for Huntington's disease.)
Due to another medical condition	Code the other medical condition first (e.g., 340 [G35] multiple sclerosis)	294.1x (F02.8x)	331.83 (G31.84) (Do not use additional codes for the presumed etiological medical conditions.)
Due to multiple etiologies	Code all of the etiological medical conditions first (with the exception of vascular disease)	294.1x (F02.8x) (Plus the code for the relevant substance/medication-induced major neurocognitive disorders if substances or medications play a role in the etiology.)	331.83 (G31.84) (Plus the code for the relevant substance/medication-induced mild neurocognitive disorders if substances or medications play a role in the etiology. Do not use additional codes for the presumed etiological medical conditions.)
Unspecified neurocognitive disorder	No additional medical code	799.59 (R41.9)	799.59 (R41.9)

[a]Code first, before code for major neurocognitive disorder.
[b]Code fifth character based on symptom specifier: .x0 without behavioral disturbance; .x1 with behavioral disturbance (e.g., psychotic symptoms, mood disturbance, agitation, apathy, or other behavioral symptoms).
[c]**Note:** Behavioral disturbance specifier cannot be coded but should still be indicated in writing.
[d]See "Substance/Medication-Induced Major or Mild Neurocognitive Disorder."

Specify:

Without behavioral disturbance: If the cognitive disturbance is not accompanied by any clinically significant behavioral disturbance.

With behavioral disturbance *(specify disturbance):* If the cognitive disturbance is accompanied by a clinically significant behavioral disturbance (e.g., psychotic symptoms, mood disturbance, agitation, apathy, or other behavioral symptoms).

Specify current severity:

Mild: Difficulties with instrumental activities of daily living (e.g., housework, managing money).

Moderate: Difficulties with basic activities of daily living (e.g., feeding, dressing).

Severe: Fully dependent.

Mild Neurocognitive Disorder

Diagnostic Criteria

A. Evidence of modest cognitive decline from a previous level of performance in one or more cognitive domains (complex attention, executive function, learning and memory, language, perceptual-motor, or social cognition) based on:

1. Concern of the individual, a knowledgeable informant, or the clinician that there has been a mild decline in cognitive function; and

2. A modest impairment in cognitive performance, preferably documented by standardized neuropsychological testing or, in its absence, another quantified clinical assessment.

B. The cognitive deficits do not interfere with capacity for independence in everyday activities (i.e., complex instrumental activities of daily living such as paying bills or managing medications are preserved, but greater effort, compensatory strategies, or accommodation may be required).

C. The cognitive deficits do not occur exclusively in the context of a delirium.

D. The cognitive deficits are not better explained by another mental disorder (e.g., major depressive disorder, schizophrenia).

Specify whether due to:

Alzheimer's disease (pp. 611–614)

Frontotemporal lobar degeneration (pp. 614–618)

Lewy body disease (pp. 618–621)

Vascular disease (pp. 621–624)

Traumatic brain injury (pp. 624–627)

Substance/medication use (pp. 627–632)

HIV infection (pp. 632–634)

Prion disease (pp. 634–636)

Parkinson's disease (pp. 636–638)

Huntington's disease (pp. 638–641)

Another medical condition (pp. 641–642)

Multiple etiologies (pp. 642–643)

Unspecified (p. 643)

Coding note: For mild neurocognitive disorder due to any of the medical etiologies listed above, code **331.83 (G31.84).** Do *not* use additional codes for the presumed etiological medical conditions. For substance/medication-induced mild neurocognitive disorder, code based on type of substance; see "Substance/Medication-Induced Major or Mild Neurocognitive Disorder." For unspecified mild neurocognitive disorder, code **799.59 (R41.9).**

Specify:
  Without behavioral disturbance: If the cognitive disturbance is not accompanied by any clinically significant behavioral disturbance.
  With behavioral disturbance *(specify disturbance):* If the cognitive disturbance is accompanied by a clinically significant behavioral disturbance (e.g., psychotic symptoms, mood disturbance, agitation, apathy, or other behavioral symptoms).

Subtypes

Major and mild neurocognitive disorders (NCDs) are primarily subtyped according to the known or presumed etiological/pathological entity or entities underlying the cognitive decline. These subtypes are distinguished on the basis of a combination of time course, characteristic domains affected, and associated symptoms. For certain etiological subtypes, the diagnosis depends substantially on the presence of a potentially causative entity, such as Parkinson's or Huntington's disease, or a traumatic brain injury or stroke in the appropriate time period. For other etiological subtypes (generally the neurodegenerative diseases like Alzheimer's disease, frontotemporal lobar degeneration, and Lewy body disease), the diagnosis is based primarily on the cognitive, behavioral, and functional symptoms. Typically, the differentiation among these syndromes that lack an independently recognized etiological entity is clearer at the level of major NCD than at the level of mild NCD, but sometimes characteristic symptoms and associated features are present at the mild level as well.

NCDs are frequently managed by clinicians in multiple disciplines. For many subtypes, multidisciplinary international expert groups have developed specialized consensus criteria based on clinicopathological correlation with underlying brain pathology. The subtype criteria here have been harmonized with those expert criteria.

Specifiers

Evidence for distinct behavioral features in NCDs has been recognized, particularly in the areas of psychotic symptoms and depression. Psychotic features are common in many NCDs, particularly at the mild-to-moderate stage of major NCDs due to Alzheimer's disease, Lewy body disease, and frontotemporal lobar degeneration. Paranoia and other delusions are common features, and often a persecutory theme may be a prominent aspect of delusional ideation. In contrast to psychotic disorders with onset in earlier life (e.g., schizophrenia), disorganized speech and disorganized behavior are not characteristic of psychosis in NCDs. Hallucinations may occur in any modality, although visual hallucinations are more common in NCDs than in depressive, bipolar, or psychotic disorders.

Mood disturbances, including depression, anxiety, and elation, may occur. Depression is common early in the course (including at the mild NCD level) of NCD due to Alzheimer's disease and Parkinson's disease, while elation may occur more commonly in frontotemporal lobar degeneration. When a full affective syndrome meeting diagnostic criteria for a depressive or bipolar disorder is present, that diagnosis should be coded as well. Mood symptoms are increasingly recognized to be a significant feature in the earliest stages of mild NCDs such that clinical recognition and intervention may be important.

Agitation is common in a wide variety of NCDs, particularly in major NCD of moderate to severe severity, and often occurs in the setting of confusion or frustration. It may arise as combative behaviors, particularly in the context of resisting caregiving duties such as bathing and dressing. Agitation is characterized as disruptive motor or vocal activity and tends to occur with advanced stages of cognitive impairment across all of the NCDs.

Individuals with NCD can present with a wide variety of behavioral symptoms that are the focus of treatment. Sleep disturbance is a common symptom that can create a need for clinical attention and may include symptoms of insomnia, hypersomnia, and circadian rhythm disturbances.

Apathy is common in mild and mild major NCD. It is observed particularly in NCD due to Alzheimer's disease and may be a prominent feature of NCD due to frontotemporal lobar degeneration. Apathy is typically characterized by diminished motivation and reduced goal-directed behavior accompanied by decreased emotional responsiveness. Symptoms of apathy may manifest early in the course of NCDs when a loss of motivation to pursue daily activities or hobbies may be observed.

Other important behavioral symptoms include wandering, disinhibition, hyperphagia, and hoarding. Some of these symptoms are characteristic of specific disorders, as discussed in the relevant sections. When more than one behavioral disturbance is observed, each type should be noted in writing with the specifier "with behavioral symptoms."

Diagnostic Features

Major and mild NCDs exist on a spectrum of cognitive and functional impairment. Major NCD corresponds to the condition referred to in DSM-IV as *dementia*, retained as an alternative in this volume. The core feature of NCDs is acquired cognitive decline in one or more cognitive domains (Criterion A) based on both 1) a concern about cognition on the part of the individual, a knowledgeable informant, or the clinician, and 2) performance on an objective assessment that falls below the expected level or that has been observed to decline over time. Both a concern and objective evidence are required because they are complementary. When there is an exclusive focus on objective testing, a disorder may go undiagnosed in high-functioning individuals whose currently "normal" performance actually represents a substantial decline in abilities, or an illness may be incorrectly diagnosed in individuals whose currently "low" performance does not represent a change from their own baseline or is a result of extraneous factors like test conditions or a passing illness. Alternatively, excessive focus on subjective symptoms may fail to diagnose illness in individuals with poor insight, or whose informants deny or fail to notice their symptoms, or it may be overly sensitive in the so-called worried well.

A cognitive concern differs from a complaint in that it may or may not be voiced spontaneously. Rather, it may need to be elicited by careful questioning about specific symptoms that commonly occur in individuals with cognitive deficits (see Table 1 in the introduction to this chapter). For example, memory concerns include difficulty remembering a short grocery list or keeping track of the plot of a television program; executive concerns include difficulty resuming a task when interrupted, organizing tax records, or planning a holiday meal. At the mild NCD level, the individual is likely to describe these tasks as being more difficult or as requiring extra time or effort or compensatory strategies. At the major NCD level, such tasks may only be completed with assistance or may be abandoned altogether. At the mild NCD level, individuals and their families may not notice such symptoms or may view them as normal, particularly in the elderly; thus, careful history taking is of paramount importance. The difficulties must represent changes rather than lifelong patterns: the individual or informant may clarify this issue, or the clinician can infer change from prior experience with the patient or from occupational or other clues. It is also critical to determine that the difficulties are related to cognitive loss rather than to motor or sensory limitations.

Neuropsychological testing, with performance compared with norms appropriate to the patient's age, educational attainment, and cultural background, is part of the standard evaluation of NCDs and is particularly critical in the evaluation of mild NCD. For major NCD, performance is typically 2 or more standard deviations below appropriate norms (3rd percentile or below). For mild NCD, performance typically lies in the 1–2 standard deviation range (between the 3rd and 16th percentiles). However, neuropsychological testing is not available in all settings, and neuropsychological thresholds are sensitive to the specific test(s) and norms employed, as well as to test conditions, sensory limitations, and intercurrent illness. A variety of brief office-based or "bedside" assessments, as described in Table 1, can also supply objective data in settings where such testing is unavailable or infeasible. In any case, as with cognitive concerns, objective performance must be interpreted in light of the individual's prior performance. Optimally, this information would be available from a prior administration of the same test, but often it must be inferred based on appropriate norms, along with the individual's educational history, occupation, and other factors. Norms are more challenging to interpret in individuals with very high or very low levels of education and in individuals being tested outside their own language or cultural background.

Criterion B relates to the individual's level of independence in everyday functioning. Individuals with major NCD will have impairment of sufficient severity so as to interfere with independence, such that others will have to take over tasks that the individuals were previously able to complete on their own. Individuals with mild NCD will have preserved independence, although there may be subtle interference with function or a report that tasks require more effort or take more time than previously.

The distinction between major and mild NCD is inherently arbitrary, and the disorders exist along a continuum. Precise thresholds are therefore difficult to determine. Careful history taking, observation, and integration with other findings are required, and the implications of diagnosis should be considered when an individual's clinical manifestations lie at a boundary.

Associated Features Supporting Diagnosis

Typically the associated features that support a diagnosis of major or mild NCD will be specific to the etiological subtype (e.g., neuroleptic sensitivity and visual hallucinations in NCD due to Lewy body disease). Diagnostic features specific to each of the subtypes are found in the relevant sections.

Prevalence

The prevalence of NCD varies widely by age and by etiological subtype. Overall prevalence estimates are generally only available for older populations. Among individuals older than 60 years, prevalence increases steeply with age, so prevalence estimates are more accurate for narrow age bands than for broad categories such as "over 65" (where the mean age can vary greatly with the life expectancy of the given population). For those etiological subtypes occurring across the lifespan, prevalence estimates for NCD are likely to be available, if at all, only as the fraction of individuals who develop NCD among those with the relevant condition (e.g., traumatic brain injury, HIV infection).

Overall prevalence estimates for dementia (which is largely congruent with major NCD) are approximately 1%–2% at age 65 years and as high as 30% by age 85 years. The prevalence of mild NCD is very sensitive to the definition of the disorder, particularly in community settings, where evaluations are less detailed. In addition, in contrast with clinical settings, where cognitive concern must be high to seek and locate care, there may be a less clear decline from baseline functioning. Estimates of the prevalence of mild cognitive impairment (which is substantially congruent with mild NCD) among older individuals are fairly variable, ranging from 2% to 10% at age 65 and 5% to 25% by age 85.

Development and Course

The course of NCD varies across etiological subtypes, and this variation can be useful in differential diagnosis. Some subtypes (e.g., those related to traumatic brain injury or stroke) typically begin at a specific time and (at least after initial symptoms related to inflammation or swelling subside) remain static. Others may fluctuate over time (although if this occurs, the possibility of delirium superimposed on NCD should be considered). NCDs due to neurodegenerative diseases like Alzheimer's disease or frontotemporal lobar degeneration typically are marked by insidious onset and gradual progression, and the pattern of onset of cognitive deficits and associated features helps to distinguish among them.

NCDs with onset in childhood and adolescence may have broad repercussions for social and intellectual development, and in this setting intellectual disability (intellectual developmental disorder) and/or other neurodevelopmental disorders may also be diagnosed to capture the full diagnostic picture and ensure the provision of a broad range of services. In older individuals, NCDs often occur in the setting of medical illnesses, frailty, and sensory loss, which complicate the clinical picture for diagnosis and treatment.

When cognitive loss occurs in youth to midlife, individuals and families are likely to seek care. NCDs are typically easiest to identify at younger ages, although in some settings malingering or other factitious disorders may be a concern. Very late in life, cognitive symptoms may not cause concern or may go unnoticed. In late life, mild NCD must also be distinguished from the more modest deficits associated with "normal aging," although a substantial fraction of what has been ascribed to normal aging likely represents prodromal phases of various NCDs. In addition, it becomes harder to recognize mild NCD with age because of the increasing prevalence of medical illness and sensory deficits. It becomes harder to differentiate among subtypes with age because there are multiple potential sources of neurocognitive decline.

Risk and Prognostic Factors

Risk factors vary not only by etiological subtype but also by age at onset within etiological subtypes. Some subtypes are distributed throughout the lifespan, whereas others occur exclusively or primarily in late life. Even within the NCDs of aging, the relative prevalence varies with age: Alzheimer's disease is uncommon before age 60 years, and the prevalence increases steeply thereafter, while the overall less common frontotemporal lobar degeneration has earlier onset and represents a progressively smaller fraction of NCDs with age.

Genetic and physiological. The strongest risk factor for major and mild NCDs is age, primarily because age increases the risk of neurodegenerative and cerebrovascular disease. Female gender is associated with higher prevalence of dementia overall, and especially Alzheimer's disease, but this difference is largely, if not wholly, attributable to greater longevity in females.

Culture-Related Diagnostic Issues

Individuals' and families' level of awareness and concern about neurocognitive symptoms may vary across ethnic and occupational groups. Neurocognitive symptoms are more likely to be noticed, particularly at the mild level, in individuals who engage in complex occupational, domestic, or recreational activities. In addition, norms for neuropsychological testing tend to be available only for broad populations, and thus they may not be easily applicable to individuals with less than high school education or those being evaluated outside their primary language or culture.

Gender-Related Diagnostic Issues

Like age, culture, and occupation, gender issues may affect the level of concern and awareness of cognitive symptoms. In addition, for late-life NCDs, females are likely to be older, to have more medical comorbidity, and to live alone, which can complicate evaluation and treatment. In addition, there are gender differences in the frequency of some of the etiological subtypes.

Diagnostic Markers

In addition to a careful history, neuropsychological assessments are the key measures for diagnosis of NCDs, particularly at the mild level, where functional changes are minimal and symptoms more subtle. Ideally, individuals will be referred for formal neuropsychological testing, which will provide a quantitative assessment of all relevant domains and thus help with diagnosis; provide guidance to the family on areas where the individual may require more support; and serve as a benchmark for further decline or response to therapies. When such testing is unavailable or not feasible, the brief assessments in Table 1 can provide insight into each domain. More global brief mental status tests may be helpful but may be insensitive, particularly to modest changes in a single domain or in those with high premorbid abilities, and may be overly sensitive in those with low premorbid abilities.

In distinguishing among etiological subtypes, additional diagnostic markers may come into play, particularly neuroimaging studies such as magnetic resonance imaging scans and positron emission tomography scans. In addition, specific markers may be involved in the assessment of specific subtypes and may become more important as additional research findings accumulate over time, as discussed in the relevant sections.

Functional Consequences of Major and Mild Neurocognitive Disorders

By definition, major and mild NCDs affect functioning, given the central role of cognition in human life. Thus, the criteria for the disorders, and the threshold for differentiating mild from major NCD, are based in part on functional assessment. Within major NCD there is a broad range of functional impairment, as implemented in the severity specifiers. In addition, the specific functions that are compromised can help identify the cognitive domains affected, particularly when neuropsychological testing is not available or is difficult to interpret.

Differential Diagnosis

Normal cognition.   The differential diagnosis between normal cognition and mild NCD, as between mild and major NCD, is challenging because the boundaries are inherently arbitrary. Careful history taking and objective assessment are critical to these distinctions. A longitudinal evaluation using quantified assessments may be key in detecting mild NCD.

Delirium.   Both mild and major NCD may be difficult to distinguish from a persistent delirium, which can co-occur. Careful assessment of attention and arousal will help to make the distinction.

Major depressive disorder.   The distinction between mild NCD and major depressive disorder, which may co-occur with NCD, can also be challenging. Specific patterns of cognitive deficits may be helpful. For example, consistent memory and executive function deficits are typical of Alzheimer's disease, whereas nonspecific or more variable performance is seen in major depression. Alternatively, treatment of the depressive disorder with repeated observation over time may be required to make the diagnosis.

Specific learning disorder and other neurodevelopmental disorders.   A careful clarification of the individual's baseline status will help distinguish an NCD from a specific learning disorder or other neurodevelopmental disorders. Additional issues may enter the differential for specific etiological subtypes, as described in the relevant sections.

Comorbidity

NCDs are common in older individuals and thus often co-occur with a wide variety of age-related diseases that may complicate diagnosis or treatment. Most notable of these is delirium, for which NCD increases the risk. In older individuals, a delirium during hospitalization is, in many cases, the first time that an NCD is noticed, although a careful history will often reveal evidence of earlier decline. Mixed NCDs are also common in older individuals, as many etiological entities increase in prevalence with age. In younger individuals, NCD often co-occurs with neurodevelopmental disorders; for example, a head injury in a preschool child may also lead to significant developmental and learning issues. Additional comorbidity of NCD is often related to the etiological subtype, as discussed in the relevant sections.

Major or Mild Neurocognitive Disorder Due to Alzheimer's Disease

Diagnostic Criteria

A. The criteria are met for major or mild neurocognitive disorder.

B. There is insidious onset and gradual progression of impairment in one or more cognitive domains (for major neurocognitive disorder, at least two domains must be impaired).

C. Criteria are met for either probable or possible Alzheimer's disease as follows:

For major neurocognitive disorder:

Probable Alzheimer's disease is diagnosed if either of the following is present; otherwise, **possible Alzheimer's disease** should be diagnosed.

1. Evidence of a causative Alzheimer's disease genetic mutation from family history or genetic testing.
2. All three of the following are present:
   a. Clear evidence of decline in memory and learning and at least one other cognitive domain (based on detailed history or serial neuropsychological testing).
   b. Steadily progressive, gradual decline in cognition, without extended plateaus.
   c. No evidence of mixed etiology (i.e., absence of other neurodegenerative or cerebrovascular disease, or another neurological, mental, or systemic disease or condition likely contributing to cognitive decline).

For mild neurocognitive disorder:

Probable Alzheimer's disease is diagnosed if there is evidence of a causative Alzheimer's disease genetic mutation from either genetic testing or family history.

Possible Alzheimer's disease is diagnosed if there is no evidence of a causative Alzheimer's disease genetic mutation from either genetic testing or family history, and all three of the following are present:

1. Clear evidence of decline in memory and learning.
2. Steadily progressive, gradual decline in cognition, without extended plateaus.
3. No evidence of mixed etiology (i.e., absence of other neurodegenerative or cerebrovascular disease, or another neurological or systemic disease or condition likely contributing to cognitive decline).

D. The disturbance is not better explained by cerebrovascular disease, another neurodegenerative disease, the effects of a substance, or another mental, neurological, or systemic disorder.

Coding note: For probable major neurocognitive disorder due to Alzheimer's disease, with behavioral disturbance, code first **331.0 (G30.9)** Alzheimer's disease, followed by **294.11 (F02.81)** major neurocognitive disorder due to Alzheimer's disease. For probable major neurocognitive disorder due to Alzheimer's disease, without behavioral disturbance, code first **331.0 (G30.9)** Alzheimer's disease, followed by **294.10 (F02.80)** major neurocognitive disorder due to Alzheimer's disease, without behavioral disturbance.

For possible major neurocognitive disorder due to Alzheimer's disease, code **331.9 (G31.9)** possible major neurocognitive disorder due to Alzheimer's disease. (**Note:** Do *not* use the additional code for Alzheimer's disease. Behavioral disturbance cannot be coded but should still be indicated in writing.)

For mild neurocognitive disorder due to Alzheimer's disease, code **331.83 (G31.84).**
(**Note:** Do *not* use the additional code for Alzheimer's disease. Behavioral disturbance
cannot be coded but should still be indicated in writing.)

Diagnostic Features

Beyond the neurocognitive disorder (NCD) syndrome (Criterion A), the core features of major or mild NCD due to Alzheimer's disease include an insidious onset and gradual progression of cognitive and behavioral symptoms (Criterion B). The typical presentation is
amnestic (i.e., with impairment in memory and learning). Unusual nonamnestic presentations, particularly visuospatial and logopenic aphasic variants, also exist. At the mild
NCD phase, Alzheimer's disease manifests typically with impairment in memory and learning, sometimes accompanied by deficits in executive function. At the major NCD phase,
visuoconstructional/perceptual-motor ability and language will also be impaired, particularly when the NCD is moderate to severe. Social cognition tends to be preserved until
late in the course of the disease.

A level of diagnostic certainty must be specified denoting Alzheimer's disease as the
"probable" or "possible" etiology (Criterion C). *Probable Alzheimer's disease* is diagnosed in
both major and mild NCD if there is evidence of a causative Alzheimer's disease gene, either from genetic testing or from an autosomal dominant family history coupled with autopsy confirmation or a genetic test in an affected family member. For major NCD, a
typical clinical picture, without extended plateaus or evidence of mixed etiology, can also
be diagnosed as due to probable Alzheimer's disease. For mild NCD, given the lesser degree of certainty that the deficits will progress, these features are only sufficient for a
possible Alzheimer's etiology. If the etiology appears mixed, mild NCD due to multiple etiologies should be diagnosed. In any case, for both mild and major NCD due to Alzheimer's disease, the clinical features must not suggest another primary etiology for the NCD
(Criterion D).

Associated Features Supporting Diagnosis

In specialty clinical settings, approximately 80% of individuals with major NCD due to
Alzheimer's disease have behavioral and psychological manifestations; these features are
also frequent at the mild NCD stage of impairment. These symptoms are as or more distressing than cognitive manifestations and are frequently the reason that health care is
sought. At the mild NCD stage or the mildest level of major NCD, depression and/or apathy are often seen. With moderately severe major NCD, psychotic features, irritability,
agitation, combativeness, and wandering are common. Late in the illness, gait disturbance, dysphagia, incontinence, myoclonus, and seizures are observed.

Prevalence

The prevalence of overall dementia (major NCD) rises steeply with age. In high-income
countries, it ranges from 5% to 10% in the seventh decade to at least 25% thereafter. U.S.
census data estimates suggest that approximately 7% of individuals diagnosed with Alzheimer's disease are between ages 65 and 74 years, 53% are between ages 75 and 84 years,
and 40% are 85 years and older. The percentage of dementias attributable to Alzheimer's
disease ranges from about 60% to over 90%, depending on the setting and diagnostic criteria. Mild NCD due to Alzheimer's disease is likely to represent a substantial fraction of
mild cognitive impairment (MCI) as well.

Development and Course

Major or mild NCD due to Alzheimer's disease progresses gradually, sometimes with
brief plateaus, through severe dementia to death. The mean duration of survival after di-

agnosis is approximately 10 years, reflecting the advanced age of the majority of individuals rather than the course of the disease; some individuals can live with the disease for as long as 20 years. Late-stage individuals are eventually mute and bedbound. Death most commonly results from aspiration in those who survive through the full course. In mild NCD due to Alzheimer's disease, impairments increase over time, and functional status gradually declines until symptoms reach the threshold for the diagnosis of major NCD.

The onset of symptoms is usually in the eighth and ninth decades; early-onset forms seen in the fifth and sixth decades are often related to known causative mutations. Symptoms and pathology do not differ markedly at different onset ages. However, younger individuals are more likely to survive the full course of the disease, while older individuals are more likely to have numerous medical comorbidities that affect the course and management of the illness. Diagnostic complexity is higher in older adults because of the increased likelihood of comorbid medical illness and mixed pathology.

Risk and Prognostic Factors

Environmental.   Traumatic brain injury increases risk for major or mild NCD due to Alzheimer's disease.

Genetic and physiological.   Age is the strongest risk factor for Alzheimer's disease. The genetic susceptibility polymorphism apolipoprotein E4 increases risk and decreases age at onset, particularly in homozygous individuals. There are also extremely rare causative Alzheimer's disease genes. Individuals with Down syndrome (trisomy 21) develop Alzheimer's disease if they survive to midlife. Multiple vascular risk factors influence risk for Alzheimer's disease and may act by increasing cerebrovascular pathology or also through direct effects on Alzheimer pathology.

Culture-Related Diagnostic Issues

Detection of an NCD may be more difficult in cultural and socioeconomic settings where memory loss is considered normal in old age, where older adults face fewer cognitive demands in everyday life, or where very low educational levels pose greater challenges to objective cognitive assessment.

Diagnostic Markers

Cortical atrophy, amyloid-predominant neuritic plaques, and tau-predominant neurofibrillary tangles are hallmarks of the pathological diagnosis of Alzheimer's disease and may be confirmed via postmortem histopathological examination. For early-onset cases with autosomal dominant inheritance, a mutation in one of the known causative Alzheimer's disease genes—amyloid precursor protein (APP), presenilin 1 (PSEN1), or presenilin 2 (PSEN2)—may be involved, and genetic testing for such mutations is commercially available, at least for PSEN1. Apolipoprotein E4 cannot serve as a diagnostic marker because it is only a risk factor and neither necessary nor sufficient for disease occurrence.

Since amyloid beta-42 deposition in the brain occurs early in the pathophysiological cascade, amyloid-based diagnostic tests such as amyloid imaging on brain positron emission tomography (PET) scans and reduced levels of amyloid beta-42 in the cerebrospinal fluid (CSF) may have diagnostic value. Signs of neuronal injury, such as hippocampal and temporoparietal cortical atrophy on a magnetic resonance image scan, temporoparietal hypometabolism on a fluorodeoxyglucose PET scan, and evidence for elevated total tau and phospho-tau levels in CSF, provide evidence of neuronal damage but are less specific for Alzheimer's disease. At present, these biomarkers are not fully validated, and many are available only in tertiary care settings. However, some of them, along with novel biomarkers, will likely move into wider clinical practice in the coming years.

Functional Consequences of Major or Mild Neurocognitive Disorder Due to Alzheimer's Disease

The prominence of memory loss can cause significant difficulties relatively early in the course. Social cognition (and thus social functioning) and procedural memory (e.g., dancing, playing musical instruments) may be relatively preserved for extended periods.

Differential Diagnosis

Other neurocognitive disorders.   Major and mild NCDs due to other neurodegenerative processes (e.g., Lewy body disease, frontotemporal lobar degeneration) share the insidious onset and gradual decline caused by Alzheimer's disease but have distinctive core features of their own. In major or mild vascular NCD, there is typically history of stroke temporally related to the onset of cognitive impairment, and infarcts or white matter hyperintensities are judged sufficient to account for the clinical picture. However, particularly when there is no clear history of stepwise decline, major or mild vascular NCD can share many clinical features with Alzheimer's disease.

Other concurrent, active neurological or systemic illness.   Other neurological or systemic illness should be considered if there is an appropriate temporal relationship and severity to account for the clinical picture. At the mild NCD level, it may be difficult to distinguish an Alzheimer's disease etiology from that of another medical condition (e.g., thyroid disorders, vitamin B_{12} deficiency).

Major depressive disorder.   Particularly at the mild NCD level, the differential diagnosis also includes major depression. The presence of depression may be associated with reduced daily functioning and poor concentration that may resemble an NCD, but improvement with treatment of depression may be useful in making the distinction.

Comorbidity

Most individuals with Alzheimer's disease are elderly and have multiple medical conditions that can complicate diagnosis and influence the clinical course. Major or mild NCD due to Alzheimer's disease commonly co-occurs with cerebrovascular disease, which contributes to the clinical picture. When a comorbid condition contributes to the NCD in an individual with Alzheimer's disease, then NCD due to multiple etiologies should be diagnosed.

Major or Mild Frontotemporal Neurocognitive Disorder

Diagnostic Criteria

A. The criteria are met for major or mild neurocognitive disorder.

B. The disturbance has insidious onset and gradual progression.

C. Either (1) or (2):

1. Behavioral variant:
    a. Three or more of the following behavioral symptoms:
        i. Behavioral disinhibition.
        ii. Apathy or inertia.
        iii. Loss of sympathy or empathy.
        iv. Perseverative, stereotyped or compulsive/ritualistic behavior.
        v. Hyperorality and dietary changes.
    b. Prominent decline in social cognition and/or executive abilities.

 2. Language variant:

 a. Prominent decline in language ability, in the form of speech production, word finding, object naming, grammar, or word comprehension.

D. Relative sparing of learning and memory and perceptual-motor function.

E. The disturbance is not better explained by cerebrovascular disease, another neurodegenerative disease, the effects of a substance, or another mental, neurological, or systemic disorder.

Probable frontotemporal neurocognitive disorder is diagnosed if either of the following is present; otherwise, **possible frontotemporal neurocognitive disorder** should be diagnosed:

1. Evidence of a causative frontotemporal neurocognitive disorder genetic mutation, from either family history or genetic testing.

2. Evidence of disproportionate frontal and/or temporal lobe involvement from neuroimaging.

Possible frontotemporal neurocognitive disorder is diagnosed if there is no evidence of a genetic mutation, and neuroimaging has not been performed.

Coding note: For probable major neurocognitive disorder due to frontotemporal lobar degeneration, with behavioral disturbance, code first **331.19 (G31.09)** frontotemporal disease, followed by **294.11 (F02.81)** probable major neurocognitive disorder due to frontotemporal lobar degeneration, with behavioral disturbance. For probable major neurocognitive disorder due to frontotemporal lobar degeneration, without behavioral disturbance, code first **331.19 (G31.09)** frontotemporal disease, followed by **294.10 (F02.80)** probable major neurocognitive disorder due to frontotemporal lobar degeneration, without behavioral disturbance.

For possible major neurocognitive disorder due to frontotemporal lobar degeneration, code **331.9 (G31.9)** possible major neurocognitive disorder due to frontotemporal lobar degeneration. (**Note:** Do *not* use the additional code for frontotemporal disease. Behavioral disturbance cannot be coded but should still be indicated in writing.)

For mild neurocognitive disorder due to frontotemporal lobar degeneration, code **331.83 (G31.84)**. (**Note:** Do *not* use the additional code for frontotemporal disease. Behavioral disturbance cannot be coded but should still be indicated in writing.)

Diagnostic Features

Major or mild frontotemporal neurocognitive disorder (NCD) comprises a number of syndromic variants characterized by the progressive development of behavioral and personality change and/or language impairment. The behavioral variant and three language variants (semantic, agrammatic/nonfluent, and logopenic) exhibit distinct patterns of brain atrophy and some distinctive neuropathology. The criteria must be met for either the behavioral or the language variant to make the diagnosis, but many individuals present with features of both.

Individuals with behavioral-variant major or mild frontotemporal NCD present with varying degrees of apathy or disinhibition. They may lose interest in socialization, self-care, and personal responsibilities, or display socially inappropriate behaviors. Insight is usually impaired, and this often delays medical consultation. The first referral is often to a psychiatrist. Individuals may develop changes in social style, and in religious and political beliefs, with repetitive movements, hoarding, changes in eating behavior, and hyperorality. In later stages, loss of sphincter control may occur. Cognitive decline is less prominent, and formal testing may show relatively few deficits in the early stages. Common neurocognitive symptoms are lack of planning and organization, distractibility, and poor judgment. Deficits in executive function, such as poor performance on tests of mental flexibility, abstract reasoning, and response inhibition, are present, but learning and memory are relatively spared, and perceptual-motor abilities are almost always preserved in the early stages.

Individuals with language-variant major or mild frontotemporal NCD present with primary progressive aphasia with gradual onset, with three subtypes commonly described: semantic variant, agrammatic/nonfluent variant, and logopenic variant, and each variant has distinctive features and corresponding neuropathology.

"Probable" is distinguished from "possible" frontotemporal NCD by the presence of causative genetic factors (e.g., mutations in the gene coding for microtubule-associated protein tau) or by the presence of distinctive atrophy or reduced activity in frontotemporal regions on structural or functional imaging.

Associated Features Supporting Diagnosis

Extrapyramidal features may be prominent in some cases, with an overlap with syndromes such as progressive supranuclear palsy and corticobasal degeneration. Features of motor neuron disease may be present in some cases (e.g., muscle atrophy, weakness). A subset of individuals develop visual hallucinations.

Prevalence

Major or mild frontotemporal NCD is a common cause of early-onset NCD in individuals younger than 65 years. Population prevalence estimates are in the range of 2–10 per 100,000. Approximately 20%–25% of cases of frontotemporal NCD occur in individuals older than 65 years. Frontotemporal NCD accounts for about 5% of all cases of dementia in unselected autopsy series. Prevalence estimates of behavioral variant and semantic language variant are higher among males, and prevalence estimates of nonfluent language variant are higher among females.

Development and Course

Individuals with major or mild frontotemporal NCD commonly present in the sixth decade of life, although the age at onset varies from the third to the ninth decades. The disease is gradually progressive, with median survival being 6–11 years after symptom onset and 3–4 years after diagnosis. Survival is shorter and decline is faster in major or mild frontotemporal NCD than in typical Alzheimer's disease.

Risk and Prognostic Factors

Genetic and physiological.   Approximately 40% of individuals with major or mild frontotemporal NCD have a family history of early-onset NCD, and approximately 10% show an autosomal dominant inheritance pattern. A number of genetic factors have been identified, such as mutations in the gene encoding the microtubule associated protein tau (MAPT), the granulin gene (GRN), and the C9ORF72 gene. A number of families with causative mutations have been identified (see the section "Diagnostic Markers" for this disorder), but many individuals with known familial transmission do not have a known mutation. The presence of motor neuron disease is associated with a more rapid deterioration.

Diagnostic Markers

Computed tomography (CT) or structural magnetic resonance imaging (MRI) may show distinct patterns of atrophy. In behavioral-variant major or mild frontotemporal NCD, both frontal lobes (especially the medial frontal lobes) and the anterior temporal lobes are atrophic. In semantic language–variant major or mild frontotemporal NCD, the middle, inferior, and anterior temporal lobes are atrophic bilaterally but asymmetrically, with the left side usually being more affected. Nonfluent language–variant major or mild fronto-temporal NCD is associated with predominantly left posterior frontal-insular atrophy. The logopenic variant of major or mild frontotemporal NCD is associated with predominantly left posterior perisylvian or parietal atrophy. Functional imaging demonstrates hypoperfusion and/or cortical hypometabolism in the corresponding brain regions, which may be present in the early stages in the absence of structural abnormality. Emerging biomarkers for Alzheimer's disease (e.g., cerebrospinal fluid amyloid-beta and tau levels, and amyloid imaging) may help in the differential diagnosis, but the distinction from Alzheimer's disease can remain difficult (the logopenic variant is in fact often a manifestation of Alzheimer's disease).

In familial cases of frontotemporal NCD, the identification of genetic mutations may help confirm the diagnosis. Mutations associated with frontotemporal NCD include the genes encoding microtubule-associated protein tau (MAPT) and granulin (GRN), C9ORF72, transactive response DNA-binding protein of 43 kDa (TDP-43, or TARDBP), valosin-containing protein (VCP), chromatin modifying protein 2B (CHMP2B), and fused in sarcoma protein (FUS).

Functional Consequences of Major or Mild Frontotemporal Neurocognitive Disorder

Because of the relative early age at onset of the disorder, the disorder often affects workplace and family life. Because of the involvement of language and/or behavior, function is often more severely impaired relatively early in the course. For individuals with the behavioral variant, prior to diagnostic clarification there may be significant family disruption, legal involvement, and problems in the workplace because of socially inappropriate behaviors. The functional impairment due to behavioral change and language dysfunction, which can include hyperorality, impulsive wandering, and other disinhibited behaviors, may far exceed that due to the cognitive disturbance and may lead to nursing home placement or institutionalization. These behaviors can be severely disruptive, even in structured care settings, particularly when the individuals are otherwise healthy, nonfrail, and free of other medical comorbidities.

Differential Diagnosis

Other neurocognitive disorders. Other neurodegenerative diseases may be distinguished from major or mild frontotemporal NCD by their characteristic features. In major or mild NCD due to Alzheimer's disease, decline in learning and memory is an early feature. However, 10%–30% of patients presenting with a syndrome suggestive of major or mild frontotemporal NCD are found at autopsy to have Alzheimer's disease pathology. This occurs more frequently in individuals who present with progressive dysexecutive syndromes in the absence of behavioral changes or movement disorder or in those with the logopenic variant.

In major or mild NCD with Lewy bodies, core and suggestive features of Lewy bodies must be present. In major or mild NCD due to Parkinson's disease, spontaneous parkinsonism emerges well before the cognitive decline. In major or mild vascular NCD, depending on affected brain regions, there may also be loss of executive ability and behavioral changes such as apathy, and this disorder should be considered in the differential diagnosis. However, history of a cerebrovascular event is temporally related to the onset of cognitive impairment in major or mild vascular NCD, and neuroimaging reveals infarctions or white matter lesions sufficient to account for the clinical picture.

Other neurological conditions. Major or mild frontotemporal NCD overlaps with progressive supranuclear palsy, corticobasal degeneration, and motor neuron disease clinically as well as pathologically. Progressive supranuclear palsy is characterized by supranuclear gaze palsies and axial-predominant parkinsonism. Pseudobulbar signs may be present, and retropulsion is often prominent. Neurocognitive assessment shows psychomotor slowing, poor working memory, and executive dysfunction. Corticobasal degeneration presents with asymmetric rigidity, limb apraxia, postural instability, myoclonus, alien limb phenomenon, and cortical sensory loss. Many individuals with behavioral-variant major or mild frontotemporal NCD show features of motor neuron disease, which tend to be mixed upper and predominantly lower motor neuron disease.

Other mental disorders and medical conditions.   Behavioral-variant major or mild frontotemporal NCD may be mistaken for a primary mental disorder, such as major depression, bipolar disorders, or schizophrenia, and individuals with this variant often present initially to psychiatry. Over time, the development of progressive neurocognitive difficulties will help to make the distinction. A careful medical evaluation will help to exclude treatable causes of NCDs, such as metabolic disturbances, nutritional deficiencies, and infections.

Major or Mild Neurocognitive Disorder With Lewy Bodies

Diagnostic Criteria

A. The criteria are met for major or mild neurocognitive disorder.

B. The disorder has an insidious onset and gradual progression.

C. The disorder meets a combination of core diagnostic features and suggestive diagnostic features for either probable or possible neurocognitive disorder with Lewy bodies.

  For probable major or mild neurocognitive disorder with Lewy bodies, the individual has two core features, or one suggestive feature with one or more core features.

  For **possible major or mild neurocognitive disorder with Lewy bodies,** the individual has only one core feature, or one or more suggestive features.

  1. Core diagnostic features:

     a. Fluctuating cognition with pronounced variations in attention and alertness.

     b. Recurrent visual hallucinations that are well formed and detailed.

     c. Spontaneous features of parkinsonism, with onset subsequent to the development of cognitive decline.

  2. Suggestive diagnostic features:

     a. Meets criteria for rapid eye movement sleep behavior disorder.

     b. Severe neuroleptic sensitivity.

D. The disturbance is not better explained by cerebrovascular disease, another neurodegenerative disease, the effects of a substance, or another mental, neurological, or systemic disorder.

Coding note: For probable major neurocognitive disorder with Lewy bodies, with behavioral disturbance, code first **331.82 (G31.83)** Lewy body disease, followed by **294.11 (F02.81)** probable major neurocognitive disorder with Lewy bodies, with behavioral disturbance. For probable major neurocognitive disorder with Lewy bodies, without behavioral disturbance, code first **331.82 (G31.83)** Lewy body disease, followed by **294.10 (F02.80)** probable major neurocognitive disorder with Lewy bodies, without behavioral disturbance.

For possible major neurocognitive disorder with Lewy bodies, code **331.9 (G31.9)** possible major neurocognitive disorder with Lewy bodies. (**Note:** Do *not* use the additional code for Lewy body disease. Behavioral disturbance cannot be coded but should still be indicated in writing.)

For mild neurocognitive disorder with Lewy bodies, code **331.83 (G31.84). (Note:** Do *not* use the additional code for Lewy body disease. Behavioral disturbance cannot be coded but should still be indicated in writing.)

Diagnostic Features

Major or mild neurocognitive disorder with Lewy bodies (NCDLB), in the case of major neurocognitive disorder (NCD), corresponds to the condition known as dementia with Lewy bodies (DLB). The disorder includes not only progressive cognitive impairment (with early changes in complex attention and executive function rather than learning and memory) but also recurrent complex visual hallucinations; and concurrent symptoms of rapid eye movement (REM) sleep behavior disorder (which can be a very early manifestation); as well as hallucinations in other sensory modalities, depression, and delusions. The symptoms fluctuate in a pattern that can resemble a delirium, but no adequate underlying cause can be found. The variable presentation of NCDLB symptoms reduces the likelihood of all symptoms being observed in a brief clinic visit and necessitates a thorough assessment of caregiver observations. The use of assessment scales specifically designed to assess fluctuation may aid in diagnosis. Another core feature is spontaneous parkinsonism, which must begin after the onset of cognitive decline; by convention, major cognitive deficits are observed at least 1 year before the motor symptoms. The parkinsonism must also be distinguished from neuroleptic-induced extrapyramidal signs. Accurate diagnosis is essential to safe treatment planning, as up to 50% of individuals with NCDLB have severe sensitivity to neuroleptic drugs, and these medications should be used with extreme caution in managing the psychotic manifestations.

The diagnosis of mild NCDLB is appropriate for individuals who present with the core or suggestive features at a stage when cognitive or functional impairments are not of sufficient severity to fulfill criteria for major NCD. However, as for all mild NCDs, there will often be insufficient evidence to justify any single etiology, and use of the unspecified diagnosis is most appropriate.

Associated Features Supporting Diagnosis

Individuals with NCDLB frequently experience repeated falls and syncope and transient episodes of unexplained loss of consciousness. Autonomic dysfunction, such as orthostatic hypotension and urinary incontinence, may be observed. Auditory and other nonvisual hallucinations are common, as are systematized delusions, delusional misidentification, and depression.

Prevalence

The few population-based prevalence estimates for NCDLB available range from 0.1% to 5% of the general elderly population, and from 1.7% to 30.5% of all dementia cases. In brain bank (autopsy) series, the pathological lesions known as Lewy bodies are present in 20%–35% of cases of dementia. The male-to-female ratio is approximately 1.5:1.

Development and Course

NCDLB is a gradually progressive disorder with insidious onset. However, there is often a prodromal history of confusional episodes (delirium) of acute onset, often precipitated by illness or surgery. The distinction between NCDLB, in which Lewy bodies are primarily cortical in location, and major or mild NCD due to Parkinson's disease, in which the pathology is primarily in the basal ganglia, is the order in which the cognitive and motor symptoms emerge. In NCDLB, the cognitive decline is manifested early in the course of illness, at least a year before the onset of motor symptoms (see the section "Differential Diagnosis" for this disorder). Disease course may be characterized by occasional plateaus but eventually progresses through severe dementia to death. Average duration of survival is 5–7 years in clinical series. Onset of symptoms is typically observed from the sixth through the ninth decades of life, with most cases having their onset when affected individuals are in their mid-70s.

Risk and Prognostic Factors

Genetic and physiological.   Familial aggregation may occur, and several risk genes have been identified, but in most cases of NCDLB, there is no family history.

Diagnostic Markers

The underlying neurodegenerative disease is primarily a synucleinopathy due to alpha-synuclein misfolding and aggregation. Cognitive testing beyond the use of a brief screening instrument may be necessary to define deficits clearly. Assessment scales developed to measure fluctuation can be useful. The associated condition REM sleep behavior disorder may be diagnosed through a formal sleep study or identified by questioning the patient or informant about relevant symptoms. Neuroleptic sensitivity (challenge) is not recommended as a diagnostic marker but raises suspicion of NCDLB if it occurs. A diagnostically suggestive feature is low striatal dopamine transporter uptake on single photon emission computed tomography (SPECT) or positron emission tomography (PET) scan. Other clinically useful markers potentially include relative preservation of medial temporal structures on computed tomography (CT)/magnetic resonance imaging (MRI) brain scan; reduced striatal dopamine transporter uptake on SPECT/PET scan; generalized low uptake on SPECT/PET perfusion scan with reduced occipital activity; abnormal (low uptake) MIBG myocardial scintigraphy suggesting sympathetic denervation; and prominent slow-wave activity on the electroencephalogram with temporal lobe transient waves.

Functional Consequences of Major or Mild Neurocognitive Disorder With Lewy Bodies

Individuals with NCDLB are more functionally impaired than would be expected for their cognitive deficits when contrasted to individuals with other neurodegenerative diseases, such as Alzheimer's disease. This is largely a result of motor and autonomic impairments, which cause problems with toileting, transferring, and eating. Sleep disorders and prominent psychiatric symptoms may also add to functional difficulties. Consequently, the quality of life of individuals with NCDLB is often significantly worse than that of individuals with Alzheimer's disease.

Differential Diagnosis

Major or mild neurocognitive disorder due to Parkinson's disease.   A key differentiating feature in clinical diagnosis is the temporal sequence in which the parkinsonism and the NCD appear. For NCD due to Parkinson's disease, the individual must develop cognitive decline in the context of established Parkinson's disease; by convention, the decline should not reach the stage of major NCD until at least 1 year after Parkinson's is diagnosed. If less than a year has passed since the onset of motor symptoms, the diagnosis is NCDLB. This distinction is clearer at the major NCD level than at the mild NCD level.

The timing and sequence of parkinsonism and mild NCD may be more difficult to determine because the onset and clinical presentation can be ambiguous, and unspecified mild NCD should be diagnosed if the other core and suggestive features are absent.

Comorbidity

Lewy body pathology frequently coexists with Alzheimer's disease and cerebrovascular disease pathology, particularly among the oldest age groups. In Alzheimer's disease, there is concomitant synuclein pathology in 60% of cases (if amygdala-restricted cases are included). In general, there is a higher rate of Lewy body pathology in individuals with dementia than in older individuals without dementia.

Major or Mild Vascular Neurocognitive Disorder

Diagnostic Criteria

A. The criteria are met for major or mild neurocognitive disorder.

B. The clinical features are consistent with a vascular etiology, as suggested by either of the following:

   1. Onset of the cognitive deficits is temporally related to one or more cerebrovascular events.
   2. Evidence for decline is prominent in complex attention (including processing speed) and frontal-executive function.

C. There is evidence of the presence of cerebrovascular disease from history, physical examination, and/or neuroimaging considered sufficient to account for the neurocognitive deficits.

D. The symptoms are not better explained by another brain disease or systemic disorder.

Probable vascular neurocognitive disorder is diagnosed if one of the following is present; otherwise **possible vascular neurocognitive disorder** should be diagnosed:

1. Clinical criteria are supported by neuroimaging evidence of significant parenchymal injury attributed to cerebrovascular disease (neuroimaging-supported).
2. The neurocognitive syndrome is temporally related to one or more documented cerebrovascular events.
3. Both clinical and genetic (e.g., cerebral autosomal dominant arteriopathy with subcortical infarcts and leukoencephalopathy) evidence of cerebrovascular disease is present.

Possible vascular neurocognitive disorder is diagnosed if the clinical criteria are met but neuroimaging is not available and the temporal relationship of the neurocognitive syndrome with one or more cerebrovascular events is not established.

Coding note: For probable major vascular neurocognitive disorder, with behavioral disturbance, code **290.40 (F01.51).** For probable major vascular neurocognitive disorder, without behavioral disturbance, code **290.40 (F01.50).** For possible major vascular neurocognitive disorder, with or without behavioral disturbance, code **331.9 (G31.9).** An additional medical code for the cerebrovascular disease is not needed.

For mild vascular neurocognitive disorder, code **331.83 (G31.84).** (**Note:** Do *not* use an additional code for the vascular disease. Behavioral disturbance cannot be coded but should still be indicated in writing.)

Diagnostic Features

The diagnosis of major or mild vascular neurocognitive disorder (NCD) requires the establishment of an NCD (Criterion A) and the determination that cerebrovascular disease is the dominant if not exclusive pathology that accounts for the cognitive deficits (Criteria B and C). Vascular etiology may range from large vessel stroke to microvascular disease; the presentation is therefore very heterogeneous, stemming from the types of vascular lesions and their extent and location. The lesions may be focal, multifocal, or diffuse and occur in various combinations.

Many individuals with major or mild vascular NCD present with multiple infarctions, with an acute stepwise or fluctuating decline in cognition, and intervening periods of stability and even some improvement. Others may have gradual onset with slow progression, a rapid development of deficits followed by relative stability, or another complex presentation. Major or mild vascular NCD with a gradual onset and slow progression is generally due to small vessel disease leading to lesions in the white matter, basal ganglia, and/or thalamus. The gradual progression in these cases is often punctuated by acute events that leave subtle neurological deficits. The cognitive deficits in these cases can be attributed to disruption of cortical-subcortical circuits, and complex attention, particularly speed of information processing, and executive ability are likely to be affected.

Assessing for the presence of sufficient cerebrovascular disease relies on history, physical examination, and neuroimaging (Criterion C). Etiological certainty requires the demonstration of abnormalities on neuroimaging. The lack of neuroimaging can result in significant diagnostic inaccuracy by overlooking "silent" brain infarction and white matter lesions. However, if the neurocognitive impairment is temporally associated with one or more well-documented strokes, a probable diagnosis can be made in the absence of neuroimaging. Clinical evidence of cerebrovascular disease includes documented history of stroke, with cognitive decline temporally associated with the event, or physical signs consistent with stroke (e.g., hemiparesis; pseudobulbar syndrome, visual field defect). Neuroimaging (magnetic resonance imaging [MRI] or computed tomography [CT]) evidence of cerebrovascular disease comprises one or more of the following: one or more large vessel infarcts or hemorrhages, a strategically placed single infarct or hemorrhage (e.g., in angular gyrus, thalamus, basal forebrain), two or more lacunar infarcts outside the brain stem, or extensive and confluent white matter lesions. The latter is often termed *small vessel disease* or *subcortical ischemic changes* on clinical neuroimaging evaluations.

For mild vascular NCD, history of a single stroke or extensive white matter disease is generally sufficient. For major vascular NCD, two or more strokes, a strategically placed stroke, or a combination of white matter disease and one or more lacunes is generally necessary.

The disorder must not be better explained by another disorder. For example, prominent memory deficit early in the course might suggest Alzheimer's disease, early and prominent parkinsonian features would suggest Parkinson's disease, and a close association between onset and depression would suggest depression.

Associated Features Supporting Diagnosis

A neurological assessment often reveals history of stroke and/or transient ischemic episodes, and signs indicative of brain infarctions. Also commonly associated are personality and mood changes, abulia, depression, and emotional lability. The development of late-onset depressive symptoms accompanied by psychomotor slowing and executive dysfunction is a common presentation among older adults with progressive small vessel ischemic disease ("vascular depression").

Prevalence

Major or mild vascular NCD is the second most common cause of NCD after Alzheimer's disease. In the United States, population prevalence estimates for vascular dementia range from 0.2% in the 65–70 years age group to 16% in individuals 80 years and older. Within 3 months following stroke, 20%–30% of individuals are diagnosed with dementia. In neuropathology series, the prevalence of vascular dementia increases from 13% at age 70 years to 44.6% at age 90 years or older, in comparison with Alzheimer's disease (23.6%–51%) and combined vascular dementia and Alzheimer's disease (2%–46.4%). Higher prevalence has been reported in African Americans compared with Caucasians, and in East Asian countries (e.g., Japan, China). Prevalence is higher in males than in females.

Development and Course

Major or mild vascular NCD can occur at any age, although the prevalence increases exponentially after age 65 years. In older individuals, additional pathologies may partly account for the neurocognitive deficits. The course may vary from acute onset with partial improvement to stepwise decline to progressive decline, with fluctuations and plateaus of varying durations. Pure subcortical major or mild vascular NCD can have a slowly progressive course that simulates major or mild NCD due to Alzheimer's disease.

Risk and Prognostic Factors

Environmental.   The neurocognitive outcomes of vascular brain injury are influenced by neuroplasticity factors such as education, physical exercise, and mental activity.

Genetic and physiological.   The major risk factors for major or mild vascular NCD are the same as those for cerebrovascular disease, including hypertension, diabetes, smoking, obesity, high cholesterol levels, high homocysteine levels, other risk factors for atherosclerosis and arteriolosclerosis, atrial fibrillation, and other conditions increasing the risk of cerebral emboli. Cerebral amyloid angiopathy is an important risk factor in which amyloid deposits occur within arterial vessels. Another key risk factor is the hereditary condition cerebral autosomal dominant arteriopathy with subcortical infarcts and leukoencephalopathy, or CADASIL.

Diagnostic Markers

Structural neuroimaging, using MRI or CT, has an important role in the diagnostic process. There are no other established biomarkers of major or mild vascular NCD.

Functional Consequences of Major or Mild Vascular Neurocognitive Disorder

Major or mild vascular NCD is commonly associated with physical deficits that cause additional disability.

Differential Diagnosis

Other neurocognitive disorders.   Since incidental brain infarctions and white matter lesions are common in older individuals, it is important to consider other possible etiologies when an NCD is present. A history of memory deficit early in the course, and progressive worsening of memory, language, executive function, and perceptual-motor abilities in the absence of corresponding focal lesions on brain imaging, are suggestive of Alzheimer's disease as the primary diagnosis. Potential biomarkers currently being validated for Alzheimer's disease, such as cerebrospinal fluid levels of beta-amyloid and phosphorylated tau, and amyloid imaging, may prove to be helpful in the differential diagnosis. NCD with Lewy bodies is distinguished from major or mild vascular NCD by its core features of fluctuating cognition, visual hallucinations, and spontaneous parkinsonism. While deficits in executive function and language occur in major or mild vascular NCD, the insidious onset and gradual progression of behavioral features or language impairment are characteristic of frontotemporal NCD and are not typical of vascular etiology.

Other medical conditions.   A diagnosis of major or mild vascular NCD is not made if other diseases (e.g., brain tumor, multiple sclerosis, encephalitis, toxic or metabolic disorders) are present and are of sufficient severity to account for the cognitive impairment.

Other mental disorders.   A diagnosis of major or mild vascular NCD is inappropriate if the symptoms can be entirely attributed to delirium, although delirium may sometimes be superimposed on a preexisting major or mild vascular NCD, in which case both diagnoses can be made. If the criteria for major depressive disorder are met and the cognitive impairment is temporally related to the likely onset of the depression, major or mild vascular NCD should not be diagnosed. However, if the NCD preceded the development of the depression, or the severity of the cognitive impairment is out of proportion to the severity of the depression, both should be diagnosed.

Comorbidity

Major or mild NCD due to Alzheimer's disease commonly co-occurs with major or mild vascular NCD, in which case both diagnoses should be made. Major or mild vascular NCD and depression frequently co-occur.

Major or Mild Neurocognitive Disorder Due to Traumatic Brain Injury

Diagnostic Criteria

A. The criteria are met for major or mild neurocognitive disorder.

B. There is evidence of a traumatic brain injury—that is, an impact to the head or other mechanisms of rapid movement or displacement of the brain within the skull, with one or more of the following:

1. Loss of consciousness.
2. Posttraumatic amnesia.
3. Disorientation and confusion.
4. Neurological signs (e.g., neuroimaging demonstrating injury; a new onset of seizures; a marked worsening of a preexisting seizure disorder; visual field cuts; anosmia; hemiparesis).

C. The neurocognitive disorder presents immediately after the occurrence of the traumatic brain injury or immediately after recovery of consciousness and persists past the acute post-injury period.

Coding note: For major neurocognitive disorder due to traumatic brain injury, with behavioral disturbance: For ICD-9-CM, first code **907.0** late effect of intracranial injury without skull fracture, followed by **294.11** major neurocognitive disorder due to traumatic brain injury, with behavioral disturbance. For ICD-10-CM, first code **S06.2X9S** diffuse traumatic brain injury with loss of consciousness of unspecified duration, sequela; followed by **F02.81** major neurocognitive disorder due to traumatic brain injury, with behavioral disturbance.

For major neurocognitive disorder due to traumatic brain injury, without behavioral disturbance: For ICD-9-CM, first code **907.0** late effect of intracranial injury without skull fracture, followed by **294.10** major neurocognitive disorder due to traumatic brain injury, without behavioral disturbance. For ICD-10-CM, first code **S06.2X9S** diffuse traumatic brain injury with loss of consciousness of unspecified duration, sequela; followed by **F02.80** major neurocognitive disorder due to traumatic brain injury, without behavioral disturbance.

For mild neurocognitive disorder due to traumatic brain injury, code **331.83 (G31.84).** (**Note:** Do *not* use the additional code for traumatic brain injury. Behavioral disturbance cannot be coded but should still be indicated in writing.)

Specifiers

Rate the severity of the neurocognitive disorder (NCD), not the underlying traumatic brain injury (see the section "Development and Course" for this disorder).

Diagnostic Features

Major or mild NCD due to traumatic brain injury (TBI) is caused by an impact to the head, or other mechanisms of rapid movement or displacement of the brain within the skull, as can happen with blast injuries. *Traumatic brain injury* is defined as brain trauma with specific characteristics that include at least one of the following: loss of consciousness, post-traumatic amnesia, disorientation and confusion, or, in more severe cases, neurological signs (e.g., positive neuroimaging, a new onset of seizures or a marked worsening of a preexisting seizure disorder, visual field cuts, anosmia, hemiparesis) (Criterion B). To be attributable to TBI, the NCD must present either immediately after the brain injury occurs or immediately after the individual recovers consciousness after the injury and persist past the acute post-injury period (Criterion C).

The cognitive presentation is variable. Difficulties in the domains of complex attention, executive ability, learning, and memory are common as well as slowing in speed of information processing and disturbances in social cognition. In more severe TBI in which there is brain contusion, intracranial hemorrhage, or penetrating injury, there may be additional neurocognitive deficits, such as aphasia, neglect, and constructional dyspraxia.

Associated Features Supporting Diagnosis

Major or mild NCD due to TBI may be accompanied by disturbances in emotional function (e.g., irritability, easy frustration, tension and anxiety, affective lability); personality changes (e.g., disinhibition, apathy, suspiciousness, aggression); physical disturbances (e.g., headache, fatigue, sleep disorders, vertigo or dizziness, tinnitus or hyperacusis, photosensitivity, anosmia, reduced tolerance to psychotropic medications); and, particularly in more severe TBI, neurological symptoms and signs (e.g., seizures, hemiparesis, visual disturbances, cranial nerve deficits) and evidence of orthopedic injuries.

Prevalence

In the United States, 1.7 million TBIs occur annually, resulting in 1.4 million emergency department visits, 275,000 hospitalizations, and 52,000 deaths. About 2% of the population lives with TBI-associated disability. Males account for 59% of TBIs in the United States. The most common etiologies of TBI in the United States are falls, vehicular accidents, and being struck on the head. Collisions and blows to the head that occur in the course of contact sports are increasingly recognized as sources of mild TBI, with a concern that repeated mild TBI may have cumulatively persisting sequelae.

Development and Course

The severity of a TBI is rated at the time of injury/initial assessment as mild, moderate, or severe according to the thresholds in Table 2.

The severity rating of the TBI itself does not necessarily correspond to the severity of the resulting NCD. The course of recovery from TBI is variable, depending not only on the specifics of the injury but also on cofactors, such as age, prior history of brain damage, or substance abuse, that may favor or impede recovery.

TABLE 2   Severity ratings for traumatic brain injury

Injury characteristic	Mild TBI	Moderate TBI	Severe TBI
Loss of consciousness	<30 min	30 minutes–24 hours	>24 hours
Posttraumatic amnesia	<24 hours	24 hours–7 days	>7 days
Disorientation and confusion at initial assessment (Glasgow Coma Scale Score)	13–15 (not below 13 at 30 minutes)	9–12	3–8

Neurobehavioral symptoms tend to be most severe in the immediate aftermath of the TBI. Except in the case of severe TBI, the typical course is that of complete or substantial improvement in associated neurocognitive, neurological, and psychiatric symptoms and signs. Neurocognitive symptoms associated with mild TBI tend to resolve within days to weeks after the injury with complete resolution typical by 3 months. Other symptoms that may potentially co-occur with the neurological symptoms (e.g., depression, irritability, fatigue, headache, photosensitivity, sleep disturbance) also tend to resolve in the weeks following mild TBI. Substantial subsequent deterioration in these areas should trigger consideration of additional diagnoses. However, repeated mild TBI may be associated with persisting neurocognitive disturbance.

With moderate and severe TBI, in addition to persistence of neurocognitive deficits, there may be associated neurophysiological, emotional, and behavioral complications. These include seizures (particularly in the first year), photosensitivity, hyperacusis, irritability, aggression, depression, sleep disturbance, fatigue, apathy, inability to resume occupational and social functioning at pre-injury level, and deterioration in interpersonal relationships. Moderate and severe TBI have been associated with increased risk of depression, aggression, and possibly neurodegenerative diseases such as Alzheimer's disease.

The features of persisting major or mild NCD due to TBI will vary by age, specifics of the injury, and cofactors. Persisting TBI-related impairment in an infant or child may be reflected in delays in reaching developmental milestones (e.g., language acquisition), worse academic performance, and possibly impaired social development. Among older teenagers and adults, persisting symptoms may include various neurocognitive deficits, irritability, hypersensitivity to light and sound, easy fatigability, and mood changes, including depression, anxiety, hostility, or apathy. In older individuals with depleted cognitive reserve, mild TBI is more likely to result in incomplete recoveries.

Risk and Prognostic Factors

Risk factors for traumatic brain injury.   Traumatic brain injury rates vary by age, with the highest prevalence among individuals younger than 4 years, older adolescents, and individuals older than 65 years. Falls are the most common cause of TBI, with motor vehicle accidents being second. Sports concussions are frequent causes of TBI in older children, teenagers, and young adults.

Risk factors for neurocognitive disorder after traumatic brain injury.   Repeated concussions can lead to persistent NCD and neuropathological evidence of traumatic encephalopathy. Co-occurring intoxication with a substance may increase the severity of a TBI from a motor vehicle accident, but whether intoxication at the time of injury worsens neurocognitive outcome is unknown.

Course modifiers.   Mild TBI generally resolves within a few weeks to months, although resolution may be delayed or incomplete in the context of repeated TBI. Worse outcome from moderate to severe TBI is associated with older age (older than 40 years) and initial clinical parameters, such as low Glasgow Coma Scale score; worse motor function; pupillary nonreactivity; and computed tomography (CT) evidence of brain injury (e.g., petechial hemorrhages, subarachnoid hemorrhage, midline shift, obliteration of third ventricle).

Diagnostic Markers

Beyond neuropsychological testing, CT scanning may reveal petechial hemorrhages, subarachnoid hemorrhage, or evidence of contusion. Magnetic resonance image scanning may also reveal hyperintensities suggestive of microhemorrhages.

Functional Consequences of Major or Mild Neurocognitive Disorder Due to Traumatic Brain Injury

With mild NCD due to TBI, individuals may report reduced cognitive efficiency, difficulty concentrating, and lessened ability to perform usual activities. With major NCD due to TBI, an individual may have difficulty in independent living and self-care. Prominent neuromotor features, such as severe incoordination, ataxia, and motor slowing, may be present in major NCD due to TBI and may add to functional difficulties. Individuals with TBI histories report more depressive symptoms, and these can amplify cognitive complaints and worsen functional outcome. Additionally, loss of emotional control, including aggressive or inappropriate affect and apathy, may be present after more severe TBI with greater neurocognitive impairment. These features may compound difficulties with independent living and self-care.

Differential Diagnosis

In some instances, severity of neurocognitive symptoms may appear to be inconsistent with the severity of the TBI. After previously undetected neurological complications (e.g., chronic hematoma) are excluded, the possibility of diagnoses such as somatic symptom disorder or factitious disorder need to be considered. Posttraumatic stress disorder (PTSD) can co-occur with the NCD and have overlapping symptoms (e.g., difficulty concentrating, depressed mood, aggressive behavioral disinhibition).

Comorbidity

Among individuals with substance use disorders, the neurocognitive effects of the substance contribute to or compound the TBI-associated neurocognitive change. Some symptoms associated with TBI may overlap with symptoms found in cases of PTSD, and the two disorders may co-occur, especially in military populations.

Substance/Medication-Induced Major or Mild Neurocognitive Disorder

Diagnostic Criteria

A. The criteria are met for major or mild neurocognitive disorder.
B. The neurocognitive impairments do not occur exclusively during the course of a delirium and persist beyond the usual duration of intoxication and acute withdrawal.
C. The involved substance or medication and duration and extent of use are capable of producing the neurocognitive impairment.
D. The temporal course of the neurocognitive deficits is consistent with the timing of substance or medication use and abstinence (e.g., the deficits remain stable or improve after a period of abstinence).

E. The neurocognitive disorder is not attributable to another medical condition or is not better explained by another mental disorder.

Coding note: The ICD-9-CM and ICD-10-CM codes for the [specific substance/medication]-induced neurocognitive disorders are indicated in the table below. Note that the ICD-10-CM code depends on whether or not there is a comorbid substance use disorder present for the same class of substance. If a mild substance use disorder is comorbid with the substance-induced neurocognitive disorder, the 4th position character is "1," and the clinician should record "mild [substance] use disorder" before the substance-induced neurocognitive disorder (e.g., "mild inhalant use disorder with inhalant-induced major neurocognitive disorder"). If a moderate or severe substance use disorder is comorbid with the substance-induced neurocognitive disorder, the 4th position character is "2," and the clinician should record "moderate [substance] use disorder" or "severe [substance] use disorder," depending on the severity of the comorbid substance use disorder. If there is no comorbid substance use disorder, then the 4th position character is "9," and the clinician should record only the substance-induced neurocognitive disorder. For some classes of substances (i.e., alcohol; sedatives, hypnotics, anxiolytics), it is not permissible to code a comorbid mild substance use disorder with a substance-induced neurocognitive disorder; only a comorbid moderate or severe substance use disorder, or no substance use disorder, can be diagnosed. Behavioral disturbance cannot be coded but should still be indicated in writing.

		ICD-10-CM		
	ICD-9-CM	With use disorder, mild	With use disorder, moderate or severe	Without use disorder
Alcohol (major neurocognitive disorder), nonamnestic-confabulatory type	291.2	NA	F10.27	F10.97
Alcohol (major neurocognitive disorder), amnestic-confabulatory type	291.1	NA	F10.26	F10.96
Alcohol (mild neurocognitive disorder)	291.89	NA	F10.288	F10.988
Inhalant (major neurocognitive disorder)	292.82	F18.17	F18.27	F18.97
Inhalant (mild neurocognitive disorder)	292.89	F18.188	F18.288	F18.988
Sedative, hypnotic, or anxiolytic (major neurocognitive disorder)	292.82	NA	F13.27	F13.97
Sedative, hypnotic, or anxiolytic (mild neurocognitive disorder)	292.89	NA	F13.288	F13.988
Other (or unknown) substance (major neurocognitive disorder)	292.82	F19.17	F19.27	F19.97
Other (or unknown) substance (mild neurocognitive disorder)	292.89	F19.188	F19.288	F19.988

Specify if:

Persistent: Neurocognitive impairment continues to be significant after an extended period of abstinence.

Recording Procedures

ICD-9-CM.   The name of the substance/medication-induced neurocognitive disorder begins with the specific substance/medication (e.g., alcohol) that is presumed to be causing the neurocognitive symptoms. The diagnostic code is selected from the table included in the criteria set, which is based on the drug class. For substances that do not fit into any of the classes, the code for "other substance" should be used; and in cases in which a substance is judged to be an etiological factor but the specific class of substance is unknown, the category "unknown substance" should be used.

The name of the disorder (i.e., [specific substance]-induced major neurocognitive disorder or [specific substance]-induced mild neurocognitive disorder) is followed by the type in the case of alcohol (i.e., nonamnestic-confabulatory type, amnestic-confabulatory type), followed by specification of duration (i.e., persistent). Unlike the recording procedures for ICD-10-CM, which combine the substance/medication-induced disorder and substance use disorder into a single code, for ICD-9-CM a separate diagnostic code is given for the substance use disorder. For example, in the case of persistent amnestic-confabulatory symptoms in a man with a severe alcohol use disorder, the diagnosis is 291.1 alcohol-induced major neurocognitive disorder, amnestic-confabulatory type, persistent. An additional diagnosis of 303.90 severe alcohol use disorder is also given. If the substance/medication-induced neurocognitive disorder occurs without a comorbid substance use disorder (e.g., after a sporadic heavy use of inhalants), no accompanying substance use disorder is noted (e.g., 292.82 inhalant-induced mild neurocognitive disorder).

ICD-10-CM.   The name of the substance/medication-induced neurocognitive disorder begins with the specific substance (e.g., alcohol) that is presumed to be causing the neurocognitive symptoms. The diagnostic code is selected from the table included in the criteria set, which is based on the drug class and presence or absence of a comorbid substance use disorder. For substances that do not fit into any of the classes, the code for "other substance" should be used; and in cases in which a substance is judged to be an etiological factor but the specific class of substance is unknown, the category "unknown substance" should be used.

When recording the name of the disorder, the comorbid substance use disorder (if any) is listed first, followed by the word "with," followed by the name of the disorder (i.e., [specific substance]-induced major neurocognitive disorder or [specific substance]-induced mild neurocognitive disorder), followed by the type in the case of alcohol (i.e., nonamnestic-confabulatory type, amnestic-confabulatory type), followed by specification of duration (i.e., persistent). For example, in the case of persistent amnestic-confabulatory symptoms in a man with a severe alcohol use disorder, the diagnosis is F10.26 severe alcohol use disorder with alcohol-induced major neurocognitive disorder, amnestic-confabulatory type, persistent. A separate diagnosis of the comorbid severe alcohol use disorder is not given. If the substance-induced neurocognitive disorder occurs without a comorbid substance use disorder (e.g., after a sporadic heavy use of inhalants), no accompanying substance use disorder is noted (e.g., F18.988 inhalant-induced mild neurocognitive disorder).

Diagnostic Features

Substance/medication-induced major or mild NCD is characterized by neurocognitive impairments that persist beyond the usual duration of intoxication and acute withdrawal (Criterion B). Initially, these manifestations can reflect slow recovery of brain functions from a period of prolonged substance use, and improvements in neurocognitive as well as brain imaging indicators may be seen over many months. If the disorder continues for an extended period, *persistent* should be specified. The given substance and its use must be known to be capable of causing the observed impairments (Criterion C). While nonspecific decrements in a range of cognitive abilities can occur with nearly any substance of abuse and a variety of medications, some patterns occur more frequently with selected drug classes. For example, NCD due to sedative, hypnotic, or anxiolytic drugs (e.g., benzodiazepines, barbiturates) may show greater disturbances in memory than in other cognitive functions. NCD induced by alcohol frequently manifests with a combination of impairments in executive-function and memory and learning domains. The temporal course of the substance-induced NCD must be consistent with that of use of the given substance (Criterion D). In alcohol-induced amnestic confabulatory (Korsakoff's) NCD, the features include prominent amnesia (severe difficulty learning new information with rapid forgetting) and a tendency to confabulate. These manifestations may co-occur with signs of thiamine encephalopathy (Wernicke's encephalopathy) with associated features such as nystagmus and ataxia. Ophthalmoplegia of Wernicke's encephalopathy is typically characterized by a lateral gaze paralysis.

In addition to or independent of the more common neurocognitive symptoms related to methamphetamine use (e.g., difficulties with learning and memory; executive function), methamphetamine use can also be associated with evidence of vascular injury (e.g., focal weakness, unilateral incoordination, asymmetrical reflexes). The most common neurocognitive profile approximates that seen in vascular NCD.

Associated Features Supporting Diagnosis

Intermediate-duration NCD induced by drugs with central nervous system depressant effects may manifest with added symptoms of increased irritability, anxiety, sleep disturbance, and dysphoria. Intermediate-duration NCD induced by stimulant drugs may manifest with rebound depression, hypersomnia, and apathy. In severe forms of substance/medication-induced major NCD (e.g., associated with long-term alcohol use), there may be prominent neuromotor features, such as incoordination, ataxia, and motor slowing. There may also be loss of emotional control, including aggressive or inappropriate affect, or apathy.

Prevalence

The prevalence of these conditions is not known. Prevalence figures for substance abuse are available, and substance/medication-induced major or mild NCDs are more likely in those who are older, have longer use, and have other risk factors such as nutritional deficits.

For alcohol abuse, the rate of mild NCD of intermediate duration is approximately 30%–40% in the first 2 months of abstinence. Mild NCD may persist, particularly in those who do not achieve stable abstinence until after age 50 years. Major NCD is rare and may result from concomitant nutritional deficits, as in alcohol-induced amnestic confabulatory NCD.

For individuals quitting cocaine, methamphetamine, opioids, phencyclidine, and sedative, hypnotics, or anxiolytics, substance/medication-induced mild NCD of intermediate duration may occur in one-third or more, and there is some evidence that these substances may also be associated with persistent mild NCD. Major NCD associated with these substances is rare, if it occurs at all. In the case of methamphetamine, cerebrovascular disease can also occur, resulting in diffuse or focal brain injury that can be of mild or major neurocognitive levels. Solvent exposure has been linked to both major and mild NCD of both intermediate and persistent duration.

The presence of NCD induced by cannabis and various hallucinogens is controversial. With cannabis, intoxication is accompanied by various neurocognitive disturbances, but these tend to clear with abstinence.

Development and Course

Substance use disorders tend to commence during adolescence and peak in the 20s and 30s. Although longer history of severe substance use disorder is associated with greater likelihood of NCD, the relationships are not straightforward, with substantial and even complete recovery of neurocognitive functions being common among individuals who achieve stable abstinence prior to age 50 years. Substance/medication-induced major or mild NCD is most likely to become persistent in individuals who continue abuse of substances past age 50 years, presumably because of a combination of lessened neural plasticity and beginnings of other age-related brain changes. Earlier commencement of abuse, particularly of alcohol, may lead to defects in later neural development (e.g., later stages of maturation of frontal circuitries), which may have effects on social cognition as well as other neurocognitive abilities. For alcohol-induced NCD, there may be an additive effect of aging and alcohol-induced brain injury.

Risk and Prognostic Factors

Risk factors for substance/medication-induced NCDs include older age, longer use, and persistent use past age 50 years. In addition, for alcohol-induced NCD, long-term nutritional deficiencies, liver disease, vascular risk factors, and cardiovascular and cerebrovascular disease may contribute to risk.

Diagnostic Markers

Magnetic resonance imaging (MRI) of individuals with chronic alcohol abuse frequently reveals cortical thinning, white matter loss, and enlargement of sulci and ventricles. While neuroimaging abnormalities are more common in those with NCDs, it is possible to observe NCDs without neuroimaging abnormalities, and vice versa. Specialized techniques (e.g., diffusion tensor imaging) may reveal damage to specific white matter tracts. Magnetic resonance spectroscopy may reveal reduction in N-acetylaspartate, and increase in markers of inflammation (e.g., myoinositol) or white matter injury (e.g., choline). Many of these brain imaging changes and neurocognitive manifestations reverse following successful abstinence. In individuals with methamphetamine use disorder, MRI may also reveal hyperintensities suggestive of microhemorrhages or larger areas of infarction.

Functional Consequences of Substance/Medication-Induced Major or Mild Neurocognitive Disorder

The functional consequences of substance/medication-induced mild NCD are sometimes augmented by reduced cognitive efficiency and difficulty concentrating beyond that seen in many other NCDs. In addition, at both major and mild levels, substance/medication-induced NCDs may have associated motor syndromes that increase the level of functional impairment.

Differential Diagnosis

Individuals with substance use disorders, substance intoxication, and substance withdrawal are at increased risk for other conditions that may independently, or through a compounding effect, result in neurocognitive disturbance. These include history of traumatic brain injury and infections that can accompany substance use disorder (e.g., HIV, hepatitis C virus, syphilis). Therefore, presence of substance/medication-induced major or mild NCD should be differentiated from NCDs arising outside the context of substance use, intoxication, and withdrawal, including these accompanying conditions (e.g., traumatic brain injury).

Comorbidity

Substance use disorders, substance intoxication, and substance withdrawal are highly co-morbid with other mental disorders. Comorbid posttraumatic stress disorder, psychotic disorders, depressive and bipolar disorders, and neurodevelopmental disorders can contribute to neurocognitive impairment in substance users. Traumatic brain injury occurs more frequently with substance use, complicating efforts to determine the etiology of NCD in such cases. Severe, long-term alcohol use disorder can be associated with major organ system disease, including cerebrovascular disease and cirrhosis. Amphetamine-induced NCD may be accompanied by major or mild vascular NCD, also secondary to amphetamine use.

Major or Mild Neurocognitive Disorder Due to HIV Infection

Diagnostic Criteria

A. The criteria are met for major or mild neurocognitive disorder.

B. There is documented infection with human immunodeficiency virus (HIV).

C. The neurocognitive disorder is not better explained by non-HIV conditions, including secondary brain diseases such as progressive multifocal leukoencephalopathy or cryptococcal meningitis.

D. The neurocognitive disorder is not attributable to another medical condition and is not better explained by a mental disorder.

Coding note: For major neurocognitive disorder due to HIV infection, with behavioral disturbance, code first **042 (B20)** HIV infection, followed by **294.11 (F02.81)** major neurocognitive disorder due to HIV infection, with behavioral disturbance. For major neurocognitive disorder due to HIV infection, without behavioral disturbance, code first **042 (B20)** HIV infection, followed by **294.10 (F02.80)** major neurocognitive disorder due to HIV infection, without behavioral disturbance.

For mild neurocognitive disorder due to HIV infection, code **331.83 (G31.84)**. (**Note:** Do *not* use the additional code for HIV infection. Behavioral disturbance cannot be coded but should still be indicated in writing.)

Diagnostic Features

HIV disease is caused by infection with human immunodeficiency virus type-1 (HIV-1), which is acquired through exposure to bodily fluids of an infected person through injection drug use, unprotected sexual contact, or accidental or iatrogenic exposure (e.g., contaminated blood supply, needle puncture injury to medical personnel). HIV infects several types of cells, most particularly immune cells. Over time, the infection can cause severe depletion of "T-helper" (CD4) lymphocytes, resulting in severe immunocompromise, often leading to opportunistic infections and neoplasms. This advanced form of HIV infection is termed *acquired immune deficiency syndrome* (AIDS). Diagnosis of HIV is confirmed by established laboratory methods such as enzyme-linked immunosorbent assay for HIV antibody with Western blot confirmation and/or polymerase chain reaction–based assays for HIV.

Some individuals with HIV infection develop an NCD, which generally shows a "subcortical pattern" with prominently impaired executive function, slowing of processing speed, problems with more demanding attentional tasks, and difficulty in learning new information, but fewer problems with recall of learned information. In major NCD, slowing may be prominent. Language difficulties, such as aphasia, are uncommon, although reductions in fluency may be observed. HIV pathogenic processes can affect any part of the brain; therefore, other patterns are possible.

Associated Features Supporting Diagnosis

Major or mild NCD due to HIV infection is usually more prevalent in individuals with prior episodes of severe immunosuppression, high viral loads in the cerebrospinal fluid, and indicators of advanced HIV disease such as anemia and hypoalbuminemia. Individuals with advanced NCD may experience prominent neuromotor features such as severe incoordination, ataxia, and motor slowing. There may be loss of emotional control, including aggressive or inappropriate affect or apathy.

Prevalence

Depending on stage of HIV disease, approximately one-third to over one-half of HIV-infected individuals have at least mild neurocognitive disturbance, but some of these disturbances may not meet the full criteria for mild NCD. An estimated 25% of individuals with HIV will have signs and symptoms that meet criteria for mild NCD, and in fewer than 5% would criteria for major NCD be met.

Development and Course

An NCD due to HIV infection can resolve, improve, slowly worsen, or have a fluctuating course. Rapid progression to profound neurocognitive impairment is uncommon in the context of currently available combination antiviral treatment; consequently, an abrupt change in mental status in an individual with HIV may prompt an evaluation of other medical sources for the cognitive change, including secondary infections. Because HIV infection preferentially affects subcortical regions over the course of illness, including deep white matter, the progression of the disorder follows a "subcortical" pattern. Since HIV can affect a variety of brain regions, and the illness can take on many different trajectories depending on associated comorbidities and consequences of HIV, the overall course of an NCD due to HIV infection has considerable heterogeneity. A subcortical neurocognitive profile may interact with age over the life course, when psychomotor slowing and motor impairments such as slowed gait may occur as a consequence of other age-related conditions so that the overall progression may appear more pronounced in later life.

In developed countries, HIV disease is primarily a condition of adults, with acquisition via risky behaviors (e.g., unprotected sex, injection drug use) beginning in late adolescence and peaking during young and middle adulthood. In developing countries, particularly sub-Saharan Africa, where HIV testing and antiretroviral treatments for pregnant women are not readily available, perinatal transmission is common. The NCD in such infants and children may present primarily as neurodevelopmental delay. As individuals treated for HIV survive into older age, additive and interactive neurocognitive effects of HIV and aging, including other NCDs (e.g., due to Alzheimer's disease, due to Parkinson's disease), are possible.

Risk and Prognostic Factors

Risk and prognostic factors for HIV infection. Risk factors for HIV infection include injection drug use, unprotected sex, and unprotected blood supply and other iatrogenic factors.

Risk and prognostic factors for major or mild neurocognitive disorder due to HIV infection. Paradoxically, NCD due to HIV infection has not declined significantly with the advent of combined antiretroviral therapy, although the most severe presentations (consistent with the diagnosis of major NCD) have decreased sharply. Contributory factors may include inadequate control of HIV in the central nervous system (CNS), the evolution of drug-resistant viral strains, the effects of chronic long-term systemic and brain inflammation, and the effects of comorbid factors such as aging, drug abuse, past history of CNS trauma, and co-infections, such as with the hepatitis C virus. Chronic exposure to antiretroviral drugs also raises the possibility of neurotoxicity, although this has not been definitively established.

Diagnostic Markers

Serum HIV testing is required for the diagnosis. In addition, HIV characterization of the cerebrospinal fluid may be helpful if it reveals a disproportionately high viral load in cerebrospinal fluid versus in the plasma. Neuroimaging (i.e., magnetic resonance imaging [MRI]) may reveal reduction in total brain volume, cortical thinning, reduction in white matter volume, and patchy areas of abnormal white matter (hyperintensities). MRI or lumbar puncture may be helpful to exclude a specific medical condition such as cryptococcus infection or herpes encephalitis that may contribute to CNS changes in the context of AIDS. Specialized techniques such as diffusion tensor imaging may reveal damage to specific white matter tracts.

Functional Consequences of Major or Mild Neurocognitive Disorder Due to HIV Infection

Functional consequences of major or mild NCD due to HIV infection are variable across individuals. Thus, impaired executive abilities and slowed information processing may substantially interfere with the complex disease management decisions required for adherence to the combined antiretroviral therapy regimen. The likelihood of comorbid disease may further create functional challenges.

Differential Diagnosis

In the presence of comorbidities, such as other infections (e.g., hepatitis C virus, syphilis), drug abuse (e.g., methamphetamine abuse), or prior head injury or neurodevelopmental conditions, major or mild NCD due to HIV infection can be diagnosed provided there is evidence that infection with HIV has worsened any NCDs due to such preexisting or comorbid conditions. Among older adults, onset of neurocognitive decline related to cerebrovascular disease or neurodegeneration (e.g., major or mild NCD due to Alzheimer's disease) may need to be differentiated. In general, stable, fluctuating (without progression) or improving neurocognitive status would favor an HIV etiology, whereas steady or stepwise deterioration would suggest neurodegenerative or vascular etiology. Because more severe immunodeficiency can result in opportunistic infections of the brain (e.g., toxoplasmosis; cryptococcosis) and neoplasia (e.g., CNS lymphoma), sudden onset of an NCD or sudden worsening of that disorder demands active investigation of non-HIV etiologies.

Comorbidity

HIV disease is accompanied by chronic systemic and neuro-inflammation that can be associated with cerebrovascular disease and metabolic syndrome. These complications can be part of the pathogenesis of major or mild NCD due to HIV infection. HIV frequently co-occurs with conditions such as substance use disorders when the substance has been injected and other sexually transmitted disorders.

Major or Mild Neurocognitive Disorder Due to Prion Disease

Diagnostic Criteria

A. The criteria are met for major or mild neurocognitive disorder.
B. There is insidious onset, and rapid progression of impairment is common.
C. There are motor features of prion disease, such as myoclonus or ataxia, or biomarker evidence.

D. The neurocognitive disorder is not attributable to another medical condition and is not better explained by another mental disorder.

Coding note: For major neurocognitive disorder due to prion disease, with behavioral disturbance, code first **046.79 (A81.9)** prion disease, followed by **294.11 (F02.81)** major neurocognitive disorder due to prion disease, with behavioral disturbance. For major neurocognitive disorder due to prion disease, without behavioral disturbance, code first **046.79 (A81.9)** prion disease, followed by **294.10 (F02.80)** major neurocognitive disorder due to prion disease, without behavioral disturbance.

For mild neurocognitive disorder due to prion disease, code **331.83 (G31.84)**. (**Note:** Do *not* use the additional code for prion disease. Behavioral disturbance cannot be coded but should still be indicated in writing.)

Diagnostic Features

The classification of major or mild neurocognitive disorder (NCD) due to prion disease includes NCDs due to a group of subacute spongiform encephalopathies (including Creutzfeldt-Jakob disease, variant Creutzfeldt-Jakob disease, kuru, Gerstmann-Sträussler-Scheinker syndrome, and fatal insomnia) caused by transmissible agents known as *prions*. The most common type is sporadic Creutzfeldt-Jakob disease, typically referred to as Creutzfeldt-Jakob disease (CJD). Variant CJD is much rarer and is associated with transmission of bovine spongiform encephalopathy, also called "mad cow disease." Typically, individuals with CJD present with neurocognitive deficits, ataxia, and abnormal movements such as myoclonus, chorea, or dystonia; a startle reflex is also common. Typically, the history reveals rapid progression to major NCD over as little as 6 months, and thus the disorder is typically seen only at the major level. However, many individuals with the disorder may have atypical presentations, and the disease can be confirmed only by biopsy or at autopsy. Individuals with variant CJD may present with a greater preponderance of psychiatric symptoms, characterized a by low mood, withdrawal, and anxiety. Prion disease is typically not diagnosed without at least one of the characteristic biomarker features: recognized lesions on magnetic resonance imaging with DWI (diffusion-weighted imaging) or FLAIR (fluid-attenuated inversion recovery), tau or 14-3-3 protein in cerebrospinal fluid, characteristic triphasic waves on electroencephalogram, or, for rare familial forms, family history or genetic testing.

Prevalence

The annual incidence of sporadic CJD is approximately one or two cases per million people. Prevalence is unknown but very low given the short survival.

Development and Course

Prion disease may develop at any age in adults—the peak age for the sporadic CJD is approximately 67 years—although it has been reported to occur in individuals spanning the teenage years to late life. Prodromal symptoms of prion disease may include fatigue, anxiety, problems with appetite or sleeping, or difficulties with concentration. After several weeks, these symptoms may be followed by incoordination, altered vision, or abnormal gait or other movements that may be myoclonic, choreoathetoid, or ballistic, along with a rapidly progressive dementia. The disease typically progresses very rapidly to the major level of impairment over several months. More rarely, it can progress over 2 years and appear similar in its course to other NCDs.

Risk Factors and Prognosis

Environmental.   Cross-species transmission of prion infections, with agents that are closely related to the human form, has been demonstrated (e.g., the outbreak of bovine spongiform encephalopathy inducing variant CJD in the United Kingdom during the mid-1990s). Transmission by corneal transplantation and by human growth factor injection has been documented, and anecdotal cases of transmission to health care workers have been reported.

Genetic and physiological.   There is a genetic component in up to 15% of cases, associated with an autosomal dominant mutation.

Diagnostic Markers

Prion disease can be definitively confirmed only by biopsy or at autopsy. Although there are no distinctive findings on cerebrospinal fluid analysis across the prion diseases, reliable biomarkers are being developed and include 14-3-3 protein (particularly for sporadic CJD) as well as tau protein. Magnetic resonance brain imaging is currently considered the most sensitive diagnostic test when DWI is performed, with the most common finding being multifocal gray matter hyperintensities in subcortical and cortical regions. In some individuals, the electroencephalogram reveals periodic sharp, often triphasic and synchronous discharges at a rate of 0.5–2 Hz at some point during the course of the disorder.

Differential Diagnosis

Other major neurocognitive disorders.   Major NCD due to prion disease may appear similar in its course to other NCDs, but prion diseases are typically distinguished by their rapid progression and prominent cerebellar and motor symptoms.

Major or Mild Neurocognitive Disorder Due to Parkinson's Disease

Diagnostic Criteria

A. The criteria are met for major or mild neurocognitive disorder.
B. The disturbance occurs in the setting of established Parkinson's disease.
C. There is insidious onset and gradual progression of impairment.
D. The neurocognitive disorder is not attributable to another medical condition and is not better explained by another mental disorder.

Major or mild neurocognitive disorder probably due to Parkinson's disease should be diagnosed if 1 and 2 are both met. **Major or mild neurocognitive disorder possibly due to Parkinson's disease** should be diagnosed if 1 or 2 is met:

1. There is no evidence of mixed etiology (i.e., absence of other neurodegenerative or cerebrovascular disease or another neurological, mental, or systemic disease or condition likely contributing to cognitive decline).
2. The Parkinson's disease clearly precedes the onset of the neurocognitive disorder.

Coding note: For major neurocognitive disorder probably due to Parkinson's disease, with behavioral disturbance, code first **332.0 (G20)** Parkinson's disease, followed by **294.11 (F02.81)** major neurocognitive disorder probably due to Parkinson's disease, with behavioral disturbance. For major neurocognitive disorder probably due to Parkinson's disease, without behavioral disturbance, code first **332.0 (G20)** Parkinson's disease, followed by **294.10 (F02.80)** major neurocognitive disorder probably due to Parkinson's disease, without behavioral disturbance.

For major neurocognitive disorder possibly due to Parkinson's disease, code **331.9 (G31.9)** major neurocognitive disorder possibly due to Parkinson's disease. (**Note:** Do *not* use the additional code for Parkinson's disease. Behavioral disturbance cannot be coded but should still be indicated in writing.)

For mild neurocognitive disorder due to Parkinson's disease, code **331.83 (G31.84)**. (**Note:** Do *not* use the additional code for Parkinson's disease. Behavioral disturbance cannot be coded but should still be indicated in writing.)

Diagnostic Features

The essential feature of major or mild neurocognitive disorder (NCD) due to Parkinson's disease is cognitive decline following the onset of Parkinson's disease. The disturbance must occur in the setting of established Parkinson's disease (Criterion B), and deficits must have developed gradually (Criterion C). The NCD is viewed as *probably* due to Parkinson's disease when there is no evidence of another disorder that might be contributing to the cognitive decline *and* when the Parkinson's disease clearly precedes onset of the NCD. The NCD is considered *possibly* due to Parkinson's disease *either* when there is no evidence of another disorder that might be contributing to the cognitive decline *or* when the Parkinson's disease precedes onset of the NCD, but not both.

Associated Features Supporting Diagnosis

Frequently present features include apathy, depressed mood, anxious mood, hallucinations, delusions, personality changes, rapid eye movement sleep behavior disorder, and excessive daytime sleepiness.

Prevalence

The prevalence of Parkinson's disease in the United States steadily increases with age from approximately 0.5% between ages 65 and 69 to 3% at age 85 years and older. Parkinson's disease is more common in males than in females. Among individuals with Parkinson's disease, as many as 75% will develop a major NCD sometime in the course of their disease. The prevalence of mild NCD in Parkinson's disease has been estimated at 27%.

Development and Course

Onset of Parkinson's disease is typically between the sixth and ninth decades of life, with most expression in the early 60s. Mild NCD often develops relatively early in the course of Parkinson's disease, whereas major impairment typically does not occur until late.

Risk and Prognostic Factors

Environmental. Risk factors for Parkinson's disease include exposure to herbicides and pesticides.

Genetic and physiological. Potential risk factors for NCD among individuals with Parkinson's disease include older age at disease onset and increasing duration of disease.

Diagnostic Markers

Neuropsychological testing, with a focus on tests that do not rely on motor function, is critical in detecting the core cognitive deficits, particularly at the mild NCD phase. Structural neuroimaging and dopamine transporter scans, such as DaT scans, may differentiate Lewy body–related dementias (Parkinson's and dementia with Lewy bodies) from non–

Lewy body–related dementias (e.g., Alzheimer's disease) and can sometimes be helpful in the evaluation of major or mild NCD due to Parkinson's disease.

Differential Diagnosis

Major or mild neurocognitive disorder with Lewy bodies.   This distinction is based substantially on the timing and sequence of motor and cognitive symptoms. For NCD to be attributed to Parkinson's disease, the motor and other symptoms of Parkinson's disease must be present well before (by convention, at least 1 year prior) cognitive decline has reached the level of major NCD, whereas in major or mild NCD with Lewy bodies, cognitive symptoms begin shortly before, or concurrent with, motor symptoms. For mild NCD, the timing is harder to establish because the diagnosis itself is less clear and the two disorders exist on a continuum. Unless Parkinson's disease has been established for some time prior to the onset of cognitive decline, or typical features of major or mild NCD with Lewy bodies are present, it is preferable to diagnose unspecified mild NCD.

Major or mild neurocognitive disorder due to Alzheimer's disease.   The motor features are the key to distinguishing major or mild NCD due to Parkinson's disease from major or mild NCD due to Alzheimer's disease. However, the two disorders can co-occur.

Major or mild vascular neurocognitive disorder.   Major or mild vascular NCD may present with parkinsonian features such as psychomotor slowing that may occur as a consequence of subcortical small vessel disease. However, the parkinsonian features typically are not sufficient for a diagnosis of Parkinson's disease, and the course of the NCD usually has a clear association with cerebrovascular changes.

Neurocognitive disorder due to another medical condition (e.g., neurodegenerative disorders).   When a diagnosis of major or mild NCD due to Parkinson's disease is being considered, the distinction must also be made from other brain disorders, such as progressive supranuclear palsy, corticobasal degeneration, multiple system atrophy, tumors, and hydrocephalus.

Neuroleptic-induced parkinsonism.   Neuroleptic-induced parkinsonism can occur in individuals with other NCDs, particularly when dopamine-blocking drugs are prescribed for the behavioral manifestations of such disorders

Other medical conditions.   Delirium and NCDs due to side effects of dopamine-blocking drugs and other medical conditions (e.g., sedation or impaired cognition, severe hypothyroidism, B_{12} deficiency) must also be ruled out.

Comorbidity

Parkinson's disease may coexist with Alzheimer's disease and cerebrovascular disease, especially in older individuals. The compounding of multiple pathological features may diminish the functional abilities of individuals with Parkinson's disease. Motor symptoms and frequent co-occurrence of depression or apathy can make functional impairment worse.

Major or Mild Neurocognitive Disorder Due to Huntington's Disease

Diagnostic Criteria

A. The criteria are met for major or mild neurocognitive disorder.
B. There is insidious onset and gradual progression.
C. There is clinically established Huntington's disease, or risk for Huntington's disease based on family history or genetic testing.

D. The neurocognitive disorder is not attributable to another medical condition and is not better explained by another mental disorder.

Coding note: For major neurocognitive disorder due to Huntington's disease, with behavioral disturbance, code first **333.4 (G10)** Huntington's disease, followed by **294.11 (F02.81)** major neurocognitive disorder due to Huntington's disease, with behavioral disturbance. For major neurocognitive disorder due to Huntington's disease, without behavioral disturbance, code first **333.4 (G10)** Huntington's disease, followed by **294.10 (F02.80)** major neurocognitive disorder due to Huntington's disease, without behavioral disturbance.

For mild neurocognitive disorder due to Huntington's disease, code **331.83 (G31.84)**. (**Note:** Do *not* use the additional code for Huntington's disease. Behavioral disturbance cannot be coded but should still be indicated in writing.)

Diagnostic Features

Progressive cognitive impairment is a core feature of Huntington's disease, with early changes in executive function (i.e., processing speed, organization, and planning) rather than learning and memory. Cognitive and associated behavioral changes often precede the emergence of the typical motor abnormalities of bradykinesia (i.e., slowing of voluntary movement) and chorea (i.e., involuntary jerking movements). A diagnosis of definite Huntington's disease is given in the presence of unequivocal, extrapyramidal motor abnormalities in an individual with either a family history of Huntington's disease or genetic testing showing a CAG trinucleotide repeat expansion in the HTT gene, located on chromosome 4.

Associated Features Supporting Diagnosis

Depression, irritability, anxiety, obsessive-compulsive symptoms, and apathy are frequently, and psychosis more rarely, associated with Huntington's disease and often precede the onset of motor symptoms.

Prevalence

Neurocognitive deficits are an eventual outcome of Huntington's disease; the worldwide prevalence is estimated to be 2.7 per 100,000. The prevalence of Huntington's disease in North America, Europe, and Australia is 5.7 per 100,000, with a much lower prevalence of 0.40 per 100,000 in Asia.

Development and Course

The average age at diagnosis of Huntington's disease is approximately 40 years, although this varies widely. Age at onset is inversely correlated with CAG expansion length. Juvenile Huntington's disease (onset before age 20) may present more commonly with bradykinesia, dystonia, and rigidity than with the choreic movements characteristic of the adult-onset disorder. The disease is gradually progressive, with median survival approximately 15 years after motor symptom diagnosis.

Phenotypic expression of Huntington's disease varies by presence of motor, cognitive, and psychiatric symptoms. Psychiatric and cognitive abnormalities can predate the motor abnormality by at least 15 years. Initial symptoms requiring care often include irritability, anxiety, or depressed mood. Other behavioral disturbances may include pronounced apathy, disinhibition, impulsivity, and impaired insight, with apathy often becoming more progressive over time. Early movement symptoms may involve the appearance of fidgetiness of the extremities as well as mild *apraxia* (i.e., difficulty with purposeful movements), particularly with fine motor tasks. As the disorder progresses, other motor problems include impaired gait (*ataxia*) and postural instability. Motor impairment eventually affects speech production (*dysarthria*) such that the speech becomes very difficult to understand, which may result in significant distress resulting from the communication barrier in the context of comparatively intact cognition. Advanced motor disease severely affects gait with progressive ataxia. Eventually individuals become nonambulatory. End-stage motor disease impairs motor control of eating and swallowing, typically a major contributor to the death of the individual from aspiration pneumonia.

Risk and Prognostic Factors

Genetic and physiological.   The genetic basis of Huntington's disease is a fully penetrant autosomal dominant expansion of the CAG trinucleotide, often called a *CAG repeat* in the huntingtin gene. A repeat length of 36 or more is invariably associated with Huntington's disease, with longer repeat lengths associated with early age at onset. A CAG repeat length of 36 or more is invariably associated with Huntington's disease.

Diagnostic Markers

Genetic testing is the primary laboratory test for the determination of Huntington's disease, which is an autosomal dominant disorder with complete penetrance. The trinucleotide CAG is observed to have a repeat expansion in the gene that encodes huntingtin protein on chromosome 4. A diagnosis of Huntington's disease is not made in the presence of the gene expansion alone, but the diagnosis is made only after symptoms become manifest. Some individuals with a positive family history request genetic testing in a presymptomatic stage. Associated features may also include neuroimaging changes; volume loss in the basal ganglia, particularly the caudate nucleus and putamen, is well known to occur and progresses over the course of illness. Other structural and functional changes have been observed in brain imaging but remain research measures.

Functional Consequences of Major or Mild Neurocognitive Disorder Due to Huntington's Disease

In the prodromal phase of illness and at early diagnosis, occupational decline is most common, with most individuals reporting some loss of ability to engage in their typical work. The emotional, behavioral, and cognitive aspects of Huntington's disease, such as disinhibition and personality changes, are highly associated with functional decline. Cognitive deficits that contribute most to functional decline may include speed of processing, initiation, and attention rather than memory impairment. Given that Huntington's disease onset occurs in productive years of life, it may have a very disruptive effect on performance in the work setting as well as social and family life. As the disease progresses, disability from problems such as impaired gait, dysarthria, and impulsive or irritable behaviors may substantially add to the level of impairment and daily care needs, over and above the care needs attributable to the cognitive decline. Severe choreic movements may substantially interfere with provision of care such as bathing, dressing, and toileting.

Differential Diagnosis

Other mental disorders.   Early symptoms of Huntington's disease may include instability of mood, irritability, or compulsive behaviors that may suggest another mental disorder. However, genetic testing or the development of motor symptoms will distinguish the presence of Huntington's disease.

Other neurocognitive disorders.   The early symptoms of Huntington's disease, particularly symptoms of executive dysfunction and impaired psychomotor speed, may resemble other neurocognitive disorders (NCDs), such as major or mild vascular NCD.

Other movement disorders. Huntington's disease must also be differentiated from other disorders or conditions associated with chorea, such as Wilson's disease, drug-induced tardive dyskinesia, Sydenham's chorea, systemic lupus erythematosus, or senile chorea. Rarely, individuals may present with a course similar to that of Huntington's disease but without positive genetic testing; this is considered to be a Huntington's disease pheno-copy that results from a variety of potential genetic factors.

Major or Mild Neurocognitive Disorder Due to Another Medical Condition

Diagnostic Criteria

A. The criteria are met for major or mild neurocognitive disorder.

B. There is evidence from the history, physical examination, or laboratory findings that the neurocognitive disorder is the pathophysiological consequence of another medical condition.

C. The cognitive deficits are not better explained by another mental disorder or another specific neurocognitive disorder (e.g., Alzheimer's disease, HIV infection).

Coding note: For major neurocognitive disorder due to another medical condition, with behavioral disturbance, code first the other medical condition, followed by the major neurocognitive disorder due to another medical condition, with behavioral disturbance (e.g., 340 [G35] multiple sclerosis, **294.11 [F02.81]** major neurocognitive disorder due to multiple sclerosis, with behavioral disturbance). For major neurocognitive disorder due to another medical condition, without behavioral disturbance, code first the other medical condition, followed by the major neurocognitive disorder due to another medical condition, without behavioral disturbance (e.g., 340 [G35] multiple sclerosis, **294.10 [F02.80]** major neurocognitive disorder due to multiple sclerosis, without behavioral disturbance).

For mild neurocognitive disorder due to another medical condition, code **331.83 (G31.84).** (**Note:** Do *not* use the additional code for the other medical condition. Behavioral disturbance cannot be coded but should still be indicated in writing.)

Diagnostic Features

A number of other medical conditions can cause neurocognitive disorders (NCDs). These conditions include structural lesions (e.g., primary or secondary brain tumors, subdural hematoma, slowly progressive or normal-pressure hydrocephalus), hypoxia related to hypoperfusion from heart failure, endocrine conditions (e.g., hypothyroidism, hypercalcemia, hypoglycemia), nutritional conditions (e.g., deficiencies of thiamine or niacin), other infectious conditions (e.g., neurosyphilis, cryptococcosis), immune disorders (e.g., temporal arteritis, systemic lupus erythematosus), hepatic or renal failure, metabolic conditions (e.g., Kufs' disease, adrenoleukodystrophy, metachromatic leukodystrophy, other storage diseases of adulthood and childhood), and other neurological conditions (e.g., epilepsy, multiple sclerosis). Unusual causes of central nervous system injury, such as electrical shock or intracranial radiation, are generally evident from the history. The temporal association between the onset or exacerbation of the medical condition and the development of the cognitive deficit offers the greatest support that the NCD is induced by the medical condition. Diagnostic certainty regarding this relationship may be increased if the neurocognitive deficits ameliorate partially or stabilize in the context of treatment of the medical condition.

Development and Course

Typically the course of the NCD progresses in a manner that is commensurate with progression of the underlying medical disorder. In circumstances where the medical disorder is treatable (e.g., hypothyroidism), the neurocognitive deficit may improve or at least not progress. When the medical condition has a deteriorative course (e.g., secondary progressive multiple sclerosis), the neurocognitive deficits will progress along with the temporal course of illness.

Diagnostic Markers

Associated physical examination and laboratory findings and other clinical features depend on the nature and severity of the medical condition.

Differential Diagnosis

Other major or mild neurocognitive disorder.   The presence of an attributable medical condition does not entirely exclude the possibility of another major or mild NCD. If cognitive deficits persist following successful treatment of an associated medical condition, then another etiology may be responsible for the cognitive decline.

Major or Mild Neurocognitive Disorder Due to Multiple Etiologies

Diagnostic Criteria

A. The criteria are met for major or mild neurocognitive disorder.
B. There is evidence from the history, physical examination, or laboratory findings that the neurocognitive disorder is the pathophysiological consequence of more than one etiological process, excluding substances (e.g., neurocognitive disorder due to Alzheimer's disease with subsequent development of vascular neurocognitive disorder).
   Note: Please refer to the diagnostic criteria for the various neurocognitive disorders due to specific medical conditions for guidance on establishing the particular etiologies.
C. The cognitive deficits are not better explained by another mental disorder and do not occur exclusively during the course of a delirium.

Coding note: For major neurocognitive disorder due to multiple etiologies, with behavioral disturbance, code **294.11 (F02.81)**; for major neurocognitive disorder due to multiple etiologies, without behavioral disturbance, code **294.10 (F02.80)**. All of the etiological medical conditions (with the exception of vascular disease) should be coded and listed separately immediately before major neurocognitive disorder due to multiple etiologies (e.g., **331.0 [G30.9]** Alzheimer's disease; **331.82 [G31.83]** Lewy body disease; **294.11 [F02.81]** major neurocognitive disorder due to multiple etiologies, with behavioral disturbance).

When a cerebrovascular etiology is contributing to the neurocognitive disorder, the diagnosis of vascular neurocognitive disorder should be listed in addition to major neurocognitive disorder due to multiple etiologies. For example, for a presentation of major neurocognitive disorder due to both Alzheimer's disease and vascular disease, with behavioral disturbance, code the following: **331.0 (G30.9)** Alzheimer's disease; **294.11 (F02.81)** major neurocognitive disorder due to multiple etiologies, with behavioral disturbance; **290.40 (F01.51)** major vascular neurocognitive disorder, with behavioral disturbance.

For mild neurocognitive disorder due to multiple etiologies, code **331.83 (G31.84)**. (**Note:** Do *not* use the additional codes for the etiologies. Behavioral disturbance cannot be coded but should still be indicated in writing.)

This category is included to cover the clinical presentation of a neurocognitive disorder (NCD) for which there is evidence that multiple medical conditions have played a probable role in the development of the NCD. In addition to evidence indicative of the presence of multiple medical conditions that are known to cause NCD (i.e., findings from the history and physical examination, and laboratory findings), it may be helpful to refer to the diagnostic criteria and text for the various medical etiologies (e.g., NCD due to Parkinson's disease) for more information on establishing the etiological connection for that particular medical condition.

Unspecified Neurocognitive Disorder

799.59 (R41.9)

This category applies to presentations in which symptoms characteristic of a neurocognitive disorder that cause clinically significant distress or impairment in social, occupational, or other important areas of functioning predominate but do not meet the full criteria for any of the disorders in the neurocognitive disorders diagnostic class. The unspecified neurocognitive disorder category is used in situations in which the precise etiology cannot be determined with sufficient certainty to make an etiological attribution.

Coding note: For unspecified major or mild neurocognitive disorder, code 799.59 (R41.9). (**Note:** Do *not* use additional codes for any presumed etiological medical conditions. Behavioral disturbance cannot be coded but may be indicated in writing.)

Personality Disorders

This chapter begins with a general definition of personality disorder that applies to each of the 10 specific personality disorders. A *personality disorder* is an enduring pattern of inner experience and behavior that deviates markedly from the expectations of the individual's culture, is pervasive and inflexible, has an onset in adolescence or early adulthood, is stable over time, and leads to distress or impairment.

With any ongoing review process, especially one of this complexity, different viewpoints emerge, and an effort was made to accommodate them. Thus, personality disorders are included in both Sections II and III. The material in Section II represents an update of text associated with the same criteria found in DSM-IV-TR, whereas Section III includes the proposed research model for personality disorder diagnosis and conceptualization developed by the DSM-5 Personality and Personality Disorders Work Group. As this field evolves, it is hoped that both versions will serve clinical practice and research initiatives, respectively.

The following personality disorders are included in this chapter.

- **Paranoid personality disorder** is a pattern of distrust and suspiciousness such that others' motives are interpreted as malevolent.
- **Schizoid personality disorder** is a pattern of detachment from social relationships and a restricted range of emotional expression.
- **Schizotypal personality disorder** is a pattern of acute discomfort in close relationships, cognitive or perceptual distortions, and eccentricities of behavior.
- **Antisocial personality disorder** is a pattern of disregard for, and violation of, the rights of others.
- **Borderline personality disorder** is a pattern of instability in interpersonal relationships, self-image, and affects, and marked impulsivity.
- **Histrionic personality disorder** is a pattern of excessive emotionality and attention seeking.
- **Narcissistic personality disorder** is a pattern of grandiosity, need for admiration, and lack of empathy.
- **Avoidant personality disorder** is a pattern of social inhibition, feelings of inadequacy, and hypersensitivity to negative evaluation.
- **Dependent personality disorder** is a pattern of submissive and clinging behavior related to an excessive need to be taken care of.
- **Obsessive-compulsive personality disorder** is a pattern of preoccupation with orderliness, perfectionism, and control.
- **Personality change due to another medical condition** is a persistent personality disturbance that is judged to be due to the direct physiological effects of a medical condition (e.g., frontal lobe lesion).
- **Other specified personality disorder and unspecified personality disorder** is a category provided for two situations: 1) the individual's personality pattern meets the general criteria for a personality disorder, and traits of several different personality disorders are present, but the criteria for any specific personality disorder are not met;

or 2) the individual's personality pattern meets the general criteria for a personality disorder, but the individual is considered to have a personality disorder that is not included in the DSM-5 classification (e.g., passive-aggressive personality disorder).

The personality disorders are grouped into three clusters based on descriptive similarities. Cluster A includes paranoid, schizoid, and schizotypal personality disorders. Individuals with these disorders often appear odd or eccentric. Cluster B includes antisocial, borderline, histrionic, and narcissistic personality disorders. Individuals with these disorders often appear dramatic, emotional, or erratic. Cluster C includes avoidant, dependent, and obsessive-compulsive personality disorders. Individuals with these disorders often appear anxious or fearful. It should be noted that this clustering system, although useful in some research and educational situations, has serious limitations and has not been consistently validated.

Moreover, individuals frequently present with co-occurring personality disorders from different clusters. Prevalence estimates for the different clusters suggest 5.7% for disorders in Cluster A, 1.5% for disorders in Cluster B, 6.0% for disorders in Cluster C, and 9.1% for any personality disorder, indicating frequent co-occurrence of disorders from different clusters. Data from the 2001–2002 National Epidemiologic Survey on Alcohol and Related Conditions suggest that approximately 15% of U.S. adults have at least one personality disorder.

Dimensional Models for Personality Disorders

The diagnostic approach used in this manual represents the categorical perspective that personality disorders are qualitatively distinct clinical syndromes. An alternative to the categorical approach is the dimensional perspective that personality disorders represent maladaptive variants of personality traits that merge imperceptibly into normality and into one another. See Section III for a full description of a dimensional model for personality disorders. The DSM-IV personality disorder clusters (i.e., odd-eccentric, dramatic-emotional, and anxious-fearful) may also be viewed as dimensions representing spectra of personality dysfunction on a continuum with other mental disorders. The alternative dimensional models have much in common and together appear to cover the important areas of personality dysfunction. Their integration, clinical utility, and relationship with the personality disorder diagnostic categories and various aspects of personality dysfunction are under active investigation.

General Personality Disorder

Criteria

A. An enduring pattern of inner experience and behavior that deviates markedly from the expectations of the individual's culture. This pattern is manifested in two (or more) of the following areas:

    1. Cognition (i.e., ways of perceiving and interpreting self, other people, and events).
    2. Affectivity (i.e., the range, intensity, lability, and appropriateness of emotional response).
    3. Interpersonal functioning.
    4. Impulse control.

B. The enduring pattern is inflexible and pervasive across a broad range of personal and social situations.

C. The enduring pattern leads to clinically significant distress or impairment in social, occupational, or other important areas of functioning.

D. The pattern is stable and of long duration, and its onset can be traced back at least to adolescence or early adulthood.
E. The enduring pattern is not better explained as a manifestation or consequence of another mental disorder.
F. The enduring pattern is not attributable to the physiological effects of a substance (e.g., a drug of abuse, a medication) or another medical condition (e.g., head trauma).

Diagnostic Features

Personality traits are enduring patterns of perceiving, relating to, and thinking about the environment and oneself that are exhibited in a wide range of social and personal contexts. Only when personality traits are inflexible and maladaptive and cause significant functional impairment or subjective distress do they constitute personality disorders. The essential feature of a personality disorder is an enduring pattern of inner experience and behavior that deviates markedly from the expectations of the individual's culture and is manifested in at least two of the following areas: cognition, affectivity, interpersonal functioning, or impulse control (Criterion A). This enduring pattern is inflexible and pervasive across a broad range of personal and social situations (Criterion B) and leads to clinically significant distress or impairment in social, occupational, or other important areas of functioning (Criterion C). The pattern is stable and of long duration, and its onset can be traced back at least to adolescence or early adulthood (Criterion D). The pattern is not better explained as a manifestation or consequence of another mental disorder (Criterion E) and is not attributable to the physiological effects of a substance (e.g., a drug of abuse, a medication, exposure to a toxin) or another medical condition (e.g., head trauma) (Criterion F). Specific diagnostic criteria are also provided for each of the personality disorders included in this chapter.

The diagnosis of personality disorders requires an evaluation of the individual's long-term patterns of functioning, and the particular personality features must be evident by early adulthood. The personality traits that define these disorders must also be distinguished from characteristics that emerge in response to specific situational stressors or more transient mental states (e.g., bipolar, depressive, or anxiety disorders; substance intoxication). The clinician should assess the stability of personality traits over time and across different situations. Although a single interview with the individual is sometimes sufficient for making the diagnosis, it is often necessary to conduct more than one interview and to space these over time. Assessment can also be complicated by the fact that the characteristics that define a personality disorder may not be considered problematic by the individual (i.e., the traits are often ego-syntonic). To help overcome this difficulty, supplementary information from other informants may be helpful.

Development and Course

The features of a personality disorder usually become recognizable during adolescence or early adult life. By definition, a personality disorder is an enduring pattern of thinking, feeling, and behaving that is relatively stable over time. Some types of personality disorder (notably, antisocial and borderline personality disorders) tend to become less evident or to remit with age, whereas this appears to be less true for some other types (e.g., obsessive-compulsive and schizotypal personality disorders).

Personality disorder categories may be applied with children or adolescents in those relatively unusual instances in which the individual's particular maladaptive personality traits appear to be pervasive, persistent, and unlikely to be limited to a particular developmental stage or another mental disorder. It should be recognized that the traits of a personality disorder that appear in childhood will often not persist unchanged into adult life. For a personality disorder to be diagnosed in an individual younger than 18 years, the features must have been present for at least 1 year. The one exception to this is antisocial personality disorder, which cannot be diagnosed in individuals younger than 18 years. Although, by definition, a personality disorder requires an onset no later than early adulthood, individuals may not come to clinical attention until relatively late in life. A personality disorder may be exacerbated following the loss of significant supporting persons (e.g., a spouse) or previously stabilizing social situations (e.g., a job). However, the development of a change in personality in middle adulthood or later life warrants a thorough evaluation to determine the possible presence of a personality change due to another medical condition or an unrecognized substance use disorder.

Culture-Related Diagnostic Issues

Judgments about personality functioning must take into account the individual's ethnic, cultural, and social background. Personality disorders should not be confused with problems associated with acculturation following immigration or with the expression of habits, customs, or religious and political values professed by the individual's culture of origin. It is useful for the clinician, especially when evaluating someone from a different background, to obtain additional information from informants who are familiar with the person's cultural background.

Gender-Related Diagnostic Issues

Certain personality disorders (e.g., antisocial personality disorder) are diagnosed more frequently in males. Others (e.g., borderline, histrionic, and dependent personality disorders) are diagnosed more frequently in females. Although these differences in prevalence probably reflect real gender differences in the presence of such patterns, clinicians must be cautious not to overdiagnose or underdiagnose certain personality disorders in females or in males because of social stereotypes about typical gender roles and behaviors.

Differential Diagnosis

Other mental disorders and personality traits.   Many of the specific criteria for the personality disorders describe features (e.g., suspiciousness, dependency, insensitivity) that are also characteristic of episodes of other mental disorders. A personality disorder should be diagnosed only when the defining characteristics appeared before early adulthood, are typical of the individual's long-term functioning, and do not occur exclusively during an episode of another mental disorder. It may be particularly difficult (and not particularly useful) to distinguish personality disorders from persistent mental disorders such as persistent depressive disorder that have an early onset and an enduring, relatively stable course. Some personality disorders may have a "spectrum" relationship to other mental disorders (e.g., schizotypal personality disorder with schizophrenia; avoidant personality disorder with social anxiety disorder [social phobia]) based on phenomenological or biological similarities or familial aggregation.

Personality disorders must be distinguished from personality traits that do not reach the threshold for a personality disorder. Personality traits are diagnosed as a personality disorder only when they are inflexible, maladaptive, and persisting and cause significant functional impairment or subjective distress.

Psychotic disorders.   For the three personality disorders that may be related to the psychotic disorders (i.e., paranoid, schizoid, and schizotypal), there is an exclusion criterion stating that the pattern of behavior must not have occurred exclusively during the course of schizophrenia, a bipolar or depressive disorder with psychotic features, or another psychotic disorder. When an individual has a persistent mental disorder (e.g., schizophrenia) that was preceded by a preexisting personality disorder, the personality disorder should also be recorded, followed by "premorbid" in parentheses.

Anxiety and depressive disorders.   The clinician must be cautious in diagnosing personality disorders during an episode of a depressive disorder or an anxiety disorder, because these conditions may have cross-sectional symptom features that mimic personality traits and may make it more difficult to evaluate retrospectively the individual's long-term patterns of functioning.

Posttraumatic stress disorder. When personality changes emerge and persist after an individual has been exposed to extreme stress, a diagnosis of posttraumatic stress disorder should be considered.

Substance use disorders. When an individual has a substance use disorder, it is important not to make a personality disorder diagnosis based solely on behaviors that are consequences of substance intoxication or withdrawal or that are associated with activities in the service of sustaining substance use (e.g., antisocial behavior).

Personality change due to another medical condition. When enduring changes in personality arise as a result of the physiological effects of another medical condition (e.g., brain tumor), a diagnosis of personality change due to another medical condition should be considered.

Cluster A Personality Disorders

Paranoid Personality Disorder

Diagnostic Criteria   301.0 (F60.0)

A. A pervasive distrust and suspiciousness of others such that their motives are interpreted as malevolent, beginning by early adulthood and present in a variety of contexts, as indicated by four (or more) of the following:

1. Suspects, without sufficient basis, that others are exploiting, harming, or deceiving him or her.
2. Is preoccupied with unjustified doubts about the loyalty or trustworthiness of friends or associates.
3. Is reluctant to confide in others because of unwarranted fear that the information will be used maliciously against him or her.
4. Reads hidden demeaning or threatening meanings into benign remarks or events.
5. Persistently bears grudges (i.e., is unforgiving of insults, injuries, or slights).
6. Perceives attacks on his or her character or reputation that are not apparent to others and is quick to react angrily or to counterattack.
7. Has recurrent suspicions, without justification, regarding fidelity of spouse or sexual partner.

B. Does not occur exclusively during the course of schizophrenia, a bipolar disorder or depressive disorder with psychotic features, or another psychotic disorder and is not attributable to the physiological effects of another medical condition.

Note: If criteria are met prior to the onset of schizophrenia, add "premorbid," i.e., "paranoid personality disorder (premorbid)."

Diagnostic Features

The essential feature of paranoid personality disorder is a pattern of pervasive distrust and suspiciousness of others such that their motives are interpreted as malevolent. This pattern begins by early adulthood and is present in a variety of contexts.

Individuals with this disorder assume that other people will exploit, harm, or deceive them, even if no evidence exists to support this expectation (Criterion A1). They suspect on the basis of little or no evidence that others are plotting against them and may attack them suddenly, at any time and without reason. They often feel that they have been deeply and irreversibly injured by another person or persons even when there is no objective evidence for this. They are preoccupied with unjustified doubts about the loyalty or trustworthiness of their friends and associates, whose actions are minutely scrutinized for evidence of hostile intentions (Criterion A2). Any perceived deviation from trustworthiness or loyalty serves to support their underlying assumptions. They are so amazed when a friend or associate shows loyalty that they cannot trust or believe it. If they get into trouble, they expect that friends and associates will either attack or ignore them.

Individuals with paranoid personality disorder are reluctant to confide in or become close to others because they fear that the information they share will be used against them (Criterion A3). They may refuse to answer personal questions, saying that the information is "nobody's business." They read hidden meanings that are demeaning and threatening into benign remarks or events (Criterion A4). For example, an individual with this disorder may misinterpret an honest mistake by a store clerk as a deliberate attempt to short-change, or view a casual humorous remark by a co-worker as a serious character attack. Compliments are often misinterpreted (e.g., a compliment on a new acquisition is misinterpreted as a criticism for selfishness; a compliment on an accomplishment is misinterpreted as an attempt to coerce more and better performance). They may view an offer of help as a criticism that they are not doing well enough on their own.

Individuals with this disorder persistently bear grudges and are unwilling to forgive the insults, injuries, or slights that they think they have received (Criterion A5). Minor slights arouse major hostility, and the hostile feelings persist for a long time. Because they are constantly vigilant to the harmful intentions of others, they very often feel that their character or reputation has been attacked or that they have been slighted in some other way. They are quick to counterattack and react with anger to perceived insults (Criterion A6). Individuals with this disorder may be pathologically jealous, often suspecting that their spouse or sexual partner is unfaithful without any adequate justification (Criterion A7). They may gather trivial and circumstantial "evidence" to support their jealous beliefs. They want to maintain complete control of intimate relationships to avoid being betrayed and may constantly question and challenge the whereabouts, actions, intentions, and fidelity of their spouse or partner.

Paranoid personality disorder should not be diagnosed if the pattern of behavior occurs exclusively during the course of schizophrenia, a bipolar disorder or depressive disorder with psychotic features, or another psychotic disorder, or if it is attributable to the physiological effects of a neurological (e.g., temporal lobe epilepsy) or another medical condition (Criterion B).

Associated Features Supporting Diagnosis

Individuals with paranoid personality disorder are generally difficult to get along with and often have problems with close relationships. Their excessive suspiciousness and hostility may be expressed in overt argumentativeness, in recurrent complaining, or by quiet, apparently hostile aloofness. Because they are hypervigilant for potential threats, they may act in a guarded, secretive, or devious manner and appear to be "cold" and lacking in tender feelings. Although they may appear to be objective, rational, and unemotional, they more often display a labile range of affect, with hostile, stubborn, and sarcastic expressions predominating. Their combative and suspicious nature may elicit a hostile response in others, which then serves to confirm their original expectations.

Because individuals with paranoid personality disorder lack trust in others, they have an excessive need to be self-sufficient and a strong sense of autonomy. They also need to have a high degree of control over those around them. They are often rigid, critical of others, and unable to collaborate, although they have great difficulty accepting criticism themselves. They may blame others for their own shortcomings. Because of their quickness to counterattack in response to the threats they perceive around them, they may be litigious and frequently become involved in legal disputes. Individuals with this disorder seek to confirm their preconceived negative notions regarding people or situations they encounter, attributing malevolent motivations to others that are projections of their own fears. They may exhibit thinly hidden, unrealistic grandiose fantasies, are often attuned to issues of power and rank, and tend to develop negative stereotypes of others, particularly those from population groups distinct from their own. Attracted by simplistic formulations of the world, they are often wary of ambiguous situations. They may be perceived as "fanatics" and form tightly knit "cults" or groups with others who share their paranoid belief systems.

Particularly in response to stress, individuals with this disorder may experience very brief psychotic episodes (lasting minutes to hours). In some instances, paranoid personality disorder may appear as the premorbid antecedent of delusional disorder or schizophrenia. Individuals with paranoid personality disorder may develop major depressive disorder and may be at increased risk for agoraphobia and obsessive-compulsive disorder. Alcohol and other substance use disorders frequently occur. The most common co-occurring personality disorders appear to be schizotypal, schizoid, narcissistic, avoidant, and borderline.

Prevalence

A prevalence estimate for paranoid personality based on a probability subsample from Part II of the National Comorbidity Survey Replication suggests a prevalence of 2.3%, while the National Epidemiologic Survey on Alcohol and Related Conditions data suggest a prevalence of paranoid personality disorder of 4.4%.

Development and Course

Paranoid personality disorder may be first apparent in childhood and adolescence with solitariness, poor peer relationships, social anxiety, underachievement in school, hypersensitivity, peculiar thoughts and language, and idiosyncratic fantasies. These children may appear to be "odd" or "eccentric" and attract teasing. In clinical samples, this disorder appears to be more commonly diagnosed in males.

Risk and Prognostic Factors

Genetic and physiological.   There is some evidence for an increased prevalence of paranoid personality disorder in relatives of probands with schizophrenia and for a more specific familial relationship with delusional disorder, persecutory type.

Culture-Related Diagnostic Issues

Some behaviors that are influenced by sociocultural contexts or specific life circumstances may be erroneously labeled paranoid and may even be reinforced by the process of clinical evaluation. Members of minority groups, immigrants, political and economic refugees, or individuals of different ethnic backgrounds may display guarded or defensive behaviors because of unfamiliarity (e.g., language barriers or lack of knowledge of rules and regulations) or in response to the perceived neglect or indifference of the majority society. These behaviors can, in turn, generate anger and frustration in those who deal with these individuals, thus setting up a vicious cycle of mutual mistrust, which should not be confused with paranoid personality disorder. Some ethnic groups also display culturally related behaviors that can be misinterpreted as paranoid.

Differential Diagnosis

Other mental disorders with psychotic symptoms.   Paranoid personality disorder can be distinguished from delusional disorder, persecutory type; schizophrenia; and a bipolar or depressive disorder with psychotic features because these disorders are all characterized by a period of persistent psychotic symptoms (e.g., delusions and hallucinations). For an additional diagnosis of paranoid personality disorder to be given, the personality disorder must have been present before the onset of psychotic symptoms and must persist when the psychotic symptoms are in remission. When an individual has another persistent mental disorder (e.g., schizophrenia) that was preceded by paranoid personality disorder, paranoid personality disorder should also be recorded, followed by "premorbid" in parentheses.

Personality change due to another medical condition.   Paranoid personality disorder must be distinguished from personality change due to another medical condition, in which the traits that emerge are attributable to the direct effects of another medical condition on the central nervous system.

Substance use disorders.   Paranoid personality disorder must be distinguished from symptoms that may develop in association with persistent substance use.

Paranoid traits associated with physical handicaps.   The disorder must also be distinguished from paranoid traits associated with the development of physical handicaps (e.g., a hearing impairment).

Other personality disorders and personality traits.   Other personality disorders may be confused with paranoid personality disorder because they have certain features in common. It is therefore important to distinguish among these disorders based on differences in their characteristic features. However, if an individual has personality features that meet criteria for one or more personality disorders in addition to paranoid personality disorder, all can be diagnosed. Paranoid personality disorder and schizotypal personality disorder share the traits of suspiciousness, interpersonal aloofness, and paranoid ideation, but schizotypal personality disorder also includes symptoms such as magical thinking, unusual perceptual experiences, and odd thinking and speech. Individuals with behaviors that meet criteria for schizoid personality disorder are often perceived as strange, eccentric, cold, and aloof, but they do not usually have prominent paranoid ideation. The tendency of individuals with paranoid personality disorder to react to minor stimuli with anger is also seen in borderline and histrionic personality disorders. However, these disorders are not necessarily associated with pervasive suspiciousness. People with avoidant personality disorder may also be reluctant to confide in others, but more from fear of being embarrassed or found inadequate than from fear of others' malicious intent. Although antisocial behavior may be present in some individuals with paranoid personality disorder, it is not usually motivated by a desire for personal gain or to exploit others as in antisocial personality disorder, but rather is more often attributable to a desire for revenge. Individuals with narcissistic personality disorder may occasionally display suspiciousness, social withdrawal, or alienation, but this derives primarily from fears of having their imperfections or flaws revealed.

Paranoid traits may be adaptive, particularly in threatening environments. Paranoid personality disorder should be diagnosed only when these traits are inflexible, maladaptive, and persisting and cause significant functional impairment or subjective distress.

Schizoid Personality Disorder

Diagnostic Criteria   **301.20 (F60.1)**

A. A pervasive pattern of detachment from social relationships and a restricted range of expression of emotions in interpersonal settings, beginning by early adulthood and present in a variety of contexts, as indicated by four (or more) of the following:

1. Neither desires nor enjoys close relationships, including being part of a family.
2. Almost always chooses solitary activities.
3. Has little, if any, interest in having sexual experiences with another person.
4. Takes pleasure in few, if any, activities.
5. Lacks close friends or confidants other than first-degree relatives.
6. Appears indifferent to the praise or criticism of others.
7. Shows emotional coldness, detachment, or flattened affectivity.

B. Does not occur exclusively during the course of schizophrenia, a bipolar disorder or depressive disorder with psychotic features, another psychotic disorder, or autism spectrum disorder and is not attributable to the physiological effects of another medical condition.

Note: If criteria are met prior to the onset of schizophrenia, add "premorbid," i.e., "schizoid personality disorder (premorbid)."

Diagnostic Features

The essential feature of schizoid personality disorder is a pervasive pattern of detachment from social relationships and a restricted range of expression of emotions in interpersonal settings. This pattern begins by early adulthood and is present in a variety of contexts.

Individuals with schizoid personality disorder appear to lack a desire for intimacy, seem indifferent to opportunities to develop close relationships, and do not seem to derive much satisfaction from being part of a family or other social group (Criterion A1). They prefer spending time by themselves, rather than being with other people. They often appear to be socially isolated or "loners" and almost always choose solitary activities or hobbies that do not include interaction with others (Criterion A2). They prefer mechanical or abstract tasks, such as computer or mathematical games. They may have very little interest in having sexual experiences with another person (Criterion A3) and take pleasure in few, if any, activities (Criterion A4). There is usually a reduced experience of pleasure from sensory, bodily, or interpersonal experiences, such as walking on a beach at sunset or having sex. These individuals have no close friends or confidants, except possibly a first-degree relative (Criterion A5).

Individuals with schizoid personality disorder often seem indifferent to the approval or criticism of others and do not appear to be bothered by what others may think of them (Criterion A6). They may be oblivious to the normal subtleties of social interaction and often do not respond appropriately to social cues so that they seem socially inept or superficial and self-absorbed. They usually display a "bland" exterior without visible emotional reactivity and rarely reciprocate gestures or facial expressions, such as smiles or nods (Criterion A7). They claim that they rarely experience strong emotions such as anger and joy. They often display a constricted affect and appear cold and aloof. However, in those very unusual circumstances in which these individuals become at least temporarily comfortable in revealing themselves, they may acknowledge having painful feelings, particularly related to social interactions.

Schizoid personality disorder should not be diagnosed if the pattern of behavior occurs exclusively during the course of schizophrenia, a bipolar or depressive disorder with psychotic features, another psychotic disorder, or autism spectrum disorder, or if it is attributable to the physiological effects of a neurological (e.g., temporal lobe epilepsy) or another medical condition (Criterion B).

Associated Features Supporting Diagnosis

Individuals with schizoid personality disorder may have particular difficulty expressing anger, even in response to direct provocation, which contributes to the impression that they lack emotion. Their lives sometimes seem directionless, and they may appear to "drift" in their goals. Such individuals often react passively to adverse circumstances and have difficulty responding appropriately to important life events. Because of their lack of social skills and lack of desire for sexual experiences, individuals with this disorder have few friendships, date infrequently, and often do not marry. Occupational functioning may be impaired, particularly if interpersonal involvement is required, but individuals with this disorder may do well when they work under conditions of social isolation. Particularly in response to stress, individuals with this disorder may experience very brief psychotic episodes (lasting minutes to hours). In some instances, schizoid personality disorder may appear as the premorbid antecedent of delusional disorder or schizophrenia. Individuals with this disorder may sometimes develop major depressive disorder. Schizoid personality disorder most often co-occurs with schizotypal, paranoid, and avoidant personality disorders.

Prevalence

Schizoid personality disorder is uncommon in clinical settings. A prevalence estimate for schizoid personality based on a probability subsample from Part II of the National Comorbidity Survey Replication suggests a prevalence of 4.9%. Data from the 2001–2002 National Epidemiologic Survey on Alcohol and Related Conditions suggest a prevalence of 3.1%.

Development and Course

Schizoid personality disorder may be first apparent in childhood and adolescence with solitariness, poor peer relationships, and underachievement in school, which mark these children or adolescents as different and make them subject to teasing.

Risk and Prognostic Factors

Genetic and physiological.   Schizoid personality disorder may have increased prevalence in the relatives of individuals with schizophrenia or schizotypal personality disorder.

Culture-Related Diagnostic Issues

Individuals from a variety of cultural backgrounds sometimes exhibit defensive behaviors and interpersonal styles that may be erroneously labeled as "schizoid." For example, those who have moved from rural to metropolitan environments may react with "emotional freezing" that may last for several months and manifest as solitary activities, constricted affect, and other deficits in communication. Immigrants from other countries are sometimes mistakenly perceived as cold, hostile, or indifferent.

Gender-Related Diagnostic Issues

Schizoid personality disorder is diagnosed slightly more often in males and may cause more impairment in them.

Differential Diagnosis

Other mental disorders with psychotic symptoms.   Schizoid personality disorder can be distinguished from delusional disorder, schizophrenia, and a bipolar or depressive disorder with psychotic features because these disorders are all characterized by a period of persistent psychotic symptoms (e.g., delusions and hallucinations). To give an additional diagnosis of schizoid personality disorder, the personality disorder must have been present before the onset of psychotic symptoms and must persist when the psychotic symptoms are in remission. When an individual has a persistent psychotic disorder (e.g., schizophrenia) that was preceded by schizoid personality disorder, schizoid personality disorder should also be recorded, followed by "premorbid" in parentheses.

Autism spectrum disorder.   There may be great difficulty differentiating individuals with schizoid personality disorder from those with milder forms of autism spectrum disorder, which may be differentiated by more severely impaired social interaction and stereotyped behaviors and interests.

Personality change due to another medical condition.   Schizoid personality disorder must be distinguished from personality change due to another medical condition, in which the traits that emerge are attributable to the effects of another medical condition on the central nervous system.

Substance use disorders.   Schizoid personality disorder must also be distinguished from symptoms that may develop in association with persistent substance use.

Other personality disorders and personality traits.   Other personality disorders may be confused with schizoid personality disorder because they have certain features in common. It is, therefore, important to distinguish among these disorders based on differences in their characteristic features. However, if an individual has personality features that meet criteria for one or more personality disorders in addition to schizoid personality disorder, all can be diagnosed. Although characteristics of social isolation and restricted affectivity are common to schizoid, schizotypal, and paranoid personality disorders, schizoid personality disorder can be distinguished from schizotypal personality disorder by the lack of cognitive and perceptual distortions and from paranoid personality disorder by the lack of suspiciousness and paranoid ideation. The social isolation of schizoid personality disorder can be distinguished from that of avoidant personality disorder, which is attributable to fear of being embarrassed or found inadequate and excessive anticipation of rejection. In contrast, people with schizoid personality disorder have a more pervasive detachment and limited desire for social intimacy. Individuals with obsessive-compulsive personality disorder may also show an apparent social detachment stemming from devotion to work and discomfort with emotions, but they do have an underlying capacity for intimacy.

Individuals who are "loners" may display personality traits that might be considered schizoid. Only when these traits are inflexible and maladaptive and cause significant functional impairment or subjective distress do they constitute schizoid personality disorder.

Schizotypal Personality Disorder

Diagnostic Criteria   301.22 (F21)

A. A pervasive pattern of social and interpersonal deficits marked by acute discomfort with, and reduced capacity for, close relationships as well as by cognitive or perceptual distortions and eccentricities of behavior, beginning by early adulthood and present in a variety of contexts, as indicated by five (or more) of the following:

   1. Ideas of reference (excluding delusions of reference).
   2. Odd beliefs or magical thinking that influences behavior and is inconsistent with subcultural norms (e.g., superstitiousness, belief in clairvoyance, telepathy, or "sixth sense"; in children and adolescents, bizarre fantasies or preoccupations).
   3. Unusual perceptual experiences, including bodily illusions.
   4. Odd thinking and speech (e.g., vague, circumstantial, metaphorical, overelaborate, or stereotyped).
   5. Suspiciousness or paranoid ideation.

6. Inappropriate or constricted affect.
7. Behavior or appearance that is odd, eccentric, or peculiar.
8. Lack of close friends or confidants other than first-degree relatives.
9. Excessive social anxiety that does not diminish with familiarity and tends to be associated with paranoid fears rather than negative judgments about self.

B. Does not occur exclusively during the course of schizophrenia, a bipolar disorder or depressive disorder with psychotic features, another psychotic disorder, or autism spectrum disorder.

Note: If criteria are met prior to the onset of schizophrenia, add "premorbid," e.g., "schizotypal personality disorder (premorbid)."

Diagnostic Features

The essential feature of schizotypal personality disorder is a pervasive pattern of social and interpersonal deficits marked by acute discomfort with, and reduced capacity for, close relationships as well as by cognitive or perceptual distortions and eccentricities of behavior. This pattern begins by early adulthood and is present in a variety of contexts.

Individuals with schizotypal personality disorder often have ideas of reference (i.e., incorrect interpretations of casual incidents and external events as having a particular and unusual meaning specifically for the person) (Criterion A1). These should be distinguished from delusions of reference, in which the beliefs are held with delusional conviction. These individuals may be superstitious or preoccupied with paranormal phenomena that are outside the norms of their subculture (Criterion A2). They may feel that they have special powers to sense events before they happen or to read others' thoughts. They may believe that they have magical control over others, which can be implemented directly (e.g., believing that their spouse's taking the dog out for a walk is the direct result of thinking an hour earlier it should be done) or indirectly through compliance with magical rituals (e.g., walking past a specific object three times to avoid a certain harmful outcome). Perceptual alterations may be present (e.g., sensing that another person is present or hearing a voice murmuring his or her name) (Criterion A3). Their speech may include unusual or idiosyncratic phrasing and construction. It is often loose, digressive, or vague, but without actual derailment or incoherence (Criterion A4). Responses can be either overly concrete or overly abstract, and words or concepts are sometimes applied in unusual ways (e.g., the individual may state that he or she was not "talkable" at work).

Individuals with this disorder are often suspicious and may have paranoid ideation (e.g., believing their colleagues at work are intent on undermining their reputation with the boss) (Criterion A5). They are usually not able to negotiate the full range of affects and interpersonal cuing required for successful relationships and thus often appear to interact with others in an inappropriate, stiff, or constricted fashion (Criterion A6). These individuals are often considered to be odd or eccentric because of unusual mannerisms, an often unkempt manner of dress that does not quite "fit together," and inattention to the usual social conventions (e.g., the individual may avoid eye contact, wear clothes that are ink stained and ill-fitting, and be unable to join in the give-and-take banter of co-workers) (Criterion A7).

Individuals with schizotypal personality disorder experience interpersonal relatedness as problematic and are uncomfortable relating to other people. Although they may express unhappiness about their lack of relationships, their behavior suggests a decreased desire for intimate contacts. As a result, they usually have no or few close friends or confidants other than a first-degree relative (Criterion A8). They are anxious in social situations, particularly those involving unfamiliar people (Criterion A9). They will interact with other individuals when they have to but prefer to keep to themselves because they feel that they are different and just do not "fit in." Their social anxiety does not easily abate, even when they spend more time in the setting or become more familiar with the other people, because their anxiety tends to be associated with suspiciousness regarding others' motivations. For example, when attending a dinner party, the individual with schizotypal personality disorder will not become more relaxed as time goes on, but rather may become increasingly tense and suspicious.

Schizotypal personality disorder should not be diagnosed if the pattern of behavior occurs exclusively during the course of schizophrenia, a bipolar or depressive disorder with psychotic features, another psychotic disorder, or autism spectrum disorder (Criterion B).

Associated Features Supporting Diagnosis

Individuals with schizotypal personality disorder often seek treatment for the associated symptoms of anxiety or depression rather than for the personality disorder features per se. Particularly in response to stress, individuals with this disorder may experience transient psychotic episodes (lasting minutes to hours), although they usually are insufficient in duration to warrant an additional diagnosis such as brief psychotic disorder or schizophreniform disorder. In some cases, clinically significant psychotic symptoms may develop that meet criteria for brief psychotic disorder, schizophreniform disorder, delusional disorder, or schizophrenia. Over half may have a history of at least one major depressive episode. From 30% to 50% of individuals diagnosed with this disorder have a concurrent diagnosis of major depressive disorder when admitted to a clinical setting. There is considerable co-occurrence with schizoid, paranoid, avoidant, and borderline personality disorders.

Prevalence

In community studies of schizotypal personality disorder, reported rates range from 0.6% in Norwegian samples to 4.6% in a U.S. community sample. The prevalence of schizotypal personality disorder in clinical populations seems to be infrequent (0%–1.9%), with a higher estimated prevalence in the general population (3.9%) found in the National Epidemiologic Survey on Alcohol and Related Conditions.

Development and Course

Schizotypal personality disorder has a relatively stable course, with only a small proportion of individuals going on to develop schizophrenia or another psychotic disorder. Schizotypal personality disorder may be first apparent in childhood and adolescence with solitariness, poor peer relationships, social anxiety, underachievement in school, hypersensitivity, peculiar thoughts and language, and bizarre fantasies. These children may appear "odd" or "eccentric" and attract teasing.

Risk and Prognostic Factors

Genetic and physiological.   Schizotypal personality disorder appears to aggregate familially and is more prevalent among the first-degree biological relatives of individuals with schizophrenia than among the general population. There may also be a modest increase in schizophrenia and other psychotic disorders in the relatives of probands with schizotypal personality disorder.

Cultural-Related Diagnostic Issues

Cognitive and perceptual distortions must be evaluated in the context of the individual's cultural milieu. Pervasive culturally determined characteristics, particularly those regarding religious beliefs and rituals, can appear to be schizotypal to the uninformed outsider (e.g., voodoo, speaking in tongues, life beyond death, shamanism, mind reading, sixth sense, evil eye, magical beliefs related to health and illness).

Gender-Related Diagnostic Issues

Schizotypal personality disorder may be slightly more common in males.

Differential Diagnosis

Other mental disorders with psychotic symptoms.   Schizotypal personality disorder can be distinguished from delusional disorder, schizophrenia, and a bipolar or depressive disorder with psychotic features because these disorders are all characterized by a period of persistent psychotic symptoms (e.g., delusions and hallucinations). To give an additional diagnosis of schizotypal personality disorder, the personality disorder must have been present before the onset of psychotic symptoms and persist when the psychotic symptoms are in remission. When an individual has a persistent psychotic disorder (e.g., schizophrenia) that was preceded by schizotypal personality disorder, schizotypal personality disorder should also be recorded, followed by "premorbid" in parentheses.

Neurodevelopmental disorders.   There may be great difficulty differentiating children with schizotypal personality disorder from the heterogeneous group of solitary, odd children whose behavior is characterized by marked social isolation, eccentricity, or peculiarities of language and whose diagnoses would probably include milder forms of autism spectrum disorder or language communication disorders. Communication disorders may be differentiated by the primacy and severity of the disorder in language and by the characteristic features of impaired language found in a specialized language assessment. Milder forms of autism spectrum disorder are differentiated by the even greater lack of social awareness and emotional reciprocity and stereotyped behaviors and interests.

Personality change due to another medical condition.   Schizotypal personality disorder must be distinguished from personality change due to another medical condition, in which the traits that emerge are attributable to the effects of another medical condition on the central nervous system.

Substance use disorders.   Schizotypal personality disorder must also be distinguished from symptoms that may develop in association with persistent substance use.

Other personality disorders and personality traits.   Other personality disorders may be confused with schizotypal personality disorder because they have certain features in common. It is, therefore, important to distinguish among these disorders based on differences in their characteristic features. However, if an individual has personality features that meet criteria for one or more personality disorders in addition to schizotypal personality disorder, all can be diagnosed. Although paranoid and schizoid personality disorders may also be characterized by social detachment and restricted affect, schizotypal personality disorder can be distinguished from these two diagnoses by the presence of cognitive or perceptual distortions and marked eccentricity or oddness. Close relationships are limited in both schizotypal personality disorder and avoidant personality disorder; however, in avoidant personality disorder an active desire for relationships is constrained by a fear of rejection, whereas in schizotypal personality disorder there is a lack of desire for relationships and persistent detachment. Individuals with narcissistic personality disorder may also display suspiciousness, social withdrawal, or alienation, but in narcissistic personality disorder these qualities derive primarily from fears of having imperfections or flaws revealed. Individuals with borderline personality disorder may also have transient, psychotic-like symptoms, but these are usually more closely related to affective shifts in response to stress (e.g., intense anger, anxiety, disappointment) and are usually more dissociative (e.g., derealization, depersonalization). In contrast, individuals with schizotypal personality disorder are more likely to have enduring psychotic-like symptoms that may worsen under stress but are less likely to be invariably associated with pronounced affective symptoms. Although social isolation may occur in borderline personality disorder, it is usually secondary to repeated interpersonal failures due to angry outbursts and frequent mood shifts, rather than a result of a persistent lack of social contacts and desire for intimacy. Furthermore, individuals with schizotypal personality disorder do not usually demonstrate the impulsive or manipulative behaviors of the individual with borderline personality disorder. However, there is a high rate of co-occurrence between the two disorders, so that making such distinctions is not always feasible. Schizotypal features during adolescence may be reflective of transient emotional turmoil, rather than an enduring personality disorder.

Cluster B Personality Disorders

Antisocial Personality Disorder

Diagnostic Criteria   301.7 (F60.2)

A. A pervasive pattern of disregard for and violation of the rights of others, occurring since age 15 years, as indicated by three (or more) of the following:

   1. Failure to conform to social norms with respect to lawful behaviors, as indicated by repeatedly performing acts that are grounds for arrest.
   2. Deceitfulness, as indicated by repeated lying, use of aliases, or conning others for personal profit or pleasure.
   3. Impulsivity or failure to plan ahead.
   4. Irritability and aggressiveness, as indicated by repeated physical fights or assaults.
   5. Reckless disregard for safety of self or others.
   6. Consistent irresponsibility, as indicated by repeated failure to sustain consistent work behavior or honor financial obligations.
   7. Lack of remorse, as indicated by being indifferent to or rationalizing having hurt, mistreated, or stolen from another.

B. The individual is at least age 18 years.
C. There is evidence of conduct disorder with onset before age 15 years.
D. The occurrence of antisocial behavior is not exclusively during the course of schizophrenia or bipolar disorder.

Diagnostic Features

The essential feature of antisocial personality disorder is a pervasive pattern of disregard for, and violation of, the rights of others that begins in childhood or early adolescence and continues into adulthood. This pattern has also been referred to as *psychopathy, sociopathy,* or *dyssocial personality disorder*. Because deceit and manipulation are central features of antisocial personality disorder, it may be especially helpful to integrate information acquired from systematic clinical assessment with information collected from collateral sources.

For this diagnosis to be given, the individual must be at least age 18 years (Criterion B) and must have had a history of some symptoms of conduct disorder before age 15 years (Criterion C). Conduct disorder involves a repetitive and persistent pattern of behavior in which the basic rights of others or major age-appropriate societal norms or rules are violated. The specific behaviors characteristic of conduct disorder fall into one of four categories: aggression to people and animals, destruction of property, deceitfulness or theft, or serious violation of rules.

The pattern of antisocial behavior continues into adulthood. Individuals with antisocial personality disorder fail to conform to social norms with respect to lawful behavior (Criterion A1). They may repeatedly perform acts that are grounds for arrest (whether they are arrested or not), such as destroying property, harassing others, stealing, or pursuing illegal occupations. Persons with this disorder disregard the wishes, rights, or feelings of others. They are frequently deceitful and manipulative in order to gain personal profit or pleasure (e.g., to obtain money, sex, or power) (Criterion A2). They may repeatedly lie, use an alias, con others, or malinger. A pattern of impulsivity may be manifested by a failure to plan ahead (Criterion A3). Decisions are made on the spur of the moment, without forethought and without consideration for the consequences to self or others; this may lead to sudden changes of jobs, residences, or relationships. Individuals with antisocial personality disorder tend to be irritable and aggressive and may repeatedly get into physical fights or commit acts of physical assault (including spouse beating or child beating) (Criterion A4). (Aggressive acts that are required to defend oneself or someone else are not considered to be evidence for this item.) These individuals also display a reckless disregard for the safety of themselves or others (Criterion A5). This may be evidenced in their driving behavior (i.e., recurrent speeding, driving while intoxicated, multiple accidents). They may engage in sexual behavior or substance use that has a high risk for harmful consequences. They may neglect or fail to care for a child in a way that puts the child in danger.

Individuals with antisocial personality disorder also tend to be consistently and extremely irresponsible (Criterion A6). Irresponsible work behavior may be indicated by significant periods of unemployment despite available job opportunities, or by abandonment of several jobs without a realistic plan for getting another job. There may also be a pattern of repeated absences from work that are not explained by illness either in themselves or in their family. Financial irresponsibility is indicated by acts such as defaulting on debts, failing to provide child support, or failing to support other dependents on a regular basis. Individuals with antisocial personality disorder show little remorse for the consequences of their acts (Criterion A7). They may be indifferent to, or provide a superficial rationalization for, having hurt, mistreated, or stolen from someone (e.g., "life's unfair," "losers deserve to lose"). These individuals may blame the victims for being foolish, helpless, or deserving their fate (e.g., "he had it coming anyway"); they may minimize the harmful consequences of their actions; or they may simply indicate complete indifference. They generally fail to compensate or make amends for their behavior. They may believe that everyone is out to "help number one" and that one should stop at nothing to avoid being pushed around.

The antisocial behavior must not occur exclusively during the course of schizophrenia or bipolar disorder (Criterion D).

Associated Features Supporting Diagnosis

Individuals with antisocial personality disorder frequently lack empathy and tend to be callous, cynical, and contemptuous of the feelings, rights, and sufferings of others. They may have an inflated and arrogant self-appraisal (e.g., feel that ordinary work is beneath them or lack a realistic concern about their current problems or their future) and may be excessively opinionated, self-assured, or cocky. They may display a glib, superficial charm and can be quite voluble and verbally facile (e.g., using technical terms or jargon that might impress someone who is unfamiliar with the topic). Lack of empathy, inflated self-appraisal, and superficial charm are features that have been commonly included in traditional conceptions of psychopathy that may be particularly distinguishing of the disorder and more predictive of recidivism in prison or forensic settings, where criminal, delinquent, or aggressive acts are likely to be nonspecific. These individuals may also be irresponsible and exploitative in their sexual relationships. They may have a history of many sexual partners and may never have sustained a monogamous relationship. They may be irresponsible as parents, as evidenced by malnutrition of a child, an illness in the child resulting from a lack of minimal hygiene, a child's dependence on neighbors or nonresident relatives for food or shelter, a failure to arrange for a caretaker for a young child when the individual is away from home, or repeated squandering of money required for household necessities. These individuals may receive dishonorable discharges from the armed services, may fail to be self-supporting, may become impoverished or even homeless, or may spend many years in penal institutions. Individuals with antisocial personality disorder are more likely than people in the general population to die prematurely by violent means (e.g., suicide, accidents, homicides).

Individuals with antisocial personality disorder may also experience dysphoria, including complaints of tension, inability to tolerate boredom, and depressed mood. They may have associated anxiety disorders, depressive disorders, substance use disorders, somatic symptom disorder, gambling disorder, and other disorders of impulse control. Individuals with antisocial personality disorder also often have personality features that meet criteria for other personality disorders, particularly borderline, histrionic, and narcissistic personality disorders. The likelihood of developing antisocial personality disorder in adult life is increased if the individual experienced childhood onset of conduct disorder (before age 10 years) and accompanying attention-deficit/hyperactivity disorder. Child abuse or neglect, unstable or erratic parenting, or inconsistent parental discipline may increase the likelihood that conduct disorder will evolve into antisocial personality disorder.

Prevalence

Twelve-month prevalence rates of antisocial personality disorder, using criteria from previous DSMs, are between 0.2% and 3.3%. The highest prevalence of antisocial personality disorder (greater than 70%) is among most severe samples of males with alcohol use disorder and from substance abuse clinics, prisons, or other forensic settings. Prevalence is higher in samples affected by adverse socioeconomic (i.e., poverty) or sociocultural (i.e., migration) factors.

Development and Course

Antisocial personality disorder has a chronic course but may become less evident or remit as the individual grows older, particularly by the fourth decade of life. Although this remission tends to be particularly evident with respect to engaging in criminal behavior, there is likely to be a decrease in the full spectrum of antisocial behaviors and substance use. By definition, antisocial personality cannot be diagnosed before age 18 years.

Risk and Prognostic Factors

Genetic and physiological. Antisocial personality disorder is more common among the first-degree biological relatives of those with the disorder than in the general population. The risk to biological relatives of females with the disorder tends to be higher than the risk to biological relatives of males with the disorder. Biological relatives of individuals with this disorder are also at increased risk for somatic symptom disorder and substance use disorders. Within a family that has a member with antisocial personality disorder, males more often have antisocial personality disorder and substance use disorders, whereas females more often have somatic symptom disorder. However, in such families, there is an increase in prevalence of all of these disorders in both males and females compared with the general population. Adoption studies indicate that both genetic and environmental factors contribute to the risk of developing antisocial personality disorder. Both adopted and biological children of parents with antisocial personality disorder have an increased risk of developing antisocial personality disorder, somatic symptom disorder, and substance use disorders. Adopted-away children resemble their biological parents more than their adoptive parents, but the adoptive family environment influences the risk of developing a personality disorder and related psychopathology.

Culture-Related Diagnostic Issues

Antisocial personality disorder appears to be associated with low socioeconomic status and urban settings. Concerns have been raised that the diagnosis may at times be misapplied to individuals in settings in which seemingly antisocial behavior may be part of a protective survival strategy. In assessing antisocial traits, it is helpful for the clinician to consider the social and economic context in which the behaviors occur.

Gender-Related Diagnostic Issues

Antisocial personality disorder is much more common in males than in females. There has been some concern that antisocial personality disorder may be underdiagnosed in females, particularly because of the emphasis on aggressive items in the definition of conduct disorder.

Differential Diagnosis

The diagnosis of antisocial personality disorder is not given to individuals younger than 18 years and is given only if there is a history of some symptoms of conduct disorder before age 15 years. For individuals older than 18 years, a diagnosis of conduct disorder is given only if the criteria for antisocial personality disorder are not met.

Substance use disorders.   When antisocial behavior in an adult is associated with a substance use disorder, the diagnosis of antisocial personality disorder is not made unless the signs of antisocial personality disorder were also present in childhood and have continued into adulthood. When substance use and antisocial behavior both began in childhood and continued into adulthood, both a substance use disorder and antisocial personality disorder should be diagnosed if the criteria for both are met, even though some antisocial acts may be a consequence of the substance use disorder (e.g., illegal selling of drugs, thefts to obtain money for drugs).

Schizophrenia and bipolar disorders.   Antisocial behavior that occurs exclusively during the course of schizophrenia or a bipolar disorder should not be diagnosed as antisocial personality disorder.

Other personality disorders.   Other personality disorders may be confused with antisocial personality disorder because they have certain features in common. It is therefore important to distinguish among these disorders based on differences in their characteristic features. However, if an individual has personality features that meet criteria for one or more personality disorders in addition to antisocial personality disorder, all can be diagnosed. Individuals with antisocial personality disorder and narcissistic personality disorder share a tendency to be tough-minded, glib, superficial, exploitative, and lack empathy. However, narcissistic personality disorder does not include characteristics of impulsivity, aggression, and deceit. In addition, individuals with antisocial personality disorder may not be as needy of the admiration and envy of others, and persons with narcissistic personality disorder usually lack the history of conduct disorder in childhood or criminal behavior in adulthood. Individuals with antisocial personality disorder and histrionic personality disorder share a tendency to be impulsive, superficial, excitement seeking, reckless, seductive, and manipulative, but persons with histrionic personality disorder tend to be more exaggerated in their emotions and do not characteristically engage in antisocial behaviors. Individuals with histrionic and borderline personality disorders are manipulative to gain nurturance, whereas those with antisocial personality disorder are manipulative to gain profit, power, or some other material gratification. Individuals with antisocial personality disorder tend to be less emotionally unstable and more aggressive than those with borderline personality disorder. Although antisocial behavior may be present in some individuals with paranoid personality disorder, it is not usually motivated by a desire for personal gain or to exploit others as in antisocial personality disorder, but rather is more often attributable to a desire for revenge.

Criminal behavior not associated with a personality disorder.   Antisocial personality disorder must be distinguished from criminal behavior undertaken for gain that is not accompanied by the personality features characteristic of this disorder. Only when antisocial personality traits are inflexible, maladaptive, and persistent and cause significant functional impairment or subjective distress do they constitute antisocial personality disorder.

Borderline Personality Disorder

Diagnostic Criteria   **301.83 (F60.3)**

A pervasive pattern of instability of interpersonal relationships, self-image, and affects, and marked impulsivity, beginning by early adulthood and present in a variety of contexts, as indicated by five (or more) of the following:

1. Frantic efforts to avoid real or imagined abandonment. (**Note:** Do not include suicidal or self-mutilating behavior covered in Criterion 5.)
2. A pattern of unstable and intense interpersonal relationships characterized by alternating between extremes of idealization and devaluation.
3. Identity disturbance: markedly and persistently unstable self-image or sense of self.
4. Impulsivity in at least two areas that are potentially self-damaging (e.g., spending, sex, substance abuse, reckless driving, binge eating). (**Note:** Do not include suicidal or self-mutilating behavior covered in Criterion 5.)
5. Recurrent suicidal behavior, gestures, or threats, or self-mutilating behavior.
6. Affective instability due to a marked reactivity of mood (e.g., intense episodic dysphoria, irritability, or anxiety usually lasting a few hours and only rarely more than a few days).
7. Chronic feelings of emptiness.
8. Inappropriate, intense anger or difficulty controlling anger (e.g., frequent displays of temper, constant anger, recurrent physical fights).
9. Transient, stress-related paranoid ideation or severe dissociative symptoms.

Diagnostic Features

The essential feature of borderline personality disorder is a pervasive pattern of instability of interpersonal relationships, self-image, and affects, and marked impulsivity that begins by early adulthood and is present in a variety of contexts.

Individuals with borderline personality disorder make frantic efforts to avoid real or imagined abandonment (Criterion 1). The perception of impending separation or rejection, or the loss of external structure, can lead to profound changes in self-image, affect, cognition, and behavior. These individuals are very sensitive to environmental circumstances. They experience intense abandonment fears and inappropriate anger even when faced with a realistic time-limited separation or when there are unavoidable changes in plans (e.g., sudden despair in reaction to a clinician's announcing the end of the hour; panic or fury when someone important to them is just a few minutes late or must cancel an appointment). They may believe that this "abandonment" implies they are "bad." These abandonment fears are related to an intolerance of being alone and a need to have other people with them. Their frantic

efforts to avoid abandonment may include impulsive actions such as self-mutilating or suicidal behaviors, which are described separately in Criterion 5.

Individuals with borderline personality disorder have a pattern of unstable and intense
relationships (Criterion 2). They may idealize potential caregivers or lovers at the first or
second meeting, demand to spend a lot of time together, and share the most intimate details
early in a relationship. However, they may switch quickly from idealizing other people to
devaluing them, feeling that the other person does not care enough, does not give enough,
or is not "there" enough. These individuals can empathize with and nurture other people,
but only with the expectation that the other person will "be there" in return to meet their
own needs on demand. These individuals are prone to sudden and dramatic shifts in their
view of others, who may alternatively be seen as beneficent supports or as cruelly punitive.
Such shifts often reflect disillusionment with a caregiver whose nurturing qualities had
been idealized or whose rejection or abandonment is expected.

There may be an identity disturbance characterized by markedly and persistently unstable self-image or sense of self (Criterion 3). There are sudden and dramatic shifts in self-
image, characterized by shifting goals, values, and vocational aspirations. There may be
sudden changes in opinions and plans about career, sexual identity, values, and types of
friends. These individuals may suddenly change from the role of a needy supplicant for
help to that of a righteous avenger of past mistreatment. Although they usually have a self-
image that is based on being bad or evil, individuals with this disorder may at times have
feelings that they do not exist at all. Such experiences usually occur in situations in which
the individual feels a lack of a meaningful relationship, nurturing, and support. These individuals may show worse performance in unstructured work or school situations.

Individuals with borderline personality disorder display impulsivity in at least two areas
that are potentially self-damaging (Criterion 4). They may gamble, spend money irrespon-
sibly, binge eat, abuse substances, engage in unsafe sex, or drive recklessly. Individuals
with this disorder display recurrent suicidal behavior, gestures, or threats, or self-mutilating behavior (Criterion 5). Completed suicide occurs in 8%–10% of such individuals, and
self-mutilative acts (e.g., cutting or burning) and suicide threats and attempts are very
common. Recurrent suicidality is often the reason that these individuals present for help.
These self-destructive acts are usually precipitated by threats of separation or rejection or
by expectations that the individual assumes increased responsibility. Self-mutilation may
occur during dissociative experiences and often brings relief by reaffirming the ability to
feel or by expiating the individual's sense of being evil.

Individuals with borderline personality disorder may display affective instability that
is due to a marked reactivity of mood (e.g., intense episodic dysphoria, irritability, or anxiety usually lasting a few hours and only rarely more than a few days) (Criterion 6). The
basic dysphoric mood of those with borderline personality disorder is often disrupted by
periods of anger, panic, or despair and is rarely relieved by periods of well-being or satisfaction. These episodes may reflect the individual's extreme reactivity to interpersonal
stresses. Individuals with borderline personality disorder may be troubled by chronic feelings of emptiness (Criterion 7). Easily bored, they may constantly seek something to do.
Individuals with this disorder frequently express inappropriate, intense anger or have difficulty controlling their anger (Criterion 8). They may display extreme sarcasm, enduring
bitterness, or verbal outbursts. The anger is often elicited when a caregiver or lover is seen
as neglectful, withholding, uncaring, or abandoning. Such expressions of anger are often
followed by shame and guilt and contribute to the feeling they have of being evil. During
periods of extreme stress, transient paranoid ideation or dissociative symptoms (e.g., depersonalization) may occur (Criterion 9), but these are generally of insufficient severity or
duration to warrant an additional diagnosis. These episodes occur most frequently in response to a real or imagined abandonment. Symptoms tend to be transient, lasting minutes or hours. The real or perceived return of the caregiver's nurturance may result in a
remission of symptoms.

Associated Features Supporting Diagnosis

Individuals with borderline personality disorder may have a pattern of undermining themselves at the moment a goal is about to be realized (e.g., dropping out of school just before graduation; regressing severely after a discussion of how well therapy is going; destroying a good relationship just when it is clear that the relationship could last). Some individuals develop psychotic-like symptoms (e.g., hallucinations, body-image distortions, ideas of reference, hypnagogic phenomena) during times of stress. Individuals with this disorder may feel more secure with transitional objects (i.e., a pet or inanimate possession) than in interpersonal relationships. Premature death from suicide may occur in individuals with this disorder, especially in those with co-occurring depressive disorders or substance use disorders. Physical handicaps may result from self-inflicted abuse behaviors or failed suicide attempts. Recurrent job losses, interrupted education, and separation or divorce are common. Physical and sexual abuse, neglect, hostile conflict, and early parental loss are more common in the childhood histories of those with borderline personality disorder. Common co-occurring disorders include depressive and bipolar disorders, substance use disorders, eating disorders (notably bulimia nervosa), posttraumatic stress disorder, and attention-deficit/hyperactivity disorder. Borderline personality disorder also frequently co-occurs with the other personality disorders.

Prevalence

The median population prevalence of borderline personality disorder is estimated to be 1.6% but may be as high as 5.9%. The prevalence of borderline personality disorder is about 6% in primary care settings, about 10% among individuals seen in outpatient mental health clinics, and about 20% among psychiatric inpatients. The prevalence of borderline personality disorder may decrease in older age groups.

Development and Course

There is considerable variability in the course of borderline personality disorder. The most common pattern is one of chronic instability in early adulthood, with episodes of serious affective and impulsive dyscontrol and high levels of use of health and mental health resources. The impairment from the disorder and the risk of suicide are greatest in the young-adult years and gradually wane with advancing age. Although the tendency toward intense emotions, impulsivity, and intensity in relationships is often lifelong, individuals who engage in therapeutic intervention often show improvement beginning sometime during the first year. During their 30s and 40s, the majority of individuals with this disorder attain greater stability in their relationships and vocational functioning. Follow-up studies of individuals identified through outpatient mental health clinics indicate that after about 10 years, as many as half of the individuals no longer have a pattern of behavior that meets full criteria for borderline personality disorder.

Risk and Prognostic Factors

Genetic and physiological. Borderline personality disorder is about five times more common among first-degree biological relatives of those with the disorder than in the general population. There is also an increased familial risk for substance use disorders, antisocial personality disorder, and depressive or bipolar disorders.

Culture-Related Diagnostic Issues

The pattern of behavior seen in borderline personality disorder has been identified in many settings around the world. Adolescents and young adults with identity problems (especially when accompanied by substance use) may transiently display behaviors that misleadingly give the impression of borderline personality disorder. Such situations are characterized by emotional instability, "existential" dilemmas, uncertainty, anxiety-provoking choices, conflicts about sexual orientation, and competing social pressures to decide on careers.

Gender-Related Diagnostic Issues

Borderline personality disorder is diagnosed predominantly (about 75%) in females.

Differential Diagnosis

Depressive and bipolar disorders.   Borderline personality disorder often co-occurs with depressive or bipolar disorders, and when criteria for both are met, both may be diagnosed. Because the cross-sectional presentation of borderline personality disorder can be mimicked by an episode of depressive or bipolar disorder, the clinician should avoid giving an additional diagnosis of borderline personality disorder based only on cross-sectional presentation without having documented that the pattern of behavior had an early onset and a long-standing course.

Other personality disorders.   Other personality disorders may be confused with borderline personality disorder because they have certain features in common. It is therefore important to distinguish among these disorders based on differences in their characteristic features. However, if an individual has personality features that meet criteria for one or more personality disorders in addition to borderline personality disorder, all can be diagnosed. Although histrionic personality disorder can also be characterized by attention seeking, manipulative behavior, and rapidly shifting emotions, borderline personality disorder is distinguished by self-destructiveness, angry disruptions in close relationships, and chronic feelings of deep emptiness and loneliness. Paranoid ideas or illusions may be present in both borderline personality disorder and schizotypal personality disorder, but these symptoms are more transient, interpersonally reactive, and responsive to external structuring in borderline personality disorder. Although paranoid personality disorder and narcissistic personality disorder may also be characterized by an angry reaction to minor stimuli, the relative stability of self-image, as well as the relative lack of self-destructiveness, impulsivity, and abandonment concerns, distinguishes these disorders from borderline personality disorder. Although antisocial personality disorder and borderline personality disorder are both characterized by manipulative behavior, individuals with antisocial personality disorder are manipulative to gain profit, power, or some other material gratification, whereas the goal in borderline personality disorder is directed more toward gaining the concern of caretakers. Both dependent personality disorder and borderline personality disorder are characterized by fear of abandonment; however, the individual with borderline personality disorder reacts to abandonment with feelings of emotional emptiness, rage, and demands, whereas the individual with dependent personality disorder reacts with increasing appeasement and submissiveness and urgently seeks a replacement relationship to provide caregiving and support. Borderline personality disorder can further be distinguished from dependent personality disorder by the typical pattern of unstable and intense relationships.

Personality change due to another medical condition.   Borderline personality disorder must be distinguished from personality change due to another medical condition, in which the traits that emerge are attributable to the effects of another medical condition on the central nervous system.

Substance use disorders.   Borderline personality disorder must also be distinguished from symptoms that may develop in association with persistent substance use.

Identity problems.   Borderline personality disorder should be distinguished from an identity problem, which is reserved for identity concerns related to a developmental phase (e.g., adolescence) and does not qualify as a mental disorder.

Histrionic Personality Disorder

Diagnostic Criteria	**301.50** (F60.4)

A pervasive pattern of excessive emotionality and attention seeking, beginning by early adulthood and present in a variety of contexts, as indicated by five (or more) of the following:

1. Is uncomfortable in situations in which he or she is not the center of attention.
2. Interaction with others is often characterized by inappropriate sexually seductive or provocative behavior.
3. Displays rapidly shifting and shallow expression of emotions.
4. Consistently uses physical appearance to draw attention to self.
5. Has a style of speech that is excessively impressionistic and lacking in detail.
6. Shows self-dramatization, theatricality, and exaggerated expression of emotion.
7. Is suggestible (i.e., easily influenced by others or circumstances).
8. Considers relationships to be more intimate than they actually are.

Diagnostic Features

The essential feature of histrionic personality disorder is pervasive and excessive emotionality and attention-seeking behavior. This pattern begins by early adulthood and is present in a variety of contexts.

Individuals with histrionic personality disorder are uncomfortable or feel unappreciated when they are not the center of attention (Criterion 1). Often lively and dramatic, they tend to draw attention to themselves and may initially charm new acquaintances by their enthusiasm, apparent openness, or flirtatiousness. These qualities wear thin, however, as these individuals continually demand to be the center of attention. They commandeer the role of "the life of the party." If they are not the center of attention, they may do something dramatic (e.g., make up stories, create a scene) to draw the focus of attention to themselves. This need is often apparent in their behavior with a clinician (e.g., being flattering, bringing gifts, providing dramatic descriptions of physical and psychological symptoms that are replaced by new symptoms each visit).

The appearance and behavior of individuals with this disorder are often inappropriately sexually provocative or seductive (Criterion 2). This behavior not only is directed toward persons in whom the individual has a sexual or romantic interest but also occurs in a wide variety of social, occupational, and professional relationships beyond what is appropriate for the social context. Emotional expression may be shallow and rapidly shifting (Criterion 3). Individuals with this disorder consistently use physical appearance to draw attention to themselves (Criterion 4). They are overly concerned with impressing others by their appearance and expend an excessive amount of time, energy, and money on clothes and grooming. They may "fish for compliments" regarding appearance and may be easily and excessively upset by a critical comment about how they look or by a photograph that they regard as unflattering.

These individuals have a style of speech that is excessively impressionistic and lacking in detail (Criterion 5). Strong opinions are expressed with dramatic flair, but underlying reasons are usually vague and diffuse, without supporting facts and details. For example, an individual with histrionic personality disorder may comment that a certain individual is a wonderful human being, yet be unable to provide any specific examples of good qualities to support this opinion. Individuals with this disorder are characterized by self-dramatization, theatricality, and an exaggerated expression of emotion (Criterion 6). They may embarrass friends and acquaintances by an excessive public display of emotions (e.g., embracing casual acquaintances with excessive ardor, sobbing uncontrollably on minor sentimental occasions, having temper tantrums). However, their emotions often seem to be turned on and off too quickly to be deeply felt, which may lead others to accuse the individual of faking these feelings.

Individuals with histrionic personality disorder have a high degree of suggestibility (Criterion 7). Their opinions and feelings are easily influenced by others and by current fads. They may be overly trusting, especially of strong authority figures whom they see as magically solving their problems. They have a tendency to play hunches and to adopt convictions quickly. Individuals with this disorder often consider relationships more intimate than they actually are, describing almost every acquaintance as "my dear, dear friend" or referring to physicians met only once or twice under professional circumstances by their first names (Criterion 8).

Associated Features Supporting Diagnosis

Individuals with histrionic personality disorder may have difficulty achieving emotional intimacy in romantic or sexual relationships. Without being aware of it, they often act out a role (e.g., "victim" or "princess") in their relationships to others. They may seek to control their partner through emotional manipulation or seductiveness on one level, while displaying a marked dependency on them at another level. Individuals with this disorder often have impaired relationships with same-sex friends because their sexually provocative interpersonal style may seem a threat to their friends' relationships. These individuals may also alienate friends with demands for constant attention. They often become depressed and upset when they are not the center of attention. They may crave novelty, stimulation, and excitement and have a tendency to become bored with their usual routine. These individuals are often intolerant of, or frustrated by, situations that involve delayed gratification, and their actions are often directed at obtaining immediate satisfaction. Although they often initiate a job or project with great enthusiasm, their interest may lag quickly. Longer-term relationships may be neglected to make way for the excitement of new relationships.

The actual risk of suicide is not known, but clinical experience suggests that individuals with this disorder are at increased risk for suicidal gestures and threats to get attention and coerce better caregiving. Histrionic personality disorder has been associated with higher rates of somatic symptom disorder, conversion disorder (functional neurological symptom disorder), and major depressive disorder. Borderline, narcissistic, antisocial, and dependent personality disorders often co-occur.

Prevalence

Data from the 2001–2002 National Epidemiologic Survey on Alcohol and Related Conditions suggest a prevalence of histrionic personality of 1.84%.

Culture-Related Diagnostic Issues

Norms for interpersonal behavior, personal appearance, and emotional expressiveness vary widely across cultures, genders, and age groups. Before considering the various traits (e.g., emotionality, seductiveness, dramatic interpersonal style, novelty seeking, sociability, charm, impressionability, a tendency to somatization) to be evidence of histrionic personality disorder, it is important to evaluate whether they cause clinically significant impairment or distress.

Gender-Related Diagnostic Issues

In clinical settings, this disorder has been diagnosed more frequently in females; however, the sex ratio is not significantly different from the sex ratio of females within the respective clinical setting. In contrast, some studies using structured assessments report similar prevalence rates among males and females.

Differential Diagnosis

Other personality disorders and personality traits.   Other personality disorders may be confused with histrionic personality disorder because they have certain features in common. It is therefore important to distinguish among these disorders based on differences in their characteristic features. However, if an individual has personality features that meet criteria for one or more personality disorders in addition to histrionic personality disorder, all can be diagnosed. Although borderline personality disorder can also be characterized by attention seeking, manipulative behavior, and rapidly shifting emotions, it is distinguished by self-destructiveness, angry disruptions in close relationships, and chronic feelings of deep emptiness and identity disturbance. Individuals with antisocial personality disorder and histrionic personality disorder share a tendency to be impulsive, superficial, excitement seeking, reckless, seductive, and manipulative, but persons with histrionic personality disorder tend to be more exaggerated in their emotions and do not characteristically engage in antisocial behaviors. Individuals with histrionic personality disorder are manipulative to gain nurturance, whereas those with antisocial personality disorder are manipulative to gain profit, power, or some other material gratification. Although individuals with narcissistic personality disorder also crave attention from others, they usually want praise for their "superiority," whereas individuals with histrionic personality disorder are willing to be viewed as fragile or dependent if this is instrumental in getting attention. Individuals with narcissistic personality disorder may exaggerate the intimacy of their relationships with other people, but they are more apt to emphasize the "VIP" status or wealth of their friends. In dependent personality disorder, the individual is excessively dependent on others for praise and guidance, but is without the flamboyant, exaggerated, emotional features of individuals with histrionic personality disorder.

Many individuals may display histrionic personality traits. Only when these traits are inflexible, maladaptive, and persisting and cause significant functional impairment or subjective distress do they constitute histrionic personality disorder.

Personality change due to another medical condition.   Histrionic personality disorder must be distinguished from personality change due to another medical condition, in which the traits that emerge are attributable to the effects of another medical condition on the central nervous system.

Substance use disorders.   The disorder must also be distinguished from symptoms that may develop in association with persistent substance use.

Narcissistic Personality Disorder

Diagnostic Criteria	**301.81 (F60.81)**

A pervasive pattern of grandiosity (in fantasy or behavior), need for admiration, and lack of empathy, beginning by early adulthood and present in a variety of contexts, as indicated by five (or more) of the following:

1. Has a grandiose sense of self-importance (e.g., exaggerates achievements and talents, expects to be recognized as superior without commensurate achievements).
2. Is preoccupied with fantasies of unlimited success, power, brilliance, beauty, or ideal love.
3. Believes that he or she is "special" and unique and can only be understood by, or should associate with, other special or high-status people (or institutions).
4. Requires excessive admiration.
5. Has a sense of entitlement (i.e., unreasonable expectations of especially favorable treatment or automatic compliance with his or her expectations).

6. Is interpersonally exploitative (i.e., takes advantage of others to achieve his or her own ends).
7. Lacks empathy: is unwilling to recognize or identify with the feelings and needs of others.
8. Is often envious of others or believes that others are envious of him or her.
9. Shows arrogant, haughty behaviors or attitudes.

Diagnostic Features

The essential feature of narcissistic personality disorder is a pervasive pattern of grandiosity, need for admiration, and lack of empathy that begins by early adulthood and is present in a variety of contexts.

Individuals with this disorder have a grandiose sense of self-importance (Criterion 1). They routinely overestimate their abilities and inflate their accomplishments, often appearing boastful and pretentious. They may blithely assume that others attribute the same value to their efforts and may be surprised when the praise they expect and feel they deserve is not forthcoming. Often implicit in the inflated judgments of their own accomplishments is an underestimation (devaluation) of the contributions of others. Individuals with narcissistic personality disorder are often preoccupied with fantasies of unlimited success, power, brilliance, beauty, or ideal love (Criterion 2). They may ruminate about "long overdue" admiration and privilege and compare themselves favorably with famous or privileged people.

Individuals with narcissistic personality disorder believe that they are superior, special, or unique and expect others to recognize them as such (Criterion 3). They may feel that they can only be understood by, and should only associate with, other people who are special or of high status and may attribute "unique," "perfect," or "gifted" qualities to those with whom they associate. Individuals with this disorder believe that their needs are special and beyond the ken of ordinary people. Their own self-esteem is enhanced (i.e., "mirrored") by the idealized value that they assign to those with whom they associate. They are likely to insist on having only the "top" person (doctor, lawyer, hairdresser, instructor) or being affiliated with the "best" institutions but may devalue the credentials of those who disappoint them.

Individuals with this disorder generally require excessive admiration (Criterion 4). Their self-esteem is almost invariably very fragile. They may be preoccupied with how well they are doing and how favorably they are regarded by others. This often takes the form of a need for constant attention and admiration. They may expect their arrival to be greeted with great fanfare and are astonished if others do not covet their possessions. They may constantly fish for compliments, often with great charm. A sense of entitlement is evident in these individuals' unreasonable expectation of especially favorable treatment (Criterion 5). They expect to be catered to and are puzzled or furious when this does not happen. For example, they may assume that they do not have to wait in line and that their priorities are so important that others should defer to them, and then get irritated when others fail to assist "in their very important work." This sense of entitlement, combined with a lack of sensitivity to the wants and needs of others, may result in the conscious or unwitting exploitation of others (Criterion 6). They expect to be given whatever they want or feel they need, no matter what it might mean to others. For example, these individuals may expect great dedication from others and may overwork them without regard for the impact on their lives. They tend to form friendships or romantic relationships only if the other person seems likely to advance their purposes or otherwise enhance their self-esteem. They often usurp special privileges and extra resources that they believe they deserve because they are so special.

Individuals with narcissistic personality disorder generally have a lack of empathy and have difficulty recognizing the desires, subjective experiences, and feelings of others (Criterion 7). They may assume that others are totally concerned about their welfare. They tend to discuss their own concerns in inappropriate and lengthy detail, while failing to recognize that others also have feelings and needs. They are often contemptuous and impatient with others who talk about their own problems and concerns. These individuals may be oblivious to the hurt their remarks may inflict (e.g., exuberantly telling a former lover that "I am now in the relationship of a lifetime!"; boasting of health in front of someone who is sick). When recognized, the needs, desires, or feelings of others are likely to be viewed disparagingly as signs of weakness or vulnerability. Those who relate to individuals with narcissistic personality disorder typically find an emotional coldness and lack of reciprocal interest.

These individuals are often envious of others or believe that others are envious of them (Criterion 8). They may begrudge others their successes or possessions, feeling that they better deserve those achievements, admiration, or privileges. They may harshly devalue the contributions of others, particularly when those individuals have received acknowledgment or praise for their accomplishments. Arrogant, haughty behaviors characterize these individuals; they often display snobbish, disdainful, or patronizing attitudes (Criterion 9). For example, an individual with this disorder may complain about a clumsy waiter's "rudeness" or "stupidity" or conclude a medical evaluation with a condescending evaluation of the physician.

Associated Features Supporting Diagnosis

Vulnerability in self-esteem makes individuals with narcissistic personality disorder very sensitive to "injury" from criticism or defeat. Although they may not show it outwardly, criticism may haunt these individuals and may leave them feeling humiliated, degraded, hollow, and empty. They may react with disdain, rage, or defiant counterattack. Such experiences often lead to social withdrawal or an appearance of humility that may mask and protect the grandiosity. Interpersonal relations are typically impaired because of problems derived from entitlement, the need for admiration, and the relative disregard for the sensitivities of others. Though overweening ambition and confidence may lead to high achievement, performance may be disrupted because of intolerance of criticism or defeat. Sometimes vocational functioning can be very low, reflecting an unwillingness to take a risk in competitive or other situations in which defeat is possible. Sustained feelings of shame or humiliation and the attendant self-criticism may be associated with social withdrawal, depressed mood, and persistent depressive disorder (dysthymia) or major depressive disorder. In contrast, sustained periods of grandiosity may be associated with a hypomanic mood. Narcissistic personality disorder is also associated with anorexia nervosa and substance use disorders (especially related to cocaine). Histrionic, borderline, antisocial, and paranoid personality disorders may be associated with narcissistic personality disorder.

Prevalence

Prevalence estimates for narcissistic personality disorder, based on DSM-IV definitions, range from 0% to 6.2% in community samples.

Development and Course

Narcissistic traits may be particularly common in adolescents and do not necessarily indicate that the individual will go on to have narcissistic personality disorder. Individuals with narcissistic personality disorder may have special difficulties adjusting to the onset of physical and occupational limitations that are inherent in the aging process.

Gender-Related Diagnostic Issues

Of those diagnosed with narcissistic personality disorder, 50%–75% are male.

Differential Diagnosis

Other personality disorders and personality traits. Other personality disorders may be confused with narcissistic personality disorder because they have certain features in common. It is, therefore, important to distinguish among these disorders based on differences in their characteristic features. However, if an individual has personality features that meet criteria for one or more personality disorders in addition to narcissistic personality disorder, all can be diagnosed. The most useful feature in discriminating narcissistic personality disorder from histrionic, antisocial, and borderline personality disorders, in which the interactive styles are coquettish, callous, and needy, respectively, is the grandiosity characteristic of narcissistic personality disorder. The relative stability of self-image as well as the relative lack of self-destructiveness, impulsivity, and abandonment concerns also help distinguish narcissistic personality disorder from borderline personality disorder. Excessive pride in achievements, a relative lack of emotional display, and disdain for others' sensitivities help distinguish narcissistic personality disorder from histrionic personality disorder. Although individuals with borderline, histrionic, and narcissistic personality disorders may require much attention, those with narcissistic personality disorder specifically need that attention to be admiring. Individuals with antisocial and narcissistic personality disorders share a tendency to be tough-minded, glib, superficial, exploitative, and unempathic. However, narcissistic personality disorder does not necessarily include characteristics of impulsivity, aggression, and deceit. In addition, individuals with antisocial personality disorder may not be as needy of the admiration and envy of others, and persons with narcissistic personality disorder usually lack the history of conduct disorder in childhood or criminal behavior in adulthood. In both narcissistic personality disorder and obsessive-compulsive personality disorder, the individual may profess a commitment to perfectionism and believe that others cannot do things as well. In contrast to the accompanying self-criticism of those with obsessive-compulsive personality disorder, individuals with narcissistic personality disorder are more likely to believe that they have achieved perfection. Suspiciousness and social withdrawal usually distinguish those with schizotypal or paranoid personality disorder from those with narcissistic personality disorder. When these qualities are present in individuals with narcissistic personality disorder, they derive primarily from fears of having imperfections or flaws revealed.

Many highly successful individuals display personality traits that might be considered narcissistic. Only when these traits are inflexible, maladaptive, and persisting and cause significant functional impairment or subjective distress do they constitute narcissistic personality disorder.

Mania or hypomania.   Grandiosity may emerge as part of manic or hypomanic episodes, but the association with mood change or functional impairments helps distinguish these episodes from narcissistic personality disorder.

Substance use disorders.   Narcissistic personality disorder must also be distinguished from symptoms that may develop in association with persistent substance use.

Cluster C Personality Disorders

Avoidant Personality Disorder

Diagnostic Criteria   **301.82 (F60.6)**

A pervasive pattern of social inhibition, feelings of inadequacy, and hypersensitivity to negative evaluation, beginning by early adulthood and present in a variety of contexts, as indicated by four (or more) of the following:

1. Avoids occupational activities that involve significant interpersonal contact because of fears of criticism, disapproval, or rejection.

2. Is unwilling to get involved with people unless certain of being liked.
3. Shows restraint within intimate relationships because of the fear of being shamed or ridiculed.
4. Is preoccupied with being criticized or rejected in social situations.
5. Is inhibited in new interpersonal situations because of feelings of inadequacy.
6. Views self as socially inept, personally unappealing, or inferior to others.
7. Is unusually reluctant to take personal risks or to engage in any new activities because they may prove embarrassing.

Diagnostic Features

The essential feature of avoidant personality disorder is a pervasive pattern of social inhibition, feelings of inadequacy, and hypersensitivity to negative evaluation that begins by early adulthood and is present in a variety of contexts.

Individuals with avoidant personality disorder avoid work activities that involve significant interpersonal contact because of fears of criticism, disapproval, or rejection (Criterion 1). Offers of job promotions may be declined because the new responsibilities might result in criticism from co-workers. These individuals avoid making new friends unless they are certain they will be liked and accepted without criticism (Criterion 2). Until they pass stringent tests proving the contrary, other people are assumed to be critical and disapproving. Individuals with this disorder will not join in group activities unless there are repeated and generous offers of support and nurturance. Interpersonal intimacy is often difficult for these individuals, although they are able to establish intimate relationships when there is assurance of uncritical acceptance. They may act with restraint, have difficulty talking about themselves, and withhold intimate feelings for fear of being exposed, ridiculed, or shamed (Criterion 3).

Because individuals with this disorder are preoccupied with being criticized or rejected in social situations, they may have a markedly low threshold for detecting such reactions (Criterion 4). If someone is even slightly disapproving or critical, they may feel extremely hurt. They tend to be shy, quiet, inhibited, and "invisible" because of the fear that any attention would be degrading or rejecting. They expect that no matter what they say, others will see it as "wrong," and so they may say nothing at all. They react strongly to subtle cues that are suggestive of mockery or derision. Despite their longing to be active participants in social life, they fear placing their welfare in the hands of others. Individuals with avoidant personality disorder are inhibited in new interpersonal situations because they feel inadequate and have low self-esteem (Criterion 5). Doubts concerning social competence and personal appeal become especially manifest in settings involving interactions with strangers. These individuals believe themselves to be socially inept, personally unappealing, or inferior to others (Criterion 6). They are unusually reluctant to take personal risks or to engage in any new activities because these may prove embarrassing (Criterion 7). They are prone to exaggerate the potential dangers of ordinary situations, and a restricted lifestyle may result from their need for certainty and security. Someone with this disorder may cancel a job interview for fear of being embarrassed by not dressing appropriately. Marginal somatic symptoms or other problems may become the reason for avoiding new activities.

Associated Features Supporting Diagnosis

Individuals with avoidant personality disorder often vigilantly appraise the movements and expressions of those with whom they come into contact. Their fearful and tense demeanor may elicit ridicule and derision from others, which in turn confirms their self-doubts. These individuals are very anxious about the possibility that they will react to criticism with blushing or crying. They are described by others as being "shy," "timid," "lonely," and "isolated." The major problems associated with this disorder occur in social and occupational functioning. The low self-esteem and hypersensitivity to rejection are associated with restricted interpersonal contacts. These individuals may become relatively isolated and usually do not have a large social support network that can help them weather crises. They desire affection and acceptance and may fantasize about idealized relationships with others. The avoidant behaviors can also adversely affect occupational functioning because these individuals try to avoid the types of social situations that may be important for meeting the basic demands of the job or for advancement.

Other disorders that are commonly diagnosed with avoidant personality disorder include depressive, bipolar, and anxiety disorders, especially social anxiety disorder (social phobia). Avoidant personality disorder is often diagnosed with dependent personality disorder, because individuals with avoidant personality disorder become very attached to and dependent on those few other people with whom they are friends. Avoidant personality disorder also tends to be diagnosed with borderline personality disorder and with the Cluster A personality disorders (i.e., paranoid, schizoid, or schizotypal personality disorders).

Prevalence

Data from the 2001–2002 National Epidemiologic Survey on Alcohol and Related Conditions suggest a prevalence of about 2.4% for avoidant personality disorder.

Development and Course

The avoidant behavior often starts in infancy or childhood with shyness, isolation, and fear of strangers and new situations. Although shyness in childhood is a common precursor of avoidant personality disorder, in most individuals it tends to gradually dissipate as they get older. In contrast, individuals who go on to develop avoidant personality disorder may become increasingly shy and avoidant during adolescence and early adulthood, when social relationships with new people become especially important. There is some evidence that in adults, avoidant personality disorder tends to become less evident or to remit with age. This diagnosis should be used with great caution in children and adolescents, for whom shy and avoidant behavior may be developmentally appropriate.

Culture-Related Diagnostic Issues

There may be variation in the degree to which different cultural and ethnic groups regard diffidence and avoidance as appropriate. Moreover, avoidant behavior may be the result of problems in acculturation following immigration.

Gender-Related Diagnostic Issues

Avoidant personality disorder appears to be equally frequent in males and females.

Differential Diagnosis

Anxiety disorders. There appears to be a great deal of overlap between avoidant personality disorder and social anxiety disorder (social phobia), so much so that they may be alternative conceptualizations of the same or similar conditions. Avoidance also characterizes both avoidant personality disorder and agoraphobia, and they often co-occur.

Other personality disorders and personality traits. Other personality disorders may be confused with avoidant personality disorder because they have certain features in common. It is, therefore, important to distinguish among these disorders based on differences in their characteristic features. However, if an individual has personality features that meet criteria for one or more personality disorders in addition to avoidant personality disorder, all can be diagnosed. Both avoidant personality disorder and dependent personality disorder are characterized by feelings of inadequacy, hypersensitivity to criticism, and a need for reassurance. Although the primary focus of concern in avoidant personality disorder is avoidance of humiliation and rejection, in dependent personality disorder the focus is on being taken care of. However, avoidant personality disorder and dependent personality disorder are particularly likely to co-occur. Like avoidant personality disorder, schizoid personality disorder and schizotypal personality disorder are characterized by social isolation. However, individuals with avoidant personality disorder want to have relationships with others and feel their loneliness deeply, whereas those with schizoid or schizotypal personality disorder may be content with and even prefer their social isolation. Paranoid personality disorder and avoidant personality disorder are both characterized by a reluctance to confide in others. However, in avoidant personality disorder, this reluctance is attributable more to a fear of being embarrassed or being found inadequate than to a fear of others' malicious intent.

Many individuals display avoidant personality traits. Only when these traits are inflexible, maladaptive, and persisting and cause significant functional impairment or subjective distress do they constitute avoidant personality disorder.

Personality change due to another medical condition.   Avoidant personality disorder must be distinguished from personality change due to another medical condition, in which the traits that emerge are attributable to the effects of another medical condition on the central nervous system.

Substance use disorders.   Avoidant personality disorder must also be distinguished from symptoms that may develop in association with persistent substance use.

Dependent Personality Disorder

Diagnostic Criteria   301.6 (F60.7)

A pervasive and excessive need to be taken care of that leads to submissive and clinging behavior and fears of separation, beginning by early adulthood and present in a variety of contexts, as indicated by five (or more) of the following:

1. Has difficulty making everyday decisions without an excessive amount of advice and reassurance from others.
2. Needs others to assume responsibility for most major areas of his or her life.
3. Has difficulty expressing disagreement with others because of fear of loss of support or approval. (**Note:** Do not include realistic fears of retribution.)
4. Has difficulty initiating projects or doing things on his or her own (because of a lack of self-confidence in judgment or abilities rather than a lack of motivation or energy).
5. Goes to excessive lengths to obtain nurturance and support from others, to the point of volunteering to do things that are unpleasant.
6. Feels uncomfortable or helpless when alone because of exaggerated fears of being unable to care for himself or herself.
7. Urgently seeks another relationship as a source of care and support when a close relationship ends.
8. Is unrealistically preoccupied with fears of being left to take care of himself or herself.

Diagnostic Features

The essential feature of dependent personality disorder is a pervasive and excessive need to be taken care of that leads to submissive and clinging behavior and fears of separation. This pattern begins by early adulthood and is present in a variety of contexts. The dependent and submissive behaviors are designed to elicit caregiving and arise from a self-perception of being unable to function adequately without the help of others.

Individuals with dependent personality disorder have great difficulty making everyday decisions (e.g., what color shirt to wear to work or whether to carry an umbrella) without an excessive amount of advice and reassurance from others (Criterion 1). These individuals tend to be passive and to allow other people (often a single other person) to take the initiative and assume responsibility for most major areas of their lives (Criterion 2). Adults with this disorder typically depend on a parent or spouse to decide where they should live, what kind of job they should have, and which neighbors to befriend. Adolescents with this disorder may allow their parent(s) to decide what they should wear, with whom they should associate, how they should spend their free time, and what school or college they should attend. This need for others to assume responsibility goes beyond age-appropriate and situation-appropriate requests for assistance from others (e.g., the specific needs of children, elderly persons, and handicapped persons). Dependent personality disorder may occur in an individual who has a serious medical condition or disability, but in such cases the difficulty in taking responsibility must go beyond what would normally be associated with that condition or disability.

Because they fear losing support or approval, individuals with dependent personality disorder often have difficulty expressing disagreement with other individuals, especially those on whom they are dependent (Criterion 3). These individuals feel so unable to function alone that they will agree with things that they feel are wrong rather than risk losing the help of those to whom they look for guidance. They do not get appropriately angry at others whose support and nurturance they need for fear of alienating them. If the individual's concerns regarding the consequences of expressing disagreement are realistic (e.g., realistic fears of retribution from an abusive spouse), the behavior should not be considered to be evidence of dependent personality disorder.

Individuals with this disorder have difficulty initiating projects or doing things independently (Criterion 4). They lack self-confidence and believe that they need help to begin and carry through tasks. They will wait for others to start things because they believe that as a rule others can do them better. These individuals are convinced that they are incapable of functioning independently and present themselves as inept and requiring constant assistance. They are, however, likely to function adequately if given the assurance that someone else is supervising and approving. There may be a fear of becoming or appearing to be more competent, because they may believe that this will lead to abandonment. Because they rely on others to handle their problems, they often do not learn the skills of independent living, thus perpetuating dependency.

Individuals with dependent personality disorder may go to excessive lengths to obtain nurturance and support from others, even to the point of volunteering for unpleasant tasks if such behavior will bring the care they need (Criterion 5). They are willing to submit to what others want, even if the demands are unreasonable. Their need to maintain an important bond will often result in imbalanced or distorted relationships. They may make extraordinary self-sacrifices or tolerate verbal, physical, or sexual abuse. (It should be noted that this behavior should be considered evidence of dependent personality disorder only when it can clearly be established that other options are available to the individual.) Individuals with this disorder feel uncomfortable or helpless when alone, because of their exaggerated fears of being unable to care for themselves (Criterion 6). They will "tag along" with important others just to avoid being alone, even if they are not interested or involved in what is happening.

When a close relationship ends (e.g., a breakup with a lover; the death of a caregiver), individuals with dependent personality disorder may urgently seek another relationship to provide the care and support they need (Criterion 7). Their belief that they are unable to function in the absence of a close relationship motivates these individuals to become quickly and indiscriminately attached to another individual. Individuals with this disorder are often preoccupied with fears of being left to care for themselves (Criterion 8). They see themselves as so totally dependent on the advice and help of an important other person that they worry about being abandoned by that person when there are no grounds to justify such fears. To be considered as evidence of this criterion, the fears must be excessive and unrealistic. For example, an elderly man with cancer who moves into his son's household for care is exhibiting dependent behavior that is appropriate given this person's life circumstances.

Associated Features Supporting Diagnosis

Individuals with dependent personality disorder are often characterized by pessimism and self-doubt, tend to belittle their abilities and assets, and may constantly refer to themselves as "stupid." They take criticism and disapproval as proof of their worthlessness and lose faith in themselves. They may seek overprotection and dominance from others. Occupational functioning may be impaired if independent initiative is required. They may avoid positions of responsibility and become anxious when faced with decisions. Social relations tend to be limited to those few people on whom the individual is dependent. There may be an increased risk of depressive disorders, anxiety disorders, and adjustment disorders. Dependent personality disorder often co-occurs with other personality disorders, especially borderline, avoidant, and histrionic personality disorders. Chronic physical illness or separation anxiety disorder in childhood or adolescence may predispose the individual to the development of this disorder.

Prevalence

Data from the 2001–2002 National Epidemiologic Survey on Alcohol and Related Conditions yielded an estimated prevalence of dependent personality disorder of 0.49%, and dependent personality was estimated, based on a probability subsample from Part II of the National Comorbidity Survey Replication, to be 0.6%.

Development and Course

This diagnosis should be used with great caution, if at all, in children and adolescents, for whom dependent behavior may be developmentally appropriate.

Culture-Related Diagnostic Issues

The degree to which dependent behaviors are considered to be appropriate varies substantially across different age and sociocultural groups. Age and cultural factors need to be considered in evaluating the diagnostic threshold of each criterion. Dependent behavior should be considered characteristic of the disorder only when it is clearly in excess of the individual's cultural norms or reflects unrealistic concerns. An emphasis on passivity, politeness, and deferential treatment is characteristic of some societies and may be misinterpreted as traits of dependent personality disorder. Similarly, societies may differentially foster and discourage dependent behavior in males and females.

Gender-Related Diagnostic Issues

In clinical settings, dependent personality disorder has been diagnosed more frequently in females, although some studies report similar prevalence rates among males and females.

Differential Diagnosis

Other mental disorders and medical conditions. Dependent personality disorder must be distinguished from dependency arising as a consequence of other mental disorders (e.g., depressive disorders, panic disorder, agoraphobia) and as a result of other medical conditions.

Other personality disorders and personality traits.   Other personality disorders may be confused with dependent personality disorder because they have certain features in common. It is therefore important to distinguish among these disorders based on differences in their characteristic features. However, if an individual has personality features that meet criteria for one or more personality disorders in addition to dependent personality disorder, all can be diagnosed. Although many personality disorders are characterized by dependent features, dependent personality disorder can be distinguished by its predominantly submissive, reactive, and clinging behavior. Both dependent personality disorder and borderline personality disorder are characterized by fear of abandonment; however, the individual with borderline personality disorder reacts to abandonment with feelings of emotional emptiness, rage, and demands, whereas the individual with dependent personality disorder reacts with increasing appeasement and submissiveness and urgently seeks a replacement relationship to provide caregiving and support. Borderline personality disorder can further be distinguished from dependent personality disorder by a typical pattern of unstable and intense relationships. Individuals with histrionic personality disorder, like those with dependent personality disorder, have a strong need for reassurance and approval and may appear childlike and clinging. However, unlike dependent personality disorder, which is characterized by self-effacing and docile behavior, histrionic personality disorder is characterized by gregarious flamboyance with active demands for attention. Both dependent personality disorder and avoidant personality disorder are characterized by feelings of inadequacy, hypersensitivity to criticism, and a need for reassurance; however, individuals with avoidant personality disorder have such a strong fear of humiliation and rejection that they withdraw until they are certain they will be accepted. In contrast, individuals with dependent personality disorder have a pattern of seeking and maintaining connections to important others, rather than avoiding and withdrawing from relationships.

Many individuals display dependent personality traits. Only when these traits are inflexible, maladaptive, and persisting and cause significant functional impairment or subjective distress do they constitute dependent personality disorder.

Personality change due to another medical condition.   Dependent personality disorder must be distinguished from personality change due to another medical condition, in which the traits that emerge are attributable to the effects of another medical condition on the central nervous system.

Substance use disorders.   Dependent personality disorder must also be distinguished from symptoms that may develop in association with persistent substance use.

Obsessive-Compulsive Personality Disorder

Diagnostic Criteria   **301.4 (F60.5)**

A pervasive pattern of preoccupation with orderliness, perfectionism, and mental and interpersonal control, at the expense of flexibility, openness, and efficiency, beginning by early adulthood and present in a variety of contexts, as indicated by four (or more) of the following:

1. Is preoccupied with details, rules, lists, order, organization, or schedules to the extent that the major point of the activity is lost.
2. Shows perfectionism that interferes with task completion (e.g., is unable to complete a project because his or her own overly strict standards are not met).
3. Is excessively devoted to work and productivity to the exclusion of leisure activities and friendships (not accounted for by obvious economic necessity).
4. Is overconscientious, scrupulous, and inflexible about matters of morality, ethics, or values (not accounted for by cultural or religious identification).

5. Is unable to discard worn-out or worthless objects even when they have no sentimental value.
6. Is reluctant to delegate tasks or to work with others unless they submit to exactly his or her way of doing things.
7. Adopts a miserly spending style toward both self and others; money is viewed as something to be hoarded for future catastrophes.
8. Shows rigidity and stubbornness.

Diagnostic Features

The essential feature of obsessive-compulsive personality disorder is a preoccupation with orderliness, perfectionism, and mental and interpersonal control, at the expense of flexibility, openness, and efficiency. This pattern begins by early adulthood and is present in a variety of contexts.

Individuals with obsessive-compulsive personality disorder attempt to maintain a sense of control through painstaking attention to rules, trivial details, procedures, lists, schedules, or form to the extent that the major point of the activity is lost (Criterion 1). They are excessively careful and prone to repetition, paying extraordinary attention to detail and repeatedly checking for possible mistakes. They are oblivious to the fact that other people tend to become very annoyed at the delays and inconveniences that result from this behavior. For example, when such individuals misplace a list of things to be done, they will spend an inordinate amount of time looking for the list rather than spending a few moments re-creating it from memory and proceeding to accomplish the tasks. Time is poorly allocated, and the most important tasks are left to the last moment. The perfectionism and self-imposed high standards of performance cause significant dysfunction and distress in these individuals. They may become so involved in making every detail of a project absolutely perfect that the project is never finished (Criterion 2). For example, the completion of a written report is delayed by numerous time-consuming rewrites that all come up short of "perfection." Deadlines are missed, and aspects of the individual's life that are not the current focus of activity may fall into disarray.

Individuals with obsessive-compulsive personality disorder display excessive devotion to work and productivity to the exclusion of leisure activities and friendships (Criterion 3). This behavior is not accounted for by economic necessity. They often feel that they do not have time to take an evening or a weekend day off to go on an outing or to just relax. They may keep postponing a pleasurable activity, such as a vacation, so that it may never occur. When they do take time for leisure activities or vacations, they are very uncomfortable unless they have taken along something to work on so they do not "waste time." There may be a great concentration on household chores (e.g., repeated excessive cleaning so that "one could eat off the floor"). If they spend time with friends, it is likely to be in some kind of formally organized activity (e.g., sports). Hobbies or recreational activities are approached as serious tasks requiring careful organization and hard work to master. The emphasis is on perfect performance. These individuals turn play into a structured task (e.g., correcting an infant for not putting rings on the post in the right order; telling a toddler to ride his or her tricycle in a straight line; turning a baseball game into a harsh "lesson").

Individuals with obsessive-compulsive personality disorder may be excessively conscientious, scrupulous, and inflexible about matters of morality, ethics, or values (Criterion 4). They may force themselves and others to follow rigid moral principles and very strict standards of performance. They may also be mercilessly self-critical about their own mistakes. Individuals with this disorder are rigidly deferential to authority and rules and insist on quite literal compliance, with no rule bending for extenuating circumstances. For example, the individual will not lend a quarter to a friend who needs one to make a telephone call because "neither a borrower nor a lender be" or because it would be "bad" for the person's character. These qualities should not be accounted for by the individual's cultural or religious identification.

Individuals with this disorder may be unable to discard worn-out or worthless objects, even when they have no sentimental value (Criterion 5). Often these individuals will admit to being "pack rats." They regard discarding objects as wasteful because "you never know when you might need something" and will become upset if someone tries to get rid of the things they have saved. Their spouses or roommates may complain about the amount of space taken up by old parts, magazines, broken appliances, and so on.

Individuals with obsessive-compulsive personality disorder are reluctant to delegate tasks or to work with others (Criterion 6). They stubbornly and unreasonably insist that everything be done their way and that people conform to their way of doing things. They often give very detailed instructions about how things should be done (e.g., there is one and only one way to mow the lawn, wash the dishes, build a doghouse) and are surprised and irritated if others suggest creative alternatives. At other times they may reject offers of help even when behind schedule because they believe no one else can do it right.

Individuals with this disorder may be miserly and stingy and maintain a standard of living far below what they can afford, believing that spending must be tightly controlled to provide for future catastrophes (Criterion 7). Obsessive-compulsive personality disorder is characterized by rigidity and stubbornness (Criterion 8). Individuals with this disorder are so concerned about having things done the one "correct" way that they have trouble going along with anyone else's ideas. These individuals plan ahead in meticulous detail and are unwilling to consider changes. Totally wrapped up in their own perspective, they have difficulty acknowledging the viewpoints of others. Friends and colleagues may become frustrated by this constant rigidity. Even when individuals with obsessive-compulsive personality disorder recognize that it may be in their interest to compromise, they may stubbornly refuse to do so, arguing that it is "the principle of the thing."

Associated Features Supporting Diagnosis

When rules and established procedures do not dictate the correct answer, decision making may become a time-consuming, often painful process. Individuals with obsessive-compulsive personality disorder may have such difficulty deciding which tasks take priority or what is the best way of doing some particular task that they may never get started on anything. They are prone to become upset or angry in situations in which they are not able to maintain control of their physical or interpersonal environment, although the anger is typically not expressed directly. For example, an individual may be angry when service in a restaurant is poor, but instead of complaining to the management, the individual ruminates about how much to leave as a tip. On other occasions, anger may be expressed with righteous indignation over a seemingly minor matter. Individuals with this disorder may be especially attentive to their relative status in dominance-submission relationships and may display excessive deference to an authority they respect and excessive resistance to authority they do not respect.

Individuals with this disorder usually express affection in a highly controlled or stilted fashion and may be very uncomfortable in the presence of others who are emotionally expressive. Their everyday relationships have a formal and serious quality, and they may be stiff in situations in which others would smile and be happy (e.g., greeting a lover at the airport). They carefully hold themselves back until they are sure that whatever they say will be perfect. They may be preoccupied with logic and intellect, and intolerant of affective behavior in others. They often have difficulty expressing tender feelings, rarely paying compliments. Individuals with this disorder may experience occupational difficulties and distress, particularly when confronted with new situations that demand flexibility and compromise.

Individuals with anxiety disorders, including generalized anxiety disorder, social anxiety disorder (social phobia), and specific phobias, and obsessive-compulsive disorder (OCD) have an increased likelihood of having a personality disturbance that meets criteria for obsessive-compulsive personality disorder. Even so, it appears that the majority of individuals with OCD do not have a pattern of behavior that meets criteria for this personality disorder. Many of the features of obsessive-compulsive personality disorder overlap with "type A" personality characteristics (e.g., preoccupation with work, competitiveness, time urgency), and these features may be present in people at risk for myocardial infarction. There may be an association between obsessive-compulsive personality disorder and depressive and bipolar disorders and eating disorders.

Prevalence

Obsessive-compulsive personality disorder is one of the most prevalent personality disorders in the general population, with estimated prevalence ranging from 2.1% to 7.9%.

Culture-Related Diagnostic Issues

In assessing an individual for obsessive-compulsive personality disorder, the clinician should not include those behaviors that reflect habits, customs, or interpersonal styles that are culturally sanctioned by the individual's reference group. Certain cultures place substantial emphasis on work and productivity; the resulting behaviors in members of those societies need not be considered indications of obsessive-compulsive personality disorder.

Gender-Related Diagnostic Issues

In systematic studies, obsessive-compulsive personality disorder appears to be diagnosed about twice as often among males.

Differential Diagnosis

Obsessive-compulsive disorder.   Despite the similarity in names, OCD is usually easily distinguished from obsessive-compulsive personality disorder by the presence of true obsessions and compulsions in OCD. When criteria for both obsessive-compulsive personality disorder and OCD are met, both diagnoses should be recorded.

Hoarding disorder.   A diagnosis of hoarding disorder should be considered especially when hoarding is extreme (e.g., accumulated stacks of worthless objects present a fire hazard and make it difficult for others to walk through the house). When criteria for both obsessive-compulsive personality disorder and hoarding disorder are met, both diagnoses should be recorded.

Other personality disorders and personality traits.   Other personality disorders may be confused with obsessive-compulsive personality disorder because they have certain features in common. It is, therefore, important to distinguish among these disorders based on differences in their characteristic features. However, if an individual has personality features that meet criteria for one or more personality disorders in addition to obsessive-compulsive personality disorder, all can be diagnosed. Individuals with narcissistic personality disorder may also profess a commitment to perfectionism and believe that others cannot do things as well, but these individuals are more likely to believe that they have achieved perfection, whereas those with obsessive-compulsive personality disorder are usually self-critical. Individuals with narcissistic or antisocial personality disorder lack generosity but will indulge themselves, whereas those with obsessive-compulsive personality disorder adopt a miserly spending style toward both self and others. Both schizoid personality disorder and obsessive-compulsive personality disorder may be characterized by an apparent formality and social detachment. In obsessive-compulsive personality disorder, this stems from discomfort with emotions and excessive devotion to work, whereas in schizoid personality disorder there is a fundamental lack of capacity for intimacy.

Obsessive-compulsive personality traits in moderation may be especially adaptive, particularly in situations that reward high performance. Only when these traits are inflexible, maladaptive, and persisting and cause significant functional impairment or subjective distress do they constitute obsessive-compulsive personality disorder.

Personality change due to another medical condition.   Obsessive-compulsive personality disorder must be distinguished from personality change due to another medical condition, in which the traits emerge attributable to the effects of another medical condition on the central nervous system.

Substance use disorders.   Obsessive-compulsive personality disorder must also be distinguished from symptoms that may develop in association with persistent substance use.

Other Personality Disorders

Personality Change
Due to Another Medical Condition

Diagnostic Criteria   **310.1 (F07.0)**

A. A persistent personality disturbance that represents a change from the individual's previous characteristic personality pattern.

   Note: In children, the disturbance involves a marked deviation from normal development or a significant change in the child's usual behavior patterns, lasting at least 1 year.

B. There is evidence from the history, physical examination, or laboratory findings that the disturbance is the direct pathophysiological consequence of another medical condition.

C. The disturbance is not better explained by another mental disorder (including another mental disorder due to another medical condition).

D. The disturbance does not occur exclusively during the course of a delirium.

E. The disturbance causes clinically significant distress or impairment in social, occupational, or other important areas of functioning.

Specify whether:
   Labile type: If the predominant feature is affective lability.
   Disinhibited type: If the predominant feature is poor impulse control as evidenced by sexual indiscretions, etc.
   Aggressive type: If the predominant feature is aggressive behavior.
   Apathetic type: If the predominant feature is marked apathy and indifference.
   Paranoid type: If the predominant feature is suspiciousness or paranoid ideation.
   Other type: If the presentation is not characterized by any of the above subtypes.
   Combined type: If more than one feature predominates in the clinical picture.
   Unspecified type

Coding note: Include the name of the other medical condition (e.g., 310.1 [F07.0] personality change due to temporal lobe epilepsy). The other medical condition should be coded and listed separately immediately before the personality disorder due to another medical condition (e.g., 345.40 [G40.209] temporal lobe epilepsy; 310.1 [F07.0] personality change due to temporal lobe epilepsy).

Subtypes

The particular personality change can be specified by indicating the symptom presentation that predominates in the clinical presentation.

Diagnostic Features

The essential feature of a personality change due to another medical condition is a persistent personality disturbance that is judged to be due to the direct pathophysiological effects of a medical condition. The personality disturbance represents a change from the individual's previous characteristic personality pattern. In children, this condition may be manifested as a marked deviation from normal development rather than as a change in a stable personality pattern (Criterion A). There must be evidence from the history, physical examination, or laboratory findings that the personality change is the direct physiological consequence of another medical condition (Criterion B). The diagnosis is not given if the disturbance is better explained by another mental disorder (Criterion C). The diagnosis is not given if the disturbance occurs exclusively during the course of a delirium (Criterion D). The disturbance must also cause clinically significant distress or impairment in social, occupational, or other important areas of functioning (Criterion E).

Common manifestations of the personality change include affective instability, poor impulse control, outbursts of aggression or rage grossly out of proportion to any precipitating psychosocial stressor, marked apathy, suspiciousness, or paranoid ideation. The phenomenology of the change is indicated using the subtypes listed in the criteria set. An individual with the disorder is often characterized by others as "not himself [or herself]." Although it shares the term "personality" with the other personality disorders, this diagnosis is distinct by virtue of its specific etiology, different phenomenology, and more variable onset and course.

The clinical presentation in a given individual may depend on the nature and localization of the pathological process. For example, injury to the frontal lobes may yield symptoms such as lack of judgment or foresight, facetiousness, disinhibition, and euphoria. Right hemisphere strokes have often been shown to evoke personality changes in association with unilateral spatial neglect, anosognosia (i.e., inability of the individual to recognize a bodily or functional deficit, such as the existence of hemiparesis), motor impersistence, and other neurological deficits.

Associated Features Supporting Diagnosis

A variety of neurological and other medical conditions may cause personality changes, including central nervous system neoplasms, head trauma, cerebrovascular disease, Huntington's disease, epilepsy, infectious conditions with central nervous system involvement (e.g., HIV), endocrine conditions (e.g., hypothyroidism, hypo- and hyperadrenocorticism), and autoimmune conditions with central nervous system involvement (e.g., systemic lupus erythematosus). The associated physical examination findings, laboratory findings, and patterns of prevalence and onset reflect those of the neurological or other medical condition involved.

Differential Diagnosis

Chronic medical conditions associated with pain and disability.   Chronic medical conditions associated with pain and disability can also be associated with changes in personality. The diagnosis of personality change due to another medical condition is given only if a direct pathophysiological mechanism can be established. This diagnosis is not given if the change is due to a behavioral or psychological adjustment or response to another medical condition (e.g., dependent behaviors that result from a need for the assistance of others following a severe head trauma, cardiovascular disease, or dementia).

Delirium or major neurocognitive disorder.   Personality change is a frequently associated feature of a delirium or major neurocognitive disorder. A separate diagnosis of personality change due to another medical condition is not given if the change occurs exclusively during the course of a delirium. However, the diagnosis of personality change due to another medical condition may be given in addition to the diagnosis of major neurocognitive disorder if the personality change is a prominent part of the clinical presentation.

Another mental disorder due to another medical condition.   The diagnosis of personality change due to another medical condition is not given if the disturbance is better explained by another mental disorder due to another medical condition (e.g., depressive disorder due to brain tumor).

Substance use disorders.   Personality changes may also occur in the context of substance use disorders, especially if the disorder is long-standing. The clinician should inquire carefully about the nature and extent of substance use. If the clinician wishes to indicate an etiological relationship between the personality change and substance use, the unspecified category for the specific substance (e.g., unspecified stimulant-related disorder) can be used.

Other mental disorders.   Marked personality changes may also be an associated feature of other mental disorders (e.g., schizophrenia; delusional disorder; depressive and bipolar disorders; other specified and unspecified disruptive behavior, impulse-control, and conduct disorders; panic disorder). However, in these disorders, no specific physiological factor is judged to be etiologically related to the personality change.

Other personality disorders.   Personality change due to another medical condition can be distinguished from a personality disorder by the requirement for a clinically significant change from baseline personality functioning and the presence of a specific etiological medical condition.

Other Specified Personality Disorder

301.89 (F60.89)

This category applies to presentations in which symptoms characteristic of a personality disorder that cause clinically significant distress or impairment in social, occupational, or other important areas of functioning predominate but do not meet the full criteria for any of the disorders in the personality disorders diagnostic class. The other specified personality disorder category is used in situations in which the clinician chooses to communicate the specific reason that the presentation does not meet the criteria for any specific personality disorder. This is done by recording "other specified personality disorder" followed by the specific reason (e.g., "mixed personality features").

Unspecified Personality Disorder

301.9 (F60.9)

This category applies to presentations in which symptoms characteristic of a personality disorder that cause clinically significant distress or impairment in social, occupational, or other important areas of functioning predominate but do not meet the full criteria for any of the disorders in the personality disorders diagnostic class. The unspecified personality disorder category is used in situations in which the clinician chooses *not* to specify the reason that the criteria are not met for a specific personality disorder, and includes presentations in which there is insufficient information to make a more specific diagnosis.

Paraphilic Disorders

Paraphilic disorders included in this manual are voyeuristic disorder (spying on others in private activities), exhibitionistic disorder (exposing the genitals), frotteuristic disorder (touching or rubbing against a nonconsenting individual), sexual masochism disorder (undergoing humiliation, bondage, or suffering), sexual sadism disorder (inflicting humiliation, bondage, or suffering), pedophilic disorder (sexual focus on children), fetishistic disorder (using nonliving objects or having a highly specific focus on nongenital body parts), and transvestic disorder (engaging in sexually arousing cross-dressing). These disorders have traditionally been selected for specific listing and assignment of explicit diagnostic criteria in DSM for two main reasons: they are relatively common, in relation to other paraphilic disorders, and some of them entail actions for their satisfaction that, because of their noxiousness or potential harm to others, are classed as criminal offenses. The eight listed disorders do not exhaust the list of possible paraphilic disorders. Many dozens of distinct paraphilias have been identified and named, and almost any of them could, by virtue of its negative consequences for the individual or for others, rise to the level of a paraphilic disorder. The diagnoses of the other specified and unspecified paraphilic disorders are therefore indispensable and will be required in many cases.

In this chapter, the order of presentation of the listed paraphilic disorders generally corresponds to common classification schemes for these conditions. The first group of disorders is based on *anomalous activity preferences.* These disorders are subdivided into *courtship disorders,* which resemble distorted components of human courtship behavior (voyeuristic disorder, exhibitionistic disorder, and frotteuristic disorder), and *algolagnic disorders,* which involve pain and suffering (sexual masochism disorder and sexual sadism disorder). The second group of disorders is based on *anomalous target preferences.* These disorders include one directed at other humans (pedophilic disorder) and two directed elsewhere (fetishistic disorder and transvestic disorder).

The term *paraphilia* denotes any intense and persistent sexual interest other than sexual interest in genital stimulation or preparatory fondling with phenotypically normal, physically mature, consenting human partners. In some circumstances, the criteria "intense and persistent" may be difficult to apply, such as in the assessment of persons who are very old or medically ill and who may not have "intense" sexual interests of any kind. In such circumstances, the term *paraphilia* may be defined as any sexual interest greater than or equal to normophilic sexual interests. There are also specific paraphilias that are generally better described as *preferential* sexual interests than as intense sexual interests.

Some paraphilias primarily concern the individual's erotic activities, and others primarily concern the individual's erotic targets. Examples of the former would include intense and persistent interests in spanking, whipping, cutting, binding, or strangulating another person, or an interest in these activities that equals or exceeds the individual's interest in copulation or equivalent interaction with another person. Examples of the latter would include intense or preferential sexual interest in children, corpses, or amputees (as a class), as well as intense or preferential interest in nonhuman animals, such as horses or dogs, or in inanimate objects, such as shoes or articles made of rubber.

A *paraphilic disorder* is a paraphilia that is currently causing distress or impairment to the individual or a paraphilia whose satisfaction has entailed personal harm, or risk of harm, to others. A paraphilia is a necessary but not a sufficient condition for having a paraphilic disorder, and a paraphilia by itself does not necessarily justify or require clinical intervention.

In the diagnostic criteria set for each of the listed paraphilic disorders, Criterion A specifies the qualitative nature of the paraphilia (e.g., an erotic focus on children or on exposing the genitals to strangers), and Criterion B specifies the negative consequences of the paraphilia (i.e., distress, impairment, or harm to others). In keeping with the distinction between paraphilias and paraphilic disorders, the term *diagnosis* should be reserved for individuals who meet both Criteria A and B (i.e., individuals who have a paraphilic disorder). If an individual meets Criterion A but not Criterion B for a particular paraphilia—a circumstance that might arise when a benign paraphilia is discovered during the clinical investigation of some other condition—then the individual may be said to have that paraphilia but not a paraphilic disorder.

It is not rare for an individual to manifest two or more paraphilias. In some cases, the paraphilic foci are closely related and the connection between the paraphilias is intuitively comprehensible (e.g., foot fetishism and shoe fetishism). In other cases, the connection between the paraphilias is not obvious, and the presence of multiple paraphilias may be coincidental or else related to some generalized vulnerability to anomalies of psychosexual development. In any event, comorbid diagnoses of separate paraphilic disorders may be warranted if more than one paraphilia is causing suffering to the individual or harm to others.

Because of the two-pronged nature of diagnosing paraphilic disorders, clinician-rated or self-rated measures and severity assessments could address either the strength of the paraphilia itself or the seriousness of its consequences. Although the distress and impairment stipulated in the Criterion B are special in being the immediate or ultimate result of the paraphilia and not primarily the result of some other factor, the phenomena of reactive depression, anxiety, guilt, poor work history, impaired social relations, and so on are not unique in themselves and may be quantified with multipurpose measures of psychosocial functioning or quality of life.

The most widely applicable framework for assessing the strength of a paraphilia itself is one in which examinees' paraphilic sexual fantasies, urges, or behaviors are evaluated in relation to their normophilic sexual interests and behaviors. In a clinical interview or on self-administered questionnaires, examinees can be asked whether their paraphilic sexual fantasies, urges, or behaviors are weaker than, approximately equal to, or stronger than their normophilic sexual interests and behaviors. This same type of comparison can be, and usually is, employed in psychophysiological measures of sexual interest, such as penile plethysmography in males or viewing time in males and females.

Voyeuristic Disorder

Diagnostic Criteria   **302.82** (F65.3)

A. Over a period of at least 6 months, recurrent and intense sexual arousal from observing an unsuspecting person who is naked, in the process of disrobing, or engaging in sexual activity, as manifested by fantasies, urges, or behaviors.

B. The individual has acted on these sexual urges with a nonconsenting person, or the sexual urges or fantasies cause clinically significant distress or impairment in social, occupational, or other important areas of functioning.

C. The individual experiencing the arousal and/or acting on the urges is at least 18 years of age.

Specify if:

In a controlled environment: This specifier is primarily applicable to individuals living in institutional or other settings where opportunities to engage in voyeuristic behavior are restricted.

In full remission: The individual has not acted on the urges with a nonconsenting person, and there has been no distress or impairment in social, occupational, or other areas of functioning, for at least 5 years while in an uncontrolled environment.

Specifiers

The "in full remission" specifier does not address the continued presence or absence of voyeurism per se, which may still be present after behaviors and distress have remitted.

Diagnostic Features

The diagnostic criteria for voyeuristic disorder can apply both to individuals who more or less freely disclose this paraphilic interest and to those who categorically deny any sexual arousal from observing an unsuspecting person who is naked, disrobing, or engaged in sexual activity despite substantial objective evidence to the contrary. If disclosing individuals also report distress or psychosocial problems because of their voyeuristic sexual preferences, they could be diagnosed with voyeuristic disorder. On the other hand, if they declare no distress, demonstrated by lack of anxiety, obsessions, guilt, or shame, about these paraphilic impulses and are not impaired in other important areas of functioning because of this sexual interest, and their psychiatric or legal histories indicate that they do not act on it, they could be ascertained as having voyeuristic sexual interest but should *not* be diagnosed with voyeuristic disorder.

Nondisclosing individuals include, for example, individuals known to have been spying repeatedly on unsuspecting persons who are naked or engaging in sexual activity on separate occasions but who deny any urges or fantasies concerning such sexual behavior, and who may report that known episodes of watching unsuspecting naked or sexually active persons were all accidental and nonsexual. Others may disclose past episodes of observing unsuspecting naked or sexually active persons but contest any significant or sustained sexual interest in this behavior. Since these individuals deny having fantasies or impulses about watching others nude or involved in sexual activity, it follows that they would also reject feeling subjectively distressed or socially impaired by such impulses. Despite their nondisclosing stance, such individuals may be diagnosed with voyeuristic disorder. Recurrent voyeuristic behavior constitutes sufficient support for voyeurism (by fulfilling Criterion A) and simultaneously demonstrates that this paraphilically motivated behavior is causing harm to others (by fulfilling Criterion B).

"Recurrent" spying on unsuspecting persons who are naked or engaging in sexual activity (i.e., multiple victims, each on a separate occasion) may, as a general rule, be interpreted as three or more victims on separate occasions. Fewer victims can be interpreted as satisfying this criterion if there were multiple occasions of watching the same victim or if there is corroborating evidence of a distinct or preferential interest in secret watching of naked or sexually active unsuspecting persons. Note that multiple victims, as suggested earlier, are a sufficient but not a necessary condition for diagnosis; the criteria may also be met if the individual acknowledges intense voyeuristic sexual interest.

The Criterion A time frame, indicating that signs or symptoms of voyeurism must have persisted for at least 6 months, should also be understood as a general guideline, not a strict threshold, to ensure that the sexual interest in secretly watching unsuspecting naked or sexually active others is not merely transient.

Adolescence and puberty generally increase sexual curiosity and activity. To alleviate the risk of pathologizing normative sexual interest and behavior during pubertal adolescence, the minimum age for the diagnosis of voyeuristic disorder is 18 years (Criterion C).

Prevalence

Voyeuristic acts are the most common of potentially law-breaking sexual behaviors. The population prevalence of voyeuristic disorder is unknown. However, based on voyeuristic sexual acts in nonclinical samples, the highest possible lifetime prevalence for voyeuristic disorder is approximately 12% in males and 4% in females.

Development and Course

Adult males with voyeuristic disorder often first become aware of their sexual interest in secretly watching unsuspecting persons during adolescence. However, the minimum age for a diagnosis of voyeuristic disorder is 18 years because there is substantial difficulty in differentiating it from age-appropriate puberty-related sexual curiosity and activity. The persistence of voyeurism over time is unclear. Voyeuristic disorder, however, per definition requires one or more contributing factors that may change over time with or without treatment: subjective distress (e.g., guilt, shame, intense sexual frustration, loneliness), psychiatric morbidity, hypersexuality, and sexual impulsivity; psychosocial impairment; and/or the propensity to act out sexually by spying on unsuspecting naked or sexually active persons. Therefore, the course of voyeuristic disorder is likely to vary with age.

Risk and Prognostic Factors

Temperamental.   Voyeurism is a necessary precondition for voyeuristic disorder; hence, risk factors for voyeurism should also increase the rate of voyeuristic disorder.

Environmental.   Childhood sexual abuse, substance misuse, and sexual preoccupation/hypersexuality have been suggested as risk factors, although the causal relationship to voyeurism is uncertain and the specificity unclear.

Gender-Related Diagnostic Issues

Voyeuristic disorder is very uncommon among females in clinical settings, while the male-to-female ratio for single sexually arousing voyeuristic acts might be 3:1.

Differential Diagnosis

Conduct disorder and antisocial personality disorder.   Conduct disorder in adolescents and antisocial personality disorder would be characterized by additional norm-breaking and antisocial behaviors, and the specific sexual interest in secretly watching unsuspecting others who are naked or engaging in sexual activity should be lacking.

Substance use disorders.   Substance use disorders might involve single voyeuristic episodes by intoxicated individuals but should not involve the typical sexual interest in secretly watching unsuspecting persons being naked or engaging in sexual activity. Hence, recurrent voyeuristic sexual fantasies, urges, or behaviors that occur also when the individual is not intoxicated suggest that voyeuristic disorder might be present.

Comorbidity

Known comorbidities in voyeuristic disorder are largely based on research with males suspected of or convicted for acts involving the secret watching of unsuspecting nude or sexually active persons. Hence, these comorbidities might not apply to all individuals with voyeuristic disorder. Conditions that occur comorbidly with voyeuristic disorder include hypersexuality and other paraphilic disorders, particularly exhibitionistic disorder. Depressive, bipolar, anxiety, and substance use disorders; attention-deficit/hyperactivity disorder; and conduct disorder and antisocial personality disorder are also frequent comorbid conditions.

Exhibitionistic Disorder

Diagnostic Criteria	302.4 (F65.2)

A. Over a period of at least 6 months, recurrent and intense sexual arousal from the exposure of one's genitals to an unsuspecting person, as manifested by fantasies, urges, or behaviors.

B. The individual has acted on these sexual urges with a nonconsenting person, or the sexual urges or fantasies cause clinically significant distress or impairment in social, occupational, or other important areas of functioning.

Specify whether:

Sexually aroused by exposing genitals to prepubertal children
Sexually aroused by exposing genitals to physically mature individuals
Sexually aroused by exposing genitals to prepubertal children and to physically mature individuals

Specify if:

In a controlled environment: This specifier is primarily applicable to individuals living in institutional or other settings where opportunities to expose one's genitals are restricted.

In full remission: The individual has not acted on the urges with a nonconsenting person, and there has been no distress or impairment in social, occupational, or other areas of functioning, for at least 5 years while in an uncontrolled environment.

Subtypes

The subtypes for exhibitionistic disorder are based on the age or physical maturity of the nonconsenting individuals to whom the individual prefers to expose his or her genitals. The nonconsenting individuals could be prepubescent children, adults, or both. This specifier should help draw adequate attention to characteristics of victims of individuals with exhibitionistic disorder to prevent co-occurring pedophilic disorder from being overlooked. However, indications that the individual with exhibitionistic disorder is sexually attracted to exposing his or her genitals to children should not preclude a diagnosis of pedophilic disorder.

Specifiers

The "in full remission" specifier does not address the continued presence or absence of exhibitionism per se, which may still be present after behaviors and distress have remitted.

Diagnostic Features

The diagnostic criteria for exhibitionistic disorder can apply both to individuals who more or less freely disclose this paraphilia and to those who categorically deny any sexual attraction to exposing their genitals to unsuspecting persons despite substantial objective evidence to the contrary. If disclosing individuals also report psychosocial difficulties because of their sexual attractions or preferences for exposing, they may be diagnosed with exhibitionistic disorder. In contrast, if they declare no distress (exemplified by absence of anxiety, obsessions, and guilt or shame about these paraphilic impulses) and are not impaired by this sexual interest in other important areas of functioning, and their self-reported, psychiatric, or legal histories indicate that they do not act on them, they could be ascertained as having exhibitionistic sexual interest but *not* be diagnosed with exhibitionistic disorder.

Examples of nondisclosing individuals include those who have exposed themselves repeatedly to unsuspecting persons on separate occasions but who deny any urges or fantasies about such sexual behavior and who report that known episodes of exposure were all accidental and nonsexual. Others may disclose past episodes of sexual behavior involving genital exposure but refute any significant or sustained sexual interest in such behavior. Since these individuals deny having urges or fantasies involving genital exposure, it follows that they would also deny feeling subjectively distressed or socially impaired by such impulses. Such individuals may be diagnosed with exhibitionistic disorder despite their negative self-report. Recurrent exhibitionistic behavior constitutes sufficient support for exhibitionism (Criterion A) and simultaneously demonstrates that this paraphilically motivated behavior is causing harm to others (Criterion B).

"Recurrent" genital exposure to unsuspecting others (i.e., multiple victims, each on a separate occasion) may, as a general rule, be interpreted as three or more victims on separate occasions. Fewer victims can be interpreted as satisfying this criterion if there were multiple occasions of exposure to the same victim, or if there is corroborating evidence of a strong or preferential interest in genital exposure to unsuspecting persons. Note that multiple victims, as suggested earlier, are a sufficient but not a necessary condition for diagnosis, as criteria may be met by an individual's acknowledging intense exhibitionistic sexual interest with distress and/or impairment.

The Criterion A time frame, indicating that signs or symptoms of exhibitionism must have persisted for at least 6 months, should also be understood as a general guideline, not a strict threshold, to ensure that the sexual interest in exposing one's genitals to unsuspecting others is not merely transient. This might be expressed in clear evidence of repeated behaviors or distress over a nontransient period shorter than 6 months.

Prevalence

The prevalence of exhibitionistic disorder is unknown. However, based on exhibitionistic sexual acts in nonclinical or general populations, the highest possible prevalence for exhibitionistic disorder in the male population is 2%–4%. The prevalence of exhibitionistic disorder in females is even more uncertain but is generally believed to be much lower than in males.

Development and Course

Adult males with exhibitionistic disorder often report that they first became aware of sexual interest in exposing their genitals to unsuspecting persons during adolescence, at a somewhat later time than the typical development of normative sexual interest in women or men. Although there is no minimum age requirement for the diagnosis of exhibitionistic disorder, it may be difficult to differentiate exhibitionistic behaviors from age-appropriate sexual curiosity in adolescents. Whereas exhibitionistic impulses appear to emerge in adolescence or early adulthood, very little is known about persistence over time. By definition, exhibitionistic disorder requires one or more contributing factors, which may change over time with or without treatment; subjective distress (e.g., guilt, shame, intense sexual frustration, loneliness), mental disorder comorbidity, hypersexuality, and sexual impulsivity; psychosocial impairment; and/or the propensity to act out sexually by exposing the genitals to unsuspecting persons. Therefore, the course of exhibitionistic disorder is likely to vary with age. As with other sexual preferences, advancing age may be associated with decreasing exhibitionistic sexual preferences and behavior.

Risk and Prognostic Factors

Temperamental.   Since exhibitionism is a necessary precondition for exhibitionistic disorder, risk factors for exhibitionism should also increase the rate of exhibitionistic disorder. Antisocial history, antisocial personality disorder, alcohol misuse, and pedophilic sexual preference might increase risk of sexual recidivism in exhibitionistic offenders.

Hence, antisocial personality disorder, alcohol use disorder, and pedophilic interest may be considered risk factors for exhibitionistic disorder in males with exhibitionistic sexual preferences.

Environmental. Childhood sexual and emotional abuse and sexual preoccupation/hypersexuality have been suggested as risk factors for exhibitionism, although the causal relationship to exhibitionism is uncertain and the specificity unclear.

Gender-Related Diagnostic Issues

Exhibitionistic disorder is highly unusual in females, whereas single sexually arousing exhibitionistic acts might occur up to half as often among women compared with men.

Functional Consequences of Exhibitionistic Disorder

The functional consequences of exhibitionistic disorder have not been addressed in research involving individuals who have not acted out sexually by exposing their genitals to unsuspecting strangers but who fulfill Criterion B by experiencing intense emotional distress over these preferences.

Differential Diagnosis

Potential differential diagnoses for exhibitionistic disorder sometimes occur also as comorbid disorders. Therefore, it is generally necessary to evaluate the evidence for exhibitionistic disorder and other possible conditions as separate questions.

Conduct disorder and antisocial personality disorder. Conduct disorder in adolescents and antisocial personality disorder would be characterized by additional norm-breaking and antisocial behaviors, and the specific sexual interest in exposing the genitals should be lacking.

Substance use disorders. Alcohol and substance use disorders might involve single exhibitionistic episodes by intoxicated individuals but should not involve the typical sexual interest in exposing the genitals to unsuspecting persons. Hence, recurrent exhibitionistic sexual fantasies, urges, or behaviors that occur also when the individual is not intoxicated suggest that exhibitionistic disorder might be present.

Comorbidity

Known comorbidities in exhibitionistic disorder are largely based on research with individuals (almost all males) convicted for criminal acts involving genital exposure to nonconsenting individuals. Hence, these comorbidities might not apply to all individuals who qualify for a diagnosis of exhibitionistic disorder. Conditions that occur comorbidly with exhibitionistic disorder at high rates include depressive, bipolar, anxiety, and substance use disorders; hypersexuality; attention-deficit/hyperactivity disorder; other paraphilic disorders; and antisocial personality disorder.

Frotteuristic Disorder

Diagnostic Criteria   **302.89 (F65.81)**

A. Over a period of at least 6 months, recurrent and intense sexual arousal from touching or rubbing against a nonconsenting person, as manifested by fantasies, urges, or behaviors.

B. The individual has acted on these sexual urges with a nonconsenting person, or the sexual urges or fantasies cause clinically significant distress or impairment in social, occupational, or other important areas of functioning.

Specify if:

In a controlled environment: This specifier is primarily applicable to individuals living in institutional or other settings where opportunities to touch or rub against a nonconsenting person are restricted.

In full remission: The individual has not acted on the urges with a nonconsenting person, and there has been no distress or impairment in social, occupational, or other areas of functioning, for at least 5 years while in an uncontrolled environment.

Specifiers

The "in remission" specifier does not address the continued presence or absence of frotteurism per se, which may still be present after behaviors and distress have remitted.

Diagnostic Features

The diagnostic criteria for frotteuristic disorder can apply both to individuals who relatively freely disclose this paraphilia and to those who firmly deny any sexual attraction from touching or rubbing against a nonconsenting individual regardless of considerable objective evidence to the contrary. If disclosing individuals also report psychosocial impairment due to their sexual preferences for touching or rubbing against a nonconsenting individual, they could be diagnosed with frotteuristic disorder. In contrast, if they declare no distress (demonstrated by lack of anxiety, obsessions, guilt, or shame) about these paraphilic impulses and are not impaired in other important areas of functioning because of this sexual interest, and their psychiatric or legal histories indicate that they do not act on it, they could be ascertained as having frotteuristic sexual interest but should *not* be diagnosed with frotteuristic disorder.

Nondisclosing individuals include, for instance, individuals known to have been touching or rubbing against nonconsenting individuals on separate occasions but who contest any urges or fantasies concerning such sexual behavior. Such individuals may report that identified episodes of touching or rubbing against an unwilling individual were all unintentional and nonsexual. Others may disclose past episodes of touching or rubbing against nonconsenting individuals but contest any major or persistent sexual interest in this. Since these individuals deny having fantasies or impulses about touching or rubbing, they would consequently reject feeling distressed or psychosocially impaired by such impulses. Despite their nondisclosing position, such individuals may be diagnosed with frotteuristic disorder. *Recurrent* frotteuristic behavior constitutes satisfactory support for frotteurism (by fulfilling Criterion A) and concurrently demonstrates that this paraphilically motivated behavior is causing harm to others (by fulfilling Criterion B).

"Recurrent" touching or rubbing against a nonconsenting individual (i.e., multiple victims, each on a separate occasion) may, as a general rule, be interpreted as three or more victims on separate occasions. Fewer victims can be interpreted as satisfying this criterion if there were multiple occasions of touching or rubbing against the same unwilling individual, or corroborating evidence of a strong or preferential interest in touching or rubbing against nonconsenting individuals. Note that multiple victims are a sufficient but not a necessary condition for diagnosis; criteria may also be met if the individual acknowledges intense frotteuristic sexual interest with clinically significant distress and/or impairment.

The Criterion A time frame, indicating that signs or symptoms of frotteurism must persist for at least 6 months, should also be interpreted as a general guideline, not a strict threshold, to ensure that the sexual interest in touching or rubbing against a nonconsenting individual is not transient. Hence, the duration part of Criterion A may also be met if there is clear evidence of recurrent behaviors or distress over a shorter but nontransient time period.

Prevalence

Frotteuristic acts, including the uninvited sexual touching of or rubbing against another individual, may occur in up to 30% of adult males in the general population. Approximately

10%–14% of adult males seen in outpatient settings for paraphilic disorders and hypersexuality have a presentation that meets diagnostic criteria for frotteuristic disorder. Hence, whereas the population prevalence of frotteuristic *disorder* is unknown, it is not likely that it exceeds the rate found in selected clinical settings.

Development and Course

Adult males with frotteuristic disorder often report first becoming aware of their sexual interest in surreptitiously touching unsuspecting persons during late adolescence or emerging adulthood. However, children and adolescents may also touch or rub against unwilling others in the absence of a diagnosis of frotteuristic disorder. Although there is no minimum age for the diagnosis, frotteuristic disorder can be difficult to differentiate from conduct-disordered behavior without sexual motivation in individuals at younger ages. The persistence of frotteurism over time is unclear. Frotteuristic disorder, however, by definition requires one or more contributing factors that may change over time with or without treatment: subjective distress (e.g., guilt, shame, intense sexual frustration, loneliness); psychiatric morbidity; hypersexuality and sexual impulsivity; psychosocial impairment; and/or the propensity to act out sexually by touching or rubbing against unconsenting persons. Therefore, the course of frotteuristic disorder is likely to vary with age. As with other sexual preferences, advancing age may be associated with decreasing frotteuristic sexual preferences and behavior.

Risk and Prognostic Factors

Temperamental.   Nonsexual antisocial behavior and sexual preoccupation/hypersexuality might be nonspecific risk factors, although the causal relationship to frotteurism is uncertain and the specificity unclear. However, frotteurism is a necessary precondition for frotteuristic disorder, so risk factors for frotteurism should also increase the rate of frotteuristic disorder.

Gender-Related Diagnostic Issues

There appear to be substantially fewer females with frotteuristic sexual preferences than males.

Differential Diagnosis

Conduct disorder and antisocial personality disorder.   Conduct disorder in adolescents and antisocial personality disorder would be characterized by additional norm-breaking and antisocial behaviors, and the specific sexual interest in touching or rubbing against a nonconsenting individual should be lacking.

Substance use disorders.   Substance use disorders, particularly those involving stimulants such as cocaine and amphetamines, might involve single frotteuristic episodes by intoxicated individuals but should not involve the typical sustained sexual interest in touching or rubbing against unsuspecting persons. Hence, recurrent frotteuristic sexual fantasies, urges, or behaviors that occur also when the individual is not intoxicated suggest that frotteuristic disorder might be present.

Comorbidity

Known comorbidities in frotteuristic disorder are largely based on research with males suspected of or convicted for criminal acts involving sexually motivated touching of or rubbing against a nonconsenting individual. Hence, these comorbidities might not apply to other individuals with a diagnosis of frotteuristic disorder based on subjective distress over their sexual interest. Conditions that occur comorbidly with frotteuristic disorder include hypersexuality and other paraphilic disorders, particularly exhibitionistic disorder and voyeuristic disorder. Conduct disorder, antisocial personality disorder, depressive disorders, bipolar disorders, anxiety disorders, and substance use disorders also co-occur. Potential differential diagnoses for frotteuristic disorder sometimes occur also as comorbid disorders. Therefore, it is generally necessary to evaluate the evidence for frotteuristic disorder and possible comorbid conditions as separate questions.

Sexual Masochism Disorder

Diagnostic Criteria   302.83 (F65.51)

A. Over a period of at least 6 months, recurrent and intense sexual arousal from the act of being humiliated, beaten, bound, or otherwise made to suffer, as manifested by fantasies, urges, or behaviors.

B. The fantasies, sexual urges, or behaviors cause clinically significant distress or impairment in social, occupational, or other important areas of functioning.

Specify if:
   With asphyxiophilia: If the individual engages in the practice of achieving sexual arousal related to restriction of breathing.

Specify if:
   In a controlled environment: This specifier is primarily applicable to individuals living in institutional or other settings where opportunities to engage in masochistic sexual behaviors are restricted.
   In full remission: There has been no distress or impairment in social, occupational, or other areas of functioning for at least 5 years while in an uncontrolled environment.

Diagnostic Features

The diagnostic criteria for sexual masochism disorder are intended to apply to individuals who freely admit to having such paraphilic interests. Such individuals openly acknowledge intense sexual arousal from the act of being humiliated, beaten, bound, or otherwise made to suffer, as manifested by fantasies, urges, or behaviors. If these individuals also report psychosocial difficulties because of their sexual attractions or preferences for being humiliated, beaten, bound, or otherwise made to suffer, they may be diagnosed with sexual masochism disorder. In contrast, if they declare no distress, exemplified by anxiety, obsessions, guilt, or shame, about these paraphilic impulses, and are not hampered by them in pursuing other personal goals, they could be ascertained as having masochistic sexual interest but should *not* be diagnosed with sexual masochism disorder.

The Criterion A time frame, indicating that the signs or symptoms of sexual masochism must have persisted for at least 6 months, should be understood as a general guideline, not a strict threshold, to ensure that the sexual interest in being humiliated, beaten, bound, or otherwise made to suffer is not merely transient. However, the disorder can be diagnosed in the context of a clearly sustained but shorter time period.

Associated Features Supporting Diagnosis

The extensive use of pornography involving the act of being humiliated, beaten, bound, or otherwise made to suffer is sometimes an associated feature of sexual masochism disorder.

Prevalence

The population prevalence of sexual masochism disorder is unknown. In Australia, it has been estimated that 2.2% of males and 1.3% of females had been involved in bondage and discipline, sadomasochism, or dominance and submission in the past 12 months.

Development and Course

Community individuals with paraphilias have reported a mean age at onset for masochism of 19.3 years, although earlier ages, including puberty and childhood, have also been reported for the onset of masochistic fantasies. Very little is known about persistence over time. Sexual masochism disorder per definition requires one or more contributing factors, which may change over time with or without treatment. These include subjective distress (e.g., guilt, shame, intense sexual frustration, loneliness), psychiatric morbidity, hypersexuality and sexual impulsivity, and psychosocial impairment. Therefore, the course of sexual masochism disorder is likely to vary with age. Advancing age is likely to have the same reducing effect on sexual preference involving sexual masochism as it has on other paraphilic or normophilic sexual behavior.

Functional Consequences of Sexual Masochism Disorder

The functional consequences of sexual masochism disorder are unknown. However, masochists are at risk of accidental death while practicing asphyxiophilia or other autoerotic procedures.

Differential Diagnosis

Many of the conditions that could be differential diagnoses for sexual masochism disorder (e.g., transvestic fetishism, sexual sadism disorder, hypersexuality, alcohol and substance use disorders) sometimes occur also as comorbid diagnoses. Therefore, it is necessary to carefully evaluate the evidence for sexual masochism disorder, keeping the possibility of other paraphilias or other mental disorders as part of the differential diagnosis. Sexual masochism in the absence of distress (i.e., no disorder) is also included in the differential, as individuals who conduct the behaviors may be satisfied with their masochistic interest.

Comorbidity

Known comorbidities with sexual masochism disorder are largely based on individuals in treatment. Disorders that occur comorbidly with sexual masochism disorder typically include other paraphilic disorders, such as transvestic fetishism.

Sexual Sadism Disorder

Diagnostic Criteria	**302.84 (F65.52)**

A. Over a period of at least 6 months, recurrent and intense sexual arousal from the physical or psychological suffering of another person, as manifested by fantasies, urges, or behaviors.
B. The individual has acted on these sexual urges with a nonconsenting person, or the sexual urges or fantasies cause clinically significant distress or impairment in social, occupational, or other important areas of functioning.

Specify if:

In a controlled environment: This specifier is primarily applicable to individuals living in institutional or other settings where opportunities to engage in sadistic sexual behaviors are restricted.

In full remission: The individual has not acted on the urges with a nonconsenting person, and there has been no distress or impairment in social, occupational, or other areas of functioning, for at least 5 years while in an uncontrolled environment.

Diagnostic Features

The diagnostic criteria for sexual sadism disorder are intended to apply both to individuals who freely admit to having such paraphilic interests and to those who deny any sexual interest in the physical or psychological suffering of another individual despite substantial objective evidence to the contrary. Individuals who openly acknowledge intense sexual interest in the physical or psychological suffering of others are referred to as "admitting individuals." If these individuals also report psychosocial difficulties because of their sexual attractions or preferences for the physical or psychological suffering of another individual, they may be diagnosed with sexual sadism disorder. In contrast, if admitting individuals declare no distress, exemplified by anxiety, obsessions, guilt, or shame, about these paraphilic impulses, and are not hampered by them in pursuing other goals, and their self-reported, psychiatric, or legal histories indicate that they do not act on them, then they could be ascertained as having sadistic sexual interest but they would *not* meet criteria for sexual sadism disorder.

Examples of individuals who deny any interest in the physical or psychological suffering of another individual include individuals known to have inflicted pain or suffering on multiple victims on separate occasions but who deny any urges or fantasies about such sexual behavior and who may further claim that known episodes of sexual assault were either unintentional or nonsexual. Others may admit past episodes of sexual behavior involving the infliction of pain or suffering on a nonconsenting individual but do not report any significant or sustained sexual interest in the physical or psychological suffering of another individual. Since these individuals deny having urges or fantasies involving sexual arousal to pain and suffering, it follows that they would also deny feeling subjectively distressed or socially impaired by such impulses. Such individuals may be diagnosed with sexual sadism disorder despite their negative self-report. Their recurrent behavior constitutes clinical support for the presence of the paraphilia of sexual sadism (by satisfying Criterion A) and simultaneously demonstrates that their paraphilically motivated behavior is causing clinically significant distress, harm, or risk of harm to others (satisfying Criterion B).

"Recurrent" sexual sadism involving nonconsenting others (i.e., multiple victims, each on a separate occasion) may, as general rule, be interpreted as three or more victims on separate occasions. Fewer victims can be interpreted as satisfying this criterion, if there are multiple instances of infliction of pain and suffering to the same victim, or if there is corroborating evidence of a strong or preferential interest in pain and suffering involving multiple victims. Note that multiple victims, as suggested earlier, are a sufficient but not a necessary condition for diagnosis, as the criteria may be met if the individual acknowledges intense sadistic sexual interest.

The Criterion A time frame, indicating that the signs or symptoms of sexual sadism must have persisted for at least 6 months, should also be understood as a general guideline, not a strict threshold, to ensure that the sexual interest in inflicting pain and suffering on nonconsenting victims is not merely transient. However, the diagnosis may be met if there is a clearly sustained but shorter period of sadistic behaviors.

Associated Features Supporting Diagnosis

The extensive use of pornography involving the infliction of pain and suffering is sometimes an associated feature of sexual sadism disorder.

Prevalence

The population prevalence of sexual sadism disorder is unknown and is largely based on individuals in forensic settings. Depending on the criteria for sexual sadism, prevalence varies widely, from 2% to 30%. Among civilly committed sexual offenders in the United States, less than 10% have sexual sadism. Among individuals who have committed sexually motivated homicides, rates of sexual sadism disorder range from 37% to 75%.

Development and Course

Individuals with sexual sadism in forensic samples are almost exclusively male, but a representative sample of the population in Australia reported that 2.2% of men and 1.3% of women said they had been involved in bondage and discipline, "sadomasochism," or dominance and submission in the previous year. Information on the development and course of sexual sadism disorder is extremely limited. One study reported that females became aware of their sadomasochistic interest as young adults, and another reported that the mean age at onset of sadism in a group of males was 19.4 years. Whereas sexual sadism per se is probably a lifelong characteristic, sexual sadism disorder may fluctuate according to the individual's subjective distress or his or her propensity to harm nonconsenting others. Advancing age is likely to have the same reducing effect on this disorder as it has on other paraphilic or normophilic sexual behavior.

Differential Diagnosis

Many of the conditions that could be differential diagnoses for sexual sadism disorder (e.g., antisocial personality disorder, sexual masochism disorder, hypersexuality, substance use disorders) sometimes occur also as comorbid diagnoses. Therefore, it is necessary to carefully evaluate the evidence for sexual sadism disorder, keeping the possibility of other paraphilias or mental disorders as part of the differential diagnosis. The majority of individuals who are active in community networks that practice sadistic and masochistic behaviors do not express any dissatisfaction with their sexual interests, and their behavior would not meet DSM-5 criteria for sexual sadism disorder. Sadistic interest, but not the disorder, may be considered in the differential diagnosis.

Comorbidity

Known comorbidities with sexual sadism disorder are largely based on individuals (almost all males) convicted for criminal acts involving sadistic acts against nonconsenting victims. Hence, these comorbidities might not apply to all individuals who never engaged in sadistic activity with a nonconsenting victim but who qualify for a diagnosis of sexual sadism disorder based on subjective distress over their sexual interest. Disorders that are commonly comorbid with sexual sadism disorder include other paraphilic disorders.

Pedophilic Disorder

Diagnostic Criteria	302.2 (F65.4)

A. Over a period of at least 6 months, recurrent, intense sexually arousing fantasies, sexual urges, or behaviors involving sexual activity with a prepubescent child or children (generally age 13 years or younger).
B. The individual has acted on these sexual urges, or the sexual urges or fantasies cause marked distress or interpersonal difficulty.
C. The individual is at least age 16 years and at least 5 years older than the child or children in Criterion A.

   Note: Do not include an individual in late adolescence involved in an ongoing sexual relationship with a 12- or 13-year-old.

Specify whether:

   Exclusive type (attracted only to children)
   Nonexclusive type

Specify if:
    Sexually attracted to males
    Sexually attracted to females
    Sexually attracted to both
Specify if:
    Limited to incest

Diagnostic Features

The diagnostic criteria for pedophilic disorder are intended to apply both to individuals who freely disclose this paraphilia and to individuals who deny any sexual attraction to prepubertal children (generally age 13 years or younger), despite substantial objective evidence to the contrary. Examples of disclosing this paraphilia include candidly acknowledging an intense sexual interest in children and indicating that sexual interest in children is greater than or equal to sexual interest in physically mature individuals. If individuals also complain that their sexual attractions or preferences for children are causing psychosocial difficulties, they may be diagnosed with pedophilic disorder. However, if they report an absence of feelings of guilt, shame, or anxiety about these impulses and are not functionally limited by their paraphilic impulses (according to self-report, objective assessment, or both), and their self-reported and legally recorded histories indicate that they have never acted on their impulses, then these individuals have a pedophilic sexual interest but not pedophilic disorder.

Examples of individuals who deny attraction to children include individuals who are known to have sexually approached multiple children on separate occasions but who deny any urges or fantasies about sexual behavior involving children, and who may further claim that the known episodes of physical contact were all unintentional and nonsexual. Other individuals may acknowledge past episodes of sexual behavior involving children but deny any significant or sustained sexual interest in children. Since these individuals may deny experiences impulses or fantasies involving children, they may also deny feeling subjectively distressed. Such individuals may still be diagnosed with pedophilic disorder despite the absence of self-reported distress, provided that there is evidence of recurrent behaviors persisting for 6 months (Criterion A) and evidence that the individual has acted on sexual urges or experienced interpersonal difficulties as a consequence of the disorder (Criterion B).

Presence of multiple victims, as discussed above, is sufficient but not necessary for diagnosis; that is, the individual can still meet Criterion A by merely acknowledging intense or preferential sexual interest in children.

The Criterion A clause, indicating that the signs or symptoms of pedophilia have persisted for 6 months or longer, is intended to ensure that the sexual attraction to children is not merely transient. However, the diagnosis may be made if there is clinical evidence of sustained persistence of the sexual attraction to children even if the 6-month duration cannot be precisely determined.

Associated Features Supporting Diagnosis

The extensive use of pornography depicting prepubescent children is a useful diagnostic indicator of pedophilic disorder. This is a specific instance of the general case that individuals are likely to choose the kind of pornography that corresponds to their sexual interests.

Prevalence

The population prevalence of pedophilic disorder is unknown. The highest possible prevalence for pedophilic disorder in the male population is approximately 3%–5%. The population prevalence of pedophilic disorder in females is even more uncertain, but it is likely a small fraction of the prevalence in males.

Development and Course

Adult males with pedophilic disorder may indicate that they become aware of strong or preferential sexual interest in children around the time of puberty—the same time frame in which males who later prefer physically mature partners became aware of their sexual interest in women or men. Attempting to diagnose pedophilic disorder at the age at which it first manifests is problematic because of the difficulty during adolescent development in differentiating it from age-appropriate sexual interest in peers or from sexual curiosity. Hence, Criterion C requires for diagnosis a minimum age of 16 years and at least 5 years older than the child or children in Criterion A.

Pedophilia per se appears to be a lifelong condition. Pedophilic disorder, however, necessarily includes other elements that may change over time with or without treatment: subjective distress (e.g., guilt, shame, intense sexual frustration, or feelings of isolation) or psychosocial impairment, or the propensity to act out sexually with children, or both. Therefore, the course of pedophilic disorder may fluctuate, increase, or decrease with age.

Adults with pedophilic disorder may report an awareness of sexual interest in children that preceded engaging in sexual behavior involving children or self-identification as a pedophile. Advanced age is as likely to similarly diminish the frequency of sexual behavior involving children as it does other paraphilically motivated and normophilic sexual behavior.

Risk and Prognostic Factors

Temperamental.   There appears to be an interaction between pedophilia and antisociality, such that males with both traits are more likely to act out sexually with children. Thus, antisocial personality disorder may be considered a risk factor for pedophilic disorder in males with pedophilia.

Environmental.   Adult males with pedophilia often report that they were sexually abused as children. It is unclear, however, whether this correlation reflects a causal influence of childhood sexual abuse on adult pedophilia.

Genetic and physiological.   Since pedophilia is a necessary condition for pedophilic disorder, any factor that increases the probability of pedophilia also increases the risk of pedophilic disorder. There is some evidence that neurodevelopmental perturbation in utero increases the probability of development of a pedophilic interest.

Gender-Related Diagnostic Issues

Psychophysiological laboratory measures of sexual interest, which are sometimes useful in diagnosing pedophilic disorder in males, are not necessarily useful in diagnosing this disorder in females, even when an identical procedure (e.g., viewing time) or analogous procedures (e.g., penile plethysmography and vaginal photoplethysmography) are available.

Diagnostic Markers

Psychophysiological measures of sexual interest may sometimes be useful when an individual's history suggests the possible presence of pedophilic disorder but the individual denies strong or preferential attraction to children. The most thoroughly researched and longest used of such measures is *penile plethysmography*, although the sensitivity and specificity of diagnosis may vary from one site to another. *Viewing time*, using photographs of nude or minimally clothed persons as visual stimuli, is also used to diagnose pedophilic disorder, especially in combination with self-report measures. Mental health professionals in the United States, however, should be aware that possession of such visual stimuli, even for diagnostic purposes, may violate American law regarding possession of child pornography and leave the mental health professional susceptible to criminal prosecution.

Differential Diagnosis

Many of the conditions that could be differential diagnoses for pedophilic disorder also sometimes occur as comorbid diagnoses. It is therefore generally necessary to evaluate the evidence for pedophilic disorder and other possible conditions as separate questions.

Antisocial personality disorder.   This disorder increases the likelihood that a person who is primarily attracted to the mature physique will approach a child, on one or a few occasions, on the basis of relative availability. The individual often shows other signs of this personality disorder, such as recurrent law-breaking.

Alcohol and substance use disorders.   The disinhibiting effects of intoxication may also increase the likelihood that a person who is primarily attracted to the mature physique will sexually approach a child.

Obsessive-compulsive disorder.   There are occasional individuals who complain about ego-dystonic thoughts and worries about possible attraction to children. Clinical interviewing usually reveals an absence of sexual thoughts about children during high states of sexual arousal (e.g., approaching orgasm during masturbation) and sometimes additional ego-dystonic, intrusive sexual ideas (e.g., concerns about homosexuality).

Comorbidity

Psychiatric comorbidity of pedophilic disorder includes substance use disorders; depressive, bipolar, and anxiety disorders; antisocial personality disorder; and other paraphilic disorders. However, findings on comorbid disorders are largely among individuals convicted for sexual offenses involving children (almost all males) and may not be generalizable to other individuals with pedophilic disorder (e.g., individuals who have never approached a child sexually but who qualify for the diagnosis of pedophilic disorder on the basis of subjective distress).

Fetishistic Disorder

Diagnostic Criteria   **302.81 (F65.0)**

A. Over a period of at least 6 months, recurrent and intense sexual arousal from either the use of nonliving objects or a highly specific focus on nongenital body part(s), as manifested by fantasies, urges, or behaviors.
B. The fantasies, sexual urges, or behaviors cause clinically significant distress or impairment in social, occupational, or other important areas of functioning.
C. The fetish objects are not limited to articles of clothing used in cross-dressing (as in transvestic disorder) or devices specifically designed for the purpose of tactile genital stimulation (e.g., vibrator).

Specify:
  Body part(s)
  Nonliving object(s)
  Other

Specify if:
  In a controlled environment: This specifier is primarily applicable to individuals living in institutional or other settings where opportunities to engage in fetishistic behaviors are restricted.
  In full remission: There has been no distress or impairment in social, occupational, or other areas of functioning for at least 5 years while in an uncontrolled environment.

Specifiers

Although individuals with fetishistic disorder may report intense and recurrent sexual arousal to inanimate objects or a specific body part, it is not unusual for non–mutually exclusive combinations of fetishes to occur. Thus, an individual may have fetishistic disorder associated with an inanimate object (e.g., female undergarments) or an exclusive focus on an intensely eroticized body part (e.g., feet, hair), or their fetishistic interest may meet criteria for various combinations of these specifiers (e.g., socks, shoes and feet).

Diagnostic Features

The paraphilic focus of fetishistic disorder involves the persistent and repetitive use of or dependence on nonliving objects or a highly specific focus on a (typically nongenital) body part as primary elements associated with sexual arousal (Criterion A). A diagnosis of fetishistic disorder must include clinically significant personal distress or psychosocial role impairment (Criterion B). Common fetish objects include female undergarments, male or female footwear, rubber articles, leather clothing, or other wearing apparel. Highly eroticized body parts associated with fetishistic disorder include feet, toes, and hair. It is not uncommon for sexualized fetishes to include both inanimate objects and body parts (e.g., dirty socks and feet), and for this reason the definition of fetishistic disorder now re-incorporates *partialism* (i.e., an exclusive focus on a body part) into its boundaries. Partialism, previously considered a paraphilia not otherwise specified disorder, had historically been subsumed in fetishism prior to DSM-III.

Many individuals who self-identify as fetishist practitioners do not necessarily report clinical impairment in association with their fetish-associated behaviors. Such individuals could be considered as having a fetish but not fetishistic disorder. A diagnosis of fetishistic disorder requires concurrent fulfillment of both the behaviors in Criterion A and the clinically significant distress or impairment in functioning noted in Criterion B.

Associated Features Supporting Diagnosis

Fetishistic disorder can be a multisensory experience, including holding, tasting, rubbing, inserting, or smelling the fetish object while masturbating, or preferring that a sexual partner wear or utilize a fetish object during sexual encounters. Some individuals may acquire extensive collections of highly desired fetish objects.

Development and Course

Usually paraphilias have an onset during puberty, but fetishes can develop prior to adolescence. Once established, fetishistic disorder tends to have a continuous course that fluctuates in intensity and frequency of urges or behavior.

Culture-Related Diagnostic Issues

Knowledge of and appropriate consideration for normative aspects of sexual behavior are important factors to explore to establish a clinical diagnosis of fetishistic disorder and to distinguish a clinical diagnosis from a socially acceptable sexual behavior.

Gender-Related Diagnostic Issues

Fetishistic disorder has not been systematically reported to occur in females. In clinical samples, fetishistic disorder is nearly exclusively reported in males.

Functional Consequences of Fetishistic Disorder

Typical impairments associated with fetishistic disorder include sexual dysfunction during romantic reciprocal relationships when the preferred fetish object or body part is unavailable during foreplay or coitus. Some individuals with fetishistic disorder may prefer solitary sexual activity associated with their fetishistic preference(s) even while involved in a meaningful reciprocal and affectionate relationship.

Although fetishistic disorder is relatively uncommon among arrested sexual offenders with paraphilias, males with fetishistic disorder may steal and collect their particular fetishistic objects of desire. Such individuals have been arrested and charged for nonsexual antisocial behaviors (e.g., breaking and entering, theft, burglary) that are primarily motivated by the fetishistic disorder.

Differential Diagnosis

Transvestic disorder. The nearest diagnostic neighbor of fetishistic disorder is transvestic disorder. As noted in the diagnostic criteria, fetishistic disorder is not diagnosed when fetish objects are limited to articles of clothing exclusively worn during cross-dressing (as in transvestic disorder), or when the object is genitally stimulating because it has been designed for that purpose (e.g., a vibrator).

Sexual masochism disorder or other paraphilic disorders. Fetishes can co-occur with other paraphilic disorders, especially "sadomasochism" and transvestic disorder. When an individual fantasizes about or engages in "forced cross-dressing" and is primarily sexually aroused by the domination or humiliation associated with such fantasy or repetitive activity, the diagnosis of sexual masochism disorder should be made.

Fetishistic behavior without fetishistic disorder. Use of a fetish object for sexual arousal without any associated distress or psychosocial role impairment or other adverse consequence would not meet criteria for fetishistic disorder, as the threshold required by Criterion B would not be met. For example, an individual whose sexual partner either shares or can successfully incorporate his interest in caressing, smelling, or licking feet or toes as an important element of foreplay would not be diagnosed with fetishistic disorder; nor would an individual who prefers, and is not distressed or impaired by, solitary sexual behavior associated with wearing rubber garments or leather boots.

Comorbidity

Fetishistic disorder may co-occur with other paraphilic disorders as well as hypersexuality. Rarely, fetishistic disorder may be associated with neurological conditions.

Transvestic Disorder

Diagnostic Criteria	302.3 (F65.1)

A. Over a period of at least 6 months, recurrent and intense sexual arousal from cross-dressing, as manifested by fantasies, urges, or behaviors.

B. The fantasies, sexual urges, or behaviors cause clinically significant distress or impairment in social, occupational, or other important areas of functioning.

Specify if:
  With fetishism: If sexually aroused by fabrics, materials, or garments.
  With autogynephilia: If sexually aroused by thoughts or images of self as female.

Specify if:
  In a controlled environment: This specifier is primarily applicable to individuals living in institutional or other settings where opportunities to cross-dress are restricted.
  In full remission: There has been no distress or impairment in social, occupational, or other areas of functioning for at least 5 years while in an uncontrolled environment.

Specifiers

The presence of fetishism decreases the likelihood of gender dysphoria in men with transvestic disorder. The presence of autogynephilia increases the likelihood of gender dysphoria in men with transvestic disorder.

Diagnostic Features

The diagnosis of transvestic disorder does not apply to all individuals who dress as the opposite sex, even those who do so habitually. It applies to individuals whose cross-dressing or thoughts of cross-dressing are always or often accompanied by sexual excitement (Criterion A) and who are emotionally distressed by this pattern or feel it impairs social or interpersonal functioning (Criterion B). The cross-dressing may involve only one or two articles of clothing (e.g., for men, it may pertain only to women's undergarments), or it may involve dressing completely in the inner and outer garments of the other sex and (in men) may include the use of women's wigs and make-up. Transvestic disorder is nearly exclusively reported in males. Sexual arousal, in its most obvious form of penile erection, may co-occur with cross-dressing in various ways. In younger males, cross-dressing often leads to masturbation, following which any female clothing is removed. Older males often learn to avoid masturbating or doing anything to stimulate the penis so that the avoidance of ejaculation allows them to prolong their cross-dressing session. Males with female partners sometimes complete a cross-dressing session by having intercourse with their partners, and some have difficulty maintaining a sufficient erection for intercourse without cross-dressing (or private fantasies of cross-dressing).

Clinical assessment of distress or impairment, like clinical assessment of transvestic sexual arousal, is usually dependent on the individual's self-report. The pattern of behavior "purging and acquisition" often signifies the presence of distress in individuals with transvestic disorder. During this behavioral pattern, an individual (usually a man) who has spent a great deal of money on women's clothes and other apparel (e.g., shoes, wigs) discards the items (i.e., purges them) in an effort to overcome urges to cross-dress, and then begins acquiring a woman's wardrobe all over again.

Associated Features Supporting Diagnosis

Transvestic disorder in men is often accompanied by *autogynephilia* (i.e., a male's paraphilic tendency to be sexually aroused by the thought or image of himself as a woman). Autogynephilic fantasies and behaviors may focus on the idea of exhibiting female physiological functions (e.g., lactation, menstruation), engaging in stereotypically feminine behavior (e.g., knitting), or possessing female anatomy (e.g., breasts).

Prevalence

The prevalence of transvestic disorder is unknown. Transvestic disorder is rare in males and extremely rare in females. Fewer than 3% of males report having ever been sexually aroused by dressing in women's attire. The percentage of individuals who have cross-dressed with sexual arousal more than once or a few times in their lifetimes would be even lower. The majority of males with transvestic disorder identify as heterosexual, although some individuals have occasional sexual interaction with other males, especially when they are cross-dressed.

Development and Course

In males, the first signs of transvestic disorder may begin in childhood, in the form of strong fascination with a particular item of women's attire. Prior to puberty, cross-dressing produces generalized feelings of pleasurable excitement. With the arrival of puberty, dressing in women's clothes begins to elicit penile erection and, in some cases, leads directly to first ejaculation. In many cases, cross-dressing elicits less and less sexual excitement as the individual grows older; eventually it may produce no discernible penile response at all. The desire to cross-dress, at the same time, remains the same or grows even stronger. Individuals who report such a diminution of sexual response typically report that the sexual excitement of cross-dressing has been replaced by feelings of comfort or well-being.

In some cases, the course of transvestic disorder is continuous, and in others it is episodic. It is not rare for men with transvestic disorder to lose interest in cross-dressing when they first fall in love with a woman and begin a relationship, but such abatement usually proves temporary. When the desire to cross-dress returns, so does the associated distress.

Some cases of transvestic disorder progress to gender dysphoria. The males in these cases, who may be indistinguishable from others with transvestic disorder in adolescence or early childhood, gradually develop desires to remain in the female role for longer periods and to feminize their anatomy. The development of gender dysphoria is usually accompanied by a (self-reported) reduction or elimination of sexual arousal in association with cross-dressing.

The manifestation of transvestism in penile erection and stimulation, like the manifestation of other paraphilic as well as normophilic sexual interests, is most intense in adolescence and early adulthood. The severity of transvestic disorder is highest in adulthood, when the transvestic drives are most likely to conflict with performance in heterosexual intercourse and desires to marry and start a family. Middle-age and older men with a history of transvestism are less likely to present with transvestic disorder than with gender dysphoria.

Functional Consequences of Transvestic Disorder

Engaging in transvestic behaviors can interfere with, or detract from, heterosexual relationships. This can be a source of distress to men who wish to maintain conventional marriages or romantic partnerships with women.

Differential Diagnosis

Fetishistic disorder.   This disorder may resemble transvestic disorder, in particular, in men with fetishism who put on women's undergarments while masturbating with them. Distinguishing transvestic disorder depends on the individual's specific thoughts during such activity (e.g., are there any ideas of being a woman, being like a woman, or being dressed as a woman?) and on the presence of other fetishes (e.g., soft, silky fabrics, whether these are used for garments or for something else).

Gender dysphoria.   Individuals with transvestic disorder do not report an incongruence between their experienced gender and assigned gender nor a desire to be of the other gender; and they typically do not have a history of childhood cross-gender behaviors, which would be present in individuals with gender dysphoria. Individuals with a presentation that meets full criteria for transvestic disorder as well as gender dysphoria should be given both diagnoses.

Comorbidity

Transvestism (and thus transvestic disorder) is often found in association with other paraphilias. The most frequently co-occurring paraphilias are fetishism and masochism. One particularly dangerous form of masochism, *autoerotic asphyxia,* is associated with transvestism in a substantial proportion of fatal cases.

Other Specified Paraphilic Disorder

302.89 (F65.89)

This category applies to presentations in which symptoms characteristic of a paraphilic disorder that cause clinically significant distress or impairment in social, occupational, or other important areas of functioning predominate but do not meet the full criteria for any of the disorders in the paraphilic disorders diagnostic class. The other specified paraphilic disorder category is used in situations in which the clinician chooses to communicate the specific reason that the presentation does not meet the criteria for any specific paraphilic disorder. This is done by recording "other specified paraphilic disorder" followed by the specific reason (e.g., "zoophilia").

Examples of presentations that can be specified using the "other specified" designation include, but are not limited to, recurrent and intense sexual arousal involving *telephone scatologia* (obscene phone calls), *necrophilia* (corpses), *zoophilia* (animals), *coprophilia* (feces), *klismaphilia* (enemas), or *urophilia* (urine) that has been present for at least 6 months and causes marked distress or impairment in social, occupational, or other important areas of functioning. Other specified paraphilic disorder can be specified as in remission and/or as occurring in a controlled environment.

Unspecified Paraphilic Disorder

302.9 (F65.9)

This category applies to presentations in which symptoms characteristic of a paraphilic disorder that cause clinically significant distress or impairment in social, occupational, or other important areas of functioning predominate but do not meet the full criteria for any of the disorders in the paraphilic disorders diagnostic class. The unspecified paraphilic disorder category is used in situations in which the clinician chooses *not* to specify the reason that the criteria are not met for a specific paraphilic disorder, and includes presentations in which there is insufficient information to make a more specific diagnosis.

Other Mental Disorders

Four disorders are included in this chapter: other specified mental disorder due to another medical condition; unspecified mental disorder due to another medical condition; other specified mental disorder; and unspecified mental disorder. This residual category applies to presentations in which symptoms characteristic of a mental disorder that cause clinically significant distress or impairment in social, occupational, or other important areas of functioning predominate but do not meet the full criteria for any other mental disorder in DSM-5. For other specified and unspecified mental disorders due to another medical condition, it must be established that the disturbance is caused by the physiological effects of another medical condition. If other specified and unspecified mental disorders are due to another medical condition, it is necessary to code and list the medical condition first (e.g., 042 [B20] HIV disease), followed by the other specified or unspecified mental disorder (use appropriate code).

Other Specified Mental Disorder Due to Another Medical Condition

294.8 (F06.8)

This category applies to presentations in which symptoms characteristic of a mental disorder due to another medical condition that cause clinically significant distress or impairment in social, occupational, or other important areas of functioning predominate but do not meet the full criteria for any specific mental disorder attributable to another medical condition. The other specified mental disorder due to another medical condition category is used in situations in which the clinician chooses to communicate the specific reason that the presentation does not meet the criteria for any specific mental disorder attributable to another medical condition. This is done by recording the name of the disorder, with the specific etiological medical condition inserted in place of "another medical condition," followed by the specific symptomatic manifestation that does not meet the criteria for any specific mental disorder due to another medical condition. Furthermore, the diagnostic code for the specific medical condition must be listed immediately before the code for the other specified mental disorder due to another medical condition. For example, dissociative symptoms due to complex partial seizures would be coded and recorded as 345.40 (G40.209) complex partial seizures, 294.8 (F06.8) other specified mental disorder due to complex partial seizures, dissociative symptoms.

An example of a presentation that can be specified using the "other specified" designation is the following:

Dissociative symptoms: This includes symptoms occurring, for example, in the context of complex partial seizures.

Unspecified Mental Disorder Due to Another Medical Condition

294.9 (F09)

This category applies to presentations in which symptoms characteristic of a mental disorder due to another medical condition that cause clinically significant distress or impairment in social, occupational, or other important areas of functioning predominate but do not meet the full criteria for any specific mental disorder due to another medical condition. The unspecified mental disorder due to another medical condition category is used in situations in which the clinician chooses *not* to specify the reason that the criteria are not met for a specific mental disorder due to another medical condition, and includes presentations for which there is insufficient information to make a more specific diagnosis (e.g., in emergency room settings). This is done by recording the name of the disorder, with the specific etiological medical condition inserted in place of "another medical condition." Furthermore, the diagnostic code for the specific medical condition must be listed immediately before the code for the unspecified mental disorder due to another medical condition. For example, dissociative symptoms due to complex partial seizures would be coded and recorded as 345.40 (G40.209) complex partial seizures, 294.9 (F06.9) unspecified mental disorder due to complex partial seizures.

Other Specified Mental Disorder

300.9 (F99)

This category applies to presentations in which symptoms characteristic of a mental disorder that cause clinically significant distress or impairment in social, occupational, or other important areas of functioning predominate but do not meet the full criteria for any specific mental disorder. The other specified mental disorder category is used in situations in which the clinician chooses to communicate the specific reason that the presentation does not meet the criteria for any specific mental disorder. This is done by recording "other specified mental disorder" followed by the specific reason.

Unspecified Mental Disorder

300.9 (F99)

This category applies to presentations in which symptoms characteristic of a mental disorder that cause clinically significant distress or impairment in social, occupational, or other important areas of functioning predominate but do not meet the full criteria for any mental disorder. The unspecified mental disorder category is used in situations in which the clinician chooses *not* to specify the reason that the criteria are not met for a specific mental disorder, and includes presentations for which there is insufficient information to make a more specific diagnosis (e.g., in emergency room settings).

Medication-Induced Movement Disorders and Other Adverse Effects of Medication

Medication-induced movement disorders are included in Section II because of their frequent importance in 1) the management by medication of mental disorders or other medical conditions and 2) the differential diagnosis of mental disorders (e.g., anxiety disorder versus neuroleptic-induced akathisia; malignant catatonia versus neuroleptic malignant syndrome). Although these movement disorders are labeled "medication induced," it is often difficult to establish the causal relationship between medication exposure and the development of the movement disorder, especially because some of these movement disorders also occur in the absence of medication exposure. The conditions and problems listed in this chapter are not mental disorders.

The term *neuroleptic* is becoming outdated because it highlights the propensity of antipsychotic medications to cause abnormal movements, and it is being replaced with the term *antipsychotic* in many contexts. Nevertheless, the term *neuroleptic* remains appropriate in this context. Although newer antipsychotic medications may be less likely to cause some medication-induced movement disorders, those disorders still occur. Neuroleptic medications include so-called conventional, "typical," or first-generation antipsychotic agents (e.g., chlorpromazine, haloperidol, fluphenazine); "atypical" or second-generation antipsychotic agents (e.g., clozapine, risperidone, olanzapine, quetiapine); certain dopamine receptor–blocking drugs used in the treatment of symptoms such as nausea and gastroparesis (e.g., prochlorperazine, promethazine, trimethobenzamide, thiethylperazine, metoclopramide); and amoxapine, which is marketed as an antidepressant.

Neuroleptic-Induced Parkinsonism
Other Medication-Induced Parkinsonism

332.1 (G21.11)   Neuroleptic-Induced Parkinsonism
332.1 (G21.19)   Other Medication-Induced Parkinsonism
Parkinsonian tremor, muscular rigidity, akinesia (i.e., loss of movement or difficulty initiating movement), or bradykinesia (i.e., slowing movement) developing within a few weeks of starting or raising the dosage of a medication (e.g., a neuroleptic) or after reducing the dosage of a medication used to treat extrapyramidal symptoms.

Neuroleptic Malignant Syndrome

333.92 (G21.0)   Neuroleptic Malignant Syndrome
Although neuroleptic malignant syndrome is easily recognized in its classic full-blown form, it is often heterogeneous in onset, presentation, progression, and outcome. The clinical features described below are those considered most important in making the diagnosis of neuroleptic malignant syndrome based on consensus recommendations.

Diagnostic Features

Patients have generally been exposed to a dopamine antagonist within 72 hours prior to symptom development. Hyperthermia (>100.4°F or >38.0°C on at least two occasions, measured orally), associated with profuse diaphoresis, is a distinguishing feature of neuroleptic malignant syndrome, setting it apart from other neurological side effects of antipsychotic medications. Extreme elevations in temperature, reflecting a breakdown in central thermoregulation, are more likely to support the diagnosis of neuroleptic malignant syndrome. Generalized rigidity, described as "lead pipe" in its most severe form and usually unresponsive to antiparkinsonian agents, is a cardinal feature of the disorder and may be associated with other neurological symptoms (e.g., tremor, sialorrhea, akinesia, dystonia, trismus, myoclonus, dysarthria, dysphagia, rhabdomyolysis). Creatine kinase elevation of at least four times the upper limit of normal is commonly seen. Changes in mental status, characterized by delirium or altered consciousness ranging from stupor to coma, are often an early sign. Affected individuals may appear alert but dazed and unresponsive, consistent with catatonic stupor. Autonomic activation and instability—manifested by tachycardia (rate>25% above baseline), diaphoresis, blood pressure elevation (systolic or diastolic ≥25% above baseline) or fluctuation (≥20 mmHg diastolic change or ≥25 mmHg systolic change within 24 hours), urinary incontinence, and pallor—may be seen at any time but provide an early clue to the diagnosis. Tachypnea (rate >50% above baseline) is common, and respiratory distress—resulting from metabolic acidosis, hypermetabolism, chest wall restriction, aspiration pneumonia, or pulmonary emboli—can occur and lead to sudden respiratory arrest.

A workup, including laboratory investigation, to exclude other infectious, toxic, metabolic, and neuropsychiatric etiologies or complications is essential (see the section "Differential Diagnosis" later in this discussion). Although several laboratory abnormalities are associated with neuroleptic malignant syndrome, no single abnormality is specific to the diagnosis. Individuals with neuroleptic malignant syndrome may have leukocytosis, metabolic acidosis, hypoxia, decreased serum iron concentrations, and elevations in serum muscle enzymes and catecholamines. Findings from cerebrospinal fluid analysis and neuroimaging studies are generally normal, whereas electroencephalography shows generalized slowing. Autopsy findings in fatal cases have been nonspecific and variable, depending on complications.

Development and Course

Evidence from database studies suggests incidence rates for neuroleptic malignant syndrome of 0.01%–0.02% among individuals treated with antipsychotics. The temporal progression of signs and symptoms provides important clues to the diagnosis and prognosis of neuroleptic malignant syndrome. Alteration in mental status and other neurological signs typically precede systemic signs. The onset of symptoms varies from hours to days after drug initiation. Some cases develop within 24 hours after drug initiation, most within the first week, and virtually all cases within 30 days. Once the syndrome is diagnosed and oral antipsychotic drugs are discontinued, neuroleptic malignant syndrome is self-limited in most cases. The mean recovery time after drug discontinuation is 7–10 days, with most individuals recovering within 1 week and nearly all within 30 days. The duration may be prolonged when long-acting antipsychotics are implicated. There have been reports of individuals in whom residual neurological signs persisted for weeks after the acute hypermetabolic symptoms resolved. Total resolution of symptoms can be obtained in most cases of neuroleptic malignant syndrome; however, fatality rates of 10%–20% have been reported when the disorder is not recognized. Although many individuals do not experience a recurrence of neuroleptic malignant syndrome when rechallenged with antipsychotic medication, some do, especially when antipsychotics are reinstituted soon after an episode.

Risk and Prognostic Factors

Neuroleptic malignant syndrome is a potential risk in any individual after antipsychotic drug administration. It is not specific to any neuropsychiatric diagnosis and may occur in individuals without a diagnosable mental disorder who receive dopamine antagonists. Clinical, systemic, and metabolic factors associated with a heightened risk of neuroleptic malignant syndrome include agitation, exhaustion, dehydration, and iron deficiency. A prior episode associated with antipsychotics has been described in 15%–20% of index cases, suggesting underlying vulnerability in some patients; however, genetic findings based on neurotransmitter receptor polymorphisms have not been replicated consistently.

Nearly all dopamine antagonists have been associated with neuroleptic malignant syndrome, although high-potency antipsychotics pose a greater risk compared with low-potency agents and newer atypical antipsychotics. Partial or milder forms may be associated with newer antipsychotics, but neuroleptic malignant syndrome varies in severity even with older drugs. Dopamine antagonists used in medical settings (e.g., metoclopramide, prochlorperazine) have also been implicated. Parenteral administration routes, rapid titration rates, and higher total drug dosages have been associated with increased risk; however, neuroleptic malignant syndrome usually occurs within the therapeutic dosage range of antipsychotics.

Differential Diagnosis

Neuroleptic malignant syndrome must be distinguished from other serious neurological or medical conditions, including central nervous system infections, inflammatory or autoimmune conditions, status epilepticus, subcortical structural lesions, and systemic conditions (e.g., pheochromocytoma, thyrotoxicosis, tetanus, heat stroke).

Neuroleptic malignant syndrome also must be distinguished from similar syndromes resulting from the use of other substances or medications, such as serotonin syndrome; parkinsonian hyperthermia syndrome following abrupt discontinuation of dopamine agonists; alcohol or sedative withdrawal; malignant hyperthermia occurring during anesthesia; hyperthermia associated with abuse of stimulants and hallucinogens; and atropine poisoning from anticholinergics.

In rare instances, individuals with schizophrenia or a mood disorder may present with malignant catatonia, which may be indistinguishable from neuroleptic malignant syndrome. Some investigators consider neuroleptic malignant syndrome to be a drug-induced form of malignant catatonia.

Medication-Induced Acute Dystonia

333.72 (G24.02)   Medication-Induced Acute Dystonia
Abnormal and prolonged contraction of the muscles of the eyes (oculogyric crisis), head, neck (torticollis or retrocollis), limbs, or trunk developing within a few days of starting or raising the dosage of a medication (such as a neuroleptic) or after reducing the dosage of a medication used to treat extrapyramidal symptoms.

Medication-Induced Acute Akathisia

333.99 (G25.71)   Medication-Induced Acute Akathisia
Subjective complaints of restlessness, often accompanied by observed excessive movements (e.g., fidgety movements of the legs, rocking from foot to foot, pacing, inability to sit or stand still), developing within a few weeks of starting or raising the dosage of a medication (such as a neuroleptic) or after reducing the dosage of a medication used to treat extrapyramidal symptoms.

Tardive Dyskinesia

333.85 (G24.01)   Tardive Dyskinesia

Involuntary athetoid or choreiform movements (lasting at least a few weeks) generally of the tongue, lower face and jaw, and extremities (but sometimes involving the pharyngeal, diaphragmatic, or trunk muscles) developing in association with the use of a neuroleptic medication for at least a few months.

Symptoms may develop after a shorter period of medication use in older persons. In some patients, movements of this type may appear after discontinuation, or after change or reduction in dosage, of neuroleptic medications, in which case the condition is called *neuroleptic withdrawal-emergent dyskinesia*. Because withdrawal-emergent dyskinesia is usually time-limited, lasting less than 4–8 weeks, dyskinesia that persists beyond this window is considered to be tardive dyskinesia.

Tardive Dystonia
Tardive Akathisia

333.72 (G24.09)   Tardive Dystonia
333.99 (G25.71)   Tardive Akathisia

Tardive syndrome involving other types of movement problems, such as dystonia or akathisia, which are distinguished by their late emergence in the course of treatment and their potential persistence for months to years, even in the face of neuroleptic discontinuation or dosage reduction.

Medication-Induced Postural Tremor

333.1 (G25.1)   Medication-Induced Postural Tremor

Fine tremor (usually in the range of 8–12 Hz) occurring during attempts to maintain a posture and developing in association with the use of medication (e.g., lithium, antidepressants, valproate). This tremor is very similar to the tremor seen with anxiety, caffeine, and other stimulants.

Other Medication-Induced Movement Disorder

333.99 (G25.79)   Other Medication-Induced Movement Disorder

This category is for medication-induced movement disorders not captured by any of the specific disorders listed above. Examples include 1) presentations resembling neuroleptic malignant syndrome that are associated with medications other than neuroleptics and 2) other medication-induced tardive conditions.

Antidepressant Discontinuation Syndrome

995.29 (T43.205A)   Initial encounter

995.29 (T43.205D)   Subsequent encounter

995.29 (T43.205S)   Sequelae

Antidepressant discontinuation syndrome is a set of symptoms that can occur after an abrupt cessation (or marked reduction in dose) of an antidepressant medication that was taken continuously for at least 1 month. Symptoms generally begin within 2–4 days and typically include specific sensory, somatic, and cognitive-emotional manifestations. Frequently reported sensory and somatic symptoms include flashes of lights, "electric shock" sensations, nausea, and hyperresponsivity to noises or lights. Nonspecific anxiety and feelings of dread may also be reported. Symptoms are alleviated by restarting the same medication or starting a different medication that has a similar mechanism of action— for example, discontinuation symptoms after withdrawal from a serotonin-norepineph-rine reuptake inhibitor may be alleviated by starting a tricyclic antidepressant. To qualify as antidepressant discontinuation syndrome, the symptoms should not have been present before the antidepressant dosage was reduced and are not better explained by another mental disorder (e.g., manic or hypomanic episode, substance intoxication, substance withdrawal, somatic symptom disorder).

Diagnostic Features

Discontinuation symptoms may occur following treatment with tricyclic antidepressants (e.g., imipramine, amitriptyline, desipramine), serotonin reuptake inhibitors (e.g., fluox-etine, paroxetine, sertraline), and monoamine oxidase inhibitors (e.g., phenelzine, selegi-line, pargyline). The incidence of this syndrome depends on the dosage and half-life of the medication being taken, as well as the rate at which the medication is tapered. Short-acting medications that are stopped abruptly rather than tapered gradually may pose the great-est risk. The short-acting selective serotonin reuptake inhibitor (SSRI) paroxetine is the agent most commonly associated with discontinuation symptoms, but such symptoms oc-cur for all types of antidepressants.

Unlike withdrawal syndromes associated with opioids, alcohol, and other substances of abuse, antidepressant discontinuation syndrome has no pathognomonic symptoms. In-stead, the symptoms tend to be vague and variable and typically begin 2–4 days after the last dose of the antidepressant. For SSRIs (e.g., paroxetine), symptoms such as dizziness, ringing in the ears, "electric shocks in the head," an inability to sleep, and acute anxiety are described. The antidepressant use prior to discontinuation must not have incurred hypo-mania or euphoria (i.e., there should be confidence that the discontinuation syndrome is not the result of fluctuations in mood stability associated with the previous treatment). The antidepressant discontinuation syndrome is based solely on pharmacological factors and is not related to the reinforcing effects of an antidepressant. Also, in the case of stim-ulant augmentation of an antidepressant, abrupt cessation may result in stimulant with-drawal symptoms (see "Stimulant Withdrawal" in the chapter "Substance-Related and Addictive Disorders") rather than the antidepressant discontinuation syndrome described here.

Prevalence

The prevalence of antidepressant discontinuation syndrome is unknown but is thought to vary according to the dosage prior to discontinuation, the half-life and receptor-binding affinity of the medication, and possibly the individual's genetically influenced rate of me-tabolism for this medication.

Course and Development

Because longitudinal studies are lacking, little is known about the clinical course of anti-depressant discontinuation syndrome. Symptoms appear to abate over time with very gradual dosage reductions. After an episode, some individuals may prefer to resume med-ication indefinitely if tolerated.

Differential Diagnosis

The differential diagnosis of antidepressant discontinuation syndrome includes anxiety and depressive disorders, substance use disorders, and tolerance to medications.

Anxiety and depressive disorders.   Discontinuation symptoms often resemble symptoms of a persistent anxiety disorder or a return of somatic symptoms of depression for which the medication was initially given.

Substance use disorders.   Antidepressant discontinuation syndrome differs from substance withdrawal in that antidepressants themselves have no reinforcing or euphoric effects. The medication dosage has usually not been increased without the clinician's permission, and the individual generally does not engage in drug-seeking behavior to obtain additional medication. Criteria for a substance use disorder are not met.

Tolerance to medications.   Tolerance and discontinuation symptoms can occur as a normal physiological response to stopping medication after a substantial duration of exposure. Most cases of medication tolerance can be managed through carefully controlled tapering.

Comorbidity

Typically, the individual was initially started on the medication for a major depressive disorder; the original symptoms may return during the discontinuation syndrome.

Other Adverse Effect of Medication

995.20 (T50.905A) Initial encounter

995.20 (T50.905D) Subsequent encounter

995.20 (T50.905S) Sequelae

This category is available for optional use by clinicians to code side effects of medication (other than movement symptoms) when these adverse effects become a main focus of clinical attention. Examples include severe hypotension, cardiac arrhythmias, and priapism.

Other Conditions That May Be a Focus of Clinical Attention

This discussion covers other conditions and problems that may be a focus of clinical attention or that may otherwise affect the diagnosis, course, prognosis, or treatment of a patient's mental disorder. These conditions are presented with their corresponding codes from ICD-9-CM (usually V codes) and ICD-10-CM (usually Z codes). A condition or problem in this chapter may be coded if it is a reason for the current visit or helps to explain the need for a test, procedure, or treatment. Conditions and problems in this chapter may also be included in the medical record as useful information on circumstances that may affect the patient's care, regardless of their relevance to the current visit.

The conditions and problems listed in this chapter are not mental disorders. Their inclusion in DSM-5 is meant to draw attention to the scope of additional issues that may be encountered in routine clinical practice and to provide a systematic listing that may be useful to clinicians in documenting these issues.

Relational Problems

Key relationships, especially intimate adult partner relationships and parent/caregiver-child relationships, have a significant impact on the health of the individuals in these relationships. These relationships can be health promoting and protective, neutral, or detrimental to health outcomes. In the extreme, these close relationships can be associated with maltreatment or neglect, which has significant medical and psychological consequences for the affected individual. A relational problem may come to clinical attention either as the reason that the individual seeks health care or as a problem that affects the course, prognosis, or treatment of the individual's mental or other medical disorder.

Problems Related to Family Upbringing

V61.20 (Z62.820)   Parent-Child Relational Problem
For this category, the term *parent* is used to refer to one of the child's primary caregivers, who may be a biological, adoptive, or foster parent or may be another relative (such as a grandparent) who fulfills a parental role for the child. This category should be used when the main focus of clinical attention is to address the quality of the parent-child relationship or when the quality of the parent-child relationship is affecting the course, prognosis, or treatment of a mental or other medical disorder. Typically, the parent-child relational problem is associated with impaired functioning in behavioral, cognitive, or affective domains. Examples of behavioral problems include inadequate parental control, supervision, and involvement with the child; parental overprotection; excessive parental pressure; arguments that escalate to threats of physical violence; and avoidance without resolution of problems. Cognitive problems may include negative attributions of the other's intentions, hostility toward or scapegoating of the other, and unwarranted feelings of estrangement. Affective problems may include feelings of sadness, apathy, or anger about the other individual in the relationship. Clinicians should take into account the developmental needs of the child and the cultural context.

V61.8 (Z62.891)   Sibling Relational Problem

This category should be used when the focus of clinical attention is a pattern of interaction among siblings that is associated with significant impairment in individual or family functioning or with development of symptoms in one or more of the siblings, or when a sibling relational problem is affecting the course, prognosis, or treatment of a sibling's mental or other medical disorder. This category can be used for either children or adults if the focus is on the sibling relationship. Siblings in this context include full, half-, step-, foster, and adopted siblings.

V61.8 (Z62.29)   Upbringing Away From Parents

This category should be used when the main focus of clinical attention pertains to issues regarding a child being raised away from the parents or when this separate upbringing affects the course, prognosis, or treatment of a mental or other medical disorder. The child could be one who is under state custody and placed in kin care or foster care. The child could also be one who is living in a nonparental relative's home, or with friends, but whose out-of-home placement is not mandated or sanctioned by the courts. Problems related to a child living in a group home or orphanage are also included. This category excludes issues related to V60.6 (Z59.3) children in boarding schools.

V61.29 (Z62.898)   Child Affected by Parental Relationship Distress

This category should be used when the focus of clinical attention is the negative effects of parental relationship discord (e.g., high levels of conflict, distress, or disparagement) on a child in the family, including effects on the child's mental or other medical disorders.

Other Problems Related to Primary Support Group

V61.10 (Z63.0)   Relationship Distress With Spouse or Intimate Partner

This category should be used when the major focus of the clinical contact is to address the quality of the intimate (spouse or partner) relationship or when the quality of that relationship is affecting the course, prognosis, or treatment of a mental or other medical disorder. Partners can be of the same or different genders. Typically, the relationship distress is associated with impaired functioning in behavioral, cognitive, or affective domains. Examples of behavioral problems include conflict resolution difficulty, withdrawal, and overinvolvement. Cognitive problems can manifest as chronic negative attributions of the other's intentions or dismissals of the partner's positive behaviors. Affective problems would include chronic sadness, apathy, and/or anger about the other partner.

> **Note:** This category excludes clinical encounters for V61.1x (Z69.1x) mental health services for spousal or partner abuse problems and V65.49 (Z70.9) sex counseling.

V61.03 (Z63.5)   Disruption of Family by Separation or Divorce

This category should be used when partners in an intimate adult couple are living apart due to relationship problems or are in the process of divorce.

V61.8 (Z63.8)   High Expressed Emotion Level Within Family

Expressed emotion is a construct used as a qualitative measure of the "amount" of emotion—in particular, hostility, emotional overinvolvement, and criticism directed toward a family member who is an identified patient—displayed in the family environment. This category should be used when a family's high level of expressed emotion is the focus of clinical attention or is affecting the course, prognosis, or treatment of a family member's mental or other medical disorder.

V62.82 (Z63.4)   Uncomplicated Bereavement

This category can be used when the focus of clinical attention is a normal reaction to the death of a loved one. As part of their reaction to such a loss, some grieving individuals present with symptoms characteristic of a major depressive episode—for example, feelings of sadness and associated symptoms such as insomnia, poor appetite, and weight loss. The bereaved individual typically regards the depressed mood as "normal," although the individual may seek professional help for relief of associated symptoms such as insomnia or anorexia. The duration and expression of "normal" bereavement vary considerably among different cultural groups. Further guidance in distinguishing grief from a major depressive episode is provided in the criteria for major depressive episode.

Abuse and Neglect

Maltreatment by a family member (e.g., caregiver, intimate adult partner) or by a nonrelative can be the area of current clinical focus, or such maltreatment can be an important factor in the assessment and treatment of patients with mental or other medical disorders. Because of the legal implications of abuse and neglect, care should be used in assessing these conditions and assigning these codes. Having a past history of abuse or neglect can influence diagnosis and treatment response in a number of mental disorders, and may also be noted along with the diagnosis.

For the following categories, in addition to listings of the confirmed or suspected event of abuse or neglect, other codes are provided for use if the current clinical encounter is to provide mental health services to either the victim or the perpetrator of the abuse or neglect. A separate code is also provided for designating a past history of abuse or neglect.

Coding Note for ICD-10-CM Abuse and Neglect Conditions
For T codes only, the 7th character should be coded as follows:

A (initial encounter)—Use while the patient is receiving active treatment for the condition (e.g., surgical treatment, emergency department encounter, evaluation and treatment by a new clinician); or

D (subsequent encounter)—Use for encounters after the patient has received active treatment for the condition and when he or she is receiving routine care for the condition during the healing or recovery phase (e.g., cast change or removal, removal of external or internal fixation device, medication adjustment, other aftercare and follow-up visits).

Child Maltreatment and Neglect Problems

Child Physical Abuse

Child physical abuse is nonaccidental physical injury to a child—ranging from minor bruises to severe fractures or death—occurring as a result of punching, beating, kicking, biting, shaking, throwing, stabbing, choking, hitting (with a hand, stick, strap, or other object), burning, or any other method that is inflicted by a parent, caregiver, or other individual who has responsibility for the child. Such injury is considered abuse regardless of whether the caregiver intended to hurt the child. Physical discipline, such as spanking or paddling, is not considered abuse as long as it is reasonable and causes no bodily injury to the child.

Child Physical Abuse, Confirmed
995.54 (T74.12XA) Initial encounter
995.54 (T74.12XD) Subsequent encounter

Child Physical Abuse, Suspected
995.54 (T76.12XA) Initial encounter
995.54 (T76.12XD) Subsequent encounter

Other Circumstances Related to Child Physical Abuse

V61.21 (Z69.010)   Encounter for mental health services for victim of child abuse by parent

V61.21 (Z69.020)   Encounter for mental health services for victim of nonparental child abuse

V15.41 (Z62.810)   Personal history (past history) of physical abuse in childhood

V61.22 (Z69.011)   Encounter for mental health services for perpetrator of parental child abuse

V62.83 (Z69.021)   Encounter for mental health services for perpetrator of nonparental child abuse

Child Sexual Abuse

Child sexual abuse encompasses any sexual act involving a child that is intended to provide sexual gratification to a parent, caregiver, or other individual who has responsibility for the child. Sexual abuse includes activities such as fondling a child's genitals, penetration, incest, rape, sodomy, and indecent exposure. Sexual abuse also includes noncontact exploitation of a child by a parent or caregiver—for example, forcing, tricking, enticing, threatening, or pressuring a child to participate in acts for the sexual gratification of others, without direct physical contact between child and abuser.

Child Sexual Abuse, Confirmed

995.53 (T74.22XA) Initial encounter

995.53 (T74.22XD) Subsequent encounter

Child Sexual Abuse, Suspected

995.53 (T76.22XA) Initial encounter

995.53 (T76.22XD) Subsequent encounter

Other Circumstances Related to Child Sexual Abuse

V61.21 (Z69.010)   Encounter for mental health services for victim of child sexual abuse by parent

V61.21 (Z69.020)   Encounter for mental health services for victim of nonparental child sexual abuse

V15.41 (Z62.810)   Personal history (past history) of sexual abuse in childhood

V61.22 (Z69.011)   Encounter for mental health services for perpetrator of parental child sexual abuse

V62.83 (Z69.021)   Encounter for mental health services for perpetrator of nonparental child sexual abuse

Child Neglect

Child neglect is defined as any confirmed or suspected egregious act or omission by a child's parent or other caregiver that deprives the child of basic age-appropriate needs and thereby results, or has reasonable potential to result, in physical or psychological harm to the child. Child neglect encompasses abandonment; lack of appropriate supervision; failure to attend to necessary emotional or psychological needs; and failure to provide necessary education, medical care, nourishment, shelter, and/or clothing.

Child Neglect, Confirmed

995.52 (T74.02XA) Initial encounter

995.52 (T74.02XD) Subsequent encounter

Child Neglect, Suspected

995.52 (T76.02XA) Initial encounter

995.52 (T76.02XD) Subsequent encounter

Other Circumstances Related to Child Neglect

V61.21 (Z69.010) Encounter for mental health services for victim of child neglect by parent

V61.21 (Z69.020) Encounter for mental health services for victim of nonparental child neglect

V15.42 (Z62.812) Personal history (past history) of neglect in childhood

V61.22 (Z69.011) Encounter for mental health services for perpetrator of parental child neglect

V62.83 (Z69.021) Encounter for mental health services for perpetrator of nonparental child neglect

Child Psychological Abuse

Child psychological abuse is nonaccidental verbal or symbolic acts by a child's parent or caregiver that result, or have reasonable potential to result, in significant psychological harm to the child. (Physical and sexual abusive acts are not included in this category.) Examples of psychological abuse of a child include berating, disparaging, or humiliating the child; threatening the child; harming/abandoning—or indicating that the alleged offender will harm/abandon—people or things that the child cares about; confining the child (as by tying a child's arms or legs together or binding a child to furniture or another object, or confining a child to a small enclosed area [e.g., a closet]); egregious scapegoating of the child; coercing the child to inflict pain on himself or herself; and disciplining the child excessively (i.e., at an extremely high frequency or duration, even if not at a level of physical abuse) through physical or nonphysical means.

Child Psychological Abuse, Confirmed

995.51 (T74.32XA) Initial encounter

995.51 (T74.32XD) Subsequent encounter

Child Psychological Abuse, Suspected

995.51 (T76.32XA) Initial encounter

995.51 (T76.32XD) Subsequent encounter

Other Circumstances Related to Child Psychological Abuse

V61.21 (Z69.010) Encounter for mental health services for victim of child psychological abuse by parent

V61.21 (Z69.020) Encounter for mental health services for victim of nonparental child psychological abuse

V15.42 (Z62.811) Personal history (past history) of psychological abuse in childhood

V61.22 (Z69.011) Encounter for mental health services for perpetrator of parental child psychological abuse

V62.83 (Z69.021) Encounter for mental health services for perpetrator of nonparental child psychological abuse

Adult Maltreatment and Neglect Problems

Spouse or Partner Violence, Physical

This category should be used when nonaccidental acts of physical force that result, or have reasonable potential to result, in physical harm to an intimate partner or that evoke significant fear in the partner have occurred during the past year. Nonaccidental acts of physical force include shoving, slapping, hair pulling, pinching, restraining, shaking, throwing, biting, kicking, hitting with the fist or an object, burning, poisoning, applying force to the throat, cutting off the air supply, holding the head under water, and using a weapon. Acts for the purpose of physically protecting oneself or one's partner are excluded.

Spouse or Partner Violence, Physical, Confirmed

995.81 (T74.11XA) Initial encounter

995.81 (T74.11XD) Subsequent encounter

Spouse or Partner Violence, Physical, Suspected

995.81 (T76.11XA) Initial encounter

995.81 (T76.11XD) Subsequent encounter

Other Circumstances Related to Spouse or Partner Violence, Physical

V61.11 (Z69.11) Encounter for mental health services for victim of spouse or partner violence, physical

V15.41 (Z91.410) Personal history (past history) of spouse or partner violence, physical

V61.12 (Z69.12) Encounter for mental health services for perpetrator of spouse or partner violence, physical

Spouse or Partner Violence, Sexual

This category should be used when forced or coerced sexual acts with an intimate partner have occurred during the past year. Sexual violence may involve the use of physical force or psychological coercion to compel the partner to engage in a sexual act against his or her will, whether or not the act is completed. Also included in this category are sexual acts with an intimate partner who is unable to consent.

Spouse or Partner Violence, Sexual, Confirmed

995.83 (T74.21XA) Initial encounter

995.83 (T74.21XD) Subsequent encounter

Spouse or Partner Violence, Sexual, Suspected

995.83 (T76.21XA) Initial encounter

995.83 (T76.21XD) Subsequent encounter

Other Circumstances Related to Spouse or Partner Violence, Sexual

V61.11 (Z69.81) Encounter for mental health services for victim of spouse or partner violence, sexual

V15.41 (Z91.410) Personal history (past history) of spouse or partner violence, sexual

V61.12 (Z69.12) Encounter for mental health services for perpetrator of spouse or partner violence, sexual

Spouse or Partner Neglect

Partner neglect is any egregious act or omission in the past year by one partner that deprives a dependent partner of basic needs and thereby results, or has reasonable potential to result, in physical or psychological harm to the dependent partner. This category is used in the context of relationships in which one partner is extremely dependent on the other partner for care or for assistance in navigating ordinary daily activities—for example, a partner who is incapable of self-care owing to substantial physical, psychological/intellectual, or cultural limitations (e.g., inability to communicate with others and manage everyday activities due to living in a foreign culture).

Spouse or Partner Neglect, Confirmed

995.85 (T74.01XA)   Initial encounter

995.85 (T74.01XD)   Subsequent encounter

Spouse or Partner Neglect, Suspected

995.85 (T76.01XA) Initial encounter

995.85 (T76.01XD) Subsequent encounter

Other Circumstances Related to Spouse or Partner Neglect

V61.11 (Z69.11)   Encounter for mental health services for victim of spouse or partner neglect

V15.42 (Z91.412)   Personal history (past history) of spouse or partner neglect

V61.12 (Z69.12)   Encounter for mental health services for perpetrator of spouse or partner neglect

Spouse or Partner Abuse, Psychological

Partner psychological abuse encompasses nonaccidental verbal or symbolic acts by one partner that result, or have reasonable potential to result, in significant harm to the other partner. This category should be used when such psychological abuse has occurred during the past year. Acts of psychological abuse include berating or humiliating the victim; interrogating the victim; restricting the victim's ability to come and go freely; obstructing the victim's access to assistance (e.g., law enforcement; legal, protective, or medical resources); threatening the victim with physical harm or sexual assault; harming, or threatening to harm, people or things that the victim cares about; unwarranted restriction of the victim's access to or use of economic resources; isolating the victim from family, friends, or social support resources; stalking the victim; and trying to make the victim think that he or she is crazy.

Spouse or Partner Abuse, Psychological, Confirmed

995.82 (T74.31XA) Initial encounter

995.82 (T74.31XD) Subsequent encounter

Spouse or Partner Abuse, Psychological, Suspected

995.82 (T76.31XA) Initial encounter

995.82 (T76.31XD) Subsequent encounter

Other Circumstances Related to Spouse or Partner Abuse, Psychological

V61.11 (Z69.11)   Encounter for mental health services for victim of spouse or partner psychological abuse

V15.42 (Z91.411) Personal history (past history) of spouse or partner psychological abuse

V61.12 (Z69.12) Encounter for mental health services for perpetrator of spouse or partner psychological abuse

Adult Abuse by Nonspouse or Nonpartner

These categories should be used when an adult has been abused by another adult who is not an intimate partner. Such maltreatment may involve acts of physical, sexual, or emotional abuse. Examples of adult abuse include nonaccidental acts of physical force (e.g., pushing/shoving, scratching, slapping, throwing something that could hurt, punching, biting) that have resulted—or have reasonable potential to result—in physical harm or have caused significant fear; forced or coerced sexual acts; and verbal or symbolic acts with the potential to cause psychological harm (e.g., berating or humiliating the person; interrogating the person; restricting the person's ability to come and go freely; obstructing the person's access to assistance; threatening the person; harming or threatening to harm people or things that the person cares about; restricting the person's access to or use of economic resources; isolating the person from family, friends, or social support resources; stalking the person; trying to make the person think that he or she is crazy). Acts for the purpose of physically protecting oneself or the other person are excluded.

Adult Physical Abuse by Nonspouse or Nonpartner, Confirmed

995.81 (T74.11XA) Initial encounter

995.81 (T74.11XD) Subsequent encounter

Adult Physical Abuse by Nonspouse or Nonpartner, Suspected

995.81 (T76.11XA) Initial encounter

995.81 (T76.11XD) Subsequent encounter

Adult Sexual Abuse by Nonspouse or Nonpartner, Confirmed

995.83 (T74.21XA) Initial encounter

995.83 (T74.21XD) Subsequent encounter

Adult Sexual Abuse by Nonspouse or Nonpartner, Suspected

995.83 (T76.21XA) Initial encounter

995.83 (T76.21XD) Subsequent encounter

Adult Psychological Abuse by Nonspouse or Nonpartner, Confirmed

995.82 (T74.31XA) Initial encounter

995.82 (T74.31XD) Subsequent encounter

Adult Psychological Abuse by Nonspouse or Nonpartner, Suspected

995.82 (T76.31XA) Initial encounter

995.82 (T76.31XD) Subsequent encounter

Other Circumstances Related to Adult Abuse by Nonspouse or Nonpartner

V65.49 (Z69.81) Encounter for mental health services for victim of nonspousal or nonpartner adult abuse

V62.83 (Z69.82) Encounter for mental health services for perpetrator of nonspousal or nonpartner adult abuse

Educational and Occupational Problems

Educational Problems

V62.3 (Z55.9)   Academic or Educational Problem

This category should be used when an academic or educational problem is the focus of clinical attention or has an impact on the individual's diagnosis, treatment, or prognosis. Problems to be considered include illiteracy or low-level literacy; lack of access to schooling owing to unavailability or unattainability; problems with academic performance (e.g., failing school examinations, receiving failing marks or grades) or underachievement (below what would be expected given the individual's intellectual capacity); discord with teachers, school staff, or other students; and any other problems related to education and/or literacy.

Occupational Problems

V62.21 (Z56.82)   Problem Related to Current Military Deployment Status

This category should be used when an occupational problem directly related to an individual's military deployment status is the focus of clinical attention or has an impact on the individual's diagnosis, treatment, or prognosis. Psychological reactions to deployment are not included in this category; such reactions would be better captured as an adjustment disorder or another mental disorder.

V62.29 (Z56.9)   Other Problem Related to Employment

This category should be used when an occupational problem is the focus of clinical attention or has an impact on the individual's treatment or prognosis. Areas to be considered include problems with employment or in the work environment, including unemployment; recent change of job; threat of job loss; job dissatisfaction; stressful work schedule; uncertainty about career choices; sexual harassment on the job; other discord with boss, supervisor, co-workers, or others in the work environment; uncongenial or hostile work environments; other psychosocial stressors related to work; and any other problems related to employment and/or occupation.

Housing and Economic Problems

Housing Problems

V60.0 (Z59.0)   Homelessness

This category should be used when lack of a regular dwelling or living quarters has an impact on an individual's treatment or prognosis. An individual is considered to be homeless if his or her primary nighttime residence is a homeless shelter, a warming shelter, a domestic violence shelter, a public space (e.g., tunnel, transportation station, mall), a building not intended for residential use (e.g., abandoned structure, unused factory), a cardboard box or cave, or some other ad hoc housing situation.

V60.1 (Z59.1)   Inadequate Housing

This category should be used when lack of adequate housing has an impact on an individual's treatment or prognosis. Examples of inadequate housing conditions include lack of heat (in cold temperatures) or electricity, infestation by insects or rodents, inadequate plumbing and toilet facilities, overcrowding, lack of adequate sleeping space, and excessive noise. It is important to consider cultural norms before assigning this category.

V60.89 (Z59.2)   Discord With Neighbor, Lodger, or Landlord

This category should be used when discord with neighbors, lodgers, or a landlord is a focus of clinical attention or has an impact on the individual's treatment or prognosis.

V60.6 (Z59.3)   Problem Related to Living in a Residential Institution
This category should be used when a problem (or problems) related to living in a residential institution is a focus of clinical attention or has an impact on the individual's treatment or prognosis. Psychological reactions to a change in living situation are not included in this category; such reactions would be better captured as an adjustment disorder.

Economic Problems

V60.2 (Z59.4)   Lack of Adequate Food or Safe Drinking Water

V60.2 (Z59.5)   Extreme Poverty

V60.2 (Z59.6)   Low Income

V60.2 (Z59.7)   Insufficient Social Insurance or Welfare Support
This category should be used for individuals who meet eligibility criteria for social or welfare support but are not receiving such support, who receive support that is insufficient to address their needs, or who otherwise lack access to needed insurance or support programs. Examples include inability to qualify for welfare support owing to lack of proper documentation or evidence of address, inability to obtain adequate health insurance because of age or a preexisting condition, and denial of support owing to excessively stringent income or other requirements.

V60.9 (Z59.9)   Unspecified Housing or Economic Problem
This category should be used when there is a problem related to housing or economic circumstances other than as specified above.

Other Problems Related to the Social Environment

V62.89 (Z60.0)   Phase of Life Problem
This category should be used when a problem adjusting to a life-cycle transition (a particular developmental phase) is the focus of clinical attention or has an impact on the individual's treatment or prognosis. Examples of such transitions include entering or completing school, leaving parental control, getting married, starting a new career, becoming a parent, adjusting to an "empty nest" after children leave home, and retiring.

V60.3 (Z60.2)   Problem Related to Living Alone
This category should be used when a problem associated with living alone is the focus of clinical attention or has an impact on the individual's treatment or prognosis. Examples of such problems include chronic feelings of loneliness, isolation, and lack of structure in carrying out activities of daily living (e.g., irregular meal and sleep schedules, inconsistent performance of home maintenance chores).

V62.4 (Z60.3)   Acculturation Difficulty
This category should be used when difficulty in adjusting to a new culture (e.g., following migration) is the focus of clinical attention or has an impact on the individual's treatment or prognosis.

V62.4 (Z60.4)   Social Exclusion or Rejection
This category should be used when there is an imbalance of social power such that there is recurrent social exclusion or rejection by others. Examples of social rejection include bullying, teasing, and intimidation by others; being targeted by others for verbal abuse and humiliation; and being purposefully excluded from the activities of peers, workmates, or others in one's social environment.

V62.4 (Z60.5)   Target of (Perceived) Adverse Discrimination or Persecution
This category should be used when there is perceived or experienced discrimination against or persecution of the individual based on his or her membership (or perceived

membership) in a specific category. Typically, such categories include gender or gender identity, race, ethnicity, religion, sexual orientation, country of origin, political beliefs, disability status, caste, social status, weight, and physical appearance.

V62.9 (Z60.9)   Unspecified Problem Related to Social Environment
This category should be used when there is a problem related to the individual's social environment other than as specified above.

Problems Related to Crime or Interaction With the Legal System

V62.89 (Z65.4)	**Victim of Crime**
V62.5 (Z65.0)	**Conviction in Civil or Criminal Proceedings Without Imprisonment**
V62.5 (Z65.1)	**Imprisonment or Other Incarceration**
V62.5 (Z65.2)	**Problems Related to Release From Prison**
V62.5 (Z65.3)	**Problems Related to Other Legal Circumstances**

Other Health Service Encounters for Counseling and Medical Advice

V65.49 (Z70.9)   Sex Counseling
This category should be used when the individual seeks counseling related to sex education, sexual behavior, sexual orientation, sexual attitudes (embarrassment, timidity), others' sexual behavior or orientation (e.g., spouse, partner, child), sexual enjoyment, or any other sex-related issue.

V65.40 (Z71.9)   Other Counseling or Consultation
This category should be used when counseling is provided or advice/consultation is sought for a problem that is not specified above or elsewhere in this chapter. Examples include spiritual or religious counseling, dietary counseling, and counseling on nicotine use.

Problems Related to Other Psychosocial, Personal, and Environmental Circumstances

V62.89 (Z65.8)   Religious or Spiritual Problem
This category can be used when the focus of clinical attention is a religious or spiritual problem. Examples include distressing experiences that involve loss or questioning of faith, problems associated with conversion to a new faith, or questioning of spiritual values that may not necessarily be related to an organized church or religious institution.

V61.7 (Z64.0)	**Problems Related to Unwanted Pregnancy**
V61.5 (Z64.1)	**Problems Related to Multiparity**
V62.89 (Z64.4)	**Discord With Social Service Provider, Including Probation Officer, Case Manager, or Social Services Worker**
V62.89 (Z65.4)	**Victim of Terrorism or Torture**
V62.22 (Z65.5)	**Exposure to Disaster, War, or Other Hostilities**
V62.89 (Z65.8)	**Other Problem Related to Psychosocial Circumstances**
V62.9 (Z65.9)	**Unspecified Problem Related to Unspecified Psychosocial Circumstances**

Other Circumstances of Personal History

V15.49 (Z91.49)   **Other Personal History of Psychological Trauma**

V15.59 (Z91.5)   **Personal History of Self-Harm**

V62.22 (Z91.82)   **Personal History of Military Deployment**

V15.89 (Z91.89)   **Other Personal Risk Factors**

V69.9 (Z72.9)   Problem Related to Lifestyle

This category should be used when a lifestyle problem is a specific focus of treatment or directly affects the course, prognosis, or treatment of a mental or other medical disorder. Examples of lifestyle problems include lack of physical exercise, inappropriate diet, high-risk sexual behavior, and poor sleep hygiene. A problem that is attributable to a symptom of a mental disorder should not be coded unless that problem is a specific focus of treatment or directly affects the course, prognosis, or treatment of the individual. In such cases, both the mental disorder and the lifestyle problem should be coded.

V71.01 (Z72.811)   Adult Antisocial Behavior

This category can be used when the focus of clinical attention is adult antisocial behavior that is not due to a mental disorder (e.g., conduct disorder, antisocial personality disorder). Examples include the behavior of some professional thieves, racketeers, or dealers in illegal substances.

V71.02 (Z72.810)   Child or Adolescent Antisocial Behavior

This category can be used when the focus of clinical attention is antisocial behavior in a child or adolescent that is not due to a mental disorder (e.g., intermittent explosive disorder, conduct disorder). Examples include isolated antisocial acts by children or adolescents (not a pattern of antisocial behavior).

Problems Related to Access to Medical and Other Health Care

V63.9 (Z75.3)   **Unavailability or Inaccessibility of Health Care Facilities**

V63.8 (Z75.4)   **Unavailability or Inaccessibility of Other Helping Agencies**

Nonadherence to Medical Treatment

V15.81 (Z91.19)   Nonadherence to Medical Treatment

This category can be used when the focus of clinical attention is nonadherence to an important aspect of treatment for a mental disorder or another medical condition. Reasons for such nonadherence may include discomfort resulting from treatment (e.g., medication side effects), expense of treatment, personal value judgments or religious or cultural beliefs about the proposed treatment, age-related debility, and the presence of a mental disorder (e.g., schizophrenia, personality disorder). This category should be used only when the problem is sufficiently severe to warrant independent clinical attention and does not meet diagnostic criteria for psychological factors affecting other medical conditions.

278.00 (E66.9)   Overweight or Obesity

This category may be used when overweight or obesity is a focus of clinical attention.

V65.2 (Z76.5)   Malingering

The essential feature of malingering is the intentional production of false or grossly exaggerated physical or psychological symptoms, motivated by external incentives such as avoiding military duty, avoiding work, obtaining financial compensation, evading criminal prosecution, or obtaining drugs. Under some circumstances, malingering may represent adaptive behavior—for example, feigning illness while a captive of the enemy during wartime. Malingering should be strongly suspected if any combination of the following is noted:

1. Medicolegal context of presentation (e.g., the individual is referred by an attorney to the clinician for examination, or the individual self-refers while litigation or criminal charges are pending).
2. Marked discrepancy between the individual's claimed stress or disability and the objective findings and observations.
3. Lack of cooperation during the diagnostic evaluation and in complying with the prescribed treatment regimen.
4. The presence of antisocial personality disorder.

Malingering differs from factitious disorder in that the motivation for the symptom production in malingering is an external incentive, whereas in factitious disorder external incentives are absent. Malingering is differentiated from conversion disorder and somatic symptom–related mental disorders by the intentional production of symptoms and by the obvious external incentives associated with it. Definite evidence of feigning (such as clear evidence that loss of function is present during the examination but not at home) would suggest a diagnosis of factitious disorder if the individual's apparent aim is to assume the sick role, or malingering if it is to obtain an incentive, such as money.

V40.31 (Z91.83)   Wandering Associated With a Mental Disorder

This category is used for individuals with a mental disorder whose desire to walk about leads to significant clinical management or safety concerns. For example, individuals with major neurocognitive or neurodevelopmental disorders may experience a restless urge to wander that places them at risk for falls and causes them to leave supervised settings without needed accompaniment. This category excludes individuals whose intent is to escape an unwanted housing situation (e.g., children who are running away from home, patients who no longer wish to remain in the hospital) or those who walk or pace as a result of medication-induced akathisia.

> **Coding note:** First code associated mental disorder (e.g., major neurocognitive disorder, autism spectrum disorder), then code V40.31 (Z91.83) wandering associated with [specific mental disorder].

V62.89 (R41.83)   Borderline Intellectual Functioning

This category can be used when an individual's borderline intellectual functioning is the focus of clinical attention or has an impact on the individual's treatment or prognosis. Differentiating borderline intellectual functioning and mild intellectual disability (intellectual developmental disorder) requires careful assessment of intellectual and adaptive functions and their discrepancies, particularly in the presence of co-occurring mental disorders that may affect patient compliance with standardized testing procedures (e.g., schizophrenia or attention-deficit/hyperactivity disorder with severe impulsivity).

SECTION III
Emerging Measures and Models

This section contains tools and techniques to enhance the clinical decision-making process, understand the cultural context of mental disorders, and recognize emerging diagnoses for further study. It provides strategies to enhance clinical practice and new criteria to stimulate future research, representing a dynamic DSM-5 that will evolve with advances in the field.

Among the tools in Section III is a Level 1 cross-cutting self/informant-rated measure that serves as a review of systems across mental disorders. A clinician-rated severity scale for schizophrenia and other psychotic disorders also is provided, as well as the World Health Organization Disability Assessment Schedule, Version 2 (WHODAS 2.0). Level 2 severity measures are available online (www.psychiatry.org/dsm5) and may be used to explore significant responses to the Level 1 screen. A comprehensive review of the cultural context of mental disorders, and the Cultural Formulation Interview (CFI) for clinical use, are provided.

Proposed disorders for future study are provided, which include a new model for the diagnosis of personality disorders as an alternative to the established diagnostic criteria; the proposed model incorporates impairments in personality functioning as well as pathological personality traits. Also included are new conditions that are the focus of active research, such as attenuated psychosis syndrome and nonsuicidal self-injury.

Assessment Measures

A growing body of scientific evidence favors dimensional concepts in the diagnosis of mental disorders. The limitations of a categorical approach to diagnosis include the failure to find zones of rarity between diagnoses (i.e., delineation of mental disorders from one another by natural boundaries), the need for intermediate categories like schizoaffective disorder, high rates of comorbidity, frequent not-otherwise-specified (NOS) diagnoses, relative lack of utility in furthering the identification of unique antecedent validators for most mental disorders, and lack of treatment specificity for the various diagnostic categories.

From both clinical and research perspectives, there is a need for a more dimensional approach that can be combined with DSM's set of categorical diagnoses. Such an approach incorporates variations of features within an individual (e.g., differential severity of individual symptoms both within and outside of a disorder's diagnostic criteria as measured by intensity, duration, or number of symptoms, along with other features such as type and severity of disabilities) rather than relying on a simple yes-or-no approach. For diagnoses for which all symptoms are needed for a diagnosis (a monothetic criteria set), different severity levels of the constituent symptoms may be noted. If a threshold endorsement of multiple symptoms is needed, such as at least five of nine symptoms for major depressive disorder (a polythetic criteria set), both severity levels and different combinations of the criteria may identify more homogeneous diagnostic groups.

A dimensional approach depending primarily on an individual's subjective reports of symptom experiences along with the clinician's interpretation is consistent with current diagnostic practice. It is expected that as our understanding of basic disease mechanisms based on pathophysiology, neurocircuitry, gene-environment interactions, and laboratory tests increases, approaches that integrate both objective and subjective patient data will be developed to supplement and enhance the accuracy of the diagnostic process.

Cross-cutting symptom measures modeled on general medicine's review of systems can serve as an approach for reviewing critical psychopathological domains. The general medical review of systems is crucial to detecting subtle changes in different organ systems that can facilitate diagnosis and treatment. A similar review of various mental functions can aid in a more comprehensive mental status assessment by drawing attention to symptoms that may not fit neatly into the diagnostic criteria suggested by the individual's presenting symptoms, but may nonetheless be important to the individual's care. The cross-cutting measures have two levels: Level 1 questions are a brief survey of 13 symptom domains for adult patients and 12 domains for child and adolescent patients. Level 2 questions provide a more in-depth assessment of certain domains. These measures were developed to be administered both at initial interview and over time to track the patient's symptom status and response to treatment.

Severity measures are disorder-specific, corresponding closely to the criteria that constitute the disorder definition. They may be administered to individuals who have received a diagnosis or who have a clinically significant syndrome that falls short of meeting full criteria for a diagnosis. Some of the assessments are self-completed by the individual, while others require a clinician to complete. As with the cross-cutting symptom measures, these measures were developed to be administered both at initial interview and over time to track the severity of the individual's disorder and response to treatment.

The World Health Organization Disability Assessment Schedule, Version 2.0 (WHODAS 2.0) was developed to assess a patient's ability to perform activities in six areas: understanding and communicating; getting around; self-care; getting along with people; life activities (e.g., household, work/school); and participation in society. The scale is self-administered and was developed to be used in patients with any medical disorder. It corresponds to concepts contained in the WHO International Classification of Functioning, Disability and Health. This assessment can also be used over time to track changes in a patient's disabilities.

This chapter focuses on the DSM-5 Level 1 Cross-Cutting Symptom Measure (adult self-rated and parent/guardian versions); the Clinician-Rated Dimensions of Psychosis Symptom Severity; and the WHODAS 2.0. Clinician instructions, scoring information, and interpretation guidelines are included for each. These measures and additional dimensional assessments, including those for diagnostic severity, can be found online at www.psychiatry.org/dsm5.

Cross-Cutting Symptom Measures

Level 1 Cross-Cutting Symptom Measure

The DSM-5 Level 1 Cross-Cutting Symptom Measure is a patient- or informant-rated measure that assesses mental health domains that are important across psychiatric diagnoses. It is intended to help clinicians identify additional areas of inquiry that may have significant impact on the individual's treatment and prognosis. In addition, the measure may be used to track changes in the individual's symptom presentation over time.

The adult version of the measure consists of 23 questions that assess 13 psychiatric domains, including depression, anger, mania, anxiety, somatic symptoms, suicidal ideation, psychosis, sleep problems, memory, repetitive thoughts and behaviors, dissociation, personality functioning, and substance use (Table 1). Each domain consists of one to three questions. Each item inquires about how much (or how often) the individual has been bothered by the specific symptom during the past 2 weeks. If the individual is of impaired capacity and unable to complete the form (e.g., an individual with dementia), a knowledgeable adult informant may complete this measure. The measure was found to be clinically useful and to have good reliability in the DSM-5 field trials that were conducted in adult clinical samples across the United States and in Canada.

The parent/guardian-rated version of the measure (for children ages 6–17) consists of 25 questions that assess 12 psychiatric domains, including depression, anger, irritability, mania, anxiety, somatic symptoms, inattention, suicidal ideation/attempt, psychosis, sleep disturbance, repetitive thoughts and behaviors, and substance use (Table 2). Each item asks the parent or guardian to rate how much (or how often) his or her child has been bothered by the specific psychiatric symptom during the past 2 weeks. The measure was also found to be clinically useful and to have good reliability in the DSM-5 field trials that were conducted in pediatric clinical samples across the United States. For children ages 11–17, along with the parent/guardian rating of the child's symptoms, the clinician may consider having the child complete the child-rated version of the measure. The child-rated version of the measure can be found online at www.psychiatry.org/dsm5.

Scoring and interpretation.   On the adult self-rated version of the measure, each item is rated on a 5-point scale (0=none or not at all; 1=slight or rare, less than a day or two; 2=mild or several days; 3=moderate or more than half the days; and 4=severe or nearly every day). The score on each item within a domain should be reviewed. However, a rating of mild (i.e., 2) or greater on any item within a domain, except for substance use, suicidal ideation, and psychosis, may serve as a guide for additional inquiry and follow-up to determine if a more detailed assessment is necessary, which may include the Level 2 cross-cutting symptom assessment for the domain (see Table 1). For substance use, suicidal ideation, and psychosis, a

TABLE 1 Adult DSM-5 Self-Rated Level 1 Cross-Cutting Symptom Measure: 13 domains, thresholds for further inquiry, and associated DSM-5 Level 2 measures

Domain	Domain name	Threshold to guide further inquiry	DSM-5 Level 2 Cross-Cutting Symptom Measure[a]
I.	Depression	Mild or greater	Level 2—Depression—Adult (PROMIS Emotional Distress—Short Form)
II.	Anger	Mild or greater	Level 2—Anger—Adult (PROMIS Emotional Distress—Anger—Short Form)
III.	Mania	Mild or greater	Level 2—Mania—Adult (Altman Self-Rating Mania Scale [ASRM])
IV.	Anxiety	Mild or greater	Level 2—Anxiety—Adult (PROMIS Emotional Distress—Anxiety—Short Form)
V.	Somatic symptoms	Mild or greater	Level 2—Somatic Symptom—Adult (Patient Health Questionnaire–15 [PHQ-15] Somatic Symptom Severity Scale)
VI.	Suicidal ideation	Slight or greater	None
VII.	Psychosis	Slight or greater	None
VIII.	Sleep problems	Mild or greater	Level 2—Sleep Disturbance—Adult (PROMIS Sleep Disturbance—Short Form)
IX.	Memory	Mild or greater	None
X.	Repetitive thoughts and behaviors	Mild or greater	Level 2—Repetitive Thoughts and Behaviors—Adult (Florida Obsessive-Compulsive Inventory [FOCI] Severity Scale)
XI.	Dissociation	Mild or greater	None
XII.	Personality functioning	Mild or greater	None
XIII.	Substance use	Slight or greater	Level 2—Substance Use—Adult (adapted from the NIDA-Modified ASSIST)

Note. NIDA=National Institute on Drug Abuse.
[a]Available at www.psychiatry.org/dsm5.

rating of slight (i.e., 1) or greater on any item within the domain may serve as a guide for additional inquiry and follow-up to determine if a more detailed assessment is needed. As such, indicate the highest score within a domain in the "Highest domain score" column. Table 1 outlines threshold scores that may guide further inquiry for the remaining domains.

On the parent/guardian-rated version of the measure (for children ages 6–17), 19 of the 25 items are each rated on a 5-point scale (0=none or not at all; 1=slight or rare, less than a day or two; 2=mild or several days; 3=moderate or more than half the days; and 4=severe or nearly every day). The suicidal ideation, suicide attempt, and substance abuse items are each rated on a "Yes, No, or Don't Know" scale. The score on each item within a domain should be reviewed. However, with the exception of inattention and psychosis, a rating of mild (i.e., 2) or greater on any item within a domain that is scored on the 5-point scale may serve as a guide for additional inquiry and follow-up to determine if a more detailed assessment is necessary, which may include the Level 2 cross-cutting symptom assessment for the domain (see Table 2). For inattention or psychosis, a rating of slight or greater (i.e., 1 or greater) may be

TABLE 2 Parent/guardian-rated DSM-5 Level 1 Cross-Cutting Symptom Measure
for child age 6–17: 12 domains, thresholds for further inquiry, and
associated Level 2 measures

Domain	Domain name	Threshold to guide further inquiry	DSM-5 Level 2 Cross-Cutting Symptom Measure[a]
I.	Somatic symptoms	Mild or greater	Level 2—Somatic Symptoms—Parent/Guardian of Child Age 6–17 (Patient Health Questionnaire–15 Somatic Symptom Severity Scale [PHQ-15])
II.	Sleep problems	Mild or greater	Level 2—Sleep Disturbance—Parent/Guardian of Child Age 6–17 (PROMIS Sleep Disturbance—Short Form)
III.	Inattention	Slight or greater	Level 2—Inattention—Parent/Guardian of Child Age 6–17 (Swanson, Nolan, and Pelham, Version IV [SNAP-IV])
IV.	Depression	Mild or greater	Level 2—Depression—Parent/Guardian of Child Age 6–17 (PROMIS Emotional Distress—Depression—Parent Item Bank)
V.	Anger	Mild or greater	Level 2—Anger—Parent/Guardian of Child (PROMIS Calibrated Anger Measure—Parent)
VI.	Irritability	Mild or greater	Level 2—Irritability—Parent/Guardian of Child (Affective Reactivity Index [ARI])
VII.	Mania	Mild or greater	Level 2—Mania—Parent/Guardian of Child Age 6–17 (Altman Self-Rating Mania Scale [ASRM])
VIII.	Anxiety	Mild or greater	Level 2—Anxiety—Parent/Guardian of Child Age 6–17 (PROMIS Emotional Distress—Anxiety—Parent Item Bank)
IX.	Psychosis	Slight or greater	None
X.	Repetitive thoughts and behaviors	Mild or greater	None
XI.	Substance use	Yes	Level 2—Substance Use—Parent/Guardian of Child Age 6–17 (adapted from the NIDA-modified ASSIST)
		Don't Know	NIDA-modified ASSIST (adapted)—Child-Rated (age 11–17 years)
XII.	Suicidal ideation/ suicide attempts	Yes	None
		Don't Know	None

Note. NIDA=National Institute on Drug Abuse.
[a]Available at www.psychiatry.org/dsm5.

used as an indicator for additional inquiry. A parent or guardian's rating of "Don't Know" on the suicidal ideation, suicide attempt, and any of the substance use items, especially for children ages 11–17 years, may result in additional probing of the issues with the child, including using the child-rated Level 2 Cross-Cutting Symptom Measure for the relevant domain. Because additional inquiry is made on the basis of the highest score on any item within a domain, clinicians should indicate that score in the "Highest Domain Score" column. Table 2 outlines threshold scores that may guide further inquiry for the remaining domains.

Level 2 Cross-Cutting Symptom Measures

Any threshold scores on the Level 1 Cross-Cutting Symptom Measure (as noted in Tables 1 and 2 and described in "Scoring and Interpretation" indicate a possible need for detailed clinical inquiry. Level 2 Cross-Cutting Symptom Measures provide one method of obtaining more in-depth information on potentially significant symptoms to inform diagnosis, treatment planning, and follow-up. They are available online at www.psychiatry.org/dsm5. Tables 1 and 2 outline each Level 1 domain and identify the domains for which DSM-5 Level 2 Cross-Cutting Symptom Measures are available for more detailed assessments. Adult and pediatric (parent and child) versions are available online for most Level 1 symptom domains at www.psychiatry.org/dsm5.

Frequency of Use of the Cross-Cutting Symptom Measures

To track change in the individual's symptom presentation over time, the Level 1 and relevant Level 2 cross-cutting symptom measures may be completed at regular intervals as clinically indicated, depending on the stability of the individual's symptoms and treatment status. For individuals with impaired capacity and for children ages 6–17 years, it is preferable for the measures to be completed at follow-up appointments by the same knowledgeable informant and by the same parent or guardian. Consistently high scores on a particular domain may indicate significant and problematic symptoms for the individual that might warrant further assessment, treatment, and follow-up. Clinical judgment should guide decision making.

DSM-5 Self-Rated Level 1 Cross-Cutting Symptom Measure—Adult

Name: _____   Age: _____   Sex: [ ] Male [ ] Female   Date: _____

If the measure is being completed by an informant, what is your relationship with the individual?: _____

In a typical week, approximately how much time do you spend with the individual? _____ hours/week

Instructions: The questions below ask about things that might have bothered you. For each question, circle the number that best describes how much (or how often) you have been bothered by each problem during the **past TWO (2) WEEKS.**

		During the past **TWO (2) WEEKS**, how much (or how often) have you been bothered by the following problems?	**None** Not at all	**Slight** Rare, less than a day or two	**Mild** Several days	**Moderate** More than half the days	**Severe** Nearly every day	**Highest Domain Score** (clinician)
I.	1.	Little interest or pleasure in doing things?	0	1	2	3	4	
	2.	Feeling down, depressed, or hopeless?	0	1	2	3	4	
II.	3.	Feeling more irritated, grouchy, angry than usual?	0	1	2	3	4	
III.	4.	Sleeping less than usual, but still have a lot of energy?	0	1	2	3	4	
	5.	Starting lots more projects than usual or doing more risky things than usual?	0	1	2	3	4	
IV.	6.	Feeling nervous, anxious, frightened, worried, or on edge?	0	1	2	3	4	
	7.	Feeling panic or being frightened?	0	1	2	3	4	
	8.	Avoiding situations that make you anxious?	0	1	2	3	4	
V.	9.	Unexplained aches and pains (e.g., head, back, joints, abdomen, legs)?	0	1	2	3	4	
	10.	Feeling that your illnesses are not being taken seriously enough?	0	1	2	3	4	
VI.	11.	Thoughts of actually hurting yourself?	0	1	2	3	4	

			0	1	2	3	4
VII.	12.	Hearing things other people couldn't hear, such as voices even when no one was around?	0	1	2	3	4
	13.	Feeling that someone could hear your thoughts, or that you could hear what another person was thinking?	0	1	2	3	4
VIII.	14.	Problems with sleep that affected your sleep quality over all?	0	1	2	3	4
IX.	15.	Problems with memory (e.g., learning new information) or with location (e.g., finding your way home)?	0	1	2	3	4
X.	16.	Unpleasant thoughts, urges, or images that repeatedly enter your mind?	0	1	2	3	4
	17.	Feeling driven to perform certain behaviors or mental acts over and over again?	0	1	2	3	4
XI.	18.	Feeling detached or distant from yourself, your body, your physical surroundings, or your memories?	0	1	2	3	4
XII.	19.	Not knowing who you really are or what you want out of life?	0	1	2	3	4
	20.	Not feeling close to other people or enjoying your relationships with them?	0	1	2	3	4
XIII.	21.	Drink at least 4 drinks of any kind of alcohol in a single day?	0	1	2	3	4
	22.	Smoke any cigarettes, a cigar, or pipe, or use snuff or chewing tobacco?	0	1	2	3	4
	23.	Use any of the following medicines ON YOUR OWN, that is, without a doctor's prescription, in greater amounts or longer than prescribed [e.g., painkillers (like Vicodin), stimulants (like Ritalin or Adderall), sedatives or tranquilizers (like sleeping pills or Valium), or drugs like marijuana, cocaine or crack, club drugs (like ecstasy), hallucinogens (like LSD), heroin, inhalants or solvents (like glue), or methamphetamine (like speed)]?	0	1	2	3	4

Parent/Guardian-Rated DSM-5 Level 1 Cross-Cutting Symptom Measure—Child Age 6–17

Child's Name: _____   Age: _____   Sex: [ ] Male [ ] Female   Date: _____

Relationship to the child: _____

Instructions (*to parent or guardian of child*): The questions below ask about things that might have bothered your child. For each question, circle the number that best describes how much (or how often) your child has been bothered by each problem during **the past TWO (2) WEEKS.**

	During the past **TWO (2) WEEKS,** how much (or how often) has your child…	**None** Not at all	**Slight** Rare, less than a day or two	**Mild** Several days	**Moderate** More than half the days	**Severe** Nearly every day	**Highest Domain Score** (clinician)
I.	1. Complained of stomachaches, headaches, or other aches and pains?	0	1	2	3	4	
	2. Said he/she was worried about his/her health or about getting sick?	0	1	2	3	4	
II.	3. Had problems sleeping—that is, trouble falling asleep, staying asleep, or waking up too early?	0	1	2	3	4	
III.	4. Had problems paying attention when he/she was in class or doing his/her homework or reading a book or playing a game?	0	1	2	3	4	
IV.	5. Had less fun doing things than he/she used to?	0	1	2	3	4	
	6. Seemed sad or depressed for several hours?	0	1	2	3	4	
V. and VI.	7. Seemed more irritated or easily annoyed than usual?	0	1	2	3	4	
	8. Seemed angry or lost his/her temper?	0	1	2	3	4	
VII.	9. Starting lots more projects than usual or doing more risky things than usual?	0	1	2	3	4	
	10. Sleeping less than usual for him/her but still has lots of energy?	0	1	2	3	4	
VIII.	11. Said he/she felt nervous, anxious, or scared?	0	1	2	3	4	
	12. Not been able to stop worrying?	0	1	2	3	4	
	13. Said he/she couldn't do things he/she wanted to or should have done because they made him/her feel nervous?	0	1	2	3	4	

			0	1	2	3	4
IX.	14.	Said that he/she heard voices—when there was no one there—speaking about him/her or telling him/her what to do or saying bad things to him/her?	0	1	2	3	4
	15.	Said that he/she had a vision when he/she was completely awake—that is, saw something or someone that no one else could see?	0	1	2	3	4
X.	16.	Said that he/she had thoughts that kept coming into his/her mind that he/she would do something bad or that something bad would happen to him/her or to someone else?	0	1	2	3	4
	17.	Said he/she felt the need to check on certain things over and over again, like whether a door was locked or whether the stove was turned off?	0	1	2	3	4
	18.	Seemed to worry a lot about things he/she touched being dirty or having germs or being poisoned?	0	1	2	3	4
	19.	Said that he/she had to do things in a certain way, like counting or saying special things out loud, in order to keep something bad from happening?	0	1	2	3	4

In the past TWO (2) WEEKS, has your child...

XI.	20.	Had an alcoholic beverage (beer, wine, liquor, etc.)?	❑ Yes	❑ No	❑ Don't Know
	21.	Smoked a cigarette, a cigar, or pipe, or used snuff or chewing tobacco?	❑ Yes	❑ No	❑ Don't Know
	22.	Used drugs like marijuana, cocaine or crack, club drugs (like ecstasy), hallucinogens (like LSD), heroin, inhalants or solvents (like glue), or methamphetamine (like speed)?	❑ Yes	❑ No	❑ Don't Know
	23.	Used any medicine without a doctor's prescription (e.g., painkillers [like Vicodin], stimulants [like Ritalin or Adderall], sedatives or tranquilizers [like sleeping pills or Valium], or steroids)?	❑ Yes	❑ No	❑ Don't Know
XII.	24.	In the **past TWO (2) WEEKS,** has he/she talked about wanting to kill himself/herself or about wanting to commit suicide?	❑ Yes	❑ No	❑ Don't Know
	25.	Has he/she EVER tried to kill himself/herself?	❑ Yes	❑ No	❑ Don't Know

Clinician-Rated Dimensions of Psychosis Symptom Severity

As described in the chapter "Schizophrenia Spectrum and Other Psychotic Disorders," psychotic disorders are heterogeneous, and symptom severity can predict important aspects of the illness, such as the degree of cognitive and/or neurobiological deficits. Dimensional assessments capture meaningful variation in the severity of symptoms, which may help with treatment planning, prognostic decision-making, and research on pathophysiological mechanisms. The Clinician-Rated Dimensions of Psychosis Symptom Severity provides scales for the dimensional assessment of the primary symptoms of psychosis, including hallucinations, delusions, disorganized speech, abnormal psychomotor behavior, and negative symptoms. A scale for the dimensional assessment of cognitive impairment is also included. Many individuals with psychotic disorders have impairments in a range of cognitive domains, which predict functional abilities. In addition, scales for dimensional assessment of depression and mania are provided, which may alert clinicians to mood pathology. The severity of mood symptoms in psychosis has prognostic value and guides treatment.

The Clinician-Rated Dimensions of Psychosis Symptom Severity is an 8-item measure that may be completed by the clinician at the time of the clinical assessment. Each item asks the clinician to rate the severity of each symptom as experienced by the individual during the past 7 days.

Scoring and Interpretation

Each item on the measure is rated on a 5-point scale (0=none; 1=equivocal; 2=present, but mild; 3=present and moderate; and 4=present and severe) with a symptom-specific definition of each rating level. The clinician may review all of the individual's available information and, based on clinical judgment, select (with checkmark) the level that most accurately describes the severity of the individual's condition. The clinician then indicates the score for each item in the "Score" column provided.

Frequency of Use

To track changes in the individual's symptom severity over time, the measure may be completed at regular intervals as clinically indicated, depending on the stability of the individual's symptoms and treatment status. Consistently high scores on a particular domain may indicate significant and problematic areas for the individual that might warrant further assessment, treatment, and follow-up. Clinical judgment should guide decision making.

Clinician-Rated Dimensions of Psychosis Symptom Severity

Name: _____ Sex: [ ] Male [ ] Female Age: _____ Date: _____

Instructions: Based on all the information you have on the individual and using your clinical judgment, please rate (with checkmark) the presence and severity of the following symptoms as experienced by the individual in the past seven (7) days.

Domain	0	1	2	3	4	Score
I. Hallucinations	☐ Not present	☐ Equivocal (severity or duration not sufficient to be considered psychosis)	☐ Present, but mild (little pressure to act upon voices, not very bothered by voices)	☐ Present and moderate (some pressure to respond to voices, or is somewhat bothered by voices)	☐ Present and severe (severe pressure to respond to voices, or is very bothered by voices)	
II. Delusions	☐ Not present	☐ Equivocal (severity or duration not sufficient to be considered psychosis)	☐ Present, but mild (little pressure to act upon delusional beliefs, not very bothered by beliefs)	☐ Present and moderate (some pressure to act upon beliefs, or is somewhat bothered by beliefs)	☐ Present and severe (severe pressure to act upon beliefs, or is very bothered by beliefs)	
III. Disorganized speech	☐ Not present	☐ Equivocal (severity or duration not sufficient to be considered disorganization)	☐ Present, but mild (some difficulty following speech)	☐ Present and moderate (speech often difficult to follow)	☐ Present and severe (speech almost impossible to follow)	
IV. Abnormal psychomotor behavior	☐ Not present	☐ Equivocal (severity or duration not sufficient to be considered abnormal psychomotor behavior)	☐ Present, but mild (occasional abnormal or bizarre motor behavior or catatonia)	☐ Present and moderate (frequent abnormal or bizarre motor behavior or catatonia)	☐ Present and severe (abnormal or bizarre motor behavior or catatonia almost constant)	
V. Negative symptoms (restricted emotional expression or avolition)	☐ Not present	☐ Equivocal decrease in facial expressivity, prosody, gestures, or self-initiated behavior	☐ Present, but mild decrease in facial expressivity, prosody, gestures, or self-initiated behavior	☐ Present and moderate decrease in facial expressivity, prosody, gestures, or self-initiated behavior	☐ Present and severe decrease in facial expressivity, prosody, gestures, or self-initiated behavior	

Domain	0	1	2	3	4	Score
VI. Impaired cognition	☐ Not present	☐ Equivocal (cognitive function not clearly outside the range expected for age or SES; i.e., within 0.5 SD of mean)	☐ Present, but mild (some reduction in cognitive function; below expected for age and SES, 0.5–1 SD from mean)	☐ Present and moderate (clear reduction in cognitive function; below expected for age and SES, 1–2 SD from mean)	☐ Present and severe (severe reduction in cognitive function; below expected for age and SES, >2 SD from mean)	
VII. Depression	☐ Not present	☐ Equivocal (occasionally feels sad, down, depressed, or hopeless; concerned about having failed someone or at something but not preoccupied)	☐ Present, but mild (frequent periods of feeling very sad, down, moderately depressed, or hopeless; concerned about having failed someone or at something, with some preoccupation)	☐ Present and moderate (frequent periods of deep depression or hopelessness; preoccupation with guilt, having done wrong)	☐ Present and severe (deeply depressed or hopeless daily; delusional guilt or unreasonable self-reproach grossly out of proportion to circumstances)	
VIII. Mania	☐ Not present	☐ Equivocal (occasional elevated, expansive, or irritable mood or some restlessness)	☐ Present, but mild (frequent periods of somewhat elevated, expansive, or irritable mood or restlessness)	☐ Present and moderate (frequent periods of extensively elevated, expansive, or irritable mood or restlessness)	☐ Present and severe (daily and extensively elevated, expansive, or irritable mood or restlessness)	

Note. SD=standard deviation; SES=socioeconomic status.

World Health Organization Disability Assessment Schedule 2.0

The adult self-administered version of the World Health Organization Disability Assessment Schedule 2.0 (WHODAS 2.0) is a 36-item measure that assesses disability in adults age 18 years and older. It assesses disability across six domains, including understanding and communicating, getting around, self-care, getting along with people, life activities (i.e., household, work, and/or school activities), and participation in society. If the adult individual is of impaired capacity and unable to complete the form (e.g., a patient with dementia), a knowledgeable informant may complete the proxy-administered version of the measure, which is available at www.psychiatry.org/dsm5. Each item on the self-administered version of the WHODAS 2.0 asks the individual to rate how much difficulty he or she has had in specific areas of functioning during the past 30 days.

WHODAS 2.0 Scoring Instructions Provided by WHO

WHODAS 2.0 summary scores.   There are two basic options for computing the summary scores for the WHODAS 2.0 36-item full version.

   Simple: The scores assigned to each of the items—"none" (1), "mild" (2), "moderate" (3), "severe" (4), and "extreme" (5)—are summed. This method is referred to as simple scoring because the scores from each of the items are simply added up without recoding or collapsing of response categories; thus, there is no weighting of individual items. This approach is practical to use as a hand-scoring approach, and may be the method of choice in busy clinical settings or in paper-and-pencil interview situations. As a result, the simple sum of the scores of the items across all domains constitutes a statistic that is sufficient to describe the degree of functional limitations.

   Complex: The more complex method of scoring is called "item-response-theory" (IRT)–based scoring. It takes into account multiple levels of difficulty for each WHODAS 2.0 item. It takes the coding for each item response as "none," "mild," "moderate," "severe," and "extreme" separately, and then uses a computer to determine the summary score by differentially weighting the items and the levels of severity. The computer program is available from the WHO Web site. The scoring has three steps:

- Step 1—Summing of recoded item scores within each domain.
- Step 2—Summing of all six domain scores.
- Step 3—Converting the summary score into a metric ranging from 0 to 100 (where 0=no disability; 100=full disability).

WHODAS 2.0 domain scores.   WHODAS 2.0 produces domain-specific scores for six different functioning domains: cognition, mobility, self-care, getting along, life activities (household and work/school), and participation.

WHODAS 2.0 population norms.   For the population norms for IRT-based scoring of the WHODAS 2.0 and for the population distribution of IRT-based scores for WHODAS 2.0, please see www.who.int/classifications/icf/Pop_norms_distrib_IRT_scores.pdf.

Additional Scoring and Interpretation Guidance for DSM-5 Users

The clinician is asked to review the individual's response on each item on the measure during the clinical interview and to indicate the self-reported score for each item in the section provided for "Clinician Use Only." However, if the clinician determines that the score on an item should be different based on the clinical interview and other information available, he or she may indicate a corrected score in the raw item score box. Based on findings from the DSM-5 Field Trials in adult patient samples across six sites in the United States and one in Canada, *DSM-5 recommends calculation and use of average scores for each domain and for general disability.* The average scores are comparable to the WHODAS 5-point scale, which allows the clinician to think of the individual's disability in terms of none (1), mild (2), moderate (3), severe (4), or extreme (5). The average domain and general disability scores were found to be reliable, easy to use, and clinically useful to the clinicians in the DSM-5 Field Trials. The *average domain score* is calculated by dividing the raw domain score by the number of items in the domain (e.g., if all the items within the "understanding and communicating" domain are rated as being moderate, then the average domain score would be 18/6=3, indicating moderate disability). The *average general disability score* is calculated by dividing the raw overall score by number of items in the measure (i.e., 36). The individual should be encouraged to complete all of the items on the WHODAS 2.0. If no response is given on 10 or more items of the measure (i.e., more than 25% of the 36 total items), calculation of the simple and average general disability scores may not be helpful. If 10 or more of the total items on the measure are missing but the items for some of the domains are 75%–100% complete, the simple or average domain scores may be used for those domains.

Frequency of use.   To track change in the individual's level of disability over time, the measure may be completed at regular intervals as clinically indicated, depending on the stability of the individual's symptoms and treatment status. Consistently high scores on a particular domain may indicate significant and problematic areas for the individual that might warrant further assessment and intervention.

WHODAS 2.0
World Health Organization Disability Assessment Schedule 2.0
36-item version, self-administered

Patient Name: _____ **Age:** _____ **Sex:** ☐ Male ☐ Female **Date:** _____

This questionnaire asks about <u>difficulties due to health/mental health conditions</u>. Health conditions include **diseases or illnesses, other health problems that may be short or long lasting, injuries, mental or emotional problems, and problems with alcohol or drugs.** Think back over the **past 30 days** and answer these questions thinking about how much difficulty you had doing the following activities. For each question, please circle only **one** response.

Numeric scores assigned to each of the items:	1	2	3	4	5	Raw Item Score	Raw Domain Score	Average Domain Score
In the <u>last 30 days</u>, how much difficulty did you have in:							*Clinician Use Only*	
Understanding and communicating								
D1.1 <u>Concentrating</u> on doing something for <u>ten minutes</u>?	None	Mild	Moderate	Severe	Extreme or cannot do			
D1.2 <u>Remembering</u> to do <u>important things</u>?	None	Mild	Moderate	Severe	Extreme or cannot do			
D1.3 <u>Analyzing and finding solutions to problems</u> in day-to-day life?	None	Mild	Moderate	Severe	Extreme or cannot do		30	5
D1.4 <u>Learning a new task</u>, for example, learning how to get to a new place?	None	Mild	Moderate	Severe	Extreme or cannot do			
D1.5 <u>Generally understanding</u> what people say?	None	Mild	Moderate	Severe	Extreme or cannot do			
D1.6 <u>Starting and maintaining</u> a <u>conversation?</u>	None	Mild	Moderate	Severe	Extreme or cannot do			
Getting around								
D2.1 <u>Standing</u> for <u>long periods</u>, such as <u>30 minutes</u>?	None	Mild	Moderate	Severe	Extreme or cannot do			
D2.2 <u>Standing up</u> from sitting down?	None	Mild	Moderate	Severe	Extreme or cannot do			
D2.3 <u>Moving</u> around <u>inside your home</u>?	None	Mild	Moderate	Severe	Extreme or cannot do		25	5
D2.4 <u>Getting out</u> of your <u>home</u>?	None	Mild	Moderate	Severe	Extreme or cannot do			
D2.5 <u>Walking a long distance</u>, such as a kilometer (or equivalent)?	None	Mild	Moderate	Severe	Extreme or cannot do			
Self-care								
D3.1 <u>Washing</u> your <u>whole body</u>?	None	Mild	Moderate	Severe	Extreme or cannot do			
D3.2 Getting <u>dressed</u>?	None	Mild	Moderate	Severe	Extreme or cannot do			
D3.3 <u>Eating</u>?	None	Mild	Moderate	Severe	Extreme or cannot do		20	5
D3.4 Staying <u>by yourself</u> for a <u>few days</u>?	None	Mild	Moderate	Severe	Extreme or cannot do			
Getting along with people								
D4.1 <u>Dealing</u> with people <u>you do not know</u>?	None	Mild	Moderate	Severe	Extreme or cannot do			
D4.2 <u>Maintaining a friendship</u>?	None	Mild	Moderate	Severe	Extreme or cannot do			
D4.3 <u>Getting along</u> with people who are <u>close</u> to you?	None	Mild	Moderate	Severe	Extreme or cannot do		25	5
D4.4 <u>Making new friends</u>?	None	Mild	Moderate	Severe	Extreme or cannot do			
D4.5 <u>Sexual</u> activities?	None	Mild	Moderate	Severe	Extreme or cannot do			

								Clinician Use Only		
	Numeric scores assigned to each of the items:	1	2	3	4	5	Raw Item Score	Raw Domain Score	Average Domain Score	
	In the last 30 days, how much difficulty did you have in:									
Life activities—Household										
D5.1	Taking care of your household responsibilities?	None	Mild	Moderate	Severe	Extreme or cannot do				
D5.2	Doing most important household tasks well?	None	Mild	Moderate	Severe	Extreme or cannot do				
D5.3	Getting all of the household work done that you needed to do?	None	Mild	Moderate	Severe	Extreme or cannot do		20	5	
D5.4	Getting your household work done as quickly as needed?	None	Mild	Moderate	Severe	Extreme or cannot do				
Life activities—School/Work										
	If you work (paid, non-paid, self-employed) or go to school, complete questions D5.5–D5.8, below. Otherwise, skip to D6.1.									
	Because of your health condition, in the past 30 days, how much difficulty did you have in:									
D5.5	Your day-to-day work/school?	None	Mild	Moderate	Severe	Extreme or cannot do				
D5.6	Doing your most important work/school tasks well?	None	Mild	Moderate	Severe	Extreme or cannot do				
D5.7	Getting all of the work done that you need to do?	None	Mild	Moderate	Severe	Extreme or cannot do		20	5	
D5.8	Getting your work done as quickly as needed?	None	Mild	Moderate	Severe	Extreme or cannot do				
Participation in society										
	In the past 30 days:									
D6.1	How much of a problem did you have in joining in community activities (for example, festivities, religious, or other activities) in the same way as anyone else can?	None	Mild	Moderate	Severe	Extreme or cannot do				
D6.2	How much of a problem did you have because of barriers or hindrances around you?	None	Mild	Moderate	Severe	Extreme or cannot do				
D6.3	How much of a problem did you have living with dignity because of the attitudes and actions of others?	None	Mild	Moderate	Severe	Extreme or cannot do				
D6.4	How much time did you spend on your health condition or its consequences?	None	Some	Moderate	A Lot	Extreme or cannot do		40	5	
D6.5	How much have you been emotionally affected by your health condition?	None	Mild	Moderate	Severe	Extreme or cannot do				
D6.6	How much has your health been a drain on the financial resources of you or your family?	None	Mild	Moderate	Severe	Extreme or cannot do				
D6.7	How much of a problem did your family have because of your health problems?	None	Mild	Moderate	Severe	Extreme or cannot do				
D6.8	How much of a problem did you have in doing things by yourself for relaxation or pleasure?	None	Mild	Moderate	Severe	Extreme or cannot do				
						General Disability Score (Total):		180	5	

Cultural Formulation

Understanding the cultural context of illness experience is essential for effective diagnostic assessment and clinical management. *Culture* refers to systems of knowledge, concepts, rules, and practices that are learned and transmitted across generations. Culture includes language, religion and spirituality, family structures, life-cycle stages, ceremonial rituals, and customs, as well as moral and legal systems. Cultures are open, dynamic systems that undergo continuous change over time; in the contemporary world, most individuals and groups are exposed to multiple cultures, which they use to fashion their own identities and make sense of experience. These features of culture make it crucial not to overgeneralize cultural information or stereotype groups in terms of fixed cultural traits.

Race is a culturally constructed category of identity that divides humanity into groups based on a variety of superficial physical traits attributed to some hypothetical intrinsic, biological characteristics. Racial categories and constructs have varied widely over history and across societies. The construct of race has no consistent biological definition, but it is socially important because it supports racial ideologies, racism, discrimination, and social exclusion, which can have strong negative effects on mental health. There is evidence that racism can exacerbate many psychiatric disorders, contributing to poor outcome, and that racial biases can affect diagnostic assessment.

Ethnicity is a culturally constructed group identity used to define peoples and communities. It may be rooted in a common history, geography, language, religion, or other shared characteristics of a group, which distinguish that group from others. Ethnicity may be self-assigned or attributed by outsiders. Increasing mobility, intermarriage, and intermixing of cultures has defined new mixed, multiple, or hybrid ethnic identities.

Culture, race, and ethnicity are related to economic inequities, racism, and discrimination that result in health disparities. Cultural, ethnic, and racial identities can be sources of strength and group support that enhance resilience, but they may also lead to psychological, interpersonal, and intergenerational conflict or difficulties in adaptation that require diagnostic assessment.

Outline for Cultural Formulation

The Outline for Cultural Formulation introduced in DSM-IV provided a framework for assessing information about cultural features of an individual's mental health problem and how it relates to a social and cultural context and history. DSM-5 not only includes an updated version of the Outline but also presents an approach to assessment, using the Cultural Formulation Interview (CFI), which has been field-tested for diagnostic usefulness among clinicians and for acceptability among patients.

The revised Outline for Cultural Formulation calls for systematic assessment of the following categories:

- **Cultural identity of the individual:** Describe the individual's racial, ethnic, or cultural reference groups that may influence his or her relationships with others, access to resources, and developmental and current challenges, conflicts, or predicaments. For immigrants and racial or ethnic minorities, the degree and kinds of involvement with both the culture of origin and the host culture or majority culture should be noted separately. Language abilities, preferences, and patterns of use are relevant for identifying difficulties with access to care, social integration, and the need for an interpreter. Other clinically relevant aspects of identity may include religious affiliation, socioeconomic background, personal and family places of birth and growing up, migrant status, and sexual orientation.

- **Cultural conceptualizations of distress:** Describe the cultural constructs that influence how the individual experiences, understands, and communicates his or her symptoms or problems to others. These constructs may include cultural syndromes, idioms of distress, and explanatory models or perceived causes. The level of severity and meaning of the distressing experiences should be assessed in relation to the norms of the individual's cultural reference groups. Assessment of coping and help-seeking patterns should consider the use of professional as well as traditional, alternative, or complementary sources of care.
- **Psychosocial stressors and cultural features of vulnerability and resilience:** Identify key stressors and supports in the individual's social environment (which may include both local and distant events) and the role of religion, family, and other social networks (e.g., friends, neighbors, coworkers) in providing emotional, instrumental, and informational support. Social stressors and social supports vary with cultural interpretations of events, family structure, developmental tasks, and social context. Levels of functioning, disability, and resilience should be assessed in light of the individual's cultural reference groups.
- **Cultural features of the relationship between the individual and the clinician:** Identify differences in culture, language, and social status between an individual and clinician that may cause difficulties in communication and may influence diagnosis and treatment. Experiences of racism and discrimination in the larger society may impede establishing trust and safety in the clinical diagnostic encounter. Effects may include problems eliciting symptoms, misunderstanding of the cultural and clinical significance of symptoms and behaviors, and difficulty establishing or maintaining the rapport needed for an effective clinical alliance.
- **Overall cultural assessment:** Summarize the implications of the components of the cultural formulation identified in earlier sections of the Outline for diagnosis and other clinically relevant issues or problems as well as appropriate management and treatment intervention.

Cultural Formulation Interview (CFI)

The Cultural Formulation Interview (CFI) is a set of 16 questions that clinicians may use to obtain information during a mental health assessment about the impact of culture on key aspects of an individual's clinical presentation and care. In the CFI, *culture* refers to

- The values, orientations, knowledge, and practices that individuals derive from membership in diverse social groups (e.g., ethnic groups, faith communities, occupational groups, veterans groups).
- Aspects of an individual's background, developmental experiences, and current social contexts that may affect his or her perspective, such as geographical origin, migration, language, religion, sexual orientation, or race/ethnicity.
- The influence of family, friends, and other community members (the individual's *social network*) on the individual's illness experience.

The CFI is a brief semistructured interview for systematically assessing cultural factors in the clinical encounter that may be used with any individual. The CFI focuses on the individual's experience and the social contexts of the clinical problem. The CFI follows a person-centered approach to cultural assessment by eliciting information from the individual about his or her own views and those of others in his or her social network. This approach is designed to avoid stereotyping, in that each individual's cultural knowledge affects how he or she interprets illness experience and guides how he or she seeks help. Because the CFI concerns the individual's personal views, there are no right or wrong answers to these questions. The interview follows and is available online at www.psychiatry.org/dsm5.

The CFI is formatted as two text columns. The left-hand column contains the instructions for administering the CFI and describes the goals for each interview domain. The questions in the right-hand column illustrate how to explore these domains, but they are not meant to be exhaustive. Follow-up questions may be needed to clarify individuals' answers. Questions may be rephrased as needed. The CFI is intended as a guide to cultural assessment and should be used flexibly to maintain a natural flow of the interview and rapport with the individual.

The CFI is best used in conjunction with demographic information obtained prior to the interview in order to tailor the CFI questions to address the individual's background and current situation. Specific demographic domains to be explored with the CFI will vary across individuals and settings. A comprehensive assessment may include place of birth, age, gender, racial/ethnic origin, marital status, family composition, education, language fluencies, sexual orientation, religious or spiritual affiliation, occupation, employment, income, and migration history.

The CFI can be used in the initial assessment of individuals in all clinical settings, regardless of the cultural background of the individual or of the clinician. Individuals and clinicians who appear to share the same cultural background may nevertheless differ in ways that are relevant to care. The CFI may be used in its entirety, or components may be incorporated into a clinical evaluation as needed. The CFI may be especially helpful when there is

- Difficulty in diagnostic assessment owing to significant differences in the cultural, religious, or socioeconomic backgrounds of clinician and the individual.
- Uncertainty about the fit between culturally distinctive symptoms and diagnostic criteria.
- Difficulty in judging illness severity or impairment.
- Disagreement between the individual and clinician on the course of care.
- Limited engagement in and adherence to treatment by the individual.

The CFI emphasizes four domains of assessment: Cultural Definition of the Problem (questions 1–3); Cultural Perceptions of Cause, Context, and Support (questions 4–10); Cultural Factors Affecting Self-Coping and Past Help Seeking (questions 11–13); and Cultural Factors Affecting Current Help Seeking (questions 14–16). Both the person-centered process of conducting the CFI and the information it elicits are intended to enhance the cultural validity of diagnostic assessment, facilitate treatment planning, and promote the individual's engagement and satisfaction. To achieve these goals, the information obtained from the CFI should be integrated with all other available clinical material into a comprehensive clinical and contextual evaluation. An Informant version of the CFI can be used to collect collateral information on the CFI domains from family members or caregivers.

Supplementary modules have been developed that expand on each domain of the CFI and guide clinicians who wish to explore these domains in greater depth. Supplementary modules have also been developed for specific populations, such as children and adolescents, elderly individuals, and immigrants and refugees. These supplementary modules are referenced in the CFI under the pertinent subheadings and are available online at www.psychiatry.org/dsm5.

Cultural Formulation Interview (CFI)

Supplementary modules used to expand each CFI subtopic are noted in parentheses.

GUIDE TO INTERVIEWER

INSTRUCTIONS TO THE INTERVIEWER ARE ITALICIZED.

The following questions aim to clarify key aspects of the presenting clinical problem from the point of view of the individual and other members of the individual's social network (i.e., family, friends, or others involved in current problem). This includes the problem's meaning, potential sources of help, and expectations for services.

INTRODUCTION FOR THE INDIVIDUAL:

I would like to understand the problems that bring you here so that I can help you more effectively. I want to know about *your* experience and ideas. I will ask some questions about what is going on and how you are dealing with it. Please remember there are no right or wrong answers.

CULTURAL DEFINITION OF THE PROBLEM

CULTURAL DEFINITION OF THE PROBLEM

(Explanatory Model, Level of Functioning)

Elicit the individual's view of core problems and key concerns.

Focus on the individual's own way of understanding the problem.

Use the term, expression, or brief description elicited in question 1 to identify the problem in subsequent questions (e.g., "your conflict with your son").

1. What brings you here today?
   IF INDIVIDUAL GIVES FEW DETAILS OR ONLY MENTIONS SYMPTOMS OR A MEDICAL DIAGNOSIS, PROBE:
   People often understand their problems in their own way, which may be similar to or different from how doctors describe the problem. How would *you* describe your problem?

Ask how individual frames the problem for members of the social network.

2. Sometimes people have different ways of describing their problem to their family, friends, or others in their community. How would you describe your problem to them?

Focus on the aspects of the problem that matter most to the individual.

3. What troubles you most about your problem?

CULTURAL PERCEPTIONS OF CAUSE, CONTEXT, AND SUPPORT

CAUSES

(Explanatory Model, Social Network, Older Adults)

This question indicates the meaning of the condition for the individual, which may be relevant for clinical care.

Note that individuals may identify multiple causes, depending on the facet of the problem they are considering.

4. Why do you think this is happening to you? What do you think are the causes of your [PROBLEM]?
   PROMPT FURTHER IF REQUIRED:
   Some people may explain their problem as the result of bad things that happen in their life, problems with others, a physical illness, a spiritual reason, or many other causes.

Focus on the views of members of the individual's social network. These may be diverse and vary from the individual's.

5. What do others in your family, your friends, or others in your community think is causing your [PROBLEM]?

Cultural Formulation Interview (CFI) *(continued)*

Supplementary modules used to expand each CFI subtopic are noted in parentheses.

GUIDE TO INTERVIEWER	INSTRUCTIONS TO THE INTERVIEWER ARE *ITALICIZED.*

STRESSORS AND SUPPORTS

(Social Network, Caregivers, Psychosocial Stressors, Religion and Spirituality, Immigrants and Refugees, Cultural Identity, Older Adults, Coping and Help Seeking)

Elicit information on the individual's life context, focusing on resources, social supports, and resilience. May also probe other supports (e.g., from co-workers, from participation in religion or spirituality).

6. Are there any kinds of support that make your [PROBLEM] better, such as support from family, friends, or others?

Focus on stressful aspects of the individual's environment. Can also probe, e.g., relationship problems, difficulties at work or school, or discrimination.

7. Are there any kinds of stresses that make your [PROBLEM] worse, such as difficulties with money, or family problems?

ROLE OF CULTURAL IDENTITY

(Cultural Identity, Psychosocial Stressors, Religion and Spirituality, Immigrants and Refugees, Older Adults, Children and Adolescents)

Sometimes, aspects of people's background or identity can make their [PROBLEM] better or worse. By **background** or **identity,** I mean, for example, the communities you belong to, the languages you speak, where you or your family are from, your race or ethnic background, your gender or sexual orientation, or your faith or religion.

Ask the individual to reflect on the most salient elements of his or her cultural identity. Use this information to tailor questions 9–10 as needed.

8. For you, what are the most important aspects of your background or identity?

Elicit aspects of identity that make the problem better or worse.

9. Are there any aspects of your background or identity that make a difference to your [PROBLEM]?

Probe as needed (e.g., clinical worsening as a result of discrimination due to migration status, race/ethnicity, or sexual orientation).

Probe as needed (e.g., migration-related problems; conflict across generations or due to gender roles).

10. Are there any aspects of your background or identity that are causing other concerns or difficulties for you?

CULTURAL FACTORS AFFECTING SELF-COPING AND PAST HELP SEEKING

SELF-COPING

(Coping and Help Seeking, Religion and Spirituality, Older Adults, Caregivers, Psychosocial Stressors)

Clarify self-coping for the problem.

11. Sometimes people have various ways of dealing with problems like [PROBLEM]. What have you done on your own to cope with your [PROBLEM]?

Cultural Formulation Interview (CFI) *(continued)*

Supplementary modules used to expand each CFI subtopic are noted in parentheses.

GUIDE TO INTERVIEWER	**INSTRUCTIONS TO THE INTERVIEWER ARE *ITALICIZED*.**

PAST HELP SEEKING

(Coping and Help Seeking, Religion and Spirituality, Older Adults, Caregivers, Psychosocial Stressors, Immigrants and Refugees, Social Network, Clinician-Patient Relationship)

Elicit various sources of help (e.g., medical care, mental health treatment, support groups, work-based counseling, folk healing, religious or spiritual counseling, other forms of traditional or alternative healing).

Probe as needed (e.g., "What other sources of help have you used?").

Clarify the individual's experience and regard for previous help.

12. Often, people look for help from many different sources, including different kinds of doctors, helpers, or healers. In the past, what kinds of treatment, help, advice, or healing have you sought for your [PROBLEM]?

    PROBE IF DOES NOT DESCRIBE USEFULNESS OF HELP RECEIVED:

    What types of help or treatment were most useful? Not useful?

BARRIERS

(Coping and Help Seeking, Religion and Spirituality, Older Adults, Psychosocial Stressors, Immigrants and Refugees, Social Network, Clinician-Patient Relationship)

Clarify the role of social barriers to help seeking, access to care, and problems engaging in previous treatment.

Probe details as needed (e.g., "What got in the way?").

13. Has anything prevented you from getting the help you need?

    PROBE AS NEEDED:

    For example, money, work or family commitments, stigma or discrimination, or lack of services that understand your language or background?

CULTURAL FACTORS AFFECTING CURRENT HELP SEEKING

PREFERENCES

(Social Network, Caregivers, Religion and Spirituality, Older Adults, Coping and Help Seeking)

Clarify individual's current perceived needs and expectations of help, broadly defined.

Probe if individual lists only one source of help (e.g., "What other kinds of help would be useful to you at this time?").

Focus on the views of the social network regarding help seeking.

Now let's talk some more about the help you need.

14. What kinds of help do you think would be most useful to you at this time for your [PROBLEM]?

15. Are there other kinds of help that your family, friends, or other people have suggested would be helpful for you now?

CLINICIAN-PATIENT RELATIONSHIP

(Clinician-Patient Relationship, Older Adults)

Elicit possible concerns about the clinic or the clinician-patient relationship, including perceived racism, language barriers, or cultural differences that may undermine goodwill, communication, or care delivery.

Probe details as needed (e.g., "In what way?").

Address possible barriers to care or concerns about the clinic and the clinician-patient relationship raised previously.

Sometimes doctors and patients misunderstand each other because they come from different backgrounds or have different expectations.

16. Have you been concerned about this and is there anything that we can do to provide you with the care you need?

Cultural Formulation Interview (CFI) — Informant Version

The CFI–Informant Version collects collateral information from an informant who is knowledgeable about the clinical problems and life circumstances of the identified individual. This version can be used to supplement information obtained from the core CFI or can be used instead of the core CFI when the individual is unable to provide information—as might occur, for example, with children or adolescents, floridly psychotic individuals, or persons with cognitive impairment.

Cultural Formulation Interview (CFI)—Informant Version

GUIDE TO INTERVIEWER	INSTRUCTIONS TO THE INTERVIEWER ARE *ITALICIZED.*
The following questions aim to clarify key aspects of the presenting clinical problem from the informant's point of view. This includes the problem's meaning, potential sources of help, and expectations for services.	*INTRODUCTION FOR THE INFORMANT:* I would like to understand the problems that bring your family member/friend here so that I can help you and him/her more effectively. I want to know about **your** experience and ideas. I will ask some questions about what is going on and how you and your family member/friend are dealing with it. There are no right or wrong answers.

RELATIONSHIP WITH THE PATIENT

Clarify the informant's relationship with the individual and/or the individual's family.	1. How would you describe your relationship to [INDIVIDUAL OR TO FAMILY]? *PROBE IF NOT CLEAR:* How often do you see [INDIVIDUAL]?

CULTURAL DEFINITION OF THE PROBLEM

Elicit the informant's view of core problems and key concerns.	2. What brings your family member/friend here today?
Focus on the informant's way of understanding the individual's problem.	*IF INFORMANT GIVES FEW DETAILS OR ONLY MENTIONS SYMPTOMS OR A MEDICAL DIAGNOSIS, PROBE:*
Use the term, expression, or brief description elicited in question 1 to identify the problem in subsequent questions (e.g., "her conflict with her son").	People often understand problems in their own way, which may be similar or different from how doctors describe the problem. How would **you** describe [INDIVIDUAL'S] problem?
Ask how informant frames the problem for members of the social network.	3. Sometimes people have different ways of describing the problem to family, friends, or others in their community. How would **you** describe [INDIVIDUAL'S] problem to them?
Focus on the aspects of the problem that matter most to the informant.	4. What troubles you most about [INDIVIDUAL'S] problem?

Cultural Formulation Interview (CFI)—Informant Version *(continued)*

GUIDE TO INTERVIEWER	INSTRUCTIONS TO THE INTERVIEWER ARE *ITALICIZED.*

CULTURAL PERCEPTIONS OF CAUSE, CONTEXT, AND SUPPORT

CAUSES

This question indicates the meaning of the condition for the informant, which may be relevant for clinical care.

Note that informants may identify multiple causes depending on the facet of the problem they are considering.

5. Why do you think this is happening to [INDIVIDUAL]? What do you think are the causes of his/her [PROBLEM]?

PROMPT FURTHER IF REQUIRED:

Some people may explain the problem as the result of bad things that happen in their life, problems with others, a physical illness, a spiritual reason, or many other causes.

Focus on the views of members of the individual's social network. These may be diverse and vary from the informant's.

6. What do others in [INDIVIDUAL'S] family, his/her friends, or others in the community think is causing [INDIVIDUAL'S] [PROBLEM]?

STRESSORS AND SUPPORTS

Elicit information on the individual's life context, focusing on resources, social supports, and resilience. May also probe other supports (e.g., from coworkers, from participation in religion or spirituality).

7. Are there any kinds of supports that make his/her [PROBLEM] better, such as from family, friends, or others?

Focus on stressful aspects of the individual's environment. Can also probe, e.g., relationship problems, difficulties at work or school, or discrimination.

8. Are there any kinds of stresses that make his/her [PROBLEM] worse, such as difficulties with money, or family problems?

ROLE OF CULTURAL IDENTITY

Sometimes, aspects of people's background or identity can make the [PROBLEM] better or worse. By ***background*** or ***identity***, I mean, for example, the communities you belong to, the languages you speak, where you or your family are from, your race or ethnic background, your gender or sexual orientation, and your faith or religion.

Ask the informant to reflect on the most salient elements of the individual's cultural identity. Use this information to tailor questions 10–11 as needed.

9. For you, what are the most important aspects of [INDIVIDUAL'S] background or identity?

Elicit aspects of identity that make the problem better or worse.

10. Are there any aspects of [INDIVIDUAL'S] background or identity that make a difference to his/her [PROBLEM]?

Probe as needed (e.g., clinical worsening as a result of discrimination due to migration status, race/ethnicity, or sexual orientation).

Probe as needed (e.g., migration-related problems; conflict across generations or due to gender roles).

11. Are there any aspects of [INDIVIDUAL'S] background or identity that are causing other concerns or difficulties for him/her?

Cultural Formulation Interview (CFI)—Informant Version *(continued)*

GUIDE TO INTERVIEWER	**INSTRUCTIONS TO THE INTERVIEWER ARE** *ITALICIZED.*

CULTURAL FACTORS AFFECTING SELF-COPING AND PAST HELP SEEKING

SELF-COPING

Clarify individual's self-coping for the problem.

12. Sometimes people have various ways of dealing with problems like [PROBLEM]. What has [INDIVIDUAL] done on his/her own to cope with his/her [PROBLEM]?

PAST HELP SEEKING

Elicit various sources of help (e.g., medical care, mental health treatment, support groups, work-based counseling, folk healing, religious or spiritual counseling, other alternative healing).

Probe as needed (e.g., "What other sources of help has he/she used?").

Clarify the individual's experience and regard for previous help.

13. Often, people also look for help from many different sources, including different kinds of doctors, helpers, or healers. In the past, what kinds of treatment, help, advice, or healing has [INDIVIDUAL] sought for his/her [PROBLEM]?

PROBE IF DOES NOT DESCRIBE USE-FULNESS OF HELP RECEIVED:

What types of help or treatment were most useful? Not useful?

BARRIERS

Clarify the role of social barriers to help-seeking, access to care, and problems engaging in previous treatment.

Probe details as needed (e.g., "What got in the way?").

14. Has anything prevented [INDIVIDUAL] from getting the help he/she needs?

PROBE AS NEEDED:

For example, money, work or family commitments, stigma or discrimination, or lack of services that understand his/her language or background?

CULTURAL FACTORS AFFECTING CURRENT HELP SEEKING

PREFERENCES

Clarify individual's current perceived needs and expectations of help, broadly defined, from the point of view of the informant.

Probe if informant lists only one source of help (e.g., "What other kinds of help would be useful to [INDIVIDUAL] at this time?").

Focus on the views of the social network regarding help seeking.

Now let's talk about the help [INDIVIDUAL] needs.

15. What kinds of help would be most useful to him/her at this time for his/her [PROBLEM]?

16. Are there other kinds of help that [INDIVIDUAL'S] family, friends, or other people have suggested would be helpful for him/her now?

CLINICIAN-PATIENT RELATIONSHIP

Elicit possible concerns about the clinic or the clinician-patient relationship, including perceived racism, language barriers, or cultural differences that may undermine goodwill, communication, or care delivery.

Probe details as needed (e.g., "In what way?").

Address possible barriers to care or concerns about the clinic and the clinician-patient relationship raised previously.

Sometimes doctors and patients misunderstand each other because they come from different backgrounds or have different expectations.

17. Have you been concerned about this, and is there anything that we can do to provide [INDIVIDUAL] with the care he/she needs?

Cultural Concepts of Distress

Cultural concepts of distress refers to ways that cultural groups experience, understand, and communicate suffering, behavioral problems, or troubling thoughts and emotions. Three main types of cultural concepts may be distinguished. *Cultural syndromes* are clusters of symptoms and attributions that tend to co-occur among individuals in specific cultural groups, communities, or contexts and that are recognized locally as coherent patterns of experience. *Cultural idioms of distress* are ways of expressing distress that may not involve specific symptoms or syndromes, but that provide collective, shared ways of experiencing and talking about personal or social concerns. For example, everyday talk about "nerves" or "depression" may refer to widely varying forms of suffering without mapping onto a discrete set of symptoms, syndrome, or disorder. *Cultural explanations* or *perceived causes* are labels, attributions, or features of an explanatory model that indicate culturally recognized meaning or etiology for symptoms, illness, or distress.

These three concepts—syndromes, idioms, and explanations—are more relevant to clinical practice than the older formulation *culture-bound syndrome*. Specifically, the term *culture-bound syndrome* ignores the fact that clinically important cultural differences often involve explanations or experience of distress rather than culturally distinctive configurations of symptoms. Furthermore, the term *culture-bound* overemphasizes the local particularity and limited distribution of cultural concepts of distress. The current formulation acknowledges that *all* forms of distress are locally shaped, including the DSM disorders. From this perspective, many DSM diagnoses can be understood as operationalized prototypes that started out as cultural syndromes, and became widely accepted as a result of their clinical and research utility. Across groups there remain culturally patterned differences in symptoms, ways of talking about distress, and locally perceived causes, which are in turn associated with coping strategies and patterns of help seeking.

Cultural concepts arise from local folk or professional diagnostic systems for mental and emotional distress, and they may also reflect the influence of biomedical concepts. Cultural concepts have four key features in relation to the DSM-5 nosology:

- There is seldom a one-to-one correspondence of any cultural concept with a DSM diagnostic entity; the correspondence is more likely to be one-to-many in either direction. Symptoms or behaviors that might be sorted by DSM-5 into several disorders may be included in a single folk concept, and diverse presentations that might be classified by DSM-5 as variants of a single disorder may be sorted into several distinct concepts by an indigenous diagnostic system.
- Cultural concepts may apply to a wide range of severity, including presentations that do not meet DSM criteria for any mental disorder. For example, an individual with acute grief or a social predicament may use the same idiom of distress or display the same cultural syndrome as another individual with more severe psychopathology.
- In common usage, the same cultural term frequently denotes more than one type of cultural concept. A familiar example may be the concept of "depression," which may be used to describe a syndrome (e.g., major depressive disorder), an idiom of distress (e.g., as in the common expression "I feel depressed"), or a perceived cause (similar to "stress").
- Like culture and DSM itself, cultural concepts may change over time in response to both local and global influences.

Cultural concepts are important to psychiatric diagnosis for several reasons:

- **To avoid misdiagnosis:** Cultural variation in symptoms and in explanatory models associated with these cultural concepts may lead clinicians to misjudge the severity of a problem or assign the wrong diagnosis (e.g., unfamiliar spiritual explanations may be misunderstood as psychosis).

- **To obtain useful clinical information:** Cultural variations in symptoms and attributions may be associated with particular features of risk, resilience, and outcome.
- **To improve clinical rapport and engagement:** "Speaking the language of the patient," both linguistically and in terms of his or her dominant concepts and metaphors, can result in greater communication and satisfaction, facilitate treatment negotiation, and lead to higher retention and adherence.
- **To improve therapeutic efficacy:** Culture influences the psychological mechanisms of disorder, which need to be understood and addressed to improve clinical efficacy. For example, culturally specific catastrophic cognitions can contribute to symptom escalation into panic attacks.
- **To guide clinical research:** Locally perceived connections between cultural concepts may help identify patterns of comorbidity and underlying biological substrates.
- **To clarify the cultural epidemiology:** Cultural concepts of distress are not endorsed uniformly by everyone in a given culture. Distinguishing syndromes, idioms, and explanations provides an approach for studying the distribution of cultural features of illness across settings and regions, and over time. It also suggests questions about cultural determinants of risk, course, and outcome in clinical and community settings to enhance the evidence base of cultural research.

DSM-5 includes information on cultural concepts in order to improve the accuracy of diagnosis and the comprehensiveness of clinical assessment. Clinical assessment of individuals presenting with these cultural concepts should determine whether they meet DSM-5 criteria for a specified disorder or an *other specified or unspecified* diagnosis. Once the disorder is diagnosed, the cultural terms and explanations should be included in case formulations; they may help clarify symptoms and etiological attributions that could otherwise be confusing. Individuals whose symptoms do not meet DSM criteria for a specific mental disorder may still expect and require treatment; this should be assessed on a case-by-case basis. In addition to the CFI and its supplementary modules, DSM-5 contains the following information and tools that may be useful when integrating cultural information in clinical practice:

- **Data in DSM-5 criteria and text for specific disorders:** The text includes information on cultural variations in prevalence, symptomatology, associated cultural concepts, and other clinical aspects. It is important to emphasize that there is no one-to-one correspondence at the categorical level between DSM disorders and cultural concepts. Differential diagnosis for individuals must therefore incorporate information on cultural variation with information elicited by the CFI.
- **Other Conditions That May Be a Focus of Clinical Attention:** Some of the clinical concerns identified by the CFI may correspond to V codes or Z codes—for example, acculturation problems, parent-child relational problems, or religious or spiritual problems.
- **Glossary of Cultural Concepts of Distress:** Located in the Appendix, this glossary provides examples of well-studied cultural concepts of distress that illustrate the relevance of cultural information for clinical diagnosis and some of the interrelationships among cultural syndromes, idioms of distress, and causal explanations.

Alternative DSM-5 Model for Personality Disorders

The current approach to personality disorders appears in Section II of DSM-5, and an alternative model developed for DSM-5 is presented here in Section III. The inclusion of both models in DSM-5 reflects the decision of the APA Board of Trustees to preserve continuity with current clinical practice, while also introducing a new approach that aims to address numerous shortcomings of the current approach to personality disorders. For example, the typical patient meeting criteria for a specific personality disorder frequently also meets criteria for other personality disorders. Similarly, other specified or unspecified personality disorder is often the correct (but mostly uninformative) diagnosis, in the sense that patients do not tend to present with patterns of symptoms that correspond with one and only one personality disorder.

In the following alternative DSM-5 model, personality disorders are characterized by impairments in personality *functioning* and pathological personality *traits*. The specific personality disorder diagnoses that may be derived from this model include antisocial, avoidant, borderline, narcissistic, obsessive-compulsive, and schizotypal personality disorders. This approach also includes a diagnosis of personality disorder—trait specified (PD-TS) that can be made when a personality disorder is considered present but the criteria for a specific disorder are not met.

General Criteria for Personality Disorder

General Criteria for Personality Disorder

The essential features of a personality disorder are

A. Moderate or greater impairment in personality (self/interpersonal) functioning.

B. One or more pathological personality traits.

C. The impairments in personality functioning and the individual's personality trait expression are relatively inflexible and pervasive across a broad range of personal and social situations.

D. The impairments in personality functioning and the individual's personality trait expression are relatively stable across time, with onsets that can be traced back to at least adolescence or early adulthood.

E. The impairments in personality functioning and the individual's personality trait expression are not better explained by another mental disorder.

F. The impairments in personality functioning and the individual's personality trait expression are not solely attributable to the physiological effects of a substance or another medical condition (e.g., severe head trauma).

G. The impairments in personality functioning and the individual's personality trait expression are not better understood as normal for an individual's developmental stage or sociocultural environment.

A diagnosis of a personality disorder requires two determinations: 1) an assessment of the level of impairment in personality functioning, which is needed for Criterion A, and 2) an evaluation of pathological personality traits, which is required for Criterion B. The impairments in personality functioning and personality trait expression are relatively inflexible and pervasive across a broad range of personal and social situations (Criterion C); relatively stable across time, with onsets that can be traced back to at least adolescence or early adulthood (Criterion D); not better explained by another mental disorder (Criterion E); not attributable to the effects of a substance or another medical condition (Criterion F); and not better understood as normal for an individual's developmental stage or sociocultural environment (Criterion G). All Section III personality disorders described by criteria sets, as well as PD-TS, meet these general criteria, by definition.

Criterion A: Level of Personality Functioning

Disturbances in **self** and **interpersonal** functioning constitute the core of personality psychopathology and in this alternative diagnostic model they are evaluated on a continuum. Self functioning involves identity and self-direction; interpersonal functioning involves empathy and intimacy (see Table 1). The Level of Personality Functioning Scale (LPFS; see Table 2, pp. 775–778) uses each of these elements to differentiate five levels of impairment, ranging from little or no impairment (i.e., healthy, adaptive functioning; Level 0) to some (Level 1), moderate (Level 2), severe (Level 3), and extreme (Level 4) impairment.

TABLE 1   **Elements of personality functioning**

Self:

1. *Identity:* Experience of oneself as unique, with clear boundaries between self and others; stability of self-esteem and accuracy of self-appraisal; capacity for, and ability to regulate, a range of emotional experience.

2. *Self-direction:* Pursuit of coherent and meaningful short-term and life goals; utilization of constructive and prosocial internal standards of behavior; ability to self-reflect productively.

Interpersonal:

1. *Empathy:* Comprehension and appreciation of others' experiences and motivations; tolerance of differing perspectives; understanding the effects of one's own behavior on others.

2. *Intimacy:* Depth and duration of connection with others; desire and capacity for closeness; mutuality of regard reflected in interpersonal behavior.

Impairment in personality functioning predicts the presence of a personality disorder, and the severity of impairment predicts whether an individual has more than one personality disorder or one of the more typically severe personality disorders. A moderate level of impairment in personality functioning is required for the diagnosis of a personality disorder; this threshold is based on empirical evidence that the moderate level of impairment maximizes the ability of clinicians to accurately and efficiently identify personality disorder pathology.

Criterion B: Pathological Personality Traits

Pathological personality traits are organized into five broad domains: Negative Affectivity, Detachment, Antagonism, Disinhibition, and Psychoticism. Within the five broad **trait domains** are 25 specific **trait facets** that were developed initially from a review of existing trait models and subsequently through iterative research with samples of persons who sought mental health services. The full trait taxonomy is presented in Table 3 (see pp. 779–781). The B criteria for the specific personality disorders comprise subsets of the 25 trait facets, based on meta-analytic reviews and empirical data on the relationships of the traits to DSM-IV personality disorder diagnoses.

Criteria C and D: Pervasiveness and Stability

Impairments in personality functioning and pathological personality traits are *relatively* pervasive across a range of personal and social contexts, as personality is defined as a pattern of perceiving, relating to, and thinking about the environment and oneself. The term *relatively* reflects the fact that all except the most extremely pathological personalities show some degree of adaptability. The pattern in personality disorders is maladaptive and relatively inflexible, which leads to disabilities in social, occupational, or other important pursuits, as individuals are unable to modify their thinking or behavior, even in the face of evidence that their approach is not working. The impairments in functioning and personality traits are also *relatively* stable. Personality traits—the dispositions to behave or feel in certain ways—are more stable than the symptomatic expressions of these dispositions, but personality traits can also change. Impairments in personality functioning are more stable than symptoms.

Criteria E, F, and G: Alternative Explanations for Personality Pathology (Differential Diagnosis)

On some occasions, what appears to be a personality disorder may be better explained by another mental disorder, the effects of a substance or another medical condition, or a normal developmental stage (e.g., adolescence, late life) or the individual's sociocultural environment. When another mental disorder is present, the diagnosis of a personality disorder is not made, if the manifestations of the personality disorder clearly are an expression of the other mental disorder (e.g., if features of schizotypal personality disorder are present only in the context of schizophrenia). On the other hand, personality disorders can be accurately diagnosed in the presence of another mental disorder, such as major depressive disorder, and patients with other mental disorders should be assessed for comorbid personality disorders because personality disorders often impact the course of other mental disorders. Therefore, it is always appropriate to assess personality functioning and pathological personality traits to provide a context for other psychopathology.

Specific Personality Disorders

Section III includes diagnostic criteria for antisocial, avoidant, borderline, narcissistic, obsessive-compulsive, and schizotypal personality disorders. Each personality disorder is defined by typical impairments in personality functioning (Criterion A) and characteristic pathological personality traits (Criterion B):

- Typical features of **antisocial personality disorder** are a failure to conform to lawful and ethical behavior, and an egocentric, callous lack of concern for others, accompanied by deceitfulness, irresponsibility, manipulativeness, and/or risk taking.
- Typical features of **avoidant personality disorder** are avoidance of social situations and inhibition in interpersonal relationships related to feelings of ineptitude and inadequacy, anxious preoccupation with negative evaluation and rejection, and fears of ridicule or embarrassment.
- Typical features of **borderline personality disorder** are instability of self-image, personal goals, interpersonal relationships, and affects, accompanied by impulsivity, risk taking, and/or hostility.
- Typical features of **narcissistic personality disorder** are variable and vulnerable self-esteem, with attempts at regulation through attention and approval seeking, and either overt or covert grandiosity.

- Typical features of **obsessive-compulsive personality disorder** are difficulties in establishing and sustaining close relationships, associated with rigid perfectionism, inflexibility, and restricted emotional expression.
- Typical features of **schizotypal personality disorder** are impairments in the capacity for social and close relationships, and eccentricities in cognition, perception, and behavior that are associated with distorted self-image and incoherent personal goals and accompanied by suspiciousness and restricted emotional expression.

The A and B criteria for the six specific personality disorders and for PD-TS follow. All personality disorders also meet criteria C through G of the General Criteria for Personality Disorder.

Antisocial Personality Disorder

Typical features of antisocial personality disorder are a failure to conform to lawful and ethical behavior, and an egocentric, callous lack of concern for others, accompanied by deceitfulness, irresponsibility, manipulativeness, and/or risk taking. Characteristic difficulties are apparent in identity, self-direction, empathy, and/or intimacy, as described below, along with specific maladaptive traits in the domains of Antagonism and Disinhibition.

Proposed Diagnostic Criteria

A. Moderate or greater impairment in personality functioning, manifested by characteristic difficulties in two or more of the following four areas:

1. *Identity:* Egocentrism; self-esteem derived from personal gain, power, or pleasure.
2. *Self-direction:* Goal setting based on personal gratification; absence of prosocial internal standards, associated with failure to conform to lawful or culturally normative ethical behavior.
3. *Empathy:* Lack of concern for feelings, needs, or suffering of others; lack of remorse after hurting or mistreating another.
4. *Intimacy:* Incapacity for mutually intimate relationships, as exploitation is a primary means of relating to others, including by deceit and coercion; use of dominance or intimidation to control others.

B. Six or more of the following seven pathological personality traits:

1. *Manipulativeness* (an aspect of **Antagonism**): Frequent use of subterfuge to influence or control others; use of seduction, charm, glibness, or ingratiation to achieve one's ends.
2. *Callousness* (an aspect of **Antagonism**): Lack of concern for feelings or problems of others; lack of guilt or remorse about the negative or harmful effects of one's actions on others; aggression; sadism.
3. *Deceitfulness* (an aspect of **Antagonism**): Dishonesty and fraudulence; misrepresentation of self; embellishment or fabrication when relating events.
4. *Hostility* (an aspect of **Antagonism**): Persistent or frequent angry feelings; anger or irritability in response to minor slights and insults; mean, nasty, or vengeful behavior.
5. *Risk taking* (an aspect of **Disinhibition**): Engagement in dangerous, risky, and potentially self-damaging activities, unnecessarily and without regard for consequences; boredom proneness and thoughtless initiation of activities to counter boredom; lack of concern for one's limitations and denial of the reality of personal danger.
6. *Impulsivity* (an aspect of **Disinhibition**): Acting on the spur of the moment in response to immediate stimuli; acting on a momentary basis without a plan or consideration of outcomes; difficulty establishing and following plans.

7. *Irresponsibility* (an aspect of **Disinhibition**): Disregard for—and failure to honor—financial and other obligations or commitments; lack of respect for—and lack of follow-through on—agreements and promises.

Note. The individual is at least 18 years of age.

Specify if:
   With psychopathic features.

Specifiers. A distinct variant often termed *psychopathy* (or "primary" psychopathy) is marked by a lack of anxiety or fear and by a bold interpersonal style that may mask maladaptive behaviors (e.g., fraudulence). This psychopathic variant is characterized by low levels of anxiousness (Negative Affectivity domain) and withdrawal (Detachment domain) and high levels of attention seeking (Antagonism domain). High attention seeking and low withdrawal capture the social potency (assertive/dominant) component of psychopathy, whereas low anxiousness captures the stress immunity (emotional stability/resilience) component.

In addition to psychopathic features, trait and personality functioning specifiers may be used to record other personality features that may be present in antisocial personality disorder but are not required for the diagnosis. For example, traits of Negative Affectivity (e.g., anxiousness), are not diagnostic criteria for antisocial personality disorder (see Criterion B) but can be specified when appropriate. Furthermore, although moderate or greater impairment in personality functioning is required for the diagnosis of antisocial personality disorder (Criterion A), the level of personality functioning can also be specified.

Avoidant Personality Disorder

Typical features of avoidant personality disorder are avoidance of social situations and inhibition in interpersonal relationships related to feelings of ineptitude and inadequacy, anxious preoccupation with negative evaluation and rejection, and fears of ridicule or embarrassment. Characteristic difficulties are apparent in identity, self-direction, empathy, and/or intimacy, as described below, along with specific maladaptive traits in the domains of Negative Affectivity and Detachment.

Proposed Diagnostic Criteria

A. Moderate or greater impairment in personality functioning, manifest by characteristic difficulties in two or more of the following four areas:

1. *Identity:* Low self-esteem associated with self-appraisal as socially inept, personally unappealing, or inferior; excessive feelings of shame.
2. *Self-direction:* Unrealistic standards for behavior associated with reluctance to pursue goals, take personal risks, or engage in new activities involving interpersonal contact.
3. *Empathy:* Preoccupation with, and sensitivity to, criticism or rejection, associated with distorted inference of others' perspectives as negative.
4. *Intimacy:* Reluctance to get involved with people unless being certain of being liked; diminished mutuality within intimate relationships because of fear of being shamed or ridiculed.

B. Three or more of the following four pathological personality traits, one of which must be (1) Anxiousness:

1. *Anxiousness* (an aspect of **Negative Affectivity**): Intense feelings of nervousness, tenseness, or panic, often in reaction to social situations; worry about the negative effects of past unpleasant experiences and future negative possibilities;

feeling fearful, apprehensive, or threatened by uncertainty; fears of embarrassment.

2. ***Withdrawal*** (an aspect of **Detachment**): Reticence in social situations; avoidance of social contacts and activity; lack of initiation of social contact.

3. ***Anhedonia*** (an aspect of **Detachment**): Lack of enjoyment from, engagement in, or energy for life's experiences; deficits in the capacity to feel pleasure or take interest in things.

4. ***Intimacy avoidance*** (an aspect of **Detachment**): Avoidance of close or romantic relationships, interpersonal attachments, and intimate sexual relationships.

Specifiers.   Considerable heterogeneity in the form of additional personality traits is found among individuals diagnosed with avoidant personality disorder. Trait and level of personality functioning specifiers can be used to record additional personality features that may be present in avoidant personality disorder. For example, other Negative Affectivity traits (e.g., depressivity, separation insecurity, submissiveness, suspiciousness, hostility) are not diagnostic criteria for avoidant personality disorder (see Criterion B) but can be specified when appropriate. Furthermore, although moderate or greater impairment in personality functioning is required for the diagnosis of avoidant personality disorder (Criterion A), the level of personality functioning also can be specified.

Borderline Personality Disorder

Typical features of borderline personality disorder are instability of self-image, personal goals, interpersonal relationships, and affects, accompanied by impulsivity, risk taking, and/or hostility. Characteristic difficulties are apparent in identity, self-direction, empathy, and/or intimacy, as described below, along with specific maladaptive traits in the domain of Negative Affectivity, and also Antagonism and/or Disinhibition.

Proposed Diagnostic Criteria

A. Moderate or greater impairment in personality functioning, manifested by characteristic difficulties in two or more of the following four areas:

1. ***Identity:*** Markedly impoverished, poorly developed, or unstable self-image, often associated with excessive self-criticism; chronic feelings of emptiness; dissociative states under stress.

2. ***Self-direction:*** Instability in goals, aspirations, values, or career plans.

3. ***Empathy:*** Compromised ability to recognize the feelings and needs of others associated with interpersonal hypersensitivity (i.e., prone to feel slighted or insulted); perceptions of others selectively biased toward negative attributes or vulnerabilities.

4. ***Intimacy:*** Intense, unstable, and conflicted close relationships, marked by mistrust, neediness, and anxious preoccupation with real or imagined abandonment; close relationships often viewed in extremes of idealization and devaluation and alternating between overinvolvement and withdrawal.

B. Four or more of the following seven pathological personality traits, at least one of which must be (5) Impulsivity, (6) Risk taking, or (7) Hostility:

1. ***Emotional lability*** (an aspect of **Negative Affectivity**): Unstable emotional experiences and frequent mood changes; emotions that are easily aroused, intense, and/or out of proportion to events and circumstances.

2. ***Anxiousness*** (an aspect of **Negative Affectivity**): Intense feelings of nervousness, tenseness, or panic, often in reaction to interpersonal stresses; worry about the negative effects of past unpleasant experiences and future negative possibili-

ties; feeling fearful, apprehensive, or threatened by uncertainty; fears of falling apart or losing control.

3. *Separation insecurity* (an aspect of **Negative Affectivity**): Fears of rejection by—and/or separation from—significant others, associated with fears of excessive dependency and complete loss of autonomy.

4. *Depressivity* (an aspect of **Negative Affectivity**): Frequent feelings of being down, miserable, and/or hopeless; difficulty recovering from such moods; pessimism about the future; pervasive shame; feelings of inferior self-worth; thoughts of suicide and suicidal behavior.

5. *Impulsivity* (an aspect of **Disinhibition**): Acting on the spur of the moment in response to immediate stimuli; acting on a momentary basis without a plan or consideration of outcomes; difficulty establishing or following plans; a sense of urgency and self-harming behavior under emotional distress.

6. *Risk taking* (an aspect of **Disinhibition**): Engagement in dangerous, risky, and potentially self-damaging activities, unnecessarily and without regard to consequences; lack of concern for one's limitations and denial of the reality of personal danger.

7. *Hostility* (an aspect of **Antagonism**): Persistent or frequent angry feelings; anger or irritability in response to minor slights and insults.

Specifiers.   Trait and level of personality functioning specifiers may be used to record additional personality features that may be present in borderline personality disorder but are not required for the diagnosis. For example, traits of Psychoticism (e.g., cognitive and perceptual dysregulation) are not diagnostic criteria for borderline personality disorder (see Criterion B) but can be specified when appropriate. Furthermore, although moderate or greater impairment in personality functioning is required for the diagnosis of borderline personality disorder (Criterion A), the level of personality functioning can also be specified.

Narcissistic Personality Disorder

Typical features of narcissistic personality disorder are variable and vulnerable self-esteem, with attempts at regulation through attention and approval seeking, and either overt or covert grandiosity. Characteristic difficulties are apparent in identity, self-direction, empathy, and/or intimacy, as described below, along with specific maladaptive traits in the domain of Antagonism.

Proposed Diagnostic Criteria

A. Moderate or greater impairment in personality functioning, manifested by characteristic difficulties in two or more of the following four areas:

1. *Identity:* Excessive reference to others for self-definition and self-esteem regulation; exaggerated self-appraisal inflated or deflated, or vacillating between extremes; emotional regulation mirrors fluctuations in self-esteem.

2. *Self-direction:* Goal setting based on gaining approval from others; personal standards unreasonably high in order to see oneself as exceptional, or too low based on a sense of entitlement; often unaware of own motivations.

3. *Empathy:* Impaired ability to recognize or identify with the feelings and needs of others; excessively attuned to reactions of others, but only if perceived as relevant to self; over- or underestimation of own effect on others.

4. *Intimacy:* Relationships largely superficial and exist to serve self-esteem regulation; mutuality constrained by little genuine interest in others' experiences and predominance of a need for personal gain.

B. Both of the following pathological personality traits:

1. *Grandiosity* (an aspect of **Antagonism**): Feelings of entitlement, either overt or covert; self-centeredness; firmly holding to the belief that one is better than others; condescension toward others.

2. *Attention seeking* (an aspect of **Antagonism**): Excessive attempts to attract and be the focus of the attention of others; admiration seeking.

Specifiers.   Trait and personality functioning specifiers may be used to record additional personality features that may be present in narcissistic personality disorder but are not required for the diagnosis. For example, other traits of Antagonism (e.g., manipulativeness, deceitfulness, callousness) are not diagnostic criteria for narcissistic personality disorder (see Criterion B) but can be specified when more pervasive antagonistic features (e.g., "malignant narcissism") are present. Other traits of Negative Affectivity (e.g., depressivity, anxiousness) can be specified to record more "vulnerable" presentations. Furthermore, although moderate or greater impairment in personality functioning is required for the diagnosis of narcissistic personality disorder (Criterion A), the level of personality functioning can also be specified.

Obsessive-Compulsive Personality Disorder

Typical features of obsessive-compulsive personality disorder are difficulties in establishing and sustaining close relationships, associated with rigid perfectionism, inflexibility, and restricted emotional expression. Characteristic difficulties are apparent in identity, self-direction, empathy, and/or intimacy, as described below, along with specific maladaptive traits in the domains of Negative Affectivity and/or Detachment.

Proposed Diagnostic Criteria

A. Moderate or greater impairment in personality functioning, manifested by characteristic difficulties in two or more of the following four areas:

1. *Identity:* Sense of self derived predominantly from work or productivity; constricted experience and expression of strong emotions.

2. *Self-direction:* Difficulty completing tasks and realizing goals, associated with rigid and unreasonably high and inflexible internal standards of behavior; overly conscientious and moralistic attitudes.

3. *Empathy:* Difficulty understanding and appreciating the ideas, feelings, or behaviors of others.

4. *Intimacy:* Relationships seen as secondary to work and productivity; rigidity and stubbornness negatively affect relationships with others.

B. Three or more of the following four pathological personality traits, one of which must be (1) Rigid perfectionism:

1. *Rigid perfectionism* (an aspect of extreme Conscientiousness [the opposite pole of Disinhibition]): Rigid insistence on everything being flawless, perfect, and without errors or faults, including one's own and others' performance; sacrificing of timeliness to ensure correctness in every detail; believing that there is only one right way to do things; difficulty changing ideas and/or viewpoint; preoccupation with details, organization, and order.

2. *Perseveration* (an aspect of **Negative Affectivity**): Persistence at tasks long after the behavior has ceased to be functional or effective; continuance of the same behavior despite repeated failures.

3. *Intimacy avoidance* (an aspect of **Detachment**): Avoidance of close or romantic relationships, interpersonal attachments, and intimate sexual relationships.

4. ***Restricted affectivity*** (an aspect of **Detachment**): Little reaction to emotionally arousing situations; constricted emotional experience and expression; indifference or coldness.

Specifiers. Trait and personality functioning specifiers may be used to record additional personality features that may be present in obsessive-compulsive personality disorder but are not required for the diagnosis. For example, other traits of Negative Affectivity (e.g., anxiousness) are not diagnostic criteria for obsessive-compulsive personality disorder (see Criterion B) but can be specified when appropriate. Furthermore, although moderate or greater impairment in personality functioning is required for the diagnosis of obsessive-compulsive personality disorder (Criterion A), the level of personality functioning can also be specified.

Schizotypal Personality Disorder

Typical features of schizotypal personality disorder are impairments in the capacity for social and close relationships and eccentricities in cognition, perception, and behavior that are associated with distorted self-image and incoherent personal goals and accompanied by suspiciousness and restricted emotional expression. Characteristic difficulties are apparent in identity, self-direction, empathy, and/or intimacy, along with specific maladaptive traits in the domains of Psychoticism and Detachment.

Proposed Diagnostic Criteria

A. Moderate or greater impairment in personality functioning, manifested by characteristic difficulties in two or more of the following four areas:

1. ***Identity:*** Confused boundaries between self and others; distorted self-concept; emotional expression often not congruent with context or internal experience.
2. ***Self-direction:*** Unrealistic or incoherent goals; no clear set of internal standards.
3. ***Empathy:*** Pronounced difficulty understanding impact of own behaviors on others; frequent misinterpretations of others' motivations and behaviors.
4. ***Intimacy:*** Marked impairments in developing close relationships, associated with mistrust and anxiety.

B. Four or more of the following six pathological personality traits:

1. ***Cognitive and perceptual dysregulation*** (an aspect of **Psychoticism**): Odd or unusual thought processes; vague, circumstantial, metaphorical, overelaborate, or stereotyped thought or speech; odd sensations in various sensory modalities.
2. ***Unusual beliefs and experiences*** (an aspect of **Psychoticism**): Thought content and views of reality that are viewed by others as bizarre or idiosyncratic; unusual experiences of reality.
3. ***Eccentricity*** (an aspect of **Psychoticism**): Odd, unusual, or bizarre behavior or appearance; saying unusual or inappropriate things.
4. ***Restricted affectivity*** (an aspect of **Detachment**): Little reaction to emotionally arousing situations; constricted emotional experience and expression; indifference or coldness.
5. ***Withdrawal*** (an aspect of **Detachment**): Preference for being alone to being with others; reticence in social situations; avoidance of social contacts and activity; lack of initiation of social contact.
6. ***Suspiciousness*** (an aspect of **Detachment**): Expectations of—and heightened sensitivity to—signs of interpersonal ill-intent or harm; doubts about loyalty and fidelity of others; feelings of persecution.

Specifiers.   Trait and personality functioning specifiers may be used to record additional personality features that may be present in schizotypal personality disorder but are not required for the diagnosis. For example, traits of Negative Affectivity (e.g., depressivity, anxiousness) are not diagnostic criteria for schizotypal personality disorder (see Criterion B) but can be specified when appropriate. Furthermore, although moderate or greater impairment in personality functioning is required for the diagnosis of schizotypal personality disorder (Criterion A), the level of personality functioning can also be specified.

Personality Disorder—Trait Specified

Proposed Diagnostic Criteria

A. Moderate or greater impairment in personality functioning, manifested by difficulties in two or more of the following four areas:
   1. **Identity**
   2. **Self-direction**
   3. **Empathy**
   4. **Intimacy**

B. One or more pathological personality trait domains OR specific trait facets within domains, considering ALL of the following domains:
   1. **Negative Affectivity** (vs. Emotional Stability): Frequent and intense experiences of high levels of a wide range of negative emotions (e.g., anxiety, depression, guilt/shame, worry, anger), and their behavioral (e.g., self-harm) and interpersonal (e.g., dependency) manifestations.
   2. **Detachment** (vs. Extraversion): Avoidance of socioemotional experience, including both withdrawal from interpersonal interactions, ranging from casual, daily interactions to friendships to intimate relationships, as well as restricted affective experience and expression, particularly limited hedonic capacity.
   3. **Antagonism** (vs. Agreeableness): Behaviors that put the individual at odds with other people, including an exaggerated sense of self-importance and a concomitant expectation of special treatment, as well as a callous antipathy toward others, encompassing both unawareness of others' needs and feelings, and a readiness to use others in the service of self-enhancement.
   4. **Disinhibition** (vs. Conscientiousness): Orientation toward immediate gratification, leading to impulsive behavior driven by current thoughts, feelings, and external stimuli, without regard for past learning or consideration of future consequences.
   5. **Psychoticism** (vs. Lucidity): Exhibiting a wide range of culturally incongruent odd, eccentric, or unusual behaviors and cognitions, including both process (e.g., perception, dissociation) and content (e.g., beliefs).

Subtypes.   Because personality features vary continuously along multiple trait dimensions, a comprehensive set of potential expressions of PD-TS can be represented by DSM-5's dimensional model of maladaptive personality trait variants (see Table 3, pp. 779–781). Thus, subtypes are unnecessary for PD-TS, and instead, the descriptive elements that constitute personality are provided, arranged in an empirically based model. This arrangement allows clinicians to tailor the description of each individual's personality disorder profile, considering all five broad domains of personality trait variation and drawing on the descriptive features of these domains as needed to characterize the individual.

Specifiers.   The specific personality features of individuals are always recorded in evaluating Criterion B, so the combination of personality features characterizing an individual directly constitutes the specifiers in each case. For example, two individuals who are both characterized by emotional lability, hostility, and depressivity may differ such that the first individual is characterized additionally by callousness, whereas the second is not.

Personality Disorder Scoring Algorithms

The requirement for any two of the four A criteria for each of the six personality disorders was based on maximizing the relationship of these criteria to their corresponding personality disorder. Diagnostic thresholds for the B criteria were also set empirically to minimize change in prevalence of the disorders from DSM-IV and overlap with other personality disorders, and to maximize relationships with functional impairment. The resulting diagnostic criteria sets represent clinically useful personality disorders with high fidelity, in terms of core impairments in personality functioning of varying degrees of severity and constellations of pathological personality traits.

Personality Disorder Diagnosis

Individuals who have a pattern of impairment in personality functioning and maladaptive traits that matches one of the six defined personality disorders should be diagnosed with that personality disorder. If an individual also has one or even several prominent traits that may have clinical relevance in addition to those required for the diagnosis (e.g., see narcissistic personality disorder), the option exists for these to be noted as specifiers. Individuals whose personality functioning or trait pattern is substantially different from that of any of the six specific personality disorders should be diagnosed with PD-TS. The individual may not meet the required number of A or B criteria and, thus, have a subthreshold presentation of a personality disorder. The individual may have a mix of features of personality disorder types or some features that are less characteristic of a type and more accurately considered a mixed or atypical presentation. The specific level of impairment in personality functioning and the pathological personality traits that characterize the individual's personality can be specified for PD-TS, using the Level of Personality Functioning Scale (Table 2) and the pathological trait taxonomy (Table 3). The current diagnoses of paranoid, schizoid, histrionic, and dependent personality disorders are represented also by the diagnosis of PD-TS; these are defined by moderate or greater impairment in personality functioning and can be specified by the relevant pathological personality trait combinations.

Level of Personality Functioning

Like most human tendencies, personality functioning is distributed on a continuum. Central to functioning and adaptation are individuals' characteristic ways of thinking about and understanding themselves and their interactions with others. An optimally functioning individual has a complex, fully elaborated, and well-integrated psychological world that includes a mostly positive, volitional, and adaptive self-concept; a rich, broad, and appropriately regulated emotional life; and the capacity to behave as a productive member of society with reciprocal and fulfilling interpersonal relationships. At the opposite end of the continuum, an individual with severe personality pathology has an impoverished, disorganized, and/or conflicted psychological world that includes a weak, unclear, and maladaptive self-concept; a propensity to negative, dysregulated emotions; and a deficient capacity for adaptive interpersonal functioning and social behavior.

Self- and *Interpersonal* Functioning

Dimensional Definition

Generalized severity may be the most important single predictor of concurrent and prospective dysfunction in assessing personality psychopathology. Personality disorders are optimally characterized by a generalized personality severity continuum with additional specification of stylistic elements, derived from personality disorder symptom constellations and personality traits. At the same time, the core of personality psychopathology is impairment in ideas and feelings regarding self and interpersonal relationships; this notion is consistent with multiple theories of personality disorder and their research bases. The components of the Level of Personality Functioning Scale—identity, self-direction, empathy, and intimacy (see Table 1)—are particularly central in describing a personality functioning continuum.

Mental representations of the self and interpersonal relationships are reciprocally influential and inextricably tied, affect the nature of interaction with mental health professionals, and can have a significant impact on both treatment efficacy and outcome, underscoring the importance of assessing an individual's characteristic self-concept as well as views of other people and relationships. Although the degree of disturbance in the self and interpersonal functioning is continuously distributed, it is useful to consider the level of impairment in functioning for clinical characterization and for treatment planning and prognosis.

Rating Level of Personality Functioning

To use the Level of Personality Functioning Scale (LPFS), the clinician selects the level that most closely captures the individual's *current overall* level of impairment in personality functioning. The rating is necessary for the diagnosis of a personality disorder (moderate or greater impairment) and can be used to specify the severity of impairment present for an individual with any personality disorder at a given point in time. The LPFS may also be used as a global indicator of personality functioning without specification of a personality disorder diagnosis, or in the event that personality impairment is subthreshold for a disorder diagnosis.

Personality Traits

Definition and Description

Criterion B in the alternative model involves assessments of personality traits that are grouped into five domains. A *personality trait* is a tendency to feel, perceive, behave, and think in relatively consistent ways across time and across situations in which the trait may manifest. For example, individuals with a high level of the personality trait of *anxiousness* would tend to *feel* anxious readily, including in circumstances in which most people would be calm and relaxed. Individuals high in trait anxiousness also would *perceive* situations to be anxiety-provoking more frequently than would individuals with lower levels of this trait, and those high in the trait would tend to *behave* so as to avoid situations that they *think* would make them anxious. They would thereby tend to *think* about the world as more anxiety provoking than other people.

Importantly, individuals high in trait anxiousness would not necessarily be anxious at all times and in all situations. Individuals' trait levels also can and do change throughout life. Some changes are very general and reflect maturation (e.g., teenagers generally are higher on trait impulsivity than are older adults), whereas other changes reflect individuals' life experiences.

Dimensionality of personality traits. All individuals can be located on the spectrum of trait dimensions; that is, personality traits apply to everyone in different degrees rather than being present versus absent. Moreover, personality traits, including those identified specifically in the Section III model, exist on a spectrum with two opposing poles. For example, the opposite of the trait of *callousness* is the tendency to be empathic and kind-hearted, even in circumstances in which most persons would not feel that way. Hence, although in Section III this trait is labeled *callousness,* because that pole of the dimension is the primary focus, it could be described in full as *callousness versus kind-heartedness.* Moreover, its opposite pole can be recognized and may not be adaptive in all circumstances (e.g., individuals who, due to extreme kind-heartedness, repeatedly allow themselves to be taken advantage of by unscrupulous others).

Hierarchical structure of personality.   Some trait terms are quite specific (e.g., "talkative") and describe a narrow range of behaviors, whereas others are quite broad (e.g., Detachment) and characterize a wide range of behavioral propensities. Broad trait dimensions are called *domains,* and specific trait dimensions are called *facets.* Personality trait *domains* comprise a spectrum of more specific personality *facets* that tend to occur together. For example, withdrawal and anhedonia are specific trait *facets* in the trait *domain* of Detachment. Despite some cross-cultural variation in personality trait facets, the broad domains they collectively comprise are relatively consistent across cultures.

The Personality Trait Model

The Section III personality trait system includes five broad domains of personality trait variation—Negative Affectivity (vs. Emotional Stability), Detachment (vs. Extraversion), Antagonism (vs. Agreeableness), Disinhibition (vs. Conscientiousness), and Psychoticism (vs. Lucidity)—comprising 25 specific personality trait facets. Table 3 provides definitions of all personality domains and facets. These five broad domains are maladaptive variants of the five domains of the extensively validated and replicated personality model known as the "Big Five", or Five Factor Model of personality (FFM), and are also similar to the domains of the Personality Psychopathology Five (PSY-5). The specific 25 facets represent a list of personality facets chosen for their clinical relevance.

Although the Trait Model focuses on personality traits associated with psychopathology, there are healthy, adaptive, and resilient personality traits identified as the polar opposites of these traits, as noted in the parentheses above (i.e., Emotional Stability, Extraversion, Agreeableness, Conscientiousness, and Lucidity). Their presence can greatly mitigate the effects of mental disorders and facilitate coping and recovery from traumatic injuries and other medical illness.

Distinguishing Traits, Symptoms, and Specific Behaviors

Although traits are by no means immutable and do change throughout the life span, they show relative consistency compared with symptoms and specific behaviors. For example, a person may behave impulsively at a specific time for a specific reason (e.g., a person who is rarely impulsive suddenly decides to spend a great deal of money on a particular item because of an unusual opportunity to purchase something of unique value), but it is only when behaviors aggregate across time and circumstance, such that a pattern of behavior distinguishes between individuals, that they reflect traits. Nevertheless, it is important to recognize, for example, that even people who are impulsive are not acting impulsively all of the time. A trait is a tendency or disposition toward specific behaviors; a specific behavior is an instance or manifestation of a trait.

Similarly, traits are distinguished from most symptoms because symptoms tend to wax and wane, whereas traits are relatively more stable. For example, individuals with higher levels of *depressivity* have a greater likelihood of experiencing discrete episodes of a depressive disorder and of showing the symptoms of these disorders, such difficulty concentrating. However, even patients who have a trait propensity to *depressivity* typically cycle through distinguishable episodes of mood disturbance, and specific symptoms such as difficulty concentrating tend to wax and wane in concert with specific episodes, so they do not form part of the trait definition. Importantly, however, symptoms and traits are both amenable to intervention, and many interventions targeted at symptoms can affect the longer term patterns of personality functioning that are captured by personality traits.

Assessment of the DSM-5 Section III Personality Trait Model

The clinical utility of the Section III multidimensional personality trait model lies in its ability to focus attention on multiple relevant areas of personality variation in each individual patient. Rather than focusing attention on the identification of one and only one optimal diagnostic label, clinical application of the Section III personality trait model involves reviewing all five broad personality domains portrayed in Table 3. The clinical approach to personality is similar to the well-known review of systems in clinical medicine. For example, an individual's presenting complaint may focus on a specific neurological symptom, yet during an initial evaluation clinicians still systematically review functioning in all relevant systems (e.g., cardiovascular, respiratory, gastrointestinal), lest an important area of diminished functioning and corresponding opportunity for effective intervention be missed.

Clinical use of the Section III personality trait model proceeds similarly. An initial inquiry reviews all five broad domains of personality. This systematic review is facilitated by the use of formal psychometric instruments designed to measure specific facets and domains of personality. For example, the personality trait model is operationalized in the Personality Inventory for DSM-5 (PID-5), which can be completed in its self-report form by patients and in its informant-report form by those who know the patient well (e.g., a spouse). A detailed clinical assessment would involve collection of both patient- and informant-report data on all 25 facets of the personality trait model. However, if this is not possible, due to time or other constraints, assessment focused at the five-domain level is an acceptable clinical option when only a general (vs. detailed) portrait of a patient's personality is needed (see Criterion B of PD-TS). However, if personality-based problems are the focus of treatment, then it will be important to assess individuals' trait facets as well as domains.

Because personality traits are continuously distributed in the population, an approach to making the judgment that a specific trait is elevated (and therefore is present for diagnostic purposes) could involve comparing individuals' personality trait levels with population norms and/or clinical judgment. If a trait is elevated—that is, formal psychometric testing and/or interview data support the clinical judgment of elevation—then it is considered as contributing to meeting Criterion B of Section III personality disorders.

Clinical Utility of the Multidimensional Personality Functioning and Trait Model

Disorder and trait constructs each add value to the other in predicting important antecedent (e.g., family history, history of child abuse), concurrent (e.g., functional impairment, medication use), and predictive (e.g., hospitalization, suicide attempts) variables. DSM-5 impairments in personality functioning and pathological personality traits each contribute independently to clinical decisions about degree of disability; risks for self-harm, violence, and criminality; recommended treatment type and intensity; and prognosis—all important aspects of the utility of psychiatric diagnoses. Notably, knowing the level of an individual's personality functioning and his or her pathological trait profile also provides the clinician with a rich base of information and is valuable in treatment planning and in predicting the course and outcome of many mental disorders in addition to personality disorders. Therefore, assessment of personality functioning and pathological personality traits may be relevant whether an individual has a personality disorder or not.

TABLE 2 Level of Personality Functioning Scale

Level of impairment	SELF		INTERPERSONAL	
	Identity	Self-direction	Empathy	Intimacy
0—Little or no impairment	Has ongoing awareness of a unique self; maintains role-appropriate boundaries. Has consistent and self-regulated positive self-esteem, with accurate self-appraisal. Is capable of experiencing, tolerating, and regulating a full range of emotions.	Sets and aspires to reasonable goals based on a realistic assessment of personal capacities. Utilizes appropriate standards of behavior, attaining fulfillment in multiple realms. Can reflect on, and make constructive meaning of, internal experience.	Is capable of accurately understanding others' experiences and motivations in most situations. Comprehends and appreciates others' perspectives, even if disagreeing. Is aware of the effect of own actions on others.	Maintains multiple satisfying and enduring relationships in personal and community life. Desires and engages in a number of caring, close, and reciprocal relationships. Strives for cooperation and mutual benefit and flexibly responds to a range of others' ideas, emotions, and behaviors.
1—Some impairment	Has relatively intact sense of self, with some decrease in clarity of boundaries when strong emotions and mental distress are experienced. Self-esteem diminished at times, with overly critical or somewhat distorted self-appraisal. Strong emotions may be distressing, associated with a restriction in range of emotional experience.	Is excessively goal-directed, somewhat goal-inhibited, or conflicted about goals. May have an unrealistic or socially inappropriate set of personal standards, limiting some aspects of fulfillment. Is able to reflect on internal experiences, but may overemphasize a single (e.g., intellectual, emotional) type of self-knowledge.	Is somewhat compromised in ability to appreciate and understand others' experiences; may tend to see others as having unreasonable expectations or a wish for control. Although capable of considering and understanding different perspectives, resists doing so. Has inconsistent awareness of effect of own behavior on others.	Is able to establish enduring relationships in personal and community life, with some limitations on degree of depth and satisfaction. Is capable of forming and desires to form intimate and reciprocal relationships, but may be inhibited in meaningful expression and sometimes constrained if intense emotions or conflicts arise. Cooperation may be inhibited by unrealistic standards; somewhat limited in ability to respect or respond to others' ideas, emotions, and behaviors.

TABLE 2 Level of Personality Functioning Scale *(continued)*

| Level of impairment | SELF | | INTERPERSONAL | |
	Identity	Self-direction	Empathy	Intimacy
2—Moderate impairment	Depends excessively on others for identity definition, with compromised boundary delineation. Has vulnerable self-esteem controlled by exaggerated concern about external evaluation, with a wish for approval. Has sense of incompleteness or inferiority, with compensatory inflated, or deflated, self-appraisal. Emotional regulation depends on positive external appraisal. Threats to self-esteem may engender strong emotions such as rage or shame.	Goals are more often a means of gaining external approval than self-generated, and thus may lack coherence and/or stability. Personal standards may be unreasonably high (e.g., a need to be special or please others) or low (e.g., not consonant with prevailing social values). Fulfillment is compromised by a sense of lack of authenticity. Has impaired capacity to reflect on internal experience.	Is hyperattuned to the experience of others, but only with respect to perceived relevance to self. Is excessively self-referential; significantly compromised ability to appreciate and understand others' experiences and to consider alternative perspectives. Is generally unaware of or unconcerned about effect of own behavior on others, or unrealistic appraisal of own effect.	Is capable of forming and desires to form relationships in personal and community life, but connections may be largely superficial. Intimate relationships are predominantly based on meeting self-regulatory and self-esteem needs, with an unrealistic expectation of being perfectly understood by others. Tends not to view relationships in reciprocal terms, and cooperates predominantly for personal gain.

TABLE 2 Level of Personality Functioning Scale (continued)

| Level of impairment | SELF | | INTERPERSONAL | |
	Identity	Self-direction	Empathy	Intimacy
3—Severe impairment	Has a weak sense of autonomy/agency; experience of a lack of identity, or emptiness. Boundary definition is poor or rigid: may show overidentification with others, overemphasis on independence from others, or vacillation between these. Fragile self-esteem is easily influenced by events, and self-image lacks coherence. Self-appraisal is un-nuanced: self-loathing, self-aggrandizing, or an illogical, unrealistic combination. Emotions may be rapidly shifting or a chronic, unwavering feeling of despair.	Has difficulty establishing and/or achieving personal goals. Internal standards for behavior are unclear or contradictory. Life is experienced as meaningless or dangerous. Has significantly compromised ability to reflect on and understand own mental processes.	Ability to consider and understand the thoughts, feelings, and behavior of other people is significantly limited; may discern very specific aspects of others' experience, particularly vulnerabilities and suffering. Is generally unable to consider alternative perspectives; highly threatened by differences of opinion or alternative viewpoints. Is confused about or unaware of impact of own actions on others; often bewildered about peoples' thoughts and actions, with destructive motivations frequently misattributed to others.	Has some desire to form relationships in community and personal life is present, but capacity for positive and enduring connections is significantly impaired. Relationships are based on a strong belief in the absolute need for the intimate other(s), and/or expectations of abandonment or abuse. Feelings about intimate involvement with others alternate between fear/rejection and desperate desire for connection. Little mutuality: others are conceptualized primarily in terms of how they affect the self (negatively or positively); cooperative efforts are often disrupted due to the perception of slights from others.

TABLE 2   Level of Personality Functioning Scale *(continued)*

| Level of impairment | SELF | | INTERPERSONAL | |
	Identity	Self-direction	Empathy	Intimacy
4—Extreme impairment	Experience of a unique self and sense of agency/autonomy are virtually absent, or are organized around perceived external persecution. Boundaries with others are confused or lacking. Has weak or distorted self-image easily threatened by interactions with others; significant distortions and confusion around self-appraisal. Emotions not congruent with context or internal experience. Hatred and aggression may be dominant affects, although they may be disavowed and attributed to others.	Has poor differentiation of thoughts from actions, so goal-setting ability is severely compromised, with unrealistic or incoherent goals. Internal standards for behavior are virtually lacking. Genuine fulfillment is virtually inconceivable. Is profoundly unable to constructively reflect on own experience. Personal motivations may be unrecognized and/or experienced as external to self.	Has pronounced inability to consider and understand others' experience and motivation. Attention to others' perspectives is virtually absent (attention is hypervigilant, focused on need fulfillment and harm avoidance). Social interactions can be confusing and disorienting.	Desire for affiliation is limited because of profound disinterest or expectation of harm. Engagement with others is detached, disorganized, or consistently negative. Relationships are conceptualized almost exclusively in terms of their ability to provide comfort or inflict pain and suffering. Social/interpersonal behavior is not reciprocal; rather, it seeks fulfillment of basic needs or escape from pain.

TABLE 3   **Definitions of DSM-5 personality disorder trait domains and facets**

DOMAINS (Polar Opposites) and Facets	Definitions
NEGATIVE AFFECTIVITY (vs. Emotional Stability)	Frequent and intense experiences of high levels of a wide range of negative emotions (e.g., anxiety, depression, guilt/ shame, worry, anger) and their behavioral (e.g., self-harm) and interpersonal (e.g., dependency) manifestations.
Emotional lability	Instability of emotional experiences and mood; emotions that are easily aroused, intense, and/or out of proportion to events and circumstances.
Anxiousness	Feelings of nervousness, tenseness, or panic in reaction to diverse situations; frequent worry about the negative effects of past unpleasant experiences and future negative possibilities; feeling fearful and apprehensive about uncertainty; expecting the worst to happen.
Separation insecurity	Fears of being alone due to rejection by—and/or separation from—significant others, based in a lack of confidence in one's ability to care for oneself, both physically and emotionally.
Submissiveness	Adaptation of one's behavior to the actual or perceived interests and desires of others even when doing so is antithetical to one's own interests, needs, or desires.
Hostility	Persistent or frequent angry feelings; anger or irritability in response to minor slights and insults; mean, nasty, or vengeful behavior. *See also* Antagonism.
Perseveration	Persistence at tasks or in a particular way of doing things long after the behavior has ceased to be functional or effective; continuance of the same behavior despite repeated failures or clear reasons for stopping.
Depressivity	*See* Detachment.
Suspiciousness	*See* Detachment.
Restricted affectivity (lack of)	The **lack of** this facet characterizes **low levels** of Negative Affectivity. *See* Detachment for definition of this facet.
DETACHMENT (vs. Extraversion)	Avoidance of socioemotional experience, including both withdrawal from interpersonal interactions (ranging from casual, daily interactions to friendships to intimate relationships) and restricted affective experience and expression, particularly limited hedonic capacity.
Withdrawal	Preference for being alone to being with others; reticence in social situations; avoidance of social contacts and activity; lack of initiation of social contact.
Intimacy avoidance	Avoidance of close or romantic relationships, interpersonal attachments, and intimate sexual relationships.
Anhedonia	Lack of enjoyment from, engagement in, or energy for life's experiences; deficits in the capacity to feel pleasure and take interest in things.
Depressivity	Feelings of being down, miserable, and/or hopeless; difficulty recovering from such moods; pessimism about the future; pervasive shame and/or guilt; feelings of inferior self-worth; thoughts of suicide and suicidal behavior.
Restricted affectivity	Little reaction to emotionally arousing situations; constricted emotional experience and expression; indifference and aloofness in normatively engaging situations.
Suspiciousness	Expectations of—and sensitivity to—signs of interpersonal ill-intent or harm; doubts about loyalty and fidelity of others; feelings of being mistreated, used, and/or persecuted by others.

TABLE 3   Definitions of DSM-5 personality disorder trait domains and facets (*continued*)

DOMAINS (Polar Opposites) and Facets	Definitions
ANTAGONISM (vs. Agreeableness)	Behaviors that put the individual at odds with other people, including an exaggerated sense of self-importance and a concomitant expectation of special treatment, as well as a callous antipathy toward others, encompassing both an unawareness of others' needs and feelings and a readiness to use others in the service of self-enhancement.
Manipulativeness	Use of subterfuge to influence or control others; use of seduction, charm, glibness, or ingratiation to achieve one's ends.
Deceitfulness	Dishonesty and fraudulence; misrepresentation of self; embellishment or fabrication when relating events.
Grandiosity	Believing that one is superior to others and deserves special treatment; self-centeredness; feelings of entitlement; condescension toward others.
Attention seeking	Engaging in behavior designed to attract notice and to make oneself the focus of others' attention and admiration.
Callousness	Lack of concern for the feelings or problems of others; lack of guilt or remorse about the negative or harmful effects of one's actions on others.
Hostility	*See* Negative Affectivity.
DISINHIBITION (vs. Conscientiousness)	Orientation toward immediate gratification, leading to impulsive behavior driven by current thoughts, feelings, and external stimuli, without regard for past learning or consideration of future consequences.
Irresponsibility	Disregard for—and failure to honor—financial and other obligations or commitments; lack of respect for—and lack of follow-through on—agreements and promises; carelessness with others' property.
Impulsivity	Acting on the spur of the moment in response to immediate stimuli; acting on a momentary basis without a plan or consideration of outcomes; difficulty establishing and following plans; a sense of urgency and self-harming behavior under emotional distress.
Distractibility	Difficulty concentrating and focusing on tasks; attention is easily diverted by extraneous stimuli; difficulty maintaining goal-focused behavior, including both planning and completing tasks.
Risk taking	Engagement in dangerous, risky, and potentially self-damaging activities, unnecessarily and without regard to consequences; lack of concern for one's limitations and denial of the reality of personal danger; reckless pursuit of goals regardless of the level of risk involved.
Rigid perfectionism (lack of)	Rigid insistence on everything being flawless, perfect, and without errors or faults, including one's own and others' performance; sacrificing of timeliness to ensure correctness in every detail; believing that there is only one right way to do things; difficulty changing ideas and/or viewpoint; preoccupation with details, organization, and order. The *lack of* this facet characterizes *low levels* of Disinhibition.

TABLE 3 Definitions of DSM-5 personality disorder trait domains
and facets *(continued)*

DOMAINS (Polar Opposites) and Facets	Definitions
PSYCHOTICISM (vs. Lucidity)	Exhibiting a wide range of culturally incongruent odd, eccentric, or unusual behaviors and cognitions, including both process (e.g., perception, dissociation) and content (e.g., beliefs).
Unusual beliefs and experiences	Belief that one has unusual abilities, such as mind reading, telekinesis, thought-action fusion, unusual experiences of reality, including hallucination-like experiences.
Eccentricity	Odd, unusual, or bizarre behavior, appearance, and/or speech; having strange and unpredictable thoughts; saying unusual or inappropriate things.
Cognitive and perceptual dysregulation	Odd or unusual thought processes and experiences, including depersonalization, derealization, and dissociative experiences; mixed sleep-wake state experiences; thought-control experiences.

Conditions for Further Study

Proposed criteria sets are presented for conditions on which future research is encouraged. The specific items, thresholds, and durations contained in these research criteria sets were set by expert consensus—informed by literature review, data reanalysis, and field trial results, where available—and are intended to provide a common language for researchers and clinicians who are interested in studying these disorders. It is hoped that such research will allow the field to better understand these conditions and will inform decisions about possible placement in forthcoming editions of DSM. The DSM-5 Task Force and Work Groups subjected each of these proposed criteria sets to a careful empirical review and invited wide commentary from the field as well as from the general public. The Task Force determined that there was insufficient evidence to warrant inclusion of these proposals as official mental disorder diagnoses in Section II. *These proposed criteria sets are not intended for clinical use; only the criteria sets and disorders in Section II of DSM-5 are officially recognized and can be used for clinical purposes.*

Attenuated Psychosis Syndrome

Proposed Criteria

A. At least one of the following symptoms is present in attenuated form, with relatively intact reality testing, and is of sufficient severity or frequency to warrant clinical attention:

 1. Delusions.
 2. Hallucinations.
 3. Disorganized speech.

B. Symptom(s) must have been present at least once per week for the past month.

C. Symptom(s) must have begun or worsened in the past year.

D. Symptom(s) is sufficiently distressing and disabling to the individual to warrant clinical attention.

E. Symptom(s) is not better explained by another mental disorder, including a depressive or bipolar disorder with psychotic features, and is not attributable to the physiological effects of a substance or another medical condition.

F. Criteria for any psychotic disorder have never been met.

Diagnostic Features

Attenuated psychotic symptoms, as defined in Criterion A, are psychosis-like but below the threshold for a full psychotic disorder. Compared with psychotic disorders, the symptoms are less severe and more transient, and insight is relatively maintained. A diagnosis of attenuated psychosis syndrome requires state psychopathology associated with functional impairment rather than long-standing trait pathology. The psychopathology has not progressed to full psychotic severity. Attenuated psychosis syndrome is a disorder based on the manifest pathology and impaired function and distress. Changes in experiences and behaviors are noted by the individual and/or others, suggesting a change in mental state (i.e., the symptoms are of sufficient severity or frequency to warrant clinical attention) (Criterion A). Attenuated delusions (Criterion A1) may have suspiciousness/persecutory ideational content, including persecutory ideas of reference. The individual may have a guarded, distrustful attitude. When the delusions are moderate in severity, the individual views others as untrustworthy and may be hypervigilant or sense ill will in others. When the delusions are severe but still within the attenuated range, the individual entertains loosely organized beliefs about danger or hostile intention, but the delusions do not have the fixed nature that is necessary for the diagnosis of a psychotic disorder. Guarded behavior in the interview can interfere with the ability to gather information. Reality testing and perspective can be elicited with nonconfirming evidence, but the propensity for viewing the world as hostile and dangerous remains strong. Attenuated delusions may have grandiose content presenting as an unrealistic sense of superior capacity. When the delusions are moderate, the individual harbors notions of being gifted, influential, or special. When the delusions are severe, the individual has beliefs of superiority that often alienate friends and worry relatives. Thoughts of being special may lead to unrealistic plans and investments, yet skepticism about these attitudes can be elicited with persistent questioning and confrontation.

Attenuated hallucinations (Criterion A2) include alterations in sensory perceptions, usually auditory and/or visual. When the hallucinations are moderate, the sounds and images are often unformed (e.g., shadows, trails, halos, murmurs, rumbling), and they are experienced as unusual or puzzling. When the hallucinations are severe, these experiences become more vivid and frequent (i.e., recurring illusions or hallucinations that capture attention and affect thinking and concentration). These perceptual abnormalities may disrupt behavior, but skepticism about their reality can still be induced.

Disorganized communication (Criterion A3) may manifest as odd speech (vague, metaphorical, overelaborate, stereotyped), unfocused speech (confused, muddled, too fast or too slow, wrong words, irrelevant context, off track), or meandering speech (circumstantial, tangential). When the disorganization is moderately severe, the individual frequently gets into irrelevant topics but responds easily to clarifying questions. Speech may be odd but understandable. At the moderately severe level, speech becomes meandering and circumstantial, and when the disorganization is severe, the individual fails to get to the point without external guidance (tangential). At the severe level, some thought blocking and/or loose associations may occur infrequently, especially when the individual is under pressure, but reorienting questions quickly return structure and organization to the conversation.

The individual realizes that changes in mental state and/or in relationships are taking place. He or she maintains reasonable insight into the psychotic-like experiences and generally appreciates that altered perceptions are not real and magical ideation is not compelling. The individual must experience distress and/or impaired performance in social or role functioning (Criterion D), and the individual or responsible others must note the changes and express concern, such that clinical care is sought (Criterion A).

Associated Features Supporting Diagnosis

The individual may experience magical thinking, perceptual aberrations, difficulty in concentration, some disorganization in thought or behavior, excessive suspiciousness, anxiety, social withdrawal, and disruption in sleep-wake cycle. Impaired cognitive function and negative symptoms are often observed. Neuroimaging variables distinguish cohorts with attenuated psychosis syndrome from normal control cohorts with patterns similar to, but less severe than, that observed in schizophrenia. However, neuroimaging data is not diagnostic at the individual level.

Prevalence

The prevalence of attenuated psychosis syndrome is unknown. Symptoms in Criterion A are not uncommon in the non-help-seeking population, ranging from 8%–13% for hallucinatory experiences and delusional thinking. There appears to be a slight male preponderance for attenuated psychosis syndrome.

Development and Course

Onset of attenuated psychosis syndrome is usually in mid-to-late adolescence or early adulthood. It may be preceded by normal development or evidence for impaired cognition, negative symptoms, and/or impaired social development. In help-seeking cohorts, approximately 18% in 1 year and 32% in 3 years may progress symptomatically and met criteria for a psychotic disorder. In some cases, the syndrome may transition to a depressive or bipolar disorder with psychotic features, but development to a schizophrenia spectrum disorder is more frequent. It appears that the diagnosis is best applied to individuals ages 15–35 years. Long-term course is not yet described beyond 7–12 years.

Risk and Prognostic Factors

Temperamental. Factors predicting prognosis of attenuated psychosis syndrome have not been definitively characterized, but the presence of negative symptoms, cognitive impairment, and poor functioning are associated with poor outcome and increase risk of transition to psychosis.

Genetic and physiological. A family history of psychosis places the individual with attenuated psychosis syndrome at increased risk for developing a full psychotic disorder. Structural, functional, and neurochemical imaging data are associated with increased risk of transition to psychosis.

Functional Consequences of Attenuated Psychosis Syndrome

Many individuals may experience functional impairments. Modest-to-moderate impairment in social and role functioning may persist even with abatement of symptoms. A substantial portion of individuals with the diagnosis will improve over time; many continue to have mild symptoms and impairment, and many others will have a full recovery.

Differential Diagnosis

Brief psychotic disorder. When symptoms of attenuated psychosis syndrome initially manifest, they may resemble symptoms of brief psychotic disorder. However, in attenuated psychosis syndrome, the symptoms do not cross the psychosis threshold and reality testing/insight remains intact.

Schizotypal personality disorder. Schizotypal personality disorder, although having symptomatic features that are similar to those of attenuated psychosis syndrome, is a relatively stable trait disorder not meeting the state-dependent aspects (Criterion C) of attenuated psychosis syndrome. In addition, a broader array of symptoms is required for schizotypal personality disorder, although in the early stages of presentation it may resemble attenuated psychosis syndrome.

Depressive or bipolar disorders. Reality distortions that are temporally limited to an episode of a major depressive disorder or bipolar disorder and are descriptively more characteristic of those disorders do not meet Criterion E for attenuated psychosis syndrome. For example, feelings of low self-esteem or attributions of low regard from others in the context of major depressive disorder would not qualify for comorbid attenuated psychosis syndrome.

Anxiety disorders. Reality distortions that are temporally limited to an episode of an anxiety disorder and are descriptively more characteristic of an anxiety disorder do not meet Criterion E for attenuated psychosis syndrome. For example, a feeling of being the focus of undesired attention in the context of social anxiety disorder would not qualify for comorbid attenuated psychosis syndrome.

Bipolar II disorder.   Reality distortions that are temporally limited to an episode of mania or hypomania and are descriptively more characteristic of bipolar disorder do not meet Criterion E for attenuated psychosis syndrome. For example, inflated self-esteem in the context of pressured speech and reduced need for sleep would not qualify for comorbid attenuated psychosis syndrome.

Borderline personality disorder.   Reality distortions that are concomitant with borderline personality disorder and are descriptively more characteristic of it do not meet Criterion E for attenuated psychosis syndrome. For example, a sense of being unable to experience feelings in the context of an intense fear of real or imagined abandonment and recurrent self-mutilation would not qualify for comorbid attenuated psychosis syndrome.

Adjustment reaction of adolescence.   Mild, transient symptoms typical of normal development and consistent with the degree of stress experienced do not qualify for attenuated psychosis syndrome.

Extreme end of perceptual aberration and magical thinking in the non-ill population.   This diagnostic possibility should be strongly entertained when reality distortions are not associated with distress and functional impairment and need for care.

Substance/medication-induced psychotic disorder.   Substance use is common among individuals whose symptoms meet attenuated psychosis syndrome criteria. When otherwise qualifying characteristic symptoms are strongly temporally related to substance use episodes, Criterion E for attenuated psychosis syndrome may not be met, and a diagnosis of substance/medication-induced psychotic disorder may be preferred.

Attention-deficit/hyperactivity disorder.   A history of attentional impairment does not exclude a current attenuated psychosis syndrome diagnosis. Earlier attentional impairment may be a prodromal condition or comorbid attention-deficit/hyperactivity disorder.

Comorbidity

Individuals with attenuated psychosis syndrome often experience anxiety and/or depression. Some individuals with an attenuated psychosis syndrome diagnosis will progress to another diagnosis, including anxiety, depressive, bipolar, and personality disorders. In such cases, the psychopathology associated with the attenuated psychosis syndrome diagnosis is reconceptualized as the prodromal phase of another disorder, not a comorbid condition.

Depressive Episodes With Short-Duration Hypomania

Proposed Criteria

Lifetime experience of at least one major depressive episode meeting the following criteria:

A. Five (or more) of the following criteria have been present during the same 2-week period and represent a change from previous functioning; at least one of the symptoms is either (1) depressed mood or (2) loss of interest or pleasure. (**Note:** Do not include symptoms that are clearly attributable to a medical condition.)

   1. Depressed mood most of the day, nearly every day, as indicated by either subjective report (e.g., feels sad, empty, or hopeless) or observation made by others (e.g., appears tearful). (**Note:** In children and adolescents, can be irritable mood.)

   2. Markedly diminished interest or pleasure in all, or almost all, activities most of the day, nearly every day (as indicated by either subjective account or observation).

3. Significant weight loss when not dieting or weight gain (e.g., a change of more than 5% of body weight in a month), or decrease or increase in appetite nearly every day. (**Note:** In children, consider failure to make expected weight gain.)
4. Insomnia or hypersomnia nearly every day.
5. Psychomotor agitation or retardation nearly every day (observable by others, not merely subjective feelings of restlessness or being slowed down).
6. Fatigue or loss of energy nearly every day.
7. Feelings of worthlessness or excessive or inappropriate guilt (which may be delusional) nearly every day (not merely self-reproach or guilt about being sick).
8. Diminished ability to think or concentrate, or indecisiveness, nearly every day (either by subjective account or as observed by others).
9. Recurrent thoughts of death (not just fear of dying), recurrent suicidal ideation without a specific plan, or a suicide attempt or a specific plan for committing suicide.

B. The symptoms cause clinically significant distress or impairment in social, occupational, or other important areas of functioning.
C. The disturbance is not attributable to the physiological effects of a substance or another medical condition.
D. The disturbance is not better explained by schizoaffective disorder and is not superimposed on schizophrenia, schizophreniform disorder, delusional disorder, or other specified or unspecified schizophrenia spectrum and other psychotic disorder.

At least two lifetime episodes of hypomanic periods that involve the required criterion symptoms below but are of insufficient duration (at least 2 days but less than 4 consecutive days) to meet criteria for a hypomanic episode. The criterion symptoms are as follows:

A. A distinct period of abnormally and persistently elevated, expansive, or irritable mood and abnormally and persistently increased activity or energy.
B. During the period of mood disturbance and increased energy and activity, three (or more) of the following symptoms have persisted (four if the mood is only irritable), represent a noticeable change from usual behavior, and have been present to a significant degree:

1. Inflated self-esteem or grandiosity.
2. Decreased need for sleep (e.g., feels rested after only 3 hours of sleep).
3. More talkative than usual or pressured to keep talking.
4. Flight of ideas or subjective experience that thoughts are racing.
5. Distractibility (i.e., attention too easily drawn to unimportant or irrelevant external stimuli), as reported or observed.
6. Increase in goal-directed activity (either socially, at work or school, or sexually) or psychomotor agitation.
7. Excessive involvement in activities that have a high potential for painful consequences (e.g., the individual engages in unrestrained buying sprees, sexual indiscretions, or foolish business investments).

C. The episode is associated with an unequivocal change in functioning that is uncharacteristic of the individual when not symptomatic.
D. The disturbance in mood and the change in functioning are observable by others.
E. The episode is not severe enough to cause marked impairment in social or occupational functioning or to necessitate hospitalization. If there are psychotic features, the episode is, by definition, manic.
F. The episode is not attributable to the physiological effects of a substance (e.g., a drug of abuse, a medication or other treatment).

Diagnostic Features

Individuals with short-duration hypomania have experienced at least one major depressive episode as well as at least two episodes of 2–3 days' duration in which criteria for a hypomanic episode were met (except for symptom duration). These episodes are of sufficient intensity to be categorized as a hypomanic episode but do not meet the 4-day duration requirement. Symptoms are present to a significant degree, such that they represent a noticeable change from the individual's normal behavior.

An individual with a history of a syndromal hypomanic episode and a major depressive episode by definition has bipolar II disorder, regardless of current duration of hypomanic symptoms.

Associated Features Supporting Diagnosis

Individuals who have experienced both short-duration hypomania and a major depressive episode, with their increased comorbidity with substance use disorders and a greater family history of bipolar disorder, more closely resemble individuals with bipolar disorder than those with major depressive disorder.

Differences have also been found between individuals with short-duration hypomania and those with syndromal bipolar disorder. Work impairment was greater for individuals with syndromal bipolar disorder, as was the estimated average number of episodes. Individuals with short-duration hypomania may exhibit less severity than individuals with syndromal hypomanic episodes, including less mood lability.

Prevalence

The prevalence of short-duration hypomania is unclear, since the criteria are new as of this edition of the manual. Using somewhat different criteria, however, it has been estimated that short-duration hypomania occurs in 2.8% of the population (compared with hypomania or mania in 5.5% of the population). Short-duration hypomania may be more common in females, who may present with more features of atypical depression.

Risk and Prognostic Factors

Genetic and physiological.   A family history of mania is two to three times more common in individuals with short-duration hypomania compared with the general population, but less than half as common as in individuals with a history of syndromal mania or hypomania.

Suicide Risk

Individuals with short-duration hypomania have higher rates of suicide attempts than healthy individuals, although not as high as the rates in individuals with syndromal bipolar disorder.

Functional Consequences of Short-Duration Hypomania

Functional impairments associated specifically with short-duration hypomania are as yet not fully determined. However, research suggests that individuals with this disorder have less work impairment than individuals with syndromal bipolar disorder but more comorbid substance use disorders, particularly alcohol use disorder, than individuals with major depressive disorder.

Differential Diagnosis

Bipolar II disorder.   Bipolar II disorder is characterized by a period of at least 4 days of hypomanic symptoms, whereas short-duration hypomania is characterized by periods of

2–3 days of hypomanic symptoms. Once an individual has experienced a hypomanic episode (4 days or more), the diagnosis becomes and remains bipolar II disorder regardless of future duration of hypomanic symptom periods.

Major depressive disorder. Major depressive disorder is also characterized by at least one lifetime major depressive episode. However, the additional presence of at least two lifetime periods of 2–3 days of hypomanic symptoms leads to a diagnosis of short-duration hypomania rather than to major depressive disorder.

Major depressive disorder with mixed features. Both major depressive disorder with mixed features and short-duration hypomania are characterized by the presence of some hypomanic symptoms and a major depressive episode. However, major depressive disorder with mixed features is characterized by hypomanic features present *concurrently* with a major depressive episode, while individuals with short-duration hypomania experience subsyndromal hypomania and fully syndromal major depression at different times.

Bipolar I disorder. Bipolar I disorder is differentiated from short-duration hypomania by at least one lifetime manic episode, which is longer (at least 1 week) and more severe (causes more impaired social functioning) than a hypomanic episode. An episode (of any duration) that involves psychotic symptoms or necessitates hospitalization is by definition a manic episode rather than a hypomanic one.

Cyclothymic disorder. While cyclothymic disorder is characterized by periods of depressive symptoms and periods of hypomanic symptoms, the lifetime presence of a major depressive episode precludes the diagnosis of cyclothymic disorder.

Comorbidity

Short-duration hypomania, similar to full hypomanic episodes, has been associated with higher rates of comorbid anxiety disorders and substance use disorders than are found in the general population.

Persistent Complex Bereavement Disorder

Proposed Criteria

A. The individual experienced the death of someone with whom he or she had a close relationship.

B. Since the death, at least one of the following symptoms is experienced on more days than not and to a clinically significant degree and has persisted for at least 12 months after the death in the case of bereaved adults and 6 months for bereaved children:

1. Persistent yearning/longing for the deceased. In young children, yearning may be expressed in play and behavior, including behaviors that reflect being separated from, and also reuniting with, a caregiver or other attachment figure.
2. Intense sorrow and emotional pain in response to the death.
3. Preoccupation with the deceased.
4. Preoccupation with the circumstances of the death. In children, this preoccupation with the deceased may be expressed through the themes of play and behavior and may extend to preoccupation with possible death of others close to them.

C. Since the death, at least six of the following symptoms are experienced on more days than not and to a clinically significant degree, and have persisted for at least 12 months after the death in the case of bereaved adults and 6 months for bereaved children:

Reactive distress to the death

1. Marked difficulty accepting the death. In children, this is dependent on the child's capacity to comprehend the meaning and permanence of death.
2. Experiencing disbelief or emotional numbness over the loss.
3. Difficulty with positive reminiscing about the deceased.
4. Bitterness or anger related to the loss.
5. Maladaptive appraisals about oneself in relation to the deceased or the death (e.g., self-blame).
6. Excessive avoidance of reminders of the loss (e.g., avoidance of individuals, places, or situations associated with the deceased; in children, this may include avoidance of thoughts and feelings regarding the deceased).

Social/identity disruption

7. A desire to die in order to be with the deceased.
8. Difficulty trusting other individuals since the death.
9. Feeling alone or detached from other individuals since the death.
10. Feeling that life is meaningless or empty without the deceased, or the belief that one cannot function without the deceased.
11. Confusion about one's role in life, or a diminished sense of one's identity (e.g., feeling that a part of oneself died with the deceased).
12. Difficulty or reluctance to pursue interests since the loss or to plan for the future (e.g., friendships, activities).

D. The disturbance causes clinically significant distress or impairment in social, occupational, or other important areas of functioning.

E. The bereavement reaction is out of proportion to or inconsistent with cultural, religious, or age-appropriate norms.

Specify if:

With traumatic bereavement: Bereavement due to homicide or suicide with persistent distressing preoccupations regarding the traumatic nature of the death (often in response to loss reminders), including the deceased's last moments, degree of suffering and mutilating injury, or the malicious or intentional nature of the death.

Diagnostic Features

Persistent complex bereavement disorder is diagnosed only if at least 12 months (6 months in children) have elapsed since the death of someone with whom the bereaved had a close relationship (Criterion A). This time frame discriminates normal grief from persistent grief. The condition typically involves a persistent yearning/longing for the deceased (Criterion B1), which may be associated with intense sorrow and frequent crying (Criterion B2) or preoccupation with the deceased (Criterion B3). The individual may also be preoccupied with the manner in which the person died (Criterion B4).

Six additional symptoms are required, including marked difficulty accepting that the individual has died (Criterion C1) (e.g., preparing meals for them), disbelief that the individual is dead (Criterion C2), distressing memories of the deceased (Criterion C3), anger over the loss (Criterion C4), maladaptive appraisals about oneself in relation to the deceased or the death (Criterion C5), and excessive avoidance of reminders of the loss (Criterion C6). Individuals may also report a desire to die because they wish to be with the deceased (Criterion C7); be distrustful of others (Criterion C8); feel isolated (Criterion C9); believe that life has no meaning or purpose without the deceased (Criterion C10); experience a diminished sense of identity in which they feel a part of themselves has died or been lost (Criterion C11); or have difficulty engaging in activities, pursuing relationships, or planning for the future (Criterion C12).

Persistent complex bereavement disorder requires clinically significant distress or impairment in psychosocial functioning (Criterion D). The nature and severity of grief must be beyond expected norms for the relevant cultural setting, religious group, or developmental stage (Criterion E). Although there are variations in how grief can manifest, the symptoms of persistent complex bereavement disorder occur in both genders and in diverse social and cultural groups.

Associated Features Supporting Diagnosis

Some individuals with persistent complex bereavement disorder experience hallucinations of the deceased (auditory or visual) in which they temporarily perceive the deceased's presence (e.g., seeing the deceased sitting in his or her favorite chair). They may also experience diverse somatic complaints (e.g., digestive complaints, pain, fatigue), including symptoms experienced by the deceased.

Prevalence

The prevalence of persistent complex bereavement disorder is approximately 2.4%–4.8%. The disorder is more prevalent in females than in males.

Development and Course

Persistent complex bereavement disorder can occur at any age, beginning after the age of 1 year. Symptoms usually begin within the initial months after the death, although there may be a delay of months, or even years, before the full syndrome appears. Although grief responses commonly appear immediately following bereavement, these reactions are not diagnosed as persistent complex bereavement disorder unless the symptoms persist beyond 12 months (6 months for children).

Young children may experience the loss of a primary caregiver as traumatic, given the disorganizing effects the caregiver's absence can have on a child's coping response. In children, the distress may be expressed in play and behavior, developmental regressions, and anxious or protest behavior at times of separation and reunion. Separation distress may be predominant in younger children, and social/identity distress and risk for comorbid depression can increasingly manifest in older children and adolescents.

Risk and Prognostic Factors

Environmental. Risk for persistent complex bereavement disorder is heightened by increased dependency on the deceased person prior to the death and by the death of a child. Disturbances in caregiver support increase the risk for bereaved children.

Genetic and physiological. Risk for the disorder is heightened by the bereaved individual being female.

Culture-Related Diagnostic Issues

The symptoms of persistent complex bereavement disorder are observed across cultural settings, but grief responses may manifest in culturally specific ways. Diagnosis of the disorder requires that the persistent and severe responses go beyond cultural norms of grief responses and not be better explained by culturally specific mourning rituals.

Suicide Risk

Individuals with persistent complex bereavement disorder frequently report suicidal ideation.

Functional Consequences of Persistent Complex Bereavement Disorder

Persistent complex bereavement disorder is associated with deficits in work and social functioning and with harmful health behaviors, such as increased tobacco and alcohol use. It is also associated with marked increases in risks for serious medical conditions, including cardiac disease, hypertension, cancer, immunological deficiency, and reduced quality of life.

Differential Diagnosis

Normal grief.   Persistent complex bereavement disorder is distinguished from normal grief by the presence of severe grief reactions that persist at least 12 months (or 6 months in children) after the death of the bereaved. It is only when severe levels of grief response persist at least 12 months following the death and interfere with the individual's capacity to function that persistent complex bereavement disorder is diagnosed.

Depressive disorders.   Persistent complex bereavement disorder, major depressive disorder, and persistent depressive disorder (dysthymia) share sadness, crying, and suicidal thinking. Whereas major depressive disorder and persistent depressive disorder can share depressed mood with persistent complex bereavement disorder, the latter is characterized by a focus on the loss.

Posttraumatic stress disorder.   Individuals who experience bereavement as a result of traumatic death may develop both posttraumatic stress disorder (PTSD) and persistent complex bereavement disorder. Both conditions can involve intrusive thoughts and avoidance. Whereas intrusions in PTSD revolve around the traumatic event, intrusive memories in persistent complex bereavement disorder focus on thoughts about many aspects of the relationship with the deceased, including positive aspects of the relationship and distress over the separation. In individuals with the traumatic bereavement specifier of persistent complex bereavement disorder, the distressing thoughts or feelings may be more overtly related to the manner of death, with distressing fantasies of what happened. Both persistent complex bereavement disorder and PTSD can involve avoidance of reminders of distressing events. Whereas avoidance in PTSD is characterized by consistent avoidance of internal and external reminders of the traumatic experience, in persistent complex bereavement disorder, there is also a preoccupation with the loss and yearning for the deceased, which is absent in PTSD.

Separation anxiety disorder.   Separation anxiety disorder is characterized by anxiety about separation from current attachment figures, whereas persistent complex bereavement disorder involves distress about separation from a deceased individual.

Comorbidity

The most common comorbid disorders with persistent complex bereavement disorder are major depressive disorder, PTSD, and substance use disorders. PTSD is more frequently comorbid with persistent complex bereavement disorder when the death occurred in traumatic or violent circumstances.

Caffeine Use Disorder

Proposed Criteria

A problematic pattern of caffeine use leading to clinically significant impairment or distress, as manifested by at least the first three of the following criteria occurring within a 12-month period:

1. A persistent desire or unsuccessful efforts to cut down or control caffeine use.
2. Continued caffeine use despite knowledge of having a persistent or recurrent physical or psychological problem that is likely to have been caused or exacerbated by caffeine.

3. Withdrawal, as manifested by either of the following:

   a. The characteristic withdrawal syndrome for caffeine.

   b. Caffeine (or a closely related) substance is taken to relieve or avoid withdrawal symptoms.

4. Caffeine is often taken in larger amounts or over a longer period than was intended.

5. Recurrent caffeine use resulting in a failure to fulfill major role obligations at work, school, or home (e.g., repeated tardiness or absences from work or school related to caffeine use or withdrawal).

6. Continued caffeine use despite having persistent or recurrent social or interpersonal problems caused or exacerbated by the effects of caffeine (e.g., arguments with spouse about consequences of use, medical problems, cost).

7. Tolerance, as defined by either of the following:

   a. A need for markedly increased amounts of caffeine to achieve desired effect.

   b. Markedly diminished effect with continued use of the same amount of caffeine.

8. A great deal of time is spent in activities necessary to obtain caffeine, use caffeine, or recover from its effects.

9. Craving or a strong desire or urge to use caffeine.

A diagnosis of substance dependence due to caffeine is recognized by the World Health Organization in ICD-10. Since the publication of DSM-IV in 1994, considerable research on caffeine dependence has been published, and several recent reviews provide a current analysis of this literature. There is now sufficient evidence to warrant inclusion of caffeine use disorder as a research diagnosis in DSM-5 to encourage additional research. The working diagnostic algorithm proposed for the study of caffeine use disorder differs from that of the other substance use disorders, reflecting the need to identify only cases that have sufficient clinical importance to warrant the labeling of a mental disorder. A key goal of including caffeine use disorder in this section of DSM-5 is to stimulate research that will determine the reliability, validity, and prevalence of caffeine use disorder based on the proposed diagnostic schema, with particular attention to the association of the diagnosis with functional impairments as part of validity testing.

The proposed criteria for caffeine use disorder reflect the need for a diagnostic threshold higher than that used for the other substance use disorders. Such a threshold is intended to prevent overdiagnosis of caffeine use disorder due to the high rate of habitual nonproblematic daily caffeine use in the general population.

Diagnostic Features

Caffeine use disorder is characterized by the continued use of caffeine and failure to control use despite negative physical and/or psychological consequences. In a survey of the general population, 14% of caffeine users met the criterion of use despite harm, with most reporting that a physician or counselor had advised them to stop or reduce caffeine use within the last year. Medical and psychological problems attributed to caffeine included heart, stomach, and urinary problems, and complaints of anxiety, depression, insomnia, irritability, and difficulty thinking. In the same survey, 45% of caffeine users reported desire or unsuccessful efforts to control caffeine use, 18% reported withdrawal, 8% reported tolerance, 28% used more than intended, and 50% reported spending a great deal of time using caffeine. In addition, 19% reported a strong desire for caffeine that they could not resist, and less than 1% reported that caffeine had interfered with social activities.

Among those seeking treatment for quitting problematic caffeine use, 88% reported having made prior serious attempts to modify caffeine use, and 43% reported having been advised by a medical professional to reduce or eliminate caffeine. Ninety-three percent endorsed signs and symptoms meeting DSM-IV criteria for caffeine dependence, with the most commonly endorsed criteria being withdrawal (96%), persistent desire or unsuccessful efforts to control use (89%), and use despite knowledge of physical or psychological problems caused by caffeine (87%). The most common reasons for wanting to modify caffeine use were health-related (59%) and a desire to not be dependent on caffeine (35%).

The DSM-5 discussion of caffeine withdrawal in the Section II chapter "Substance-Related and Addictive Disorders" provides information on the features of the withdrawal criterion. It is well documented that habitual caffeine users can experience a well-defined withdrawal syndrome upon acute abstinence from caffeine, and many caffeine-dependent individuals report continued use of caffeine to avoid experiencing withdrawal symptoms.

Prevalence

The prevalence of caffeine use disorder in the general population is unclear. Based on all seven generic DSM-IV-TR criteria for dependence, 30% of current caffeine users may have met DSM-IV criteria for a diagnosis of caffeine dependence, with endorsement of three or more dependence criteria, during the past year. When only four of the seven criteria (the three primary criteria proposed above plus tolerance) are used, the prevalence appears to drop to 9%. Thus, the expected prevalence of caffeine use disorder among regular caffeine users is likely less than 9%. Given that approximately 75%–80% of the general population uses caffeine regularly, the estimated prevalence would be less than 7%. Among regular caffeine drinkers at higher risk for caffeine use problems (e.g., high school and college students, individuals in drug treatment, and individuals at pain clinics who have recent histories of alcohol or illicit drug misuse), approximately 20% may have a pattern of use that meets all three of the proposed criteria in Criterion A.

Development and Course

Individuals whose pattern of use meets criteria for a caffeine use disorder have shown a wide range of daily caffeine intake and have been consumers of various types of caffeinated products (e.g., coffee, soft drinks, tea) and medications. A diagnosis of caffeine use disorder has been shown to prospectively predict a greater incidence of caffeine reinforcement and more severe withdrawal.

There has been no longitudinal or cross-sectional lifespan research on caffeine use disorder. Caffeine use disorder has been identified in both adolescents and adults. Rates of caffeine consumption and overall level of caffeine consumption tend to increase with age until the early to mid-30s and then level off. Age-related factors for caffeine use disorder are unknown, although concern is growing related to excessive caffeine consumption among adolescents and young adults through use of caffeinated energy drinks.

Risk and Prognostic Factors

Genetic and physiological.   Heritabilities of heavy caffeine use, caffeine tolerance, and caffeine withdrawal range from 35% to 77%. For caffeine use, alcohol use, and cigarette smoking, a common genetic factor (polysubstance use) underlies the use of these three substances, with 28%–41% of the heritable effects of caffeine use (or heavy use) shared with alcohol and smoking. Caffeine and tobacco use disorders are associated and substantially influenced by genetic factors unique to these licit drugs. The magnitude of heritability for caffeine use disorder markers appears to be similar to that for alcohol and tobacco use disorder markers.

Functional Consequences of Caffeine Use Disorder

Caffeine use disorder may predict greater use of caffeine during pregnancy. Caffeine withdrawal, a key feature of caffeine use disorder, has been shown to produce functional impairment in normal daily activities. Caffeine intoxication may include symptoms of nausea and vomiting, as well as impairment of normal activities. Significant disruptions in normal daily activities may occur during caffeine abstinence.

Differential Diagnosis

Nonproblematic use of caffeine. The distinction between nonproblematic use of caffeine and caffeine use disorder can be difficult to make because social, behavioral, or psychological problems may be difficult to attribute to the substance, especially in the context of use of other substances. Regular, heavy caffeine use that can result in tolerance and withdrawal is relatively common, which by itself should not be sufficient for making a diagnosis.

Other stimulant use disorder. Problems related to use of other stimulant medications or substances may approximate the features of caffeine use disorder.

Anxiety disorders. Chronic heavy caffeine use may mimic generalized anxiety disorder, and acute caffeine consumption may produce and mimic panic attacks.

Comorbidity

There may be comorbidity between caffeine use disorder and daily cigarette smoking, a family or personal history of alcohol use disorder. Features of caffeine use disorder (e.g., tolerance, caffeine withdrawal) may be positively associated with several diagnoses: major depression, generalized anxiety disorder, panic disorder, adult antisocial personality disorder, and alcohol, cannabis, and cocaine use disorders.

Internet Gaming Disorder

Proposed Criteria

Persistent and recurrent use of the Internet to engage in games, often with other players, leading to clinically significant impairment or distress as indicated by five (or more) of the following in a 12-month period:

1. Preoccupation with Internet games. (The individual thinks about previous gaming activity or anticipates playing the next game; Internet gaming becomes the dominant activity in daily life.)
   Note: This disorder is distinct from Internet gambling, which is included under gambling disorder.
2. Withdrawal symptoms when Internet gaming is taken away. (These symptoms are typically described as irritability, anxiety, or sadness, but there are no physical signs of pharmacological withdrawal.)
3. Tolerance—the need to spend increasing amounts of time engaged in Internet games.
4. Unsuccessful attempts to control the participation in Internet games.
5. Loss of interests in previous hobbies and entertainment as a result of, and with the exception of, Internet games.
6. Continued excessive use of Internet games despite knowledge of psychosocial problems.
7. Has deceived family members, therapists, or others regarding the amount of Internet gaming.
8. Use of Internet games to escape or relieve a negative mood (e.g., feelings of helplessness, guilt, anxiety).
9. Has jeopardized or lost a significant relationship, job, or educational or career opportunity because of participation in Internet games.

Note: Only nongambling Internet games are included in this disorder. Use of the Internet for required activities in a business or profession is not included; nor is the disorder intended to include other recreational or social Internet use. Similarly, sexual Internet sites are excluded.

Specify current severity:
> Internet gaming disorder can be mild, moderate, or severe depending on the degree of disruption of normal activities. Individuals with less severe Internet gaming disorder may exhibit fewer symptoms and less disruption of their lives. Those with severe Internet gaming disorder will have more hours spent on the computer and more severe loss of relationships or career or school opportunities.

Subtypes

There are no well-researched subtypes for Internet gaming disorder to date. Internet gaming disorder most often involves specific Internet games, but it could involve non-Internet computerized games as well, although these have been less researched. It is likely that preferred games will vary over time as new games are developed and popularized, and it is unclear if behaviors and consequence associated with Internet gaming disorder vary by game type.

Diagnostic Features

Gambling disorder is currently the only non-substance-related disorder proposed for inclusion with DSM-5 substance-related and addictive disorders. However, there are other behavioral disorders that show some similarities to substance use disorders and gambling disorder for which the word *addiction* is commonly used in nonmedical settings, and the one condition with a considerable literature is the compulsive playing of Internet games. Internet gaming has been reportedly defined as an "addiction" by the Chinese government, and a treatment system has been set up. Reports of treatment of this condition have appeared in medical journals, mostly from Asian countries and some in the United States.

The DSM-5 work group reviewed more than 240 articles and found some behavioral similarities of Internet gaming to gambling disorder and to substance use disorders. The literature suffers, however, from lack of a standard definition from which to derive prevalence data. An understanding of the natural histories of cases, with or without treatment, is also missing. The literature does describe many underlying similarities to substance addictions, including aspects of tolerance, withdrawal, repeated unsuccessful attempts to cut back or quit, and impairment in normal functioning. Further, the seemingly high prevalence rates, both in Asian countries and, to a lesser extent, in the West, justified inclusion of this disorder in Section III of DSM-5.

Internet gaming disorder has significant public health importance, and additional research may eventually lead to evidence that Internet gaming disorder (also commonly referred to as *Internet use disorder, Internet addiction,* or *gaming addiction*) has merit as an independent disorder. As with gambling disorder, there should be epidemiological studies to determine prevalence, clinical course, possible genetic influence, and potential biological factors based on, for example, brain imaging data.

Internet gaming disorder is a pattern of excessive and prolonged Internet gaming that results in a cluster of cognitive and behavioral symptoms, including progressive loss of control over gaming, tolerance, and withdrawal symptoms, analogous to the symptoms of substance use disorders. As with substance-related disorders, individuals with Internet gaming disorder continue to sit at a computer and engage in gaming activities despite neglect of other activities. They typically devote 8–10 hours or more per day to this activity and at least 30 hours per week. If they are prevented from using a computer and returning to the game, they become agitated and angry. They often go for long periods without food or sleep. Normal obligations, such as school or work, or family obligations are neglected. This condition is separate from gambling disorder involving the Internet because money is not at risk.

The essential feature of Internet gaming disorder is persistent and recurrent participation in computer gaming, typically group games, for many hours. These games involve competition between groups of players (often in different global regions, so that duration of play is encouraged by the time-zone independence) participating in complex structured activities that include a significant aspect of social interactions during play. Team aspects appear to be a key motivation. Attempts to direct the individual toward schoolwork or interpersonal activities are strongly resisted. Thus personal, family, or vocational pursuits are neglected. When individuals are asked, the major reasons given for using the computer are more likely to be "avoiding boredom" rather than communicating or searching for information.

The description of criteria related to this condition is adapted from a study in China. Until the optimal criteria and threshold for diagnosis are determined empirically, conservative definitions ought to be used, such that diagnoses are considered for endorsement of five or more of nine criteria.

Associated Features Supporting Diagnosis

No consistent personality types associated with Internet gaming disorder have been identified. Some authors describe associated diagnoses, such as depressive disorders, attention-deficit/hyperactivity disorder (ADHD), or obsessive-compulsive disorder (OCD). Individuals with compulsive Internet gaming have demonstrated brain activation in specific regions triggered by exposure to the Internet game but not limited to reward system structures

Prevalence

The prevalence of Internet gaming disorder is unclear because of the varying questionnaires, criteria and thresholds employed, but it seems to be highest in Asian countries and in male adolescents 12–20 years of age. There is an abundance of reports from Asian countries, especially China and South Korea, but fewer from Europe and North America, from which prevalence estimates are highly variable. The point prevalence in adolescents (ages 15–19 years) in one Asian study using a threshold of five criteria was 8.4% for males and 4.5% for females.

Risk and Prognostic Factors

Environmental. Computer availability with Internet connection allows access to the types of games with which Internet gaming disorder is most often associated.

Genetic and physiological. Adolescent males seem to be at greatest risk of developing Internet gaming disorder, and it has been speculated that Asian environmental and/or genetic background is another risk factor, but this remains unclear.

Functional Consequences of Internet Gaming Disorder

Internet gaming disorder may lead to school failure, job loss, or marriage failure. The compulsive gaming behavior tends to crowd out normal social, scholastic, and family activities. Students may show declining grades and eventually failure in school. Family responsibilities may be neglected.

Differential Diagnosis

Excessive use of the Internet not involving playing of online games (e.g., excessive use of social media, such as Facebook; viewing pornography online) is not considered analogous to Internet gaming disorder, and future research on other excessive uses of the Internet would need to follow similar guidelines as suggested herein. Excessive gambling online may qualify for a separate diagnosis of gambling disorder.

Comorbidity

Health may be neglected due to compulsive gaming. Other diagnoses that may be associated with Internet gaming disorder include major depressive disorder, ADHD, and OCD.

Neurobehavioral Disorder Associated With Prenatal Alcohol Exposure

Proposed Criteria

A. More than minimal exposure to alcohol during gestation, including prior to pregnancy recognition. Confirmation of gestational exposure to alcohol may be obtained from maternal self-report of alcohol use in pregnancy, medical or other records, or clinical observation.

B. Impaired neurocognitive functioning as manifested by one or more of the following:

1. Impairment in global intellectual performance (i.e., IQ of 70 or below, or a standard score of 70 or below on a comprehensive developmental assessment).

2. Impairment in executive functioning (e.g., poor planning and organization; inflexibility; difficulty with behavioral inhibition).

3. Impairment in learning (e.g., lower academic achievement than expected for intellectual level; specific learning disability).

4. Memory impairment (e.g., problems remembering information learned recently; repeatedly making the same mistakes; difficulty remembering lengthy verbal instructions).

5. Impairment in visual-spatial reasoning (e.g., disorganized or poorly planned drawings or constructions; problems differentiating left from right).

C. Impaired self-regulation as manifested by one or more of the following:

1. Impairment in mood or behavioral regulation (e.g., mood lability; negative affect or irritability; frequent behavioral outbursts).

2. Attention deficit (e.g., difficulty shifting attention; difficulty sustaining mental effort).

3. Impairment in impulse control (e.g., difficulty waiting turn; difficulty complying with rules).

D. Impairment in adaptive functioning as manifested by two or more of the following, one of which must be (1) or (2):

1. Communication deficit (e.g., delayed acquisition of language; difficulty understanding spoken language).

2. Impairment in social communication and interaction (e.g., overly friendly with strangers; difficulty reading social cues; difficulty understanding social consequences).

3. Impairment in daily living skills (e.g., delayed toileting, feeding, or bathing; difficulty managing daily schedule).

4. Impairment in motor skills (e.g., poor fine motor development; delayed attainment of gross motor milestones or ongoing deficits in gross motor function; deficits in coordination and balance).

E. Onset of the disorder (symptoms in Criteria B, C, and D) occurs in childhood.

F. The disturbance causes clinically significant distress or impairment in social, academic, occupational, or other important areas of functioning.

G. The disorder is not better explained by the direct physiological effects associated with postnatal use of a substance (e.g., a medication, alcohol or other drugs), a general medical condition (e.g., traumatic brain injury, delirium, dementia), another known teratogen (e.g., fetal hydantoin syndrome), a genetic condition (e.g., Williams syndrome, Down syndrome, Cornelia de Lange syndrome), or environmental neglect.

Alcohol is a neurobehavioral teratogen, and prenatal alcohol exposure has teratogenic effects on central nervous system (CNS) development and subsequent function. *Neurobehavioral disorder associated with prenatal alcohol exposure* (ND-PAE) is a new clarifying term, intended to encompass the full range of developmental disabilities associated with exposure to alcohol in utero. The current diagnostic guidelines allow ND-PAE to be diagnosed both in the absence and in the presence of the physical effects of prenatal alcohol exposure (e.g., facial dysmorphology required for a diagnosis of fetal alcohol syndrome).

Diagnostic Features

The essential features of ND-PAE are the manifestation of impairment in neurocognitive, behavioral, and adaptive functioning associated with prenatal alcohol exposure. Impairment can be documented based on past diagnostic evaluations (e.g., psychological or educational assessments) or medical records, reports by the individual or informants, and/or observation by a clinician.

A clinical diagnosis of fetal alcohol syndrome, including specific prenatal alcohol-related facial dysmorphology and growth retardation, can be used as evidence of significant levels of prenatal alcohol exposure. Although both animal and human studies have documented adverse effects of lower levels of drinking, identifying how much prenatal exposure is needed to significantly impact neurodevelopmental outcome remains challenging. Data suggest that a history of more than minimal gestational exposure (e.g., more than light drinking) prior to pregnancy recognition and/or following pregnancy recognition may be required. Light drinking is defined as 1–13 drinks per month during pregnancy with no more than 2 of these drinks consumed on any 1 drinking occasion. Identifying a minimal threshold of drinking during pregnancy will require consideration of a variety of factors known to affect exposure and/or interact to influence developmental outcomes, including stage of prenatal development, gestational smoking, maternal and fetal genetics, and maternal physical status (i.e., age, health, and certain obstetric problems).

Symptoms of ND-PAE include marked impairment in global intellectual performance (IQ) or neurocognitive impairments in any of the following areas: executive functioning, learning, memory, and/or visual-spatial reasoning. Impairments in self-regulation are present and may include impairment in mood or behavioral regulation, attention deficit, or impairment in impulse control. Finally, impairments in adaptive functioning include communication deficits and impairment in social communication and interaction. Impairment in daily living (self-help) skills and impairment in motor skills may be present. As it may be difficult to obtain an accurate assessment of the neurocognitive abilities of very young children, it is appropriate to defer a diagnosis for children 3 years of age and younger.

Associated Features Supporting Diagnosis

Associated features vary depending on age, degree of alcohol exposure, and the individual's environment. An individual can be diagnosed with this disorder regardless of socioeconomic or cultural background. However, ongoing parental alcohol/substance misuse, parental mental illness, exposure to domestic or community violence, neglect or abuse, disrupted caregiving relationships, multiple out-of-home placements, and lack of continuity in medical or mental health care are often present.

Prevalence

The prevalence rates of ND-PAE are unknown. However, estimated prevalence rates of clinical conditions associated with prenatal alcohol exposure are 2%–5% in the United States.

Development and Course

Among individuals with prenatal alcohol exposure, evidence of CNS dysfunction varies according to developmental stage. Although about one-half of young children prenatally exposed to alcohol show marked developmental delay in the first 3 years of life, other children affected by prenatal alcohol exposure may not exhibit signs of CNS dysfunction until they are preschool- or school-age. Additionally, impairments in higher order cognitive processes (i.e., executive functioning), which are often associated with prenatal alcohol exposure, may be more easily assessed in older children. When children reach school age, learning difficulties, impairment in executive function, and problems with integrative language functions usually emerge more clearly, and both social skills deficits and challenging behavior may become more evident. In particular, as school and other requirements become more complex, greater deficits are noted. Because of this, the school years represent the ages at which a diagnosis of ND-PAE would be most likely.

Suicide Risk

Suicide is a high-risk outcome, with rates increasing significantly in late adolescence and early adulthood.

Functional Consequences of Neurobehavioral Disorder Associated With Prenatal Alcohol Exposure

The CNS dysfunction seen in individuals with ND-PAE often leads to decrements in adaptive behavior and to maladaptive behavior with lifelong consequences. Individuals affected by prenatal alcohol exposure have a higher prevalence of disrupted school experiences, poor employment records, trouble with the law, confinement (legal or psychiatric), and dependent living conditions.

Differential Diagnosis

Disorders that are attributable to the physiological effects associated with postnatal use of a substance, another medical condition, or environmental neglect.   Other considerations include the physiological effects of postnatal substance use, such as a medication, alcohol, or other substances; disorders due to another medical condition, such as traumatic brain injury or other neurocognitive disorders (e.g., delirium, major neurocognitive disorder [dementia]); or environmental neglect.

Genetic and teratogenic conditions.   Genetic conditions such as Williams syndrome, Down syndrome, or Cornelia de Lange syndrome and other teratogenic conditions such as fetal hydantoin syndrome and maternal phenylketonuria may have similar physical and behavioral characteristics. A careful review of prenatal exposure history is needed to clarify the teratogenic agent, and an evaluation by a clinical geneticist may be needed to distinguish physical characteristics associated with these and other genetic conditions.

Comorbidity

Mental health problems have been identified in more than 90% of individuals with histories of significant prenatal alcohol exposure. The most common co-occurring diagnosis is attention-deficit/hyperactivity disorder, but research has shown that individuals with ND-PAE differ in neuropsychological characteristics and in their responsiveness to pharmacological interventions. Other high- probability co-occurring disorders include oppositional defiant disorder and conduct disorder, but the appropriateness of these diagnoses should be weighed in the context of the significant impairments in general intellectual and executive functioning that are often associated with prenatal alcohol exposure. Mood symptoms, including symptoms of bipolar disorder and depressive disorders, have been described. History of prenatal alcohol exposure is associated with an increased risk for later tobacco, alcohol, and other substance use disorders.

Suicidal Behavior Disorder

Proposed Criteria

A. Within the last 24 months, the individual has made a suicide attempt.

Note: A suicide attempt is a self-initiated sequence of behaviors by an individual who, at the time of initiation, expected that the set of actions would lead to his or her own death. (The "time of initiation" is the time when a behavior took place that involved applying the method.)

B. The act does not meet criteria for nonsuicidal self-injury—that is, it does not involve self-injury directed to the surface of the body undertaken to induce relief from a negative feeling/cognitive state or to achieve a positive mood state.

C. The diagnosis is not applied to suicidal ideation or to preparatory acts.

D. The act was not initiated during a state of delirium or confusion.

E. The act was not undertaken solely for a political or religious objective.

Specify if:

Current: Not more than 12 months since the last attempt.

In early remission: 12–24 months since the last attempt.

Specifiers

Suicidal behavior is often categorized in terms of violence of the method. Generally, overdoses with legal or illegal substances are considered nonviolent in method, whereas jumping, gunshot wounds, and other methods are considered violent. Another dimension for classification is medical consequences of the behavior, with high-lethality attempts being defined as those requiring medical hospitalization beyond a visit to an emergency department. An additional dimension considered includes the degree of planning versus impulsiveness of the attempt, a characteristic that might have consequences for the medical outcome of a suicide attempt.

If the suicidal behavior occurred 12–24 months prior to evaluation, the condition is considered to be in early remission. Individuals remain at higher risk for further suicide attempts and death in the 24 months after a suicide attempt, and the period 12–24 months after the behavior took place is specified as "early remission."

Diagnostic Features

The essential manifestation of suicidal behavior disorder is a suicide attempt. A *suicide attempt* is a behavior that the individual has undertaken with at least some intent to die. The behavior might or might not lead to injury or serious medical consequences. Several factors can influence the medical consequences of the suicide attempt, including poor planning, lack of knowledge about the lethality of the method chosen, low intentionality or ambivalence, or chance intervention by others after the behavior has been initiated. These should not be considered in assigning the diagnosis.

Determining the degree of intent can be challenging. Individuals might not acknowledge intent, especially in situations where doing so could result in hospitalization or cause distress to loved ones. Markers of risk include degree of planning, including selection of a time and place to minimize rescue or interruption; the individual's mental state at the time of the behavior, with acute agitation being especially concerning; recent discharge from inpatient care; or recent discontinuation of a mood stabilizer such as lithium or an antipsychotic such as clozapine in the case of schizophrenia. Examples of environmental "triggers" include recently learning of a potentially fatal medical diagnosis such as cancer, experiencing the sudden and unexpected loss of a close relative or partner, loss of employment, or displacement from housing. Conversely, features such as talking to others about future events or preparedness to sign a contract for safety are less reliable indicators.

In order for the criteria to be met, the individual must have made at least one suicide attempt. Suicide attempts can include behaviors in which, after initiating the suicide attempt, the individual changed his or her mind or someone intervened. For example, an individual might intend to ingest a given amount of medication or poison, but either stop or be stopped by another before ingesting the full amount. If the individual is dissuaded by another or changes his or her mind before initiating the behavior, the diagnosis should not be made. The act must not meet criteria for nonsuicidal self-injury—that is, it should not involve repeated (at least five times within the past 12 months) self-injurious episodes undertaken to induce relief from a negative feeling/cognitive state or to achieve a positive mood state. The act should not have been initiated during a state of delirium or confusion. If the individual deliberately became intoxicated before initiating the behavior, to reduce anticipatory anxiety and to minimize interference with the intended behavior, the diagnosis should be made.

Development and Course

Suicidal behavior can occur at any time in the lifespan but is rarely seen in children under the age of 5. In prepubertal children, the behavior will often consist of a behavior (e.g., sitting on a ledge) that a parent has forbidden because of the risk of accident. Approximately 25%–30% of persons who attempt suicide will go on to make more attempts. There is significant variability in terms of frequency, method, and lethality of attempts. However, this is not different from what is observed in other illnesses, such as major depressive disorder, in which frequency of episode, subtype of episode, and impairment for a given episode can vary significantly.

Culture-Related Diagnostic Issues

Suicidal behavior varies in frequency and form across cultures. Cultural differences might be due to method availability (e.g., poisoning with pesticides in developing countries; gunshot wounds in the southwestern United States) or the presence of culturally specific syndromes (e.g., *ataques de nervios,* which in some Latino groups might lead to behaviors that closely resemble suicide attempts or might facilitate suicide attempts).

Diagnostic Markers

Laboratory abnormalities consequent to the suicidal attempt are often evident. Suicidal behavior that leads to blood loss can be accompanied by anemia, hypotension, or shock. Overdoses might lead to coma or obtundation and associated laboratory abnormalities such as electrolyte imbalances.

Functional Consequences of Suicidal Behavior Disorder

Medical conditions (e.g., lacerations or skeletal trauma, cardiopulmonary instability, inhalation of vomit and suffocation, hepatic failure consequent to use of paracetamol) can occur as a consequence of suicidal behavior.

Comorbidity

Suicidal behavior is seen in the context of a variety of mental disorders, most commonly bipolar disorder, major depressive disorder, schizophrenia, schizoaffective disorder, anxiety disorders (in particular, panic disorders associated with catastrophic content and PTSD flashbacks), substance use disorders (especially alcohol use disorders), borderline personality disorder, antisocial personality disorder, eating disorders, and adjustment disorders. It is rarely manifested by individuals with no discernible pathology, unless it is undertaken because of a painful medical condition with the intention of drawing attention to martyrdom for political or religious reasons, or in partners in a suicide pact, both of which are excluded from this diagnosis, or when third-party informants wish to conceal the nature of the behavior.

Nonsuicidal Self-Injury

Proposed Criteria

A. In the last year, the individual has, on 5 or more days, engaged in intentional self-inflicted damage to the surface of his or her body of a sort likely to induce bleeding, bruising, or pain (e.g., cutting, burning, stabbing, hitting, excessive rubbing), with the expectation that the injury will lead to only minor or moderate physical harm (i.e., there is no suicidal intent).

   Note: The absence of suicidal intent has either been stated by the individual or can be inferred by the individual's repeated engagement in a behavior that the individual knows, or has learned, is not likely to result in death.

B. The individual engages in the self-injurious behavior with one or more of the following expectations:

   1. To obtain relief from a negative feeling or cognitive state.
   2. To resolve an interpersonal difficulty.
   3. To induce a positive feeling state.

   Note: The desired relief or response is experienced during or shortly after the self-injury, and the individual may display patterns of behavior suggesting a dependence on repeatedly engaging in it.

C. The intentional self-injury is associated with at least one of the following:

   1. Interpersonal difficulties or negative feelings or thoughts, such as depression, anxiety, tension, anger, generalized distress, or self-criticism, occurring in the period immediately prior to the self-injurious act.
   2. Prior to engaging in the act, a period of preoccupation with the intended behavior that is difficult to control.
   3. Thinking about self-injury that occurs frequently, even when it is not acted upon.

D. The behavior is not socially sanctioned (e.g., body piercing, tattooing, part of a religious or cultural ritual) and is not restricted to picking a scab or nail biting.

E. The behavior or its consequences cause clinically significant distress or interference in interpersonal, academic, or other important areas of functioning.

F. The behavior does not occur exclusively during psychotic episodes, delirium, substance intoxication, or substance withdrawal. In individuals with a neurodevelopmental disorder, the behavior is not part of a pattern of repetitive stereotypies. The behavior is not better explained by another mental disorder or medical condition (e.g., psychotic disorder, autism spectrum disorder, intellectual disability, Lesch-Nyhan syndrome, stereotypic movement disorder with self-injury, trichotillomania [hair-pulling disorder], excoriation [skin-picking] disorder).

Diagnostic Features

The essential feature of nonsuicidal self-injury is that the individual repeatedly inflicts shallow, yet painful injuries to the surface of his or her body. Most commonly, the purpose is to reduce negative emotions, such as tension, anxiety, and self-reproach, and/or to resolve an interpersonal difficulty. In some cases, the injury is conceived of as a deserved self-punishment. The individual will often report an immediate sensation of relief that occurs during the process. When the behavior occurs frequently, it might be associated with a sense of urgency and craving, the resultant behavioral pattern resembling an addiction. The inflicted wounds can become deeper and more numerous.

The injury is most often inflicted with a knife, needle, razor, or other sharp object. Common areas for injury include the frontal area of the thighs and the dorsal side of the forearm. A single session of injury might involve a series of superficial, parallel cuts—separated by 1 or 2 centimeters—on a visible or accessible location. The resulting cuts will often bleed and will eventually leave a characteristic pattern of scars.

Other methods used include stabbing an area, most often the upper arm, with a needle or sharp, pointed knife; inflicting a superficial burn with a lit cigarette end; or burning the skin by repeated rubbing with an eraser. Engagement in nonsuicidal self-injury with multiple methods is associated with more severe psychopathology, including engagement in suicide attempts.

The great majority of individuals who engage in nonsuicidal self-injury do not seek clinical attention. It is not known if this reflects frequency of engagement in the disorder, because accurate reporting is seen as stigmatizing, or because the behaviors are experienced positively by the individual who engages in them, who is unmotivated to receive treatment. Young children might experiment with these behaviors but not experience relief. In such cases, youths often report that the procedure is painful or distressing and might then discontinue the practice.

Development and Course

Nonsuicidal self-injury most often starts in the early teen years and can continue for many years. Admission to hospital for nonsuicidal self-injury reaches a peak at 20–29 years of age and then declines. However, research that has examined age at hospitalization did not provide information on age at onset of the behavior, and prospective research is needed to outline the natural history of nonsuicidal self-injury and the factors that promote or inhibit its course. Individuals often learn of the behavior on the recommendation or observation of another. Research has shown that when an individual who engages in nonsuicidal self-injury is admitted to an inpatient unit, other individuals may begin to engage in the behavior.

Risk and Prognostic Factors

Male and female prevalence rates of nonsuicidal self-injury are closer to each other than in suicidal behavior disorder, in which the female-to-male ratio is about 3:1 or 4:1.

Two theories of psychopathology—based on functional behavioral analyses—have been proposed: In the first, based on learning theory, either positive or negative reinforcement sustains the behavior. Positive reinforcement might result from punishing oneself in a way that the individual feels is deserved, with the behavior inducing a pleasant and relaxed state or generating attention and help from a significant other, or as an expression of anger. Negative reinforcement results from affect regulation and the reduction of unpleasant emotions or avoiding distressing thoughts, including thinking about suicide. In the second theory, nonsuicidal self-injury is thought to be a form of self-punishment, in which self-punitive actions are engaged in to make up for acts that caused distress or harm to others.

Functional Consequences of Nonsuicidal Self-Injury

The act of cutting might be performed with shared implements, raising the possibility of blood-borne disease transmission.

Differential Diagnosis

Borderline personality disorder. As indicated, nonsuicidal self-injury has long been re-garded as a "symptom" of borderline personality disorder, even though comprehensive clinical evaluations have found that most individuals with nonsuicidal self-injury have symptoms that also meet criteria for other diagnoses, with eating disorders and substance use disorders being especially common. Historically, nonsuicidal self-injury was regarded as pathognomonic of borderline personality disorder. Both conditions are associated with several other diagnoses. Although frequently associated, borderline personality disorder is not invariably found in individuals with nonsuicidal self-injury. The two conditions dif-fer in several ways. Individuals with borderline personality disorder often manifest dis-turbed aggressive and hostile behaviors, whereas nonsuicidal self-injury is more often associated with phases of closeness, collaborative behaviors, and positive relationships. At a more fundamental level, there are differences in the involvement of different neurotrans-mitter systems, but these will not be apparent on clinical examination.

Suicidal behavior disorder. The differentiation between nonsuicidal self-injury and sui-cidal behavior disorder is based either on the stated goal of the behavior being a wish to die (suicidal behavior disorder) or, in nonsuicidal self-injury, to experience relief as de-scribed in the criteria. Depending on the circumstances, individuals may provide reports of convenience, and several studies report high rates of false intent declaration. Individu-als with a history of frequent nonsuicidal self-injury episodes have learned that a session of cutting, while painful, is, in the short-term, largely benign. Because individuals with nonsuicidal self-injury can and do attempt and commit suicide, it is important to check past history of suicidal behavior and to obtain information from a third party concerning any recent change in stress exposure and mood. Likelihood of suicide intent has been as-sociated with the use of multiple previous methods of self-harm.

In a follow-up study of cases of "self-harm" in males treated at one of several multiple emergency centers in the United Kingdom, individuals with nonsuicidal self-injury were significantly more likely to commit suicide than other teenage individuals drawn from the same cohort. Studies that have examined the relationship between nonsuicidal self-injury and suicidal behavior disorder are limited by being retrospective and failing to obtain ver-ified accounts of the method used during previous "attempts." A significant proportion of those who engage in nonsuicidal self-injury have responded positively when asked if they have ever engaged in self-cutting (or their preferred means of self-injury) with an intention to die. It is reasonable to conclude that nonsuicidal self-injury, while not presenting a high risk for suicide when first manifested, is an especially dangerous form of self-injurious behavior.

This conclusion is also supported by a multisite study of depressed adolescents who had previously failed to respond to antidepressant medication, which noted that those with pre-vious nonsuicidal self-injury did not respond to cognitive-behavioral therapy, and by a study that found that nonsuicidal self-injury is a predictor of substance use/misuse.

Trichotillomania (hair-pulling disorder). Trichotillomania is an injurious behavior con-fined to pulling out one's own hair, most commonly from the scalp, eyebrows, or eyelashes. The behavior occurs in "sessions" that can last for hours. It is most likely to occur during a period of relaxation or distraction.

Stereotypic self-injury. Stereotypic self-injury, which can include head banging, self-biting, or self-hitting, is usually associated with intense concentration or under conditions of low external stimulation and might be associated with developmental delay.

Excoriation (skin-picking) disorder. Excoriation disorder occurs mainly in females and is usually directed to picking at an area of the skin that the individual feels is unsightly or a blemish, usually on the face or the scalp. As in nonsuicidal self-injury, the picking is often preceded by an urge and is experienced as pleasurable, even though the individual realizes that he or she is harming himself or herself. It is not associated with the use of any implement.

APPENDIX

Highlights of Changes From DSM-IV to DSM-5

Changes made to DSM-5 diagnostic criteria and texts are outlined in this chapter in the same order in which they appear in the DSM-5 classification. This abbreviated description is intended to orient readers to only the most significant changes in each disorder category. An expanded description of nearly all changes (e.g., except minor text or wording changes needed for clarity) is available online (www.psychiatry.org/dsm5). It should also be noted that Section I contains a description of changes pertaining to the chapter organization in DSM-5, the multiaxial system, and the introduction of dimensional assessments.

Neurodevelopmental Disorders

The term *mental retardation* was used in DSM-IV. However, **intellectual disability (intellectual developmental disorder)** is the term that has come into common use over the past two decades among medical, educational, and other professionals, and by the lay public and advocacy groups. Diagnostic criteria emphasize the need for an assessment of both cognitive capacity (IQ) and adaptive functioning. Severity is determined by adaptive functioning rather than IQ score.

The **communication disorders,** which are newly named from DSM-IV phonological disorder and stuttering, respectively, include **language disorder** (which combines the previous expressive and mixed receptive-expressive language disorders), **speech sound disorder** (previously phonological disorder), and **childhood-onset fluency disorder** (previously stuttering). Also included is **social (pragmatic) communication disorder,** a new condition involving persistent difficulties in the social uses of verbal and nonverbal communication.

Autism spectrum disorder is a new DSM-5 disorder encompassing the previous DSM-IV autistic disorder (autism), Asperger's disorder, childhood disintegrative disorder, Rett's disorder, and pervasive developmental disorder not otherwise specified. It is characterized by deficits in two core domains: 1) deficits in social communication and social interaction and 2) restricted repetitive patterns of behavior, interests, and activities.

Several changes have been made to the diagnostic criteria for **attention-deficit/hyperactivity disorder** (ADHD). Examples have been added to the criterion items to facilitate application across the life span; the age at onset description has been changed (from "some hyperactive-impulsive or inattentive symptoms that caused impairment were present before age 7 years" to "Several inattentive or hyperactive-impulsive symptoms were present prior to age 12"); subtypes have been replaced with presentation specifiers that map directly to the prior subtypes; a comorbid diagnosis with autism spectrum disorder is now allowed; and a symptom threshold change has been made for adults, to reflect the substantial evidence of clinically significant ADHD impairment, with the cutoff for ADHD of five symptoms, instead of six required for younger persons, both for inattention and for hyperactivity and impulsivity.

Specific learning disorder combines the DSM-IV diagnoses of reading disorder, mathematics disorder, disorder of written expression, and learning disorder not otherwise specified. Learning deficits in the areas of reading, written expression, and mathematics are coded as separate specifiers. Acknowledgment is made in the text that specific types of reading deficits are described internationally in various ways as *dyslexia* and specific types of mathematics deficits as *dyscalculia.*

The following **motor disorders** are included in DSM-5: developmental coordination disorder, stereotypic movement disorder, Tourette's disorder, persistent (chronic) motor or vocal tic disorder, provisional tic disorder, other specified tic disorder, and unspecified tic disorder. The tic criteria have been standardized across all of these disorders in this chapter.

Schizophrenia Spectrum and Other Psychotic Disorders

Two changes were made to Criterion A for **schizophrenia:** 1) the elimination of the special attribution of bizarre delusions and Schneiderian first-rank auditory hallucinations (e.g., two or more voices conversing), leading to the requirement of at least two Criterion A symptoms for any diagnosis of schizophrenia, and 2) the addition of the requirement that at least one of the Criterion A symptoms must be delusions, hallucinations, or disorganized speech. The DSM-IV subtypes of schizophrenia were eliminated due to their limited diagnostic stability, low reliability, and poor validity. Instead, a dimensional approach to rating severity for the core symptoms of schizophrenia is included in DSM-5 Section III to capture the important heterogeneity in symptom type and severity expressed across individuals with psychotic disorders. **Schizoaffective disorder** is reconceptualized as a longitudinal instead of a cross-sectional diagnosis—more comparable to schizophrenia, bipolar disorder, and major depressive disorder, which are bridged by this condition—and requires that a major mood episode be present for a majority of the total disorder's duration after Criterion A has been met. Criterion A for **delusional disorder** no longer has the requirement that the delusions must be nonbizarre; a specifier is now included for bizarre type delusions to provide continuity with DSM-IV. Criteria for **catatonia** are described uniformly across DSM-5. Furthermore, catatonia may be diagnosed with a specifier (for depressive, bipolar, and psychotic disorders, including schizophrenia), in the context of a known medical condition, or as an other specified diagnosis.

Bipolar and Related Disorders

Diagnostic criteria for **bipolar disorders** now include both changes in mood and changes in activity or energy. The DSM-IV diagnosis of bipolar I disorder, mixed episodes—requiring that the individual simultaneously meet full criteria for both mania and major depressive episode—is replaced with a new specifier "with mixed features." Particular conditions can now be diagnosed under **other specified bipolar and related disorder,** including categorization for individuals with a past history of a major depressive disorder whose symptoms meet all criteria for hypomania except the duration criterion is not met (i.e., the episode lasts only 2 or 3 days instead of the required 4 consecutive days or more). A second condition constituting an other specified bipolar and related disorder variant is that too few symptoms of hypomania are present to meet criteria for the full bipolar II syndrome, although the duration, at least 4 consecutive days, is sufficient. Finally, in both this chapter and in the chapter "Depressive Disorders," an anxious distress specifier is delineated.

Depressive Disorders

To address concerns about potential overdiagnosis and overtreatment of bipolar disorder in children, a new diagnosis, **disruptive mood dysregulation disorder,** is included for children up to age 18 years who exhibit persistent irritability and frequent episodes of extreme behavioral dyscontrol. **Premenstrual dysphoric disorder** is now promoted from Appendix B, "Criteria Sets and Axes Provided for Further Study," in DSM-IV to the main body of DSM-5. What was referred to as dysthymia in DSM-IV now falls under the category of **persistent depressive disorder,** which includes both chronic major depressive disorder and the previous dysthymic disorder. The coexistence within a **major depressive episode** of at least three manic symptoms (insufficient to satisfy criteria for a manic episode) is now acknowledged by the specifier "with mixed features." In DSM-IV, there was an exclusion criterion for a major depressive episode that was applied to depressive symptoms lasting less than 2 months following the death of a loved one (i.e., the bereavement exclusion). This exclusion is omitted in DSM-5 for several reasons, including the recognition that bereavement is a severe psychosocial stressor that can precipitate a major depressive episode in a vulnerable individual, generally beginning soon after the loss, and can add an additional risk for suffering, feelings of worthlessness, suicidal ideation, poorer medical health, and worse interpersonal and work functioning. It was critical to remove the implication that bereavement typically lasts only 2 months, when both physicians and grief counselors recognize that the duration is more commonly 1–2 years. A detailed footnote has replaced the more simplistic DSM-IV exclusion to aid clinicians in making the critical distinction between the symptoms characteristic of bereavement and those of a major depressive disorder. Finally, a new specifier to indicate the presence of mixed symptoms has been added across both the bipolar and the depressive disorders.

Anxiety Disorders

The chapter on anxiety disorders no longer includes obsessive-compulsive disorder (which is in the new chapter "Obsessive-Compulsive and Related Disorders") or posttraumatic stress disorder (PTSD) and acute stress disorder (which are in the new chapter "Trauma- and Stressor-Related Disorders"). Changes in criteria for **specific phobia** and **social anxiety disorder (social phobia)** include deletion of the requirement that individuals over age 18 years recognize that their anxiety is excessive or unreasonable. Instead, the anxiety must be out of proportion to the actual danger or threat in the situation, after cultural contextual factors are taken into account. In addition, the 6-month duration is now extended to all ages. **Panic attacks** can now be listed as a specifier that is applicable to all DSM-5 disorders. **Panic disorder** and **agoraphobia** are unlinked in DSM-5. Thus, the former DSM-IV diagnoses of panic disorder with agoraphobia, panic disorder without agoraphobia, and agoraphobia without history of panic disorder are now replaced by two diagnoses, panic disorder and agoraphobia, each with separate criteria. The "generalized" specifier for **social anxiety disorder** has been deleted and replaced with a "performance only" specifier. **Separation anxiety disorder** and **selective mutism** are now classified as anxiety disorders. The wording of the criteria is modified to more adequately represent the expression of separation anxiety symptoms in adulthood. Also, in contrast to DSM-IV, the diagnostic criteria no longer specify that onset must be before age 18 years, and a duration statement—"typically lasting for 6 months or more"—has been added for adults to minimize overdiagnosis of transient fears.

Obsessive-Compulsive and Related Disorders

The chapter "Obsessive-Compulsive and Related Disorders" is new in DSM-5. New disorders include **hoarding disorder, excoriation (skin-picking) disorder, substance/medication-induced obsessive-compulsive and related disorder,** and **obsessive-compulsive and related disorder due to another medical condition.** The DSM-IV diagnosis of trichotillomania is now termed **trichotillomania (hair-pulling disorder)** and has been moved from a DSM-IV classification of impulse-control disorders not elsewhere classified to obsessive-compulsive and related disorders in DSM-5. The DSM-IV "with poor insight" specifier for **obsessive-compulsive disorder** has been refined to allow a distinction between individuals with good or fair insight, poor insight, and "absent insight/delusional" obsessive-compulsive disorder beliefs (i.e., complete conviction that obsessive-compulsive disorder beliefs are true). Analogous "insight" specifiers have been included for body dysmorphic disorder and hoarding disorder. A "tic-related" specifier for obsessive-compulsive disorder has also been added, because presence of a comorbid tic disorder may have important clinical implications. A "muscle dysmorphia" specifier for **body dysmorphic disorder** is added to reflect a growing literature on the diagnostic validity and clinical utility of making this distinction in individuals with body dysmorphic disorder. The delusional variant of body dysmorphic disorder (which identifies individuals who are completely convinced that their perceived defects or flaws are truly abnormal appearing) is no longer coded as both delusional disorder, somatic type, and body dysmorphic disorder; in DSM-5, this presentation is designated only as body dysmorphic disorder with the absent insight/delusional specifier. Individuals can also be diagnosed with **other specified obsessive-compulsive and related disorder,** which can include conditions such as body-focused repetitive behavior disorder and obsessional jealousy, or **unspecified obsessive-compulsive and related disorder.**

Trauma- and Stressor-Related Disorders

For a diagnosis of **acute stress disorder,** qualifying traumatic events are now explicit as to whether they were experienced directly, witnessed, or experienced indirectly. Also, the DSM-IV Criterion A2 regarding the subjective reaction to the traumatic event (e.g., experiencing "fear, helplessness, or horror") has been eliminated. **Adjustment disorders** are reconceptualized as a heterogeneous array of stress-response syndromes that occur after exposure to a distressing (traumatic or nontraumatic) event, rather than as a residual category for individuals who exhibit clinically significant distress but whose symptoms do not meet criteria for a more discrete disorder (as in DSM-IV).

DSM-5 criteria for **PTSD** differ significantly from the DSM-IV criteria. The stressor criterion (Criterion A) is more explicit with regard to events that qualify as "traumatic" experiences. Also, DSM-IV Criterion A2 (subjective reaction) has been eliminated. Whereas there were three major symptom clusters in DSM-IV—reexperiencing, avoidance/numbing, and arousal—there are now four symptom clusters in DSM-5, because the avoidance/numbing cluster is divided into two distinct clusters: avoidance and persistent negative alterations in cognitions and mood. This latter category, which retains most of the DSM-IV numbing symptoms, also includes new or reconceptualized symptoms, such as persistent negative emotional states. The final cluster—alterations in arousal and reactivity—retains most of the DSM-IV arousal symptoms. It also includes irritable behavior or angry outbursts and reckless or self-destructive behavior. PTSD is now developmentally sensitive in that diagnostic thresholds have been lowered for children and adolescents. Furthermore, separate criteria have been added for children age 6 years or younger with this disorder.

The DSM-IV childhood diagnosis reactive attachment disorder had two subtypes: emotionally withdrawn/inhibited and indiscriminately social/disinhibited. In DSM-5, these subtypes are defined as distinct disorders: **reactive attachment disorder** and **disinhibited social engagement disorder.**

Dissociative Disorders

Major changes in dissociative disorders in DSM-5 include the following: 1) derealization is included in the name and symptom structure of what previously was called depersonalization disorder (**depersonalization/derealization disorder**); 2) dissociative fugue is now a specifier of **dissociative amnesia** rather than a separate diagnosis, and 3) the criteria for **dissociative identity disorder** have been changed to indicate that symptoms of disruption of identity may be reported as well as observed, and that gaps in the recall of events may occur for everyday and not just traumatic events. Also, experiences of pathological possession in some cultures are included in the description of identity disruption.

Somatic Symptom and Related Disorders

In DSM-5, somatoform disorders are now referred to as **somatic symptom and related disorders.** The DSM-5 classification reduces the number of these disorders and subcategories to avoid problematic overlap. Diagnoses of somatization disorder, hypochondriasis, pain disorder, and undifferentiated somatoform disorder have been removed. Individuals previously diagnosed with somatization disorder will usually have symptoms that meet DSM-5 criteria for **somatic symptom disorder,** but only if they have the maladaptive thoughts, feelings, and behaviors that define the disorder, in addition to their somatic symptoms. Because the distinction between somatization disorder and undifferentiated somatoform disorder was arbitrary, they are merged in DSM-5 under somatic symptom disorder. Individuals previously diagnosed with hypochondriasis who have high health anxiety but no somatic symptoms would receive a DSM-5 diagnosis of **illness anxiety disorder** (unless their health anxiety was better explained by a primary anxiety disorder, such as generalized anxiety disorder). Some individuals with chronic pain would be appropriately diagnosed as having somatic symptom disorder, with predominant pain. For others, psychological factors affecting other medical conditions or an adjustment disorder would be more appropriate.

   Psychological factors affecting other medical conditions is a new mental disorder in DSM-5, having formerly been listed in the DSM-IV chapter "Other Conditions That May Be a Focus of Clinical Attention." This disorder and **factitious disorder** are placed among the somatic symptom and related disorders because somatic symptoms are predominant in both disorders, and both are most often encountered in medical settings. The variants of psychological factors affecting other medical conditions are removed in favor of the stem diagnosis. Criteria for **conversion disorder (functional neurological symptom disorder)** have been modified to emphasize the essential importance of the neurological examination, and in recognition that relevant psychological factors may not be demonstrable at the time of diagnosis. Other specified somatic symptom disorder, other specified illness anxiety disorder, and pseudocyesis are now the only exemplars of the **other specified somatic symptom and related disorder** classification.

Feeding and Eating Disorders

Because of the elimination of the DSM-IV-TR chapter "Disorders Usually First Diagnosed During Infancy, Childhood, or Adolescence," this chapter describes several disorders found in the DSM-IV section "Feeding and Eating Disorders of Infancy or Early Childhood," such as **pica** and **rumination disorder.** The DSM-IV category feeding disorder of infancy or early childhood has been renamed **avoidant/restrictive food intake disorder,** and the criteria are significantly expanded. The core diagnostic criteria for **anorexia nervosa** are conceptually unchanged from DSM-IV with one exception: the requirement for amenorrhea is eliminated. As in DSM-IV, individuals with this disorder are required by Criterion A to be at a significantly low body weight for their developmental stage. The wording of the criterion is changed for clarification, and guidance regarding how to judge whether an individual is at or below a significantly low weight is provided in the text. In DSM-5, Criterion B is expanded to include not only overtly expressed fear of weight gain but also persistent behavior that interferes with weight gain. The only change in the DSM-IV criteria for **bulimia nervosa** is a reduction in the required minimum average frequency of binge eating and inappropriate compensatory behavior frequency from twice to once weekly. The extensive research that followed the promulgation of preliminary criteria for **binge-eating disorder** in Appendix B of DSM-IV documented the clinical utility and validity of binge-eating disorder. The only significant difference from the preliminary criteria is that the minimum average frequency of binge eating required for diagnosis is once weekly over the last 3 months, identical to the frequency criterion for bulimia nervosa (rather than at least 2 days a week for 6 months in DSM-IV).

Elimination Disorders

There have been no significant changes in this diagnostic class from DSM-IV to DSM-5. The disorders in this chapter were previously classified under disorders usually first diagnosed in infancy, childhood, or adolescence in DSM-IV and exist now as an independent classification in DSM-5.

Sleep-Wake Disorders

In DSM-5, the DSM-IV diagnoses named sleep disorder related to another mental disorder and sleep disorder related to another medical condition have been removed, and instead greater specification of coexisting conditions is provided for each sleep-wake disorder. The diagnosis of primary insomnia has been renamed **insomnia disorder** to avoid the differentiation between primary and secondary insomnia. DSM-5 also distinguishes **narcolepsy**—now known to be associated with hypocretin deficiency—from other forms of hypersomnolence (hypersomnolence disorder). Finally, throughout the DSM-5 classification of sleep-wake disorders, pediatric and developmental criteria and text are integrated where existing science and considerations of clinical utility support such integration. **Breathing-related sleep disorders** are divided into three relatively distinct disorders: obstructive sleep apnea hypopnea, central sleep apnea, and sleep-related hypoventilation. The subtypes of **circadian rhythm sleep disorders** are expanded to include advanced sleep phase type and irregular sleep-wake type, whereas the jet lag type has been removed. The use of the former "not otherwise specified" diagnoses in DSM-IV have been reduced by elevating **rapid eye movement sleep behavior disorder** and **restless legs syndrome** to independent disorders.

Sexual Dysfunctions

In DSM-5, some gender-specific sexual dysfunctions have been added, and, for females, sexual desire and arousal disorders have been combined into one disorder: **female sexual interest/arousal disorder.** All of the sexual dysfunctions (except **substance/medication-induced sexual dysfunction**) now require a minimum duration of approximately 6 months and more precise severity criteria. **Genito-pelvic pain/penetration disorder** has been added to DSM-5 and represents a merging of vaginismus and dyspareunia, which were highly comorbid and difficult to distinguish. The diagnosis of sexual aversion disorder has been removed due to rare use and lack of supporting research.

There are now only two subtypes for sexual dysfunctions: **lifelong** versus **acquired** and **generalized** versus **situational.** To indicate the presence and degree of medical and other nonmedical correlates, the following **associated features** have been added to the text: partner factors, relationship factors, individual vulnerability factors, cultural or religious factors, and medical factors.

Gender Dysphoria

Gender dysphoria is a new diagnostic class in DSM-5 and reflects a change in conceptualization of the disorder's defining features by emphasizing the phenomenon of "gender incongruence" rather than cross-gender identification per se, as was the case in DSM-IV gender identity disorder. Gender dysphoria includes separate sets of criteria: for children and for adults and adolescents. For the adolescents and adults criteria, the previous Criterion A (cross-gender identification) and Criterion B (aversion toward one's gender) are merged. In the wording of the criteria, "the other sex" is replaced by "the other gender" (or "some alternative gender")." *Gender* instead of *sex* is used systematically because the concept "sex" is inadequate when referring to individuals with a disorder of sex development. In the child criteria, "strong desire to be of the other gender" replaces the previous "repeatedly stated desire to be...the other sex" to capture the situation of some children who, in a coercive environment, may not verbalize the desire to be of another gender. For children, Criterion A1 ("a strong desire to be of the other gender or an insistence that one is the other gender...)" is now necessary (but not sufficient), which makes the diagnosis more restrictive and conservative. The subtyping on the basis of sexual orientation is removed because the distinction is no longer considered clinically useful. A **posttransition specifier** has been added to identify individuals who have undergone at least one medical procedure or treatment to support the new gender assignment (e.g., cross-sex hormone treatment). Although the concept of post-transition is modeled on the concept of full or partial remission, the term *remission* has implications in terms of symptom reduction that do not apply directly to gender dysphoria.

Disruptive, Impulse-Control, and Conduct Disorders

The chapter "Disruptive, Impulse-Control, and Conduct Disorders" is new to DSM-5 and combines disorders that were previously included in the chapter "Disorders Usually First Diagnosed in Infancy, Childhood, or Adolescence" (i.e., oppositional defiant disorder; conduct disorder; and disruptive behavior disorder not otherwise specified, now categorized as other specified and unspecified disruptive, impulse-control, and conduct disorders) and the chapter "Impulse-Control Disorders Not Elsewhere Classified" (i.e., intermittent explosive disorder, pyromania, and kleptomania). These disorders are all characterized by problems in emotional and behavioral self-control. Notably, ADHD is frequently comorbid with the disorders in this chapter but is listed with the neurodevelopmental disorders. Because of its close association with conduct disorder, antisocial personality disorder is listed both in this chapter and in the chapter "Personality Disorders," where it is described in detail.

The criteria for **oppositional defiant disorder** are now grouped into three types: angry/irritable mood, argumentative/defiant behavior, and vindictiveness. Additionally, the exclusionary criterion for conduct disorder has been removed. The criteria for **conduct disorder** include a descriptive features specifier for individuals who meet full criteria for the disorder but also present with **limited prosocial emotions.** The primary change in **intermittent explosive disorder** is in the type of aggressive outbursts that should be considered: DSM-IV required physical aggression, whereas in DSM-5 verbal aggression and nondestructive/noninjurious physical aggression also meet criteria. DSM-5 also provides more specific criteria defining frequency needed to meet the criteria and specifies that the aggressive outbursts are impulsive and/or anger based in nature, and must cause marked distress, cause impairment in occupational or interpersonal functioning, or be associated with negative financial or legal consequences. Furthermore, a minimum age of 6 years (or equivalent developmental level) is now required.

Substance-Related and Addictive Disorders

An important departure from past diagnostic manuals is that the chapter on substance-related disorders has been expanded to include **gambling disorder**. Another key change is that DSM-5 does not separate the diagnoses of substance *abuse* and *dependence* as in DSM-IV. Rather criteria are provided for **substance use disorder,** accompanied by criteria for intoxication, withdrawal, substance-induced disorders, and unspecified substance-related disorders, where relevant. Within substance use disorders, the DSM-IV recurrent substance-related legal problems criterion has been deleted from DSM-5, and a new criterion—craving, or a strong desire or urge to use a substance—has been added. In addition, the threshold for substance use disorder diagnosis in DSM-5 is set at two or more criteria, in contrast to a threshold of one or more criteria for a diagnosis of DSM-IV substance abuse and three or more for DSM-IV dependence. **Cannabis withdrawal** and **caffeine withdrawal** are new disorders (the latter was in DSM-IV Appendix B, "Criteria Sets and Axes Provided for Further Study").

Severity of the DSM-5 substance use disorders is based on the number of criteria endorsed. The DSM-IV specifier for a physiological subtype is eliminated in DSM-5, as is the DSM-IV diagnosis of polysubstance dependence. Early remission from a DSM-5 substance use disorder is defined as at least 3 but less than 12 months without meeting substance use disorder criteria (except craving), and sustained remission is defined as at least 12 months without meeting criteria (except craving). Additional new DSM-5 specifiers include **"in a controlled environment"** and **"on maintenance therapy"** as the situation warrants.

Neurocognitive Disorders

The DSM-IV diagnoses of dementia and amnestic disorder are subsumed under the newly named entity **major neurocognitive disorder** (NCD). The term *dementia* is not precluded from use in the etiological subtypes where that term is standard. Furthermore, DSM-5 now recognizes a less severe level of cognitive impairment, **mild NCD,** which is a new disorder that permits the diagnosis of less disabling syndromes that may nonetheless be the focus of concern and treatment. Diagnostic criteria are provided for both of these disorders, followed by diagnostic criteria for different **etiological subtypes.** In DSM-IV, individual diagnoses were designated for dementia of the Alzheimer's type, vascular dementia, and substance-induced dementia, whereas the other neurodegenerative disorders were classified as dementia due to another medical condition, with HIV, head trauma, Parkinson's disease, Huntington's disease, Pick's disease, Creutzfeldt-Jakob disease, and other medical conditions specified. In DSM-5, major or mild NCD due to Alzheimer's disease and major or mild vascular NCD have been retained, while new separate criteria are now presented for major or mild frontotemporal NCD, NCD with Lewy bodies, and NCDs due to traumatic brain injury, a substance/medication, HIV infection, prion disease, Parkinson's disease, Huntington's disease, another medical condition, and multiple etiologies, respectively. Unspecified NCD is also included as a diagnosis.

Personality Disorders

The criteria for personality disorders in Section II of DSM-5 have not changed from those in DSM-IV. An alternative approach to the diagnosis of personality disorders was developed for DSM-5 for further study and can be found in Section III (see "Alternative DSM-5 Model for Personality Disorders"). For the **general criteria for personality disorder,** presented in Section III, a revised personality functioning criterion (Criterion A) has been developed based on a literature review of reliable clinical measures of core impairments central to personality pathology. A diagnosis of **personality disorder—trait specified,** based on moderate or greater impairment in personality functioning and the presence of pathological personality traits, replaces personality disorder not otherwise specified and provides a much more informative diagnosis for individuals who are not optimally described as having a specific personality disorder. A greater emphasis on personality functioning and trait-based criteria increases the stability and empirical bases of the disorders. **Personality functioning** and **personality traits** also can be assessed whether or not the individual has a personality disorder—a feature that provides clinically useful information about all individuals.

Paraphilic Disorders

An overarching change from DSM-IV is the addition of the course specifiers **"in a controlled environment"** and **"in remission"** to the diagnostic criteria sets for all the paraphilic disorders. These specifiers are added to indicate important changes in an individual's status. In DSM-5, paraphilias are not *ipso facto* mental disorders. There is a distinction between paraphilias and paraphilic disorders. A *paraphilic disorder* is a paraphilia that is currently causing distress or impairment to the individual or a paraphilia whose satisfaction has entailed personal harm, or risk of harm, to others. A paraphilia is a necessary but not a sufficient condition for having a paraphilic disorder, and a paraphilia by itself does not automatically justify or require clinical intervention. The **distinction between paraphilias and paraphilic disorders** was implemented without making any changes to the basic structure of the diagnostic criteria as they had existed since DSM-III-R. The change proposed for DSM-5 is that individuals who meet both Criterion A and Criterion B would now be diagnosed as having a paraphilic disorder. A diagnosis would not be given to individuals whose symptoms meet Criterion A but not Criterion B—that is, to individuals who have a paraphilia but not a paraphilic disorder.

Glossary of Technical Terms

affect   A pattern of observable behaviors that is the expression of a subjectively experienced feeling state (emotion). Examples of affect include sadness, elation, and anger. In contrast to *mood*, which refers to a pervasive and sustained emotional "climate," *affect* refers to more fluctuating changes in emotional "weather." What is considered the normal range of the expression of affect varies considerably, both within and among different cultures. Disturbances in affect include

> **blunted** Significant reduction in the intensity of emotional expression.
>
> **flat** Absence or near absence of any sign of affective expression.
>
> **inappropriate** Discordance between affective expression and the content of speech or ideation.
>
> **labile** Abnormal variability in affect with repeated, rapid, and abrupt shifts in affective expression.
>
> **restricted or constricted** Mild reduction in the range and intensity of emotional expression.

affective blunting   *See* AFFECT.

agitation (psychomotor)   *See* PSYCHOMOTOR AGITATION.

agnosia   Loss of ability to recognize objects, persons, sounds, shapes, or smells that occurs in the absence of either impairment of the specific sense or significant memory loss.

alogia   An impoverishment in thinking that is inferred from observing speech and language behavior. There may be brief and concrete replies to questions and restriction in the amount of spontaneous speech (termed *poverty of speech*). Sometimes the speech is adequate in amount but conveys little information because it is overconcrete, overabstract, repetitive, or stereotyped (termed *poverty of content*).

amnesia   An inability to recall important autobiographical information that is inconsistent with ordinary forgetting.

anhedonia   Lack of enjoyment from, engagement in, or energy for life's experiences; deficits in the capacity to feel pleasure and take interest in things. Anhedonia is a facet of the broad personality trait domain DETACHMENT.

anosognosia   A condition in which a person with an illness seems unaware of the existence of his or her illness.

antagonism   Behaviors that put an individual at odds with other people, such as an exaggerated sense of self-importance with a concomitant expectation of special treatment, as well as a callous antipathy toward others, encompassing both unawareness of others' needs and feelings, and a readiness to use others in the service of self-enhancement. Antagonism is one of the five broad PERSONALITY TRAIT DOMAINS defined in Section III "Alternative DSM-5 Model for Personality Disorders."

SMALL CAPS indicate term found elsewhere in this glossary. Glossary definitions were informed by DSM-5 Work Groups, publicly available Internet sources, and previously published glossaries for mental disorders (World Health Organization and American Psychiatric Association).

antidepressant discontinuation syndrome A set of symptoms that can occur after abrupt cessation, or marked reduction in dose, of an antidepressant medication that had been taken continuously for at least 1 month.

anxiety The apprehensive anticipation of future danger or misfortune accompanied by a feeling of worry, distress, and/or somatic symptoms of tension. The focus of anticipated danger may be internal or external.

anxiousness Feelings of nervousness or tenseness in reaction to diverse situations; frequent worry about the negative effects of past unpleasant experiences and future negative possibilities; feeling fearful and apprehensive about uncertainty; expecting the worst to happen. Anxiousness is a facet of the broad personality trait domain NEGATIVE AFFECTIVITY.

arousal The physiological and psychological state of being awake or reactive to stimuli.

asociality A reduced initiative for interacting with other people.

attention The ability to focus in a sustained manner on a particular stimulus or activity. A disturbance in attention may be manifested by easy DISTRACTIBILITY or difficulty in finishing tasks or in concentrating on work.

attention seeking Engaging in behavior designed to attract notice and to make oneself the focus of others' attention and admiration. Attention seeking is a facet of the broad personality trait domain ANTAGONISM.

autogynephilia Sexual arousal of a natal male associated with the idea or image of being a woman.

avoidance The act of keeping away from stress-related circumstances; a tendency to circumvent cues, activities, and situations that remind the individual of a stressful event experienced.

avolition An inability to initiate and persist in goal-directed activities. When severe enough to be considered pathological, avolition is pervasive and prevents the person from completing many different types of activities (e.g., work, intellectual pursuits, self-care).

bereavement The state of having lost through death someone with whom one has had a close relationship. This state includes a range of grief and mourning responses.

biological rhythms See CIRCADIAN RHYTHMS.

callousness Lack of concern for the feelings or problems of others; lack of guilt or remorse about the negative or harmful effects of one's actions on others. Callousness is a facet of the broad personality trait domain ANTAGONISM.

catalepsy Passive induction of a posture held against gravity. Compare with WAXY FLEXIBILITY.

cataplexy Episodes of sudden bilateral loss of muscle tone resulting in the individual collapsing, often occurring in association with intense emotions such as laughter, anger, fear, or surprise.

circadian rhythms Cyclical variations in physiological and biochemical function, level of sleep-wake activity, and emotional state. Circadian rhythms have a cycle of about 24 hours, *ultradian* rhythms have a cycle that is shorter than 1 day, and *infradian* rhythms have a cycle that may last weeks or months.

cognitive and perceptual dysregulation Odd or unusual thought processes and experiences, including DEPERSONALIZATION, DEREALIZATION, and DISSOCIATION; mixed sleep-wake state experiences; and thought-control experiences. Cognitive and perceptual dysregulation is a facet of the broad personality trait domain PSYCHOTICISM.

coma State of complete loss of consciousness.

compulsion   Repetitive behaviors (e.g., hand washing, ordering, checking) or mental acts (e.g., praying, counting, repeating words silently) that the individual feels driven to perform in response to an obsession, or according to rules that must be applied rigidly. The behaviors or mental acts are aimed at preventing or reducing anxiety or distress, or preventing some dreaded event or situation; however, these behaviors or mental acts are not connected in a realistic way with what they are designed to neutralize or prevent or are clearly excessive.

conversion symptom   A loss of, or alteration in, voluntary motor or sensory functioning, with or without apparent impairment of consciousness. The symptom is not fully explained by a neurological or another medical condition or the direct effects of a substance and is not intentionally produced or feigned.

deceitfulness   Dishonesty and fraudulence; misrepresentation of self; embellishment or fabrication when relating events. Deceitfulness is a facet of the broad personality trait domain ANTAGONISM.

defense mechanism   Mechanisms that mediate the individual′s reaction to emotional conflicts and to external stressors. Some defense mechanisms (e.g., projection, splitting, acting out) are almost invariably maladaptive. Others (e.g., suppression, denial) may be either maladaptive or adaptive, depending on their severity, their inflexibility, and the context in which they occur.

delusion   A false belief based on incorrect inference about external reality that is firmly held despite what almost everyone else believes and despite what constitutes incontrovertible and obvious proof or evidence to the contrary. The belief is not ordinarily accepted by other members of the person's culture or subculture (i.e., it is not an article of religious faith). When a false belief involves a value judgment, it is regarded as a delusion only when the judgment is so extreme as to defy credibility. Delusional conviction can sometimes be inferred from an overvalued idea (in which case the individual has an unreasonable belief or idea but does not hold it as firmly as is the case with a delusion). Delusions are subdivided according to their content. Common types are listed below:

    bizarre   A delusion that involves a phenomenon that the person's culture would regard as physically impossible.

    delusional jealousy   A delusion that one's sexual partner is unfaithful.

    erotomanic   A delusion that another person, usually of higher status, is in love with the individual.

    grandiose   A delusion of inflated worth, power, knowledge, identity, or special relationship to a deity or famous person.

    mixed type   Delusions of more than one type (e.g., EROTOMANIC, GRANDIOSE, PERSECUTORY, SOMATIC) in which no one theme predominates.

    mood-congruent   *See* MOOD-CONGRUENT PSYCHOTIC FEATURES.

    mood-incongruent   *See* MOOD-INCONGRUENT PSYCHOTIC FEATURES.

    of being controlled   A delusion in which feelings, impulses, thoughts, or actions are experienced as being under the control of some external force rather than being under one's own control.

    of reference   A delusion in which events, objects, or other persons in one's immediate environment are seen as having a particular and unusual significance. These delusions are usually of a negative or pejorative nature but also may be grandiose in content. A delusion of reference differs from an *idea of reference,* in which the false belief is not as firmly held nor as fully organized into a true belief.

    persecutory   A delusion in which the central theme is that one (or someone to whom one is close) is being attacked, harassed, cheated, persecuted, or conspired against.

somatic A delusion whose main content pertains to the appearance or functioning of one's body.

thought broadcasting A delusion that one's thoughts are being broadcast out loud so that they can be perceived by others.

thought insertion A delusion that certain of one's thoughts are not one's own, but rather are inserted into one's mind.

depersonalization The experience of feeling detached from, and as if one is an outside observer of, one's mental processes, body, or actions (e.g., feeling like one is in a dream; a sense of unreality of self, perceptual alterations; emotional and/or physical numbing; temporal distortions; sense of unreality).

depressivity Feelings of being intensely sad, miserable, and/or hopeless. Some patients describe an absence of feelings and/or dysphoria; difficulty recovering from such moods; pessimism about the future; pervasive shame and/or guilt; feelings of inferior self-worth; and thoughts of suicide and suicidal behavior. Depressivity is a facet of the broad personality trait domain DETACHMENT.

derealization The experience of feeling detached from, and as if one is an outside observer of, one's surroundings (e.g., individuals or objects are experienced as unreal, dreamlike, foggy, lifeless, or visually distorted).

detachment Avoidance of socioemotional experience, including both WITHDRAWAL from interpersonal interactions (ranging from casual, daily interactions to friendships and intimate relationships [i.e., INTIMACY AVOIDANCE]) and RESTRICTED AFFECTIVITY, particularly limited hedonic capacity. Detachment is one of the five pathological PERSONALITY TRAIT DOMAINS defined in Section III "Alternative DSM-5 Model for Personality Disorders."

disinhibition Orientation toward immediate gratification, leading to impulsive behavior driven by current thoughts, feelings, and external stimuli, without regard for past learning or consideration of future consequences. RIGID PERFECTIONISM, the opposite pole of this domain, reflects excessive constraint of impulses, risk avoidance, hyperresponsibility, hyperperfectionism, and rigid, rule-governed behavior. Disinhibition is one of the five pathological PERSONALITY TRAIT DOMAINS defined in Section III "Alternative DSM-5 Model for Personality Disorders."

disorder of sex development Condition of significant inborn somatic deviations of the reproductive tract from the norm and/or of discrepancies among the biological indicators of male and female.

disorientation Confusion about the time of day, date, or season (time); where one is (place); or who one is (person).

dissociation The splitting off of clusters of mental contents from conscious awareness. Dissociation is a mechanism central to dissociative disorders. The term is also used to describe the separation of an idea from its emotional significance and affect, as seen in the inappropriate affect in schizophrenia. Often a result of psychic trauma, dissociation may allow the individual to maintain allegiance to two contradictory truths while remaining unconscious of the contradiction. An extreme manifestation of dissociation is dissociative identity disorder, in which a person may exhibit several independent personalities, each unaware of the others.

distractibility Difficulty concentrating and focusing on tasks; attention is easily diverted by extraneous stimuli; difficulty maintaining goal-focused behavior, including both planning and completing tasks. Distractibility is a facet of the broad personality trait domain DISINHIBITION.

dysarthria A disorder of speech sound production due to structural or motor impairment affecting the articulatory apparatus. Such disorders include cleft palate, muscle disorders, cranial nerve disorders, and cerebral palsy affecting bulbar structures (i.e., lower and upper motor neuron disorders).

dyskinesia Distortion of voluntary movements with involuntary muscle activity.

dysphoria (dysphoric mood) A condition in which a person experiences intense feelings of depression, discontent, and in some cases indifference to the world around them.

dyssomnias Primary disorders of sleep or wakefulness characterized by INSOMNIA or HYPERSOMNIA as the major presenting symptom. Dyssomnias are disorders of the amount, quality, or timing of sleep. Compare with PARASOMNIAS.

dysthymia Presence, while depressed, of two or more of the following: 1) poor appetite or overeating, 2) insomnia or hypersomnia, 3) low energy or fatigue, 4) low self-esteem, 5) poor concentration or difficulty making decisions, or 6) feelings of hopelessness.

dystonia Disordered tonicity of muscles.

eccentricity Odd, unusual, or bizarre behavior, appearance, and/or speech having strange and unpredictable thoughts; saying unusual or inappropriate things. Eccentricity is a facet of the broad personality trait domain PSYCHOTICISM.

echolalia The pathological, parrotlike, and apparently senseless repetition (echoing) of a word or phrase just spoken by another person.

echopraxia Mimicking the movements of another.

emotional lability Instability of emotional experiences and mood; emotions that are easily aroused, intense, and/or out of proportion to events and circumstances. Emotional lability is a facet of the broad personality trait domain NEGATIVE AFFECTIVITY.

empathy Comprehension and appreciation of others' experiences and motivations; tolerance of differing perspectives; understanding the effects of own behavior on others.

episode (episodic) A specified duration of time during which the patient has developed or experienced symptoms that meet the diagnostic criteria for a given mental disorder. Depending on the type of mental disorder, *episode* may denote a certain number of symptoms or a specified severity or frequency of symptoms. Episodes may be further differentiated as a single (first) episode or a recurrence or relapse of multiple episodes if appropriate.

euphoria A mental and emotional condition in which a person experiences intense feelings of well-being, elation, happiness, excitement, and joy.

fatigability Tendency to become easily fatigued. *See also* FATIGUE.

fatigue A state (also called exhaustion, tiredness, lethargy, languidness, languor, lassitude, and listlessness) usually associated with a weakening or depletion of one's physical and/or mental resources, ranging from a general state of lethargy to a specific, work-induced burning sensation within one's muscles. Physical fatigue leads to an inability to continue functioning at one's normal level of activity. Although widespread in everyday life, this state usually becomes particularly noticeable during heavy exercise. Mental fatigue, by contrast, most often manifests as SOMNOLENCE (sleepiness).

fear An emotional response to perceived imminent threat or danger associated with urges to flee or fight.

flashback A dissociative state during which aspects of a traumatic event are reexperienced as though they were occurring at that moment.

flight of ideas A nearly continuous flow of accelerated speech with abrupt changes from topic to topic that are usually based on understandable associations, distracting stimuli, or plays on words. When the condition is severe, speech may be disorganized and incoherent.

gender   The public (and usually legally recognized) lived role as boy or girl, man or woman. Biological factors are seen as contributing in interaction with social and psychological factors to gender development.

gender assignment   The initial assignment as male or female, which usually occurs at birth and is subsequently referred to as the "natal gender."

gender dysphoria   Distress that accompanies the incongruence between one's experienced and expressed gender and one's assigned or natal gender.

gender experience   The unique and personal ways in which individuals experience their gender in the context of the gender roles provided by their societies.

gender expression   The specific ways in which individuals enact gender roles provided in their societies.

gender identity   A category of social identity that refers to an individual's identification as male, female or, occasionally, some category other than male or female.

gender reassignment   A change of gender that can be either medical (hormones, surgery) or legal (government recognition), or both. In case of medical interventions, often referred to as *sex reassignment.*

geometric hallucination   See HALLUCINATION.

grandiosity   Believing that one is superior to others and deserves special treatment; self-centeredness; feelings of entitlement; condescension toward others. Grandiosity is a facet of the broad personality trait domain ANTAGONISM.

grimace (grimacing)   Odd and inappropriate facial expressions unrelated to situation (as seen in individuals with CATATONIA).

hallucination   A perception-like experience with the clarity and impact of a true perception but without the external stimulation of the relevant sensory organ. Hallucinations should be distinguished from ILLUSIONS, in which an actual external stimulus is misperceived or misinterpreted. The person may or may not have insight into the non-veridical nature of the hallucination. One hallucinating person may recognize the false sensory experience, whereas another may be convinced that the experience is grounded in reality. The term *hallucination* is not ordinarily applied to the false perceptions that occur during dreaming, while falling asleep (*hypnagogic*), or upon awakening (*hypno-pompic*). Transient hallucinatory experiences may occur without a mental disorder.

  auditory   A hallucination involving the perception of sound, most commonly of voice.

  geometric   Visual hallucinations involving geometric shapes such as tunnels and funnels, spirals, lattices, or cobwebs.

  gustatory   A hallucination involving the perception of taste (usually unpleasant).

  mood-congruent   *See* MOOD-CONGRUENT PSYCHOTIC FEATURES.

  mood-incongruent   *See* MOOD-INCONGRUENT PSYCHOTIC FEATURES.

  olfactory   A hallucination involving the perception of odor, such as of burning rubber or decaying fish.

  somatic   A hallucination involving the perception of physical experience localized within the body (e.g., a feeling of electricity). A somatic hallucination is to be distinguished from physical sensations arising from an as-yet-undiagnosed general medical condition, from hypochondriacal preoccupation with normal physical sensations, or from a tactile hallucination.

  tactile   A hallucination involving the perception of being touched or of something being under one's skin. The most common tactile hallucinations are the sensation of electric shocks and formication (the sensation of something creeping or crawling on or under the skin).

visual A hallucination involving sight, which may consist of formed images, such as of people, or of unformed images, such as flashes of light. Visual hallucinations should be distinguished from ILLUSIONS, which are misperceptions of real external stimuli.

hostility Persistent or frequent angry feelings; anger or irritability in response to minor slights and insults; mean, nasty, or vengeful behavior. Hostility is a facet of the broad personality trait domain ANTAGONISM.

hyperacusis Increased auditory perception.

hyperorality A condition in which inappropriate objects are placed in the mouth.

hypersexuality A stronger than usual urge to have sexual activity.

hypersomnia Excessive sleepiness, as evidenced by prolonged nocturnal sleep, difficulty maintaining an alert awake state during the day, or undesired daytime sleep episodes. See also SOMNOLENCE.

hypervigilance An enhanced state of sensory sensitivity accompanied by an exaggerated intensity of behaviors whose purpose is to detect threats. Hypervigilance is also accompanied by a state of increased anxiety which can cause exhaustion. Other symptoms include abnormally increased arousal, a high responsiveness to stimuli, and a continual scanning of the environment for threats. In hypervigilance, there is a perpetual scanning of the environment to search for sights, sounds, people, behaviors, smells, or anything else that is reminiscent of threat or trauma. The individual is placed on high alert in order to be certain danger is not near. Hypervigilance can lead to a variety of obsessive behavior patterns, as well as producing difficulties with social interaction and relationships.

hypomania An abnormality of mood resembling mania but of lesser intensity. *See also* MANIA.

hypopnea Episodes of overly shallow breathing or an abnormally low respiratory rate.

ideas of reference The feeling that causal incidents and external events have a particular and unusual meaning that is specific to the person. An idea of reference is to be distinguished from a DELUSION OF REFERENCE, in which there is a belief that is held with delusional conviction.

identity Experience of oneself as unique, with clear boundaries between self and others; stability of self-esteem and accuracy of self-appraisal; capacity for, and ability to regulate, a range of emotional experience.

illusion A misperception or misinterpretation of a real external stimulus, such as hearing the rustling of leaves as the sound of voices. *See also* HALLUCINATION.

impulsivity Acting on the spur of the moment in response to immediate stimuli; acting on a momentary basis without a plan or consideration of outcomes; difficulty establishing and following plans; a sense of urgency and self-harming behavior under emotional distress. Impulsivity is a facet of the broad personality trait domain DISINHIBITION.

incoherence Speech or thinking that is essentially incomprehensible to others because word or phrases are joined together without a logical or meaningful connection. This disturbance occurs *within* clauses, in contrast to derailment, in which the disturbance is *between* clauses. This has sometimes been referred to a "word salad" to convey the degree of linguistic disorganization. Mildly ungrammatical constructions or idiomatic usages characteristic of a particular regional or cultural backgrounds, lack of education, or low intelligence should not be considered incoherence. The term is generally not applied when there is evidence that the disturbance in speech is due to an aphasia.

insomnia A subjective complaint of difficulty falling or staying asleep or poor sleep quality.

intersex condition   A condition in which individuals have conflicting or ambiguous biological indicators of sex.

intimacy   Depth and duration of connection with others; desire and capacity for closeness; mutuality of regard reflected in interpersonal behavior.

intimacy avoidance   Avoidance of close or romantic relationships, interpersonal attachments, and intimate sexual relationships. Intimacy avoidance is a facet of the broad personality trait domain DETACHMENT.

irresponsibility   Disregard for—and failure to honor—financial and other obligations or commitments; lack of respect for—and lack of follow-through on—agreements and promises; carelessness with others' property. Irresponsibility is a facet of the broad personality trait domain DISINHIBITION.

language pragmatics   The understanding and use of language in a given context. For example, the warning "Watch your hands" when issued to a child who is dirty is intended not only to prompt the child to look at his or her hands but also to communicate the admonition "Don't get anything dirty."

lethargy   A state of decreased mental activity, characterized by sluggishness, drowsiness, inactivity, and reduced alertness.

macropsia   The visual perception that objects are larger than they actually are. Compare with MICROPSIA.

magical thinking   The erroneous belief that one's thoughts, words, or actions will cause or prevent a specific outcome in some way that defies commonly understood laws of cause and effect. Magical thinking may be a part of normal child development.

mania   A mental state of elevated, expansive, or irritable mood and persistently increased level of activity or energy. *See also* HYPOMANIA.

manipulativeness   Use of subterfuge to influence or control others; use of seduction, charm, glibness, or ingratiation to achieve one's ends. Manipulativeness is a facet of the broad personality trait domain ANTAGONISM.

mannerism   A peculiar and characteristic individual style of movement, action, thought, or speech.

melancholia (melancholic)   A mental state characterized by very severe depression.

micropsia   The visual perception that objects are smaller than they actually are. Compare with MACROPSIA.

mixed symptoms   The specifier "with mixed features" is applied to mood episodes during which subthreshold symptoms from the opposing pole are present. Whereas these concurrent "mixed" symptoms are relatively simultaneous, they may also occur closely juxtaposed in time as a waxing and waning of individual symptoms of the opposite pole (i.e., depressive symptoms during hypomanic or manic episodes, and vice versa).

mood   A pervasive and sustained emotion that colors the perception of the world. Common examples of mood include depression, elation, anger, and anxiety. In contrast to *affect,* which refers to more fluctuating changes in emotional "weather," mood refers to a pervasive and sustained emotional "climate." Types of mood include

> **dysphoric**   An unpleasant mood, such as sadness, anxiety, or irritability.
>
> **elevated**   An exaggerated feeling of well-being, or euphoria or elation. A person with elevated mood may describe feeling "high," "ecstatic," "on top of the world," or "up in the clouds."
>
> **euthymic**   Mood in the "normal" range, which implies the absence of depressed or elevated mood.

expansive Lack of restraint in expressing one's feelings, frequently with an overvaluation of one's significance or importance.

irritable Easily annoyed and provoked to anger.

mood-congruent psychotic features Delusions or hallucinations whose content is entirely consistent with the typical themes of a depressed or manic mood. If the mood is depressed, the content of the delusions or hallucinations would involve themes of personal inadequacy, guilt, disease, death, nihilism, or deserved punishment. The content of the delusion may include themes of persecution if these are based on self-derogatory concepts such as deserved punishment. If the mood is manic, the content of the delusions or hallucinations would involve themes of inflated worth, power, knowledge, or identity, or a special relationship to a deity or a famous person. The content of the delusion may include themes of persecution if these are based on concepts such as inflated worth or deserved punishment.

mood-incongruent psychotic features Delusions or hallucinations whose content is not consistent with the typical themes of a depressed or manic mood. In the case of depression, the delusions or hallucinations would not involve themes of personal inadequacy, guilt, disease, death, nihilism, or deserved punishment. In the case of mania, the delusions or hallucinations would not involve themes of inflated worth, power, knowledge, or identity, or a special relationship to a deity or a famous person.

multiple sleep latency test Polysomnographic assessment of the sleep-onset period, with several short sleep-wake cycles assessed during a single session. The test repeatedly measures the time to daytime sleep onset ("sleep latency") and occurrence of and time to onset of the rapid eye movement sleep phase.

mutism No, or very little, verbal response (in the absence of known aphasia).

narcolepsy Sleep disorder characterized by periods of extreme drowsiness and frequent daytime lapses into sleep (sleep attacks). These must have been occurring at least three times per week over the last 3 months (in the absence of treatment).

negative affectivity Frequent and intense experiences of high levels of a wide range of negative emotions (e.g., anxiety, depression, guilt/shame, worry, anger), and their behavioral (e.g., self-harm) and interpersonal (e.g., dependency) manifestations. Negative Affectivity is one of the five pathological PERSONALITY TRAIT DOMAINS defined in Section III "Alternative DSM-5 Model for Personality Disorders."

negativism Opposition to suggestion or advice; behavior opposite to that appropriate to a specific situation or against the wishes of others, including direct resistance to efforts to be moved.

night eating syndrome Recurrent episodes of night eating, as manifested by eating after awakening from sleep or excessive food consumption after the evening meal. There is awareness and recall of the eating. The night eating is not better accounted for by external influences such as changes in the individual's sleep-wake cycle or by local social norms.

nightmare disorder Repeated occurrences of extended, extremely dysphoric, and well-remembered dreams that usually involve efforts to avoid threats to survival, security or physical integrity and that generally occur during the second half of the major sleep episode. On awakening from the dysphoric dreams, the individual rapidly becomes oriented and alert.

nonsubstance addiction(s) Behavioral disorder (also called *behavioral addiction*) not related to any substance of abuse that shares some features with substance-induced addiction.

obsession   Recurrent and persistent thoughts, urges, or images that are experienced, at some time during the disturbance, as intrusive and unwanted and that in most individuals cause marked anxiety or distress. The individual attempts to ignore or suppress such thoughts, urges, or images, or to neutralize them with some other thought or action (i.e., by performing a compulsion).

overeating   Eating too much food too quickly.

overvalued idea   An unreasonable and sustained belief that is maintained with less than delusional intensity (i.e., the person is able to acknowledge the possibility that the belief may not be true). The belief is not one that is ordinarily accepted by other members of the person's culture or subculture.

panic attacks   Discrete periods of sudden onset of intense fear or terror, often associated with feelings of impending doom. During these attacks there are symptoms such as shortness of breath or smothering sensations; palpitations, pounding heart, or accelerated heart rate; chest pain or discomfort; choking; and fear of going crazy or losing control. Panic attacks may be unexpected, in which the onset of the attack is not associated with an obvious trigger and instead occurs "out of the blue," or expected, in which the panic attack is associated with an obvious trigger, either internal or external.

paranoid ideation   Ideation, of less than delusional proportions, involving suspiciousness or the belief that one is being harassed, persecuted, or unfairly treated.

parasomnias   Disorders of sleep involving abnormal behaviors or physiological events occurring during sleep or sleep-wake transitions. Compare with DYSSOMNIAS.

perseveration   Persistence at tasks or in particular way of doing things long after the behavior has ceased to be functional or effective; continuance of the same behavior despite repeated failures or clear reasons for stopping. Perseveration is a facet of the broad personality trait domain NEGATIVE AFFECTIVITY.

personality   Enduring patterns of perceiving, relating to, and thinking about the environment and oneself. PERSONALITY TRAITS are prominent aspects of personality that are exhibited in relatively consistent ways across time and across situations. Personality traits influence self and interpersonal functioning. Depending on their severity, impairments in personality functioning and personality trait expression may reflect the presence of a personality disorder.

personality disorder—trait specified   In Section III "Alternative DSM-5 Model for Personality Disorders," a proposed diagnostic category for use when a personality disorder is considered present but the criteria for a specific disorder are not met. Personality disorder—trait specified (PD-TS) is defined by significant impairment in personality functioning, as measured by the Level of Personality Functioning Scale and one or more pathological PERSONALITY TRAIT DOMAINS or PERSONALITY TRAIT FACETS. PD-TS is proposed in DSM-5 Section III for further study as a possible future replacement for other specified personality disorder and unspecified personality disorder.

personality functioning   Cognitive models of self and others that shape patterns of emotional and affiliative engagement.

personality trait   A tendency to behave, feel, perceive, and think in relatively consistent ways across time and across situations in which the trait may be manifest.

personality trait facets   Specific personality components that make up the five broad personality trait domains in the dimensional taxonomy of Section III "Alternative DSM-5 Model for Personality Disorders." For example, the broad domain antagonism has the following component facets: MANIPULATIVENESS, DECEITFULNESS, GRANDIOSITY, ATTENTION SEEKING, CALLOUSNESS, and HOSTILITY.

personality trait domains   In the dimensional taxonomy of Section III "Alternative DSM-5 Model for Personality Disorders," personality traits are organized into five broad domains: NEGATIVE AFFECTIVITY, DETACHMENT, ANTAGONISM, DISINHIBITION, and PSYCHOTICISM. Within these five broad trait domains are 25 specific personality trait facets (e.g., IMPULSIVITY, RIGID PERFECTIONISM).

phobia   A persistent fear of a specific object, activity, or situation (i.e., the phobic stimulus) out of proportion to the actual danger posed by the specific object or situation that results in a compelling desire to avoid it. If it cannot be avoided, the phobic stimulus is endured with marked distress.

pica   Persistent eating of nonnutritive nonfood substances over a period of at least 1 month. The eating of nonnutritive nonfood substances is inappropriate to the developmental level of the individual (a minimum age of 2 years is suggested for diagnosis). The eating behavior is not part of a culturally supported or socially normative practice.

polysomnography   Polysomnography (PSG), also known as a sleep study, is a multiparametric test used in the study of sleep and as a diagnostic tool in sleep medicine. The test result is called a *polysomnogram*, also abbreviated PSG. PSG monitors many body functions, including brain (electroencephalography), eye movements (electro-oculography), muscle activity or skeletal muscle activation (electromyography), and heart rhythm (electrocardiography).

posturing   Spontaneous and active maintenance of a posture against gravity (as seen in CATATONIA). Abnormal posturing may also be a sign of certain injuries to the brain or spinal cord, including the following:

> **decerebrate posture**   The arms and legs are out straight and rigid, the toes point downward, and the head is arched backward.

> **decorticate posture**   The body is rigid, the arms are stiff and bent, the fists are tight, and the legs are straight out.

> **opisthotonus**   The back is rigid and arching, and the head is thrown backward.

An affected person may alternate between different postures as the condition changes.

pressured speech   Speech that is increased in amount, accelerated, and difficult or impossible to interrupt. Usually it is also loud and emphatic. Frequently the person talks without any social stimulation and may continue to talk even though no one is listening.

prodrome   An early or premonitory sign or symptom of a disorder.

pseudocyesis   A false belief of being pregnant that is associated with objective signs and reported symptoms of pregnancy.

psychological distress   A range of symptoms and experiences of a person's internal life that are commonly held to be troubling, confusing, or out of the ordinary.

psychometric measures   Standardized instruments such as scales, questionnaires, tests, and assessments that are designed to measure human knowledge, abilities, attitudes, or personality traits.

psychomotor agitation   Excessive motor activity associated with a feeling of inner tension. The activity is usually nonproductive and repetitious and consists of behaviors such as pacing, fidgeting, wringing of the hands, pulling of clothes, and inability to sit still.

psychomotor retardation   Visible generalized slowing of movements and speech.

psychotic features   Features characterized by delusions, hallucinations, and formal thought disorder.

psychoticism   Exhibiting a wide range of culturally incongruent odd, eccentric, or unusual behaviors and cognitions, including both process (e.g., perception, dissociation) and content (e.g., beliefs). Psychoticism is one of the five broad PERSONALITY TRAIT DO-MAINS defined in Section III "Alternative DSM-5 Model for Personality Disorders."

purging disorder   Eating disorder characterized by recurrent purging behavior to influence weight or shape, such as self-induced vomiting, misuse of laxatives, diuretics, or other medications, in the absence of binge eating.

racing thoughts   A state in which the mind uncontrollably brings up random thoughts and memories and switches between them very quickly. Sometimes the thoughts are related, with one thought leading to another; other times they are completely random. A person experiencing an episode of racing thoughts has no control over them and is unable to focus on a single topic or to sleep.

rapid cycling   Term referring to bipolar disorder characterized by the presence of at least four mood episodes in the previous 12 months that meet the criteria for a manic, hypomanic, or major depressive episode. Episodes are demarcated either by partial or full remissions of at least 2 months or by a switch to an episode of the opposite polarity (e.g., major depressive episode to manic episode). The rapid cycling specifier can be applied to bipolar I or bipolar II disorder.

rapid eye movement (REM)   A behavioral sign of the phase of sleep during which the sleeper is likely to be experiencing dreamlike mental activity.

repetitive speech   Morphologically heterogeneous iterations of speech.

residual phase   Period after an episode of schizophrenia that has partly or completed remitted but in which some symptoms may remain, and symptoms such as listlessness, problems with concentrating, and withdrawal from social activities may predominate.

restless legs syndrome   An urge to move the legs, usually accompanied or caused by uncomfortable and unpleasant sensations in the legs (for pediatric restless legs syndrome, the description of these symptoms should be in the child's own words). The symptoms begin or worsen during periods of rest or inactivity. Symptoms are partially or totally relieved by movement. Symptoms are worse in the evening or at night than during the day or occur only in the night/evening.

restricted affectivity   Little reaction to emotionally arousing situations; constricted emotional experience and expression; indifference and aloofness in normatively engaging situations. Restricted affectivity is a facet of the broad personality trait domain DETACH-MENT.

rigid perfectionism   Rigid insistence on everything being flawless, perfect, and without errors or faults, including one's own and others' performance; sacrificing of timeliness to ensure correctness in every detail; believing that there is only one right way to do things; difficulty changing ideas and/or viewpoint; preoccupation with details, organization, and order. Lack of rigid perfectionism is a facet of the broad personality trait domain DISINHIBITION.

risk taking   Engagement in dangerous, risky, and potentially self-damaging activities, unnecessarily and without regard to consequences; lack of concern for one's limitations and denial of the reality of personal danger; reckless pursuit of goals regardless of the level of risk involved. Risk taking is a facet of the broad personality trait domain DISINHIBITION.

rumination (rumination disorders)   Repeated regurgitation of food over a period of at least 1 month. Regurgitated food may be re-chewed, re-swallowed, or spit out. In rumination disorders, there is no evidence that an associated gastrointestinal or another medical condition (e.g., gastroesophageal reflux) is sufficient to account for the repeated regurgitation.

seasonal pattern   A pattern of the occurrence of a specific mental disorder in selected seasons of the year.

self-directedness, self-direction   Pursuit of coherent and meaningful short-term and life goals; utilization of constructive and prosocial internal standards of behavior; ability to self-reflect productively.

separation insecurity   Fears of being alone due to rejection by and/or separation from significant others, based in a lack of confidence in one's ability to care for oneself, both physically and emotionally. Separation insecurity is a facet of the broad personality trait domain NEGATIVE AFFECTIVITY.

sex   Biological indication of male and female (understood in the context of reproductive capacity), such as sex chromosomes, gonads, sex hormones, and nonambiguous internal and external genitalia.

sign   An objective manifestation of a pathological condition. Signs are observed by the examiner rather than reported by the affected individual. Compare with SYMPTOM.

sleep-onset REM   Occurrence of the rapid eye movement (REM) phase of sleep within minutes after falling asleep. Usually assessed by a polysomnographic MULTIPLE SLEEP LATENCY TEST.

sleep terrors   Recurrent episodes of abrupt terror arousals from sleep, usually occurring during the first third of the major sleep episode and beginning with a panicky scream. There is intense fear and signs of autonomic arousal, such as mydriasis, tachycardia, rapid breathing, and sweating, during each episode.

sleepwalking   Repeated episodes of rising from bed during sleep and walking about, usually occurring during the first third of the major sleep episode. While sleepwalking, the person has a blank, staring face, is relatively unresponsive to the efforts of others to communicate with him or her, and can be awakened only with great difficulty.

somnolence (or "drowsiness")   A state of near-sleep, a strong desire for sleep, or sleeping for unusually long periods. It has two distinct meanings, referring both to the usual state preceding falling asleep and to the chronic condition that involves being in that state independent of a circadian rhythm. Compare with HYPERSOMNIA.

specific food cravings   Irresistible desire for special types of food.

startle response (or "startle reaction")   An involuntary (reflexive) reaction to a sudden unexpected stimulus, such as a loud noise or sharp movement.

stereotypies, stereotyped behaviors/movements   Repetitive, abnormally frequent, non-goal-directed movements, seemingly driven, and nonfunctional motor behavior (e.g., hand shaking or waving, body rocking, head banging, self-biting).

stress   The pattern of specific and nonspecific responses a person makes to stimulus events that disturb his or her equilibrium and tax or exceed his or her ability to cope.

stressor   Any emotional, physical, social, economic, or other factor that disrupts the normal physiological, cognitive, emotional, or behavioral balance of an individual.

stressor, psychological   Any life event or life change that may be associated temporally (and perhaps causally) with the onset, occurrence, or exacerbation of a mental disorder.

stupor   Lack of psychomotor activity, which may range from not actively relating to the environment to complete immobility.

submissiveness   Adaptation of one's behavior to the actual or perceived interests and desires of others even when doing so is antithetical to one's own interests, needs, or desires. Submissiveness is a facet of the broad personality trait domain NEGATIVE AFFECTIVITY.

subsyndromal   Below a specified level or threshold required to qualify for a particular condition. Subsyndromal conditions (*formes frustes*) are medical conditions that do not meet full criteria for a diagnosis—for example, because the symptoms are fewer or less severe than a defined syndrome—but that nevertheless can be identified and related to the "full-blown" syndrome.

suicidal ideas (suicidal ideation)   Thoughts about self-harm, with deliberate consideration or planning of possible techniques of causing one's own death.

suicide   The act of intentionally causing one's own death.

suicide attempt   An attempt to end one's own life, which may lead to one's death.

suspiciousness   Expectations of—and sensitivity to—signs of interpersonal ill intent or harm; doubts about loyalty and fidelity of others; feelings of being mistreated, used, and/or persecuted by others. Suspiciousness is a facet of the broad personality trait domain DETACHMENT.

symptom   A subjective manifestation of a pathological condition. Symptoms are reported by the affected individual rather than observed by the examiner. Compare with SIGN.

syndrome   A grouping of signs and symptoms, based on their frequent co-occurrence that may suggest a common underlying pathogenesis, course, familial pattern, or treatment selection.

synesthesias   A condition in which stimulation of one sensory or cognitive pathway leads to automatic, involuntary experiences in a second sensory or cognitive pathway.

temper outburst   An emotional outburst (also called a "tantrum"), usually associated with children or those in emotional distress, and typically characterized by stubbornness, crying, screaming, defiance, angry ranting, a resistance to attempts at pacification, and in some cases hitting. Physical control may be lost, the person may be unable to remain still, and even if the "goal" of the person is met, he or she may not be calmed.

thought-action fusion   The tendency to treat thoughts and actions as equivalent.

tic   An involuntary, sudden, rapid, recurrent, nonrhythmic motor movement or vocalization.

tolerance   A situation that occurs with continued use of a drug in which an individual requires greater dosages to achieve the same effect.

transgender   The broad spectrum of individuals who transiently or permanently identify with a gender different from their natal gender.

transsexual   An individual who seeks, or has undergone, a social transition from male to female or female to male, which in many, but not all cases may also involve a somatic transition by cross-sex hormone treatment and genital surgery ("sex reassignment surgery").

traumatic stressor   Any event (or events) that may cause or threaten death, serious injury, or sexual violence to an individual, a close family member, or a close friend.

unusual beliefs and experiences   Belief that one has unusual abilities, such as mind reading, telekinesis, or THOUGHT-ACTION FUSION; unusual experiences of reality, including hallucinatory experiences. In general, the unusual beliefs are not held at the same level of conviction as DELUSIONS. Unusual beliefs and experiences are a facet of the personality trait domain PSYCHOTICISM.

waxy flexibility   Slight, even resistance to positioning by examiner. Compare with CATALEPSY.

withdrawal, social Preference for being alone to being with others; reticence in social situations; AVOIDANCE of social contacts and activity; lack of initiation of social contact. Social withdrawal is a facet of the broad personality trait domain DETACHMENT.

worry Unpleasant or uncomfortable thoughts that cannot be consciously controlled by trying to turn the attention to other subjects. The worrying is often persistent, repetitive, and out of proportion to the topic worried about (it can even be about a triviality).

Glossary of Cultural Concepts of Distress

Ataque de nervios

Ataque de nervios ("attack of nerves") is a syndrome among individuals of Latino descent, characterized by symptoms of intense emotional upset, including acute anxiety, anger, or grief; screaming and shouting uncontrollably; attacks of crying; trembling; heat in the chest rising into the head; and becoming verbally and physically aggressive. Dissociative experiences (e.g., depersonalization, derealization, amnesia), seizure-like or fainting episodes, and suicidal gestures are prominent in some *ataques* but absent in others. A general feature of an *ataque de nervios* is a sense of being out of control. Attacks frequently occur as a direct result of a stressful event relating to the family, such as news of the death of a close relative, conflicts with a spouse or children, or witnessing an accident involving a family member. For a minority of individuals, no particular social event triggers their *ataques*; instead, their vulnerability to losing control comes from the accumulated experience of suffering.

No one-to-one relationship has been found between *ataque* and any specific psychiatric disorder, although several disorders, including panic disorder, other specified or unspecified dissociative disorder, and conversion disorder, have symptomatic overlap with *ataque*.

In community samples, *ataque* is associated with suicidal ideation, disability, and outpatient psychiatric utilization, after adjustment for psychiatric diagnoses, traumatic exposure, and other covariates. However, some *ataques* represent normative expressions of acute distress (e.g., at a funeral) without clinical sequelae. The term *ataque de nervios* may also refer to an idiom of distress that includes any "fit"-like paroxysm of emotionality (e.g., hysterical laughing) and may be used to indicate an episode of loss of control in response to an intense stressor.

Related conditions in other cultural contexts: Indisposition in Haiti, blacking out in the Southern United States, and falling out in the West Indies.

Related conditions in DSM-5: Panic attack, panic disorder, other specified or unspecified dissociative disorder, conversion (functional neurologic symptom) disorder, intermittent explosive disorder, other specified or unspecified anxiety disorder, other specified or unspecified trauma and stressor-related disorder.

Dhat syndrome

Dhat syndrome is a term that was coined in South Asia little more than half a century ago to account for common clinical presentations of young male patients who attributed their various symptoms to semen loss. Despite the name, it is not a discrete syndrome but rather a cultural explanation of distress for patients who refer to diverse symptoms, such as anxiety, fatigue, weakness, weight loss, impotence, other multiple somatic complaints, and depressive mood. The cardinal feature is anxiety and distress about the loss of *dhat* in the absence of any identifiable physiological dysfunction. *Dhat* was identified by patients as a white discharge that was noted on defecation or urination. Ideas about this substance are related to the concept of *dhatu* (semen) described in the Hindu system of medicine, Ayurveda, as one of seven essential bodily fluids whose balance is necessary to maintain health.

Although *dhat syndrome* was formulated as a cultural guide to local clinical practice, related ideas about the harmful effects of semen loss have been shown to be widespread in the general population, suggesting a cultural disposition for explaining health problems and symptoms with reference to *dhat syndrome*. Research in health care settings has yielded diverse estimates of the syndrome's prevalence (e.g., 64% of men attending psychiatric clinics in India for sexual complaints; 30% of men attending general medical clinics in Pakistan). Although *dhat syndrome* is most commonly identified with young men from lower socioeconomic backgrounds, middle-aged men may also be affected. Comparable concerns about white vaginal discharge (leukorrhea) have been associated with a variant of the concept for women.

Related conditions in other cultural contexts: *koro* in Southeast Asia, particularly Singapore and *shen-k'uei* ("kidney deficiency") in China.

Related conditions in DSM-5: Major depressive disorder, persistent depressive disorder (dysthymia), generalized anxiety disorder, somatic symptom disorder, illness anxiety disorder, erectile disorder, early (premature) ejaculation, other specified or unspecified sexual dysfunction, academic problem.

Khyâl cap

"*Khyâl* attacks" (*khyâl cap*), or "wind attacks," is a syndrome found among Cambodians in the United States and Cambodia. Common symptoms include those of panic attacks, such as dizziness, palpitations, shortness of breath, and cold extremities, as well as other symptoms of anxiety and autonomic arousal (e.g., tinnitus and neck soreness). *Khyâl* attacks include catastrophic cognitions centered on the concern that *khyâl* (a windlike substance) may rise in the body—along with blood—and cause a range of serious effects (e.g., compressing the lungs to cause shortness of breath and asphyxia; entering the cranium to cause tinnitus, dizziness, blurry vision, and a fatal syncope). *Khyâl* attacks may occur without warning, but are frequently brought about by triggers such as worrisome thoughts, standing up (i.e., orthostasis), specific odors with negative associations, and agoraphobic-type cues like going to crowded spaces or riding in a car. *Khyâl* attacks usually meet panic attack criteria and may shape the experience of other anxiety and trauma- and stressor-related disorders. *Khyâl* attacks may be associated with considerable disability.

Related conditions in other cultural contexts: Laos (*pen lom*), Tibet (*srog rlung gi nad*), Sri Lanka (*vata*), and Korea (*hwa byung*).

Related conditions in DSM-5: Panic attack, panic disorder, generalized anxiety disorder, agoraphobia, posttraumatic stress disorder, illness anxiety disorder.

Kufungisisa

Kufungisisa ("thinking too much" in Shona) is an idiom of distress and a cultural explanation among the Shona of Zimbabwe. As an explanation, it is considered to be causative of anxiety, depression, and somatic problems (e.g., "my heart is painful because I think too much"). As an idiom of psychosocial distress, it is indicative of interpersonal and social difficulties (e.g., marital problems, having no money to take care of children). *Kufungisisa* involves ruminating on upsetting thoughts, particularly worries.

Kufungisisa is associated with a range of psychopathology, including anxiety symptoms, excessive worry, panic attacks, depressive symptoms, and irritability. In a study of a random community sample, two-thirds of the cases identified by a general psychopathology measure were of this complaint.

In many cultures, "thinking too much" is considered to be damaging to the mind and body and to cause specific symptoms like headache and dizziness. "Thinking too much" may also be a key component of cultural syndromes such as "brain fag" in Nigeria. In the case of brain fag, "thinking too much" is primarily attributed to excessive study, which is considered to damage the brain in particular, with symptoms including feelings of heat or crawling sensations in the head.

Related conditions in other cultural contexts: "Thinking too much" is a common idiom of distress and cultural explanation across many countries and ethnic groups. It has been described in Africa, the Caribbean and Latin America, and among East Asian and Native American groups.

Related conditions in DSM-5: Major depressive disorder, persistent depressive disorder (dysthymia), generalized anxiety disorder, posttraumatic stress disorder, obsessive-compulsive disorder, persistent complex bereavement disorder (see "Conditions for Further Study").

Maladi moun

Maladi moun (literally "humanly caused illness," also referred to as "sent sickness") is a cultural explanation in Haitian communities for diverse medical and psychiatric disorders. In this explanatory model, interpersonal envy and malice cause people to harm their enemies by sending illnesses such as psychosis, depression, social or academic failure, and inability to perform activities of daily living. The etiological model assumes that illness may be caused by others' envy and hatred, provoked by the victim's economic success as evidenced by a new job or expensive purchase. One person's gain is assumed to produce another person's loss, so visible success makes one vulnerable to attack. Assigning the label of sent sickness depends on mode of onset and social status more than presenting symptoms. The acute onset of new symptoms or an abrupt behavioral change raises suspicions of a spiritual attack. Someone who is attractive, intelligent, or wealthy is perceived as especially vulnerable, and even young healthy children are at risk.

Related conditions in other cultural contexts: Concerns about illness (typically, physical illness) caused by envy or social conflict are common across cultures and often expressed in the form of "evil eye" (e.g., in Spanish, *mal de ojo*; in Italian, *mal'occhiu*).

Related conditions in DSM-5: Delusional disorder, persecutory type; schizophrenia with paranoid features.

Nervios

Nervios ("nerves") is a common idiom of distress among Latinos in the United States and Latin America. *Nervios* refers to a general state of vulnerability to stressful life experiences and to difficult life circumstances. The term *nervios* includes a wide range of symptoms of emotional distress, somatic disturbance, and inability to function. The most common symptoms attributed to *nervios* include headaches and "brain aches" (occipital neck tension), irritability, stomach disturbances, sleep difficulties, nervousness, easy tearfulness, inability to concentrate, trembling, tingling sensations, and *mareos* (dizziness with occasional vertigo-like exacerbations). *Nervios* is a broad idiom of distress that spans the range of severity from cases with no mental disorder to presentations resembling adjustment, anxiety, depressive, dissociative, somatic symptom, or psychotic disorders. "Being nervous since childhood" appears to be more of a trait and may precede social anxiety disorder, while "being ill with nerves" is more related than other forms of *nervios* to psychiatric problems, especially dissociation and depression.

Related conditions in other cultural contexts: *Nevra* among Greeks in North America, *nierbi* among Sicilians in North America, and *nerves* among whites in Appalachia and Newfoundland.

Related conditions in DSM-5: Major depressive disorder, persistent depressive disorder (dysthymia), generalized anxiety disorder, social anxiety disorder, other specified or unspecified dissociative disorder, somatic symptom disorder, schizophrenia.

Shenjing shuairuo

Shenjing shuairuo ("weakness of the nervous system" in Mandarin Chinese) is a cultural syndrome that integrates conceptual categories of traditional Chinese medicine with the

Western diagnosis of neurasthenia. In the second, revised edition of the *Chinese Classification of Mental Disorders* (CCMD-2-R), *shenjing shuairuo* is defined as a syndrome composed of three out of five nonhierarchical symptom clusters: weakness (e.g., mental fatigue), emotions (e.g., feeling vexed), excitement (e.g., increased recollections), nervous pain (e.g., headache), and sleep (e.g., insomnia). *Fan nao* (feeling vexed) is a form of irritability mixed with worry and distress over conflicting thoughts and unfulfilled desires. The third edition of the CCMD retains *shenjing shuairuo* as a somatoform diagnosis of exclusion. Salient precipitants of *shenjing shuairuo* include work- or family-related stressors, loss of face (*mianzi, lianzi*), and an acute sense of failure (e.g., in academic performance). *Shenjing shuairuo* is related to traditional concepts of weakness (*xu*) and health imbalances related to deficiencies of a vital essence (e.g., the depletion of *qi* [vital energy] following overstraining or stagnation of *qi* due to excessive worry). In the traditional interpretation, *shenjing shuairuo* results when bodily channels (*jing*) conveying vital forces (*shen*) become dysregulated as a result of various social and interpersonal stressors, such as the inability to change a chronically frustrating and distressing situation. Various psychiatric disorders are associated with *shenjing shuairuo*, notably mood, anxiety, and somatic symptom disorders. In medical clinics in China, however, up to 45% of patients with *shenjing shuairuo* do not meet criteria for any DSM-IV disorder.

Related conditions in other cultural contexts: Neurasthenia-spectrum idioms and syndromes are present in India (*ashaktapanna*) and Japan (*shinkei-suijaku*), among other settings. Other conditions, such as brain fag syndrome, burnout syndrome, and chronic fatigue syndrome, are also closely related.

Related conditions in DSM-5: Major depressive disorder, persistent depressive disorder (dysthymia), generalized anxiety disorder, somatic symptom disorder, social anxiety disorder, specific phobia, posttraumatic stress disorder.

Susto

Susto ("fright") is a cultural explanation for distress and misfortune prevalent among some Latinos in the United States and among people in Mexico, Central America, and South America. It is not recognized as an illness category among Latinos from the Caribbean. *Susto* is an illness attributed to a frightening event that causes the soul to leave the body and results in unhappiness and sickness, as well as difficulties functioning in key social roles. Symptoms may appear any time from days to years after the fright is experienced. In extreme cases, *susto* may result in death. There are no specific defining symptoms for *susto*; however, symptoms that are often reported by people with *susto* include appetite disturbances, inadequate or excessive sleep, troubled sleep or dreams, feelings of sadness, low self-worth or dirtiness, interpersonal sensitivity, and lack of motivation to do anything. Somatic symptoms accompanying *susto* may include muscle aches and pains, cold in the extremities, pallor, headache, stomachache, and diarrhea. Precipitating events are diverse, and include natural phenomena, animals, interpersonal situations, and supernatural agents, among others.

Three syndromic types of *susto* (referred to as *cibih* in the local Zapotec language) have been identified, each having different relationships with psychiatric diagnoses. An interpersonal *susto* characterized by feelings of loss, abandonment, and not being loved by family, with accompanying symptoms of sadness, poor self-image, and suicidal ideation, seemed to be closely related to major depressive disorder. When *susto* resulted from a traumatic event that played a major role in shaping symptoms and in emotional processing of the experience, the diagnosis of posttraumatic stress disorder appeared more appropriate. *Susto* characterized by various recurrent somatic symptoms—for which the person sought health care from several practitioners—was thought to resemble a somatic symptom disorder.

Related conditions in other cultural contexts: Similar etiological concepts and symptom configurations are found globally. In the Andean region, *susto* is referred to as *espanto*.

Related conditions in DSM-5: Major depressive disorder, posttraumatic stress disorder, other specified or unspecified trauma and stressor-related disorder, somatic symptom disorders.

Taijin kyofusho

Taijin kyofusho ("interpersonal fear disorder" in Japanese) is a cultural syndrome characterized by anxiety about and avoidance of interpersonal situations due to the thought, feeling, or conviction that one's appearance and actions in social interactions are inadequate or offensive to others. In the United States, the variant involves having an offensive body odor and is termed *olfactory reference syndrome*. Individuals with *taijin kyofusho* tend to focus on the impact of their symptoms and behaviors on others. Variants include major concerns about facial blushing (erythrophobia), having an offensive body odor (olfactory reference syndrome), inappropriate gaze (too much or too little eye contact), stiff or awkward facial expression or bodily movements (e.g., stiffening, trembling), or body deformity.

Taijin kyofusho is a broader construct than social anxiety disorder in DSM-5. In addition to performance anxiety, *taijin kyofusho* includes two culture-related forms: a "sensitive type," with extreme social sensitivity and anxiety about interpersonal interactions, and an "offensive type," in which the major concern is offending others. As a category, *taijin kyofusho* thus includes syndromes with features of body dysmorphic disorder as well as delusional disorder. Concerns may have a delusional quality, responding poorly to simple reassurance or counterexample.

The distinctive symptoms of *taijin kyofusho* occur in specific cultural contexts and, to some extent, with more severe social anxiety across cultures. Similar syndromes are found in Korea and other societies that place a strong emphasis on the self-conscious maintenance of appropriate social behavior in hierarchical interpersonal relationships. *Taijin kyofusho*–like symptoms have also been described in other cultural contexts, including the United States, Australia, and New Zealand.

Related conditions in other cultural contexts: *Taein kong po* in Korea.

Related conditions in DSM-5: Social anxiety disorder, body dysmorphic disorder, delusional disorder, obsessive-compulsive disorder, olfactory reference syndrome (a type of other specified obsessive-compulsive and related disorder). Olfactory reference syndrome is related specifically to the *jikoshu-kyofu* variant of *taijin kyofusho*, whose core symptom is the concern that the person emits an offensive body odor. This presentation is seen in various cultures outside Japan.

Alphabetical Listing of DSM-5 Diagnoses and Codes (ICD-9-CM and ICD-10-CM)

ICD-9-CM codes are to be used for coding purposes in the United States through September 30, 2015. ICD-10-CM codes are to be used starting October 1, 2015. For DSM-5 coding and other updates, see the DSM-5® Update on www.PsychiatryOnline.org.

ICD-9-CM	ICD-10-CM	Disorder, condition, or problem
V62.3	Z55.9	Academic or educational problem
V62.4	Z60.3	Acculturation difficulty
308.3	F43.0	Acute stress disorder
		Adjustment disorders
309.24	F43.22	With anxiety
309.0	F43.21	With depressed mood
309.3	F43.24	With disturbance of conduct
309.28	F43.23	With mixed anxiety and depressed mood
309.4	F43.25	With mixed disturbance of emotions and conduct
309.9	F43.20	Unspecified
V71.01	Z72.811	Adult antisocial behavior
307.0	F98.5	Adult-onset fluency disorder
		Adult physical abuse by nonspouse or nonpartner, Confirmed
995.81	T74.11XA	Initial encounter
995.81	T74.11XD	Subsequent encounter
		Adult physical abuse by nonspouse or nonpartner, Suspected
995.81	T76.11XA	Initial encounter
995.81	T76.11XD	Subsequent encounter
		Adult psychological abuse by nonspouse or nonpartner, Confirmed
995.82	T74.31XA	Initial encounter
995.82	T74.31XD	Subsequent encounter
		Adult psychological abuse by nonspouse or nonpartner, Suspected
995.82	T76.31XA	Initial encounter
995.82	T76.31XD	Subsequent encounter
		Adult sexual abuse by nonspouse or nonpartner, Confirmed
995.83	T74.21XA	Initial encounter
995.83	T74.21XD	Subsequent encounter
		Adult sexual abuse by nonspouse or nonpartner, Suspected
995.83	T76.21XA	Initial encounter
995.83	T76.21XD	Subsequent encounter

ICD-9-CM	ICD-10-CM	Disorder, condition, or problem
300.22	F40.00	Agoraphobia
291.89		Alcohol-induced anxiety disorder
	F10.180	With mild use disorder
	F10.280	With moderate or severe use disorder
	F10.980	Without use disorder
291.89		Alcohol-induced bipolar and related disorder
	F10.14	With mild use disorder
	F10.24	With moderate or severe use disorder
	F10.94	Without use disorder
291.89		Alcohol-induced depressive disorder
	F10.14	With mild use disorder
	F10.24	With moderate or severe use disorder
	F10.94	Without use disorder
291.1		Alcohol-induced major neurocognitive disorder, Amnestic confabulatory type
	F10.26	With moderate or severe use disorder
	F10.96	Without use disorder
291.2		Alcohol-induced major neurocognitive disorder, Nonamnestic confabulatory type
	F10.27	With moderate or severe use disorder
	F10.97	Without use disorder
291.89		Alcohol-induced mild neurocognitive disorder
	F10.288	With moderate or severe use disorder
	F10.988	Without use disorder
291.9		Alcohol-induced psychotic disorder
	F10.159	With mild use disorder
	F10.259	With moderate or severe use disorder
	F10.959	Without use disorder
291.89		Alcohol-induced sexual dysfunction
	F10.181	With mild use disorder
	F10.281	With moderate or severe use disorder
	F10.981	Without use disorder
291.82		Alcohol-induced sleep disorder
	F10.182	With mild use disorder
	F10.282	With moderate or severe use disorder
	F10.982	Without use disorder
303.00		Alcohol intoxication
	F10.129	With mild use disorder
	F10.229	With moderate or severe use disorder
	F10.929	Without use disorder
291.0		Alcohol intoxication delirium
	F10.121	With mild use disorder
	F10.221	With moderate or severe use disorder
	F10.921	Without use disorder

ICD-9-CM	ICD-10-CM	Disorder, condition, or problem
		Alcohol use disorder
305.00	F10.10	Mild
303.90	F10.20	Moderate
303.90	F10.20	Severe
291.81		Alcohol withdrawal
	F10.232	With perceptual disturbances
	F10.239	Without perceptual disturbances
291.0	F10.231	Alcohol withdrawal delirium
292.89		Amphetamine (or other stimulant)–induced anxiety disorder
	F15.180	With mild use disorder
	F15.280	With moderate or severe use disorder
	F15.980	Without use disorder
292.84		Amphetamine (or other stimulant)–induced bipolar and related disorder
	F15.14	With mild use disorder
	F15.24	With moderate or severe use disorder
	F15.94	Without use disorder
	F15.921	Amphetamine (or other stimulant)–induced delirium
292.84		Amphetamine (or other stimulant)–induced depressive disorder
	F15.14	With mild use disorder
	F15.24	With moderate or severe use disorder
	F15.94	Without use disorder
292.89		Amphetamine (or other stimulant)–induced obsessive-compulsive and related disorder
	F15.188	With mild use disorder
	F15.288	With moderate or severe use disorder
	F15.988	Without use disorder
292.9		Amphetamine (or other stimulant)–induced psychotic disorder
	F15.159	With mild use disorder
	F15.259	With moderate or severe use disorder
	F15.959	Without use disorder
292.89		Amphetamine (or other stimulant)–induced sexual dysfunction
	F15.181	With mild use disorder
	F15.281	With moderate or severe use disorder
	F15.981	Without use disorder
292.85		Amphetamine (or other stimulant)–induced sleep disorder
	F15.182	With mild use disorder
	F15.282	With moderate or severe use disorder
	F15.982	Without use disorder
292.89		Amphetamine or other stimulant intoxication
		Amphetamine or other stimulant intoxication, With perceptual disturbances
	F15.122	With mild use disorder
	F15.222	With moderate or severe use disorder
	F15.922	Without use disorder

ICD-9-CM	ICD-10-CM	Disorder, condition, or problem
		Amphetamine or other stimulant intoxication, Without perceptual disturbances
	F15.129	With mild use disorder
	F15.229	With moderate or severe use disorder
	F15.929	Without use disorder
292.81		Amphetamine (or other stimulant) intoxication delirium
	F15.121	With mild use disorder
	F15.221	With moderate or severe use disorder
	F15.921	Without use disorder
292.0	F15.23	Amphetamine or other stimulant withdrawal
		Amphetamine-type substance use disorder
305.70	F15.10	Mild
304.40	F15.20	Moderate
304.40	F15.20	Severe
307.1		Anorexia nervosa
	F50.02	Binge-eating/purging type
	F50.01	Restricting type
		Antidepressant discontinuation syndrome
995.29	T43.205A	Initial encounter
995.29	T43.205S	Sequelae
995.29	T43.205D	Subsequent encounter
301.7	F60.2	Antisocial personality disorder
293.84	F06.4	Anxiety disorder due to another medical condition
		Attention-deficit/hyperactivity disorder
314.01	F90.2	Combined presentation
314.01	F90.1	Predominantly hyperactive/impulsive presentation
314.00	F90.0	Predominantly inattentive presentation
299.00	F84.0	Autism spectrum disorder
301.82	F60.6	Avoidant personality disorder
307.59	F50.89	Avoidant/restrictive food intake disorder
307.51	F50.81	Binge-eating disorder
		Bipolar I disorder, Current or most recent episode depressed
296.56	F31.76	In full remission
296.55	F31.75	In partial remission
296.51	F31.31	Mild
296.52	F31.32	Moderate
296.53	F31.4	Severe
296.54	F31.5	With psychotic features
296.50	F31.9	Unspecified
296.40	F31.0	Bipolar I disorder, Current or most recent episode hypomanic
296.46	F31.72	In full remission
296.45	F31.71	In partial remission
296.40	F31.9	Unspecified

ICD-9-CM	ICD-10-CM	Disorder, condition, or problem
		Bipolar I disorder, Current or most recent episode manic
296.46	F31.74	In full remission
296.45	F31.73	In partial remission
296.41	F31.11	Mild
296.42	F31.12	Moderate
296.43	F31.13	Severe
296.44	F31.2	With psychotic features
296.40	F31.9	Unspecified
296.7	F31.9	Bipolar I disorder, Current or most recent episode unspecified
296.89	F31.81	Bipolar II disorder
293.83		Bipolar and related disorder due to another medical condition
	F06.33	With manic features
	F06.33	With manic- or hypomanic-like episodes
	F06.34	With mixed features
300.7	F45.22	Body dysmorphic disorder
V62.89	R41.83	Borderline intellectual functioning
301.83	F60.3	Borderline personality disorder
298.8	F23	Brief psychotic disorder
307.51	F50.2	Bulimia nervosa
292.89		Caffeine-induced anxiety disorder
	F15.180	With mild use disorder
	F15.280	With moderate or severe use disorder
	F15.980	Without use disorder
292.85		Caffeine-induced sleep disorder
	F15.182	With mild use disorder
	F15.282	With moderate or severe use disorder
	F15.982	Without use disorder
305.90	F15.929	Caffeine intoxication
292.0	F15.93	Caffeine withdrawal
292.89		Cannabis-induced anxiety disorder
	F12.180	With mild use disorder
	F12.280	With moderate or severe use disorder
	F12.980	Without use disorder
292.9		Cannabis-induced psychotic disorder
	F12.159	With mild use disorder
	F12.259	With moderate or severe use disorder
	F12.959	Without use disorder
292.85		Cannabis-induced sleep disorder
	F12.188	With mild use disorder
	F12.288	With moderate or severe use disorder
	F12.988	Without use disorder
292.89		Cannabis intoxication

ICD-9-CM	ICD-10-CM	Disorder, condition, or problem
		Cannabis intoxication, With perceptual disturbances
	F12.122	With mild use disorder
	F12.222	With moderate or severe use disorder
	F12.922	Without use disorder
		Cannabis intoxication, Without perceptual disturbances
	F12.129	With mild use disorder
	F12.229	With moderate or severe use disorder
	F12.929	Without use disorder
292.81		Cannabis intoxication delirium
	F12.121	With mild use disorder
	F12.221	With moderate or severe use disorder
	F12.921	Without use disorder
		Cannabis use disorder
305.20	F12.10	Mild
304.30	F12.20	Moderate
304.30	F12.20	Severe
292.0	F12.288	Cannabis withdrawal
293.89	F06.1	Catatonia associated with another mental disorder (catatonia specifier)
293.89	F06.1	Catatonic disorder due to another medical condition
		Central sleep apnea
780.57	G47.37	Central sleep apnea comorbid with opioid use
786.04	R06.3	Cheyne-Stokes breathing
327.21	G47.31	Idiopathic central sleep apnea
V61.29	Z62.898	Child affected by parental relationship distress
		Child neglect, Confirmed
995.52	T74.02XA	Initial encounter
995.52	T74.02XD	Subsequent encounter
		Child neglect, Suspected
995.52	T76.02XA	Initial encounter
995.52	T76.02XD	Subsequent encounter
V71.02	Z72.810	Child or adolescent antisocial behavior
		Child physical abuse, Confirmed
995.54	T74.12XA	Initial encounter
995.54	T74.12XD	Subsequent encounter
		Child physical abuse, Suspected
995.54	T76.12XA	Initial encounter
995.54	T76.12XD	Subsequent encounter
		Child psychological abuse, Confirmed
995.51	T74.32XA	Initial encounter
995.51	T74.32XD	Subsequent encounter
		Child psychological abuse, Suspected
995.51	T76.32XA	Initial encounter
995.51	T76.32XD	Subsequent encounter

ICD-9-CM	ICD-10-CM	Disorder, condition, or problem
		Child sexual abuse, Confirmed
995.53	T74.22XA	Initial encounter
995.53	T74.22XD	Subsequent encounter
		Child sexual abuse, Suspected
995.53	T76.22XA	Initial encounter
995.53	T76.22XD	Subsequent encounter
315.35	F80.81	Childhood-onset fluency disorder (stuttering)
		Circadian rhythm sleep-wake disorders
307.45	G47.22	Advanced sleep phase type
307.45	G47.21	Delayed sleep phase type
307.45	G47.23	Irregular sleep-wake type
307.45	G47.24	Non-24-hour sleep-wake type
307.45	G47.26	Shift work type
307.45	G47.20	Unspecified type
292.89		Cocaine-induced anxiety disorder
	F14.180	With mild use disorder
	F14.280	With moderate or severe use disorder
	F14.980	Without use disorder
292.84		Cocaine-induced bipolar and related disorder
	F14.14	With mild use disorder
	F14.24	With moderate or severe use disorder
	F14.94	Without use disorder
292.84		Cocaine-induced depressive disorder
	F14.14	With mild use disorder
	F14.24	With moderate or severe use disorder
	F14.94	Without use disorder
292.89		Cocaine-induced obsessive-compulsive and related disorder
	F14.188	With mild use disorder
	F14.288	With moderate or severe use disorder
	F14.988	Without use disorder
292.9		Cocaine-induced psychotic disorder
	F14.159	With mild use disorder
	F14.259	With moderate or severe use disorder
	F14.959	Without use disorder
292.89		Cocaine-induced sexual dysfunction
	F14.181	With mild use disorder
	F14.281	With moderate or severe use disorder
	F14.981	Without use disorder
292.85		Cocaine-induced sleep disorder
	F14.182	With mild use disorder
	F14.282	With moderate or severe use disorder
	F14.982	Without use disorder

ICD-9-CM	ICD-10-CM	Disorder, condition, or problem
292.89		Cocaine intoxication
		Cocaine intoxication, With perceptual disturbances
	F14.122	With mild use disorder
	F14.222	With moderate or severe use disorder
	F14.922	Without use disorder
		Cocaine intoxication, Without perceptual disturbances
	F14.129	With mild use disorder
	F14.229	With moderate or severe use disorder
	F14.929	Without use disorder
292.81		Cocaine intoxication delirium
	F14.121	With mild use disorder
	F14.221	With moderate or severe use disorder
	F14.921	Without use disorder
		Cocaine use disorder
305.60	F14.10	Mild
304.20	F14.20	Moderate
304.20	F14.20	Severe
292.0	F14.23	Cocaine withdrawal
		Conduct disorder
312.82	F91.2	Adolescent-onset type
312.81	F91.1	Childhood-onset type
312.89	F91.9	Unspecified onset
300.11		Conversion disorder (functional neurological symptom disorder)
	F44.4	With abnormal movement
	F44.6	With anesthesia or sensory loss
	F44.5	With attacks or seizures
	F44.7	With mixed symptoms
	F44.6	With special sensory symptoms
	F44.4	With speech symptoms
	F44.4	With swallowing symptoms
	F44.4	With weakness/paralysis
V62.5	Z65.0	Conviction in civil or criminal proceedings without imprisonment
301.13	F34.0	Cyclothymic disorder
302.74	F52.32	Delayed ejaculation
		Delirium
293.0	F05	Delirium due to another medical condition
293.0	F05	Delirium due to multiple etiologies
292.81		Medication-induced delirium (*for ICD-10-CM codes, see specific substances*)
		Substance intoxication delirium (*see specific substances for codes*)
		Substance withdrawal delirium (*see specific substances for codes*)
297.1	F22	Delusional disorder
301.6	F60.7	Dependent personality disorder

ICD-9-CM	ICD-10-CM	Disorder, condition, or problem
300.6	F48.1	Depersonalization/derealization disorder
293.83		Depressive disorder due to another medical condition
	F06.31	With depressive features
	F06.32	With major depressive–like episode
	F06.34	With mixed features
315.4	F82	Developmental coordination disorder
V60.89	Z59.2	Discord with neighbor, lodger, or landlord
V62.89	Z64.4	Discord with social service provider, including probation officer, case manager, or social services worker
313.89	F94.2	Disinhibited social engagement disorder
V61.03	Z63.5	Disruption of family by separation or divorce
296.99	F34.81	Disruptive mood dysregulation disorder
300.12	F44.0	Dissociative amnesia
300.13	F44.1	Dissociative amnesia, with dissociative fugue
300.14	F44.81	Dissociative identity disorder
307.7	F98.1	Encopresis
307.6	F98.0	Enuresis
302.72	F52.21	Erectile disorder
698.4	F42.4	Excoriation (skin-picking) disorder
302.4	F65.2	Exhibitionistic disorder
V62.22	Z65.5	Exposure to disaster, war, or other hostilities
V60.2	Z59.5	Extreme poverty
300.19	F68.10	Factitious disorder
302.73	F52.31	Female orgasmic disorder
302.72	F52.22	Female sexual interest/arousal disorder
302.81	F65.0	Fetishistic disorder
302.89	F65.81	Frotteuristic disorder
312.31	F63.0	Gambling disorder
302.85	F64.0	Gender dysphoria in adolescents and adults
302.6	F64.2	Gender dysphoria in children
300.02	F41.1	Generalized anxiety disorder
302.76	F52.6	Genito-pelvic pain/penetration disorder
315.8	F88	Global developmental delay
292.89	F16.983	Hallucinogen persisting perception disorder
V61.8	Z63.8	High expressed emotion level within family
301.50	F60.4	Histrionic personality disorder
300.3	F42.3	Hoarding disorder
V60.0	Z59.0	Homelessness
307.44	F51.11	Hypersomnolence disorder
300.7	F45.21	Illness anxiety disorder
V62.5	Z65.1	Imprisonment or other incarceration
V60.1	Z59.1	Inadequate housing

ICD-9-CM	ICD-10-CM	Disorder, condition, or problem
292.89		Inhalant-induced anxiety disorder
	F18.180	With mild use disorder
	F18.280	With moderate or severe use disorder
	F18.980	Without use disorder
292.84		Inhalant-induced depressive disorder
	F18.14	With mild use disorder
	F18.24	With moderate or severe use disorder
	F18.94	Without use disorder
292.82		Inhalant-induced major neurocognitive disorder
	F18.17	With mild use disorder
	F18.27	With moderate or severe use disorder
	F18.97	Without use disorder
292.89		Inhalant-induced mild neurocognitive disorder
	F18.188	With mild use disorder
	F18.288	With moderate or severe use disorder
	F18.988	Without use disorder
292.9		Inhalant-induced psychotic disorder
	F18.159	With mild use disorder
	F18.259	With moderate or severe use disorder
	F18.959	Without use disorder
292.89		Inhalant intoxication
	F18.129	With mild use disorder
	F18.229	With moderate or severe use disorder
	F18.929	Without use disorder
292.81		Inhalant intoxication delirium
	F18.121	With mild use disorder
	F18.221	With moderate or severe use disorder
	F18.921	Without use disorder
		Inhalant use disorder
305.90	F18.10	Mild
304.60	F18.20	Moderate
304.60	F18.20	Severe
307.42	F51.01	Insomnia disorder
V60.2	Z59.7	Insufficient social insurance or welfare support
		Intellectual disability (intellectual developmental disorder)
317	F70	Mild
318.0	F71	Moderate
318.1	F72	Severe
318.2	F73	Profound
312.34	F63.81	Intermittent explosive disorder
312.32	F63.2	Kleptomania
V60.2	Z59.4	Lack of adequate food or safe drinking water
315.32	F80.2	Language disorder
V60.2	Z59.6	Low income

ICD-9-CM	ICD-10-CM	Disorder, condition, or problem
		Major depressive disorder, Recurrent episode
296.36	F33.42	In full remission
296.35	F33.41	In partial remission
296.31	F33.0	Mild
296.32	F33.1	Moderate
296.33	F33.2	Severe
296.34	F33.3	With psychotic features
296.30	F33.9	Unspecified
		Major depressive disorder, Single episode
296.26	F32.5	In full remission
296.25	F32.4	In partial remission
296.21	F32.0	Mild
296.22	F32.1	Moderate
296.23	F32.2	Severe
296.24	F32.3	With psychotic features
296.20	F32.9	Unspecified
331.9	G31.9	Major frontotemporal neurocognitive disorder, Possible
		Major frontotemporal neurocognitive disorder, Probable (*code first* 331.19 [G31.09] frontotemporal disease)
294.11	F02.81	With behavioral disturbance
294.10	F02.80	Without behavioral disturbance
331.9	G31.9	Major neurocognitive disorder due to Alzheimer's disease, Possible
		Major neurocognitive disorder due to Alzheimer's disease, Probable (*code first* 331.0 [G30.9] Alzheimer's disease)
294.11	F02.81	With behavioral disturbance
294.10	F02.80	Without behavioral disturbance
		Major neurocognitive disorder due to another medical condition
294.11	F02.81	With behavioral disturbance
294.10	F02.80	Without behavioral disturbance
		Major neurocognitive disorder due to HIV infection (*code first* 042 [B20] HIV infection)
294.11	F02.81	With behavioral disturbance
294.10	F02.80	Without behavioral disturbance
		Major neurocognitive disorder due to Huntington's disease (*code first* 333.4 [G10] Huntington's disease)
294.11	F02.81	With behavioral disturbance
294.10	F02.80	Without behavioral disturbance
331.9	G31.9	Major neurocognitive disorder with Lewy bodies, Possible
		Major neurocognitive disorder with Lewy bodies, Probable (*code first* 331.82 [G31.83] Lewy body disease)
294.11	F02.81	With behavioral disturbance
294.10	F02.80	Without behavioral disturbance
		Major neurocognitive disorder due to multiple etiologies
294.11	F02.81	With behavioral disturbance
294.10	F02.80	Without behavioral disturbance

ICD-9-CM	ICD-10-CM	Disorder, condition, or problem
331.9	G31.9	Major neurocognitive disorder due to Parkinson's disease, Possible
		Major neurocognitive disorder due to Parkinson's disease, Probable (*code first* 332.0 [G20] Parkinson's disease)
294.11	F02.81	With behavioral disturbance
294.10	F02.80	Without behavioral disturbance
		Major neurocognitive disorder due to prion disease (*code first* 046.79 [A81.9] prion disease)
294.11	F02.81	With behavioral disturbance
294.10	F02.80	Without behavioral disturbance
		Major neurocognitive disorder due to traumatic brain injury (*code first* 907.0 late effect of intracranial injury without skull fracture [S06.2X9S diffuse traumatic brain injury with loss of consciousness of unspecified duration, sequela])
294.11	F02.81	With behavioral disturbance
294.10	F02.80	Without behavioral disturbance
331.9	G31.9	Major vascular neurocognitive disorder, Possible
		Major vascular neurocognitive disorder, Probable
290.40	F01.51	With behavioral disturbance
290.40	F01.50	Without behavioral disturbance
302.71	F52.0	Male hypoactive sexual desire disorder
V65.2	Z76.5	Malingering
333.99	G25.71	Medication-induced acute akathisia
333.72	G24.02	Medication-induced acute dystonia
292.81		Medication-induced delirium (*for ICD-10-CM codes, see specific substances*)
333.1	G25.1	Medication-induced postural tremor
331.83	G31.84	Mild frontotemporal neurocognitive disorder
331.83	G31.84	Mild neurocognitive disorder due to Alzheimer's disease
331.83	G31.84	Mild neurocognitive disorder due to another medical condition
331.83	G31.84	Mild neurocognitive disorder due to HIV infection
331.83	G31.84	Mild neurocognitive disorder due to Huntington's disease
331.83	G31.84	Mild neurocognitive disorder due to multiple etiologies
331.83	G31.84	Mild neurocognitive disorder due to Parkinson's disease
331.83	G31.84	Mild neurocognitive disorder due to prion disease
331.83	G31.84	Mild neurocognitive disorder due to traumatic brain injury
331.83	G31.84	Mild neurocognitive disorder with Lewy bodies
331.83	G31.84	Mild vascular neurocognitive disorder
301.81	F60.81	Narcissistic personality disorder
		Narcolepsy
347.00	G47.419	Autosomal dominant cerebellar ataxia, deafness, and narcolepsy
347.00	G47.419	Autosomal dominant narcolepsy, obesity, and type 2 diabetes
347.10	G47.429	Narcolepsy secondary to another medical condition
347.01	G47.411	Narcolepsy with cataplexy but without hypocretin deficiency
347.00	G47.419	Narcolepsy without cataplexy but with hypocretin deficiency
332.1	G21.11	Neuroleptic-induced parkinsonism

ICD-9-CM	ICD-10-CM	Disorder, condition, or problem
333.92	G21.0	Neuroleptic malignant syndrome
307.47	F51.5	Nightmare disorder
V15.81	Z91.19	Nonadherence to medical treatment
		Non–rapid eye movement sleep arousal disorders
307.46	F51.4	Sleep terror type
307.46	F51.3	Sleepwalking type
300.3	F42.2	Obsessive-compulsive disorder
301.4	F60.5	Obsessive-compulsive personality disorder
294.8	F06.8	Obsessive-compulsive and related disorder due to another medical condition
327.23	G47.33	Obstructive sleep apnea hypopnea
292.89		Opioid-induced anxiety disorder
	F11.188	With mild use disorder
	F11.288	With moderate or severe use disorder
	F11.988	Without use disorder
	F11.921	Opioid-induced delirium
292.84		Opioid-induced depressive disorder
	F11.14	With mild use disorder
	F11.24	With moderate or severe use disorder
	F11.94	Without use disorder
292.89		Opioid-induced sexual dysfunction
	F11.181	With mild use disorder
	F11.281	With moderate or severe use disorder
	F11.981	Without use disorder
292.85		Opioid-induced sleep disorder
	F11.182	With mild use disorder
	F11.282	With moderate or severe use disorder
	F11.982	Without use disorder
292.89		Opioid intoxication
		Opioid intoxication, With perceptual disturbances
	F11.122	With mild use disorder
	F11.222	With moderate or severe use disorder
	F11.922	Without use disorder
		Opioid intoxication, Without perceptual disturbances
	F11.129	With mild use disorder
	F11.229	With moderate or severe use disorder
	F11.929	Without use disorder
292.81		Opioid intoxication delirium
	F11.121	With mild use disorder
	F11.221	With moderate or severe use disorder
	F11.921	Without use disorder
		Opioid use disorder
305.50	F11.10	Mild
304.00	F11.20	Moderate
304.00	F11.20	Severe

ICD-9-CM	ICD-10-CM	Disorder, condition, or problem
292.0	F11.23	Opioid withdrawal
292.0	F11.23	Opioid withdrawal delirium
313.81	F91.3	Oppositional defiant disorder
		Other adverse effect of medication
995.20	T50.905A	Initial encounter
995.20	T50.905S	Sequelae
995.20	T50.905D	Subsequent encounter
		Other circumstances related to adult abuse by nonspouse or nonpartner
V62.83	Z69.82	Encounter for mental health services for perpetrator of nonspousal adult abuse
V65.49	Z69.81	Encounter for mental health services for victim of nonspousal adult abuse
		Other circumstances related to child neglect
V62.83	Z69.021	Encounter for mental health services for perpetrator of nonparental child neglect
V61.22	Z69.011	Encounter for mental health services for perpetrator of parental child neglect
V61.21	Z69.010	Encounter for mental health services for victim of child neglect by parent
V61.21	Z69.020	Encounter for mental health services for victim of nonparental child neglect
V15.42	Z62.812	Personal history (past history) of neglect in childhood
		Other circumstances related to child physical abuse
V62.83	Z69.021	Encounter for mental health services for perpetrator of nonparental child abuse
V61.22	Z69.011	Encounter for mental health services for perpetrator of parental child abuse
V61.21	Z69.010	Encounter for mental health services for victim of child abuse by parent
V61.21	Z69.020	Encounter for mental health services for victim of nonparental child abuse
V15.41	Z62.810	Personal history (past history) of physical abuse in childhood
		Other circumstances related to child psychological abuse
V62.83	Z69.021	Encounter for mental health services for perpetrator of nonparental child psychological abuse
V61.22	Z69.011	Encounter for mental health services for perpetrator of parental child psychological abuse
V61.21	Z69.010	Encounter for mental health services for victim of child psychological abuse by parent
V61.21	Z69.020	Encounter for mental health services for victim of nonparental child psychological abuse
V15.42	Z62.811	Personal history (past history) of psychological abuse in childhood
		Other circumstances related to child sexual abuse
V62.83	Z69.021	Encounter for mental health services for perpetrator of nonparental child sexual abuse
V61.22	Z69.011	Encounter for mental health services for perpetrator of parental child sexual abuse

ICD-9-CM	ICD-10-CM	Disorder, condition, or problem
V61.21	Z69.010	Encounter for mental health services for victim of child sexual abuse by parent
V61.21	Z69.020	Encounter for mental health services for victim of nonparental child sexual abuse
V15.41	Z62.810	Personal history (past history) of sexual abuse in childhood
		Other circumstances related to spouse or partner abuse, Psychological
V61.12	Z69.12	Encounter for mental health services for perpetrator of spouse or partner psychological abuse
V61.11	Z69.11	Encounter for mental health services for victim of spouse or partner psychological abuse
V15.42	Z91.411	Personal history (past history) of spouse or partner psychological abuse
		Other circumstances related to spouse or partner neglect
V61.12	Z69.12	Encounter for mental health services for perpetrator of spouse or partner neglect
V61.11	Z69.11	Encounter for mental health services for victim of spouse or partner neglect
V15.42	Z91.412	Personal history (past history) of spouse or partner neglect
		Other circumstances related to spouse or partner violence, Physical
V61.12	Z69.12	Encounter for mental health services for perpetrator of spouse or partner violence, Physical
V61.11	Z69.11	Encounter for mental health services for victim of spouse or partner violence, Physical
V15.41	Z91.410	Personal history (past history) of spouse or partner violence, Physical
		Other circumstances related to spouse or partner violence, Sexual
V61.12	Z69.12	Encounter for mental health services for perpetrator of spouse or partner violence, Sexual
V61.11	Z69.81	Encounter for mental health services for victim of spouse or partner violence, Sexual
V15.41	Z91.410	Personal history (past history) of spouse or partner violence, Sexual
V65.40	Z71.9	Other counseling or consultation
292.89		Other hallucinogen–induced anxiety disorder
	F16.180	With mild use disorder
	F16.280	With moderate or severe use disorder
	F16.980	Without use disorder
292.84		Other hallucinogen–induced bipolar and related disorder
	F16.14	With mild use disorder
	F16.24	With moderate or severe use disorder
	F16.94	Without use disorder
292.84		Other hallucinogen–induced depressive disorder
	F16.14	With mild use disorder
	F16.24	With moderate or severe use disorder
	F16.94	Without use disorder

ICD-9-CM	ICD-10-CM	Disorder, condition, or problem
292.9		Other hallucinogen–induced psychotic disorder
	F16.159	With mild use disorder
	F16.259	With moderate or severe use disorder
	F16.959	Without use disorder
292.89		Other hallucinogen intoxication
	F16.129	With mild use disorder
	F16.229	With moderate or severe use disorder
	F16.929	Without use disorder
292.81		Other hallucinogen intoxication delirium
	F16.121	With mild use disorder
	F16.221	With moderate or severe use disorder
	F16.921	Without use disorder
		Other hallucinogen use disorder
305.30	F16.10	Mild
304.50	F16.20	Moderate
304.50	F16.20	Severe
333.99	G25.79	Other medication-induced movement disorder
332.1	G21.19	Other medication-induced parkinsonism
V15.49	Z91.49	Other personal history of psychological trauma
V15.89	Z91.89	Other personal risk factors
V62.29	Z56.9	Other problem related to employment
V62.89	Z65.8	Other problem related to psychosocial circumstances
300.09	F41.8	Other specified anxiety disorder
314.01	F90.8	Other specified attention-deficit/hyperactivity disorder
296.89	F31.89	Other specified bipolar and related disorder
780.09	R41.0	Other specified delirium
311	F32.89	Other specified depressive disorder
312.89	F91.8	Other specified disruptive, impulse-control, and conduct disorder
300.15	F44.89	Other specified dissociative disorder
		Other specified elimination disorder
787.60	R15.9	With fecal symptoms
788.39	N39.498	With urinary symptoms
307.59	F50.89	Other specified feeding or eating disorder
302.6	F64.8	Other specified gender dysphoria
780.54	G47.19	Other specified hypersomnolence disorder
780.52	G47.09	Other specified insomnia disorder
300.9	F99	Other specified mental disorder
294.8	F06.8	Other specified mental disorder due to another medical condition
315.8	F88	Other specified neurodevelopmental disorder
300.3	F42.8	Other specified obsessive-compulsive and related disorder
302.89	F65.89	Other specified paraphilic disorder
301.89	F60.89	Other specified personality disorder
298.8	F28	Other specified schizophrenia spectrum and other psychotic disorder
302.79	F52.8	Other specified sexual dysfunction

ICD-9-CM	ICD-10-CM	Disorder, condition, or problem
780.59	G47.8	Other specified sleep-wake disorder
300.89	F45.8	Other specified somatic symptom and related disorder
307.20	F95.8	Other specified tic disorder
309.89	F43.8	Other specified trauma- and stressor-related disorder
292.89		Other (or unknown) substance–induced anxiety disorder
	F19.180	With mild use disorder
	F19.280	With moderate or severe use disorder
	F19.980	Without use disorder
292.84		Other (or unknown) substance–induced bipolar and related disorder
	F19.14	With mild use disorder
	F19.24	With moderate or severe use disorder
	F19.94	Without use disorder
	F19.921	Other (or unknown) substance–induced delirium
292.84		Other (or unknown) substance–induced depressive disorder
	F19.14	With mild use disorder
	F19.24	With moderate or severe use disorder
	F19.94	Without use disorder
292.82		Other (or unknown) substance–induced major neurocognitive disorder
	F19.17	With mild use disorder
	F19.27	With moderate or severe use disorder
	F19.97	Without use disorder
292.89		Other (or unknown) substance–induced mild neurocognitive disorder
	F19.188	With mild use disorder
	F19.288	With moderate or severe use disorder
	F19.988	Without use disorder
292.89		Other (or unknown) substance–induced obsessive-compulsive and related disorder
	F19.188	With mild use disorder
	F19.288	With moderate or severe use disorder
	F19.988	Without use disorder
292.9		Other (or unknown) substance–induced psychotic disorder
	F19.159	With mild use disorder
	F19.259	With moderate or severe use disorder
	F19.959	Without use disorder
292.89		Other (or unknown) substance–induced sexual dysfunction
	F19.181	With mild use disorder
	F19.281	With moderate or severe use disorder
	F19.981	Without use disorder
292.85		Other (or unknown) substance–induced sleep disorder
	F19.182	With mild use disorder
	F19.282	With moderate or severe use disorder
	F19.982	Without use disorder

ICD-9-CM	ICD-10-CM	Disorder, condition, or problem
292.89		Other (or unknown) substance intoxication
	F19.129	With mild use disorder
	F19.229	With moderate or severe use disorder
	F19.929	Without use disorder
292.81		Other (or unknown) substance intoxication delirium
	F19.121	With mild use disorder
	F19.221	With moderate or severe use disorder
	F19.921	Without use disorder
		Other (or unknown) substance use disorder
305.90	F19.10	Mild
304.90	F19.20	Moderate
304.90	F19.20	Severe
292.0	F19.239	Other (or unknown) substance withdrawal
292.0	F19.231	Other (or unknown) substance withdrawal delirium
		Other or unspecified stimulant use disorder
305.70	F15.10	Mild
304.40	F15.20	Moderate
304.40	F15.20	Severe
278.00	E66.9	Overweight or obesity
		Panic attack specifier
300.01	F41.0	Panic disorder
301.0	F60.0	Paranoid personality disorder
V61.20	Z62.820	Parent-child relational problem
302.2	F65.4	Pedophilic disorder
307.22	F95.1	Persistent (chronic) motor or vocal tic disorder
300.4	F34.1	Persistent depressive disorder (dysthymia)
V62.22	Z91.82	Personal history of military deployment
V15.59	Z91.5	Personal history of self-harm
310.1	F07.0	Personality change due to another medical condition
V62.89	Z60.0	Phase of life problem
292.89		Phencyclidine-induced anxiety disorder
	F16.180	With mild use disorder
	F16.280	With moderate or severe use disorder
	F16.980	Without use disorder
292.84		Phencyclidine-induced bipolar and related disorder
	F16.14	With mild use disorder
	F16.24	With moderate or severe use disorder
	F16.94	Without use disorder
292.84		Phencyclidine-induced depressive disorder
	F16.14	With mild use disorder
	F16.24	With moderate or severe use disorder
	F16.94	Without use disorder

ICD-9-CM	ICD-10-CM	Disorder, condition, or problem
292.9		Phencyclidine-induced psychotic disorder
	F16.159	With mild use disorder
	F16.259	With moderate or severe use disorder
	F16.959	Without use disorder
292.89		Phencyclidine intoxication
	F16.129	With mild use disorder
	F16.229	With moderate or severe use disorder
	F16.929	Without use disorder
292.81		Phencyclidine intoxication delirium
	F16.121	With mild use disorder
	F16.221	With moderate or severe use disorder
	F16.921	Without use disorder
		Phencyclidine use disorder
305.90	F16.10	Mild
304.60	F16.20	Moderate
304.60	F16.20	Severe
307.52		Pica
	F50.89	In adults
	F98.3	In children
309.81	F43.10	Posttraumatic stress disorder
302.75	F52.4	Premature (early) ejaculation
625.4	F32.81	Premenstrual dysphoric disorder
V62.21	Z56.82	Problem related to current military deployment status
V69.9	Z72.9	Problem related to lifestyle
V60.3	Z60.2	Problem related to living alone
V60.6	Z59.3	Problem related to living in a residential institution
V61.5	Z64.1	Problems related to multiparity
V62.5	Z65.3	Problems related to other legal circumstances
V62.5	Z65.2	Problems related to release from prison
V61.7	Z64.0	Problems related to unwanted pregnancy
307.21	F95.0	Provisional tic disorder
316	F54	Psychological factors affecting other medical conditions
		Psychotic disorder due to another medical condition
293.81	F06.2	With delusions
293.82	F06.0	With hallucinations
312.33	F63.1	Pyromania
327.42	G47.52	Rapid eye movement sleep behavior disorder
313.89	F94.1	Reactive attachment disorder
V61.10	Z63.0	Relationship distress with spouse or intimate partner
V62.89	Z65.8	Religious or spiritual problem
333.94	G25.81	Restless legs syndrome
307.53	F98.21	Rumination disorder

ICD-9-CM	ICD-10-CM	Disorder, condition, or problem
		Schizoaffective disorder
295.70	F25.0	Bipolar type
295.70	F25.1	Depressive type
301.20	F60.1	Schizoid personality disorder
295.90	F20.9	Schizophrenia
295.40	F20.81	Schizophreniform disorder
301.22	F21	Schizotypal personality disorder
292.89		Sedative-, hypnotic-, or anxiolytic-induced anxiety disorder
	F13.180	With mild use disorder
	F13.280	With moderate or severe use disorder
	F13.980	Without use disorder
292.84		Sedative-, hypnotic-, or anxiolytic-induced bipolar and related disorder
	F13.14	With mild use disorder
	F13.24	With moderate or severe use disorder
	F13.94	Without use disorder
	F13.921	Sedative-, hypnotic-, or anxiolytic-induced delirium
292.84		Sedative-, hypnotic-, or anxiolytic-induced depressive disorder
	F13.14	With mild use disorder
	F13.24	With moderate or severe use disorder
	F13.94	Without use disorder
292.82		Sedative-, hypnotic-, or anxiolytic-induced major neurocognitive disorder
	F13.27	With moderate or severe use disorder
	F13.97	Without use disorder
292.89		Sedative-, hypnotic-, or anxiolytic-induced mild neurocognitive disorder
	F13.288	With moderate or severe use disorder
	F13.988	Without use disorder
292.9		Sedative-, hypnotic-, or anxiolytic-induced psychotic disorder
	F13.159	With mild use disorder
	F13.259	With moderate or severe use disorder
	F13.959	Without use disorder
292.89		Sedative-, hypnotic-, or anxiolytic-induced sexual dysfunction
	F13.181	With mild use disorder
	F13.281	With moderate or severe use disorder
	F13.981	Without use disorder
292.85		Sedative-, hypnotic-, or anxiolytic-induced sleep disorder
	F13.182	With mild use disorder
	F13.282	With moderate or severe use disorder
	F13.982	Without use disorder
292.89		Sedative, hypnotic, or anxiolytic intoxication
	F13.129	With mild use disorder
	F13.229	With moderate or severe use disorder
	F13.929	Without use disorder

ICD-9-CM	ICD-10-CM	Disorder, condition, or problem
292.81		Sedative, hypnotic, or anxiolytic intoxication delirium
	F13.121	With mild use disorder
	F13.221	With moderate or severe use disorder
	F13.921	Without use disorder
		Sedative, hypnotic, or anxiolytic use disorder
305.40	F13.10	Mild
304.10	F13.20	Moderate
304.10	F13.20	Severe
292.0		Sedative, hypnotic, or anxiolytic withdrawal
	F13.232	With perceptual disturbances
	F13.239	Without perceptual disturbances
292.0	F13.231	Sedative, hypnotic, or anxiolytic withdrawal delirium
313.23	F94.0	Selective mutism
309.21	F93.0	Separation anxiety disorder
V65.49	Z70.9	Sex counseling
302.83	F65.51	Sexual masochism disorder
302.84	F65.52	Sexual sadism disorder
V61.8	Z62.891	Sibling relational problem
		Sleep-related hypoventilation
327.26	G47.36	Comorbid sleep-related hypoventilation
327.25	G47.35	Congenital central alveolar hypoventilation
327.24	G47.34	Idiopathic hypoventilation
300.23	F40.10	Social anxiety disorder (social phobia)
V62.4	Z60.4	Social exclusion or rejection
315.39	F80.82	Social (pragmatic) communication disorder
300.82	F45.1	Somatic symptom disorder
		Specific learning disorder
315.1	F81.2	With impairment in mathematics
315.00	F81.0	With impairment in reading
315.2	F81.81	With impairment in written expression
		Specific phobia
300.29	F40.218	Animal
300.29		Blood-injection-injury
	F40.230	Fear of blood
	F40.231	Fear of injections and transfusions
	F40.233	Fear of injury
	F40.232	Fear of other medical care
300.29	F40.228	Natural environment
300.29	F40.298	Other
300.29	F40.248	Situational
315.39	F80.0	Speech sound disorder
		Spouse or partner abuse, Psychological, Confirmed
995.82	T74.31XA	Initial encounter
995.82	T74.31XD	Subsequent encounter

ICD-9-CM	ICD-10-CM	Disorder, condition, or problem
		Spouse or partner abuse, Psychological, Suspected
995.82	T76.31XA	Initial encounter
995.82	T76.31XD	Subsequent encounter
		Spouse or partner neglect, Confirmed
995.85	T74.01XA	Initial encounter
995.85	T74.01XD	Subsequent encounter
		Spouse or partner neglect, Suspected
995.85	T76.01XA	Initial encounter
995.85	T76.01XD	Subsequent encounter
		Spouse or partner violence, Physical, Confirmed
995.81	T74.11XA	Initial encounter
995.81	T74.11XD	Subsequent encounter
		Spouse or partner violence, Physical, Suspected
995.81	T76.11XA	Initial encounter
995.81	T76.11XD	Subsequent encounter
		Spouse or partner violence, Sexual, Confirmed
995.83	T74.21XA	Initial encounter
995.83	T74.21XD	Subsequent encounter
		Spouse or partner violence, Sexual, Suspected
995.83	T76.21XA	Initial encounter
995.83	T76.21XD	Subsequent encounter
307.3	F98.4	Stereotypic movement disorder
		Stimulant intoxication *(see amphetamine or cocaine intoxication for specific codes)*
		Stimulant use disorder *(see amphetamine or cocaine use disorder for specific codes)*
		Stimulant withdrawal *(see amphetamine or cocaine withdrawal for specific codes)*
		Substance intoxication delirium *(see specific substances for codes)*
		Substance withdrawal delirium *(see specific substances for codes)*
		Substance/medication-induced anxiety disorder *(see specific substances for codes)*
		Substance/medication-induced bipolar and related disorder *(see specific substances for codes)*
		Substance/medication-induced depressive disorder *(see specific substances for codes)*
		Substance/medication-induced major or mild neurocognitive disorder *(see specific substances for codes)*
		Substance/medication-induced obsessive-compulsive and related disorder *(see specific substances for codes)*
		Substance/medication-induced psychotic disorder *(see specific substances for codes)*
		Substance/medication-induced sexual dysfunction *(see specific substances for codes)*
		Substance/medication-induced sleep disorder *(see specific substances for codes)*

ICD-9-CM	ICD-10-CM	Disorder, condition, or problem
333.99	G25.71	Tardive akathisia
333.85	G24.01	Tardive dyskinesia
333.72	G24.09	Tardive dystonia
V62.4	Z60.5	Target of (perceived) adverse discrimination or persecution
292.85		Tobacco-induced sleep disorder
	F17.208	With moderate or severe use disorder
		Tobacco use disorder
305.1	Z72.0	Mild
305.1	F17.200	Moderate
305.1	F17.200	Severe
292.0	F17.203	Tobacco withdrawal
307.23	F95.2	Tourette's disorder
302.3	F65.1	Transvestic disorder
312.39	F63.3	Trichotillomania (hair-pulling disorder)
V63.9	Z75.3	Unavailability or inaccessibility of health care facilities
V63.8	Z75.4	Unavailability or inaccessibility of other helping agencies
V62.82	Z63.4	Uncomplicated bereavement
291.9	F10.99	Unspecified alcohol-related disorder
300.00	F41.9	Unspecified anxiety disorder
314.01	F90.9	Unspecified attention-deficit/hyperactivity disorder
296.80	F31.9	Unspecified bipolar and related disorder
292.9	F15.99	Unspecified caffeine-related disorder
292.9	F12.99	Unspecified cannabis-related disorder
293.89	F06.1	Unspecified catatonia (*code first* 781.99 [R29.818] other symptoms involving nervous and musculoskeletal systems)
307.9	F80.9	Unspecified communication disorder
780.09	R41.0	Unspecified delirium
311	F32.9	Unspecified depressive disorder
312.9	F91.9	Unspecified disruptive, impulse-control, and conduct disorder
300.15	F44.9	Unspecified dissociative disorder
		Unspecified elimination disorder
787.60	R15.9	With fecal symptoms
788.30	R32	With urinary symptoms
307.50	F50.9	Unspecified feeding or eating disorder
302.6	F64.9	Unspecified gender dysphoria
292.9	F16.99	Unspecified hallucinogen-related disorder
V60.9	Z59.9	Unspecified housing or economic problem
780.54	G47.10	Unspecified hypersomnolence disorder
292.9	F18.99	Unspecified inhalant-related disorder
780.52	G47.00	Unspecified insomnia disorder
319	F79	Unspecified intellectual disability (intellectual developmental disorder)
300.9	F99	Unspecified mental disorder
294.9	F09	Unspecified mental disorder due to another medical condition
799.59	R41.9	Unspecified neurocognitive disorder

ICD-9-CM	ICD-10-CM	Disorder, condition, or problem
315.9	F89	Unspecified neurodevelopmental disorder
300.3	F42.9	Unspecified obsessive-compulsive and related disorder
292.9	F11.99	Unspecified opioid-related disorder
292.9	F19.99	Unspecified other (or unknown) substance–related disorder
302.9	F65.9	Unspecified paraphilic disorder
301.9	F60.9	Unspecified personality disorder
292.9	F16.99	Unspecified phencyclidine-related disorder
V62.9	Z60.9	Unspecified problem related to social environment
V62.9	Z65.9	Unspecified problem related to unspecified psychosocial circumstances
298.9	F29	Unspecified schizophrenia spectrum and other psychotic disorder
292.9	F13.99	Unspecified sedative-, hypnotic-, or anxiolytic-related disorder
302.70	F52.9	Unspecified sexual dysfunction
780.59	G47.9	Unspecified sleep-wake disorder
300.82	F45.9	Unspecified somatic symptom and related disorder
292.9		Unspecified stimulant-related disorder
	F15.99	Unspecified amphetamine or other stimulant-related disorder
	F14.99	Unspecified cocaine-related disorder
307.20	F95.9	Unspecified tic disorder
292.9	F17.209	Unspecified tobacco-related disorder
309.9	F43.9	Unspecified trauma- and stressor-related disorder
V61.8	Z62.29	Upbringing away from parents
V62.89	Z65.4	Victim of crime
V62.89	Z65.4	Victim of terrorism or torture
302.82	F65.3	Voyeuristic disorder
V40.31	Z91.83	Wandering associated with a mental disorder

Numerical Listing of DSM-5 Diagnoses and Codes (ICD-9-CM)

ICD-9-CM codes are to be used for coding purposes in the United States through September 30, 2015. ICD-10-CM codes are to be used starting October 1, 2015. For DSM-5 coding and other updates, see the DSM-5® Update on www.PsychiatryOnline.org.

ICD-9-CM	Disorder, condition, or problem
278.00	Overweight or obesity
290.40	Probable major vascular neurocognitive disorder, With behavioral disturbance
290.40	Probable major vascular neurocognitive disorder, Without behavioral disturbance
291.0	Alcohol intoxication delirium
291.0	Alcohol withdrawal delirium
291.1	Alcohol-induced major neurocognitive disorder, Amnestic confabulatory type
291.2	Alcohol-induced major neurocognitive disorder, Nonamnestic confabulatory type
291.81	Alcohol withdrawal
291.82	Alcohol-induced sleep disorder
291.89	Alcohol-induced anxiety disorder
291.89	Alcohol-induced bipolar and related disorder
291.89	Alcohol-induced depressive disorder
291.89	Alcohol-induced mild neurocognitive disorder
291.89	Alcohol-induced sexual dysfunction
291.9	Alcohol-induced psychotic disorder
291.9	Unspecified alcohol-related disorder
292.0	Amphetamine or other stimulant withdrawal
292.0	Caffeine withdrawal
292.0	Cannabis withdrawal
292.0	Cocaine withdrawal
292.0	Opioid withdrawal
292.0	Opioid withdrawal delirium
292.0	Other (or unknown) substance withdrawal
292.0	Other (or unknown) substance withdrawal delirium
292.0	Sedative, hypnotic, or anxiolytic withdrawal
292.0	Sedative, hypnotic, or anxiolytic withdrawal delirium
292.0	Tobacco withdrawal
292.81	Amphetamine (or other stimulant) intoxication delirium
292.81	Cannabis intoxication delirium
292.81	Cocaine intoxication delirium

ICD-9-CM	Disorder, condition, or problem
292.81	Inhalant intoxication delirium
292.81	Medication-induced delirium
292.81	Opioid intoxication delirium
292.81	Other hallucinogen intoxication delirium
292.81	Other (or unknown) substance intoxication delirium
292.81	Phencyclidine intoxication delirium
292.81	Sedative, hypnotic, or anxiolytic intoxication delirium
292.82	Inhalant-induced major neurocognitive disorder
292.82	Other (or unknown) substance–induced major neurocognitive disorder
292.82	Sedative-, hypnotic-, or anxiolytic-induced major neurocognitive disorder
292.84	Amphetamine (or other stimulant)–induced bipolar and related disorder
292.84	Amphetamine (or other stimulant)–induced depressive disorder
292.84	Cocaine-induced bipolar and related disorder
292.84	Cocaine-induced depressive disorder
292.84	Inhalant-induced depressive disorder
292.84	Opioid-induced depressive disorder
292.84	Other hallucinogen–induced bipolar and related disorder
292.84	Other hallucinogen–induced depressive disorder
292.84	Other (or unknown) substance–induced bipolar and related disorder
292.84	Other (or unknown) substance–induced depressive disorder
292.84	Phencyclidine-induced bipolar and related disorder
292.84	Phencyclidine-induced depressive disorder
292.84	Sedative-, hypnotic-, or anxiolytic-induced bipolar and related disorder
292.84	Sedative-, hypnotic-, or anxiolytic-induced depressive disorder
292.85	Amphetamine (or other stimulant)–induced sleep disorder
292.85	Caffeine-induced sleep disorder
292.85	Cannabis-induced sleep disorder
292.85	Cocaine-induced sleep disorder
292.85	Opioid-induced sleep disorder
292.85	Other (or unknown) substance–induced sleep disorder
292.85	Sedative-, hypnotic-, or anxiolytic-induced sleep disorder
292.85	Tobacco-induced sleep disorder
292.89	Amphetamine (or other stimulant)–induced anxiety disorder
292.89	Amphetamine (or other stimulant)–induced obsessive-compulsive and related disorder
292.89	Amphetamine (or other stimulant)–induced sexual dysfunction
292.89	Amphetamine or other stimulant intoxication
292.89	Caffeine-induced anxiety disorder
292.89	Cannabis-induced anxiety disorder
292.89	Cannabis intoxication
292.89	Cocaine-induced anxiety disorder
292.89	Cocaine-induced obsessive-compulsive and related disorder
292.89	Cocaine-induced sexual dysfunction
292.89	Cocaine intoxication
292.89	Hallucinogen persisting perception disorder

ICD-9-CM	Disorder, condition, or problem
292.89	Inhalant-induced anxiety disorder
292.89	Inhalant-induced mild neurocognitive disorder
292.89	Inhalant intoxication
292.89	Opioid-induced anxiety disorder
292.89	Opioid-induced sexual dysfunction
292.89	Opioid intoxication
292.89	Other hallucinogen–induced anxiety disorder
292.89	Other hallucinogen intoxication
292.89	Other (or unknown) substance–induced anxiety disorder
292.89	Other (or unknown) substance–induced mild neurocognitive disorder
292.89	Other (or unknown) substance–induced obsessive-compulsive and related disorder
292.89	Other (or unknown) substance–induced sexual dysfunction
292.89	Other (or unknown) substance intoxication
292.89	Phencyclidine-induced anxiety disorder
292.89	Phencyclidine intoxication
292.89	Sedative-, hypnotic-, or anxiolytic-induced anxiety disorder
292.89	Sedative-, hypnotic-, or anxiolytic-induced mild neurocognitive disorder
292.89	Sedative-, hypnotic-, or anxiolytic-induced sexual dysfunction
292.89	Sedative, hypnotic, or anxiolytic intoxication
292.9	Amphetamine (or other stimulant)–induced psychotic disorder
292.9	Cannabis-induced psychotic disorder
292.9	Cocaine-induced psychotic disorder
292.9	Inhalant-induced psychotic disorder
292.9	Other hallucinogen–induced psychotic disorder
292.9	Other (or unknown) substance–induced psychotic disorder
292.9	Phencyclidine-induced psychotic disorder
292.9	Sedative-, hypnotic-, or anxiolytic-induced psychotic disorder
292.9	Unspecified caffeine-related disorder
292.9	Unspecified cannabis-related disorder
292.9	Unspecified hallucinogen-related disorder
292.9	Unspecified inhalant-related disorder
292.9	Unspecified opioid-related disorder
292.9	Unspecified other (or unknown) substance–related disorder
292.9	Unspecified phencyclidine-related disorder
292.9	Unspecified sedative-, hypnotic-, or anxiolytic-related disorder
292.9	Unspecified stimulant-related disorder
292.9	Unspecified tobacco-related disorder
293.0	Delirium due to another medical condition
293.0	Delirium due to multiple etiologies
293.81	Psychotic disorder due to another medical condition, With delusions
293.82	Psychotic disorder due to another medical condition, With hallucinations
293.83	Bipolar and related disorder due to another medical condition
293.83	Depressive disorder due to another medical condition
293.84	Anxiety disorder due to another medical condition
293.89	Catatonia associated with another mental disorder (catatonia specifier)

ICD-9-CM	Disorder, condition, or problem
293.89	Catatonic disorder due to another medical condition
293.89	Unspecified catatonia (*code first* 781.99 other symptoms involving nervous and musculoskeletal systems)
294.10	Major neurocognitive disorder due to another medical condition, Without behavioral disturbance
294.10	Major neurocognitive disorder due to HIV infection, Without behavioral disturbance (*code first* 042 HIV infection)
294.10	Major neurocognitive disorder due to Huntington's disease, Without behavioral disturbance (*code first* 333.4 Huntington's disease)
294.10	Major neurocognitive disorder due to multiple etiologies, Without behavioral disturbance
294.10	Major neurocognitive disorder probably due to Parkinson's disease, Without behavioral disturbance (*code first* 332.0 Parkinson's disease)
294.10	Major neurocognitive disorder due to prion disease, Without behavioral disturbance (*code first* 046.79 prion disease)
294.10	Major neurocognitive disorder due to traumatic brain injury, Without behavioral disturbance (*code first* 907.0 late effect of intracranial injury without skull fracture)
294.10	Probable major frontotemporal neurocognitive disorder, Without behavioral disturbance (*code first* 331.19 frontotemporal disease)
294.10	Probable major neurocognitive disorder due to Alzheimer's disease, Without behavioral disturbance (*code first* 331.0 Alzheimer's disease)
294.10	Probable major neurocognitive disorder with Lewy bodies, Without behavioral disturbance (*code first* 331.82 Lewy body disease)
294.11	Major neurocognitive disorder due to another medical condition, With behavioral disturbance
294.11	Major neurocognitive disorder due to HIV infection, With behavioral disturbance (*code first* 042 HIV infection)
294.11	Major neurocognitive disorder due to Huntington's disease, With behavioral disturbance (*code first* 333.4 Huntington's disease)
294.11	Major neurocognitive disorder due to multiple etiologies, With behavioral disturbance
294.11	Major neurocognitive disorder probably due to Parkinson's disease, With behavioral disturbance (*code first* 332.0 Parkinson's disease)
294.11	Major neurocognitive disorder due to prion disease, With behavioral disturbance (*code first* 046.79 prion disease)
294.11	Major neurocognitive disorder due to traumatic brain injury, With behavioral disturbance (*code first* 907.0 late effect of intracranial injury without skull fracture)
294.11	Probable major frontotemporal neurocognitive disorder, With behavioral disturbance (*code first* 331.19 frontotemporal disease)
294.11	Probable major neurocognitive disorder due to Alzheimer's disease, With behavioral disturbance (*code first* 331.0 Alzheimer's disease)
294.11	Probable major neurocognitive disorder with Lewy bodies, With behavioral disturbance (*code first* 331.82 Lewy body disease)
294.8	Obsessive-compulsive and related disorder due to another medical condition
294.8	Other specified mental disorder due to another medical condition
294.9	Unspecified mental disorder due to another medical condition

ICD-9-CM	Disorder, condition, or problem
295.40	Schizophreniform disorder
295.70	Schizoaffective disorder, Bipolar type
295.70	Schizoaffective disorder, Depressive type
295.90	Schizophrenia
296.20	Major depressive disorder, Single episode, Unspecified
296.21	Major depressive disorder, Single episode, Mild
296.22	Major depressive disorder, Single episode, Moderate
296.23	Major depressive disorder, Single episode, Severe
296.24	Major depressive disorder, Single episode, With psychotic features
296.25	Major depressive disorder, Single episode, In partial remission
296.26	Major depressive disorder, Single episode, In full remission
296.30	Major depressive disorder, Recurrent episode, Unspecified
296.31	Major depressive disorder, Recurrent episode, Mild
296.32	Major depressive disorder, Recurrent episode, Moderate
296.33	Major depressive disorder, Recurrent episode, Severe
296.34	Major depressive disorder, Recurrent episode, With psychotic features
296.35	Major depressive disorder, Recurrent episode, In partial remission
296.36	Major depressive disorder, Recurrent episode, In full remission
296.40	Bipolar I disorder, Current or most recent episode hypomanic
296.40	Bipolar I disorder, Current or most recent episode hypomanic, Unspecified
296.40	Bipolar I disorder, Current or most recent episode manic, Unspecified
296.41	Bipolar I disorder, Current or most recent episode manic, Mild
296.42	Bipolar I disorder, Current or most recent episode manic, Moderate
296.43	Bipolar I disorder, Current or most recent episode manic, Severe
296.44	Bipolar I disorder, Current or most recent episode manic, With psychotic features
296.45	Bipolar I disorder, Current or most recent episode hypomanic, In partial remission
296.45	Bipolar I disorder, Current or most recent episode manic, In partial remission
296.46	Bipolar I disorder, Current or most recent episode hypomanic, In full remission
296.46	Bipolar I disorder, Current or most recent episode manic, In full remission
296.50	Bipolar I disorder, Current or most recent episode depressed, Unspecified
296.51	Bipolar I disorder, Current or most recent episode depressed, Mild
296.52	Bipolar I disorder, Current or most recent episode depressed, Moderate
296.53	Bipolar I disorder, Current or most recent episode depressed, Severe
296.54	Bipolar I disorder, Current or most recent episode depressed, With psychotic features
296.55	Bipolar I disorder, Current or most recent episode depressed, In partial remission
296.56	Bipolar I disorder, Current or most recent episode depressed, In full remission
296.7	Bipolar I disorder, Current or most recent episode unspecified
296.80	Unspecified bipolar and related disorder
296.89	Bipolar II disorder
296.89	Other specified bipolar and related disorder
296.99	Disruptive mood dysregulation disorder
297.1	Delusional disorder
298.8	Brief psychotic disorder
298.8	Other specified schizophrenia spectrum and other psychotic disorder

ICD-9-CM	Disorder, condition, or problem
298.9	Unspecified schizophrenia spectrum and other psychotic disorder
299.00	Autism spectrum disorder
300.00	Unspecified anxiety disorder
300.01	Panic disorder
300.02	Generalized anxiety disorder
300.09	Other specified anxiety disorder
300.11	Conversion disorder (functional neurological symptom disorder)
300.12	Dissociative amnesia
300.13	Dissociative amnesia, With dissociative fugue
300.14	Dissociative identity disorder
300.15	Other specified dissociative disorder
300.15	Unspecified dissociative disorder
300.19	Factitious disorder
300.22	Agoraphobia
300.23	Social anxiety disorder (social phobia)
300.29	Specific phobia, Animal
300.29	Specific phobia, Blood-injection-injury
300.29	Specific phobia, Natural environment
300.29	Specific phobia, Other
300.29	Specific phobia, Situational
300.3	Hoarding disorder
300.3	Obsessive-compulsive disorder
300.3	Other specified obsessive-compulsive and related disorder
300.3	Unspecified obsessive-compulsive and related disorder
300.4	Persistent depressive disorder (dysthymia)
300.6	Depersonalization/derealization disorder
300.7	Body dysmorphic disorder
300.7	Illness anxiety disorder
300.82	Somatic symptom disorder
300.82	Unspecified somatic symptom and related disorder
300.89	Other specified somatic symptom and related disorder
300.9	Other specified mental disorder
300.9	Unspecified mental disorder
301.0	Paranoid personality disorder
301.13	Cyclothymic disorder
301.20	Schizoid personality disorder
301.22	Schizotypal personality disorder
301.4	Obsessive-compulsive personality disorder
301.50	Histrionic personality disorder
301.6	Dependent personality disorder
301.7	Antisocial personality disorder
301.81	Narcissistic personality disorder
301.82	Avoidant personality disorder
301.83	Borderline personality disorder
301.89	Other specified personality disorder

ICD-9-CM	Disorder, condition, or problem
301.9	Unspecified personality disorder
302.2	Pedophilic disorder
302.3	Transvestic disorder
302.4	Exhibitionistic disorder
302.6	Gender dysphoria in children
302.6	Other specified gender dysphoria
302.6	Unspecified gender dysphoria
302.70	Unspecified sexual dysfunction
302.71	Male hypoactive sexual desire disorder
302.72	Erectile disorder
302.72	Female sexual interest/arousal disorder
302.73	Female orgasmic disorder
302.74	Delayed ejaculation
302.75	Premature (early) ejaculation
302.76	Genito-pelvic pain/penetration disorder
302.79	Other specified sexual dysfunction
302.81	Fetishistic disorder
302.82	Voyeuristic disorder
302.83	Sexual masochism disorder
302.84	Sexual sadism disorder
302.85	Gender dysphoria in adolescents and adults
302.89	Frotteuristic disorder
302.89	Other specified paraphilic disorder
302.9	Unspecified paraphilic disorder
303.00	Alcohol intoxication
303.90	Alcohol use disorder, Moderate
303.90	Alcohol use disorder, Severe
304.00	Opioid use disorder, Moderate
304.00	Opioid use disorder, Severe
304.10	Sedative, hypnotic, or anxiolytic use disorder, Moderate
304.10	Sedative, hypnotic, or anxiolytic use disorder, Severe
304.20	Cocaine use disorder, Moderate
304.20	Cocaine use disorder, Severe
304.30	Cannabis use disorder, Moderate
304.30	Cannabis use disorder, Severe
304.40	Amphetamine-type substance use disorder, Moderate
304.40	Amphetamine-type substance use disorder, Severe
304.40	Other or unspecified stimulant use disorder, Moderate
304.40	Other or unspecified stimulant use disorder, Severe
304.50	Other hallucinogen use disorder, Moderate
304.50	Other hallucinogen use disorder, Severe
304.60	Inhalant use disorder, Moderate
304.60	Inhalant use disorder, Severe
304.60	Phencyclidine use disorder, Moderate
304.60	Phencyclidine use disorder, Severe

ICD-9-CM	Disorder, condition, or problem
304.90	Other (or unknown) substance use disorder, Moderate
304.90	Other (or unknown) substance use disorder, Severe
305.00	Alcohol use disorder, Mild
305.1	Tobacco use disorder, Mild
305.1	Tobacco use disorder, Moderate
305.1	Tobacco use disorder, Severe
305.20	Cannabis use disorder, Mild
305.30	Other hallucinogen use disorder, Mild
305.40	Sedative, hypnotic, or anxiolytic use disorder, Mild
305.50	Opioid use disorder, Mild
305.60	Cocaine use disorder, Mild
305.70	Amphetamine-type substance use disorder, Mild
305.70	Other or unspecified stimulant use disorder, Mild
305.90	Caffeine intoxication
305.90	Inhalant use disorder, Mild
305.90	Other (or unknown) substance use disorder, Mild
305.90	Phencyclidine use disorder, Mild
307.0	Adult-onset fluency disorder
307.1	Anorexia nervosa
307.20	Other specified tic disorder
307.20	Unspecified tic disorder
307.21	Provisional tic disorder
307.22	Persistent (chronic) motor or vocal tic disorder
307.23	Tourette's disorder
307.3	Stereotypic movement disorder
307.42	Insomnia disorder
307.44	Hypersomnolence disorder
307.45	Circadian rhythm sleep-wake disorders, Advanced sleep phase type
307.45	Circadian rhythm sleep-wake disorders, Delayed sleep phase type
307.45	Circadian rhythm sleep-wake disorders, Irregular sleep-wake type
307.45	Circadian rhythm sleep-wake disorders, Non-24-hour sleep-wake type
307.45	Circadian rhythm sleep-wake disorders, Shift work type
307.45	Circadian rhythm sleep-wake disorders, Unspecified type
307.46	Non–rapid eye movement sleep arousal disorders, Sleep terror type
307.46	Non–rapid eye movement sleep arousal disorders, Sleepwalking type
307.47	Nightmare disorder
307.50	Unspecified feeding or eating disorder
307.51	Binge-eating disorder
307.51	Bulimia nervosa
307.52	Pica
307.53	Rumination disorder
307.59	Avoidant/restrictive food intake disorder
307.59	Other specified feeding or eating disorder
307.6	Enuresis
307.7	Encopresis
307.9	Unspecified communication disorder

ICD-9-CM	Disorder, condition, or problem
308.3	Acute stress disorder
309.0	Adjustment disorders, With depressed mood
309.21	Separation anxiety disorder
309.24	Adjustment disorders, With anxiety
309.28	Adjustment disorders, With mixed anxiety and depressed mood
309.3	Adjustment disorders, With disturbance of conduct
309.4	Adjustment disorders, With mixed disturbance of emotions and conduct
309.81	Posttraumatic stress disorder
309.89	Other specified trauma- and stressor-related disorder
309.9	Adjustment disorders, Unspecified
309.9	Unspecified trauma- and stressor-related disorder
310.1	Personality change due to another medical condition
311	Other specified depressive disorder
311	Unspecified depressive disorder
312.31	Gambling disorder
312.32	Kleptomania
312.33	Pyromania
312.34	Intermittent explosive disorder
312.39	Trichotillomania (hair-pulling disorder)
312.81	Conduct disorder, Childhood-onset type
312.82	Conduct disorder, Adolescent-onset type
312.89	Conduct disorder, Unspecified onset
312.89	Other specified disruptive, impulse-control, and conduct disorder
312.9	Unspecified disruptive, impulse-control, and conduct disorder
313.23	Selective mutism
313.81	Oppositional defiant disorder
313.89	Disinhibited social engagement disorder
313.89	Reactive attachment disorder
314.00	Attention-deficit/hyperactivity disorder, Predominantly inattentive presentation
314.01	Attention-deficit/hyperactivity disorder, Combined presentation
314.01	Attention-deficit/hyperactivity disorder, Predominantly hyperactive/ impulsive presentation
314.01	Other specified attention-deficit/hyperactivity disorder
314.01	Unspecified attention-deficit/hyperactivity disorder
315.00	Specific learning disorder, With impairment in reading
315.1	Specific learning disorder, With impairment in mathematics
315.2	Specific learning disorder, With impairment in written expression
315.32	Language disorder
315.35	Childhood-onset fluency disorder (stuttering)
315.39	Social (pragmatic) communication disorder
315.39	Speech sound disorder
315.4	Developmental coordination disorder
315.8	Global developmental delay
315.8	Other specified neurodevelopmental disorder
315.9	Unspecified neurodevelopmental disorder
316	Psychological factors affecting other medical conditions

ICD-9-CM	Disorder, condition, or problem
317	Intellectual disability (intellectual developmental disorder), Mild
318.0	Intellectual disability (intellectual developmental disorder), Moderate
318.1	Intellectual disability (intellectual developmental disorder), Severe
318.2	Intellectual disability (intellectual developmental disorder), Profound
319	Unspecified intellectual disability (intellectual developmental disorder)
327.21	Central sleep apnea, Idiopathic central sleep apnea
327.23	Obstructive sleep apnea hypopnea
327.24	Sleep-related hypoventilation, Idiopathic hypoventilation
327.25	Sleep-related hypoventilation, Congenital central alveolar hypoventilation
327.26	Sleep-related hypoventilation, Comorbid sleep-related hypoventilation
327.42	Rapid eye movement sleep behavior disorder
331.83	Mild frontotemporal neurocognitive disorder
331.83	Mild neurocognitive disorder due to Alzheimer's disease
331.83	Mild neurocognitive disorder due to another medical condition
331.83	Mild neurocognitive disorder due to HIV infection
331.83	Mild neurocognitive disorder due to Huntington's disease
331.83	Mild neurocognitive disorder with Lewy bodies
331.83	Mild neurocognitive disorder due to multiple etiologies
331.83	Mild neurocognitive disorder due to Parkinson's disease
331.83	Mild neurocognitive disorder due to prion disease
331.83	Mild neurocognitive disorder due to traumatic brain injury
331.83	Mild vascular neurocognitive disorder
331.9	Major neurocognitive disorder possibly due to Parkinson's disease
331.9	Possible major frontotemporal neurocognitive disorder
331.9	Possible major neurocognitive disorder due to Alzheimer's disease
331.9	Possible major neurocognitive disorder with Lewy bodies
331.9	Possible major vascular neurocognitive disorder
333.1	Medication-induced postural tremor
332.1	Neuroleptic-induced parkinsonism
332.1	Other medication-induced parkinsonism
333.72	Medication-induced acute dystonia
333.72	Tardive dystonia
333.85	Tardive dyskinesia
333.92	Neuroleptic malignant syndrome
333.94	Restless legs syndrome
333.99	Medication-induced acute akathisia
333.99	Other medication-induced movement disorder
333.99	Tardive akathisia
347.00	Autosomal dominant cerebellar ataxia, deafness, and narcolepsy
347.00	Autosomal dominant narcolepsy, obesity, and type 2 diabetes
347.00	Narcolepsy without cataplexy but with hypocretin deficiency
347.01	Narcolepsy with cataplexy but without hypocretin deficiency
347.10	Narcolepsy secondary to another medical condition
625.4	Premenstrual dysphoric disorder
698.4	Excoriation (skin-picking) disorder

ICD-9-CM	Disorder, condition, or problem
780.09	Other specified delirium
780.09	Unspecified delirium
780.52	Other specified insomnia disorder
780.52	Unspecified insomnia disorder
780.54	Other specified hypersomnolence disorder
780.54	Unspecified hypersomnolence disorder
780.57	Central sleep apnea, Central sleep apnea comorbid with opioid use
780.59	Other specified sleep-wake disorder
780.59	Unspecified sleep-wake disorder
786.04	Central sleep apnea, Cheyne-Stokes breathing
787.60	Other specified elimination disorder, With fecal symptoms
787.60	Unspecified elimination disorder, With fecal symptoms
788.30	Unspecified elimination disorder, With urinary symptoms
788.39	Other specified elimination disorder, With urinary symptoms
799.59	Unspecified neurocognitive disorder
995.20	Other adverse effect of medication, Initial encounter
995.20	Other adverse effect of medication, Sequelae
995.20	Other adverse effect of medication, Subsequent encounter
995.29	Antidepressant discontinuation syndrome, Initial encounter
995.29	Antidepressant discontinuation syndrome, Sequelae
995.29	Antidepressant discontinuation syndrome, Subsequent encounter
995.51	Child psychological abuse, Confirmed, Initial encounter
995.51	Child psychological abuse, Confirmed, Subsequent encounter
995.51	Child psychological abuse, Suspected, Initial encounter
995.51	Child psychological abuse, Suspected, Subsequent encounter
995.52	Child neglect, Confirmed, Initial encounter
995.52	Child neglect, Confirmed, Subsequent encounter
995.52	Child neglect, Suspected, Initial encounter
995.52	Child neglect, Suspected, Subsequent encounter
995.53	Child sexual abuse, Confirmed, Initial encounter
995.53	Child sexual abuse, Confirmed, Subsequent encounter
995.53	Child sexual abuse, Suspected, Initial encounter
995.53	Child sexual abuse, Suspected, Subsequent encounter
995.54	Child physical abuse, Confirmed, Initial encounter
995.54	Child physical abuse, Confirmed, Subsequent encounter
995.54	Child physical abuse, Suspected, Initial encounter
995.54	Child physical abuse, Suspected, Subsequent encounter
995.81	Adult physical abuse by nonspouse or nonpartner, Confirmed, Initial encounter
995.81	Adult physical abuse by nonspouse or nonpartner, Confirmed, Subsequent encounter
995.81	Adult physical abuse by nonspouse or nonpartner, Suspected, Initial encounter
995.81	Adult physical abuse by nonspouse or nonpartner, Suspected, Subsequent encounter

ICD-9-CM	Disorder, condition, or problem
995.81	Spouse or partner violence, Physical, Confirmed, Initial encounter
995.81	Spouse or partner violence, Physical, Confirmed, Subsequent encounter
995.81	Spouse or partner violence, Physical, Suspected, Initial encounter
995.81	Spouse or partner violence, Physical, Suspected, Subsequent encounter
995.82	Adult psychological abuse by nonspouse or nonpartner, Confirmed, Initial encounter
995.82	Adult psychological abuse by nonspouse or nonpartner, Confirmed, Subsequent encounter
995.82	Adult psychological abuse by nonspouse or nonpartner, Suspected, Initial encounter
995.82	Adult psychological abuse by nonspouse or nonpartner, Suspected, Subsequent encounter
995.82	Spouse or partner abuse, Psychological, Confirmed, Initial encounter
995.82	Spouse or partner abuse, Psychological, Confirmed, Subsequent encounter
995.82	Spouse or partner abuse, Psychological, Suspected, Initial encounter
995.82	Spouse or partner abuse, Psychological, Suspected, Subsequent encounter
995.83	Adult sexual abuse by nonspouse or nonpartner, Confirmed, Initial encounter
995.83	Adult sexual abuse by nonspouse or nonpartner, Confirmed, Subsequent encounter
995.83	Adult sexual abuse by nonspouse or nonpartner, Suspected, Initial encounter
995.83	Adult sexual abuse by nonspouse or nonpartner, Suspected, Subsequent encounter
995.83	Spouse or partner violence, Sexual, Confirmed, Initial encounter
995.83	Spouse or partner violence, Sexual, Confirmed, Subsequent encounter
995.83	Spouse or partner violence, Sexual, Suspected, Initial encounter
995.83	Spouse or partner violence, Sexual, Suspected, Subsequent encounter
995.85	Spouse or partner neglect, Confirmed, Initial encounter
995.85	Spouse or partner neglect, Confirmed, Subsequent encounter
995.85	Spouse or partner neglect, Suspected, Initial encounter
995.85	Spouse or partner neglect, Suspected, Subsequent encounter
V15.41	Personal history (past history) of physical abuse in childhood
V15.41	Personal history (past history) of sexual abuse in childhood
V15.41	Personal history (past history) of spouse or partner violence, Physical
V15.41	Personal history (past history) of spouse or partner violence, Sexual
V15.42	Personal history (past history) of neglect in childhood
V15.42	Personal history (past history) of psychological abuse in childhood
V15.42	Personal history (past history) of spouse or partner neglect
V15.42	Personal history (past history) of spouse or partner psychological abuse
V15.49	Other personal history of psychological trauma
V15.59	Personal history of self-harm
V15.81	Nonadherence to medical treatment
V15.89	Other personal risk factors
V40.31	Wandering associated with a mental disorder
V60.0	Homelessness
V60.1	Inadequate housing
V60.2	Extreme poverty

ICD-9-CM	Disorder, condition, or problem
V60.2	Insufficient social insurance or welfare support
V60.2	Lack of adequate food or safe drinking water
V60.2	Low income
V60.3	Problem related to living alone
V60.6	Problem related to living in a residential institution
V60.89	Discord with neighbor, lodger, or landlord
V60.9	Unspecified housing or economic problem
V61.03	Disruption of family by separation or divorce
V61.10	Relationship distress with spouse or intimate partner
V61.11	Encounter for mental health services for victim of spouse or partner neglect
V61.11	Encounter for mental health services for victim of spouse or partner psychological abuse
V61.11	Encounter for mental health services for victim of spouse or partner violence, Physical
V61.11	Encounter for mental health services for victim of spouse or partner violence, Sexual
V61.12	Encounter for mental health services for perpetrator of spouse or partner neglect
V61.12	Encounter for mental health services for perpetrator of spouse or partner psychological abuse
V61.12	Encounter for mental health services for perpetrator of spouse or partner violence, Physical
V61.12	Encounter for mental health services for perpetrator of spouse or partner violence, Sexual
V61.20	Parent-child relational problem
V61.21	Encounter for mental health services for victim of child abuse by parent
V61.21	Encounter for mental health services for victim of child neglect by parent
V61.21	Encounter for mental health services for victim of child psychological abuse by parent
V61.21	Encounter for mental health services for victim of child sexual abuse by parent
V61.21	Encounter for mental health services for victim of nonparental child abuse
V61.21	Encounter for mental health services for victim of nonparental child neglect
V61.21	Encounter for mental health services for victim of nonparental child psychological abuse
V61.21	Encounter for mental health services for victim of nonparental child sexual abuse
V61.22	Encounter for mental health services for perpetrator of parental child abuse
V61.22	Encounter for mental health services for perpetrator of parental child neglect
V61.22	Encounter for mental health services for perpetrator of parental child psychological abuse
V61.22	Encounter for mental health services for perpetrator of parental child sexual abuse
V61.29	Child affected by parental relationship distress
V61.5	Problems related to multiparity
V61.7	Problems related to unwanted pregnancy
V61.8	High expressed emotion level within family
V61.8	Sibling relational problem

ICD-9-CM	Disorder, condition, or problem
V61.8	Upbringing away from parents
V62.21	Problem related to current military deployment status
V62.22	Exposure to disaster, war, or other hostilities
V62.22	Personal history of military deployment
V62.29	Other problem related to employment
V62.3	Academic or educational problem
V62.4	Acculturation difficulty
V62.4	Social exclusion or rejection
V62.4	Target of (perceived) adverse discrimination or persecution
V62.5	Conviction in civil or criminal proceedings without imprisonment
V62.5	Imprisonment or other incarceration
V62.5	Problems related to other legal circumstances
V62.5	Problems related to release from prison
V62.82	Uncomplicated bereavement
V62.83	Encounter for mental health services for perpetrator of nonparental child abuse
V62.83	Encounter for mental health services for perpetrator of nonparental child neglect
V62.83	Encounter for mental health services for perpetrator of nonparental child psychological abuse
V62.83	Encounter for mental health services for perpetrator of nonparental child sexual abuse
V62.83	Encounter for mental health services for perpetrator of nonspousal adult abuse
V62.89	Borderline intellectual functioning
V62.89	Discord with social service provider, including probation officer, case manager, or social services worker
V62.89	Other problem related to psychosocial circumstances
V62.89	Phase of life problem
V62.89	Religious or spiritual problem
V62.89	Victim of crime
V62.89	Victim of terrorism or torture
V62.9	Unspecified problem related to social environment
V62.9	Unspecified problem related to unspecified psychosocial circumstances
V63.8	Unavailability or inaccessibility of other helping agencies
V63.9	Unavailability or inaccessibility of health care facilities
V65.2	Malingering
V65.40	Other counseling or consultation
V65.49	Encounter for mental health services for victim of nonspousal adult abuse
V65.49	Sex counseling
V69.9	Problem related to lifestyle
V71.01	Adult antisocial behavior
V71.02	Child or adolescent antisocial behavior

Numerical Listing of DSM-5 Diagnoses and Codes (ICD-10-CM)

ICD-10-CM codes are to be used for coding purposes in the United States starting October 1, 2015. For DSM-5 coding and other updates, see the DSM-5® Update on www.PsychiatryOnline.org.

ICD-10-CM	Disorder, condition, or problem
E66.9	Overweight or obesity
F01.50	Probable major vascular neurocognitive disorder, Without behavioral disturbance
F01.51	Probable major vascular neurocognitive disorder, With behavioral disturbance
F02.80	Major neurocognitive disorder due to another medical condition, Without behavioral disturbance
F02.80	Major neurocognitive disorder due to HIV infection, Without behavioral disturbance (*code first* B20 HIV infection)
F02.80	Major neurocognitive disorder due to Huntington's disease, Without behavioral disturbance (*code first* G10 Huntington's disease)
F02.80	Major neurocognitive disorder due to multiple etiologies, Without behavioral disturbance
F02.80	Major neurocognitive disorder probably due to Parkinson's disease, Without behavioral disturbance (*code first* G20 Parkinson's disease)
F02.80	Major neurocognitive disorder due to prion disease, Without behavioral disturbance (*code first* A81.9 prion disease)
F02.80	Major neurocognitive disorder due to traumatic brain injury, Without behavioral disturbance (*code first* S06.2X9S diffuse traumatic brain injury with loss of consciousness of unspecified duration, sequela)
F02.80	Probable major frontotemporal neurocognitive disorder, Without behavioral disturbance (*code first* G31.09 frontotemporal disease)
F02.80	Probable major neurocognitive disorder due to Alzheimer's disease, Without behavioral disturbance (*code first* G30.9 Alzheimer's disease)
F02.80	Probable major neurocognitive disorder with Lewy bodies, Without behavioral disturbance (*code first* G31.83 Lewy body disease)
F02.81	Major neurocognitive disorder due to another medical condition, With behavioral disturbance
F02.81	Major neurocognitive disorder due to HIV infection, With behavioral disturbance (*code first* B20 HIV infection)
F02.81	Major neurocognitive disorder due to Huntington's disease, With behavioral disturbance (*code first* G10 Huntington's disease)
F02.81	Major neurocognitive disorder due to multiple etiologies, With behavioral disturbance

ICD-10-CM	Disorder, condition, or problem
F02.81	Major neurocognitive disorder probably due to Parkinson's disease, With behavioral disturbance (*code first* G20 Parkinson's disease)
F02.81	Major neurocognitive disorder due to prion disease, With behavioral disturbance (*code first* A81.9 prion disease)
F02.81	Major neurocognitive disorder due to traumatic brain injury, With behavioral disturbance (*code first* S06.2X9S diffuse traumatic brain injury with loss of consciousness of unspecified duration, sequela)
F02.81	Probable major frontotemporal neurocognitive disorder, With behavioral disturbance (*code first* G31.09 frontotemporal disease)
F02.81	Probable major neurocognitive disorder due to Alzheimer's disease, With behavioral disturbance (*code first* G30.9 Alzheimer's disease)
F02.81	Probable major neurocognitive disorder with Lewy bodies, With behavioral disturbance (*code first* G31.83 Lewy body disease)
F05	Delirium due to another medical condition
F05	Delirium due to multiple etiologies
F06.0	Psychotic disorder due to another medical condition, With hallucinations
F06.1	Catatonia associated with another mental disorder (catatonia specifier)
F06.1	Catatonic disorder due to another medical condition
F06.1	Unspecified catatonia (*code first* R29.818 other symptoms involving nervous and musculoskeletal systems)
F06.2	Psychotic disorder due to another medical condition, With delusions
F06.31	Depressive disorder due to another medical condition, With depressive features
F06.32	Depressive disorder due to another medical condition, With major depressive–like episode
F06.33	Bipolar and related disorder due to another medical condition, With manic features
F06.33	Bipolar and related disorder due to another medical condition, With manic- or hypomanic-like episodes
F06.34	Bipolar and related disorder due to another medical condition, With mixed features
F06.34	Depressive disorder due to another medical condition, With mixed features
F06.4	Anxiety disorder due to another medical condition
F06.8	Obsessive-compulsive and related disorder due to another medical condition
F06.8	Other specified mental disorder due to another medical condition
F07.0	Personality change due to another medical condition
F09	Unspecified mental disorder due to another medical condition
F10.10	Alcohol use disorder, Mild
F10.121	Alcohol intoxication delirium, With mild use disorder
F10.129	Alcohol intoxication, With mild use disorder
F10.14	Alcohol-induced bipolar and related disorder, With mild use disorder
F10.14	Alcohol-induced depressive disorder, With mild use disorder
F10.159	Alcohol-induced psychotic disorder, With mild use disorder
F10.180	Alcohol-induced anxiety disorder, With mild use disorder
F10.181	Alcohol-induced sexual dysfunction, With mild use disorder
F10.182	Alcohol-induced sleep disorder, With mild use disorder
F10.20	Alcohol use disorder, Moderate
F10.20	Alcohol use disorder, Severe
F10.221	Alcohol intoxication delirium, With moderate or severe use disorder

ICD-10-CM	Disorder, condition, or problem
F10.229	Alcohol intoxication, With moderate or severe use disorder
F10.231	Alcohol withdrawal delirium
F10.232	Alcohol withdrawal, With perceptual disturbances
F10.239	Alcohol withdrawal, Without perceptual disturbances
F10.24	Alcohol-induced bipolar and related disorder, With moderate or severe use disorder
F10.24	Alcohol-induced depressive disorder, With moderate or severe use disorder
F10.259	Alcohol-induced psychotic disorder, With moderate or severe use disorder
F10.26	Alcohol-induced major neurocognitive disorder, Amnestic confabulatory type, With moderate or severe use disorder
F10.27	Alcohol-induced major neurocognitive disorder, Nonamnestic confabulatory type, With moderate or severe use disorder
F10.280	Alcohol-induced anxiety disorder, With moderate or severe use disorder
F10.281	Alcohol-induced sexual dysfunction, With moderate or severe use disorder
F10.282	Alcohol-induced sleep disorder, With moderate or severe use disorder
F10.288	Alcohol-induced mild neurocognitive disorder, With moderate or severe use disorder
F10.921	Alcohol intoxication delirium, Without use disorder
F10.929	Alcohol intoxication, Without use disorder
F10.94	Alcohol-induced bipolar and related disorder, Without use disorder
F10.94	Alcohol-induced depressive disorder, Without use disorder
F10.959	Alcohol-induced psychotic disorder, Without use disorder
F10.96	Alcohol-induced major neurocognitive disorder, Amnestic confabulatory type, Without use disorder
F10.97	Alcohol-induced major neurocognitive disorder, Nonamnestic confabulatory type, Without use disorder
F10.980	Alcohol-induced anxiety disorder, Without use disorder
F10.981	Alcohol-induced sexual dysfunction, Without use disorder
F10.982	Alcohol-induced sleep disorder, Without use disorder
F10.988	Alcohol-induced mild neurocognitive disorder, Without use disorder
F10.99	Unspecified alcohol-related disorder
F11.10	Opioid use disorder, Mild
F11.121	Opioid intoxication delirium, With mild use disorder
F11.122	Opioid intoxication, With perceptual disturbances, With mild use disorder
F11.129	Opioid intoxication, Without perceptual disturbances, With mild use disorder
F11.14	Opioid-induced depressive disorder, With mild use disorder
F11.181	Opioid-induced sexual dysfunction, With mild use disorder
F11.182	Opioid-induced sleep disorder, With mild use disorder
F11.188	Opioid-induced anxiety disorder, With mild use disorder
F11.20	Opioid use disorder, Moderate
F11.20	Opioid use disorder, Severe
F11.221	Opioid intoxication delirium, With moderate or severe use disorder
F11.222	Opioid intoxication, With perceptual disturbances, With moderate or severe use disorder
F11.229	Opioid intoxication, Without perceptual disturbances, With moderate or severe use disorder
F11.23	Opioid withdrawal

ICD-10-CM	Disorder, condition, or problem
F11.23	Opioid withdrawal delirium
F11.24	Opioid-induced depressive disorder, With moderate or severe use disorder
F11.281	Opioid-induced sexual dysfunction, With moderate or severe use disorder
F11.282	Opioid-induced sleep disorder, With moderate or severe use disorder
F11.288	Opioid-induced anxiety disorder, With moderate or severe use disorder
F11.921	Opioid-induced delirium
F11.921	Opioid intoxication delirium, Without use disorder
F11.922	Opioid intoxication, With perceptual disturbances, Without use disorder
F11.929	Opioid intoxication, Without perceptual disturbances, Without use disorder
F11.94	Opioid-induced depressive disorder, Without use disorder
F11.981	Opioid-induced sexual dysfunction, Without use disorder
F11.982	Opioid-induced sleep disorder, Without use disorder
F11.988	Opioid-induced anxiety disorder, Without use disorder
F11.99	Unspecified opioid-related disorder
F12.10	Cannabis use disorder, Mild
F12.121	Cannabis intoxication delirium, With mild use disorder
F12.122	Cannabis intoxication, With perceptual disturbances, With mild use disorder
F12.129	Cannabis intoxication, Without perceptual disturbances, With mild use disorder
F12.159	Cannabis-induced psychotic disorder, With mild use disorder
F12.180	Cannabis-induced anxiety disorder, With mild use disorder
F12.188	Cannabis-induced sleep disorder, With mild use disorder
F12.20	Cannabis use disorder, Moderate
F12.20	Cannabis use disorder, Severe
F12.221	Cannabis intoxication delirium, With moderate or severe use disorder
F12.222	Cannabis intoxication, With perceptual disturbances, With moderate or severe use disorder
F12.229	Cannabis intoxication, Without perceptual disturbances, With moderate or severe use disorder
F12.259	Cannabis-induced psychotic disorder, With moderate or severe use disorder
F12.280	Cannabis-induced anxiety disorder, With moderate or severe use disorder
F12.288	Cannabis-induced sleep disorder, With moderate or severe use disorder
F12.288	Cannabis withdrawal
F12.921	Cannabis intoxication delirium, Without use disorder
F12.922	Cannabis intoxication, With perceptual disturbances, Without use disorder
F12.929	Cannabis intoxication, Without perceptual disturbances, Without use disorder
F12.959	Cannabis-induced psychotic disorder, Without use disorder
F12.980	Cannabis-induced anxiety disorder, Without use disorder
F12.988	Cannabis-induced sleep disorder, Without use disorder
F12.99	Unspecified cannabis-related disorder
F13.10	Sedative, hypnotic, or anxiolytic use disorder, Mild
F13.121	Sedative, hypnotic, or anxiolytic intoxication delirium, With mild use disorder
F13.129	Sedative, hypnotic, or anxiolytic intoxication, With mild use disorder
F13.14	Sedative-, hypnotic-, or anxiolytic-induced bipolar and related disorder, With mild use disorder
F13.14	Sedative-, hypnotic-, or anxiolytic-induced depressive disorder, With mild use disorder

ICD-10-CM	Disorder, condition, or problem
F13.159	Sedative-, hypnotic-, or anxiolytic-induced psychotic disorder, With mild use disorder
F13.180	Sedative-, hypnotic-, or anxiolytic-induced anxiety disorder, With mild use disorder
F13.181	Sedative-, hypnotic-, or anxiolytic-induced sexual dysfunction, With mild use disorder
F13.182	Sedative-, hypnotic-, or anxiolytic-induced sleep disorder, With mild use disorder
F13.20	Sedative, hypnotic, or anxiolytic use disorder, Moderate
F13.20	Sedative, hypnotic, or anxiolytic use disorder, Severe
F13.221	Sedative, hypnotic, or anxiolytic intoxication delirium, With moderate or severe use disorder
F13.229	Sedative, hypnotic, or anxiolytic intoxication, With moderate or severe use disorder
F13.231	Sedative, hypnotic, or anxiolytic withdrawal delirium
F13.232	Sedative, hypnotic, or anxiolytic withdrawal, With perceptual disturbances
F13.239	Sedative, hypnotic, or anxiolytic withdrawal, Without perceptual disturbances
F13.24	Sedative-, hypnotic-, or anxiolytic-induced bipolar and related disorder, With moderate or severe use disorder
F13.24	Sedative-, hypnotic-, or anxiolytic-induced depressive disorder, With moderate or severe use disorder
F13.259	Sedative-, hypnotic-, or anxiolytic-induced psychotic disorder, With moderate or severe use disorder
F13.27	Sedative-, hypnotic-, or anxiolytic-induced major neurocognitive disorder, With moderate or severe use disorder
F13.280	Sedative-, hypnotic-, or anxiolytic-induced anxiety disorder, With moderate or severe use disorder
F13.281	Sedative-, hypnotic-, or anxiolytic-induced sexual dysfunction, With moderate or severe use disorder
F13.282	Sedative-, hypnotic-, or anxiolytic-induced sleep disorder, With moderate or severe use disorder
F13.288	Sedative-, hypnotic-, or anxiolytic-induced mild neurocognitive disorder, With moderate or severe use disorder
F13.921	Sedative-, hypnotic-, or anxiolytic-induced delirium
F13.921	Sedative, hypnotic, or anxiolytic intoxication delirium, Without use disorder
F13.929	Sedative, hypnotic, or anxiolytic intoxication, Without use disorder
F13.94	Sedative-, hypnotic-, or anxiolytic-induced bipolar and related disorder, Without use disorder
F13.94	Sedative-, hypnotic-, or anxiolytic-induced depressive disorder, Without use disorder
F13.959	Sedative-, hypnotic-, or anxiolytic-induced psychotic disorder, Without use disorder
F13.97	Sedative-, hypnotic-, or anxiolytic-induced major neurocognitive disorder, Without use disorder
F13.980	Sedative-, hypnotic-, or anxiolytic-induced anxiety disorder, Without use disorder
F13.981	Sedative-, hypnotic-, or anxiolytic-induced sexual dysfunction, Without use disorder
F13.982	Sedative-, hypnotic-, or anxiolytic-induced sleep disorder, Without use disorder
F13.988	Sedative-, hypnotic-, or anxiolytic-induced mild neurocognitive disorder, Without use disorder

ICD-10-CM	Disorder, condition, or problem
F13.99	Unspecified sedative-, hypnotic-, or anxiolytic-related disorder
F14.10	Cocaine use disorder, Mild
F14.121	Cocaine intoxication delirium, With mild use disorder
F14.122	Cocaine intoxication, With perceptual disturbances, With mild use disorder
F14.129	Cocaine intoxication, Without perceptual disturbances, With mild use disorder
F14.14	Cocaine-induced bipolar and related disorder, With mild use disorder
F14.14	Cocaine-induced depressive disorder, With mild use disorder
F14.159	Cocaine-induced psychotic disorder, With mild use disorder
F14.180	Cocaine-induced anxiety disorder, With mild use disorder
F14.181	Cocaine-induced sexual dysfunction, With mild use disorder
F14.182	Cocaine-induced sleep disorder, With mild use disorder
F14.188	Cocaine-induced obsessive-compulsive and related disorder, With mild use disorder
F14.20	Cocaine use disorder, Moderate
F14.20	Cocaine use disorder, Severe
F14.221	Cocaine intoxication delirium, With moderate or severe use disorder
F14.222	Cocaine intoxication, With perceptual disturbances, With moderate or severe use disorder
F14.229	Cocaine intoxication, Without perceptual disturbances, With moderate or severe use disorder
F14.23	Cocaine withdrawal
F14.24	Cocaine-induced bipolar and related disorder, With moderate or severe use disorder
F14.24	Cocaine-induced depressive disorder, With moderate or severe use disorder
F14.259	Cocaine-induced psychotic disorder, With moderate or severe use disorder
F14.280	Cocaine-induced anxiety disorder, With moderate or severe use disorder
F14.281	Cocaine-induced sexual dysfunction, With moderate or severe use disorder
F14.282	Cocaine-induced sleep disorder, With moderate or severe use disorder
F14.288	Cocaine-induced obsessive-compulsive and related disorder, With moderate or severe use disorder
F14.921	Cocaine intoxication delirium, Without use disorder
F14.922	Cocaine intoxication, With perceptual disturbances, Without use disorder
F14.929	Cocaine intoxication, Without perceptual disturbances, Without use disorder
F14.94	Cocaine-induced bipolar and related disorder, Without use disorder
F14.94	Cocaine-induced depressive disorder, Without use disorder
F14.959	Cocaine-induced psychotic disorder, Without use disorder
F14.980	Cocaine-induced anxiety disorder, Without use disorder
F14.981	Cocaine-induced sexual dysfunction, Without use disorder
F14.982	Cocaine-induced sleep disorder, Without use disorder
F14.988	Cocaine-induced obsessive-compulsive and related disorder, Without use disorder
F14.99	Unspecified stimulant-related disorder, Unspecified Cocaine-related disorder
F15.10	Amphetamine-type substance use disorder, Mild
F15.10	Other or unspecified stimulant use disorder, Mild
F15.121	Amphetamine (or other stimulant) intoxication delirium, With mild use disorder
F15.122	Amphetamine or other stimulant intoxication, With perceptual disturbances, With mild use disorder

ICD-10-CM	Disorder, condition, or problem
F15.129	Amphetamine or other stimulant intoxication, Without perceptual disturbances, With mild use disorder
F15.14	Amphetamine (or other stimulant)–induced bipolar and related disorder, With mild use disorder
F15.14	Amphetamine (or other stimulant)–induced depressive disorder, With mild use disorder
F15.159	Amphetamine (or other stimulant)–induced psychotic disorder, With mild use disorder
F15.180	Amphetamine (or other stimulant)–induced anxiety disorder, With mild use disorder
F15.180	Caffeine-induced anxiety disorder, With mild use disorder
F15.181	Amphetamine (or other stimulant)–induced sexual dysfunction, With mild use disorder
F15.182	Amphetamine (or other stimulant)–induced sleep disorder, With mild use disorder
F15.182	Caffeine-induced sleep disorder, With mild use disorder
F15.188	Amphetamine (or other stimulant)–induced obsessive-compulsive and related disorder, With mild use disorder
F15.20	Amphetamine-type substance use disorder, Moderate
F15.20	Amphetamine-type substance use disorder, Severe
F15.20	Other or unspecified stimulant use disorder, Moderate
F15.20	Other or unspecified stimulant use disorder, Severe
F15.221	Amphetamine (or other stimulant) intoxication delirium, With moderate or severe use disorder
F15.222	Amphetamine or other stimulant intoxication, With perceptual disturbances, With moderate or severe use disorder
F15.229	Amphetamine or other stimulant intoxication, Without perceptual disturbances, With moderate or severe use disorder
F15.23	Amphetamine or other stimulant withdrawal
F15.24	Amphetamine (or other stimulant)–induced bipolar and related disorder, With moderate or severe use disorder
F15.24	Amphetamine (or other stimulant)–induced depressive disorder, With moderate or severe use disorder
F15.259	Amphetamine (or other stimulant)–induced psychotic disorder, With moderate or severe use disorder
F15.280	Amphetamine (or other stimulant)–induced anxiety disorder, With moderate or severe use disorder
F15.280	Caffeine-induced anxiety disorder, With moderate or severe use disorder
F15.281	Amphetamine (or other stimulant)–induced sexual dysfunction, With moderate or severe use disorder
F15.282	Amphetamine (or other stimulant)–induced sleep disorder, With moderate or severe use disorder
F15.282	Caffeine-induced sleep disorder, With moderate or severe use disorder
F15.288	Amphetamine (or other stimulant)–induced obsessive-compulsive and related disorder, With moderate or severe use disorder
F15.921	Amphetamine (or other stimulant)–induced delirium
F15.921	Amphetamine (or other stimulant) intoxication delirium, Without use disorder
F15.922	Amphetamine or other stimulant intoxication, With perceptual disturbances, Without use disorder

ICD-10-CM	Disorder, condition, or problem
F15.929	Amphetamine or other stimulant intoxication, Without perceptual disturbances, Without use disorder
F15.929	Caffeine intoxication
F15.93	Caffeine withdrawal
F15.94	Amphetamine (or other stimulant)–induced bipolar and related disorder, Without use disorder
F15.94	Amphetamine (or other stimulant)–induced depressive disorder, Without use disorder
F15.959	Amphetamine (or other stimulant)–induced psychotic disorder, Without use disorder
F15.980	Amphetamine (or other stimulant)–induced anxiety disorder, Without use disorder
F15.980	Caffeine-induced anxiety disorder, Without use disorder
F15.981	Amphetamine (or other stimulant)–induced sexual dysfunction, Without use disorder
F15.982	Amphetamine (or other stimulant)–induced sleep disorder, Without use disorder
F15.982	Caffeine-induced sleep disorder, Without use disorder
F15.988	Amphetamine (or other stimulant)–induced obsessive-compulsive and related disorder, Without use disorder
F15.99	Unspecified amphetamine or other stimulant-related disorder
F15.99	Unspecified caffeine-related disorder
F16.10	Other hallucinogen use disorder, Mild
F16.10	Phencyclidine use disorder, Mild
F16.121	Other hallucinogen intoxication delirium, With mild use disorder
F16.121	Phencyclidine intoxication delirium, With mild use disorder
F16.129	Other hallucinogen intoxication, With mild use disorder
F16.129	Phencyclidine intoxication, With mild use disorder
F16.14	Other hallucinogen–induced bipolar and related disorder, With mild use disorder
F16.14	Other hallucinogen–induced depressive disorder, With mild use disorder
F16.14	Phencyclidine-induced bipolar and related disorder, With mild use disorder
F16.14	Phencyclidine-induced depressive disorder, With mild use disorder
F16.159	Other hallucinogen–induced psychotic disorder, With mild use disorder
F16.159	Phencyclidine-induced psychotic disorder, With mild use disorder
F16.180	Other hallucinogen–induced anxiety disorder, With mild use disorder
F16.180	Phencyclidine-induced anxiety disorder, With mild use disorder
F16.20	Other hallucinogen use disorder, Moderate
F16.20	Other hallucinogen use disorder, Severe
F16.20	Phencyclidine use disorder, Moderate
F16.20	Phencyclidine use disorder, Severe
F16.221	Other hallucinogen intoxication delirium, With moderate or severe use disorder
F16.221	Phencyclidine intoxication delirium, With moderate or severe use disorder
F16.229	Other hallucinogen intoxication, With moderate or severe use disorder
F16.229	Phencyclidine intoxication, With moderate or severe use disorder
F16.24	Other hallucinogen–induced bipolar and related disorder, With moderate or severe use disorder

ICD-10-CM	Disorder, condition, or problem
F16.24	Other hallucinogen–induced depressive disorder, With moderate or severe use disorder
F16.24	Phencyclidine-induced bipolar and related disorder, With moderate or severe use disorder
F16.24	Phencyclidine-induced depressive disorder, With moderate or severe use disorder
F16.259	Other hallucinogen–induced psychotic disorder, With moderate or severe use disorder
F16.259	Phencyclidine-induced psychotic disorder, With moderate or severe use disorder
F16.280	Other hallucinogen–induced anxiety disorder, With moderate or severe use disorder
F16.280	Phencyclidine-induced anxiety disorder, With moderate or severe use disorder
F16.921	Other hallucinogen intoxication delirium, Without use disorder
F16.921	Phencyclidine intoxication delirium, Without use disorder
F16.929	Other hallucinogen intoxication, Without use disorder
F16.929	Phencyclidine intoxication, Without use disorder
F16.94	Other hallucinogen–induced bipolar and related disorder, Without use disorder
F16.94	Other hallucinogen–induced depressive disorder, Without use disorder
F16.94	Phencyclidine-induced bipolar and related disorder, Without use disorder
F16.94	Phencyclidine-induced depressive disorder, Without use disorder
F16.959	Other hallucinogen–induced psychotic disorder, Without use disorder
F16.959	Phencyclidine-induced psychotic disorder, Without use disorder
F16.980	Other hallucinogen–induced anxiety disorder, Without use disorder
F16.980	Phencyclidine-induced anxiety disorder, Without use disorder
F16.983	Hallucinogen persisting perception disorder
F16.99	Unspecified hallucinogen-related disorder
F16.99	Unspecified phencyclidine-related disorder
F17.200	Tobacco use disorder, Moderate
F17.200	Tobacco use disorder, Severe
F17.203	Tobacco withdrawal
F17.208	Tobacco-induced sleep disorder, With moderate or severe use disorder
F17.209	Unspecified tobacco-related disorder
F18.10	Inhalant use disorder, Mild
F18.121	Inhalant intoxication delirium, With mild use disorder
F18.129	Inhalant intoxication, With mild use disorder
F18.14	Inhalant-induced depressive disorder, With mild use disorder
F18.159	Inhalant-induced psychotic disorder, With mild use disorder
F18.17	Inhalant-induced major neurocognitive disorder, With mild use disorder
F18.180	Inhalant-induced anxiety disorder, With mild use disorder
F18.188	Inhalant-induced mild neurocognitive disorder, With mild use disorder
F18.20	Inhalant use disorder, Moderate
F18.20	Inhalant use disorder, Severe
F18.221	Inhalant intoxication delirium, With moderate or severe use disorder
F18.229	Inhalant intoxication, With moderate or severe use disorder
F18.24	Inhalant-induced depressive disorder, With moderate or severe use disorder
F18.259	Inhalant-induced psychotic disorder, With moderate or severe use disorder

ICD-10-CM	Disorder, condition, or problem
F18.27	Inhalant-induced major neurocognitive disorder, With moderate or severe use disorder
F18.280	Inhalant-induced anxiety disorder, With moderate or severe use disorder
F18.288	Inhalant-induced mild neurocognitive disorder, With moderate or severe use disorder
F18.921	Inhalant intoxication delirium, Without use disorder
F18.929	Inhalant intoxication, Without use disorder
F18.94	Inhalant-induced depressive disorder, Without use disorder
F18.959	Inhalant-induced psychotic disorder, Without use disorder
F18.97	Inhalant-induced major neurocognitive disorder, Without use disorder
F18.980	Inhalant-induced anxiety disorder, Without use disorder
F18.988	Inhalant-induced mild neurocognitive disorder, Without use disorder
F18.99	Unspecified inhalant-related disorder
F19.10	Other (or unknown) substance use disorder, Mild
F19.121	Other (or unknown) substance intoxication delirium, With mild use disorder
F19.129	Other (or unknown) substance intoxication, With mild use disorder
F19.14	Other (or unknown) substance–induced bipolar and related disorder, With mild use disorder
F19.14	Other (or unknown) substance–induced depressive disorder, With mild use disorder
F19.159	Other (or unknown) substance–induced psychotic disorder, With mild use disorder
F19.17	Other (or unknown) substance–induced major neurocognitive disorder, With mild use disorder
F19.180	Other (or unknown) substance–induced anxiety disorder, With mild use disorder
F19.181	Other (or unknown) substance–induced sexual dysfunction, With mild use disorder
F19.182	Other (or unknown) substance–induced sleep disorder, With mild use disorder
F19.188	Other (or unknown) substance–induced mild neurocognitive disorder, With mild use disorder
F19.188	Other (or unknown) substance–induced obsessive-compulsive and related disorder, With mild use disorder
F19.20	Other (or unknown) substance use disorder, Moderate
F19.20	Other (or unknown) substance use disorder, Severe
F19.221	Other (or unknown) substance intoxication delirium, With moderate or severe use disorder
F19.229	Other (or unknown) substance intoxication, With moderate or severe use disorder
F19.231	Other (or unknown) substance withdrawal delirium
F19.239	Other (or unknown) substance withdrawal
F19.24	Other (or unknown) substance–induced bipolar and related disorder, With moderate or severe use disorder
F19.24	Other (or unknown) substance–induced depressive disorder, With moderate or severe use disorder
F19.259	Other (or unknown) substance–induced psychotic disorder, With moderate or severe use disorder
F19.27	Other (or unknown) substance–induced major neurocognitive disorder, With moderate or severe use disorder

ICD-10-CM	Disorder, condition, or problem
F19.280	Other (or unknown) substance–induced anxiety disorder, With moderate or severe use disorder
F19.281	Other (or unknown) substance–induced sexual dysfunction, With moderate or severe use disorder
F19.282	Other (or unknown) substance–induced sleep disorder, With moderate or severe use disorder
F19.288	Other (or unknown) substance–induced mild neurocognitive disorder, With moderate or severe use disorder
F19.288	Other (or unknown) substance–induced obsessive-compulsive and related disorder, With moderate or severe use disorder
F19.921	Other (or unknown) substance–induced delirium
F19.921	Other (or unknown) substance intoxication delirium, Without use disorder
F19.929	Other (or unknown) substance intoxication, Without use disorder
F19.94	Other (or unknown) substance–induced bipolar and related disorder, Without use disorder
F19.94	Other (or unknown) substance–induced depressive disorder, Without use disorder
F19.959	Other (or unknown) substance–induced psychotic disorder, Without use disorder
F19.97	Other (or unknown) substance–induced major neurocognitive disorder, Without use disorder
F19.980	Other (or unknown) substance–induced anxiety disorder, Without use disorder
F19.981	Other (or unknown) substance–induced sexual dysfunction, Without use disorder
F19.982	Other (or unknown) substance–induced sleep disorder, Without use disorder
F19.988	Other (or unknown) substance–induced mild neurocognitive disorder, Without use disorder
F19.988	Other (or unknown) substance–induced obsessive-compulsive and related disorder, Without use disorder
F19.99	Unspecified other (or unknown) substance–related disorder
F20.81	Schizophreniform disorder
F20.9	Schizophrenia
F21	Schizotypal personality disorder
F22	Delusional disorder
F23	Brief psychotic disorder
F25.0	Schizoaffective disorder, Bipolar type
F25.1	Schizoaffective disorder, Depressive type
F28	Other specified schizophrenia spectrum and other psychotic disorder
F29	Unspecified schizophrenia spectrum and other psychotic disorder
F31.0	Bipolar I disorder, Current or most recent episode hypomanic
F31.11	Bipolar I disorder, Current or most recent episode manic, Mild
F31.12	Bipolar I disorder, Current or most recent episode manic, Moderate
F31.13	Bipolar I disorder, Current or most recent episode manic, Severe
F31.2	Bipolar I disorder, Current or most recent episode manic, With psychotic features
F31.31	Bipolar I disorder, Current or most recent episode depressed, Mild
F31.32	Bipolar I disorder, Current or most recent episode depressed, Moderate
F31.4	Bipolar I disorder, Current or most recent episode depressed, Severe
F31.5	Bipolar I disorder, Current or most recent episode depressed, With psychotic features

ICD-10-CM	Disorder, condition, or problem
F31.71	Bipolar I disorder, Current or most recent episode hypomanic, In partial remission
F31.72	Bipolar I disorder, Current or most recent episode hypomanic, In full remission
F31.73	Bipolar I disorder, Current or most recent episode manic, In partial remission
F31.74	Bipolar I disorder, Current or most recent episode manic, In full remission
F31.75	Bipolar I disorder, Current or most recent episode depressed, In partial remission
F31.76	Bipolar I disorder, Current or most recent episode depressed, In full remission
F31.81	Bipolar II disorder
F31.89	Other specified bipolar and related disorder
F31.9	Bipolar I disorder, Current or most recent episode depressed, Unspecified
F31.9	Bipolar I disorder, Current or most recent episode hypomanic, Unspecified
F31.9	Bipolar I disorder, Current or most recent episode manic, Unspecified
F31.9	Bipolar I disorder, Current or most recent episode unspecified
F31.9	Unspecified bipolar and related disorder
F32.0	Major depressive disorder, Single episode, Mild
F32.1	Major depressive disorder, Single episode, Moderate
F32.2	Major depressive disorder, Single episode, Severe
F32.3	Major depressive disorder, Single episode, With psychotic features
F32.4	Major depressive disorder, Single episode, In partial remission
F32.5	Major depressive disorder, Single episode, In full remission
F32.81	Premenstrual dysphoric disorder
F32.89	Other specified depressive disorder
F32.9	Major depressive disorder, Single episode, Unspecified
F32.9	Unspecified depressive disorder
F33.0	Major depressive disorder, Recurrent episode, Mild
F33.1	Major depressive disorder, Recurrent episode, Moderate
F33.2	Major depressive disorder, Recurrent episode, Severe
F33.3	Major depressive disorder, Recurrent episode, With psychotic features
F33.41	Major depressive disorder, Recurrent episode, In partial remission
F33.42	Major depressive disorder, Recurrent episode, In full remission
F33.9	Major depressive disorder, Recurrent episode, Unspecified
F34.0	Cyclothymic disorder
F34.1	Persistent depressive disorder (dysthymia)
F34.81	Disruptive mood dysregulation disorder
F40.00	Agoraphobia
F40.10	Social anxiety disorder (social phobia)
F40.218	Specific phobia, Animal
F40.228	Specific phobia, Natural environment
F40.230	Specific phobia, Fear of blood
F40.231	Specific phobia, Fear of injections and transfusions
F40.232	Specific phobia, Fear of other medical care
F40.233	Specific phobia, Fear of injury
F40.248	Specific phobia, Situational
F40.298	Specific phobia, Other
F41.0	Panic disorder
F41.1	Generalized anxiety disorder
F41.8	Other specified anxiety disorder

ICD-10-CM	Disorder, condition, or problem
F41.9	Unspecified anxiety disorder
F42.2	Obsessive-compulsive disorder
F42.3	Hoarding disorder
F42.4	Excoriation (skin-picking) disorder
F42.8	Other specified obsessive-compulsive and related disorder
F42.9	Unspecified obsessive-compulsive and related disorder
F43.0	Acute stress disorder
F43.10	Posttraumatic stress disorder
F43.20	Adjustment disorders, Unspecified
F43.21	Adjustment disorders, With depressed mood
F43.22	Adjustment disorders, With anxiety
F43.23	Adjustment disorders, With mixed anxiety and depressed mood
F43.24	Adjustment disorders, With disturbance of conduct
F43.25	Adjustment disorders, With mixed disturbance of emotions and conduct
F43.8	Other specified trauma- and stressor-related disorder
F43.9	Unspecified trauma- and stressor-related disorder
F44.0	Dissociative amnesia
F44.1	Dissociative amnesia, With dissociative fugue
F44.4	Conversion disorder (functional neurological symptom disorder), With abnormal movement
F44.4	Conversion disorder (functional neurological symptom disorder), With speech symptoms
F44.4	Conversion disorder (functional neurological symptom disorder), With swallowing symptoms
F44.4	Conversion disorder (functional neurological symptom disorder), With weakness/paralysis
F44.5	Conversion disorder (functional neurological symptom disorder), With attacks or seizures
F44.6	Conversion disorder (functional neurological symptom disorder), With anesthesia or sensory loss
F44.6	Conversion disorder (functional neurological symptom disorder), With special sensory symptoms
F44.7	Conversion disorder (functional neurological symptom disorder), With mixed symptoms
F44.81	Dissociative identity disorder
F44.89	Other specified dissociative disorder
F44.9	Unspecified dissociative disorder
F45.1	Somatic symptom disorder
F45.21	Illness anxiety disorder
F45.22	Body dysmorphic disorder
F45.8	Other specified somatic symptom and related disorder
F45.9	Unspecified somatic symptom and related disorder
F48.1	Depersonalization/derealization disorder
F50.01	Anorexia nervosa, Restricting type
F50.02	Anorexia nervosa, Binge-eating/purging type
F50.2	Bulimia nervosa
F50.81	Binge-eating disorder

ICD-10-CM	Disorder, condition, or problem
F50.89	Avoidant/restrictive food intake disorder
F50.89	Other specified feeding or eating disorder
F50.89	Pica, in adults
F50.9	Unspecified feeding or eating disorder
F51.01	Insomnia disorder
F51.11	Hypersomnolence disorder
F51.3	Non–rapid eye movement sleep arousal disorders, Sleepwalking type
F51.4	Non–rapid eye movement sleep arousal disorders, Sleep terror type
F51.5	Nightmare disorder
F52.0	Male hypoactive sexual desire disorder
F52.21	Erectile disorder
F52.22	Female sexual interest/arousal disorder
F52.31	Female orgasmic disorder
F52.32	Delayed ejaculation
F52.4	Premature (early) ejaculation
F52.6	Genito-pelvic pain/penetration disorder
F52.8	Other specified sexual dysfunction
F52.9	Unspecified sexual dysfunction
F54	Psychological factors affecting other medical conditions
F60.0	Paranoid personality disorder
F60.1	Schizoid personality disorder
F60.2	Antisocial personality disorder
F60.3	Borderline personality disorder
F60.4	Histrionic personality disorder
F60.5	Obsessive-compulsive personality disorder
F60.6	Avoidant personality disorder
F60.7	Dependent personality disorder
F60.81	Narcissistic personality disorder
F60.89	Other specified personality disorder
F60.9	Unspecified personality disorder
F63.0	Gambling disorder
F63.1	Pyromania
F63.2	Kleptomania
F63.3	Trichotillomania (hair-pulling disorder)
F63.81	Intermittent explosive disorder
F64.0	Gender dysphoria in adolescents and adults
F64.2	Gender dysphoria in children
F64.8	Other specified gender dysphoria
F64.9	Unspecified gender dysphoria
F65.0	Fetishistic disorder
F65.1	Transvestic disorder
F65.2	Exhibitionistic disorder
F65.3	Voyeuristic disorder
F65.4	Pedophilic disorder
F65.51	Sexual masochism disorder
F65.52	Sexual sadism disorder

ICD-10-CM	Disorder, condition, or problem
F65.81	Frotteuristic disorder
F65.89	Other specified paraphilic disorder
F65.9	Unspecified paraphilic disorder
F68.10	Factitious disorder
F70	Intellectual disability (intellectual developmental disorder), Mild
F71	Intellectual disability (intellectual developmental disorder), Moderate
F72	Intellectual disability (intellectual developmental disorder), Severe
F73	Intellectual disability (intellectual developmental disorder), Profound
F79	Unspecified intellectual disability (intellectual developmental disorder)
F80.0	Speech sound disorder
F80.2	Language disorder
F80.81	Childhood-onset fluency disorder (stuttering)
F80.82	Social (pragmatic) communication disorder
F80.9	Unspecified communication disorder
F81.0	Specific learning disorder, With impairment in reading
F81.2	Specific learning disorder, With impairment in mathematics
F81.81	Specific learning disorder, With impairment in written expression
F82	Developmental coordination disorder
F84.0	Autism spectrum disorder
F88	Global developmental delay
F88	Other specified neurodevelopmental disorder
F89	Unspecified neurodevelopmental disorder
F90.0	Attention-deficit/hyperactivity disorder, Predominantly inattentive presentation
F90.1	Attention-deficit/hyperactivity disorder, Predominantly hyperactive/impulsive presentation
F90.2	Attention-deficit/hyperactivity disorder, Combined presentation
F90.8	Other specified attention-deficit/hyperactivity disorder
F90.9	Unspecified attention-deficit/hyperactivity disorder
F91.1	Conduct disorder, Childhood-onset type
F91.2	Conduct disorder, Adolescent-onset type
F91.3	Oppositional defiant disorder
F91.8	Other specified disruptive, impulse-control, and conduct disorder
F91.9	Conduct disorder, Unspecified onset
F91.9	Unspecified disruptive, impulse-control, and conduct disorder
F93.0	Separation anxiety disorder
F94.0	Selective mutism
F94.1	Reactive attachment disorder
F94.2	Disinhibited social engagement disorder
F95.0	Provisional tic disorder
F95.1	Persistent (chronic) motor or vocal tic disorder
F95.2	Tourette's disorder
F95.8	Other specified tic disorder
F95.9	Unspecified tic disorder
F98.0	Enuresis
F98.1	Encopresis
F98.21	Rumination disorder

ICD-10-CM	Disorder, condition, or problem
F98.3	Pica, in children
F98.4	Stereotypic movement disorder
F98.5	Adult-onset fluency disorder
F99	Other specified mental disorder
F99	Unspecified mental disorder
G21.0	Neuroleptic malignant syndrome
G21.11	Neuroleptic-induced parkinsonism
G21.19	Other medication-induced parkinsonism
G24.01	Tardive dyskinesia
G24.02	Medication-induced acute dystonia
G24.09	Tardive dystonia
G25.1	Medication-induced postural tremor
G25.71	Medication-induced acute akathisia
G25.71	Tardive akathisia
G25.79	Other medication-induced movement disorder
G25.81	Restless legs syndrome
G31.84	Mild frontotemporal neurocognitive disorder
G31.84	Mild neurocognitive disorder due to Alzheimer's disease
G31.84	Mild neurocognitive disorder due to another medical condition
G31.84	Mild neurocognitive disorder due to HIV infection
G31.84	Mild neurocognitive disorder due to Huntington's disease
G31.84	Mild neurocognitive disorder with Lewy bodies
G31.84	Mild neurocognitive disorder due to multiple etiologies
G31.84	Mild neurocognitive disorder due to Parkinson's disease
G31.84	Mild neurocognitive disorder due to prion disease
G31.84	Mild neurocognitive disorder due to traumatic brain injury
G31.84	Mild vascular neurocognitive disorder
G31.9	Major neurocognitive disorder possibly due to Parkinson's disease
G31.9	Possible major frontotemporal neurocognitive disorder
G31.9	Possible major neurocognitive disorder due to Alzheimer's disease
G31.9	Possible major neurocognitive disorder with Lewy bodies
G31.9	Possible major vascular neurocognitive disorder
G47.00	Unspecified insomnia disorder
G47.09	Other specified insomnia disorder
G47.10	Unspecified hypersomnolence disorder
G47.19	Other specified hypersomnolence disorder
G47.20	Circadian rhythm sleep-wake disorders, Unspecified type
G47.21	Circadian rhythm sleep-wake disorders, Delayed sleep phase type
G47.22	Circadian rhythm sleep-wake disorders, Advanced sleep phase type
G47.23	Circadian rhythm sleep-wake disorders, Irregular sleep-wake type
G47.24	Circadian rhythm sleep-wake disorders, Non-24-hour sleep-wake type
G47.26	Circadian rhythm sleep-wake disorders, Shift work type
G47.31	Central sleep apnea, Idiopathic central sleep apnea

ICD-10-CM	Disorder, condition, or problem
G47.33	Obstructive sleep apnea hypopnea
G47.34	Sleep-related hypoventilation, Idiopathic hypoventilation
G47.35	Sleep-related hypoventilation, Congenital central alveolar hypoventilation
G47.36	Sleep-related hypoventilation, Comorbid sleep-related hypoventilation
G47.37	Central sleep apnea comorbid with opioid use
G47.411	Narcolepsy with cataplexy but without hypocretin deficiency
G47.419	Autosomal dominant cerebellar ataxia, deafness, and narcolepsy
G47.419	Autosomal dominant narcolepsy, obesity, and type 2 diabetes
G47.419	Narcolepsy without cataplexy but with hypocretin deficiency
G47.429	Narcolepsy secondary to another medical condition
G47.52	Rapid eye movement sleep behavior disorder
G47.8	Other specified sleep-wake disorder
G47.9	Unspecified sleep-wake disorder
N39.498	Other specified elimination disorder, With urinary symptoms
R06.3	Central sleep apnea, Cheyne-Stokes breathing
R15.9	Other specified elimination disorder, With fecal symptoms
R15.9	Unspecified elimination disorder, With fecal symptoms
R32	Unspecified elimination disorder, With urinary symptoms
R41.0	Other specified delirium
R41.0	Unspecified delirium
R41.83	Borderline intellectual functioning
R41.9	Unspecified neurocognitive disorder
T43.205A	Antidepressant discontinuation syndrome, Initial encounter
T43.205D	Antidepressant discontinuation syndrome, Subsequent encounter
T43.205S	Antidepressant discontinuation syndrome, Sequelae
T50.905A	Other adverse effect of medication, Initial encounter
T50.905D	Other adverse effect of medication, Subsequent encounter
T50.905S	Other adverse effect of medication, Sequelae
T74.01XA	Spouse or partner neglect, Confirmed, Initial encounter
T74.01XD	Spouse or partner neglect, Confirmed, Subsequent encounter
T74.02XA	Child neglect, Confirmed, Initial encounter
T74.02XD	Child neglect, Confirmed, Subsequent encounter
T74.11XA	Adult physical abuse by nonspouse or nonpartner, Confirmed, Initial encounter
T74.11XA	Spouse or partner violence, Physical, Confirmed, Initial encounter
T74.11XD	Adult physical abuse by nonspouse or nonpartner, Confirmed, Subsequent encounter
T74.11XD	Spouse or partner violence, Physical, Confirmed, Subsequent encounter
T74.12XA	Child physical abuse, Confirmed, Initial encounter
T74.12XD	Child physical abuse, Confirmed, Subsequent encounter
T74.21XA	Adult sexual abuse by nonspouse or nonpartner, Confirmed, Initial encounter
T74.21XA	Spouse or partner violence, Sexual, Confirmed, Initial encounter
T74.21XD	Adult sexual abuse by nonspouse or nonpartner, Confirmed, Subsequent encounter

ICD-10-CM	Disorder, condition, or problem
T74.21XD	Spouse or partner violence, Sexual, Confirmed, Subsequent encounter
T74.22XA	Child sexual abuse, Confirmed, Initial encounter
T74.22XD	Child sexual abuse, Confirmed, Subsequent encounter
T74.31XA	Adult psychological abuse by nonspouse or nonpartner, Confirmed, Initial encounter
T74.31XA	Spouse or partner abuse, Psychological, Confirmed, Initial encounter
T74.31XD	Adult psychological abuse by nonspouse or nonpartner, Confirmed, Subsequent encounter
T74.31XD	Spouse or partner abuse, Psychological, Confirmed, Subsequent encounter
T74.32XA	Child psychological abuse, Confirmed, Initial encounter
T74.32XD	Child psychological abuse, Confirmed, Subsequent encounter
T76.01XA	Spouse or partner neglect, Suspected, Initial encounter
T76.01XD	Spouse or partner neglect, Suspected, Subsequent encounter
T76.02XA	Child neglect, Suspected, Initial encounter
T76.02XD	Child neglect, Suspected, Subsequent encounter
T76.11XA	Adult physical abuse by nonspouse or nonpartner, Suspected, Initial encounter
T76.11XA	Spouse or partner violence, Physical, Suspected, Initial encounter
T76.11XD	Adult physical abuse by nonspouse or nonpartner, Suspected, Subsequent encounter
T76.11XD	Spouse or partner violence, Physical, Suspected, Subsequent encounter
T76.12XA	Child physical abuse, Suspected, Initial encounter
T76.12XD	Child physical abuse, Suspected, Subsequent encounter
T76.21XA	Adult sexual abuse by nonspouse or nonpartner, Suspected, Initial encounter
T76.21XA	Spouse or partner violence, Sexual, Suspected, Initial encounter
T76.21XD	Adult sexual abuse by nonspouse or nonpartner, Suspected, Subsequent encounter
T76.21XD	Spouse or partner violence, Sexual, Suspected, Subsequent encounter
T76.22XA	Child sexual abuse, Suspected, Initial encounter
T76.22XD	Child sexual abuse, Suspected, Subsequent encounter
T76.31XA	Adult psychological abuse by nonspouse or nonpartner, Suspected, Initial encounter
T76.31XA	Spouse or partner abuse, Psychological, Suspected, Initial encounter
T76.31XD	Adult psychological abuse by nonspouse or nonpartner, Suspected, Subsequent encounter
T76.31XD	Spouse or partner abuse, Psychological, Suspected, Subsequent encounter
T76.32XA	Child psychological abuse, Suspected, Initial encounter
T76.32XD	Child psychological abuse, Suspected, Subsequent encounter
Z55.9	Academic or educational problem
Z56.82	Problem related to current military deployment status
Z56.9	Other problem related to employment
Z59.0	Homelessness
Z59.1	Inadequate housing
Z59.2	Discord with neighbor, lodger, or landlord
Z59.3	Problem related to living in a residential institution
Z59.4	Lack of adequate food or safe drinking water
Z59.5	Extreme poverty

ICD-10-CM	Disorder, condition, or problem
Z59.6	Low income
Z59.7	Insufficient social insurance or welfare support
Z59.9	Unspecified housing or economic problem
Z60.0	Phase of life problem
Z60.2	Problem related to living alone
Z60.3	Acculturation difficulty
Z60.4	Social exclusion or rejection
Z60.5	Target of (perceived) adverse discrimination or persecution
Z60.9	Unspecified problem related to social environment
Z62.29	Upbringing away from parents
Z62.810	Personal history (past history) of physical abuse in childhood
Z62.810	Personal history (past history) of sexual abuse in childhood
Z62.811	Personal history (past history) of psychological abuse in childhood
Z62.812	Personal history (past history) of neglect in childhood
Z62.820	Parent-child relational problem
Z62.891	Sibling relational problem
Z62.898	Child affected by parental relationship distress
Z63.0	Relationship distress with spouse or intimate partner
Z63.4	Uncomplicated bereavement
Z63.5	Disruption of family by separation or divorce
Z63.8	High expressed emotion level within family
Z64.0	Problems related to unwanted pregnancy
Z64.1	Problems related to multiparity
Z64.4	Discord with social service provider, including probation officer, case manager, or social services worker
Z65.0	Conviction in civil or criminal proceedings without imprisonment
Z65.1	Imprisonment or other incarceration
Z65.2	Problems related to release from prison
Z65.3	Problems related to other legal circumstances
Z65.4	Victim of crime
Z65.4	Victim of terrorism or torture
Z65.5	Exposure to disaster, war, or other hostilities
Z65.8	Other problem related to psychosocial circumstances
Z65.8	Religious or spiritual problem
Z65.9	Unspecified problem related to unspecified psychosocial circumstances
Z69.010	Encounter for mental health services for victim of child abuse by parent
Z69.010	Encounter for mental health services for victim of child neglect by parent
Z69.010	Encounter for mental health services for victim of child psychological abuse by parent
Z69.010	Encounter for mental health services for victim of child sexual abuse by parent
Z69.011	Encounter for mental health services for perpetrator of parental child abuse
Z69.011	Encounter for mental health services for perpetrator of parental child neglect
Z69.011	Encounter for mental health services for perpetrator of parental child psychological abuse
Z69.011	Encounter for mental health services for perpetrator of parental child sexual abuse
Z69.020	Encounter for mental health services for victim of nonparental child abuse

ICD-10-CM	Disorder, condition, or problem
Z69.020	Encounter for mental health services for victim of nonparental child neglect
Z69.020	Encounter for mental health services for victim of nonparental child psychological abuse
Z69.020	Encounter for mental health services for victim of nonparental child sexual abuse
Z69.021	Encounter for mental health services for perpetrator of nonparental child abuse
Z69.021	Encounter for mental health services for perpetrator of nonparental child neglect
Z69.021	Encounter for mental health services for perpetrator of nonparental child psychological abuse
Z69.021	Encounter for mental health services for perpetrator of nonparental child sexual abuse
Z69.11	Encounter for mental health services for victim of spouse or partner neglect
Z69.11	Encounter for mental health services for victim of spouse or partner psychological abuse
Z69.11	Encounter for mental health services for victim of spouse or partner violence, Physical
Z69.12	Encounter for mental health services for perpetrator of spouse or partner neglect
Z69.12	Encounter for mental health services for perpetrator of spouse or partner psychological abuse
Z69.12	Encounter for mental health services for perpetrator of spouse or partner violence, Physical
Z69.12	Encounter for mental health services for perpetrator of spouse or partner violence, Sexual
Z69.81	Encounter for mental health services for victim of nonspousal adult abuse
Z69.81	Encounter for mental health services for victim of spouse or partner violence, Sexual
Z69.82	Encounter for mental health services for perpetrator of nonspousal adult abuse
Z70.9	Sex counseling
Z71.9	Other counseling or consultation
Z72.0	Tobacco use disorder, mild
Z72.810	Child or adolescent antisocial behavior
Z72.811	Adult antisocial behavior
Z72.9	Problem related to lifestyle
Z75.3	Unavailability or inaccessibility of health care facilities
Z75.4	Unavailability or inaccessibility of other helping agencies
Z76.5	Malingering
Z91.19	Nonadherence to medical treatment
Z91.410	Personal history (past history) of spouse or partner violence, Physical
Z91.410	Personal history (past history) of spouse or partner violence, Sexual
Z91.411	Personal history (past history) of spouse or partner psychological abuse
Z91.412	Personal history (past history) of spouse or partner neglect
Z91.49	Other personal history of psychological trauma
Z91.5	Personal history of self-harm
Z91.82	Personal history of military deployment
Z91.83	Wandering associated with a mental disorder
Z91.89	Other personal risk factors

DSM-5 Advisors and Other Contributors

Past DSM-5 APA Staff

Erin J. Dalder-Alpher
Kristin Edwards
Leah I. Engel

Lenna Jawdat
Elizabeth C. Martin
Rocio J. Salvador

Work Group Advisors

ADHD and Disruptive Behavior Disorders

Emil F. Coccaro, M.D.
Deborah Dabrick, Ph.D.
Prudence W. Fisher, Ph.D.
Benjamin B. Lahey, Ph.D.
Salvatore Mannuzza, Ph.D.
Mary Solanto, Ph.D.
J. Blake Turner, Ph.D.
Eric Youngstrom, Ph.D.

Anxiety, Obsessive-Compulsive Spectrum, Posttraumatic, and Dissociative Disorders

Lynn E. Alden, Ph.D.
David B. Arciniegas, M.D.
David H. Barlow, Ph.D.
Katja Beesdo-Baum, Ph.D.
Chris R. Brewin, Ph.D.
Richard J. Brown, Ph.D.
Timothy A. Brown, Ph.D.
Richard A. Bryant, Ph.D.
Joan M. Cook, Ph.D.
Joop de Jong, M.D., Ph.D.
Paul F. Dell, Ph.D.
Damiaan Denys, M.D.
Bruce P. Dohrenwend, Ph.D.
Brian A. Fallon, M.D., M.P.H.
Edna B. Foa, Ph.D.
Martin E. Franklin, Ph.D.
Wayne K. Goodman, M.D.
Jon E. Grant, J.D., M.D.
Bonnie L. Green, Ph.D.
Richard G. Heimberg, Ph.D.
Judith L. Herman, M.D.
Devon E. Hinton, M.D., Ph.D.
Stefan G. Hofmann, Ph.D.
Charles W. Hoge, M.D.
Terence M. Keane, Ph.D.
Nancy J. Keuthen, Ph.D.
Dean G. Kilpatrick, Ph.D.
Katharina Kircanski, Ph.D.
Laurence J. Kirmayer, M.D.
Donald F. Klein, M.D., D.Sc.
Amaro J. Laria, Ph.D.
Richard T. LeBeau, M.A.
Richard J. Loewenstein, M.D.
David Mataix-Cols, Ph.D.
Thomas W. McAllister, M.D.

Harrison G. Pope, M.D., M.P.H.
Ronald M. Rapee, Ph.D.
Steven A. Rasmussen, M.D.
Patricia A. Resick, Ph.D.
Vedat Sar, M.D.
Sanjaya Saxena, M.D.
Paula P. Schnurr, Ph.D.
M. Katherine Shear, M.D.
Daphne Simeon, M.D.
Harvey S. Singer, M.D.
Melinda A. Stanley, Ph.D.
James J. Strain, M.D.
Kate Wolitzky Taylor, Ph.D.
Onno van der Hart, Ph.D.
Eric Vermetten, M.D., Ph.D.
John T. Walkup, M.D.
Sabine Wilhelm, Ph.D.
Douglas W. Woods, Ph.D.
Richard E. Zinbarg, Ph.D.
Joseph Zohar, M.D.

Childhood and Adolescent Disorders

Adrian Angold, Ph.D.
Deborah Beidel, Ph.D.
David Brent, M.D.
John Campo, M.D.
Gabrielle Carlson, M.D.
Prudence W. Fisher, Ph.D.
David Klonsky, Ph.D.
Matthew Nock, Ph.D.
J. Blake Turner, Ph.D.

Eating Disorders

Michael J. Devlin, M.D.
Denise E. Wilfley, Ph.D.
Susan Z. Yanovski, M.D.

Mood Disorders

Boris Birmaher, M.D.
Yeates Conwell, M.D.
Ellen B. Dennehy, Ph.D.
S. Ann Hartlage, Ph.D.
Jack M. Hettema, M.D., Ph.D.
Michael C. Neale, Ph.D.
Gordon B. Parker, M.D., Ph.D., D.Sc.
Roy H. Perlis, M.D. M.Sc.
Holly G. Prigerson, Ph.D.
Norman E. Rosenthal, M.D.
Peter J. Schmidt, M.D.

Mort M. Silverman, M.D.
Meir Steiner, M.D., Ph.D.
Mauricio Tohen, M.D., Dr.P.H., M.B.A.
Sidney Zisook, M.D.

Neurocognitive Disorders

Jiska Cohen-Mansfield, Ph.D.
Vladimir Hachinski, M.D., C.M., D.Sc.
Sharon Inouye, M.D., M.P.H.
Grant Iverson, Ph.D.
Laura Marsh, M.D.
Bruce Miller, M.D.
Jacobo Mintzer, M.D., M.B.A.
Bruce Pollock, M.D., Ph.D.
George Prigatano, Ph.D.
Ron Ruff, Ph.D.
Ingmar Skoog, M.D., Ph.D.
Robert Sweet, M.D.
Paula Trzepacz, M.D.

Neurodevelopmental Disorders

Ari Ne'eman
Nickola Nelson, Ph.D.
Diane Paul, Ph.D.
Eva Petrova, Ph.D.
Andrew Pickles, Ph.D.
Jan Piek, Ph.D.
Helene Polatajko, Ph.D.
Alya Reeve, M.D.
Mabel Rice, Ph.D.
Joseph Sergeant, Ph.D.
Bennett Shaywitz, M.D.
Sally Shaywitz, M.D.
Audrey Thurm, Ph.D.
Keith Widaman, Ph.D.
Warren Zigman, Ph.D.

Personality and Personality Disorders

Eran Chemerinski, M.D.
Thomas N. Crawford, Ph.D.
Harold W. Koenigsberg, M.D.
Kristian E. Markon, Ph.D.
Rebecca L. Shiner, Ph.D.
Kenneth R. Silk, M.D.
Jennifer L. Tackett, Ph.D.
David Watson, Ph.D.

Psychotic Disorders

Kamaldeep Bhui, M.D.
Manuel J. Cuesta, M.D., Ph.D.
Richard Douyon, M.D.
Paolo Fusar-Poli, Ph.D.
John H. Krystal, M.D.
Thomas H. McGlashan, M.D.
Victor Peralta, M.D., Ph.D.
Anita Riecher-Rössler, M.D.
Mary V. Seeman, M.D.

Sexual and Gender Identity Disorders

Stan E. Althof, Ph.D.
Richard Balon, M.D.
John H.J. Bancroft, M.D., M.A., D.P.M.
Howard E. Barbaree, Ph.D., M.A.
Rosemary J. Basson, M.D.
Sophie Bergeron, Ph.D.
Anita L. Clayton, M.D.
David L. Delmonico, Ph.D.
Domenico Di Ceglie, M.D.
Esther Gomez-Gil, M.D.
Jamison Green, Ph.D.
Richard Green, M.D, J.D.
R. Karl Hanson, Ph.D.
Lawrence Hartmann, M.D.
Stephen J. Hucker, M.B.
Eric S. Janus, J.D.
Patrick M. Jern, Ph.D.
Megan S. Kaplan, Ph.D.
Raymond A. Knight, Ph.D.
Ellen T.M. Laan, Ph.D.
Stephen B. Levine, M.D.
Christopher G. McMahon, M.B.
Marta Meana, Ph.D.
Michael H. Miner, Ph.D., M.A.
William T. O'Donohue, Ph.D.
Michael A. Perelman, Ph.D.
Caroline F. Pukall, Ph.D.
Robert E. Pyke, M.D., Ph.D.
Vernon L. Quinsey, Ph.D. M.Sc.
David L. Rowland, Ph.D., M.A.
Michael Sand, Ph.D., M.P.H.
Leslie R. Schover, Ph.D., M.A.
Paul Stern, B.S, J.D.
David Thornton, Ph.D.
Leonore Tiefer, Ph.D.
Douglas E. Tucker, M.D.
Jacques van Lankveld, Ph.D.
Marcel D. Waldinger, M.D., Ph.D.

Sleep-Wake Disorders

Donald L. Bliwise, Ph.D.
Daniel J. Buysse, M.D.
Vishesh K. Kapur, M.D., M.P.H.
Sanjeeve V. Kothare, M.D.
Kenneth L. Lichstein, Ph.D.
Mark W. Mahowald, M.D.
Rachel Manber, Ph.D.
Emmanuel Mignot, M.D., Ph.D.
Timothy H. Monk, Ph.D., D.Sc.
Thomas C. Neylan, M.D.
Maurice M. Ohayon, M.D., D.Sc., Ph.D.
Judith Owens, M.D., M.P.H.
Daniel L. Picchietti, M.D.
Stuart F. Quan, M.D.
Thomas Roth, Ph.D.
Daniel Weintraub, M.D.

Theresa B. Young, Ph.D.
Phyllis C. Zee, M.D., Ph.D.

Somatic Symptom Disorders

Brenda Bursch, Ph.D.
Kurt Kroenke, M.D.
W. Curt LaFrance, Jr., M.D., M.P.H.
Jon Stone, M.B., Ch.B., Ph.D.
Lynn M. Wegner, M.D.

Substance-Related Disorders

Raymond F. Anton, Jr., M.D.
Deborah A. Dawson, Ph.D.
Roland R. Griffiths, Ph.D.
Dorothy K. Hatsukami, Ph.D.
John E. Helzer, M.D.
Marilyn A. Huestis, Ph.D.
John R. Hughes, M.D.
Laura M. Juliano, Ph.D.
Thomas R. Kosten, M.D.
Nora D. Volkow, M.D.

DSM-5 Study Group and Other DSM-5 Group Advisors

Lifespan Developmental Approaches

Christina Bryant, Ph.D.
Amber Gum, Ph.D.
Thomas Meeks, M.D.
Jan Mohlman, Ph.D.
Steven Thorp, Ph.D.
Julie Wetherell, Ph.D.

Gender and Cross-Cultural Issues

Neil K. Aggarwal, M.D., M.B.A., M.A.
Sofie Bäärnhielm, M.D., Ph.D.
José J. Bauermeister, Ph.D.
James Boehnlein, M.D., M.Sc.
Jaswant Guzder, M.D.
Alejandro Interian, Ph.D.
Sushrut S. Jadhav, M.B.B.S., M.D., Ph.D.
Laurence J. Kirmayer, M.D.
Alex J. Kopelowicz, M.D.
Amaro J. Laria, Ph.D.
Steven R. Lopez, Ph.D.
Kwame J. McKenzie, M.D.
John R. Peteet, M.D.

Hans (J.G.B.M.) Rohlof, M.D.
Cecile Rousseau, M.D.
Mitchell G. Weiss, M.D., Ph.D.

Psychiatric/General Medical Interface

Daniel L. Coury, M.D.
Bernard P. Dreyer, M.D.
Danielle Laraque, M.D.
Lynn M. Wegner, M.D.

Impairment and Disability

Prudence W. Fisher, Ph.D.
Martin Prince, M.D., M.Sc.
Michael R. Von Korff, Sc.D.

Diagnostic Assessment Instruments

Prudence W. Fisher, Ph.D.
Robert D. Gibbons, Ph.D.
Ruben Gur, Ph.D.
John E. Helzer, M.D.
John Houston, M.D., Ph.D.
Kurt Kroenke, M.D.

Other Contributors/Consultants

ADHD and Disruptive Behavior Disorders

Patrick E. Shrout, Ph.D.
Erik Willcutt, Ph.D.

Anxiety, Obsessive-Compulsive Spectrum, Posttraumatic, and Dissociative Disorders

Etzel Cardeña, Ph.D.
Richard J. Castillo, Ph.D.
Eric Hollander, M.D.
Charlie Marmar, M.D.
Alfonso Martínez-Taboas, Ph.D.
Mark W. Miller, Ph.D.
Mark H. Pollack, M.D.
Heidi S. Resnick, Ph.D.

Childhood and Adolescent Disorders

Grace T. Baranek, Ph.D.
Colleen Jacobson, Ph.D.
Maria Oquendo, M.D.
Sir Michael Rutter, M.D.

Eating Disorders

Nancy L. Zucker, Ph.D.

Mood Disorders

Keith Hawton, M.D., Ph.D.
David A. Jobes, Ph.D.
Maria A. Oquendo, M.D.
Alan C. Swann, M.D.

Neurocognitive Disorders

J. Eric Ahlskog, M.D., Ph.D.
Allen J. Aksamit, M.D.
Marilyn Albert, Ph.D.
Guy Mckhann, M.D.
Bradley Boeve, M.D.
Helena Chui, M.D.
Sureyya Dikmen, Ph.D.
Douglas Galasko, M.D.
Harvey Levin, Ph.D.
Mark Lovell, Ph.D.
Jeffery Max, M.B.B.Ch.
Ian McKeith, M.D.
Cynthia Munro, Ph.D.
Marlene Oscar-Berman, Ph.D.
Alexander Troster, Ph.D.

Neurodevelopmental Disorders

Anna Barnett, Ph.D.
Martha Denckla, M.D.
Jack M. Fletcher, Ph.D.
Dido Green, Ph.D.
Stephen Greenspan, Ph.D.
Bruce Pennington, Ph.D.
Ruth Shalev, M.D.
Larry B. Silver, M.D.
Lauren Swineford, Ph.D.
Michael Von Aster, M.D.

Personality and Personality Disorders

Patricia R. Cohen, Ph.D.
Jaime L. Derringer, Ph.D.
Lauren Helm, M.D.
Christopher J. Patrick, Ph.D.
Anthony Pinto, Ph.D.

Psychotic Disorders

Scott W. Woods, M.D.

Sexual and Gender Identity Disorders

Alan J. Riley, M.Sc.
Ray C. Rosen, Ph.D.

Sleep-Wake Disorders

Jack D. Edinger, Ph.D.
David Gozal, M.D.
Hochang B. Lee, M.D.
Tore A. Nielsen, Ph.D.
Michael J. Sateia, M.D.
Jamie M. Zeitzer, Ph.D.

Somatic Symptom Disorders

Chuck V. Ford, M.D.
Patricia I. Rosebush, M.Sc.N., M.D.

Substance-Related Disorders

Sally M. Anderson, Ph.D.
Julie A. Kable, Ph.D.
Christopher Martin, Ph.D.
Sarah N. Mattson, Ph.D.
Edward V. Nunes, Jr., M.D.
Mary J. O'Connor, Ph.D.
Heather Carmichael Olson, Ph.D.
Blair Paley, Ph.D.
Edward P. Riley, Ph.D.
Tulshi D. Saha, Ph.D.
Wim van den Brink, M.D., Ph.D.
George E. Woody, M.D.

Diagnostic Spectra and DSM/ICD Harmonization

Bruce Cuthbert, Ph.D.

Lifespan Developmental Approaches

Aartjan Beekman Ph.D.
Alistair Flint, M.B.
David Sultzer, M.D.
Ellen Whyte, M.D.

Gender and Cross-Cultural Issues

Sergio Aguilar-Gaxiola, M.D., Ph.D.
Kavoos G. Bassiri, M.S.
Venkataramana Bhat, M.D.
Marit Boiler, M.P.H.
Denise Canso, M.Sc.
Smita N. Deshpande, M.D., D.P.M.
Ravi DeSilva, M.D.
Esperanza Diaz, M.D.
Byron J. Good, Ph.D.
Simon Groen, M.A.
Ladson Hinton, M.D.
Lincoln I. Khasakhala, Ph.D.
Francis G. Lu, M.D.
Athena Madan, M.A.
Anne W. Mbwayo, Ph.D.
Oanh Meyer, Ph.D.
Victoria N. Mutiso, Ph.D., D.Sc.
David M. Ndetei, M.D.
Andel V. Nicasio, M.S.Ed.
Vasudeo Paralikar, M.D., Ph.D.
Kanak Patil, M.A.
Filipa I. Santos, H.B.Sc.
Sanjeev B. Sarmukaddam, Ph.D., M.Sc.
Monica Z. Scalco, M.D., Ph.D.
Katie Thompson, M.A.
Hendry Ton, M.D., M.Sc.
Rob C.J. van Dijk, M.Sc.
William A. Vega, Ph.D.
Johann M. Vega-Dienstmaier, M.D.
Joseph Westermeyer, M.D., Ph.D.

Psychiatric/General Medical Interface

Daniel J. Balog, M.D.
Charles C. Engel, M.D., M.P.H.
Charles D. Motsinger, M.D.

Impairment and Disability

Cille Kennedy, Ph.D.

Diagnostic Assessment Instruments

Paul J. Pikonis, Ph.D.

Other Conditions That May Be a Focus of Clinical Attention

William E. Narrow, M.D., M.P.H., *Chair*
Roger Peele, M.D.
Lawson R. Wulsin, M.D.
Charles H. Zeanah, M.D.
Prudence W. Fisher, Ph.D., *Advisor*
Stanley N. Caroff, M.D., *Contributor/Consultant*
James B. Lohr, M.D., *Contributor/Consultant*
Marianne Wambolt, Ph.D., *Contributor/Consultant*

DSM-5 Research Group

Allan Donner, Ph.D.

CPHC Peer Reviewers

Kenneth Altshuler, M.D.
Pedro G. Alvarenga, M.D.
Diana J. Antonacci, M.D.
Richard Balon, M.D.
David H. Barlow, Ph.D.
L. Jarrett Barnhill, M.D.
Katja Beesdo-Baum, Ph.D.
Marty Boman, Ed.D.
James Bourgeois, M.D.
David Braff, M.D.
Harry Brandt, M.D.
Kirk Brower, M.D.
Rachel Bryant-Waugh, Ph.D.
Jack D. Burke Jr., M.D., M.P.H.
Brenda Bursch, Ph.D.
Joseph Camilleri, M.D.
Patricia Casey, M.D.
F. Xavier Castellanos, M.D.
Eran Chemerinski, M.D.
Wai Chen, M.D.
Elie Cheniaux, M.D., D.Sc.
Cheryl Chessick, M.D,
J. Richard Ciccone, M.D.
Anita H. Clayton, M.D.
Tihalia J. Coleman, Ph.D.
John Csernansky, M.D.
Manuel J. Cuesta M.D., Ph.D.
Joanne L. Davis, M.D.
David L. Delmonico, Ph.D.
Ray J. DePaulo, M.D.
Dimitris Dikeos, M.D.
Ina E. Djonlagic, M.D.
C. Neill Epperson, M.D.
Javier I. Escobar, M.D., M.Sc.
Spencer Eth, M.D.
David Fassler, M.D.
Giovanni A. Fava, M.D.
Robert Feinstein, M.D.
Molly Finnerty, M.D.
Mark H. Fleisher, M.D.
Alessio Florentini, M.D.

Laura Fochtmann, M.D.
Marshal Forstein, M.D.
William French, M.D.
Maximillian Gahr, M.D.
Cynthia Geppert, M.D.
Ann Germaine, Ph.D.
Marcia Goin, M.D.
David A. Gorelick, M.D., Ph.D.
David Graeber, M.D.
Cynthia A. Graham, Ph.D.
Andreas Hartmann, M.D.
Victoria Hendrick, M.D.
Merrill Herman, M.D.
David Herzog, M.D.
Mardi Horowitz, M.D.
Ya-fen Huang, M.D.
Anthony Kales, M.D
Niranjan S. Karnik, M.D., Ph.D.
Jeffrey Katzman, M.D.
Bryan King, M.D.
Cecilia Kjellgren, M.D.
Harold W. Koenigsberg, M.D.
Richard B. Krueger, M.D.
Steven Lamberti, M.D.
Ruth A. Lanius, M.D.
John Lauriello, M.D.
Anthony Lehman, M.D.
Michael Linden, M.D.
Mark W. Mahowald, M.D.
Marsha D. Marcus, Ph.D.
Stephen Marder, M.D.
Wendy Marsh, M.D.
Michael S. McCloskey, Ph.D.
Jeffrey Metzner, M.D.
Robert Michels, M.D.
Laura Miller, M.D.
Michael C. Miller, M.D.
Frederick Moeller, M.D.
Peter T. Morgan, M.D., Ph.D.
Madhav Muppa, M.D.
Philip Muskin, M.D.

Joachim Nitschke, M.D.
Abraham Nussbaum, M.D.
Ann Olincy, M.D.
Mark Onslow, Ph.D.
Sally Ozonoff, Ph.D.
John R. Peteet, M.D.
Ismene L. Petrakis, M.D.
Christophe M. Pfeiffer, M.D.
Karen Pierce, M.D.
Belinda Plattner, M.D.
Franklin Putnam, M.D.
Stuart F. Quan, M.D.
John Racy, M.D.
Phillip Resnick, M.D.
Michele Riba, M.D.
Jerold Rosenbaum, M.D.
Stephen Ross, M.D.
Lawrence Scahill, M.S.N., Ph.D.
Daniel Schechter, M.D.
Mary V. Seeman, M.D.
Alessandro Serretti, M.D.
Jianhua Shen, M.D.

Ravi Kumar R. Singareddy, M.D.
Ingmar Skoog, M.D., Ph.D.
Gary Small, M.D.
Paul Soloff, M.D.
Christina Stadler, M.D., Ph.D.
Nada Stotland, M.D.
Neil Swerdlow, M.D.
Kim Tillery, Ph.D.
David Tolin, Ph.D.
Jayne Trachman, M.D.
Luke Tsai, M.D.
Ming T. Tsuang, M.D., Ph.D.
Richard Tuch, M.D.
Johan Verhulst, M.D.
B. Timothy Walsh, M.D.
Michael Weissberg, M.D.
Godehard Weniger, M.D.
Keith Widaman, Ph.D.
Thomas Wise, M.D.
George E. Woods, M.D.
Kimberly A. Yonkers, M.D.
Alexander Young, M.D.

DSM-5 Field Trials in Academic Clinical Centers— Adult Samples

David Geffen School of Medicine, University of California, Los Angeles

Investigator

Helen Lavretsky, M.D., Principal Investigator

Referring and Interviewing Clinicians

Jessica Brommelhoff, Ph.D.
Xavier Cagigas, Ph.D.
Paul Cernin, Ph.D.
Linda Ercoli, Ph.D.
Randall Espinoza, M.D.

Helen Lavretsky, M.D.
Jeanne Kim, Ph.D.
David Merrill, M.D.
Karen Miller, Ph.D.
Christopher Nunez, Ph.D.

Research Coordinators

Natalie St. Cyr, M.A., Lead Research
  Coordinator
Nora Nazarian, B.A.
Colin Shinn, M.A.

Centre for Addiction and Mental Health, Toronto, Ontario, Canada

Investigators

Bruce G. Pollock, M.D., Ph.D., Lead Principal
  Investigator
R. Michael Bagby, Ph.D., Principal Investigator
Kwame J. McKenzie, M.D., Principal
  Investigator
Tony P. George, M.D., Co-investigator
Lena C. Quilty, Ph.D., Co-investigator
Peter Voore, M.D., Co-investigator

Referring and Interviewing Clinicians

Donna E. Akman, Ph.D.
R. Michael Bagby, Ph.D.
Wayne C. V. Baici, M.D.
Crystal Baluyut, M.D.

Eva W. C. Chow, M.D., J.D., M.P.H.
Z. J. Daskalakis, M.D., Ph.D.
Pablo Diaz-Hermosillo, M.D.
George Foussias, M.Sc., M.D.
Paul A. Frewen, Ph.D.
Ariel Graff-Guerrero, M.D., M.Sc., Ph.D.
Margaret K. Hahn, M.D.
Lorena Hsu, Ph.D.
Justine Joseph, Ph.D.
Sean Kidd, Ph.D.
Kwame J. McKenzie, M.D.
Mahesh Menon, Ph.D.
Romina Mizrahi, M.D., Ph.D.
Daniel J. Mueller, M.D., Ph.D.
Lena C. Quilty, Ph.D.
Anthony C. Ruocco, Ph.D.

Jorge Soni, M.D.
Aristotle N. Voineskos, M.D., Ph.D.
George Voineskos, M.D.
Peter Voore, Ph.D.
Chris Watson, Ph.D.

Referring Clinicians
Ofer Agid, M.D.
Ash Bender, M.D.
Patricia Cavanagh, M.D.
Sarah Colman, M.D.
Vincenzo Deluca, M.D.
Justin Geagea, M.D.
David S. Goldbloom, M.D.
Daniel Greben, M.D.
Malati Gupta, M.D.
Ken Harrison, M.D.
Imraan Jeeva, M.D.
Joel Jeffries, M.B.
Judith Laposa, Ph.D.

Jan Malat, M.D.
Shelley McMain, Ph.D.
Bruce Pollock, M.D., Ph.D.
Andriy V. Samokhvalov, M.D., Ph.D.
Martin Strassnig, M.D.
Albert H. C. Wong, M.D., Ph.D.

Research Coordinators
Gloria I. Leo, M.A., Lead Research Coordinator
Anissa D. Bachan, B.A.
Bahar Haji-Khamneh, M.A.
Olga Likhodi, M.Sc.
Eleanor J. Liu, Ph.D.
Sarah A. McGee Ng, B.B.A.

Other Research Staff
Susan E. Dickens, M.A., Clinical Research
    Manager
Sandy Richards, B.Sc.N., Schizophrenia
    Research Manager

Dallas VA Medical Center, Dallas, Texas

Investigators
Carol S. North, M.D., M.P.E., Principal
    Investigator
Alina Suris, Ph.D., A.B.P.P., Principal
    Investigator

Referring and Interviewing Clinicians
Barry Ardolf, Psy.D.
Abila Awan, M.D.
Joel Baskin, M.D.
John Black, Ph.D.
Jeffrey Dodds, Ph.D.
Gloria Emmett, Ph.D.
Karma Hudson, M.D.
Jamylah Jackson, Ph.D., A.B.P.P.
Lynda Kirkland-Culp, Ph.D., A.B.P.P.
Heidi Koehler, Ph.D., A.B.P.P.
Elizabeth Lewis, Psy.D.
Aashish Parikh, M.D.
Reed Robinson, Ph.D.
Jheel Shah, M.D.
Geetha Shivakumar, M.D.
Sarah Spain, Ph.D., A.B.P.P.

Lisa Thoman, Ph.D.
Lia Thomas, M.D.
Jamie Zabukovec, Psy.D.
Mustafa Zaidi, M.D.
Andrea Zartman, Ph.D.

General Referral Sources
Robert Blake, L.M.S.W.
Evelyn Gibbs, L.M.S.W.
Michelle King-Thompson, L.M.S.W.

Research Coordinators
Jeannie B. Whitman, Ph.D., Lead Research
    Coordinator
Sunday Adewuyi, M.D.
Elizabeth Anderson, B.A.
Solaleh Azimipour, B.S.
Carissa Barney, B.S.
Kristie Cavazos, B.A.
Robert Devereaux, B.S.
Dana Downs, M.S., M.S.W.
Sharjeel Farooqui, M.D.
Julia Smith, Psy.D.
Kun-Ying H. Sung, B.S.

School of Medicine, The University of Texas San Antonio, San Antonio, Texas

Investigator
Mauricio Tohen, M.D., Dr.P.H., M.B.A.,
    Principal Investigator

Referring and Interviewing Clinicians
Suman Baddam, Psy.D.
Charles L. Bowden, M.D.

Nancy Diazgranados, M.D., M.S.
Craig A. Dike, Psy.D.
Dianne E. Dunn, Psy.D., M.P.H.
Elena Gherman, M.D.
Jodi M. Gonzalez, Ph.D.
Pablo Gonzalez, M.D.
Phillip Lai, Psy.D.

Natalie Maples-Aguilar, M.A., L.P.A.
Marlon P. Quinones, M.D.
Jeslina J. Raj, Psy.D.
David L. Roberts, Ph.D.
Nancy Sandusky, R.N., F.P.M.H.N.P.-B.C.,
　D.N.P.-C.
Donna S. Stutes, M.S., L.P.C.
Mauricio Tohen, M.D., Dr.PH, M.B.A.
Dawn I. Velligan, Ph.D.
Weiran Wu, M.D., Ph.D.

Referring Clinicians

Albana Dassori, M.D.
Megan Frederick, M.A.

Robert Gonzalez, M.D.
Uma Kasinath, M.D.
Camis Milam, M.D.
Vivek Singh, M.D.
Peter Thompson, M.D.

Research Coordinators

Melissa Hernandez, B.A., Lead Research
　Coordinator
Fermin Alejandro Carrizales, B.A.
Martha Dahl, R.N., B.S.N.
Patrick M. Smith, B.A.
Nicole B. Watson, M.A.

Michael E. DeBakey VA Medical Center and the Menninger Clinic, Houston, Texas (Joint Study Site)

Michael E. DeBakey VA Medical Center

Investigator

Laura Marsh, M.D., Principal Investigator

Referring and Interviewing Clinicians

Shalini Aggarwal, M.D.
Su Bailey, Ph.D.
Minnete (Helen) Beckner, Ph.D.
Crystal Clark, M.D.
Charles DeJohn, M.D.
Robert Garza, M.D.
Aruna Gottumakkla, M.D.
Janet Hickey, M.D.
James Ireland, M.D.
Mary Lois Lacey, A.P.R.N.
Wendy Leopoulos, M.D.
Laura Marsh, M.D.
Deleene Menefee, Ph.D.
Brian I. Miller, Ph.D.
Candy Smith, Ph.D.
Avila Steele, Ph.D.
Jill Wanner, Ph.D.
Rachel Wells, Ph.D.
Kaki York-Ward, Ph.D.

Referring Clinicians

Sara Allison, M.D.
Leonard Denney, L.C.S.W.
Catherine Flores, L.C.S.W.
Nathalie Marie, M.D.
Christopher Martin, M.D.
Sanjay Mathew, M.D.
Erica Montgomery, M.D.
Gregory Scholl, P.A.
Jocelyn Ulanday, M.D., M.P.H.

Research Coordinators

Sarah Neely Torres, B.S., Lead Research
　Coordinator
Kathleen Grout, M.A.
Lea Kiefer, M.P.H.
Jana Tran, M.A.

Volunteer Research Assistants

Catherine Clark
Linh Hoang

Menninger Clinic

Investigator

Efrain Bleiberg, M.D., Principal Investigator

Referring and Interviewing Clinicians

Jennifer Baumgardner, Ph.D.
Elizabeth Dodd Conaway, L.C.S.W., B.C.D.
Warren Christianson, D.O.
Wesley Clayton, L.M.S.W.
J. Christopher Fowler, Ph.D.
Michael Groat, Ph.D.
Edythe Harvey, M.D.
Denise Kagan, Ph.D.
Hans Meyer, L.C.S.W.

Segundo Robert-Ibarra, M.D.
Sandhya Trivedi, M.D.
Rebecca Wagner, Ph.D.
Harrell Woodson, Ph.D.
Amanda Yoder, L.C.S.W.

Referring Clinicians

James Flack, M.D.
David Ness, M.D.

Research Coordinators

Steve Herrera, B.S., M.T., Lead Research
　Coordinator
Allison Kalpakci, B.A.

Mayo Clinic, Rochester, Minnesota

Investigators

Mark A. Frye, M.D., Principal Investigator
Glenn E. Smith, Ph.D., Principal Investigator
Jeffrey P. Staab M.D., M.S., Principal
    Investigator

Referring and Interviewing Clinicians

Osama Abulseoud, M.D.
Jane Cerhan, Ph.D.
Julie Fields, Ph.D.
Mark A. Frye, M.D.
Manuel Fuentes, M.D.
Yonas Geda, M.D.
Maria Harmandayan, M.D.
Reba King, M.D.
Simon Kung, M.D.
Mary Machuda, Ph.D.
Donald McAlpine, M.D.
Alastair McKean, M.D.
Juliana Moraes, M.D.
Teresa Rummans, M.D.

James R. Rundell, M.D.
Richard Seime, Ph.D.
Glenn E. Smith, Ph.D.
Christopher Sola, D.O.
Jeffrey P. Staab M.D., M.S.
Marin Veldic, M.D.
Mark D. Williams, M.D.
Maya Yustis, Ph.D.

Research Coordinators

Lisa Seymour, B.S., Lead Research Coordinator
Scott Feeder, M.S.
Lee Gunderson, B.S.
Sherrie Hanna, M.A., L.P.
Kelly Harper, B.A.
Katie Mingo, B.A.
Cynthia Stoppel, A.S.

Other Study Staff

Anna Frye
Andrea Hogan

Perelman School of Medicine, University of Pennsylvania, Philadelphia, Pennsylvania

Investigators

Mahendra T. Bhati, M.D., Principal Investigator
Marna S. Barrett, Ph.D., Co-investigator
Michael E. Thase, M.D., Co-investigator

Referring and Interviewing Clinicians

Peter B. Bloom, M.D.
Nicole K Chalmers L.C.S.W.
Torrey A. Creed, Ph.D.
Mario Cristancho, M.D.
Amy Cunningham, Psy.D.
John P. Dennis, Ph.D.
Josephine Elia, M.D.
Peter Gariti, Ph.D., L.C.S.W.
Philip Gehrman, Ph.D.
Laurie Gray, M.D.
Emily A.P. Haigh, Ph.D.
Nora J. Johnson, M.B.A., M.S., Psy.D.
Paulo Knapp, M.D.
Yong-Tong Li, M.D.
Bill Mace, Ph.D.
Kevin S. McCarthy, Ph.D.
Dimitri Perivoliotis, Ph.D.
Luke Schultz, Ph.D.
Tracy Steen, Ph.D.
Chris Tjoa, M.D.
Nancy A. Wintering, L.C.S.W.

Referring Clinicians

Eleanor Ainslie, M.D.
Kelly C. Allison, Ph.D.

Rebecca Aspden, M.D.
Claudia F. Baldassano, M.D.
Vijayta Bansal, M.D.
Rachel A. Bennett, M.D.
Richard Bollinger, Ph.D.
Andrea Bowen, M.D.
Karla Campanella, M.D.
Anthony Carlino, M.D.
Noah Carroll, M.S.S.
Alysia Cirona, M.D.
Samuel Collier, M.D.
Andreea Crauciuc, L.C.S.W.
Pilar Cristancho, M.D.
Traci D'Almeida, M.D.
Kathleen Diller, M.D.
Benoit Dubé, M.D.
Jon Dukes, M.S.W.
Lauren Elliott, M.D.
Mira Elwell, B.A.
Mia Everett, M.D.
Lucy F. Faulconbridge, Ph.D.
Patricia Furlan, Ph.D.
Joanna Goldstein, L.C.S.W.
Paul Grant, Ph.D.
Jillian Graves, L.C.S.W.
Tamar Gur, M.D., Ph.D.
Alisa Gutman, M.D., Ph.D.
Nora Hymowitz, M.D.
Sofia Jensen, M.D.
Tiffany King, M.S.W.
Katherine Levine, M.D.

Alice Li, M.D.
Janet Light, L.C.S.W.
John Listerud, M.D., Ph.D.
Emily Malcoun, Ph.D.
Donovan Maust, M.D.
Adam Meadows, M.D.
Michelle Moyer, M.D.
Rebecca Naugle, L.C.S.W.
Cory Newman, Ph.D.
John Northrop, M.D., Ph.D.
Elizabeth A. Ellis Ohr, Psy.D.
John O'Reardon, M.D.
Abraham Pachikara, M.D.
Andrea Perelman, M.S.W.
Diana Perez, M.S.W.
Bianca Previdi, M.D.
J. Russell Ramsay, Ph.D.
Jorge Rivera-Colon, M.D.
Jan Smedley, L.C.S.W.
Katie Struble, M.S.W.
Aita Susi, M.D.
Yekaterina Tatarchuk, M.D.
Ellen Tarves, M.A.
Allison Tweedie, M.D.
Holly Valerio, M.D.

Thomas A. Wadden, Ph.D.
Joseph Wright, Ph.D.
Yan Xuan, M.D.
David Yusko, Psy.D.

Research Coordinators

Jordan A. Coello, B.A., Lead Research
    Coordinator
Eric Wang, B.S.E.

Volunteer Research Assistants/ Interns

Jeannine Barker, M.A., A.T.R.
Jacqueline Baron
Kelsey Bogue
Alexandra Ciomek
Martekuor Dodoo, B.A.
Julian Domanico
Laura Heller, B.A.
Leah Hull-Rawson, B.A.
Jacquelyn Klehm, B.A.
Christina Lam
Dante Proetto, B.S.
Molly Roy
Casey Shannon

Stanford University School of Medicine, Stanford, California

Investigators

Carl Feinstein, M.D., Principal Investigator
Debra Safer, M.D., Principal Investigator

Referring and Interviewing Clinicians

Kari Berquist, Ph.D.
Eric Clausell, Ph.D.
Danielle Colborn, Ph.D.
Whitney Daniels, M.D.
Alison Darcy, Ph.D.
Krista Fielding, M.D.
Mina Fisher, M.D.
Kara Fitzpatrick, Ph.D.
Wendy Froehlich, M.D.
Grace Gengoux, Ph.D.
Anna Cassandra Golding, Ph.D.
Lisa Groesz, Ph.D.
Kyle Hinman, M.D.
Rob Holaway, Ph.D.
Matthew Holve, M.D.
Rex Huang, M.D.
Nina Kirz, M.D.
Megan Klabunde, Ph.D.
John Leckie, Ph.D.
Naomi Leslie, M.D.
Adrianne Lona, M.D.
Ranvinder Rai, M.D.
Rebecca Rialon, Ph.D.
Beverly Rodriguez, M.D., Ph.D.
Debra Safer, M.D.
Mary Sanders, Ph.D.

Jamie Scaletta, Ph.D.
Norah Simpson, Ph.D.
Manpreet Singh, M.D.
Maria-Christina Stewart, Ph.D.
Melissa Vallas, M.D.
Patrick Whalen, Ph.D.
Sanno Zack, Ph.D.

Referring Clinicians

Robin Apple, Ph.D.
Victor Carrion, M.D.
Carl Feinstein, M.D.
Christine Gray, Ph.D.
Antonio Hardan, M.D.
Megan Jones, Psy.D.
Linda Lotspeich, M.D.
Lauren Mikula, Psy.D.
Brandyn Street, Ph.D.
Violeta Tan, M.D.
Heather Taylor, Ph.D.
Jacob Towery, M.D.
Sharon Williams, Ph.D.

Research Coordinators

Kate Arnow, B.A., Lead Research Coordinator
Nandini Datta, B.S.
Stephanie Manasse, B.A.

Volunteer Research Assistants/ Interns

Arianna Martin, M.S.
Adriana Nevado, B.A.

Children's Hospital Colorado, Aurora, Colorado

Investigator

Marianne Wamboldt, M.D., Principal
Investigator

Referring and Interviewing Clinicians

Galia Abadi, M.D.
Steven Behling, Ph.D.
Jamie Blume, Ph.D.
Adam Burstein, M.D.
Debbie Carter, M.D.
Kelly Caywood, Ph.D.
Meredith Chapman, M.D.
Paulette Christian, A.P.P.M.H.N.
Mary Cook, M.D.
Anthony Cordaro, M.D.
Audrey Dumas, M.D.
Guido Frank, M.D.
Karen Frankel, Ph.D.
Darryl Graham, Ph.D.
Yael Granader, Ph.D.
Isabelle Guillemet, M.D.
Patrece Hairston, Ph.D.
Charles Harrison, Ph.D.
Tammy Herckner, L.C.S.W.
Cassie Karlsson, M.D.
Kimberly Kelsay, M.D.
David Kieval, Ph.D.
Megan Klabunde, Ph.D.
Jaimelyn Kost, L.C.S.W.
Harrison Levine, M.D.
Raven Lipmanson, M.D.
Susan Lurie, M.D.
Asa Marokus, M.D.
Idalia Massa, Ph.D.
Christine McDunn, Ph.D.
Scot McKay, M.D.
Marissa Murgolo, L.C.S.W.
Alyssa Oland, Ph.D.
Lina Patel, Ph.D.
Rheena Pineda, Ph.D.
Gautam Rajendran, M.D.
Diane Reichmuth, Ph.D
Michael Rollin, M.D.

Marlena Romero, L.C.S.W.
Michelle Roy, Ph.D.
Celeste St. John-Larkin, M.D.
Elise Sannar, Ph.D.
Daniel Savin, M.D.
Claire Dean Sinclair, Ph.D.
Ashley Smith, L.C.S.W.
Mindy Solomon, Ph.D.
Sally Tarbell, Ph.D.
Helen Thilly, L.C.S.W.
Sara Tlustos-Carter, Ph.D.
Holly Vause, A.P.P.M.H.N
Marianne Wamboldt, M.D.
Angela Ward, L.C.S.W.
Jason Williams, Ph.D.
Jason Willoughby, Ph.D.
Brennan Young, Ph.D.

Referring Clinicians

Kelly Bhatnagar, Ph.D.
Jeffery Dolgan, Ph.D.
Jennifer Eichberg, L.C.S.W.
Jennifer Hagman, M.D.
James Masterson, L.C.S.W.
Hy Gia Park, M.D.
Tami Roblek, Ph.D.
Wendy Smith, Ph.D.
David Williams, M.D.

Research Coordinators

Laurie Burnside, M.S.M., C.C.R.C., Lead
Research Coordinator
Darci Anderson, B.A., C.C.R.C.
Heather Kennedy, M.P.H.
Amanda Millar, B.A.
Vanessa Waruinge, B.S.
Elizabeth Wallace, B.A.

Volunteer Research Assistants/ Interns

Wisdom Amouzou
Ashley Anderson
Michael Richards
Mateya Whyte

Baystate Medical Center, Springfield, Massachusetts

Investigators

Bruce Waslick, M.D., Principal Investigator
Cheryl Bonica, Ph.D., Co-investigator
John Fanton, M.D., Co-investigator
Barry Sarvet, M.D., Co-investigator

Referring and Interviewing Clinicians

Julie Bermant, R.N., M.S.N., N.P.
Cheryl Bonica, Ph.D.
Jodi Devine, L.I.C.S.W.
William Fahey, Ph.D.
John Fanton, M.D.

Stephane Jacobus, Ph.D.
Barry Sarvet, M.D.
Peter Thunfors, Ph.D.
Bruce Waslick, M.D.
Vicki Weld, L.I.C.S.W.
Sara Wiener, L.I.C.S.W.
Shadi Zaghloul, M.D.

Referring Clinicians

Sarah Detenber, L.I.C.S.W.
Gordon Garrison, L.I.C.S.W.
Jacqueline Humpreys, L.I.C.S.W.
Noreen McGirr, L.I.C.S.W.

Sarah Marcotte, L.C.S.W.
Patricia Rogowski, R.N., C.N.S.

Research Coordinators

Julie Kingsbury, C.C.R.P., Lead Research
    Coordinator
Brenda Martin, B.A.

Volunteer Research Assistant/ Intern

Liza Detenber

New York State Psychiatric Institute, New York, N.Y., Weill Cornell Medical College, Payne Whitney and Westchester Divisions, New York and White Plains, N.Y., and North Shore Child and Family Guidance Center, Roslyn Heights, N.Y. (Joint Study Site)

Investigator

Prudence W. Fisher, Ph.D., Principal
    Investigator

Research Coordinators

Julia K. Carmody, B.A., Lead Research
    Coordinator
Zvi R. Shapiro, B.A., Lead Research
    Coordinator

Volunteers

Preeya Desai
Samantha Keller
Jeremy Litfin, M.A.
Sarah L. Pearlstein, B.A.
Cedilla Sacher

New York State Psychiatric Institute

Referring and Interviewing Clinicians

Michele Cohen, L.C.S.W.
Eduvigis Cruz-Arrieta, Ph.D.
Miriam Ehrensaft, Ph.D.
Laurence Greenhill, M.D.
Schuyler Henderson, M.D., M.P.H.
Sharlene Jackson, Ph.D.
Lindsay Moskowitz, M.D.
Sweene C. Oscar, Ph.D.
Xenia Protopopescu, M.D.
James Rodriguez, Ph.D.
Gregory Tau, M.D.
Melissa Tebbs, L.C.S.W.
Carolina Velez-Grau, L.C.S.W.
Khadijah Booth Watkins, M.D.

Referring Clinicians

George Alvarado, M.D.
Alison Baker, M.D.
Elena Baron, Psy.D.
Lincoln Bickford, M.D., Ph.D.
Zachary Blumkin, Psy.D.
Colleen Cullen, L.C.S.W.
Chyristianne DeAlmeida, Ph.D.
Matthew Ehrlich, M.D.

Eve Friedl, M.D.
Clare Gaskins, Ph.D.
Alice Greenfield, L.C.S.W.
Liora Hoffman, M.D.
Kathleen Jung, M.D.
Karimi Mailutha, M.D., M.P.H.
Valentina Nikulina, Ph.D.
Tal Reis, Ph.D.
Moira Rynn, M.D.
Jasmine Sawhney, M.D.
Sarajbit Singh, M.D.
Katherine Stratigos, M.D.
Oliver Stroeh, M.D.
Russell Tobe, M.D.
Meghan Tomb, Ph.D.
Michelle Tricamo, M.D.

Research Coordinators

Angel A. Caraballo, M.D.
Erica M. Chin, Ph.D.
Daniel T. Chrzanowski, M.D.
Tess Dougherty, B.A.
Stephanie Hundt, M.A.
Moira A. Rynn, M.D.
Deborah Stedge, R.N.

Weill Cornell Medical College, Payne Whitney and Westchester Divisions

Referring and Interviewing Clinicians

Archana Basu, Ph.D.
Shannon M. Bennett, M.D.
Maria De Pena-Nowak, M.D.
Jill Feldman, L.M.S.W.
Dennis Gee, M.D.
Jo R. Hariton, Ph.D.
Lakshmi P. Reddy, M.D.
Margaret Yoon, M.D.

Referring Clinicians

Margo Benjamin, M.D.
Vanessa Bobb, M.D.
Elizabeth Bochtler, M.D.
Katie Cave, L.C.S.W.
Maalobeeka Gangopadhyay, M.D.

Jodi Gold, M.D.
Tejal Kaur, M.D.
Aaron Krasner, M.D.
Amy Miranda, L.C.S.W.
Cynthia Pfeffer, M.D.
James Rebeta, Ph.D.
Sharon Skariah, M.D.
Jeremy Stone, Ph.D.
Dirk Winter, M.D.

Research Coordinators

Alex Eve Keller, B.S., Lead Research Coordinator
Nomi Bodner (volunteer)
Barbara L. Flye, Ph.D.
Jamie S. Neiman (volunteer)
Rebecca L. Rendleman, M.D.

North Shore Child and Family Guidance Center

Referring and Interviewing Clinicians

Casye Brachfeld-Launer, L.C.S.W.
Susan Klein Cohen, Ph.D.
Amy Gelb, L.C.S.W.-R.
Jodi Glasser, L.C.S.W.
Elizabeth Goulding-Tag, L.C.S.W.
Deborah B. Kassimir, L.C.S.W.
Margo Posillico Messina, L.C.S.W.
Andréa Moullin-Heddle, L.M.S.W.
Lisa Pineda, L.C.S.W.
Elissa Smilowitz, L.C.S.W.

Referring Clinicians

Regina Barros-Rivera, L.C.S.W.-R. Assistant
  Executive Director
Maria Christiansen, B.S.
Amy Davies-Hollander, L.M.S.W.
Eartha Hackett, M.S.Ed., M.Sc., B.Sc.

Bruce Kaufstein, L.C.S.W.-R, Director of
  Clinical Services
Kathy Knaust, L.C.S.W.
John Levinson, L.C.S.W.-R, B.C.D.
Andrew Maleckoff, L.C.S.W., Executive
  Director/CEO
Sarah Rosen, L.C.S.W.-R, A.C.S.W.
Abigail Rothenberg, L.M.S.W.
Christine Scotten, A.C.S.W.
Michelle Spatano, L.C.S.W.-R.
Diane Straneri, M.S., R.N., C.S.
Rosara Torrisi, L.M.S.W.
Rob Vichnis, L.C.S.W.

Research Coordinators

Toni Kolb-Papetti, L.C.S.W.
Sheena M. Dauro (volunteer)

DSM-5 Field Trials Pilot Study, Johns Hopkins Medical Institution, Baltimore, Maryland

Adult Sample

Community Psychiatry Outpatient Program, Department of Psychiatry and Behavioral Sciences Main Campus

Investigators

Bernadette Cullen, M.B., B.Ch., B.A.O.,
  Principal Investigator
Holly C. Wilcox, Ph.D., Principal Investigator

Referring and Interviewing Clinicians

Bernadette Cullen, M.B., B.Ch., B.A.O.
Shane Grant, L.C.S.W.-C.
Charee Green, L.C.P.C.

Emily Lorensen, L.C.S.W.-C.
Kathleen Malloy, L.C.P.C.
Gary Pilarchik, L.C.S.W.-C
Holly Slater, L.C.P.C.
Stanislav Spivak, M.D.
Tarcia Spencer Turner, L.C.P.C.
Nicholas Seldes Windt, L.C.S.W.-C.

Research Coordinators

Mellisha McKitty, B.A.
Alison Newcomer, M.H.S.

Pediatric Sample

Child and Adolescent Outpatient Program, Department of Psychiatry and Behavioral Sciences Bayview Medical Center

Investigators

Joan P. Gerring, M.D., Principal Investigator
Leslie Miller, M.D., Principal Investigator
Holly C. Wilcox, Ph.D., Co-investigator

Referring and Interviewing Clinicians

Shannon Barnett, M.D.
Gwen Condon, L.C.P.C.
Brijan Fellows, L.C.S.W.-C.
Heather Garner, L.C.S.W.-C.
Joan P. Gerring, M.D.

Anna Gonzaga, M.D.
Debra Jenkins, L.C.S.W.-C.
Paige N. Johnston, L.C.P.C.
Brenda Memel, D.N.P., R.N.
Leslie Miller, M.D.
Ryan Moore, L.C.S.W.-C.
Shauna Reinblatt, M.D.
Monique Vardi, L.C.P.C.

Research Coordinators

Mellisha McKitty, B.A.
Alison Newcomer, M.H.S.

DSM-5 Field Trials in Routine Clinical Practice Settings: Collaborating Investigators

Archil Abashidze, M.D.
Francis R. Abueg, Ph.D.
Jennifer Louise Accuardi, M.S.
Balkozar S. Adam, M.D.
Miriam E. Adams, Sc.D., M.S.W., L.I.C.S.W.
Suzanna C. Adams, M.A.
Lawrence Adler, M.D.
Rownak Afroz, M.D.
Khalid I. Afzal, M.D.
Joseph Alimasuya, M.D.
Emily Allen, M.S.
Katherine A. Allen, L.M.F.T., M.A.
William D. Allen, M.S.
Jafar AlMashat, M.D.
Anthony T. Alonzo, D.M.F.T.
Guillermo Alvarez, B.A., M.A.
Angela Amoia-Lutz, L.M.F.T.
Krista A. Anderson, M.A., L.M.F.T.
Lisa R. Anderson, M.Ed., L.C.P.C.
Pamela M. Anderson, L.M.F.T.
Shannon N. Anderson, M.A., L.P.C., N.C.C.
Eric S. Andrews, M.A.
Vicki Arbuckle, M.S., Nursing(N.P.)
Namita K. Arora, M.D.
Darryl Arrington, M.A.
Bearlyn Y. Ash, M.S.
Wylie J. Bagley, Ph.D.
Kumar D. Bahl, M.D.
Deborah C. Bailey, M.A., M.S., Ph.D.
Carolyn Baird, D.N.P., M.B.A., R.N.-B.C.,
    C.A.R.N.-A.P., I.C.C.D.P.D.
Joelle Bangsund M.S.W.
Maria Baratta, M.S.W., Ph.D.
Stan Barnard, M.S.W.
Deborah Barnes, M.S.

Margaret L. Barnes, Ph.D.
David Barnum, Ph.D.
Raymond M. Baum, M.D.
Edward Wescott Beal, M.D.
Michelle Beaudoin, M.A.
Ernest E. Beckham, Ph.D.
Lori L. Beckwith, M.Ed
Emmet Bellville, M.A.
Randall E. Bennett, M.A.
Lynn Benson, Ph.D.
Robert Scott Benson, M.D.
Linda Benton, M.S.W.
Ditza D. Berger, Ph.D.
Louise I. Bertman, Ph.D.
Robin Bieber, M.S., L.M.F.T.
Diana M. Bigham, M.A.
David R. Blackburn, Ph.D.
Kelley Blackwell, L.M.F.T.
Lancia Blatchley, B.A., L.M.F.T.
Stacey L. Block, L.M.S.W., A.C.S.W.
Karen J. Bloodworth, M.S., N.C.C., L.P.C.
Lester Bloomenstiel, M.S.
Christine M. Blue, D.O.
Marina Bluvshtein, Ph.D.
Callie Gray Bobbitt, M.S.W., L.C.S.W.
Moses L. Boone, Jr., L.M.S.W., B.C.D.
Steffanie Boudreau-Thomas, M.A.-L.P.C.
Jay L. Boulter, M.A.
Aaron Daniel Bourne, M.A.
Helen F. Bowden, Ph.D.
Aryn Bowley-Safranek, B.S., M.S.
Elizabeth Boyajian, Ph.D.
Beth K. Boyarsky, M.D.
Gail M. Boyd, Ph.D.
Jeffrey M. Brandler, Ed.S., C.A.S., S.A.P.

Sandra L. Branton, Ed.D.
Karen J. Brocco-Kish, M.D.
Kristin Brooks, P.M.H.N.P.
Ann Marie Brown, M.S.W.
Philip Brown, M.S.W.
Kellie Buckner, Ed.S.
Richard Bunt, M.D.
Neil F. Buono, D.Min.
Janice Bureau, M.S.W., L.C.S.W.
Kimlee Butterfield, M.S.W.
Claudia Byrne, Ph.D.
Quinn Callicott, M.S.W., L.C.S.W.
Alvaro Camacho, M.D., M.P.H.
Sandra Cambra, Ph.D.
Heather Campbell, M.A.
Nancy Campbell, Ph.D., M.S.W.
Karen Ranee Canada, L.M.F.T.
Joseph P. Cannavo, M.D.
Catherine F. Caporale, Ph.D.
Frederick Capps, Ph.D., M.S.
Rebecca J. Carney, M.B.A., M.A., L.M.H.C.
Kelly J. Carroll, M.S.W.
Richard W. Carroll, Ph.D., L.P.C., A.C.S.
Sherry Casper, Ph.D.
Joseph A. Catania, L.I.S.W.S., L.C.D.C. III
Manisha P. Cavendish, Ph.D.
Kenneth M. Certa, M.D.
Shambhavi Chandraiah, M.D.
Calvin Chatlos, M.D.
Daniel C. Chen, M.D.
Darlene Cheryl, M.S.W.
Matthew R. Chirman, M.S.
Carole A. Chisholm, M.S.W.
Shobha A. Chottera, M.D.
Joseph Logue Christenson, M.D.
Pamela Christy, Psy.D.
Sharon M. Freeman Clevenger, Ph.D.,
    P.M.H.C.N.S.-B.C.
Mary Ann Cohen, M.D.
Mitchell J. Cohen, M.D.
Diego L. Coira, M.D.
Melinda A. Lawless Coker, Psy.D.
Carol Cole, M.S.W., L.C.S.W.
Caron Collins, M.A., L.M.F.T.
Wanda Collins, M.S.N.
Linda Cook Cason, M.A.
Ayanna Cooke-Chen, M.D., Ph.D.
Heidi B. Cooperstein, D.O.
Ileana Corbelle, M.S.W.
Kimberly Corbett, Psy.D.
Angelina Cordova, M.A.Ed.
Jennifer Carol Cox, L.P.C.
Sheree Cox, M.A., R.N., N.C.C., D.C.C.,
    L.M.H.C.
William Frederick Cox, M.D.
Sally M. Cox, M.S.Ed.
Debbie Herman Crane, M.S.W.
Arthur Ray Crawford, III, Ph.D.

Roula Creighton, M.D.
John R. Crossfield, L.M.H.C.
Sue Cutbirth, R.N., M.S.N, C.S., P.M.H.N.P.
Marco Antonio Cuyar, M.S.
Rebecca Susan Daily, M.D.
Lori S. Danenberg, Ph.D.
Chan Dang-Vu, M.D.
Mary Hynes Danielak, Psy.D.
Cynthia A. Darby, M.Ed., Ed.S.
Douglas Darnall, Ph.D.
Christopher Davidson, M.D.
Doreen Davis, Ph.D., L.C.S.W.
Sandra Davis, Ph.D., L.M.H.C., N.C.C.
Walter Pitts Davis, M.Th.
Christian J. Dean, Ph.D.
Kent Dean, Ph.D.
Elizabeth Dear, M.A.
Shelby DeBause, M.A.
Rebecca B. DeLaney, M.S.S.W., L.C.S.W., B.C.D.
John R. Delatorre, M.A.
Frank DeLaurentis, M.D.
Eric Denner, M.A., M.B.A.
Mary Dennihan, L.M.F.T.
Kenny Dennis, M.A.
Pamela L. Detrick, Ph.D., M.S., F.N.P.-B.C.,
    P.M.H.N.P.-B.C., R.N.-B.C., C.A.P.,
    G.C.A.C.
Robert Detrinis, M.D.
Daniel A. Deutschman, M.D.
Tania Diaz, Psy.D.
Sharon Dobbs, M.S.W., L.C.S.W.
David Doreau, M.Ed.
Gayle L. Dosher, M.A.
D'Ann Downey, Ph.D., M.S.W.
Beth Doyle, M.A.
Amy J. Driskill, M.S., L.C.M.F.T.
James Drury, M.D.
Brenda-Lee Duarte, M.Ed.
Shane E. Dulemba, M.S.N.
Nancy R. G. Dunbar, M.D.
Cathy Duncan, M.A.
Rebecca S. Dunn, M.S.N., A.R.N.P.
Debbie Earnshaw, M.A.
Shawna Eddy-Kissell, M.A.
Momen El Nesr, M.D.
Jeffrey Bruce Elliott, Psy.D.
Leslie Ellis, Ph.D.
Donna M. Emfield, L.C.P.C.
Gretchen S. Enright, M.D.
John C. Espy, Ph.D.
Renuka Evani, M.B.B.S., M.D.
Heather Evans, M.S.Ed, L.P.C.N.C.C.
Cesar A. Fabiani, M.D.
Fahim Fahim, M.D.
Samuel Fam, M.D.
Edward H. Fankhanel, Ph.D., Ed.D.
Tamara Farmer, M.S.N, A.R.N.P.
Farida Farzana, M.D.

Philip Fast, M.S.
Patricia Feltrup-Exum, M.A.M.F.T.
Hector J. Fernandez-Barillas, Ph.D.
Julie Ferry, M.S.W., L.I.C.S.W.
Jane Fink, Ph.D., M.S.S.A.
Kathy Finkle, L.P.C.M.H.
Steven Finlay, Ph.D.
Rik Fire, M.S.W., L.C.S.W.
Ann Flood, Ph.D.
Jeanine Lee Foreman, M.S.
Thyra Fossum, Ph.D.
Karen S. Franklin, L.I.C.S.W.
Sherre K. Franklin, M.A.
Helen R. Frey, M.A., E.D.
Michael L. Freytag, B.S., M.A.
Beth Gagnon, M.S.W.
Patrice L.R. Gallagher, Ph.D.
Angela J. Gallien, M.A.
Robert Gallo, M.S.W.
Mario Galvarino, M.D.
Vladimir I. Gasca, M.D.
Joshua Gates, Ph.D.
Anthony Gaudioso, Ph.D.
Michelle S. Gauthier, A.P.R.N., M.S.N,
    P.M.H.N.P.-B.C.
Rachel E. Gearhart, L.C.S.W.
Stephen D. Gelfond, M.D.
Nancy S. Gerow, M.S.
Michael J. Gerson, Ph.D.
Susan M. A. Geyer, L.M.S.W.
Lorrie Gfeller-Strouts, Ph.D.
Shubu Ghosh, M.D.
Richard Dorsey Gillespie, M.Div.
Stuart A. Gitlin, M.S.S.A.
Jeannette E. Given, Ph.D.
Frances Gizzi, L.C.S.W.
Stephen I. Glicksman, Ph.D.
Martha Glisky, Ph.D.
Sonia Godbole, M.D.
Howard M. Goldfischer, Psy.D.
Mary Jane Gonzalez-Huss, Ph.D.
Michael I. Good, M.D.
Dawn Goodman-Martin, M.A.-L.M.H.C.
Robert Gorkin, Ph.D., M.D.
Jeff Gorski, M.S.W.
Linda O. Graf, M.Ed., L.C.P.C.
Ona Graham, Psy.D.
Aubrie M. Graves, L.M.S.W., C.A.S.A.C.
Howard S. Green, M.D.
Karen Torry Green, M.S.W.
Gary Greenberg, Ph.D.
Marjorie Greenhut, M.A.
James L. Greenstone, Ed.D., J.D.
Raymond A. Griffin, Ph.D.
Joseph Grillo, Ph.D.
Janeane M. Grisez, A.A., B.A.
Lawrence S. Gross, M.D.
Robert J. Gross, M.D.

Sally J. Grosscup, Ph.D.
Philip A. Grossi, M.D.
Gabrielle Guedet, Ph.D.
Nicholas Guenzel, B.A., B.S., M.S.N.
Mary G. Hales, M.A.
Tara C. Haley, M.S., L.M.F.T.
John D. Hall, M.D.
Amy Hammer, M.S.W.
Michael S. Hanau, M.D.
Linda K.W. Hansen, M.A., L.P.
Genevieve R. Hansler, M.S.W.
Mary T. Harrington, L.C.S.W.
Lois Hartman, L.C.P.C.
Steven Lee Hartsock, Ph.D., M.S.W.
Victoria Ann Harwood, M.S.W., L.C.S.W.
Rossi A. Hassad, Ph.D., M.P.H.
Erin V. Hatcher, M.S.N.
Richard L. Hauger, M.D.
Kimberly M. Haverly, M.A.
Gale Eisner Heater, M.S., M.F.T.
Katlin Hecox, M.A.
Brenda Heideman, M.S.W.
Melinda Heinen, M.Sc.
Marie-Therese Heitkamp, M.S.
Melissa B. Held, M.A.
Jessica Hellings, M.D.
Bonnie Helmick-O'Brien, M.A., L.M.F.T.
MaLinda T. Henderson, M.S.N, F.P.M.H.N.P.
Gwenn Herman, M.S.W.
Martha W. Hernandez, M.S.N, A.P.R.N.,
    P.M.H.C.N.S.
Robin L. Hewitt, M.S.
Kenneth Hoffman, Ph.D.
Patricia E. Hogan, D.O.
Peggy Holcomb, Ph.D.
Garland H. Holloman, Jr., M.D.
Kimberly Huegel, M.S.W., L.C.S.W.
Jason Hughes, L.P.C.-S., N.C.C.
Jennifer C. Hughes, Ph.D., M.S.W., L.I.S.W.-S.
Michelle K. Humke, M.A.
Judith G. Hunt, L.M.F.T.
Tasneem Hussainee, M.D.
Sharlene J. Hutchinson, M.S.N.
Muhammad Ikram, M.D.
Sunday Ilechukwu, M.D., D.Psy. Cli.
Douglas H. Ingram, M.D.
Marilynn Irvine, Ph.D.
Marjorie Isaacs, Psy.D.
Raymond Isackila, Ed.S., P.C.C.-S., L.I.C.D.C.
Mohammed A. Issa, M.D.
John L. Jankord, M.A.
Barbara P. Jannah, L.C.S.W.
C. Stuart Johnson, M.S.
Dawn M. Johnson, M.A.
Deanna V. Johnson, M.S., A.P.R.N., B.C.
Eric C. Johnson, M.F.T.
Joy Johnson, Ph.D., L.C.S.W.
Willard Johnson, Ph.D.

Xenia Johnson-Bhembe, M.D.
Vann S. Joines, Ph.D.
Margaret Jones, Psy.D.
Patricia Jorgenson, M.S.W.
Steven M. Joseph, M.D.
Taylere Joseph, M.A.
Jeanette M. Joyner-Craddock, M.S.S.W.
Melissa Kachapis, M.A.
Charles T. Kaelber, M.D.
Aimee C. Kaempf, M.D.
Peter Andrew Kahn, M.D.
Robert P. Kahn-Rose, M.D.
Maher Karam-Hage, M.D.
Todd H. Kasdan, M.D.
Karen Kaufman, M.S., L.M.F.T.
Rhesa Kaulia, M.A., M.F.T.
Debbie Lynn Kelly, M.S.N, P.M.H.N.P.-B.C.
W. Stephen Kelly, Ph.D.
Selena Kennedy, M.A.
Judith A. Kenney, M.S., L.P.C.
Mark Patrick Kerekes, M.D.
Alyse Kerr, M.S., N.C.C., N.A.D.D.-C.C., L.P.C.
Karen L. Kerschmann, L.C.S.W.
Marcia Kesner, M.S.
Ashan Khan, Ph.D.
Shaukat Khan, M.D.
Audrey Khatchikian, Ph.D.
Laurie B. Kimmel, M.S.W.
Jason H. King, Ph.D.
Nancy Leigh King, M.S.W., L.C.S.W., L.C.A.S.
Kyle Kinne, M.S.C
Cassandra M. Klyman, M.D.
David R. Knapp, L.C.S.W.
Margaret Knerr, M.S.
Michael R. Knox, Ph.D.
Carolyn Koblin, M.S.
Valerie Kolbert, M.S., A.R.N.P.-B.C.
Heather Koontz, M.S.W.
Faye Koop, Ph.D., L.C.M.F.T.
Fern M. Kopakin, M.S.W., L.C.S.W.
Joel Kotin, M.D.
Sharlene K. Kraemer, M.S.E.
Marjorie Vego Krausz, M.A., Ed.D.
Nancy J. Krell, M.S.W.
Mindy E. Kronenberg, Ph.D.
Dwayne Kruse, M.S., M.F.T.
Ajay S. Kuchibhatla, M.D.
Shubha N. Kumar, M.D.
Helen H. Kyomen, M.D., M.S.
Rebecca M. Lachut, M.Ed., Ed.S.
Alexis Lake, M.S.S.
Ramaswamy Lakshmanan, M.D.
Brigitta Lalone, L.C.S.W.-R
John W. Lancaster, Ph.D.
Patience R. Land, L.I.C.S.W., M.S.W., M.P.A.
Amber Lange, M.A., Ph.D.
Jeff K. Larsen, M.A.
Nathan E. Lavid, M.D.

Michelle Leader, Ph.D.
Stephen E. Lee, M.D.
Cathryn L. Leff, Ph.D., L.M.F.T.
Rachael Kollar Leombruno, L.M.F.T.
Arlene I. Lev, M.S.W., L.C.S.W.-R
Gregory K. Lewis, M.A.-L.M.F.T.
Jane Hart Lewis, M.S.
Melissa S. Lewis, M.S.W., L.I.C.S.W.
Norman Gerald Lewis, F.R.A.N.Z.C.P.
Robin Joy Lewis, Ph.D.
Ryan Michael Ley, M.D.
Tammy R. Lias, M.A.
Russell F. Lim, M.D.
Jana Lincoln, M.D.
Ted Lindberg, L.M.S.W., L.M.F.T., M.S.W.
Peggy Solow Liss, M.S.W.
Andrea Loeb, Psy.D.
William David Lohr, M.D.
Mary L. Ludy, M.A., L.M.H.C., L.M.F.T.
Nathan Lundin, M.A., L.P.C.
Veena Luthra, M.D.
Patti Lyerly, L.C.S.W.
Denise E. Maas, M.A.
Silvia MacAllister, L.M.F.T.
Nicola MacCallum, M.S., M.F.C. Therapy
Colin N. MacKenzie, M.D.
Cynthia Mack-Ernsdorff, Ph.D.
John R. Madsen-Bibeau, M.S., M.Div
Christopher J. Maglio, Ph.D.
Deepak Mahajan, M.D.
Debra Majewski, M.A.
Harish Kumar Malhotra, M.D.
Pamela Marcus, R.N., M.S.
Mary P. Marshall, Ph.D.
Flora Lynne Martin, M.A., L.P.C., A.D.C.
Robert S. Martin, M.D.
Jennifer L. Martinez, M.S.
Ninfa Martinez-Aguilar, M.A., M.F.T.
Emily Martinsen, M.S.W.
Farhan A. Matin, M.D.
Janus Maybee, P.M.H.N.P.
Karen Mazarin-Stanek, M.A.
Eben L. McClenahan, M.D., M.S.
Jerlyn C. McCleod, M.D.
Susan E. McCue, M.S.W., L.C.S.W.
Kent D. McDonald, M.S.
Daniel McDonnell, M.S.N, P.M.H.-N.P.
Robert McElhose, Ph.D.
Lisa D. McGrath, Ph.D.
Mark McGrosky, M.S.W.
Katherine M. McKay, Ph.D.
Darren D. McKinnis, M.S.W.
Mona McNelis-Broadley, M.S.W., L.C.S.W.
Rick McQuistion, Ph.D.
Susan Joy Mendelsohn, Psy.D.
Barbara S. Menninga, M.Ed.
Hindi Mermelstein, M.D., F.A.P.M.
Rachel B. Michaelsen, M.S.W.

Thomas F. Micka, M.D.
Tonya Miles, Psy.D.
Matthew Miller, M.S.
Michael E. Miller, M.D.
Noel Miller, L.M.S.W., M.B.A., M.P.S.
Kalpana Miriyala, M.D.
Sandra Moenssens, M.S.
Erin Mokhtar, M.A.
Robert E. Montgomery, M.Ed.
Susan Moon, M.A.
Theresa K. Moon, M.D.
David B. Moore, B.A., M.Div., M.S.S.W., Ph.D.
Joanne M. Moore, M.S.
Peter I. M. Moran, M.B.B.Ch.
Anna Moriarty, M.P.S., L.P.C., L.M.H.C.
Richard Dean Morris, M.A.
Michael M. Morrison, M.A.
Carlton E. Munson, Ph.D.
Timothy A. Murphy, M.D.
Beth L. Murphy, Psy.D.
Melissa A. Myers, M.D.
Stefan Nawab, M.D.
Allyson Matney Neal, D.N.P.
Steven Nicholas, M.A.
Aurelian N. Niculescu, M.D.
Earl S. Nielsen, Ph.D.
Terry Oleson, Ph.D.
Julianne R. Oliver, B.S., M.S., Ph.D.
Robert O. Olsen, M.D.
Amy O'Neill, M.D.
Oscar H. Oo, Psy.D., A.B.P.P.
Laurie Orlando, J.D., M.A.
Jill Osborne, M.S., Ed.S.
Kimberly Overlie, M.S.
L. Kola Oyewumi, Ph.D.
Zachary J. Pacha, M.S.W.
Suzette R. Papadakis, M.S.
Amanda C. Parsons, M.A., L.P.C.C.
Lee R. Pate, B.A., M.A.
Eric L. Patterson, L.P.C.
Sherri Paulson, M.Ed., L.S.C.W.
Peter Dennis Pautz, B.A., M.S.W.
Malinda J. Perkins, M.S.W., L.C.S.W.
Eleanor F. Perlman, M.S.W.
Deborah K. Perry, M.S.W.
Amanda Peterman, L.M.F.T.
Shawn Pflugardt, Psy.D.
Robert J. Dean Phillips, M.S.
Laura Pieper, M.S.W., L.C.S.W.
Lori D. Pink, M.S.W., B.C.D
Michael G. Pipich, M.S., L.M.F.T.
Cynthia G. Pizzulli, M.S.W., Ph.D.
Kathy C. Points, M.A.
Marya E. Pollack, M.D., M.P.H.
Sanford E. Pomerantz, M.D.
Eva Ponder, M.S.W., Psy.D.
Ernest Poortinga, M.D.
David Post, M.D.

Laura L. Post, M.D., Ph.D., J.D.
Patrick W. Powell, Ed.D.
Beth M. Prewett, Psy.D.
Robert Price, D.C.C., M.Ed.
John Pruett, M.D.
Aneita S. Radov, M.A.
Dawn M. Raffa, Ph.D.
Kavitha Raja, M.D.
Ranjit Ram, M.D.
Mohamed Ibrahim Ramadan, M.D., M.S.
Christopher S. Randolph, M.D.
Nancy Rappaport, M.Ed.
John Moir Rauenhorst, M.D.
Laurel Jean Rebenstock, L.M.S.W.
Edwin Renaud, Ph.D.
Heather J. Rhodes, M.A.
Jennifer S. Ritchie-Goodline, Psy.D.
Daniel G. Roberts, M.A.
Brenda Rohren, M.A., M.F.S., L.I.M.H.P.,
    L.A.D.C., M.A.C.
Donna G. Rolin-Kenny, Ph.D., A.P.R.N.,
    P.M.H.C.N.S.-B.C.
Sylvia E. Rosario, M.Ed.
Mindy S. Rosenbloom, M.D.
Harvey A. Rosenstock, M.D.
Thalia Ross, M.S.S.W.
Fernando Rosso, M.D.
Barry H. Roth, M.D.
Thomas S. Rue, M.A., L.M.H.C.
Elizabeth Ruegg, L.C.S.W.
Diane Rullo, Ph.D.
Angie Rumaldo, Ph.D.
Eric Rutberg, M.A., D.H.Ed.
Joseph A. Sabella, L.M.H.C.
Kemal Sagduyu, M.D.
Adam H. Saltz, M.S.W.
Jennifer A. Samardak, L.I.S.W.-S.
George R. Samuels, M.A., M.S.W.
Carmen Sanjurjo, M.A.
John S. Saroyan, Ed.D.
Brigid Kathleen Sboto, M.A., M.F.T.
Lori Cluff Schade, M.S.
Joan E. Schaper, M.S.N.
Rae J. Schilling, Ph.D.
Larry Schor, Ph.D.
Donna J. Schwartz, M.S.W., L.I.C.S.W.
Amy J. Schwarzenbart, P.M.H.-C.N.S., B.C.,
    A.P.N.P.
John V. Scialli, M.D.
Chad Scott, Ph.D., L.P.C.C.
Sabine Sell, M.F.T.
Minal Shah, N.S., N.C.C., L.P.C.
Lynn Shell, M.S.N.
Dharmesh Navin Sheth, M.D.
S. Christopher Shim, M.D.
Marta M. Shinn, Ph.D.
Andreas Sidiropoulos, M.D., Ph.D.
Michael Siegell, M.D.

Michael G. Simonds, Psy.D.
Gagandeep Singh, M.D.
Melissa Rae Skrzypchak, M.S.S.W., L.C.S.W.
Paula Slater, M.D.
William Bill Slaughter, M.D., M.A.
Aki Smith, Ph.D.
Deborah L. Smith, Ed.M.
Diane E. Smith, M.A., L.M.F.T.
James S. Sommer, M.S.
J. Richard Spatafora, M.D.
Judy Splittgerber, M.S.N., C.S., N.P.
Thiruneermalai T.G. Sriram, M.D.
Martha W. St. John, M.D.
Sybil Stafford, Ph.D.
Timothy Stambaugh, M.A.
Laura A. Stamboni, M.S.W.
Carol L. R. Stark, M.D.
Stephanie Steinman, M.S.
Claudia M. Stevens, M.S.W.
Jennifer Boyer Stevens, Psy.D.
Dominique Stevens-Young, M.S.W., L.C.S.W.
Kenneth Stewart, Ph.D.
Daniel Storch, M.D.
Suzanne Straebler, A.P.R.N.
Dawn Stremel, M.A., L.M.F.T.
Emel Stroup, Psy.D.
John W. Stump, M.S., L.M.F.T.
Thomas G. Suk, M.A.
Elizabeth Sunzeri, M.S.
Linnea Swanson, M.A., Psy.D.
Patricia Swanson, M.A.
Fereidoon Taghizadeh, M.D.
Bonnie L. Tardif, L.M.H.C., N.C.C., B.C.P.C.C.
Joan Tavares, M.S.W.
Ann Taylor, M.S.W.
Dawn O'Dwyer Taylor, Ph.D.
Chanel V. Tazza, L.M.H.C.
Martha H. Teater, M.A.
Clark D. Terrell, M.D.
Mark R. Thelen, Psy.D.
Norman E. Thibault, M.S., Ph.D.
Tojuana L. Thomason, Ph.D.
Paula Thomson, Psy.D.
D. Chadwick Thompson, M.A.
Susan Thorne-Devin, A.M.
Jean Eva Thumm, M.A.P.C., M.A.T., L.M.F.T., B.C.C.
James E. Tille, Ph.D., D.Min.
Jacalyn G. Tippey, Ph.D.
Saraswathi Tirumalasetty, M.D.
Jacqueline A. Torrance, M.S.
Terrence Trobaugh, M.S.
Louisa V. Troemel, Psy.D., L.M.F.T.

Susan Ullman, M.S.W.
Jennifer M. Underwood, M.S.W., L.C.S.W.
Rodney Dale Veldhuizen, M.A.
Michelle Voegels, B.S.N., M.S.N., B.C.
Wess Vogt, M.D.
R. Christopher Votolato, Psy.D.
John W. Waid, Ph.D.
Christa A. Wallis, M.A.
Dominique Walmsley, M.A.
Bhupinder Singh Waraich, M.D.
Joseph Ward, N.C.C., L.P.C. M.Ed.
Robert Ward, M.S.W.
Marilee L. M. Wasell, Ph.D.
Gannon J. Watts, L.P.C.-S., L.A.C., N.C.C., N.C.S.C., A.A.D.C., I.C.A.A.D.C.
Sheila R. Webster, M.A., M.S.S.A.
Burton Weiss, M.D.
Dennis V. Weiss, M.D.
Jonathan S. Weiss, M.D.
Richard Wendel, Ph.D.
Paul L. West, Ed.D.
Kris Sandra Wheatley, M.A., L.C.P.C., N.C.C.
Leneigh White, M.A.
Danny R. Whitehead, L.I.C.S.W.
Jean Whitinger, M.A.
Peter D. Wilk, M.D.
Vanessa Wilkinson, L.P.C.
Tim F. Willia, M.S., M.A.Ed., L.P.C.
Cathy E. Willis, M.A., L.M.F.T., C.A.D.C.
Jeffery John Wilson, M.D.
Jacquie Wilson, M.Ed.
David D. Wines, M.S.W.
Barbara A. Wirebaugh, M.S.W.
Daniel L. Wise, Ph.D.
Christina Wong, M.S.W., L.C.S.W.
Susanna Wood, M.S.W., L.C.S.W.
Linda L. Woodall, M.D.
Leoneen Woodard-Faust, M.D.
Sheryl E. Woodhouse, L.M.F.T.
Gregory J. Worthington, Psy.D.
Tanya Wozniak, M.D.
Kimberly Isaac Wright, M.A.
Peter Yamamoto, M.D.
Maria Ruiza Ang Yee, M.D.
Michael B. Zafrani, M.D.
Jafet E. Gonzalez Zakarchenco, M.D.
John Zibert, Ph.D.
Karen Zilberstein, M.S.W.
Cathi Zillmann, C.P.N.P., N.P.P.
Gerald A. Zimmerman, Ph.D.
Michele Zimmerman, M.A., P.M.H.C.N.S.-B.C.
Judith A. Zink, M.A.

Vanderbilt University REDCap Team

Paul Harris, Ph.D.
Sudah Kashyap, B.E.
Brenda Minor

Jon Scherdin, M.A.
Rob Taylor, M.A.
Janey Wang, M.S.

Index

Page numbers printed in **boldface type** refer to tables.